Dietary Reference Intakes (DRIs): Recommended Intakes for Individuals, Elements

Food and Nutrition Board, Institute of Medicine, National Academies

Life stage group	Calcium (mg/d)	Chromium (µg/d)	Copper (µg/d)	Fluoride (mg/d)	Iodine (µg/d)	Iron (mg/d)	Magnesium (mg/d)	Manganese (mg/d)	Molybdenum (µg/d)	Phosphorus (mg/d)	Selenium (µg/d)	Zinc (mg/d)
Infants												
0–6 mo	200*	0.2*	200*	0.01*	110*	0.27*	30*	0.003*	2*	100*	15*	2*
7–12 mo	260*	5.5*	220*	0.5*	130*	**11**	75*	0.6*	3*	275*	20*	**3**
Children												
1–3 y	500*	11*	340	0.7*	90	7	80	1.2*	17	460	20	3
4–8 y	800*	15*	440	1*	90	10	130	1.5*	22	500	30	5
Males												
9–13 y	1,100*	25*	700	2*	120	8	240	1.9*	34	1,250	40	8
14–18 y	1,100*	35*	890	3*	150	11	410	2.2*	43	1,250	55	11
19–30 y	800*	35*	900	4*	150	8	400	2.3*	45	700	55	11
31–50 y	800*	35*	900	4*	150	8	420	2.3*	45	700	55	11
51–70 y	800*	30*	900	4*	150	8	420	2.3*	45	700	55	11
>70 y	1,000*	30*	900	4*	150	8	420	2.3*	45	700	55	11
Females												
9–13 y	1,000*	21*	700	2*	120	8	240	1.6*	34	1,250	40	8
14–18 y	1,100*	24*	890	3*	150	15	360	1.6*	43	1,250	55	9
19–30 y	800*	25*	900	3*	150	18	310	1.8*	45	700	55	8
31–50 y	800*	25*	900	3*	150	18	320	1.8*	45	700	55	8
51–70 y	1,000*	20*	900	3*	150	8	320	1.8*	45	700	55	8
>70 y	1,000*	20*	900	3*	150	8	320	1.8*	45	700	55	8
Pregnancy												
≤18 y	1,100*	29*	1,000	3*	220	27	400	2.0*	50	1,250	60	12
19–30 y	800*	30*	1,000	3*	220	27	350	2.0*	50	700	60	11
31–50 y	800*	30*	1,000	3*	220	27	360	2.0*	50	700	60	11
Lactation												
≤18 y	1,100*	44*	1,300	3*	290	10	360	2.6*	50	1,250	70	13
19–30 y	800*	45*	1,300	3*	290	9	310	2.6*	50	700	70	12
31–50 y	800	45*	1,300	3*	290	9	320	2.6*	50	700	70	12

NOTE: This table presents Recommended Dietary Allowances (RDAs) in **bold type** and Adequate Intakes (AIs) in ordinary type followed by an asterisk (*). RDAs and AIs may both be used as goals for individual intake. RDAs are set to meet the needs of almost all (97 to 98 percent) individuals in a group. For healthy breastfed infants, the AI is the mean intake. The AI for other life stage and gender group | to cover needs of all individuals in the group, but lack of data or uncertainty in the data prevent being able to specify with confidence the percentage of individuals covered by this intake.

SOURCES: Dietary Reference Intakes for Calcium, Phosphorus, Magnesium, Vitamin D, and Fluoride (1997); Dietary Reference Intakes for Thiamin, Riboflavin, Niacin, Vitamin B-6, Folate, Vitamin Pantothenic Acid, Biotin, and Choline (1998); Dietary Reference Intakes for Vitamin C, Vitamin E, Selenium, and Carotenoids (2000); and Dietary Reference Intakes for Vitamin A, Vitamin K, Arsenic Chromium, Copper, Iodine, Iron, Manganese, Molybdenum, Nickel, Silicon, Vanadium, and Zinc (2001). Dietary Reference Intakes for Calcium and Vitamin D. (2011). These reports may be accessed www.nap.edu.

Dietary Reference Intakes (DRIs): Recommended Intakes for Individuals, Macronutrients

Food and Nutrition Board, Institute of Medicine, National Academies

Life stage group	Carbohydrate (g/d)	Total fiber (g/d)	Fat (g/d)	Linoleic acid (g/d)	α-Linolenic acid (g/d)	Protein[a] (g/d)
Infants						
0–6 mo	60*	ND	31*	4.4*	0.5*	9.1*
7–12 mo	95*	ND	30*	4.6*	0.5*	**13.5**
Children						
1–3 y	**130**	19*	ND[b]	7*	0.7*	**13**
4–8 y	**130**	25*	ND	10*	0.9*	**19**
Males						
9–13 y	**130**	31*	ND	12*	1.2*	**34**
14–18 y	**130**	38*	ND	16*	1.6*	**52**
19–30 y	**130**	38*	ND	17*	1.6*	**56**
31–50 y	**130**	38*	ND	17*	1.6*	**56**
51–70 y	**130**	30*	ND	14*	1.6*	**56**
>70 y	**130**	30*	ND	14*	1.6*	**56**
Females						
9–13 y	**130**	26*	ND	10*	1.0*	**34**
14–18 y	**130**	26*	ND	11*	1.1*	**46**
19–30 y	**130**	25*	ND	12*	1.1*	**46**
31–50 y	**130**	25*	ND	12*	1.1*	**46**
51–70 y	**130**	21*	ND	11*	1.1*	**46**
>70 y	**130**	21*	ND	11*	1.1*	**46**
Pregnancy						
14–18 y	**175**	28*	ND	13*	1.4*	**71**
19–30 y	**175**	28*	ND	13*	1.4*	**71**
31–50 y	**175**	28*	ND	13*	1.4*	**71**
Lactation						
14–18 y	**210**	29*	ND	13*	1.3*	**71**
19–30 y	**210**	29*	ND	13*	1.3*	**71**
31–50 y	**210**	29*	ND	13*	1.3*	**71**

NOTE: This table presents Recommended Dietary Allowances (RDAs) in **bold type** and Adequate Intakes (AIs) in ordinary type followed by an asterisk (*). RDAs and AIs may both be used as goals for individual intake. RDAs are set to meet the needs of almost all (97 to 98 percent) individuals in a group. For healthy breastfed infants, the AI is the mean intake. The AI for other life stage and gender groups is believed to cover needs of all individuals in the group, but lack of data or uncertainty in the data prevent being able to specify with confidence the percentage of individuals covered by this intake.

[a]Based on 0.8 g protein/kg body weight for reference body weight.

[b]ND = not determinable at this time

SOURCE: Dietary Reference Intakes for Energy, Carbohydrate, Fiber, Fat, Fatty Acids, Cholesterol, Protein, and Amino Acids (2002). This report may be accessed via www.nap.edu.

Tenth Edition

NUTRITION

FOR HEALTH, FITNESS & SPORT

Melvin H. Williams

Old Dominion University

Dawn E. Anderson

Winona State University

Eric S. Rawson

Bloomsburg University

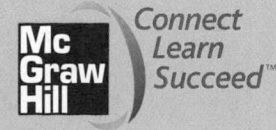

McGraw Hill

Connect
Learn
Succeed™

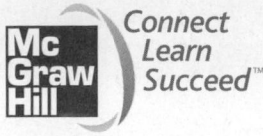

The McGraw-Hill Companies

Connect
Learn
Succeed™

NUTRITION FOR HEALTH, FITNESS AND SPORT, TENTH EDITION

Published by McGraw-Hill, a business unit of The McGraw-Hill Companies, Inc., 1221 Avenue of the Americas, New York, NY 10020. Copyright © 2013 by The McGraw-Hill Companies, Inc. All rights reserved. Printed in the United States of America. Previous editions © 2010, 2007, 2005, and 2002. No part of this publication may be reproduced or distributed in any form or by any means, or stored in a database or retrieval system, without the prior written consent of The McGraw-Hill Companies, Inc., including, but not limited to, in any network or other electronic storage or transmission, or broadcast for distance learning.

Some ancillaries, including electronic and print components, may not be available to customers outside the United States.

This book is printed on acid-free paper.

1 2 3 4 5 6 7 8 9 0 DOW/DOW 1 0 9 8 7 6 5 4 3 2

ISBN 978–0–07–131816–7
MHID 0–07–131816–X

www.mhhe.com

To Jeanne,
Sara, Nik, Katy, and Lucy May
Serena, Jeff, Daniel, and David Newsom
—*Melvin H. Williams*

To Jeff, Amanda, and Melanie
and Bill Morgan
—*Dawn E. Anderson*

To Debbie, Christopher, Matthew,
and Erica
—*Eric S. Rawson*

and

To our teachers, colleagues,
and students
Mel, Dawn, and Eric

Brief Contents

Contents

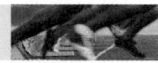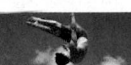

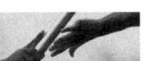

CHAPTER THREE

Human Energy 88

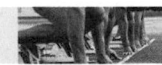

CHAPTER FOUR

Carbohydrates: The Main Energy Food 121

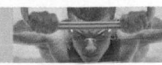

CHAPTER FIVE

Fat: An Important Energy Source During Exercise 171

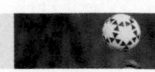

CHAPTER EIGHT

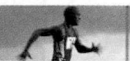

Minerals: The Inorganic Regulators 319

CHAPTER NINE

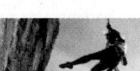

Water, Electrolytes, and Temperature Regulation 363

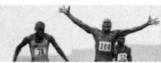

CHAPTER TEN

Body Weight and Composition for Health and Sport 416

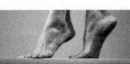

CHAPTER ELEVEN

Weight Maintenance and Loss through Proper Nutrition and Exercise 458

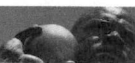

CHAPTER TWELVE

Weight Gaining through Proper Nutrition and Exercise 517

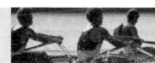

Food Drugs and Related Supplements 545

Preface

In this new millennium, our love affair with fitness and sports continues to grow. Worldwide, although physical inactivity is still very prevalent in developed nations, more of us are joining fitness facilities or initiating fitness programs, such as bicycling, running, swimming, walking, and weight training. Improvement in health and fitness is one of the major reasons that more and more people initiate an exercise program. Research has shown that adults who become physically active also may become more interested in other aspects of their lifestyles—particularly nutrition—that may affect their health in a positive way. Indeed, according to all major health organizations, proper exercise and a healthful diet are two of the most important lifestyle behaviors to help prevent chronic disease.

Nutrition is the study of foods and their effects upon health, development, and performance. Although a relatively young science, nutrition research has made a significant contribution to our knowledge of essential nutrient needs. During the first part of the twentieth century, most nutrition research focused on identification of essential nutrients and amounts needed to prevent nutrient-deficiency diseases, such as scurvy from inadequate vitamin C. As nutrition science evolved, medical researchers focused on the effects of foods and their specific constituents as a means to help prevent major chronic diseases, such as heart disease and cancer, that are epidemic in developed countries. *Nutriceutical* is a relatively new term used to characterize the drug, or medical, effects of a particular nutrient. Recent research findings continue to indicate that our diet is one of the most important determinants of our health status. Although individual nutrients are still being evaluated for possible health benefits, research is also focusing on dietary patterns, or the totality of the diet, and resultant health benefits.

Other than the health benefits of exercise and fitness, many physically active individuals also are finding the joy of athletic competition, participating in local sport events such as golf tournaments, tennis matches, triathlons, and road races. Individuals who compete athletically are always looking for a means to improve performance, be it a new piece of equipment or an improved training method. In this regard, proper nutrition may be a very important factor in improving exercise and sport performance. The United States Anti-Doping Agency (USADA), in its *Optimal Dietary Intake* guidelines for competitive athletes, notes that now more than ever, athletes need accurate sports nutrition information, indicating that optimal nutrition is an integral part of peak performance, while an inadequate diet and lack of fuel can limit an athlete's potential for maximum performance. Although the effect of diet on sport and exercise performance was studied only sporadically prior to 1970, subsequently numerous sport scientists and sport nutritionists have studied the performance-enhancing effects of nutrition, such as diet composition and dietary supplements. Results of these studies have provided nutritional guidance to enhance performance in specific athletic endeavors.

With the completion of the Human Genome Project, gene therapies are currently being developed for the medical treatment of various health problems. Moreover, some contend that genetic manipulations may be used to enhance sports performance. For example, gene doping to increase insulin-like growth factor, which can stimulate muscle growth, may be applied to sport.

Our personal genetic code plays an important role in determining our health status and our sports abilities, and futurists speculate that one day each of us will carry our own genetic chip that will enable us to tailor food selection and exercise programs to optimize our health and sport performance. Such may be the case, but for the time being we must depend on available scientific evidence to provide us with prudent guidelines.

Each year literally thousands of published studies and reviews analyze the effects of nutrition on health or exercise and sports performance. The major purpose of this text is to evaluate these scientific data and present prudent recommendations for individuals who want to modify their diet for optimal health or exercise/sport performance.

Textbook Overview

This book uses a question-answer approach, which is convenient when you may have occasional short periods to study, such as riding a bus or during a lunch break. In addition, the questions are arranged in a logical sequence, the answer to one question often leading into the question that follows. Where appropriate, cross-referencing within the text is used to expand the discussion. No deep scientific background is needed for the chemical aspects of nutrition and energy expenditure, as these have been simplified. Instructors who use this book as a course text may add details of biochemistry as they feel necessary.

Chapter 1 introduces you to the general effects of exercise and nutrition on health-related and sports-related fitness, including the importance of well-controlled scientific research. Chapter 2 provides a broad overview of sound guidelines relative to nutrition for optimal health and physical performance. Chapter 3 focuses upon energy and energy pathways in the body, the key to all exercise and sport activities.

Chapters 4 through 9 deal with the six basic nutrients—carbohydrate, fat, protein, vitamins, minerals, and water—with emphasis on the health and performance implications for the physically active individual. Chapters 10 through 12 review concepts of body composition and weight control, with suggestions on how to gain or lose body weight through diet and exercise, as well as the implications of such changes for health and athletic performance. Chapter 13 covers several drug foods, such as alcohol and caffeine, and other related dietary supplements regarding their effects on health and exercise performance. Several appendixes complement the text, providing data on caloric expenditure during exercise; detailed metabolic pathways for carbohydrate, fat, and protein, methods to determine body composition; nutritional value of fast foods; and other information pertinent to physically active individuals.

New to the Tenth Edition

The first edition of this textbook, titled *Nutrition for Fitness and Sport,* was published in 1983, and I have been the sole author for all subsequent editions. I am joined in this tenth edition by two professors who are actively involved in the disciplines of exercise physiology and sports nutrition, and who have used this text over the years to teach their university classes. Dawn Anderson is a professor in the Department of Health, Exercise, & Rehabilitative Sciences at Winona State University in Minnesota. Her email address is danderson@winona.edu. Eric Rawson is an associate professor in the Department of Exercise Science at Bloomsburg University in Pennsylvania. His email address is erawson@bloomu.edu. Dr. Anderson revised chapters 4, 5, 6, and 9; Dr. Rawson revised chapters 2, 3, 7, and 8; and I revised the remaining chapters.

The content throughout each chapter of the book has been updated, where merited, based on contemporary research findings regarding the effects of nutritional practices on health, fitness, and sport performance. More than 300 new references, including clinical studies, reviews, and meta-analyses, have been added to the text. Major changes include incorporation of the new *Dietary Guidelines for Americans* and the associated MyPlate model that has replaced the MyPyramid model. The new MyPlate model is designed to be more user friendly for the American population and is discussed in several chapters. New information from authoritative position statements dealing with exercise and nutrition issues has been incorporated in various chapters where relevant. These position statements have been developed by such prominent groups as the American College of Sports Medicine, the American Dietetic Association, Dietitians of Canada, the American Medical Association, the International Society of Sports Nutrition, the National Strength and Conditioning Association, and the American Academy of Pediatrics. Additionally, numerous Websites have been listed to help students explore various exercise and nutrition issues in more depth.

Chapter 1—Introduction to Nutrition for Health, Fitness, and Sports Performance
- New information on diet and health from the World Health Organization (WHO) report, *Global Strategy on Diet, Physical Activity and Health.*
- Introduction of the role of epigenetics in health.
- Discussion of the joint position stand by the American College of Sports Medicine and the American Diabetes Association on the role of physical activity in diabetes.
- Updated discussion of the role of myokines and adipokines on health.
- Introduction of updated government reports on diet, exercise, and health, including *Healthy People 2020, Physical Activity Guidelines for Americans,* and *Dietary Guidelines for Americans 2010,* including the new *ChooseMyPlate* model.
- Update of the position statement on *Nutrition and Athletic Performance* by the American College of Sports Medicine, the American Dietetic Association, and the Dietitians of Canada.
- Discussion of cautions on using the internet for diet and exercise information.

Chapter 2—Healthful Nutrition for Fitness and Sport: The Consumer Athlete
- Introduction and discussion of the new U.S. government nutrition education program ChooseMyPlate.
- Tips on how to use the new ChooseMyPlate.gov website.
- Update on how to increase the nutrient density of the diet, including tips from the Nutrient Rich Foods Coalition website.
- New data on whole grain and sugar consumption in American adults.
- New data on red meat consumption and morbidity and mortality.
- Updated position stand on vegetarian diets from the American Dietetic Association.
- New discussion on nutrients that were denied FDA approved qualified health claim status.

Chapter 3—Human Energy
- New data on physical activity and energy expenditure assessment using pedometers and accelerometers.
- New data on the sedentary behaviors and mortality and how to increase passive and occupational energy expenditure.
- New data on the thermic effect of food and the development of obesity.
- New discussion on the benefits of group exercise on exercise adherence.
- New data on exercising in a fasted versus fed state.
- New section and figures on the "Myth of the Fat Burning Zone" highlighting the misconceptions about exercise intensity, fat burning, energy expenditure, and weight loss.

Chapter 4—Carbohydrates: The Main Energy Food
- New information concerning carbohydrate consumption before and during an event relative to physical performance.
- Updated discussion on low-glycemic index foods and their impact on performace.
- New information on the impact of protein and carbohydrate consumption during recovery.

- Incorporation of updated government reports on diet, exercise, and health, including *Healthy People 2020* and *Dietary Guidelines for Americans 2010,* including the new *ChooseMyPlate* model.

Chapter 5—Fat: An Important Energy Source During Exercise
- Update of the position statement on *Nutrition and Athletic Performance* by the American College of Sports Medicine, the American Dietetic Association, and the Dietitians of Canada.
- Incorporation of updated government reports on diet, exercise, and health, including *Healthy People 2020* and *Dietary Guidelines for Americans 2010,* including the new *ChooseMyPlate* model.
- Updated discussion on chronic fat loading.
- New information on the impact of caloric restriction and fasting on performance.
- Updated information on the use of omega-3 fatty acids and their effects on fatigue and pulmonary function.
- Updated discussion of how to favorably modify the serum lipid profile.
- New information on the relative risk of *trans* fat intake and coronary heart disease, as well as the updated recommendation of *trans* fat intake by the American Heart Association.

Chapter 6—Protein: The Tissue Builder
- Incorporation of updated government reports on diet, exercise, and health, including *Healthy People 2020* and *Dietary Guidelines for Americans 2010,* including the new *ChooseMyPlate* model.
- Update of the position statement on *Nutrition and Athletic Performance* by the American College of Sports Medicine, the American Dietetic Association, and the Dietitians of Canada.
- New information regarding protein recommendations for active individuals from the International Society of Sports Nutrition.
- Updated information regarding protein intake prior to, and after exercise.
- New information on creatine supplementation.
- Updated discussions on Beta-Hydroxy-Beta-Methylbutyrate (IIMB), β-alanine, and taurine supplementation.
- New information on dietary nitrate supplementation.

Chapter 7—Vitamins: The Organic Regulators
- Updated dietary reference intakes for vitamin D.
- Discussion of the controversy surrounding the new vitamin D guidelines, including the discussion of vitamin D deficiency, insufficiency, and optimal level for health or performance.
- New data on vitamin D status and mortality, and prevalence and consequences of vitamin D deficiency in athletes.
- Updated website for the vitamin D Dietary Supplement Fact Sheet from the NIH Office of Dietary Supplements.
- New data on potential dangers of vitamin E supplementation in healthy and patient populations.
- New data on the effects of niacin and folic acid on disease.
- New data on the effects of antioxidant vitamins on mortality and muscle damage.
- Update on the effects of quercetin supplementation on various endurance tasks, metabolic outcomes, and perceived exertion in trained individuals.

Chapter 8—Minerals: The Inorganic Regulators
- Updated dietary reference intakes for calcium.
- New data on the role of calcium supplements in cancer and weight loss.
- Discussion of meal replacement powders and exceeding the upper tolerable limit of nutrients.
- New data on osteopenia and osteoporosis in cyclists.
- New data on creatine supplementation and bone health.
- New data on iron overload in runners.

Chapter 9—Water, Electrolytes, and Temperature Regulation
- Updated discussion on dehydration and sports specific activities.
- Updated information on carbohydrate, sodium, and potassium content of fluid replacement and high-carbohydrate beverages.
- Expanded information on hyponatremia.
- New information regarding hypertension in young people.
- Updated discussion on dietary modifications that may reduce or prevent hypertension.
- Updated information on the DASH Eating Plan.

Chapter 10—Body Weight and Composition for Health and Sport
- New data on the health risks of obesity, a global problem termed *globesity.*
- New information on calculating the Body Mass Index for children and teens.
- Update on the use of body composition analysis techniques.
- Update on the role of various genetic and environmental factors in the development of obesity.
- New data on the interactions among levels of physical activity and body weight relative to cardiovascular disease.
- Brief discussion of some of the proposed changes to forthcoming fifth edition of *Diagnostic and Statistical Manual of Mental Disorders (DSM-IV).*

Chapter 11—Weight Management and Loss through Proper Nutrition and Exercise
- New information on use of the ChooseMyPlate program for personalized diet and exercise programs for weight control.
- New information on the concept of caloric restriction and macronutrient content of the diet on weight loss.
- Updated information on the top-rated commercial weight-loss programs.
- Update on the efficacy and safety of dietary supplements for weight loss.
- Update of the American College of Sports Medicine Position Stand on physical activity for weight loss.
- Update of the Compendium of Physical Activities, which includes calculation of energy expenditure for more than 800 physical activities.

Chapter 12—Weight Gaining through Proper Nutrition and Exercise
- New data on the role of amount, timing, and quality of protein intake and increases in muscle mass associated with resistance training.
- New data on the role of eccentric exercise on development of muscle strength.

- Updates of policy and position statements by the American Academy of Pediatrics and by the National Strength and Conditioning Association regarding resistance training programs for youngsters.
- New data on the potential health benefits of resistance training.

Chapter 13—Food Drugs and Related Supplements
- New information from the *Global Status Report on Alcohol and Health* report by the World Health Organization on the adverse and positive health effects of alcohol consumption.
- Updated information on the positive ergogenic effects of caffeine, including an analysis in the position stand by the International Society of Sports Nutrition.
- Updated discussion of the potential positive and negative health effects of caffeine consumption, including a new section on energy drinks.
- Updated information on the performance-enhancing and health effects of human growth hormone and anabolic steroids.
- New information on the role of Epigallocatechin-3-gallate (EGCG), an extract from green tea, as an ergogenic aid.

Enhanced Pedagogy

Each chapter contains several features to help enhance the learning process. **Chapter Learning Objectives** are presented at the beginning of each chapter, highlighting the key points and serving as a studying guide. **Key Terms** also are listed at the beginning of each chapter, along with the page number on which they are first highlighted and defined. Although some terms may appear in the text before they are defined, a thorough glossary includes the key terms as well as other terms warranting definition. **Key Concepts** provide a summary of essential information presented throughout each chapter. Students are encouraged to participate in several practical activities to help reinforce learning. **Check for Yourself** includes individual activities, such as checking food labels at the supermarket or measuring one's own body fat percentage. The **Application Exercise** at the end of each chapter may require more extensive involvement, such as a case study in weight control involving yourself or a survey of an athletic team. Students may wish to peruse all application exercises at the beginning of the course, as some may take several weeks or months to complete.

The bibliographic references are of three types. *Books* listed provide broad coverage of the major topics in the chapter. *Reviews* are detailed analyses of selected topics, usually involving a synthesis and analysis of specific research studies. The *specific studies* listed are primary research studies. The reference lists have been completely updated for this tenth edition, with the inclusion of more than 300 new references, and provide the scientific basis for the new concepts or additional support for those concepts previously developed. These references provide greater in-depth reading materials for the interested student. Although the content of this book is based on appropriate scientific studies, a reference-citation style is not used, that is, each statement is not referenced by a bibliographic source. However, names of authors may be used to highlight a reference source where deemed appropriate.

This book is designed primarily to serve as a college text in professional preparation programs in health and physical education, exercise science, athletic training, sports medicine, and sports nutrition. It is also directed to the physically active individual interested in the nutritional aspects of physical and athletic performance.

Those who may desire to initiate a physical training program may also find the nutritional information useful, as well as the guidelines for initiating a training program. This book may serve as a handy reference for coaches, trainers, and athletes. With the tremendous expansion of youth sports programs, parents may find the information valuable relative to the nutritional requirements of their active children.

In summary, the major purpose of this book is to help provide a sound knowledge base relative to the role that nutrition, complemented by exercise, may play in the enhancement of both health and sport performance. We hope that the information provided in this text will help the reader develop a more healthful and performance-enhancing diet. Bon appetit!

Acknowledgments

This book would not be possible without the many medical/health scientists and exercise/sport scientists throughout the world who, through their numerous studies and research, have provided the scientific data that underlie its development. I am fortunate to have developed a friendship with many of you, and I extend my sincere appreciation to all of you.

The reviewers of the nine previous editions have played an integral role in the changes that are made, and this edition is no exception. We wish to extend a special note of appreciation to those who reviewed the ninth edition text and provided many valuable suggestions for improving the manuscript.

Tenth Edition:

Angela M. Alphonso
Clinton Community College

Raymond Bessinger
Winthrop University

Robert Buresh
Kennesaw State University

Cathryn Dooly
Lander University

Danielle Gandolfo
Delgado Community College

Rikki Keen
University of Alaska Anchorage

Cherie Moore
Cuesta College

Mary Pregler-Belmont
University of Dubuque

Jacquelyn Sgambati
Coastal Carolina University

Amanda Timberlake
Life University

Green T. Waggener
Valdosta State University

Brian Wallace
United States Sports Academy

Lauri Wright
University of South Florida

We would like to acknowledge deep gratitude to Darlene Schueller, Developmental Editor at McGraw-Hill, for her dedicated support throughout the revision process. Darlene was always available to address queries regarding various facets of the production process, and her responses were very prompt. We would also like to thank Anna Hoppmann, Digital Asset Librarian, for her assistance in navigating the photo database of McGraw-Hill, and Joyce Watters, our project manager. Our deep gratitude to Colin Wheatley, Executive Editor, and Lynne Meyers, Senior Developmental Editor, for their continued support. Many thanks also to Brooke Graves for her detailed review as a copyeditor.

Melvin H. Williams
Norfolk, Virginia
Dawn E. Anderson
Winona, Minnesota
Eric S. Rawson
Bloomsburg, Pennsylvania

Instructor and Student Resources

Available at www.mhhe.com/williams10e are a number of instructor and student resources to accompany the text. For students, these include a BMI calculator, animations, daily food log, and more. For instructors, resources include PPT lecture outlines, image PowerPoint files, and more.

![McGraw-Hill create logo]

McGraw-Hill Create™

Craft your teaching resources to match the way you teach! With McGraw-Hill Create, you can easily rearrange chapters, combine material from other content sources, and quickly upload content you have written, like your course syllabus or teaching notes. Find the content you need in Create by searching through thousands of leading McGraw-Hill textbooks. Arrange your book to fit your teaching style. Create even allows you to personalize your book's appearance by selecting the cover and adding your name, school, and course information. Order a Create book and you'll receive a complimentary print review copy in 3–5 business days or a complimentary electronic review copy (eComp) via email in minutes. Go to www.mcgrawhill create.com today and register to experience how McGraw-Hill Create empowers you to teach *your* students *your* way.

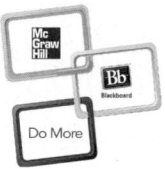

McGraw-Hill Higher Education and Blackboard® have teamed up.

Blackboard, the web-based course management system, has partnered with McGraw-Hill to better allow students and faculty to use online materials and activities to complement face-to-face teaching. Blackboard features exciting social learning and teaching tools that foster more logical, visually impactful and active learning opportunities for students. You'll transform your closed-door classrooms into communities where students remain connected to their educational experience 24 hours a day.

This partnership allows you and your students access to McGraw-Hill's Create right from within your Blackboard course—all with one single sign-on. McGraw-Hill and Blackboard can now offer you easy access to industry leading technology and content, whether your campus hosts it, or we do. Be sure to ask your local McGraw-Hill representative for details.

McGraw-Hill Connect® Nutrition

McGraw-Hill Connect Nutrition is a web-based assignment and assessment platform that gives students the means to better connect with their coursework, with their instructors, and with the important concepts that they will need to know for success now and in the future. With Connect Nutrition, instructors can deliver assignments, quizzes, and tests easily online. Students can practice important skills at their own pace and on their own schedule. Ask your McGraw-Hill representative for more details and check it out at www.mcgrawhillconnect.com.

Electronic Textbook Option

This text is offered through CourseSmart for both instructors and students. CourseSmart is an online resource where students can purchase the complete text online at almost half the cost of a traditional text. Purchasing the eTextbook allows students to take advantage of CourseSmart's web tools for learning, which include full-text search, notes and highlighting, and email tools for sharing notes between classmates. To learn more about CourseSmart options, contact your sales representative or visit www.CourseSmart.com.

Introduction to Nutrition for Health, Fitness, and Sports Performance

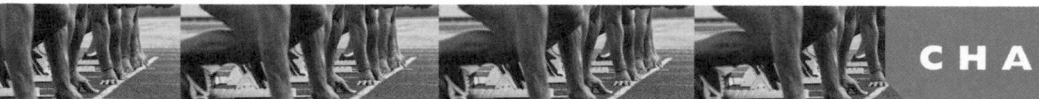

CHAPTER ONE

LEARNING OBJECTIVES

After studying this chapter, you should be able to:

1. Explain the role of both genetics and environment, particularly nutrition and exercise, in the determination of optimal health and successful sport performance.

2. List each of the components of health-related fitness, and then identify the potential health benefits of a physical fitness program designed to enhance both aerobic and musculoskeletal fitness.

3. Define sports-related fitness and compare it to health-related fitness, noting similarities and differences.

4. List the seven principles of exercise training and explain the importance of each.

5. List the twelve guidelines underlying the Prudent Healthy Diet and discuss, in general, the importance of proper nutrition to optimal health.

6. Understand the importance of proper nutrition, including the role of dietary supplements as ergogenic aids, to sports performance.

7. Define nutritional quackery and understand the various strategies you can use to determine whether claims regarding a dietary supplement are valid.

8. Explain what types of research have been used to evaluate the relationship between nutrition and health or sport performance, and evaluate the pros and cons of each type.

There are two major focal points of this book. One is the role that nutrition, complemented by physical activity and exercise, may play in the enhancement of one's health status. The other is the role that nutrition may play in the enhancement of fitness and sports performance. Many individuals today are physically active, and athletic competition spans all ages. Healthful nutrition is important throughout the life span of the physically active individual because suboptimal health status may impair training and competitive performance. In general, as we shall see, the diet that is optimal for health is also optimal for exercise and sports performance.

Nutrition, fitness, and health. Health care in most developed countries has improved tremendously over the past century. Primarily because of the dedicated work of medical researchers, we no longer fear the scourge of major acute infectious diseases such as polio, smallpox, or tuberculosis. However, we have become increasingly concerned with the treatment and prevention of chronic diseases. The World Health Organization (WHO) indicates that chronic diseases are now the major cause of death and disability worldwide. In the United States, the Centers for Disease Control and Prevention (CDC) indicates that seven of the ten leading causes of death are chronic diseases. Given with rank in parentheses, they include: (1) diseases of the heart, (2) cancer, (3) stroke, (4) chronic lung diseases, (6) Alzheimer's disease, (7) diabetes, and (9) chronic kidney diseases. These diseases cause more than 85 percent of all deaths, and this figure is destined to rise as the U.S. population becomes increasingly older, particularly during the first quarter of this century when the baby boomers of the 1940s and 1950s reach their senior years. Some epidemiologists contend that life expectancy in developed countries may start to decrease for the first time in history.

The two primary factors that influence one's health status are genetics and lifestyle. According to Simopoulos, all diseases have a genetic predisposition. The Human Genome Project, which deciphered the DNA code of our 80,000 to 100,000 genes, has identified various genes associated with many chronic diseases, such as breast and prostate cancer. Genetically, females whose mothers had breast cancer are at increased risk for breast cancer, while males whose fathers had prostate cancer are at increased risk for prostate cancer.

Completion of the Human Genome Project is believed to be one of the most significant medical advances of all time. Although multiple genes are involved in the etiology of most chronic diseases and research regarding the application of the findings of the Human Genome Project to improve health is in its initial stages, the future looks bright. For individuals with genetic profiles predisposing them to a specific chronic disease, such as cancer, genetic therapy eventually may provide an effective treatment or cure.

Although genetic influences may play an important role in the development of chronic diseases, so too does lifestyle. The CDC notes that although chronic diseases are among the most common and costly health problems, they are also among the most preventable by adopting a healthy lifestyle. Over the years, scientists in the field of epidemiology have identified a number of lifestyle factors considered to be health risks; these lifestyle factors are known as risk factors. A **risk factor** is a health behavior that has been associated with a particular disease, such as cigarette smoking being linked to lung cancer.

Kvaavik and others have identified four major risk factors for chronic diseases and premature death: physical inactivity, poor diet, excess alcohol consumption, and smoking. In a 20-year study, they found the greater the number of risk factors an individual possessed, the greater was the possibility of premature death. Individuals with all four of these poor health behaviors, compared to individuals with none, were more likely to die 12 years prematurely. Three of these major risk factors involve exercise and dietary behaviors. According to O'Gorman and Krook, physical inactivity is an independent risk factor for more than 25 chronic diseases.

The role of a healthful diet and exercise are intertwined with your genetic profile. What you eat and how you exercise may influence your genes. Epigenetics is a relatively new field of research involving the role of the **epigenome,** a structure located just outside the genome that may activate or deactivate DNA and subsequent genetic and cellular activity. In a recent review, Cloud indicated that various factors in our environment, such as substances in the foods we eat, may interact with the epigenome and thus modify cell functions—either in a positive or negative manner. Exercise, as noted later, also stimulates release of substances from muscle cells that may possibly affect the epigenome. Cloud notes that comparable to the Human Genome Project, a Human Epigenome Project is underway, and epigenetics may eventually lead to many beneficial health-related applications. For example, if personal genetic code indicates that your genetic profile predisposes you to certain forms of cancer, and if your genetic profile indicates that you will respond favorably to specific nutritional or exercise interventions, then a preventive diet and an exercise plan may be individualized for you. Genomics represents the study of genetic material in body cells, and the terms *nutrigenomics* and *exercisenomics* have been coined to identify the study of the genetic aspects of nutrition and exercise, respectively, as related to health benefits.

Treatment of chronic diseases is very expensive. Foreseeing a financial health-care crisis associated with an increasing prevalence of such diseases during the first half of this century, most private and public health professionals have advocated health promotion and disease prevention as the best approach to address this potential major health problem. For example, James Rippe, a renowned physician, has coined the term "lifestyle medicine" to characterize this focus on health promotion behaviors to help prevent disease. The United States Public Health Service, beginning in the 1980s, has published a series of reports designed to increase the nation's health; the latest version is entitled *Healthy People 2020: National Health Promotion/Disease Prevention Objectives. Physical activity/ fitness* and *overweight/obesity* are two major focus areas in *Healthy People 2020.* These reports emphasize that lifestyle behaviors that promote health and reduce the risk of chronic diseases are basically under the control of the individual. The role of diet and exercise in health promotion has become a worldwide priority, as documented in the WHO report, *Global Strategy on Diet, Physical Activity and Health.* The guidelines presented in these reports underlie the recommendations presented in this book. For both reports, see web addresses below.

As we shall see, proper exercise and proper nutrition, both individually and combined, may reduce many of the risk factors associated with the development of chronic diseases. These healthful benefits will be addressed at appropriate points throughout the book.

Nutrition, fitness, and sport. *Sport* is now most commonly defined as a competitive athletic activity requiring skill or physical prowess, for example, baseball, basketball, soccer, football, track, wrestling, tennis, and golf. As with health status, athletic ability and subsequent success in sport are based primarily upon two factors: natural genetic endowment and lifestyle, with lifestyle representing the appropriate type and amount of training.

To be successful at high levels of competition, athletes must possess the appropriate biomechanical, physiological, and psychological genetic characteristics associated with success in a given sport. International-class athletes have such genetic traits. In a recent review, Ahmetov and Rogozkin, two renowned Russian sport scientists, identified at least 36 genetic markers associated with the elite athlete. Moreover, Rankinen and others have assembled a human gene map for performance and health-related fitness.

Enhancement of athletic performance of elite athletes via genetic therapy, or genetic engineering, is a current concern among international sport organizations such as the International Olympic Committee (IOC) and the World Anti-Doping Agency (WADA). Several recent genetic engineering studies with rodents have produced "endurance" and "He-Man" mice. Although some sports scientists do not believe that genetic

engineering can be used to reliably produce champion athletes, others indicate it is only a matter of time and may even be in use now.

To be successful at high levels of competition, athletes must also develop their genetic characteristics maximally through proper biomechanical, physiological, and psychological coaching and training. Whatever the future holds for genetic enhancement of athletic performance, specialized exercise training will still be the key to maximizing genetic potential for a given sport activity. Training programs at the elite level have become more intense and individualized, sometimes based on genetic predispositions. Modern scientific training results in significant performance gains, and world records continue to improve.

Proper nutrition also is an important component in the total training program of the athlete. Certain nutrient deficiencies can seriously impair performance, whereas supplementation of other nutrients may help delay fatigue and improve performance. Over the past 50 years research has provided us with many answers about the role of nutrition in athletic performance, but unfortunately some findings have been misinterpreted or exaggerated so that a number of misconceptions still exist.

The purpose of this chapter is to provide a broad overview of the role that exercise and nutrition may play relative to health, fitness, and sport, and how prudent recommendations may be determined. More detailed information regarding specific relationships of nutritional practices to health and sports performance is provided in subsequent chapters.

www.health.gov/healthypeople   Check for the full report of *Healthy People 2020.*

http://www.who.int/dietphysicalactivity/en/   Check for the World Health Organization report on diet and physical activity for health.

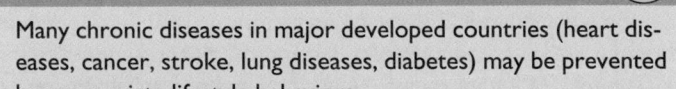

Key Concepts

▶ Many chronic diseases in major developed countries (heart diseases, cancer, stroke, lung diseases, diabetes) may be prevented by appropriate lifestyle behaviors.
▶ The two primary determinants of health status are genetics and lifestyle.

- Several of the key health promotion objectives set by the U.S. Department of Health and Human Services in *Healthy People 2020* are increased levels of physical activity, a healthier diet, and reduced levels of overweight and obesity.
- Sports success is dependent upon biomechanical, physiological, and psychological genetic characteristics specific to a given sport, but proper training, including proper nutrition, is essential to maximize one's genetic potential.

Check for Yourself

- Discuss with your parents any health problems they or your grandparents may have, such as high blood pressure or diabetes, to determine whether you may be predisposed to such health problems in the future. Having such knowledge may help you develop a preventive exercise and nutrition plan early in life. Please use the Website *www.hhs.gov/familyhistory* to create your own family history.

www.hhs.gov/familyhistory   Create your own family health history.

Health-Related Fitness: Exercise and Nutrition

Physical fitness may be defined, in general terms, as a set of abilities individuals possess to perform specific types of physical activity. The development of physical fitness is an important concern of many professional health organizations, including the American Alliance for Health, Physical Education, Recreation, and Dance (AAHPERD), which has categorized fitness components into two different categories. In general, these two categories may be referred to as health-related fitness and sports-related fitness. Both types of fitness may be influenced by nutrition and exercise.

Exercise and Health-Related Fitness

What is health-related fitness?

As mentioned previously, one's health status or wellness is influenced strongly by hereditarian predisposition and lifestyle behaviors, particularly appropriate physical activity and a high-quality diet. As we shall see in various sections of this book, one of the key factors in preventing the development of chronic disease is maintaining a healthful body weight.

Proper physical activity may certainly improve one's health status by helping to prevent excessive weight gain, but it may also enhance other facets of health-related fitness as well. **Health-related fitness** includes not only a healthy body weight and composition, but also cardiovascular-respiratory fitness, adequate muscular strength and muscular endurance, and sufficient flexibility (figure 1.1). Other measures used as markers of health-related fitness include blood pressure, bone strength, postural control and balance, and various indicators of lipid and carbohydrate metabolism. Several health professional organizations, such as

the American College of Sports Medicine (ACSM) and American Heart Association (AHA), have indicated that various forms of physical activity may be used to enhance health.

In general, **physical activity** involves any bodily movement caused by muscular contraction that results in the expenditure of energy. For purposes of studying its effects on health, epidemiologists classify physical activity as either unstructured or structured.

Unstructured physical activity includes many of the usual activities of daily living, such as leisurely walking and cycling, climbing stairs, dancing, gardening and yard work, various domestic and occupational activities, and games and other childhood pursuits. These unstructured activities are not normally planned to be exercise. However, as will be noted in chapters 2 and 10, they may play an important role in body weight control.

Structured physical activity, as the name implies, is a planned program of physical activities usually designed to improve physical fitness, including health-related fitness. For the purpose of this book, we shall refer to structured physical activity as **exercise,** particularly some form of planned vigorous exercise, such as brisk, not leisurely, walking.

What are the basic principles of exercise training?

Exercise training programs may be designed to provide specific types of health-related fitness benefits and/or enhance specific types of sports-related fitness. However, no matter what the purpose, several general principles are used in developing an appropriate exercise training program.

Principle of Overload   Overload is the basic principle of exercise training, and it represents the intensity, duration, and frequency of exercise. For example, a running program for cardiovascular-respiratory fitness could involve training at an intensity of 70 percent of maximal heart rate, a duration of 30 minutes, and a frequency of 5 times per week. The adaptations the body makes are based primarily on the specific exercise overload. The terms *moderate* exercise and *vigorous* exercise are often used to quantify exercise intensity.

Principle of Progression   Progression is an extension of the overload principle. As your body adapts to the original overload, the overload must be increased if further beneficial adaptations are desired. For example, you may start lifting a weight of 20 pounds, increase the weight to 25 pounds as you get stronger, and so forth. The overloads are progressively increased until the final health-related or sports-related goal is achieved.

Principle of Specificity   Specificity of training represents the specific adaptations the body will make in response to the type of exercise and overload. For example, running and weight lifting impose different demands, so the body adapts accordingly. Both types of exercise may provide substantial, yet different, health benefits. Exercise training programs may be designed specifically for certain health or sports-performance benefits.

Principle of Recuperation   Recuperation is an important principle of exercise training. Also known as the principle of recovery,

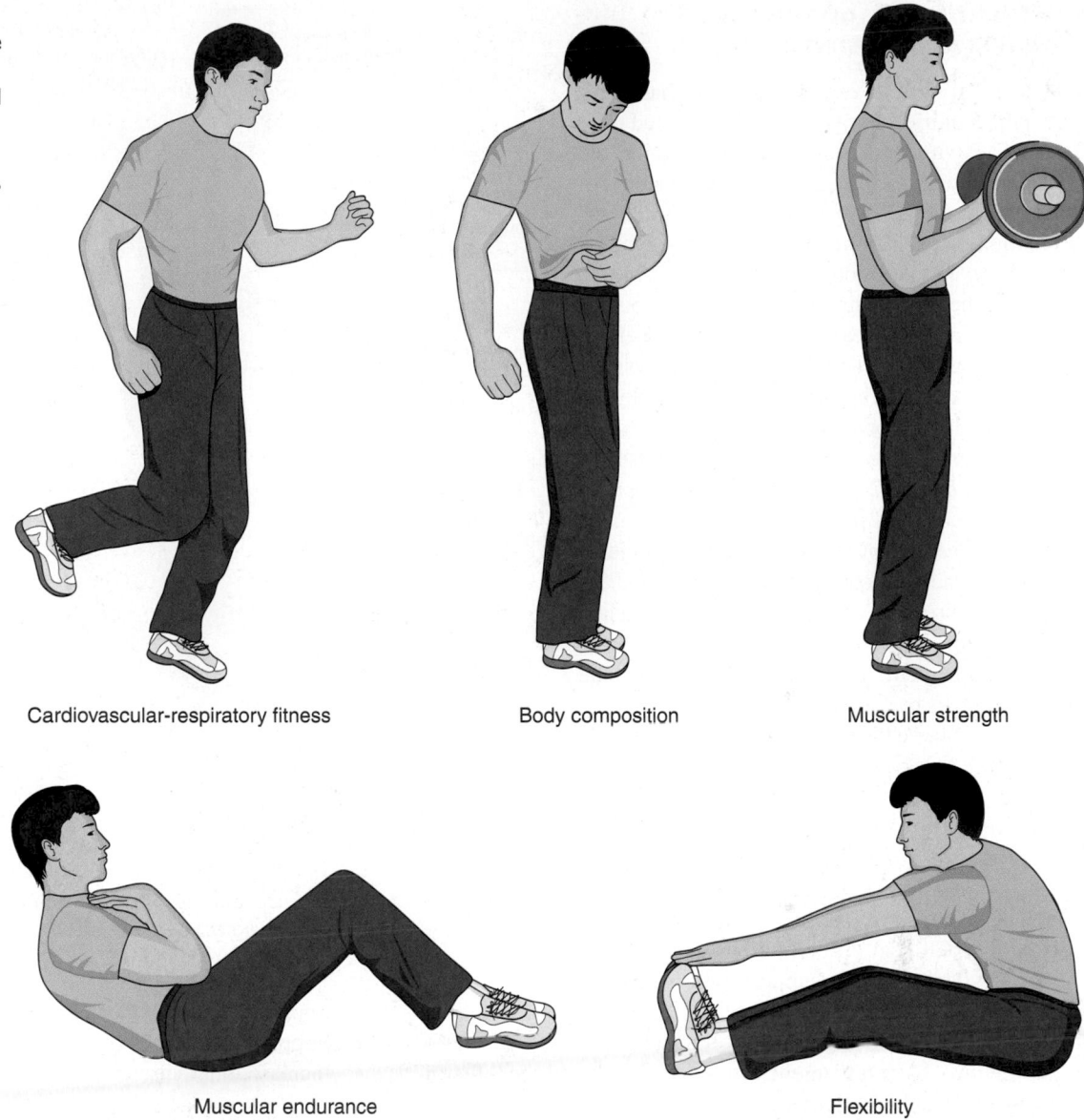

FIGURE 1.1 Health-related fitness components. The most important physical fitness components related to personal health include cardiovascular-respiratory fitness, body composition, muscular strength, muscular endurance, and flexibility.

Cardiovascular-respiratory fitness

Body composition

Muscular strength

Muscular endurance

Flexibility

it represents the time in which the body rests after exercise. This principle may apply within a specific exercise period, such as including rest periods when doing multiple sets during a weight-lifting workout. It may also apply to rest periods between bouts of exercise, such as a day of recovery between two long cardiovascular workouts.

Principle of Individuality Individuality reflects the effect exercise training will have on each given individual, as determined by genetic characteristics. The health benefits one receives from a specific exercise training program may vary tremendously among individuals. For example, although most individuals experience a reduction in blood pressure during a cardiovascular-respiratory fitness training program, some may not.

Principle of Reversibility Reversibility is also referred to as the principle of disuse, or *use it or lose it.* Without exercise, the body

will begin to lose the adaptations it has made over the course of the exercise program. Individuals who suffer a lapse in their exercise program, such as a week or so, may lose only a small amount of health-related fitness gains. However, a total relapse to a previous sedentary lifestyle can reverse all health-related fitness gains.

Principle of Overuse Overuse represents an excessive amount of exercise that may induce adverse, rather than beneficial, health effects. Overuse may be a problem during the beginning stages of an exercise program if one becomes overenthusiastic and exceeds her capacity, such as developing shin splints by running too far. Overuse may also occur in elite athletes who become overtrained, as discussed in chapter 3.

Specific exercise programs for healthy body weight and composition, cardiovascular-respiratory fitness, and muscular strength and muscular endurance are detailed in chapters 11 and 12, and several of these principles are discussed in more detail.

What is the role of exercise in health promotion?

The beneficial effect of exercise on health has been known for centuries. For example, Plato noted that "Lack of activity destroys the good condition of every human being while movement and methodical physical exercise save and preserve it." Plato's observation is even more relevant in contemporary society. Frank Booth, a prominent exercise scientist at the University of Missouri, has coined the term **Sedentary Death Syndrome, or SeDS.** Slentz and others discussed the cost of physical inactivity over time. The *short-term* cost of physical inactivity is metabolic deterioration and weight gain; the *intermediate-term* cost is an increase in disease, such as type 2 diabetes, whereas the *long-term* cost is increased premature mortality. Booth and Lees indicated that physical inactivity is cited as an actual cause of chronic disease by the U.S. Centers for Disease Control, increasing the relative risk of coronary artery disease by 45 percent, stroke by 60 percent, hypertension by 30 percent, and osteoporosis by 59 percent.

To help promote the health benefits of physical activity, the American College of Sports Medicine and the American Medical Association (AMA) recently launched a program entitled *Exercise Is Medicine™* designed to encourage physicians and other healthcare professionals to include exercise as part of the treatment for every patient. Clinical, epidemiological, and basic research evidence clearly supports the inclusion of regular physical activity as a tool for the prevention of chronic disease and the enhancement of overall health. Numerous studies and reviews have documented the manifold health benefits of exercise, which are highlighted below and in figure 1.2.

- Prevent increase in blood pressure
- Enhance blood lipid profile
- Prevent weight gain and metabolic syndrome
- Prevent type 2 diabetes
- Reduce risk of heart disease
- Promote recovery from heart disease
- Reduce risk of stroke
- Reduce risk of breast cancer
- Reduce risk of colon cancer
- Reduce risk of prostate cancer
- Improve self-image
- Reduce mental depression
- Enhance cognitive functions in the elderly
- Reduce risk of falls in the elderly
- Delay onset and severity of Alzheimer's disease
- Improve bone health
- Reduce arthritis pain
- Improve immune functions
- Promote healthy pregnancy of mother and fetus

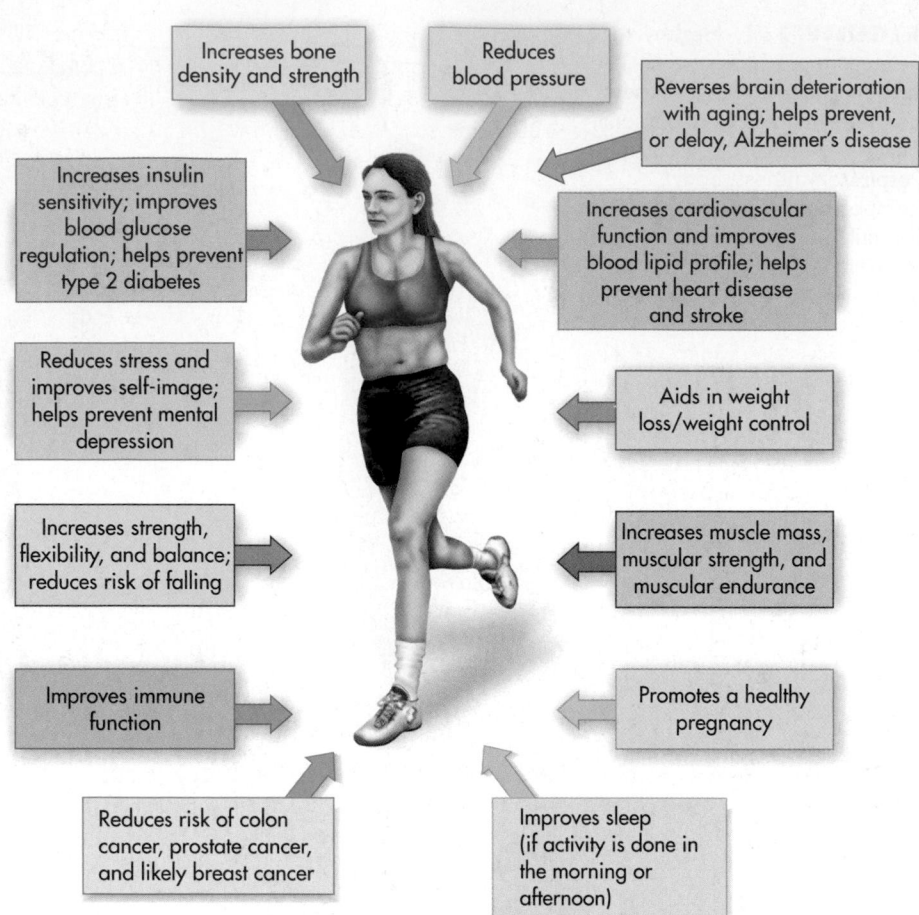

FIGURE 1.2 Exercise is medicine. Here are some of the benefits of regular, moderate physical activity and exercise. See text for discussion.

- Improve quality of sleep
- Improve quality of life
- Increase longevity

These benefits may accrue to males and females of all races across all age spans. You are never too young or too old to reap some of these health benefits of exercise.

Exercise may be especially helpful in preventing the premature development of chronic diseases. The term *predisease* recently has been used to describe several health conditions, such as a slightly elevated blood glucose, which if little is done may lead to a full-blown disease, such as diabetes. In a recent joint position stand, the American College of Sports Medicine and the American Diabetes Association concluded that it is now well established that participation in regular physical activity improves blood glucose control and can prevent or delay type 2 diabetes, along with positively affecting lipids, blood pressure, cardiovascular events, mortality, and quality of life.

In essence, physically active individuals enjoy a higher quality of life, a *joie de vivre*, because they are less likely to suffer the disabling symptoms often associated with chronic diseases, such as loss of ambulation experienced by some stroke victims. Physical activity may also increase the quantity of life. Franco and others found that a physically active lifestyle during adulthood, due to its effect of helping to prevent chronic diseases, increases life expectancy for men and women about 3.7 and 3.5 years, respectively. As James Fries, an emeritus professor who studies healthy aging at the Stanford University School of Medicine's Center on Longevity, has been quoted by Greider, "If you had to pick one thing, one single thing that came closest to the fountain of youth, it would have to be exercise."

How does exercise enhance health?

The specific mechanisms whereby exercise may help to prevent the development of various chronic diseases are not completely understood, but are involved with changes in gene expression that modify cell structure and function. Physical inactivity is a major risk factor for chronic diseases. Booth and Neufer have noted that physical inactivity causes genes to misexpress proteins, producing the metabolic dysfunctions that result in overt clinical disease if continued long enough. In contrast, exercise may cause the expression of genes with favorable health effects.

Most body cells can produce and secrete small proteins known as **cytokines,** which are similar to hormones and can affect tissues throughout the body. Cytokines enter various body tissues, influencing gene expression that may induce adaptations either favorable or unfavorable to health (figure 1.3). Two types of cytokines are of interest to us. Muscle cells produce various cytokines called *myokines,* whereas fat (adipose) cells produce cytokines called *adipokines.* The following represent several important cytokines produced in muscle and fat cells:

Muscle Cells	Fat Cells
Interleukin-6 (IL-6)	Tumor Necrosis Factor-alpha (TNF-α)
Brain-Derived Neurotropic Factor (BDNF)	Adiponectin

Muscle cells also produce *heat shock proteins* (HSPs) that may have beneficial health effects. Overall, Brandt and Pederson theorize that exercise-induced cytokine effects on genes reduce many of the traditional risk factors associated with development of chronic diseases; Geiger and others note similar effects for HSPs. For example, local inflammation is thought to promote the development of heart disease, cancer, diabetes, and dementia. Exercise produces an anti-inflammatory cytokine that may help cool inflammation and reduce such health risks. Cytokines and heat shock proteins may prevent chronic diseases in other ways as well, such as increasing the number of glucose receptors in muscle cells, improving insulin sensitivity, and helping to regulate blood glucose and prevent type 2 diabetes.

There are also other health-promoting mechanisms of exercise. Some examples include:

- Loss of excess body fat may reduce production of cytokines that may impair health.
- Loss of excess body fat may reduce estrogen levels, reducing risk of breast cancer.
- Reduction of abdominal obesity may decrease blood pressure and serum lipid levels.
- Increased mechanical stress on bone with high-impact exercise may stimulate increases in bone density.
- Production of some cytokines, such as BDNF, may enhance neurogenesis and brain functions.

Some healthful adaptations may occur with a single bout of exercise. Thompson and others have noted that a single exercise session can acutely improve the blood lipid profile, reduce blood pressure, and improve insulin sensitivity, all beneficial responses. However, such adaptations will regress unless exercise becomes habitual. Thus, to maximize health benefits, exercise should be done most days of the week because many of its benefits stem

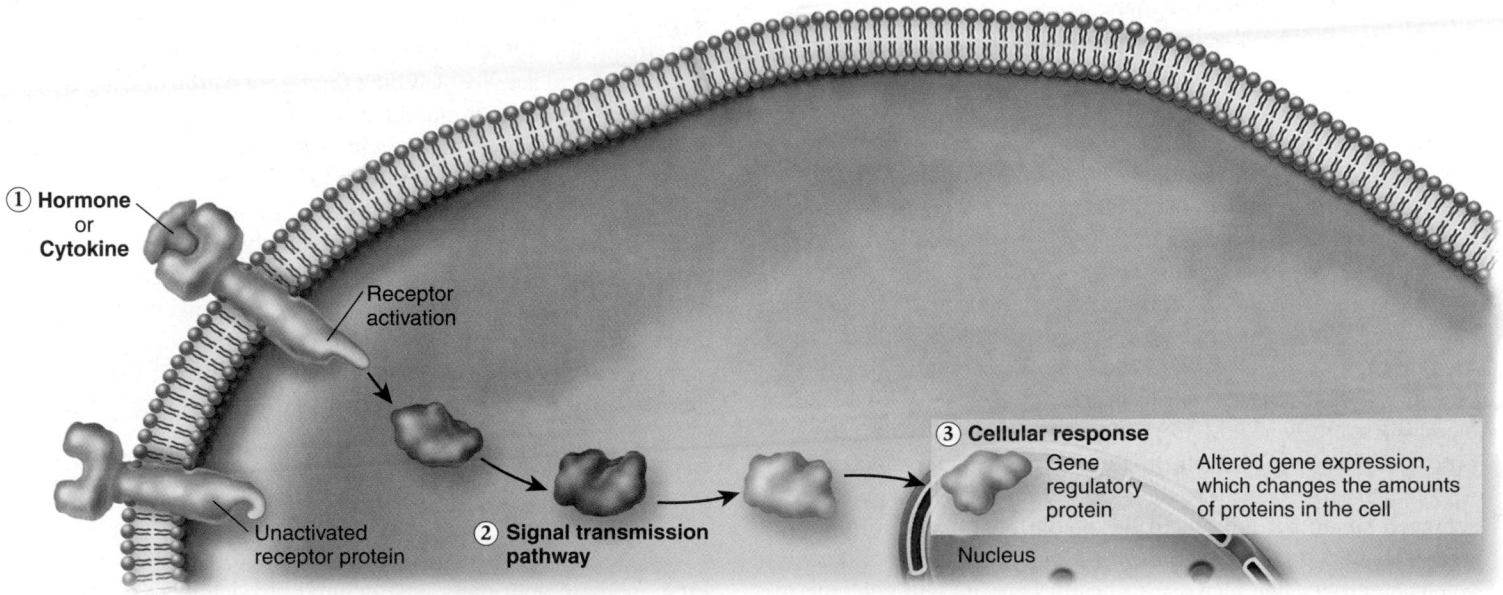

FIGURE 1.3 Exercise may induce adaptations that have favorable health effects in various body tissues. One suggested mechanism is the effect that various hormones or cytokines, which are produced during exercise, may have on gene regulation in body cells. (*1*) The hormone or cytokine binds to a cell receptor that activates a signal within the cell, (2) the signal is transmitted along a specific pathway, (3) the signal may alter gene expression and induce changes within the cell. Cell signals may also affect enzymes or other cell structures that may induce beneficial health effects.

from the most recent exercise sessions. The role that exercise may play in the prevention of some chronic diseases, such as heart disease, and associated risk factors, such as obesity, are discussed throughout this book where relevant.

Do most of us exercise enough?

In general, no. Surveys reveal that most adult Americans and Canadians have little or no physical activity in their daily lives. For example, the *Healthy People 2020* report from the United States Department of Health and Human Services indicates that more than 80 percent of adults do not meet the guidelines for both aerobic and muscle-strengthening activities. Similarly, more than 80 percent of adolescents do not do enough aerobic physical activity to meet the guidelines for youth. Other recent studies, such as those led by King and Morrow, found that 50 percent or fewer American adults engaged in sufficient physical activity for health benefits. Thus, one of the major goals of *Healthy People 2020* is to decrease the amount of physical inactivity, such as television viewing, and increase the amount of physical activity in both adults and youth.

How much physical activity is enough for health benefits?

To maximize health benefits, most health professionals recommend a comprehensive program of physical activity, including aerobic exercise, resistance training, and flexibility exercises. Aerobic exercise has been the major research focus, but resistance training also provides many health benefits, which are documented in chapter 12.

For aerobic exercise, a moderate amount of physical activity, or about 30 minutes daily of moderate-intensity exercise, is the basic recommendation. Health benefits may be achieved whether the 30 minutes of exercise is done continuously, or as three 10-minute *exercise snacks* done throughout the day. However, some exercise scientists contend that although moderate exercise is fine, more vigorous exercise can elicit additional benefits. Kuchment indicates the mechanism underlying the enhanced benefits from more vigorous exercise is not known, but one factor may be a decrease in inflammatory processes. Some guidelines to moderate-intensity and more vigorous-intensity exercise are presented under the next question.

In general, there is a curvilinear relationship between the amount of physical activity (dose) and related health benefits (response), as depicted by the dose-response graph in figure 1.4. A sedentary lifestyle has no health benefits, but health benefits increase rapidly with low to moderate levels of weekly activity. For example, Tully and others found that sedentary individuals who began an exercise program of walking just 3 days a week achieved some, but not all, of the health benefits seen by those who walked 5 days a week. Beyond moderate levels of weekly physical activity, the increase in health benefits will continue to increase gradually and then plateau. Excessive exercise may actually begin to have adverse effects on some health conditions.

However, as noted by Bouchard, there may be other specific dose-response curves. Some health conditions may improve rapidly with low to moderate weekly levels of physical activity, whereas

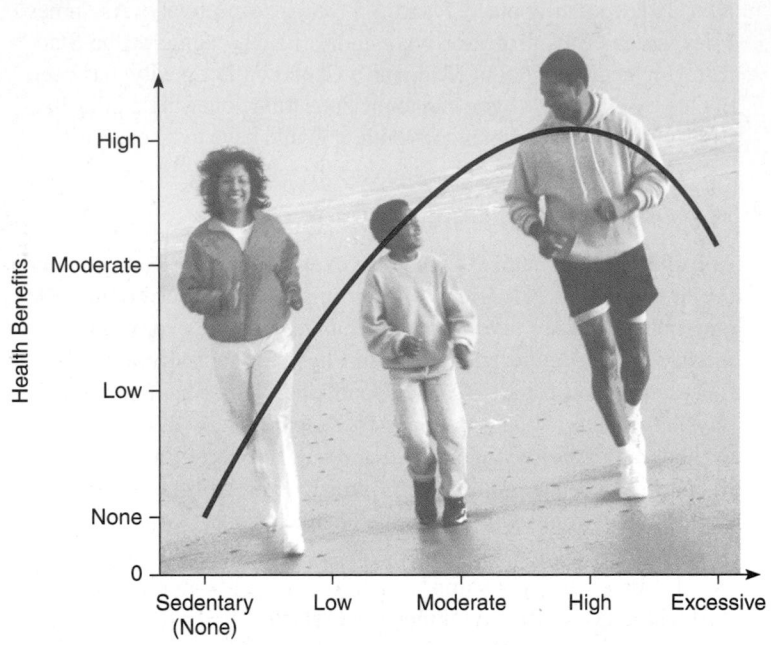

FIGURE 1.4 Significant health benefits may occur at low to moderate levels of physical activity with diminishing returns at higher levels. Excessive amounts or intensity of exercise, depending on the individual, may predispose to various types of health problems. See text for discussion.

others may necessitate increased levels. As an example of the latter, the recent ACSM Position Stand on physical activity and weight loss has noted that while moderate-intensity exercise between 150 and 250 minutes weekly will provide only modest weight loss, greater amounts of physical activity, averaging more than 250 minutes weekly, have been associated with clinically significant weight loss. Dependent on the desired health outcome, the dose (intensity, duration, frequency) of physical activity may vary accordingly, as will type of physical activity (aerobic exercise for cardiovascular fitness; resistance exercise for muscular fitness). Moreover, the response to exercise depends on the individual. Claude Bouchard, an expert in genetics, exercise, and health, noted that due to genes, physical activity may affect some, but not others. For example, although most sedentary individuals will respond favorably to an aerobic exercise training program, such as by improving insulin sensitivity, others will not respond and have no change in insulin sensitivity. Currently there is no gene profile for responders and nonresponders to exercise training, but that may change in the future so specific exercise programs may be designed for individuals.

What are some general guidelines for someone who wants to exercise properly for its health benefits?

First, increase your daily unstructured physical activity, which is a form of light exercise. One important modification to your daily lifestyle is to sit less. If your occupation is one in which you sit most of the day, take a short break every hour and walk around for several minutes. Build light physical activity into your daily schedule. For example, walk to the store instead of driving. Take

TABLE 1.1 Some examples of moderate amounts of physical activity*

Washing and waxing a car for 45–60 minutes

Washing windows or floors for 45–60 minutes

Playing various team sports for 45 minutes

Gardening for 30–45 minutes

Wheeling self in wheelchair for 30–40 minutes

Walking 2 miles in 40 minutes (20 minutes/mile)

Bicycling 5 miles in 30 minutes (10 miles/hour)

Dancing (social) fast for 30 minutes

Walking briskly 2 miles in 30 minutes (15 minutes/mile)

Water aerobics for 30 minutes

Swimming laps for 20 minutes

Bicycling 4 miles in 15 minutes (3.75 minutes/mile)

Jumping rope for 15 minutes

Running 1.5 miles in 15 minutes (10 minutes/mile)

Stairwalking for 15 minutes

*A moderate amount of physical activity is roughly equivalent to physical activity that uses about 150 Calories per day, or 1,000 Calories per week. Note that exercising at lower intensity levels requires more time (walking 2 miles in 40 minutes) than exercising at higher intensity levels (running 1.5 miles in 15 minutes). Adapted from U.S. Department of Health and Human Services. *The Surgeon General's Report on Physical Activity and Health.*

the stairs instead of the elevator. Walk your dog instead of letting him out into the backyard (your dog needs exercise, too). Accumulating more daily unstructured physical activity may be very helpful in maintaining a healthy body weight.

Second, increase your daily amount of structured physical activity. Most guidelines for structured physical activity recommend exercising at moderate or vigorous intensity.

In general, moderate-intensity exercise is defined as working at 40 to 60 percent of your aerobic capacity, which we will detail in chapter 3. You should experience noticeable increases in heart rate and breathing. Your perception of the effort needed to exercise is another gauge of its intensity. Check page 499 for the 10-point scale of perceived exertion. Moderate-intensity effort is a 5 or 6 on this scale, or the feeling that the exercise feels somewhat hard. Walking at a speed of 3 miles per hour, or 20 minutes per mile, is a good guideline to moderate-intensity exercise for most individuals. Vigorous, or high-intensity, exercise usually is defined as working at 60 percent or more of your aerobic capacity, or about a 7 or 8 on the perceived effort scale. At this level of exercise, there are large increases in heart rate and breathing, so that it should be difficult to carry on a conversation using complete sentences. Jogging or running may be considered vigorous exercise for sedentary individuals.

Both moderate and vigorous exercise, and generally a mixture of the two are recommended for health benefits. Some examples of moderate physical activity that will burn about 150 Calories in an adult male are presented in table 1.1. For individuals using exercise for body weight control, caloric expenditure is a key factor. More detailed guidelines are presented in chapter 11, but

you may want to consult appendix B to estimate Calories burned per minute for various types of physical activity and exercise. Additionally, an activity calorie calendar is available that will provide you with an estimate of caloric expenditure for a variety of daily activities and exercises. Go to *http://www.primusweb.com/fitnesspartner.*

Numerous reports providing exercise recommendations for health benefits have recently have been released by various professional and governmental health-related organizations, including the U.S. Department of Health and Human Services report, *Physical Activity Guidelines for Americans* (*www.health.gov/paguidelines/* and the *National Physical Activity Plan,* a coalition report from the American Heart Association, the ACSM, the Centers for Disease Control, the YMCA, and 15 other such organizations (*www.physicalactivityplan.org*). These exercise recommendations are above and beyond those activities of daily living, such as leisurely walking, climbing stairs, gardening, and other similar activities. The following is a summarization of these recommendations.

1. *Aerobic exercise.* Children and adolescents should do 60 minutes of moderate to vigorous physical activity daily, with vigorous activity at least 3 days per week. Short bursts of vigorous activity in games are included. Both adults and older adults should engage in moderate-intensity aerobic (endurance) exercise for a minimum of 30 minutes daily on 5 days each week, or vigorous-intensity aerobic physical activity for a minimum of 20 minutes on 3 days each week. Individuals may combine these workouts during the week, such as doing moderate-intensity exercise 2 days and vigorous-intensity on another 2 days. Moreover, the daily exercise time may be subdivided into multiple bouts, such as doing three 10-minute brisk walks to total 30 minutes over the course of a day. For additional and more extensive health benefits, adults should increase their aerobic physical activity to 300 minutes (5 hours) a week of moderate-intensity, or 150 minutes a week of vigorous activity, or an equivalent combination of moderate and vigorous exercise. Aerobic exercise programs are detailed in chapter 11.

2. *Resistance exercise.* Children and adolescents should do muscle-strengthening activity at least 3 days a week. Both adults and older adults should do exercises that maintain or increase muscular strength and endurance. The recommendation includes 8 to 10 exercises that stress the major muscle groups of the body. Individuals should perform about 8–12 repetitions of each exercise at least twice a week on nonconsecutive days. Older adults may lift lighter weights or use less resistance, but do more repetitions. Resistance exercises may include use of weights or other resistance modes, or weight-bearing activities such as stair climbing, push-ups, pull-ups, and various other calisthenics that stress major muscle groups. Resistance exercise programs will be discussed in chapter 12.

3. *Flexibility and balance exercise.* Older adults should perform activities that help maintain or increase flexibility on at least 2 days each week for at least 10 minutes daily. Flexibility exercises are designed to maintain the range of joint motion for daily activities and physical activity. Older adults should

also perform exercises that help maintain or improve balance about three times a week. Such exercises may help reduce the risk of injury from falls.

4. *Individualization.* Exercise programs, especially for older adults, should be individualized based on physical fitness level and health status. Individuals should be as active as possible for their fitness level and health status. One key component is simply to reduce the amount of daily sedentary activity. Leisure walking may be adequate physical activity for elderly individuals with compromised health status or very low fitness levels.

One of the concepts of these recommendations is *more is better*. For those who have the time and energy, exceeding the recommended amounts of physical activity may provide additional health benefits beyond those associated with the minimum recommendations. In particular, more exercise may be an important consideration to promote weight loss and prevent weight gain.

www.americanheart.org For more information on these recommendations, click on Healthy Lifestyle, and then Exercise and Fitness.

These recommendations for adults have been formatted into a MyActivity Pyramid, a graphic depicting exercise guidelines. The latest version, developed by Stephen Ball at the University of Missouri, is presented in figure 1.5.

These physical activity guidelines form the basis for designing an aerobics program for cardiovascular-respiratory fitness and proper weight control presented in chapter 11 and the principles of resistance training for muscular strength and endurance presented in chapter 12. If you are interested in starting an exercise program, you may preview those chapters or access one or more of the following excellent Websites for more detail.

http://www.health.gov/paguidelines Provides details on the Physical Activity Guidelines for Americans.

www.healthypeople.gov/hp2020 Presents details of physical activity guidelines for all Americans.

www.exerciseismedicine.org/public.htm Provides access to exercise guidelines from the American College of Sports Medicine and American Heart Association, as well as from the National Physical Activity Plan.

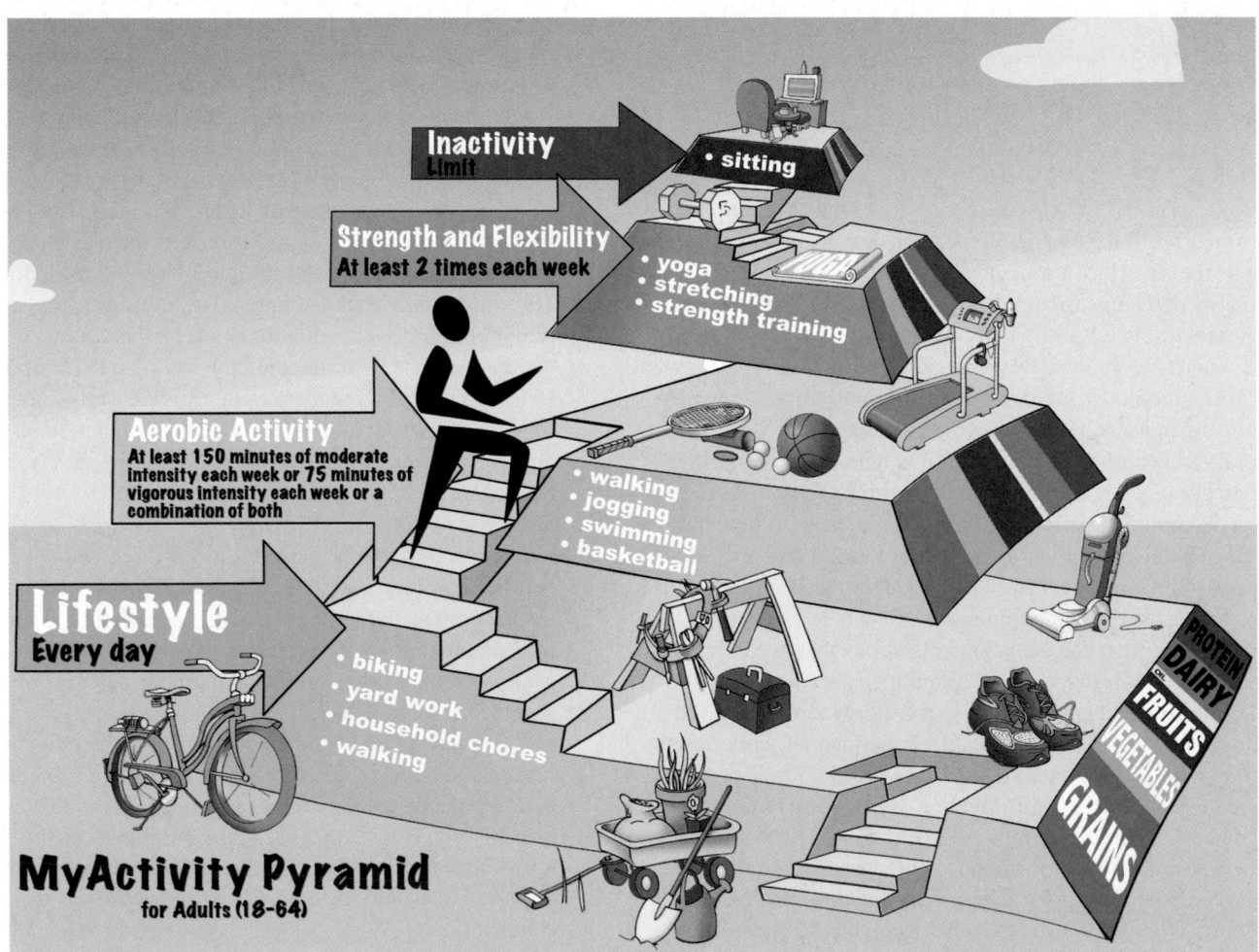

FIGURE 1.5 One version of a physical activity pyramid. See text for more specific information regarding exercise intensity and duration for adults and older adults.

Courtesy of Dr. Stephen D. Ball. Department of Nutrition and Exercise Physiology, University of Missouri, Columbia, MO.

Am I exercising enough?

Keep a record of all your physical activity for a week, such as how many minutes you walk; engage in some type of aerobic physical activity such as swimming, cycling, or jogging; or perform resistance exercise such as lifting weights. Chapter 11 contains a form you can use, modifying it as you see fit, to record your daily physical activities. Tallying your totals for the week and comparing them to the previously mentioned recommendations for aerobic and resistance exercise will give you a good idea as to whether you are meeting current recommendations. For a more detailed analysis, you can go to *www.ChooseMyPlate .gov.* Click on Interactive Tools, then Food Tracker to assess your physical activity. We will introduce ChooseMyPlate later in this and the next chapter, and also discuss using it as a guide to weight control in chapter 11.

Can too much exercise be harmful to my health?

In general, the health benefits far outweigh the risks of exercise. Although individuals training for sport may need to undergo prolonged, intense exercise training, such is not the case for those seeking health benefits of exercise. Given our current state of knowledge, adhering to the guidelines presented above, preferably at the upper time and day limits, should be safe and provide optimal health benefits associated with physical activity. However, exercise, particularly when excessive and in individuals with preexisting health problems, may increase the risk of the following health problems:

- *Orthopedic problems.* Too much exercise may lead to orthopedic problems, such as stress fractures in the lower leg in those who run, particularly in those with poor biomechanics. However, recovery from such orthopedic problems occurs with proper rest.
- *Impaired immune functions.* In a review of 30 studies, Moreira and others concluded that moderate activity may enhance immune function, whereas prolonged, high-intensity exercise may temporarily impair immune competence and cause higher rates of upper respiratory tract infection (URTI). Excessive exercise may also lead to chronic fatigue, as discussed in chapter 3.
- *Exercise-induced asthma.* Webb and Lieberman reported that in a study of more than 600 patients experiencing anaphylaxis, about 5 percent of incidents were precipitated by exercise.
- *Osteoporosis.* When coupled with inadequate dietary energy intake, exercise that leads to excessive weight loss may contribute to the menstrual irregularities in female athletes that may exacerbate loss of bone mass, or osteoporosis. This topic is discussed in chapters 8 and 10.
- *Heat illness and kidney failure.* Exercising in the heat may cause heat stroke or other heat illnesses with serious consequences, such as kidney failure and death, as discussed in chapter 9.
- *Sudden death.* Varró and Baczkó note that although sudden death among young athletes is very rare, it is still 2–4 times more frequent than in the age-matched control population, and attracts significant media attention. One cause is an enlarged heart, technically known as hypertrophic cardiomyopathy, a genetic defect that contributes to abnormal heart rhythms and subsequent heart failure. Other possible causes of sudden death include exercise-induced asthma and respiratory arrest, exercise-induced anaphylaxis, kidney failure, and head trauma. Sudden death in older athletic individuals may be associated with coronary heart disease, discussed in detail in chapter 5. Other possible causes will be discussed in later chapters, including heat stroke and use of performance-enhancing drugs.

It is important to emphasize that although a properly planned exercise program may be safe and confer multiple health benefits to most individuals, exercise may be hazardous to some. The most common concern is a heart attack. Individuals who have any concerns about their overall health, particularly those over age 35, should have a medical screening to detect risk factors for heart disease, such as high blood pressure, before increasing their level of physical activity. Such a medical screening might include an exercise stress test during which your heart rate and blood pressure are monitored for abnormal responses. Although exercise may be a temporary risk, it conveys lasting protection. The best protection for the heart is to exercise frequently, mainly because regular exercise helps prevent heart disease in the first place. Additional details are provided in subsequent chapters.

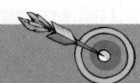

Key Concepts

▶ Health-related fitness includes a healthy body weight, cardiovascular-respiratory fitness, adequate muscular strength and muscular endurance, and sufficient flexibility.
▶ Overload is the key principle underlying the adaptations to exercise that may provide a wide array of health benefits.

- The intensity, duration, and frequency of exercise represent the means to impose an overload on body systems that enable healthful adaptations.
- ▶ Physical inactivity may be dangerous to your health. Exercise, as a form of physical activity, is becoming increasingly important as a means to achieve health benefits, by preventing the development of many chronic diseases.
- ▶ Physical activity need not be strenuous to achieve health benefits, but additional benefits may be gained through more vigorous and greater amounts of physical activity.
- ▶ Excessive exercise may cause some minor and major health problems in some individuals. You should be aware of personal health issues or other factors that may be related to exercise-associated health risks.

Check for Yourself

- ▶ As a prelude to activities presented in later chapters, make a detailed record of all your physical activities for a full day, from the moment you arise in the morning until you go to bed at night.

Nutrition and Health-Related Fitness

What is nutrition?

Nutrition usually is defined as the sum total of the processes involved in the intake and utilization of food substances by living organisms, including ingestion, digestion, absorption, transport, and metabolism of nutrients found in food. This definition stresses the biochemical or physiological functions of the food we eat, but the American Dietetic Association notes that nutrition may be interpreted in a broader sense and be affected by a variety of psychological, sociological, and economic factors.

From a standpoint of health and sport performance, it is the biochemical and physiological role or function of food that is important. However, economic factors, particularly with some college students, may influence healthful food selection. For example, healthier foods such as fresh fruits and vegetables are more expensive than highly processed food laden with highly refined grains, sugar, and fat, three inexpensive ingredients. For example, a recent government report indicated that this is what $1 can buy:

- 1,200 Calories of potato chips
- 875 Calories of soda
- 250 Calories of vegetables
- 170 Calories of fresh fruit

The primary purpose of the food we eat is to provide us with a variety of nutrients. A **nutrient** is a specific substance found in food that performs one or more physiological or biochemical functions in the body. There are six major classes of essential nutrients found in foods: carbohydrates, fats, proteins, vitamins, minerals, and water. However, as noted in chapter 2, food contains substances other than essential nutrients that may affect body functions.

As illustrated in figure 1.6, the essential nutrients perform three basic functions. First, they provide energy for human metabolism

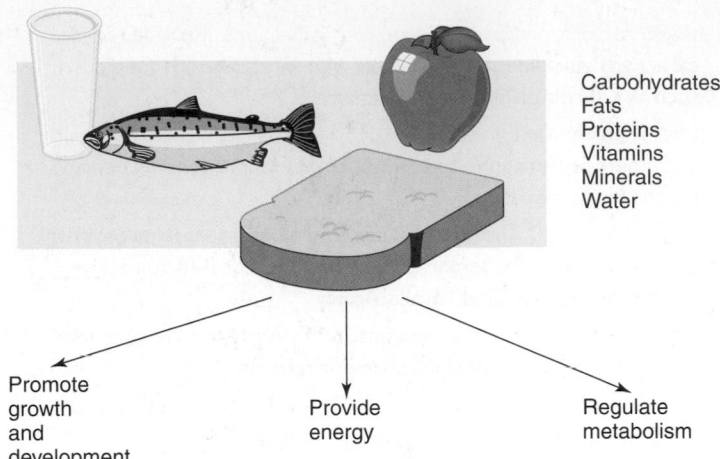

Carbohydrates
Fats
Proteins
Vitamins
Minerals
Water

Promote growth and development

Provide energy

Regulate metabolism

FIGURE 1.6 Three major functions of essential in food. Many nutrients have only one key role (e.g., glucose provides energy), whereas others have multiple roles (e.g., protein is necessary for growth and development and regulation of metabolism, and it may also be used as a source of energy).

(see chapter 3). Carbohydrates and fats are the prime sources of energy. Protein may also provide energy, but this is not its major function. Vitamins, minerals, and water are not energy sources. Second, all nutrients are used to promote growth and development by building and repairing body tissue. Protein is the major building material for muscles, other soft tissues, and enzymes, while certain minerals such as calcium and phosphorus make up the skeletal framework. Third, all nutrients are used to help regulate and maintain the diverse physiological processes of human metabolism.

In order for our bodies to function effectively, we need more than 40 specific essential nutrients, and we need these nutrients in various amounts as recommended by nutrition scientists. Dietary Reference Intakes (DRI) represent the current recommendations in the United States, and include the Recommended Dietary Allowances (RDA). These recommendations are detailed in chapter 2. Nutrient deficiencies or excesses may cause various health problems, some very serious.

What is the role of nutrition in health promotion?

As noted previously, your health is dependent upon the interaction of your genes and your environment, and the food you eat is part of your personal environment. *Let food be your medicine and medicine be your food.* This statement has been attributed to Hippocrates for over two thousand years, and it is becoming increasingly meaningful as the preventative and therapeutic health values of food relative to the development of chronic diseases are being unraveled. Nutrients and other substances in foods, similar to the aforementioned cytokines produced in muscle and fat cells, may influence gene expression, some having positive and others negative effects on our health. For example, adequate amounts of certain vitamins and minerals may help prevent damage to DNA, the functional component of your genes, while excessive alcohol may lead to DNA damage.

Most chronic diseases have a genetic basis; if one of your parents has had coronary heart disease or cancer, you have an increased probability of contracting that disease. Such diseases may go through three stages: initiation, promotion, and progression. Your genetic predisposition may lead to the initiation stage of the disease, but factors in your environment promote its development and eventual progression. In this regard, some nutrients are believed to be **promoters** that lead to progression of the disease, while other nutrients are believed to be **antipromoters** that deter the initiation process from progressing to a serious health problem.

What you eat plays an important role in the development or progression of a variety of chronic diseases. For example, the National Center for Chronic Disease Prevention and Health Promotion indicates that good nutrition lowers people's risk for many chronic diseases, including heart disease, stroke, some types of cancer, diabetes, and osteoporosis (see figure 1.7). The National Cancer Institute estimates that one-third of all cancers are linked in some way to diet, ranking just behind tobacco smoking as one of the major causes of cancer. DeMarini estimates that appropriate dietary

changes could reduce by 50 percent the deaths due to prostate, colorectal, pancreatic, and breast cancer.

As noted previously, *Exercise Is Medicine*. In a like manner, *Food Is Medicine* may also be an appropriate phrase, not only attributable to the quote from Hippocrates, but based on modern medicine as well. The types and amount of carbohydrate, fat, and protein that we eat; the amount and type of other substances such as vitamins, minerals, and phytochemicals found in our foods; the source of our food; and the method of food preparation are all factors that may influence the epigenome and subsequent gene expression or other metabolic functions that may affect our health status. The following are some of the proposed effects of various nutrients and appropriate energy intake that may help promote good health:

- Inactivate carcinogens or kill bacteria that cause cancer
- Increase insulin sensitivity
- Relax blood vessels and improve blood flow

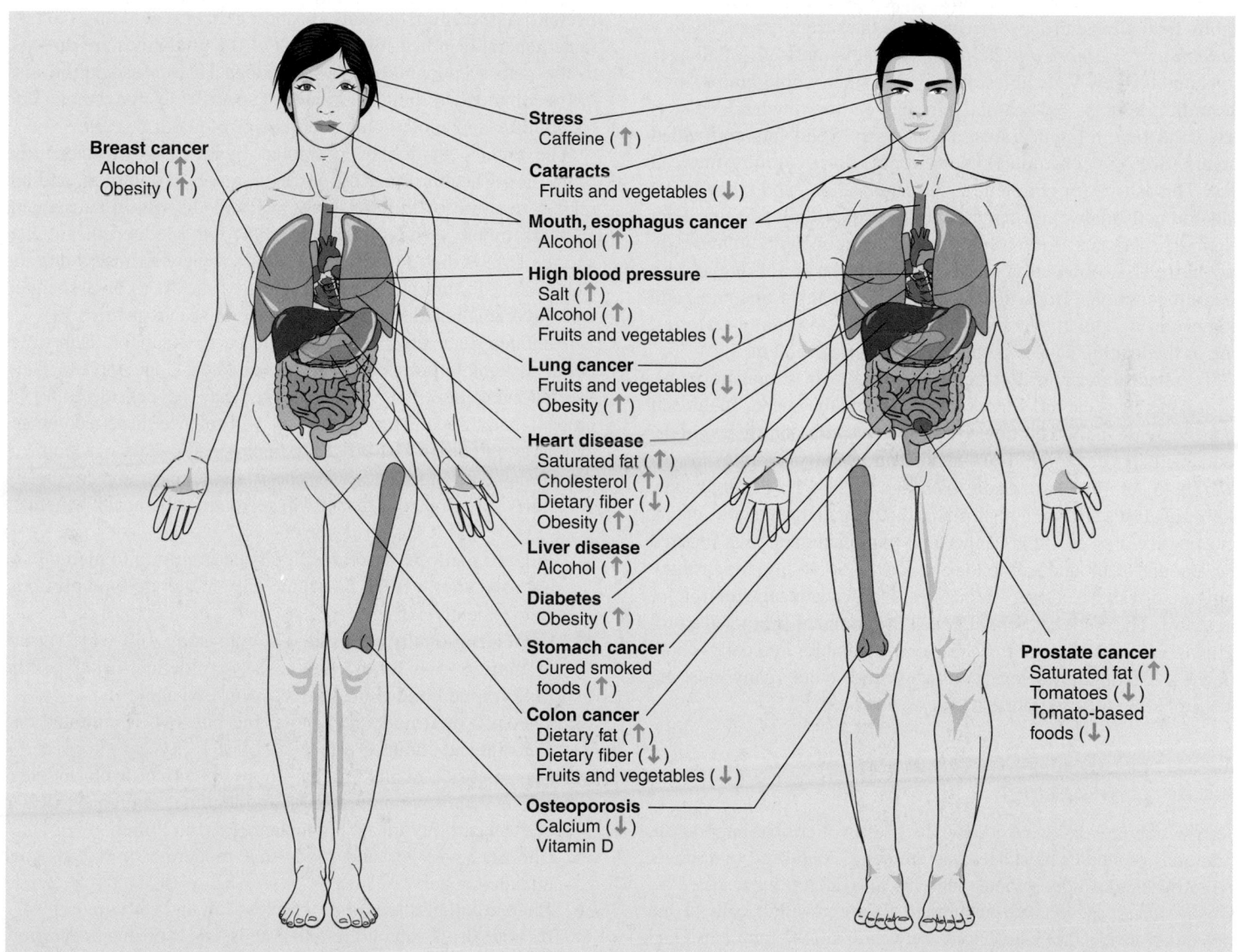

FIGURE 1.7 Some possible health problems associated with poor dietary habits. An upward arrow (↑) indicates excessive intake while a downward arrow (↓) indicates low intake or deficiency.

- Reduce blood pressure
- Optimize serum lipid levels
- Reduce inflammation
- Inhibit blood clotting
- Enhance immune system functions
- Speed up digestive processes
- Prevent damaging oxidative processes
- Reduce body fat

The beneficial, or harmful, effects of specific nutrients and various dietary practices on mechanisms underlying the development of chronic diseases will be discussed as appropriate in later sections of this book.

Do we eat right?

Surveys indicate that most people are aware of the role of nutrition in health and want to eat better for healthful purposes, but they do not translate their desires into appropriate action. Poor eating habits span all age groups. According to the recent report, *Dietary Guidelines for Americans 2010,* on average Americans of all ages consume too few vegetables, fruits, high-fiber whole grains, low-fat milk products, and seafood and they eat too much added sugars, solid fats, refined grains, and sodium. Solid fats and added sugars (SoFAS) constitute 35 percent of Calories in the American diet. This is true for children, adolescents, adults, and older adults and for both males and females. In a recent study of more than 16,000 Americans, Krebs-Smith and others concluded that nearly the entire U.S. population consumes a diet that is not on par with recommendations. In particular, many Americans, Canadians, and others throughout the world are consuming too many Calories, one of the leading causes of the global obesity problem.

To relate these nutrition findings to health in simplistic terms, most Americans eat more food (Calories) than they need, due in part to the increase in food portion sizes in recent years, and eat less of the food that they need more. The major nutrition goal of *Healthy People 2020* is to get more Americans to change their faulty dietary habits. Some advances are being made in the battle against unhealthy eating and obesity. For example, some food manufacturers have reduced the amount of fat and salt in their products. Some fast-food restaurants are offering healthier alternatives, such as oatmeal with fruit for breakfast. The National School Lunch Program has promoted a program to incorporate more fresh fruit and vegetables into daily school lunches. Although these are worthwhile endeavors, many more are needed before we can state that "We are eating right."

What are some general guidelines for healthy eating?

Because the prevention of chronic diseases is of critical importance, thousands of studies have been and are being conducted to discover the intricacies of how various nutrients may affect our health. Particular interest is focused on nutrient function within cells at the molecular level, the interactions between various nutrients, and the identification of other protective factors in certain foods. All of the answers are not in, but sufficient evidence is available to provide us with some useful, prudent guidelines for healthful eating practices.

Over the past two decades, in response to the need for healthier diets, a variety of public and private health organizations analyzed the research relating diet to health and developed some basic guidelines for the general public. The details underlying these recommendations may be found in several voluminous governmental reports, most recently the totally revamped seventh edition of *Nutrition and Your Health: Dietary Guidelines for Americans,* released by the U.S. Departments of Agriculture and Health and Human Services in 2010 and *Healthy People 2020.* These reports serve as the basis for dietary guidelines in ChooseMyPlate. Additionally, governmental health agencies in other countries, such as Britain, Canada, Germany, Japan, and Mexico, have developed dietary guidelines for health promotion in their countries, as has the WHO on a global basis. The American Heart Association released a set of dietary guidelines to help prevent heart disease, the American Cancer Society released a similar set to help prevent cancer, and the American Diabetes Association did likewise for prevention of diabetes. Other organizations, such as the American Dietetic Association, have also proposed dietary guidelines to promote general health. Although most of the guidelines are directed to the general population, the American Heart Association also has recommended dietary guidelines specifically for women and for children and adolescents over the age of about 2 years.

The dietary guidelines promoted by these government and professional health organizations have much in common, and are related to some of the diet plans we will discuss in subsequent chapters, notably the OmniHeart diet, the Mediterranean diet, and the DASH diet. For example, Sofi's review indicated that the Mediterranean diet has been consistently shown to be associated with favorable health outcomes and a better quality of life.

Although we do have considerable research to support dietary recommendations to promote health, the research is incomplete. Thus, the following dozen recommendations may be considered to be prudent, and throughout this book we will refer to these recommendations as a **Prudent Healthy Diet.** Each specific dietary recommendation may convey some health benefit, so the more of these dietary guidelines you adopt, the greater will be your overall health benefits.

1. Balance the food you eat with physical activity to maintain or improve your weight. Consume only moderate food portions. Be physically active every day.
2. Eat a nutritionally adequate diet consisting of a wide variety of nutrient-rich foods. Let healthy guidelines, such as the MyPyramid Food Guide, direct your food choices.
3. Choose a diet moderate in total fat, but low in saturated and *trans* fat and cholesterol.
4. Eat a diet rich in plant foods. Choose plenty of fruits and vegetables, whole-grain products, and legumes, which are rich in healthy carbohydrates, phytochemicals, and fiber.
5. Choose beverages and foods that moderate or reduce your intake of sugars.
6. Choose and prepare foods with less salt and sodium.
7. If you drink alcoholic beverages, do so in moderation. Pregnant women should not drink any alcohol.
8. Maintain protein intake at a moderate, yet adequate level, obtaining much of your daily protein from plant sources,

complemented with smaller amounts of fish, skinless poultry, and lean meat.

9. Choose a diet adequate in calcium and iron. Individuals susceptible to tooth decay should obtain adequate fluoride.
10. Practice food safety, including proper food storage, preservation, and preparation.
11. Eat fewer highly processed foods and more whole foods in their natural form.
12. Enjoy your food. Eat what you like, but balance it within your overall healthful diet.

An expanded discussion of these guidelines along with practical recommendations to help you implement them is presented in chapter 2. Additional details on how each specific recommendation may affect your health status, including specific considerations for women, children, and the elderly, are presented in appropriate chapters throughout this book. The following Websites present detailed information on healthy dietary guidelines:

www.dietaryguidelines.gov   The *Dietary Guidelines for Americans 2010* focus on the total diet and how to integrate all of the recommendations into practical terms, encouraging personal choice but result in an eating pattern that is nutrient dense and Calorie balanced.

www.ChooseMyPlate.gov   ChooseMyPlate offers personalized eating plans and interactive tools to help you plan your food choices based on *Dietary Guidelines for Americans.* Click on SuperTracker, a series of applications developed as this book was going to press.

www.healthcanada.gc.ca   The *Canada Food Guide, Eat Well and Be Active Educational Toolkit* provides excellent information on healthy eating. Click on Food and Nutrition.

www.eatright.org   The American Dietetic Association site provides numerous tips to eating healthy.

Am I eating right?

As part of this course, you may be required to document your actual food intake for several days and then conduct a computerized dietary analysis to determine your nutrient intake. Many computerized dietary analysis programs assess the quality of your diet from a health perspective, and make recommendations for improvement where necessary.

For the time being, you may wish to take the brief dietary inventory in the Application Exercise at the end of this chapter to provide you with a general analysis of your current eating habits. Moreover, you may also analyze your diet at the ChooseMyPlate Website. Click on Interactive Tools, then Food Tracker to assess your diet. Although more detailed information on ChooseMyPlate is presented in subsequent chapters, you may obtain some useful preliminary information on the overall healthfulness of your current diet.

Are there additional health benefits when both exercise and diet habits are improved?

A poor diet and physical inactivity are individual major risk factors for the development of chronic diseases. Collectively,

however, they may pose additional risks, particularly for the two most deadly chronic diseases—heart disease and cancer.

Heart Disease   Lloyd-Jones and others, discussing the American Heart Association's Strategic Impact Goal through 2020 and beyond, reported that ideal cardiovascular health is associated with physical activity at goal levels and pursuit of a diet consistent with current guideline recommendations. As indicated in table 1.2, which highlights risk factors for heart disease, the key lifestyle behaviors that may be effective in favorably modifying heart disease risk factors are proper nutrition and exercise. Moreover, several of the risk factors for heart disease are diseases themselves, such as diabetes, obesity, and high blood pressure, all of which may benefit from the combination of proper nutrition and exercise.

Cancer   In its recent extensive worldwide report on the means to prevent cancer, the American Institute of Cancer Research highlighted the three most important means to prevent a wide variety of cancers, and all are related to exercise and nutrition:

• Choose mostly plant foods, limit red meat, and avoid processed meat.
• Be physically active every day in any way for 30 minutes or more.
• Aim to be a healthy weight throughout life as much as possible.

Prevention of chronic diseases is a high priority for most governmental and professional health organizations, and they have developed appropriate healthy lifestyle behaviors to maximize

TABLE 1.2   Risk factors associated with coronary heart disease

Risk Factors	Classification	Positive Health Lifestyle Modification
High blood pressure	Major	Proper nutrition, aerobic exercise
High blood lipids	Major	Proper nutrition, aerobic exercise
Smoking	Major	Stop smoking
Sedentary lifestyle	Major	Aerobic exercise
ECG abnormalities	Major	Proper nutrition, aerobic exercise
Obesity	Major	Low-Calorie diet, aerobic exercise
Diabetes	Major	Proper nutrition, weight loss, aerobic exercise
Stressful lifestyle	Contributory	Stress management
Dietary intake	Contributory	Proper nutrition
Oral contraceptives	Contributory	Alternative methods of birth control
Family history	Major	Not modifiable
Gender	Contributory	Not modifiable
Race	Contributory	Not modifiable
Age	Contributory	Not modifiable

prevention efforts. Most such healthy lifestyle behaviors include exercise and healthful eating. The possible complementary effect of exercise and nutrition on chronic diseases will be presented in later chapters as appropriate. In particular, as will be discussed in chapter 10, the most significant adverse health effect resulting from the combination of a poor, hypercaloric diet and physical inactivity is obesity, which may be involved in the etiology of numerous chronic health diseases.

However, although appropriate lifestyle behaviors, such as exercise, a healthful diet, and maintaining a healthy body weight, may help prevent the development of chronic diseases, individuals with a strong genetic predisposition to various risk factors, such as high serum cholesterol levels and high blood pressure, or those who are nonresponders to exercise or diet changes, may need medication to reduce these to a level compatible with protective effects.

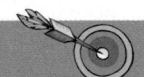

Key Concepts

▶ The primary purpose of the food we eat is to provide us with nutrients essential for the numerous physiological and biochemical functions that support life.

▶ Dietary guidelines developed by major professional health organizations are comparable, and collectively help prevent major chronic diseases such as heart disease, cancer, diabetes, high blood pressure, and obesity.

▶ Poor eating habits span all ages. The *Dietary Guidelines for Americans* and the *Healthy People 2020* report note that poor nutrition is a major health problem in the United States.

▶ Basic guidelines for a Prudent Healthy Diet include maintenance of a proper body weight and consumption of a wide variety of natural foods rich in nutrients associated with health benefits. The more healthful dietary guidelines that you adopt, the greater will be your overall health benefits.

▶ Although both proper exercise and sound nutrition habits may confer health benefits separately, health benefits may be maximized when both healthy exercise and nutrition lifestyles are adopted.

Check for Yourself

▶ As a prelude to activities presented in later chapters, make a detailed record of everything you eat for a full day, from breakfast until your late snack at night.

Sports-Related Fitness: Exercise and Nutrition

As with health, genetic endowment plays an important underlying role in the development of success in sport. Ahmetov and Rogozkin indicated that significant data confirm the influence of genes on specific characteristics necessary to become an elite athlete, such as oxygen uptake, cardiac output, and the relative proportion of fast and slow fibers in skeletal muscle. In their article entitled "What Makes a Champion?" Brutsaert and Parra also note that

genetically gifted athletes may be identified, but must optimize their athletic traits through appropriate training. Sport training will lead to improved performance, but Ahmetov and Rogozkin indicate that optimal responses to training are also dependent on possession of appropriate genes. Genes explain why some individuals benefit while others do not from the same sport training program. Elite athletes are not only born with the right genes for a given sport, but must also have the right genes to benefit from proper training. Moreover, Joyner and Coyle note that complex motivational and sociological factors also play important roles in who does or does not become a sport champion.

What is sports-related fitness?

One of the key factors determining success in sport is the ability to maximize your genetic potential with appropriate physical and mental training to prepare both mind and body for intense competition. In this regard, athletes develop **sports-related fitness,** that is, fitness components such as strength, power, speed, endurance, and neuromuscular motor skills specific to their sport.

The principles of exercise training introduced earlier, such as overload and specificity, are as applicable to sports-related fitness as they are to health-related fitness. However, training for sports performance is more intense, prolonged, and frequent than training for health, and training is specific to the energy demands and skills associated with each sport. We will discuss energy expenditure for sports performance in chapter 3, but here are some examples of sport events with varying rates of energy expenditure or energy needs:

- Explosive, power sports
  —Olympic weight lifting
- Very high-intensity sports
  —100-meter dash
- High-intensity, short duration sports
  —5,000-meter run (3.1 miles)
- Intermittent high-intensity sports
  —Soccer
- Endurance sports
  —Marathon running (26.2 miles; 42.2 kilometers)
- Low-endurance, precision skill sports
  —Golf
- Weight-control and body-image sports
  —Bodybuilding

Training of elite athletes at the United States Olympic Training Center (USOTC) focuses on three attributes:

- Physical power
- Mental strength
- Mechanical edge

Coaches and scientists work with athletes to maximize physical power production for their specific sport, to optimize mental strength in accordance with the psychological demands of the sport, and to provide the best mechanical edge by improving specific fitness and sport skills, sportswear, and sports equipment. Jay Kearney, former senior sports scientist at the USOTC, has noted that sports science

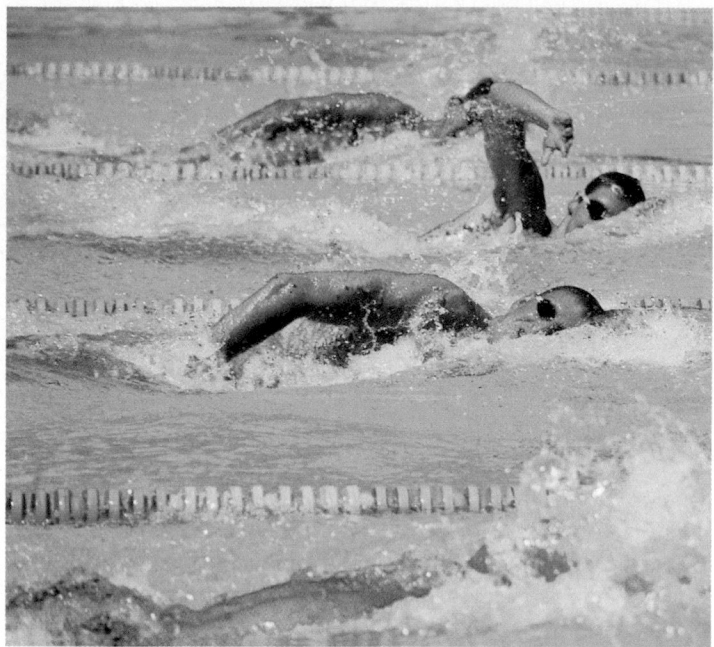

FIGURE 1.8 Elite athletes are exposed to state-of-the-art physiological, psychological, and biomechanical training that may provide an advantage measured in milliseconds, which could mean the difference between the gold and silver medal in world-class competition.

and technology provide elite competitors with the tiny margins needed to win in world-class competition (figure 1.8).

Athletes at all levels of competition, whether an elite international competitor, a college wrestler, a high school baseball player, a seniors age-group distance runner, or a youth league soccer player, can best improve their performance by intense training appropriate for their age, physical and mental development, and sport. For example, in a review as to how we should spend our time and money to improve cycling performance, Jeukendrup and Martin indicated that, of the many ways possible, training is the first and most effective means. As the saying goes, "Do the best with what you got." However, sports and exercise scientists have investigated a number of means to improve athletic performance beyond that attributable to training, and one of the most extensively investigated areas has been the effect of nutrition.

What is sports nutrition?

As noted previously, state-of-the-art physical and mental training is one of the most important factors underlying success in sports. At high levels of athletic competition, athletes generally receive excellent coaching to enhance their biomechanical skills (mechanical edge), sharpen their psychological focus (mental strength), and maximize the physiological functions (physical power) essential for optimal performance. Clyde Williams, a renowned sport scientist from England, notes that, in addition to specialized training, from earliest times certain foods were regarded as essential preparation for physical activity, including competition in the sport stadiums of ancient Greece, where the aim was to achieve greater strength, power, and stamina than one's opponent.

As we shall see, there are various dietary factors that may influence biomechanical, psychological, and physiological considerations in sport. For example, losing excess body fat will enhance biomechanical efficiency; consuming carbohydrates during exercise may maintain normal blood sugar levels and prevent psychological fatigue; and providing adequate dietary iron may ensure optimal oxygen delivery to the muscles. All these sports nutrition factors may favorably affect athletic performance.

Sports nutrition is a relatively new area of study involving the application of nutritional principles to enhance sports performance. Louise Burke, an internationally renowned sports nutritionist from Australia, defines sports nutrition as the application of eating strategies with several major objectives:

- To promote good health
- To promote adaptations to training
- To recover quickly after each training session
- To perform optimally during competition

Although investigators have studied the interactions between nutrition and various forms of sport or exercise for more than a hundred years, it is only within the past few decades that extensive research has been undertaken regarding specific recommendations for athletes.

Is sports nutrition a profession?

Sports nutrition is increasingly becoming recognized as an important factor for optimal athletic performance. Sports nutrition is sometimes referred to as *exercise nutrition* when coupled with exercise designed for health-related fitness, as discussed in the previous section, but that term is less frequently used. Several factors suggest that sports nutrition has become a profession and is a viable career opportunity.

Professional Associations Several professional associations, such as the Sports and Cardiovascular Nutritionists (SCAN) subsection of the American Dietetic Association, Professionals in Nutrition for Exercise and Sport (PINES), and the International Society of Sports Nutrition, are involved in the application of nutrition to sport, health, and wellness.

Certification Programs Several professional and sports-governing organizations have developed a recognized course of study or certification program to promote the development of professionals who can provide athletes with sound information about nutrition. For example, the American Dietetic Association has established a program for Certification as a Specialist in Sports Dietetics (CSSD), while the International Olympic Committee offers a Diploma in Sports Nutrition.

Research Productivity Numerous exercise-science/nutrition research laboratories at major universities are dedicated to sports nutrition research. Almost every scientific journal in sport/exercise science, and even in general nutrition, appears to contain at least one study or review in each issue that is related to sports nutrition.

International Meetings Numerous international meetings have focused on sports nutrition, some meetings highlighting nutritional principles for a specific sport, such as soccer or track and field.

Consensus Statements and Position Stands Several international sports-governing organizations have developed consensus statements on nutrition for their specific sport. For example, the Fédération Internationale de Football Association (FIFA), published the pamphlet, *Nutrition for Football,* which is designed to provide sound nutrition information for soccer players worldwide. A more generalized position stand entitled "Nutrition and Athletic Performance" was recently issued jointly by the American Dietetic Association, Dietitians of Canada, and the American College of Sports Medicine.

Career Opportunities Sports nutritionists are employed by professional sport teams and athletic departments of major universities to design optimal nutritional programs for their athletes. Some dietitians market themselves as full-time or part-time sports nutritionists within their communities.

Sports nutrition as we know it today has a relatively short history, but it appears to be an important aspect in the total preparation of the athlete.

---

www.acsm.org You may access the position stand entitled "Nutrition and Athletic Performance" by clicking on Publications and then Position Stands.

http://www.scandpg.org/sports-nutrition/be-a-board-certified-sports-dietitian-cssd/ Check this SCAN site to see what is necessary to become a Certified Specialist in Sports Dietetics.

www.sportsoracle.com Check this PINES site to see what is needed to become a member and the requirements for the IOC Diploma in Sports Nutrition.

Are athletes today receiving adequate nutrition?

Surveys regarding dietary intake of athletes present mixed results. Some studies find that athletes may be eating as well as or better than non-athletes and meeting or exceeding the RDA for many nutrients, while other studies reveal diets inadequate in energy intake or specific nutrients. In a study with mixed findings, Lun and others reported that many elite Canadian athletes do not consume adequate energy or carbohydrates, but their intake of micronutrients exceeds current recommended daily intakes, even when supplements are not considered, indicating that athletes make high-quality food choices. However, as Mullins and others note, even though the vitamin and mineral status of the group of athletes as a whole may appear appropriate, wide individual variability indicates that individual athletes may be undernourished. In their position statement, *Nutrition and Athletic Performance,* the American College of Sports Medicine, the American Dietetic Association, and the Dietitians of Canada indicated that athletes at greatest risk for poor vitamin and mineral status are those who restrict energy intake or have severe weight-loss practices, who eliminate one or more of the food groups from their diet, or who consume unbalanced diets. The ACSM, ADA, and DC suggest that such athletes may benefit from a daily multivitamin/mineral supplement. Many highly trained athletes do take nutritional supplements, including vitamins and minerals, according to a study by Dascombe and others.

This brief review indicates that some athletic groups are not receiving the recommended allowances for a variety of essential nutrients or may not be meeting certain recommended standards. It should be noted, however, that these surveys have analyzed the diets of the athletes only in reference to a standard, such as the RDA, and many studies have not analyzed the actual nutrient or biochemical status (such as by a blood test) of the athlete or the effects that the dietary deficiency exerted on exercise performance capacity or sport performance. The RDA for vitamins and minerals incorporates a safety factor, so an individual with a dietary intake of essential nutrients below the RDA may not necessarily suffer a true nutrient deficiency. If, however, the athlete does develop a nutrient deficiency, then athletic performance may deteriorate and health may be impaired. Examples discussed in later chapters include impaired aerobic endurance capacity associated with iron deficiency and premature decreases in bone density with calcium deficiency.

Why are some athletes malnourished? There may be various reasons, including economic factors. Part of the problem also may be that athletes do not possess sufficient knowledge to make appropriate food choices. Christine Rosenbloom, a distinguished sports nutritionist at Georgia State University, and her colleagues indicate that athletes continue to have misconceptions about the roles of specific nutrients in sport performance, and if they chose foods based on these misconceptions then sports performance may suffer.

Many athletes may not be getting sound sport nutrition information. In a survey of nutrition practices and knowledge of college varsity athletes, Jacobson and others reported that although some athletes received nutrition information from reliable sources, such as dietitians and athletic trainers (who are required to have a nutrition course for certification), considerable nutrition information was obtained from less reliable sources such as magazines. Many athletes receive nutrition information from their coaches, who may not have the background to provide proper advice, as documented by Zinn and others. Surveys of coaches indicated that 60 to 80 percent had not had a formal course in nutrition or were in need of a better nutrition background. Other constraints, such as finances and time, may limit food selection and preparation.

Given this background, Ziegler and others suggest the need to develop dietary intervention and education programs targeted at promoting optimal nutrient intakes by these athletes, not only to maintain performance, but also to improve long-term health status.

How does nutrition affect athletic performance?

The nutrients in the foods we eat can affect exercise and sports performance in accord with the three major functions of nutrients. First, nutrients may provide energy for the different energy-producing systems discussed in chapter 3. Second, nutrients also help regulate

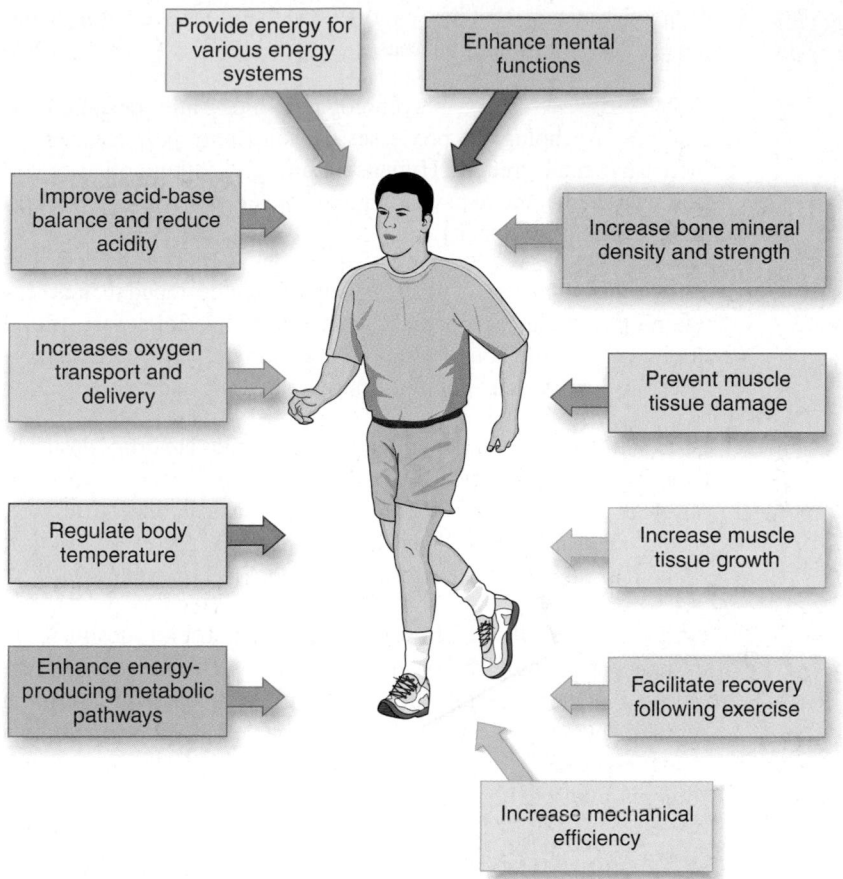

Provide energy for various energy systems

Enhance mental functions

Improve acid-base balance and reduce acidity

Increase bone mineral density and strength

Increases oxygen transport and delivery

Prevent muscle tissue damage

Regulate body temperature

Increase muscle tissue growth

Enhance energy-producing metabolic pathways

Facilitate recovery following exercise

Increase mechanical efficiency

FIGURE 1.9 Nutrients in the foods we eat and dietary strategies may influence exercise or sport performance in a variety of ways. They may provide energy for the various human energy systems, may help regulate various metabolic processes important to exercise, and may also promote the growth and development of various body tissues and organs important for energy production during exercise.

metabolic processes important to energy production and temperature regulation during exercise. Third, nutrients support the growth and development of specific body tissues and organs as they adapt to exercise training; Figure 1.9 highlights some of the roles nutrients play during exercise. A well-planned sport-specific diet will help optimize sports performance, but a poor diet plan may lead to impaired performance.

Malnutrition represents unbalanced nutrition and may exist as either undernutrition or overnutrition, that is, an individual does not receive an adequate intake (*undernutrition*) or consumes excessive amounts of single or multiple nutrients (*overnutrition*). Either condition can hamper athletic performance. An inadequate intake of certain nutrients may impair athletic performance due to an insufficient energy supply, an inability to regulate exercise metabolism at an optimal level, or a decreased synthesis of key body tissues or enzymes. In contrast, excessive intake of some nutrients may also impair athletic performance, and even the health of the athlete, by disrupting normal physiological processes or leading to undesirable changes in body composition.

What should athletes eat to help optimize sport performance?

Melinda Manore, an expert in sport nutrition, noted that there is no doubt that the type, amount, composition, and timing of food intake can dramatically affect exercise performance, recovery from exercise, body weight and composition, and health. The importance of nutrition to your athletic performance may depend on a variety of factors, including your gender, your age, your body weight status, your eating and lifestyle patterns, the environment, the type of training you do, and the type of sport or event in which you participate. As an example of the latter point, the carbohydrate needs of a golfer or baseball player may vary little from those of the nonathlete, whereas those of a marathon runner or ultraendurance triathlete may be altered significantly during training and competition.

The opinions offered by researchers in the area of exercise and nutrition relative to optimal nutrition for the athlete run the gamut. At one end, certain investigators note that the daily food requirement of athletes is quite similar to the nutritionally balanced diet for everyone else, and therefore no special recommendations are needed. On the other extreme, some state that it is almost impossible to obtain all the nutrients the athlete requires from the normal daily intake of food, and for that reason nutrient supplementation is absolutely necessary. Other reviewers advocate a compromise between these two extremes, recognizing the importance of a nutritionally balanced diet but also stressing the importance of increased consumption of specific nutrients or dietary supplements for athletes in certain situations.

The review of the scientific literature presented in this book supports the latter point of view. In general, athletes who consume enough Calories to meet their energy needs and who meet the requirements for essential nutrients should be obtaining adequate nutrition. The dietary guidelines for better health, as discussed previously and expanded upon in chapter 2, are the same for optimal physical performance. The key to sound nutrition for the athletic individual is to eat a wide variety of healthful foods.

Although a healthy diet is the foundation of a dietary plan for athletes, modifications may be important for training and competition in various sports. Some basic guidelines regarding eating for training and for competition are presented in chapter 2, whereas details regarding the use of specific nutrients, including related dietary supplements, are presented in the chapter highlighting that nutrient.

Some athletes believe that there are *super* foods or diets that may provide a competitive advantage in sports. Numerous *sports supplements* are marketed to athletes with this premise in mind, and have been the subject of considerable research by sports nutrition scientists. The following section discusses the general role of such supplements in the enhancement of sports performance.

Ergogenic Aids and Sports Performance: Beyond Training

Since time immemorial, athletes have attempted to use a wide variety of techniques or substances in attempts to enhance sports performance beyond the effects that could be obtained through training. In sport and exercise science terminology, such techniques or substances are referred to as **ergogenic aids.**

What is an ergogenic aid?

As mentioned previously, the two key factors important to athletic success are genetic endowment and state of training. At certain levels of competition, the contestants generally have similar genetic athletic abilities and have been exposed to similar training methods, and thus they are fairly evenly matched. Given the emphasis placed on winning, many athletes training for competition are always searching for the ultimate method or ingredient to provide that extra winning edge. Indeed, one report suggests that two of the key factors leading to better athletic records in recent years are improved diet and ergogenic aids.

The word *ergogenic* is derived from the Greek words *ergo* (meaning work) and *gen* (meaning production of), and is usually defined as *to increase potential for work output.* In sports, various ergogenic aids, or ergogenics, have been used for their theoretical ability to improve sports performance by enhancing physical power, mental strength, or mechanical edge. There are several different classifications of ergogenic aids, grouped according to the general nature of their application to sport. The first two classifications are often referred to as *performance-enhancing techniques,* whereas the last three classifications involve taking some substance into the body and are known as *performance-enhancing substances.* We have listed several major categories with an example of one theoretical ergogenic aid for each.

Mechanical Aids Mechanical, or biomechanical, aids are designed to increase energy efficiency, to provide a mechanical edge. Lightweight racing shoes may be used by a runner in place of heavier ones so that less energy is needed to move the legs and the economy of running increases.

Psychological Aids Psychological aids are designed to enhance psychological processes during sport performance, to increase mental strength. Hypnosis, through posthypnotic suggestion, may help remove psychological barriers that limit physiological performance capacity.

Physiological Aids Physiological aids are designed to augment natural physiological processes to increase physical power. Blood doping, or the infusion of blood into an athlete, may increase oxygen transport capacity and thus increase aerobic endurance.

Pharmacological Aids Pharmacological aids are drugs designed to influence physiological or psychological processes to increase physical power, mental strength, or mechanical edge. Caffeine, a commonly used drug, may increase physical power and mental strength to help improve performance in a variety of exercise tasks.

Nutritional Aids Nutritional aids are nutrients designed to influence physiological or psychological processes to increase physical power, mental strength, or mechanical edge. Protein supplements may be used by strength-trained athletes in attempts to increase muscle mass because protein is the major dietary constituent of muscle.

Why are nutritional ergogenics so popular?

Probably the most used ergogenic aids are dietary supplements. Dietary supplements marketed to physically active individuals are commonly known as sports nutrition supplements, or simply **sports supplements.** Companies market their products as "Supplements for the Competitive Athlete," and the overall sports supplement business is brisk. According to Dancho and Manore, sports supplements constitute approximately 10 percent of total dietary supplement sales.

Sports supplements are popular worldwide. Sports supplements are used by all types of athletes: male and female, young and old, professional and amateur. Reports indicate that 90 percent or more of elite, international-class athletes consume dietary supplements. Other surveys document significant use among high school and collegiate athletes, military personnel in elite groups such as SEALS, and fitness club members.

Sports supplements are popular for several reasons. Athletes have believed that certain foods may possess magical qualities, so it is no wonder that a wide array of nutrients or special preparations have been used since time immemorial in attempts to run faster, jump higher, or throw farther. Shrewd advertising and marketing strategies promote this belief, enticing many athletes and physically active individuals to try sports supplements. Many of these products may be endorsed by professional athletes, giving the product an aura of respectability. Specific supplements also may be recommended by coaches and fellow athletes. Additionally, as drug testing in sports gets increasingly sophisticated, leading to greater detection of pharmacological ergogenics, many athletes may resort to sports supplements, believing them to be natural, safe, and legal. However, as noted later, this may not be the case.

Are nutritional ergogenics effective?

There are a number of theoretical nutritional ergogenic aids in each of the six major classifications of nutrients, and athletes have been known to take supplements of almost every nutrient in attempts to improve performance. Here are a few examples:

Carbohydrate. Special compounds have been developed to facilitate absorption, storage, and utilization of carbohydrate during exercise.

Fats. Special fatty acids have been used in attempts to provide an alternative fuel to carbohydrate.

Protein. Special amino acids derived from protein have been developed and advertised to be more potent than anabolic steroids in stimulating muscle growth and strength development.

Vitamins. Special vitamin mixtures and even "nonvitamin vitamins," such as vitamin B_{15}, have been ascribed ergogenic qualities ranging from increases in strength to improved vision for sport.

Minerals. Special mineral supplements, such as chromium, vanadium, and boron, have been advertised to be anabolic in nature.

Water. Special oxygenated waters have been developed specifically for aerobic endurance athletes, theoretically designed to increase oxygen delivery.

In addition to essential nutrients derived from foods, there are literally hundreds of nonessential substances or compounds that are classified as food supplements and targeted to athletes as potent ergogenics, such as creatine, L-carnitine, coenzyme Q_{10}, inosine, octacosanol, and ginseng. Moreover, many products contain multiple ingredients, each purported to enhance sports performance. For example, one of the "Energy" drinks on the market includes carbohydrates, amino acids, vitamins, minerals, metabolites, herbs, and caffeine.

Nutrient supplementation above and beyond the RDA is not necessary for the vast majority of athletes. In general, consumption of specific nutrients above the RDA has not been shown to exert any ergogenic effect on human physical or athletic performance. In one review, Deldicque and Francaux indicated that the bulk of sports supplements sold on the market are labeled with various performance-enhancement claims without any scientific evidence. However, there are some exceptions. As noted in chapters 4 through 10, there may be some justification for nutrient supplementation or dietary modification in certain athletes under specific conditions, particularly in cases where nutrient deficiencies may occur. Some specific dietary supplements and food drugs may also possess ergogenic potential under certain circumstances.

The effectiveness of almost all of the popular nutritional ergogenics, including the essential nutrients, the nonessential nutrients, the food drugs caffeine and alcohol, the steroid precursor androstenedione, and other agents, will be covered in this book. A summary is presented in chapter 13.

Are nutritional ergogenics safe?

The majority of over-the-counter dietary supplements, particularly those containing essential nutrients, appear to be safe for the general population when taken in recommended dosages. However, in a *Sports Illustrated* article entitled "What You Don't Know Might Kill You," Epstein and Dohrmann indicated that sports supplements may be dangerous. Some dietary supplements, including sports supplements, may contain ingredients that pose health risks in several ways. First, using the "if one is good, then ten is better" mentality, athletes may overdose. The FDA has noted that some sports supplements contain chemicals that have been linked to numerous serious illnesses and even death, particularly when taken in excess. Second, the product label may not contain all the ingredients or may contain ingredients not listed. Several products analyzed independently have been shown to contain powerful stimulants that could have adverse effects.

Hermann Engels, a noted exercise scientist at Wayne State University, says that medical authorities are concerned about possible adverse reactions of athletes to commercially sold sports supplements, and that this may be a particular problem with young athletes. Studies indicate that adolescents are as likely to use sports supplements as adults. Young athletes, who may have a sense of invincibility, may not possess the judgment to use appropriate dosages and may overdose.

Supplements that are mislabeled and contain unlisted substances pose a serious health threat. Some companies are unscrupulous and may not list a chemical, such as ephedrine, that could provide a stimulant effect which, unknowingly, you may attribute to the *listed* ingredients and thus think the product is effective. Fortunately, the government is working to require that all ingredients be listed on dietary supplement labels, and hopefully appropriate warnings of any potential health risks will be provided as new laws take effect. Currently, some companies are voluntarily adding warnings in their advertisements and product labels.

Throughout this text, possible health risks associated with nutritional ergogenics are discussed when such information is available.

Are nutritional ergogenics legal?

The use of pharmaceutical agents to enhance performance in sport has been prohibited by the governing bodies of most organized sports. The use of drugs in sports is known as **doping,** and the World Anti-Doping Agency (WADA) has promulgated an extensive list of drugs and doping techniques that have been prohibited.

At present, all essential nutrients are not classified as drugs and are considered to be legal for use in conjunction with athletic competition. Most other food substances and constituents sold as dietary supplements are also legal. However, some dietary supplements are prohibited, such as androstenedione, because they are classified as anabolic steroids, which are prohibited drugs. Other dietary supplements may contain substances that are prohibited; for example, Chinese Ephedra and some forms of ginseng may contain ephedrine, a prohibited stimulant drug. The National Football League (NFL) has developed strict requirements for the manufacturing of dietary supplements approved for use by its players. The National Collegiate Athletic Association (NCAA) prohibits member institutions from providing ergogenic nutritional supplements to student athletes at any time, while permitting nonergogenic nutritional supplements as long as they do not contain NCAA-banned substances.

Ron Maughan, an international expert in sports nutrition, noted that contamination of sports supplements that may cause an athlete to fail a doping test is widespread. Some studies of sports supplements targeted for muscle building and marketed on the Internet have reported that up to 25 percent were contaminated with prohibited substances and note that many athletes, including Olympic champions, who have claimed they have not taken drugs, but only dietary supplements, have tested positive for doping.

It is hoped that, with pending legislation, all ingredients will be listed in correct amounts on dietary supplement labels. In the meantime, athletes should consult with appropriate authorities before using any sports nutrition supplements marketed as performance enhancers. Nevertheless, WADA notes that the use of nutritional or dietary supplements is completely at the athlete's own risk, even if the supplements are "approved" or "verified."

The following Website may be useful to evaluate the efficacy and safety of various sport supplements:

www.ais.org.au Click on Nutrition, then Supplements. The Australian Institute of Sport lists sports supplements approved for use and those that should not be used or used only under certain circumstances, along with other useful information on sport supplements.

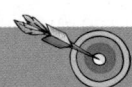

Key Concepts

▶ Probably the most prevalent ergogenic aids used to increase sport performance are those classified as nutritional, for theoretical nutritional aids may be found in all six classes of nutrients.

▶ Although most sports supplements are safe and legal, most are not effective ergogenic aids, and some are unsafe or illegal. Before using a sports supplement, athletes should try to determine if it is effective, if it is safe, and if it is legal.

Check for Yourself

▶ Go to a health food store, peruse the multiple dietary supplements available, and ask the clerk for advice on a supplement to help you enhance your sport performance, such as increasing your muscle mass or losing body fat. Write down the advice and check out advertisements on the Internet. Then, research the supplements on the Website noted above and compare the findings.

Nutritional Quackery in Health and Sports

Increasing numbers of dietary supplements are being marketed to the general population as health enhancers and to athletes as performance enhancers. Unfortunately, many of the products that advertise extravagant claims of enhanced health or performance are promoted by unscrupulous entrepreneurs, have no legitimate basis, and may be regarded as quackery.

What is nutritional quackery?

According to the Food and Drug Administration (FDA), **quackery,** as the term is used today, refers not only to the fake practitioner but also to the worthless product and the deceitful promotion of that product. Untrue or misleading claims that are deliberately or fraudulently made for any product, including food products, constitute quackery. The American Dietetic Association (ADA), in its position statement on food and nutrition misinformation, notes that such misinformation can have harmful effects on the health and economic status of consumers.

Knowledge relative to all facets of life, the science of nutrition included, has increased phenomenally in recent years. Thousands of studies have been conducted, revealing facts to help unravel some of the mysteries of human nutrition. The ADA indicates that consumers are taking greater responsibility for self-care and are eager to receive food and nutrition information. However, that creates opportunities for nutrition *mis*information, health fraud, and quackery to flourish. The ADA further notes that the media are consumers' leading source of nutrition information, but that news reports of nutrition research often provide inadequate depth for consumers to make wise decisions. Certain individuals may capitalize on these research findings for personal financial gain. For example, isolated nutritional facts may be distorted or the results of a single study will be used to market a specific nutritional product. Health hustlers will use this information to capitalize on people's fears and hopes, be it the fear that the nutritional quality of our food is being lessened by modern processing methods or the hope of improved athletic performance capacity.

Quackery is big business. A report from the U.S. National Center for Complementary and Alternative Medicine (NCAAM .NIH/gov/NEWS/CAMSTATS/COSTS) indicated that Americans spend almost $34 billion annually on questionable health practices. A substantial percentage of this amount is spent on unnecessary nutritional products. Authorities in this area have noted that the amount of misinformation about nutrition is overwhelming, and it is circulated widely, particularly by those who may profit from it. Although we may still think of quacks as sleazy individuals selling patent medicine from a covered wagon, the truth is quite different. Nutritional quacks today are super salespeople, using questionable scientific information to give their products a sense of authenticity and credibility and using sophisticated advertising and marketing techniques.

As noted previously, there are some bona fide health benefits associated with the foods we eat, but, as shall be noted in chapter 2, federal legislation establishes strict guidelines regarding the placement of health claims on food labels for most of the packaged foods that we buy. Such may not be the case, however, with dietary supplements.

Before the passage of the 1994 Dietary Supplements Health and Education Act (DSHEA), many extravagant health claims were made by some unscrupulous companies in the food supplement industry. As an example, the label of one secret formula noted that it would help you lose excess body fat while sleeping, which is untrue. Although the DSHEA was designed to eradicate such fraudulent health claims, dietary supplements today appear to have more leeway than packaged foods to imply health benefits. Technically, labels on dietary supplements are not permitted to display scientifically unsupported claims. However, companies are allowed to make general health claims like "boosts the immune system" if, for example, the product contains a nutrient, such as zinc, that has been deemed important in some way to immune functions in the body. Although companies may not claim that the product prevents diseases associated with impaired immune functions, such as the common cold, cancer, or AIDS, the consumer may erroneously make such an assumption.

Many companies now use a disclaimer for general health claims on their labels, noting that "These statements have not been evaluated by the Food and Drug Administration" and "This product is not intended to diagnose, treat, cure, or prevent any disease." Companies may also circumvent government regulations by using *freedom of the press*. They may provide information in the form of a reprint of an article, a brochure with highlighted research, or other printed materials that are distributed in connection with the sale of the product. Many dietary supplement companies also have developed infomercials for television or home pages on the Internet to provide comparable biased advertising information to potential consumers.

Although these advertising strategies may contain fraudulent information, the federal agencies that monitor such practices are understaffed and cannot litigate every case of misleading or dishonest advertising. Thus, unsuspecting consumers may be lured into buying an expensive health-food supplement that has no scientific support of its effectiveness. The FDA was to remedy this problem by 2010, but no action has been taken at the time this book went to press. A Dietary Supplement Safety Act was proposed in the Senate in 2010, but was withdrawn later that year.

Nutritional quackery is widespread, as documented in the position stand on food and nutrition misinformation by the American Dietetic Association. Years ago J.V. Durnin, an international authority on nutrition and exercise, stated that there is still no sphere of nutrition in which faddism, misconceptions, ignorance, and quackery are more obvious than in athletics, a situation that continues today.

Why is nutritional quackery so prevalent in athletics?

As with nutritional quackery in general, hope and fear are the motivating factors underlying the use of nutritional supplements by athletes. They hope that a special nutrient concoction will provide them with a slight competitive edge, and they fear losing if they do not do everything possible to win.

Various factors within the athletic environment help nurture these hopes and fears, but the most significant factor contributing to nutritional quackery in sports is direct advertising, as caricatured by the fabricated advertisement in figure 1.10. If you scan through various magazines targeted to bodybuilders or endurance athletes, you will see dozens of advertisements suggesting enhancement of strength, endurance, and sport performance. Such advertisements often use endorsements by star athletes. For example, advertisements in sports magazines and on the Internet for the

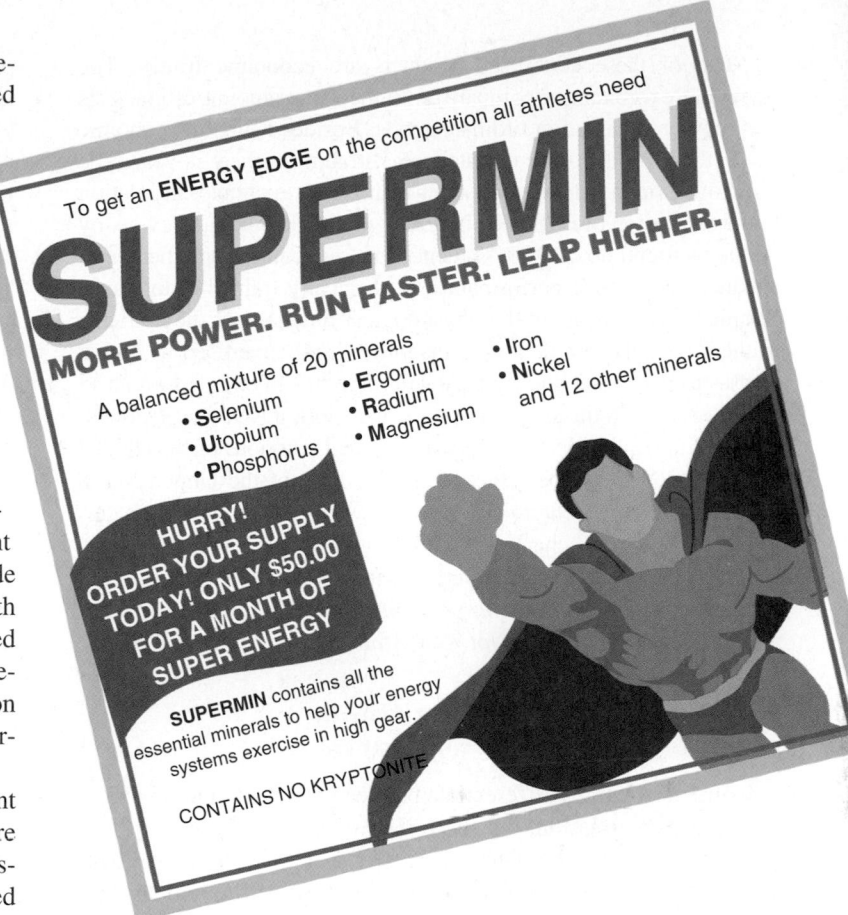

FIGURE 1.10 Simulated nutritional supplement advertisement aimed at athletes.

sports supplement FRS®Healthy Energy, endorsed by seven-time winner of the Tour de France, Lance Armstrong, suggest that its use will enhance energy and stamina. FRS is an abbreviation for Free Radical Scavenger, a topic discussed in chapter 7 relative to the putative health and performance-enhancing effects of antioxidant vitamin supplementation. FRS®Healthy Energy contains various antioxidants, but the secret antioxidant is quercetin. In general, such claims are not supported by research.

Additionally, many sports magazines will run articles on the ergogenic benefits of a particular nutrient, and in close proximity to the article place an advertisement for a product that contains that nutrient. Freedom of speech guaranteed by the First Amendment permits the author of the article to make sensational and deceptive claims about the nutrient. However, freedom of speech does not extend to advertising, so fraudulent or deceptive claims may be grounds for prosecution by the FDA or the Federal Trade Commission (FTC). Thus, by cleverly positioning the article and the advertisement, the promoter can make the desired claims about the value of the product and yet avoid any illegality. Classic examples of this technique may be found with protein and amino acid supplement advertising in magazines for bodybuilders. Moreover, many advertisements now appear in a format designed to look like a scientific review, though in actuality they are deceptive advertisements for sport supplements.

Most of these advertised products are economic frauds. The prices are exorbitant in comparison to the same amount of nutrients that may be obtained in ordinary foods. Besides being an economic fraud, these products are an intellectual fraud, for there is very little scientific evidence to support their claims. For example, in relation to the discussion of FRS® Healthy Enegry and quercetin, a review by Williams found no credible evidence that quercetin supplementation enhances endurance performance in physically trained individuals. Simple basic facts about the physiological functions of the nutrients in these products are distorted, magnified, and advertised in such a way as to make one believe they will increase athletic performance. Unfortunately, in the area of nutrition and sport, it is very easy to distort the truth and appeal to the psychological emotions of the athlete. Dr. Robert Voy, former chief medical officer of the United States Olympic Training Center, has noted that we have abandoned athletes to the hucksters and charlatans. Athletes are wasting their money on worthless, and sometimes harmful, substances, as documented by David Lightsey in his book *Muscle, Speed, and Lies: What the Sports Supplement Industry Does Not Want Athletes or Consumers to Know.*

How do I recognize nutritional quackery in health and sports?

It is often difficult to differentiate between quackery and reputable nutritional information, but the following may be used as guidelines in evaluating the claims made for a nutritional supplement or nutritional practice advertised or recommended to athletes and others. If the answer to any of these questions is yes, then one should be skeptical of such supplements and investigate their value before investing any money.

1. Does the product promise quick improvement in health or physical performance?
2. Does it contain some secret or magical ingredient or formula?
3. Is it advertised mainly by use of anecdotes, case histories, or testimonials?
4. Are currently popular personalities or star athletes featured in its advertisements?
5. Does it take a simple truth about a nutrient and exaggerate that truth in terms of health or physical performance?
6. Does it question the integrity of the scientific or medical establishment?
7. Is it advertised in a health or sports magazine whose publishers also sell nutritional aids?
8. Does the person who recommends it also sell the product?
9. Does it use the results of a single study or dated and poorly controlled research to support its claims?
10. Is it expensive, especially when compared to the cost of equivalent nutrients that may be obtained from ordinary foods?
11. Is it a recent discovery not available from any other source?
12. Is its claim too good to be true? Does it promise the impossible?

Where can I get sound nutritional information to combat quackery in health and sports?

The best means to evaluate claims of enhanced health or sport performance made by dietary supplements or other nutritional practices is to possess a good background in nutrition and a familiarity with related high-quality research. Unfortunately, most individuals, including most athletes, coaches, and physicians, have not been exposed to such an educational program, so they must either take formal course work in nutrition or sport nutrition, develop a reading program in nutrition for health and sport, or consult with an expert in the field.

This book has been designed to serve as a text for a college course in nutrition for health-related and sports-related fitness, but it may also be read independently. It is an attempt to analyze and interpret the available scientific literature as to how nutrition may affect health and sports performance, and to provide some simple guidelines for physically active individuals to help improve their health or athletic performance. It should provide the essential science-based (evidence-based) information you need to plan an effective nutritional program, either for yourself, other physically active individuals, or athletes, and to evaluate the usefulness of many nutritional supplements or practices designed to improve health or sport performance. Here are some key resources.

Books   Numerous reputable books that detail the relationship of nutrition to health and sports performance are available, and many are cited in the reference list at the end of this chapter. However, some books, such as diet books based on an author's personal experiences, may not contain reputable information. A good guide is to check the author's credentials.

Government, Health Professional, Consumer, and Commercial Organizations and Related Websites   Accurate information relating nutrition to health is published by governmental agencies such as the FDA and USDA; health professional groups such as the American Dietetic Association, Dietitians of Canada, American College of Sports Medicine, and the American Medical Association; consumer groups such as Consumers Union and Center for Science in the Public Interest; and commercial groups such as the National Dairy Council and the PepsiCo's Gatorade Sports Science Institute. Excellent materials relative to nutrition may be obtained free or at small cost from some of these organizations.

www.hsph.harvard.edu/nutritionsource   Excellent Website for nutrition information from the Harvard School of Public Health.
www.gssiweb.com   Website for the Gatorade Sports Science Institute, providing detailed reviews on various topics in sports nutrition.
www.healthfinder.gov   U.S. Department of Health and Human Services Website for information on various health topics, including nutrition.
http://medlineplus.gov   National Library of Medicine, a comprehensive health-information retrieval Website.
www.MerckSource.com   Unbiased health information, including nutrition and exercise.

Scientific Journals   Many scientific journals publish reputable findings about nutrition, exercise, and health. These technical journals may not be readily available in public libraries, but may be found in university and medical libraries. Examples of such publications include *Medicine & Science in Sports & Exercise, The Journal of the American Dietetic Association, American Journal of Clinical Nutrition, Sports Medicine,* and the *International Journal of Sport Nutrition and Exercise Metabolism.*

www.pubmed.gov National Library of Medicine Website provides abstracts of original research studies and excellent reviews and meta-analyses published in scientific medical journals. Free full-text articles are provided for some journals.

Popular Magazines Articles in popular health and sports magazines may or may not be accurate. The credentials of the author, if listed, should be a good guide to an article's authenticity. A Ph.D. listed after the author's name may not guarantee accuracy of the content of the article. Be wary of publications emanating from organizations or publishers that also sell nutritional supplements.

Consultants Nutritional consultants are another source of information. Such consultants should have a solid background in nutrition, particularly sports nutrition if they are to advise athletes. The consultant should be a registered dietitian (RD) or possess appropriate professional certification, such as the Certified Nutrition Specialist (CNS). He or she should be a member of a reputable organization of nutritionists, such as the American Dietetic Association. You may contact the ADA at its Website address and they will provide you with the name of a local dietitian. Other recognized nutritional organizations include the American Society for Nutrition Sciences, the American College of Nutrition, and the American Society for Clinical Nutrition. Qualified nutritionists are able to provide you with nutritional advice to help you meet your health goals.

www.eatright.org Contact the American Dietetic Association for the names of local dietitians, as well as other sources of sound nutrition information.

As noted previously, the American Dietetic Association's Commission on Dietetic Registration, working with members of Sports, Cardiovascular and Wellness Nutritionists (SCAN), has developed a certification program for registered dietitians (RD) who work in sports to achieve the status of Certified Specialist in Sports Dietetics (CSSD). A qualified sports nutritionist will be able to assess your nutritional status, including such variables as body composition, dietary analysis, and eating and lifestyle patterns, and relate these nutritional factors to the physiological and related nutritional demands of your sport or exercise program, providing you with a plan to help you reach your performance goals. The International Olympic Committee (IOC) also has developed a program of study leading to the IOC Diploma in Sports Nutrition.

http://www.scandpg.org/mapsearch.php Use this Website to find a sports nutritionist. Click on your state to find one closest to you. Those with the CSSD designation have earned the designation as a Certified Specialist in Sports Dietetics.

Be wary of individuals who do not possess professional degrees or appropriate certification, such as "experts" in nutrition or fitness. Many states do not have regulations restricting the use of various terms, such as *nutritionist* or *fitness professional.* Although these individuals may have some practical experience with helping people change their diets and initiate exercise programs, they normally do not have the depth of knowledge required in many cases. For proper nutritional advice, be certain to ask for proof of certification from recognized nutrition professional groups as cited previously. For fitness professionals, check for certification by such groups as the American College of Sports Medicine (ACSM), the American Council on Exercise (ACE), or the National Strength and Conditioning Association (NSCA).

Cautions on Using the Internet The U.S. Department of Health and Human Services has recommended caution in using the Internet to find health information. Along with others, here are some of its major points:

- No one regulates information on the Internet. Thus, anyone can set up a home page and claim anything.
- Some official-sounding Websites, such as Wikipedia, permit anyone to enter or modify the information presented.
- Search engines, such as Google and Yahoo, host paid advertisements that may contain biased information.
- Compare the information you find on the Internet with other resources.
- Check the author's or organization's credentials. Unfortunately, there are many so-called nutritionists and other health professionals making false claims on the Internet.
- Be wary of Websites advertising and selling products that claim to improve your health.
- Be cautious when using information found on bulletin boards or during chat sessions with others.

Several Websites listed previously provide reputable information. Although some commercial (.com) and organization (.org) Websites provide trustworthy information, and may be cited in this text, others may not be as reputable, as they may be sponsored by unethical supplement companies. In general, education (.edu) and government (.gov) Websites provide trustworthy information. The Websites cited in this text and found at *www.mhhe.com/williams* are deemed to be reliable.

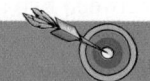

Key Concepts

▶ Nutritional quackery is widespread as related to the purported benefits of specific dietary supplements, particularly so with dietary supplements marketed to athletes.

▶ There are a number of guidelines to help identify quackery and false claims regarding dietary supplements, but one of the critical points to consider is if the claim simply appears to be too good to be true.

▶ The best means to counteract nutritional quackery is to possess a good background in nutrition. Reputable sources of information are available to help provide contemporary viewpoints on the efficacy, safety, and legality of various dietary supplements for health or sport.

Research and Prudent Recommendations

By now you should realize that nutrition and exercise may influence health and sport performance. But how do we know what effect a nutrient, food, or dietary supplement we consume or exercise program we undertake will have on *our* health or performance? To find answers to specific questions, we should rely on the findings derived from scientific research, which is the heart of *evidence-based* medicine. As sophisticated sciences, nutrition and exercise science have a relatively short history. Not too long ago, nutrition scientists were concerned primarily with identifying the major constituents of the foods we eat and their general functions in the human body, while those investigating exercise concentrated more on its application to enhance sports performance. More recently, however, numerous scientists have turned their attention to the possible health benefits of certain foods and various forms of exercise, and, in the case of sport scientists, the possible applications to athletic performance. These scientists are not only attempting to determine the general effects of diet and exercise on health and performance, but are also investigating the effects of specific nutrients at the molecular and genetic level to determine possible mechanisms of action to improve health or performance in sport.

Because this book makes a number of nutritional (and some exercise) *evidence-based* recommendations relative to sports and health, it is important to review briefly the nature and limitations of nutritional and exercise research with humans. For the purpose of this discussion, our emphasis will be on nutritional research, although the same research considerations apply to exercise as well.

What types of research provide valid information?

Several research techniques have been used to explore the effect of nutrition on health or athletic performance. The two major general categories have been epidemiological research and experimental research.

Epidemiological research, also known as *observational research,* involves studying large populations to find relationships between two or more variables, such as dietary fat and heart disease. However, the treatment of interest, such as dietary fat, is not assigned to the subjects. Their normal diet and its relationship to the development of heart disease is the main variable of interest. There are various forms of epidemiological research. One general form uses retrospective techniques. In this case, individuals who have a certain disease are identified and compared with a group of their peers, called a *cohort,* who do not have the disease. Researchers then trace the history of both groups through interviewing techniques to identify dietary practices that may have increased the risk for developing the disease. Another general form of epidemiological research uses prospective techniques. In this case, individuals who are free of a specific disease are identified and then followed for years, during which time their diets are scrutinized. As some individuals develop the disease and others do not, the investigators then attempt to determine what dietary behaviors may increase the risk for the disease.

Epidemiological research helps scientists identify important relationships between nutritional practices and health. For example, years ago several epidemiological studies reported that individuals who consumed a diet high in fat were more likely to develop heart disease. One should note that such research does not prove a cause-and-effect relationship. Although these studies did note a deleterious association between a diet high in fat and heart disease, they did not actually prove that fat consumption (possible cause) leads to heart disease (possible effect), but only that some form of relationship between the two existed. However, in some cases the relationship between a lifestyle behavior and a disease is so strong that causality is inferred. In this regard, epidemiologists often calculate and report relative risks (RR) or odds ratios (OR), which are probability estimates of getting some disease by practicing some unhealthful behavior. An RR of 1.0 is normal probability, so if a study reports an RR of 2.5 for developing heart disease in individuals who consumed a diet rich in saturated fatty acids, such diets may increase one's risk 2.5 times normal. Conversely, if a study reports an RR of 0.5 for developing heart disease by consuming a pure vegetarian diet, such diets may cut heart disease risk in half. Epidemiological research is useful in identifying relationships between variables and generating hypotheses, and is often a precursor to experimental research.

Experimental research is essential to establishing a cause-and-effect relationship (figure 1.11). In human nutrition research, experimental studies are often referred to as *randomized clinical trials (RCTs)* or *intervention studies,* usually involving a treatment group and a control, or placebo, group. RCTs may involve studying a smaller group of subjects under tightly controlled conditions for a short time frame, or larger population groups living freely over a long time frame. In RCTs an independent variable (cause) is manipulated so that changes in a dependent variable (effect) can be studied. If we continue with the example of fat and heart disease, a large (and expensive) clinical intervention study could be designed to see whether a low-fat diet could help prevent heart disease. Two groups of subjects would be matched on several risk factors associated with the development of heart disease, and over a certain time, say 10 years, one group would receive a low-fat diet (treatment, or cause) while the other would continue to consume their normal high-fat diet (control or placebo). At the end of the experiment, the differences in the incidence of heart disease (effect) between the two groups would be evaluated to determine whether or not the low-fat diet was an effective preventive strategy. Bouchard presents an excellent detailed overview of the quality of different research-based sources of evidence, noting that RCTs with large populations represent one of the richest sources of data. If the results of an RCT showed that consumption of a low-fat diet had no effect upon the incidence rate of heart disease, should you continue to consume a high-fat diet? The answer to this question, as we shall see later, is "not necessarily." The type of fat may be an important consideration.

Most of the research designed to explore the effect of nutrition on sport performance is experimental in nature, and of a much shorter duration than studies investigating the relationship

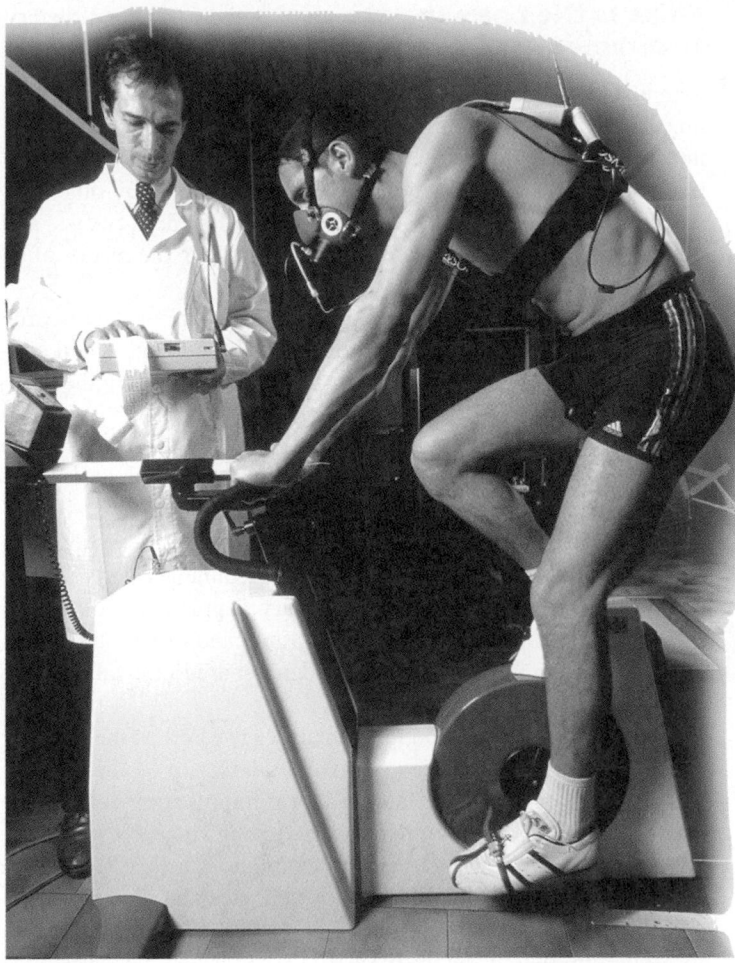

FIGURE 1.11 Well-controlled experimental research serves as the basis underlying recommendations for the use of nutritional strategies to enhance health status or sport performance.

of nutrition and health. Additionally, most sports nutrition studies are conducted in a laboratory with tight control of extraneous variables. Very few studies have actually investigated the effect of nutritional strategies on actual competitive sport performance. Nevertheless, although most of our information about the beneficial effects of various nutritional strategies on sport performance is derived from laboratory-based research, many of these studies use laboratory protocols designed to mimic the physiologic demands of a specific sport. In later chapters, as we discuss the effects of various nutritional strategies or dietary supplements on sports performance, we will often refer to studies that have problems with their experimental methodology, but we will also note studies that were well controlled. Following are some major questions you should ask when evaluating the experimental methodology of a study to see if it has been well designed. We shall use research investigating creatine supplementation as a means to increase muscular strength and power as an example.

1. Is there a legitimate reason for creatine supplementation? Theoretically, creatine may add to the stores of creatine phosphate in the muscle, an important energy source.

2. Were appropriate subjects used? As creatine phosphate may theoretically benefit power performance, trained strength athletes would be ideal subjects.

3. Are the performance tests valid? Validated tests should be used to collect data on the dependent variable, in this case valid strength and power tests.

4. Was a placebo control used? A placebo similar in appearance and taste to creatine should be used in the control trial. Ideally, a control trial in which no substance is consumed should also be incorporated into the study. Beedie and others found that inert substances could induce a positive (placebo) effect or even a negative (nocebo) effect on performance, depending on the respective perception of the subject.

5. Were the subjects randomly assigned to treatments? Subjects should be randomly assigned to separate groups, either the treatment (creatine) or the control (placebo) group. In a repeated-measures design, in which all subjects take both the creatine and the placebo in different trials, the order of administration of the creatine and placebo are counterbalanced, which is known as a *crossover design*. In general, a repeated-measures design is preferable because each subject serves as his or her own control.

6. Was the study double-blind? Neither the investigators nor the subjects should know which groups received the treatment or the placebo until the conclusion of the study.

7. Were extraneous factors controlled? Investigators should try to control other factors that may influence power, such as physical training, diet, and activity prior to testing.

8. Were the data analyzed properly? Appropriate statistical techniques should be used to reduce the risk of statistical error. Using a reasonable number of subjects also helps to minimize statistical error.

Most experienced contemporary investigators generally use similar sophisticated research designs to generate meaningful data, and their studies appear in peer-reviewed journals. A peer-reviewed journal uses a process whereby each manuscript submitted undergoes a review and critique by several experts who recommend for or against publication. However, some researchers do not apply such strict protocols, a fact that, if overlooked by reviewers, may result in publication of a faulty study.

Why do we often hear contradictory advice about the effects of nutrition on health or physical performance?

It is very difficult to conduct nutritional research about health and athletic performance with human subjects. For example, many diseases such as cancer and heart disease are caused by the interaction of multiple risk factors and may take many years to develop. It is not an easy task to control all of these risk factors in freely living human beings so that one independent variable, such as dietary fat, can be isolated to study its effect on the development of heart disease over 10 or 20 years. In a similar manner, numerous physiological, psychological, and biomechanical factors also influence athletic performance on any given day. Why can't athletes match their personal records day after day, such as the world-record 43.18-second 400-meter dash performance by Michael Johnson? Because their physiology and psychology vary from day to day, and even within the day.

Although well-designed studies in peer-reviewed scientific journals serve as the basis for making an informed decision as to whether or not to use a particular nutritional strategy or dietary supplement to enhance health or sport performance, it is important to realize that the results from one study with humans do not prove anything. For example, Ioannidis noted that even the most highly cited RCTs, particularly small ones with a limited number of subjects, may be challenged and refuted over time. Although most investigators attempt to control extraneous factors that may interfere with the interpretation of the results of their study, there may be some unknown factor that leads to an erroneous conclusion. For example, investigators studying the effect of creatine supplementation need to control dietary intake prior to testing. If not, consumption of beverages containing caffeine, an effective ergogenic aid, could confound the results. Consequently, for this and other reasons, the results of single studies, whether epidemiological or experimental, should be taken with a grain of salt—figuratively speaking of course.

The Center for Science in the Public Interest published an article entitled "Behind the Headlines," noting that headlines often neglect to consider important limitations to the study. In this regard, Wellman and others indicated that, unfortunately, all too often the media make bold headlines based on the findings of an individual study, and often these headlines may inadvertently exaggerate the findings of the study and their importance to health or physical performance. For example, a newspaper headline might blare that "Coffee drinking causes heart disease" after a study is published indicating that coffee drinking could increase blood cholesterol levels slightly. The study did *not* show that coffee drinking caused heart disease, but only that it may have adversely affected one of its risk factors. A year or so later one may read headlines that report "Coffee drinking does not cause heart disease" because a more recent individual study did not find an association between coffee use and serum cholesterol levels. Is it no wonder consumers are often confused about nutrition and its effects on health or sport performance? Wellman and others note that nutrition scientists should be more involved in helping the media accurately convey diet and health messages.

For the purpose of improving public understanding, the National Cancer Institute provided some guidelines for journalists and others in the communications business for reporting health-related nutrition research. Key points included the quality and credibility of the study; peer-reviewed study or presentation at a meeting; comparison of findings to other studies; funding sources; and putting findings in context, such as risk/benefit trade-offs. As an example of the latter point, some behavior may increase a health risk from one in a million to three in a million; if reported as a three-fold increase in risk, it may appear to be more unhealthful than it really is. Although these guidelines were presented more than 10 years ago, their use by the media does not appear to have increased appreciably.

What is the basis for the dietary recommendations presented in this book?

Scientists consider each single study as only one piece of the puzzle in attempting to find the truth. To evaluate the effects of nutritional strategies or dietary supplements on health or sport performance, individual studies should be repeated by other scientists and, if possible, a consensus developed. Reviews and meta-analyses provide a stronger foundation than the results of an individual study.

In reviews, an investigator analyzes most or all of the research on a particular topic, and usually offers a summarization and conclusion. However, the conclusion may be influenced by the studies reviewed or by the reviewer's orientation. There have been instances in which different reviewers evaluated the same studies and came up with diametrically opposed conclusions.

Meta-analysis, a review process that involves a statistical analysis of previously published studies, may actually provide a quantification and the strongest evidence available relative to the effect of nutritional strategies or dietary supplements on health or sport performance. According to Binns and others, the meta-analysis is the gold standard for evidence-based clinical practice guidelines.

The value of reviews and meta-analyses is based on the quantity and quality of studies reviewed. If the number of studies is limited and they are not well controlled, or if improper procedures are used in analyzing and comparing the findings of each study, the conclusions may be inaccurate. For example, Hart and Dey noted that three meta-analyses of the use of Echinacea for the prevention of colds had somewhat different conclusions, as selection criteria for studies used in the analysis varied. Nevertheless, well-designed reviews and, in particular, meta-analyses provide us with valuable data to make prudent decisions. In particular, position statements and position stands of various groups, such as the American College of Sports Medicine and the American Dietetic Association, are developed using an *evidence-based* approach, which includes an evaluation of the quality of the studies reviewed. Such groups normally use only RCTs to support their position on specific topics. A number of such positions are cited throughout this text where relevant.

Within the lifetime of many students, a tremendous amount of both epidemiological and experimental research has been concerned with the effect nutrition may have upon health and athletic performance. Based on evolving research findings, dietary recommendations change over time. For example, in a 25th anniversary issue, *Environmental Nutrition* compared 10 different dietary recommendations based on current research and that available 25 years ago. Here is one of the ten: Then, fat was at the root of most illnesses, including heart disease and cancer, and there was no distinction between different types of fat. Now, fat is in good favor if amounts are moderate, and unsaturated fats, especially monounsaturated, when substituted for saturated fats may even help reduce the risk of some chronic diseases.

Comparable to the science of other human behaviors, the science of human exercise and nutrition is not, as many may believe, exact. Although in many cases we still do not have absolute proof that a particular nutritional practice will produce the desired effect, we do have sufficient information to make a recommendation that is prudent, meaning that it is likely to do some good and cause no harm. Thus, the recommendations offered in this text should be considered prudent; they are based upon a careful analysis and evaluation of the available scientific literature, primarily comprehensive reviews and meta-analyses of the pertinent research by various scientists or public and private health or sports organizations. Most such organizations use RCTs as the basis for their guidelines, while some recognize possible limitations of RCTs in making specific nutrition recommendations and incorporate the totality of evidence, including epidemiological findings. In cases where the research data are limited, recommendations may be based on several individual studies if they have been well designed.

How does all this relate to me?

Remember that we all possess biological individuality and thus might react differently to a particular nutritional or exercise intervention. For example, relative to health, most of us have little or no reaction to an increase in dietary salt, but some individuals are very sensitive to salt intake and will experience a significant rise in blood pressure with increased dietary salt. Relative to athletic performance, some, but not all, individuals experience gastrointestinal distress when they ingest certain forms of carbohydrate before performing. Such individual reactions have been noted in some research studies, and are discussed where relevant in the following chapters. With advances in genetic technology, diets may one day be individualized to conform to our genetically determined favorable responses to particular dietary strategies. However, to our knowledge, individualized diets for health or sport performance based on one's genetic profile have not yet been developed.

Thus, recommendations offered in this text should not be regarded as medical advice. Individuals should consult a physician or another appropriate health professional for advice on taking any dietary supplement for health purposes. Additionally, although information presented in this book may help athletes make informed decisions regarding the use of nutritional strategies as a means to improve sport performance, athletes should confer with an appropriate health professional before using sports supplements or nutritional ergogenics.

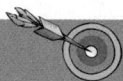

Key Concepts

► Epidemiological research helps to identify relationships between nutritional practice and health or sport performance and may be helpful in developing hypotheses for experimental research. However, experimental studies such as randomized controlled trials are needed to establish a cause-effect relationship. Such experimental studies should adhere to appropriate research design protocols.
► Prudent nutritional recommendations for enhancement of health or athletic performance are based on reputable evidence-based research.

Check for Yourself

► Obtain a scientific article from your library that involves the use of a dietary supplement to improve some facet of sport performance. To get a list of studies, you may go to www.pubmed.gov, and type in the name of the supplement and the term "exercise" in the search column, or simply scan some sports medicine journals in your library. Compare the methodology to the recommended criteria presented on page 24.
► As a student scientist, periodically check your local paper for articles that are based on a recent study about nutrition or exercise and health. Find the research study on which the newspaper article is based and compare the findings. Can you find any examples of exaggeration in the newspaper article?

APPLICATION EXERCISES

Rate and score your diet by completing the quiz on the next several pages. Keep these results until the end of the course and retake the quizzes to see if your dietary practices have changed.

Instructions
These 39 questions will give you a rough sketch of your typical eating habits. The (+) or (−) number for each answer instantly pats you on the back for good eating habits or alerts you to problems you didn't even know

you had. The quiz focuses on fat, saturated fat, cholesterol, sodium, sugar, fiber, and fruits and vegetables. It doesn't attempt to cover everything in your diet. Also, it doesn't try to measure precisely how much of the key nutrients you eat.

Next to each answer is a number with a + or − sign in front of it. **Circle the number that corresponds to the answer you choose.** That's your score for the question. If two or more answers apply, circle each one. Then average them to get your score for the question.

How to average. In answering question 19, for example, if your sandwich-eating is equally divided among tuna salad (−2), roast beef (+1), and turkey breast (+3), add the three scores (which gives you +2) and then divide by three. That gives you a score of +2/3 for the question. Round it to +1.

Pay attention to serving sizes, which we give when needed. For example, a serving of vegetables is 1/2 cup. If you usually eat one cup of vegetables at a time, count it as two servings.

The Quiz

Fruits, Vegetables, Grains, and Beans

1. How many servings of fruit or 100% fruit juice do you eat per day? *(OMIT fruit snacks like Fruit Roll-Ups and fruit-on-the-bottom yogurt. One serving = one piece or 1/2 cup of fruit or 6 oz. of fruit juice.)*
   - a. 0   −3
   - b. less than 1   −2
   - c. 1   0
   - d. 2   +1
   - e. 3   +2
   - f. 4 or more   +3

2. How many servings of non-fried vegetables do you eat per day? *(One serving = 1/2 cup. INCLUDE potatoes.)*
   - a. 0   −3
   - b. less than 1   −2
   - c. 1   0
   - d. 2   +1
   - e. 3   +2
   - f. 4 or more   +3

3. How many servings of vitamin-rich vegetables do you eat per week? *(One serving = 1/2 cup. Count ONLY broccoli, Brussels sprouts, carrots, collards, kale, red pepper, spinach, sweet potatoes, or winter squash.)*
   - a. 0   −3
   - b. 1 to 3   +1
   - c. 4 to 6   +2
   - d. 7 or more   +3

4. How many servings of leafy green vegetables do you eat per week? *(One serving = 1/2 cup cooked or 1 cup raw. Count ONLY collards, kale, mustard greens, romaine lettuce, spinach, or Swiss chard.)*
   - a. 0   −3
   - b. less than 1   −2
   - c. 1 to 2   +1
   - d. 3 to 4   +2
   - e. 5 or more   +3

5. How many times per week does your lunch or dinner contain grains, vegetables, or beans, but little or no meat, poultry, fish, eggs, or cheese?
   - a. 0   −1
   - b. 1 to 2   +1
   - c. 3 to 4   +2
   - d. 5 or more   +3

6. How many times per week do you eat beans, split peas, or lentils? *(OMIT green beans.)*
   - a. 0   −3
   - b. less than 1   −1
   - c. 1   0
   - d. 2   +1
   - e. 3   +2
   - f. 4 or more   +3

7. How many servings of grains do you eat per day? *(One serving = 1 slice of bread, 1 oz. of crackers, 1 large pancake, 1 cup pasta or cold cereal, or 1/2 cup granola, cooked cereal, rice, or bulgur. OMIT heavily sweetened cold cereals.)*
   - a. 0   −3
   - b. 1 to 2   0
   - c. 3 to 4   +1
   - d. 5 to 7   +2
   - e. 8 or more   +3

8. What type of bread, rolls, etc., do you eat?
   - a. 100% whole wheat as the only flour   +3
   - b. whole wheat flour as the 1st or 2nd flour   +2
   - c. rye, pumpernickel, or oatmeal   +1
   - d. white, French, or Italian   0

9. What kind of breakfast cereal do you eat?
   - a. whole-grain (like oatmeal or Wheaties)   +3
   - b. low-fiber (like Cream of Wheat or Corn Flakes)   0
   - c. sugary low-fiber (like Frosted Flakes) or low-fat granola   −1
   - d. regular granola   −2

Meat, Poultry, and Seafood

10. How many times per week do you eat high-fat red meats *(hamburgers, pork chops, ribs, hot dogs, pot roast, sausage, bologna, steaks other than round steak, etc.)?*
    - a. 0   +3
    - b. less than 1   +2
    - c. 1   −1
    - d. 2   −2
    - e. 3   −3
    - f. 4 or more   −4

11. How many times per week do you eat lean red meats *(hot dogs, or luncheon meats with no more than 2 grams of fat per serving, round steak, or pork tenderloin)?*
    - a. 0   +3
    - b. less than 1   +1
    - c. 1   0
    - d. 2–3   −1
    - e. 4–5   −2
    - f. 6 or more   −3

12. After cooking, how large is the serving of red meat you eat? *(To convert from raw to cooked, reduce by 25%. For example, 4 oz. of raw meat shrinks to 3 oz. after cooking. There are 16 oz. in a pound.)*
    - a. 6 oz. or more   −3
    - b. 4 to 5 oz.   −2
    - c. 3 oz. or less   0
    - d. don't eat red meat   +3

13. If you eat red meat, do you trim the visible fat when you cook or eat it?
    - a. yes   +1
    - b. no   −3

14. What kind of ground meat or poultry do you eat?
    - a. regular ground beef   −4
    - b. ground beef that's 11% to 25% fat   −3
    - c. ground chicken or 10% fat ground beef   −2
    - d. ground turkey   −1
    - e. ground turkey breast   +3
    - f. don't eat ground meat or poultry   +3

15. What chicken parts do you eat?
    - a. breast   +3
    - b. drumstick   +1
    - c. thigh   −1
    - d. wing   −2
    - e. don't eat   poultry   +3

16. If you eat poultry, do you remove the skin before eating?
    - a. yes   +2
    - b. no   −3

17. If you eat seafood, how many times per week? *(OMIT deep-fried foods, tuna packed in oil, and mayonnaise-laden tuna salad—low-fat mayo is okay.)*
    - a. less than 1   0
    - b. 1   +1
    - c. 2   +2
    - d. 3 or more   +3

Mixed Foods

18. What is your most typical breakfast? *(SUBTRACT an extra 3 points if you also eat sausage.)*
    - a. biscuit sandwich or croissant sandwich   −4
    - b. croissant, Danish, or doughnut   −3
    - c. eggs   −3
    - d. pancakes, French toast, or waffles   −1
    - e. cereal, toast, or bagel (no cream cheese)   +3
    - f. low-fat yogurt or low-fat cottage cheese   +3
    - g. don't eat breakfast   0

19. What sandwich fillings do you eat?
    - a. regular luncheon meat, cheese, or egg salad   −3
    - b. tuna or chicken salad or ham   −2
    - c. peanut butter   0
    - d. roast beef   +1
    - e. low-fat luncheon meat   +1
    - f. tuna or chicken salad made with fat-free mayo   +3
    - g. turkey breast or hummus   +3

20. What do you order on your pizza? *(Subtract 1 point if you order extra cheese, cheese-filled crust, or more than one meat topping.)*
    - a. no cheese with at least one vegetable topping   +3
    - b. cheese with at least one vegetable topping   −1
    - c. cheese   −2
    - d. cheese with one meat topping   −3
    - e. don't eat pizza   +3

21. What do you put on your pasta? *(ADD one point if you also add sautéed vegetables.)*
    - a. tomato sauce or red clam sauce   +3
    - b. meat sauce or meat balls   −1
    - c. pesto or another oily sauce   −3
    - d. Alfredo or another creamy sauce   −4

22. How many times per week do you eat deep-fried foods (*fish, chicken, french fries, potato chips, etc.*)?
    a. 0   +3   d. 3   −2
    b. 1   0   e. 4 or more −3
    c. 2   −1

23. At a salad bar, what do you choose?
    a. nothing, lemon, or vinegar   +3
    b. fat-free dressing   +2
    c. low- or reduced-Calorie dressing   +1
    d. oil and vinegar   −1
    e. regular dressing   −2
    f. cole slaw, pasta salad, or potato salad   −2
    g. cheese or eggs   −3

24. How many times per week do you eat canned or dried soups or frozen dinners? (*OMIT lower-sodium, low-fat ones.*)
    a. 0   +3   d. 3 to 4   −2
    b. 1   0   e. 5 or more −3
    c. 2   −1

25. How many servings of low-fat calcium-rich food do you eat per day? (*One serving = 2/3 cup low-fat or nonfat milk or yogurt, 1 oz. low-fat cheese, 1 1/2 oz. sardines, 3 1/2 oz. canned salmon with bones, 1 oz. tofu made with calcium sulfate, 1 cup collards or kale, or 200 mg. of a calcium supplement.*)
    a. 0   −3   d. 2   +2
    b. less than 1 −1   e. 3 or more +3
    c. 1   +1

26. How many times per week do you eat cheese? (*INCLUDE pizza, cheeseburgers, lasagna, tacos or nachos with cheese, etc. OMIT foods made with low-fat cheese.*)
    a. 0   +3   d. 3   −2
    b. 1   +1   e. 4 or more −3
    c. 2   −1

27. How many egg yolks do you eat per week? (*ADD 1 yolk for every slice of quiche you eat.*)
    a. 0   +3   d. 3   −1
    b. 1   +1   e. 4   −2
    c. 2   0   f. 5 or more −3

Fats and Oils

28. What do you put on your bread, toast, bagel, or English muffin?
    a. stick butter or cream cheese   −4
    b. stick margarine or whipped butter   −3
    c. regular tub margarine   −2
    d. light tub margarine or whipped light butter   −1

29. What do you spread on your sandwiches?
    e. jam, fat-free margarine, or fat-free cream cheese   0
    f. nothing   +3
    a. mayonnaise   −2
    b. light mayonnaise   −1
    c. catsup, mustard, or fat-free mayonnaise +1
    d. nothing   +2

30. With what do you make tuna salad, pasta salad, chicken salad, etc?
    a. mayonnaise   −2
    b. light mayonnaise   −1
    c. fat-free mayonnaise   0
    d. low-fat yogurt   +2

31. What do you use to sauté vegetables or other foods? (*Vegetable oil includes safflower, corn, sunflower, and soybean.*)
    a. butter or lard   −3
    b. margarine   −2
    c. vegetable oil or light margarine   −1
    d. olive or canola oil   +1
    e. broth   +2
    f. cooking spray   +3

Beverages

32. What do you drink on a typical day?
    a. water or club soda   +3
    b. caffeine-free coffee or tea   0
    c. diet soda   −1
    d. coffee or tea (up to 4 a day)   −1
    e. regular soda (up to 2 a day)   −2
    f. regular soda (3 or more a day)   −3
    g. coffee or tea (5 or more a day)   −3

33. What kind of "fruit" beverage do you drink?
    a. orange, grapefruit, prune, or pineapple juice   +3
    b. apple, grape, or pear juice   +1
    c. cranberry juice blend or cocktail   0
    d. fruit "drink," "ade," or "punch"   −3

34. What kind of milk do you drink?
    a. whole −3   c. 1% low-fat +2
    b. 2% fat −1   d. skim   +3

Desserts and Snacks

35. What do you eat as a snack?
    a. fruits or vegetables   +3
    b. low-fat yogurt   +2
    c. low-fat crackers   +1
    d. cookies or fried chips   −2
    e. nuts or granola bar   −2
    f. candy bar or pastry   −3

36. Which of the following "salty" snacks do you eat?
    a. potato chips, corn chips, or popcorn   −3
    b. tortilla chips   −2

c. salted pretzels or light microwave popcorn   −1
d. unsalted pretzels   +2
e. baked tortilla or potato chips or homemade air-popped popcorn   +3
f. don't eat salty snacks   +3

37. What kind of cookies do you eat?
    a. fat-free cookies   +2
    b. graham crackers or reduced-fat cookies   +1
    c. oatmeal cookies   −1
    d. sandwich cookies (like Oreos)   −2
    e. chocolate coated, chocolate chip, or peanut butter   −3
    f. don't eat cookies   +3

38. What kind of cake or pastry do you eat?
    a. cheesecake   −4
    b. pie or doughnuts   −3
    c. cake with frosting   −2
    d. cake without frosting   −1
    e. muffins   0
    f. angelfood, fat-free cake, or fat-free pastry   +1
    g. don't eat cakes or pastries   +3

39. What kind of frozen dessert do you eat? (*SUBTRACT 1 point for each of the following toppings: hot fudge, nuts, or chocolate candy bars or pieces.*)
    a. gourmet ice cream   −4
    b. regular ice cream   −3
    c. frozen yogurt or light ice cream   −1
    d. sorbet, sherbet, or ices   −1
    e. non-fat frozen yogurt or fat-free ice cream   +1
    f. don't eat frozen desserts   +3

Scoring Your Diet

Add your score for each question.

Score

0 or below	**Oops!**	We don't staple *Nutrition Action* shut, you know.
1 to 29	**Hmmm.**	Don't be discouraged. This eating business is tough.
30 to 59	**Yesss!**	Congratulations. You can invite us over to eat any day.
60 or above	**C-o-o-o-l.**	Our photographer should be at your door any second.

1. Which of the following would not be regarded as unstructured physical activity, sometimes referred to as activities of daily living?

   a. gardening
   b. housework
   c. jogging
   d. leisurely walking
   e. driving the car

2. Which basic principle of exercise training is associated with the concept that cardiovascular-respiratory training will enhance adaptations primarily in the heart whereas resistance training will enhance adaptations primarily in the skeletal muscles?

   a. overuse
   b. overload
   c. specificity
   d. progression
   e. reversibility

3. Increased levels of both aerobic and musculoskeletal fitness through physical activity may produce numerous health benefits. Which of the following is least likely to occur from a combined aerobic and resistance exercise training program?

   a. prevention of heart disease
   b. building of bone density
   c. prevention of weight gain
   d. prevention of type 1 diabetes
   e. improvement of life expectancy

4. Which of the following is not a recommended dietary guideline associated with the Prudent Healthy Diet?

   a. Maintain a healthy body weight.
   b. Eat a variety of wholesome, natural foods.
   c. Choose a diet with plenty of simple, refined carbohydrates.
   d. Abstain from alcohol if you are pregnant.
   e. Choose a diet low in saturated fat.

5. Poor nutrition may contribute to the development of numerous chronic diseases. For example, obesity, high blood pressure, diabetes, and heart disease are most associated with which of the following nutritional problems?

   a. diets rich in vitamins and minerals
   b. diets rich in dietary fiber
   c. diets rich in fat and Calories
   d. diets rich in complex carbohydrates
   e. diets rich in plant proteins

6. Which group of athletes is most likely to suffer from nutritional inadequacies?

   a. male baseball players
   b. female gymnasts
   c. male tennis players
   d. female basketball players
   e. male football players

7. Based on recent recommendations of the American College of Sports Medicine and the American Heart Association relative to exercise and health benefits for adults, which of the following statements is false?

   a. Moderate-intensity aerobic exercise should be done for a minimum of 30 minutes daily on 5 days each week.
   b. Vigorous-intensity exercise may be done for a minimum of 20 minutes on 3 days each week.
   c. Each daily exercise bout of aerobic exercise may be done continuously or in smaller segments, such as three 10-minute bouts.
   d. In general, more is better, as exceeding the minimum recommended amounts of exercise may provide additional health benefits.
   e. Resistance exercise, including exercises for the major muscle groups in the body, is recommended at least 5, and preferably 7, days per week.

8. Which of the following statements regarding ergogenic aids is false?

   a. They are designed to enhance sports performance.
   b. Use of any aid that enhances sport performance is illegal and is grounds for disqualification.
   c. Although most nutritional ergogenics are safe, some dietary supplements pose significant health risks.
   d. Endorsement of a nutritional ergogenic by a professional athlete does not necessarily mean that it is effective as advertised.
   e. Some nutritional supplements marketed as ergogenics may contain prohibited drugs.

9. In an experimental study to evaluate the effect of creatine supplementation on muscular power for sport, which of the following would not be considered acceptable for the research methodology to be followed in the conduct of the study?

   a. Use well-trained power sport athletes.
   b. Use a double-blind protocol.
   c. Use a placebo control group.
   d. Use a sport-related performance task.
   e. Use caffeine as the placebo.

10. A meta-analysis is

    a. an ergogenic aid for mathematicians.
    b. a technique to evaluate the presence of drug metabolites in athletes.
    c. a statistical evaluation of a collection of studies in order to derive a conclusion.
    d. an evaluation of the daily metabolic rate.
    e. an analytical technique to evaluate biomechanics in athletes.

Answers to multiple choice questions:
1. c; 2. c; 3. d; 4. c; 5. c; 6. b; 7. e; 8. b; 9. e; 10. c.

1. Describe the possible mechanisms whereby exercise may enhance health status, and list at least eight of the potential health benefits of a regular, comprehensive exercise program.
2. Name and describe the various principles of exercise.
3. Define the term *sports nutrition* and explain how appropriate eating strategies may enhance sports performance.
4. List at least five guideline questions one may use to evaluate advertised claims for nutritional supplements.
5. Differentiate between epidemiological research and experimental research, discussing the protocols used in each and the pros and cons of each.

References

Books

American Institute of Cancer Research. 2007. *Food, Nutrition, Physical Activity, and the Prevention of Cancer: A Global Perspective.* Washington, DC: AICR.

Antonio, J., and Stout, J. 2001. *Sports Supplements.* Philadelphia: Lippincott Williams & Wilkins.

Bahrke, M., and Yesalis, C. 2002. *Performance-Enhancing Substances in Sport and Exercise.* Champaign, IL: Human Kinetics.

Benardot, D. 2006. *Advanced Sport Nutrition.* Champaign, IL: Human Kinetics.

Burke, L. 2007. *Practical Sports Nutrition.* Champaign, IL: Human Kinetics.

Clark, N. 2008. *Nancy Clark's Sports Nutrition Guidebook: Eating to Fuel Your Active Lifestyle.* Champaign, IL: Human Kinetics.

Dunford, M. 2010. *Fundamentals of Sport and Exercise Nutrition.* Champaign, IL: Human Kinetics.

Dunford, M. 2006. *Sports Nutrition: A Practice Manual for Professionals.* Chicago: SCAN and the American Dietetic Association.

Duyff, R. 2006. *The American Dietetic Association's Complete Food and Nutrition Guide.* New York: Wiley.

Institute of Medicine, Food and Nutrition Board. 2005. *Dietary Reference Intakes for Energy, Carbohydrates, Fiber, Fat, Protein and Amino Acids (Macronutrients).* Washington, DC: National Academy Press.

Ivy, J., and Portman, R. 2004. *Nutrient Timing: The Future of Sports Nutrition.* North Bergen, NJ: Basic Health Publications.

Jeukendrup, A., and Gleeson, M. 2010. *Sport Nutrition.* Champaign, IL: Human Kinetics.

Kreider, R. B., et al. (eds.) 2009. *Exercise & Sport Nutrition: Principles, Promises, Science & Recommendations.* Santa Barbara: Fitness Technologies Press.

Lightsey, D. 2006. *Muscle, Speed, and Lies: What the Sports Supplement Industry Does Not Want Athletes or Consumers to Know.* Guilford, CT: Globe Pequot Press.

Manore, M., Meyer, N., and Thompson, J. 2009. *Sport Nutrition for Health and Performance.* Champaign, IL: Human Kinetics.

Maughan, R. J. 2000. *Nutrition in Sport.* Oxford: Blackwell Science.

McArdle, W. D., et al. 2009. *Sports and Exercise Nutrition.* Baltimore: Lippincott Williams & Wilkins.

Mooren, F., and Völker, K. 2005. *Molecular and Cellular Exercise Physiology.* Champaign, IL: Human Kinetics.

National Institutes of Health. 2002. *The Interaction of Physical Activity and Nutrition: Biological Remodeling and Plasticity.* Bethesda, MD: NIH.

Rippe, J. M. 1999. *Lifestyle Medicine.* Boston: Blackwell Science.

Shils, M., et al. 2006. *Modern Nutrition in Health and Disease.* Philadelphia: Lippincott Williams & Wilkins.

United States Anti-Doping Agency. 2005. *Optimal Dietary Intake.* Colorado Springs, CO: USADA.

U.S. Department of Agriculture and U.S. Department of Health and Human Services. 2005. *Nutrition and Your Health: Dietary Guidelines for Americans.* Washington, DC: U.S. Government Printing Office.

U.S. Department of Health and Human Services, Public Health Service. 1996. *The Surgeon General's Report on Physical Activity and Health.* Washington, DC: U.S. Government Printing Office.

U.S. Department of Health and Human Services. 2010. *Healthy People 2020.* Washington, DC: U.S. Government Printing Office.

Voy, R. 1991. *Drugs, Sports, and Politics.* Champaign, IL: Leisure Press.

Wardlaw, G., and Hampf, J. 2007. *Perspectives in Nutrition.* Boston: McGraw-Hill.

Wolinsky, I., and Driskell, J. 2008. *Sports Nutrition: Energy Metabolism and Exercise.* Boca Raton, FL: CRC Press.

Reviews

Ahmetov, I., and Rogozkin, V. 2009. Genes, athlete status and training—An overview. *Medicine and Sport Science* 54:43–71.

American Cancer Society. 2002. Nutrition and Physical Activity Guidelines Advisory Committee. American Cancer Society guidelines on nutrition and physical activity for cancer prevention: Reducing the risk of cancer with healthy food choices and physical activity. *CA: A Cancer Journal for Clinicians* 52:92–119.

American College of Sports Medicine. 2009. Position of the American Dietetic Association, Dietitians of Canada, and the American College of Sports Medicine: Nutrition and athletic performance. *Medicine & Science in Sports & Exercise* 41:709–31.

American College of Sports Medicine and American Heart Association. 2007. Exercise and acute cardiovascular events: Placing the risks into perspective. *Medicine & Science in Sports & Exercise* 39:886–97.

American Diabetes Association. 2003. Evidence-based nutrition principles and recommendations for the treatment and prevention of diabetes and related complications. *Diabetes Care* 26:S51–61.

American Dietetic Association. 2000. *10 Tips to Healthy Eating.* Chicago: The American Dietetic Association.

American Dietetic Association, Dietitians of Canada, and American College of Sports Medicine. 2000. Nutrition and athletic performance. *Journal of the American Dietetic Association* 100:1543–56.

American Heart Association Nutrition Committee. 2006. Diet and lifestyle recommendations revision 2006: A scientific statement from the American Heart Association Nutrition Committee. *Circulation* 114:82–96.

Ames, B. 2001. DNA damage from micronutrient deficiencies is likely to be a major cause of cancer. *Mutation Research* 475:7–20.

Angevaren, M., et al. 2008. Physical activity and enhanced fitness to improve cognitive function in older people without known cognitive impairment. *Cochrane Database of Systematic Reviews* April 16: (2): CD005381.

Bauman, A. 2004. Updating the evidence that physical activity is good for health: An epidemiological review 2000–2003. *Journal of Science and Medicine in Sport* 7:6–19.

Binns, C., et al. Tea or coffee? 2008. A case study on evidence for dietary advice. *Public Health Nutrition* 11:1132–41.

Blair, S., et al. 2004. The evolution of physical activity recommendations: How much is enough? *American Journal of Clinical Nutrition* 79:919S–920S.

Booth, F., and Chakravarthy, M. 2002. Cost and consequences of sedentary living: New battleground for an old enemy. *President's Council on Physical Fitness and Sports Research Digest* 3 (13):1–8.

Booth, F., and Lees, S. 2007. Fundamental questions about genes, inactivity, and chronic diseases. *Physiological Genomics* 28:146–57.

Booth, F. W., and Neufer, P. D. 2006. Exercise genomics and proteomics. In *ACSM's Advanced Exercise Physiology*, ed. C.M. Tipton. Philadelphia: Lippincott Williams & Wilkins.

Bouchard, C. 2006. Are people physically active because of their genes? *President's Council on Physical Fitness and Sports Research Digest* 7 (2):1–8.

Bouchard, C. 2001. Physical activity and health: Introduction to the dose-response symposium. *Medicine & Science in Sports & Exercise* 33:S347–50.

Brandt, C., and Pedersen, B. 2010. The role of exercise-induced myokines in muscle homeostasis and the defense against chronic diseases. *Journal of Biomedicine & Biotechnology* 520258.

Brutsaert, T., and Parra, B. 2006. What makes a champion? Explaining variation in human athletic performance. *Respiratory Physiology & Neurobiology* 151:109–23.

Burke, L. 2001. Nutritional practices of male and female endurance cyclists. *Sports Medicine* 31:521–32.

Burke, L. 1999. Nutrition for sport: Getting the most out of training. *Australian Family Physician* 28:561–7.

Carmichael, M. 2007. Stronger, faster, smarter. *Newsweek* 156 (13):38–47.

Center for Science in the Public Interest. 2006. Behind the headlines. *Nutrition Action Health Letter* 33 (3):3–7.

Cloud, J. 2010. Why genes aren't destiny. *Time* 175 (2):49–53.

Colberg, S., et al. 2010. Exercise and type 2 diabetes: American College of Sports Medicine and the American Diabetes Association: Joint Position Statement. Exercise and type 2 diabetes. *Medicine & Science in Sports & Exercise* 42:2282–303.

Consumers Union. 2007. Simple steps may slow aging. *Consumer Reports on Health* 19 (4):1, 4–5.

Cordain, L., et al. 2005. Origins and evolution of the Western diet: Healthy implications for the 21st century. *American Journal of Clinical Nutrition* 81:341–54.

Dancho, C., and Manore, M. 2001. Dietary supplement information on the World Wide Web. *ACSM's Health & Fitness Journal* 5 (6):7–12.

Deldicque, L., and Francaux, M. 2008. Functional food for exercise performance: Fact or foe? *Current Opinion in Clinical Nutrition & Metabolic Care* 11:774–81.

DeMarini, D. M. 1998. Dietary interventions and human carcinogenesis. *Mutation Research* 400:457–65.

Donnelly, J., et al. 2009. American College of Sports Medicine Position Stand. Appropriate physical activity intervention strategies for weight loss and prevention of weight regain for adults. *Medicine & Science in Sports & Exercise* 41:459–71.

Durnin, J.V. 1967. The influence of nutrition. *Canadian Medical Association Journal* 96:715–20.

Engels, H. J. 1999. Publication of adverse events in exercise studies involving nutritional agents. *International Journal of Sport Nutrition* 9:89–91.

Environmental Nutrition Editors. 2002. Celebrating 25 years of *Environmental Nutrition*: What we believed then, what we think we know now. *Environmental Nutrition* 25 (1):8.

Epstein, D., and Dohrmann, G. 2010. What you don't know might kill you. *Sports Illustrated* 110 (20):54–63.

Fédération Internationale de Football Association (FIFA). 2006. *Nutrition for Football* [pamphlet]. Altstätten, Switzerland: Druck und Medun, AG.

Febbraio, M., and Pedersen, B. 2005. Contraction-induced myokine production and release: Is skeletal muscle an endocrine organ? *Exercise and Sport Sciences Reviews* 33:114–19.

Franco, O., et al. 2005. Effects of physical activity on life expectancy with cardiovascular disease. *Archives of Internal Medicine* 165:2355–60.

Friedenreich, C., and Orenstein, M. 2002. Physical activity and cancer prevention: Etiologic evidence and biological mechanisms. *Journal of Nutrition* 132:3456S–64S.

Geiger, P., et al. 2011. Heat shock proteins are important mediators of skeletal muscle insulin sensitivity. *Exercise and Sport Sciences Reviews* 39:34–42.

Greider, K. 2011. The real fountain of youth: Exercise. *AARP Bulletin*. 12(1):10.

Hart, A., and Dey, P. 2009. Echinacea for prevention of the common cold: An illustrative overview of how information from different systematic reviews is summarised on the internet. *Preventive Medicine* 49:78–82.

Haskell, W., et al. 2007. Physical activity and public health: Updated recommendation for adults from the American College of Sports Medicine and the American Heart Association. *Medicine & Science in Sports & Exercise* 39:1423–34.

Jakicic, J., and Otto, A. 2006. Treatment and prevention of obesity: What is the role of exercise? *Nutrition Reviews* 64:S57–61.

Jeukendrup, A., and Martin, J. 2001. Improving cycling performance: How should we spend our time and money. *Sports Medicine* 31:559–69.

Joyner, M., and Coyle, E. 2008. Endurance exercise performance: The physiology of champions. *Journal of Physiology* 586:35–44.

Kearney, J. 1996. Training the Olympic athlete. *Scientific American* 274 (June):52–63.

Kuchment, A. 2007. On your marks . . . *Newsweek* 156 (13):56–59.

Kushi, L., et al. 2006. American Cancer Society Guidelines on Nutrition and Physical Activity for cancer prevention: Reducing the risk of cancer with healthy food choices and physical activity. *CA Cancer Journal for Clinicians* 56:254–81.

Lawrence, M., and Kirby, D. 2002. Nutrition and sports supplements: Fact or fiction. *Journal of Clinical Gastroenterology* 35:299–306.

LeLorier, J., et al. 1997. Discrepancies between meta-analyses and subsequent large, randomized, controlled trials. *New England Journal of Medicine* 337:559–61.

Liebman, B. 2007. Staying sharp. *Nutrition Action Health Letter* 34 (5):1, 3–7.

Lloyd-Jones, D., et al. 2010. Defining and setting national goals for cardiovascular health promotion and disease reduction: The American Heart Association's strategic Impact Goal through 2020 and beyond. *Circulation* 121:586–613.

Manore, M. 2004. Nutrition and physical activity: Fueling the active individual. *President's Council on Physical Fitness and Sports Research Digest* 5(1):1–8.

Maughan, R., et al. 2004. Dietary supplements. *Journal of Sports Sciences* 22:95–113.

Maughan, R. 2002. The athlete's diet: Nutritional goals and dietary strategies. *Proceedings of the Nutrition Society* 61:87–96.

Meadows, M. 2005. Genomics and personalized medicine. *FDA Consumer* 39(6):12–17.

Melzer, K., et al. 2004. Physical activity: The health benefits outweigh the risks. *Current Opinion in Clinical Nutrition and Metabolic Care* 7:641–47.

Mooren, F., et al. 2005. Inter- and intracellular signaling. In *Molecular and Cellular*

Exercise Physiology, eds. F. Mooren and K. Völker. Champaign, IL: Human Kinetics.

Moreira, A. et al. 2009. Does exercise increase the risk of upper respiratory tract infections? *British Medical Bulletin* 90:111–31.

Mosca, L. 2007. Evidence-based recommendations for cardiovascular disease prevention in women. 2007 Update. *Circulation* 115:1481–501.

National Cancer Institute. 1998. Commentary: Improving Public Understanding: Guidelines for communicating emerging science on nutrition, food safety, and health. *Journal of National Cancer Institute* 90 (3): 194–99.

National Institutes of Health. 2006. National Institutes of Health State-of-the-Science conference statement: Multivitamin/mineral supplements and chronic disease prevention. *Annals of Internal Medicine* 145:364–71.

Nieman, D. 2000. Is infection risk linked to exercise workload? *Medicine & Science in Sports & Exercise* 32:S406–11.

O'Gorman, D., and Krook, A. 2008. Exercise and the treatment of diabetes and obesity. *Endocrinology & Metabolism Clinics of North America* 37:887–903.

Østergård, T., et al. 2007. The effect of exercise, training, and inactivity on insulin sensitivity in diabetics and their relatives: What is new? *Applied Physiology, Nutrition, and Metabolism* 32:541–48.

Rankinen, T., et al. 2010. Advances in exercise, fitness, and performance genomics. *Medicine & Science in Sports & Exercise* 42:835–846.

Rogers, C., et al. 2008. Physical activity and cancer prevention: Pathways and targets for intervention. *Sports Medicine* 38:271–96.

Simopoulos, A. 2010. Nutrigenetics/Nutrigenomics. *Annual Review Public Health* 21:53–68.

Slentz, C., et al. 2007. Modest exercise prevents the progressive disease associated with physical inactivity. *Exercise and Sport Sciences Reviews* 35:18–23.

Sofi, F., et al. 2010. Effectiveness of the Mediterranean diet: can it help delay or prevent Alzheimer's disease? *Journal of Alzheimers Disease.* 20:795–801.

Thompson, P., et al. 2001. The acute versus the chronic response to exercise. *Medicine & Science in Sports & Exercise* 33:S438–45.

Tufts University. 2008. Moderate exercise can cut stroke risk 40%. *Health & Nutrition Letter* 26 (1):1–2.

Varró, A., and Baczkó, I. 2010. Possible mechanisms of sudden cardiac death in top athletes: A basic cardiac electrophysiological point of view. *Pflugers Archiv* 460:31–40.

Vuori, I. 2001. Health benefits of physical activity with special reference to interaction with diet. *Public Health Nutrition* 4:517–28.

Webb, L., and Lieberman, P. 2006. Anaphylaxis: A review of 601 cases. *Annals of Allergy, Asthma & Immunology* 97:39–43.

Weissgerber, T., et al. 2006. Exercise in the prevention and treatment of maternal-fetal disease: A review of the literature. *Applied Physiology, Nutrition and Metabolism* 31:661–74.

Wellman, N., et al. 1999. Do we facilitate the scientific process and the development of dietary guidance when findings from single studies are publicized? An American Society for Nutritional Sciences controversy session report. *American Journal of Clinical Nutrition* 70:802–5.

Williams, C. 1998. Diet and sports performance. In *Oxford Textbook of Sports Medicine,* eds. M. Harries et al. Oxford: Oxford University Press.

Williams, M. 2011. Sports supplements: Quercetin. *ACSM's Health & Fitness Journal* 15 (5):17–20.

Williams, M. 2006. Sports nutrition. In *Modern Nutrition in Health and Disease,* eds. M. Shils et al. Philadelphia: Lippincott Williams & Wilkins.

Williams, M., and Branch, J. D. 2000. Ergogenic aids for improved performance. In *Exercise and Sport Science,* eds. W. E. Garrett and D. T. Kirkendall. Philadelphia: Lippincott Williams & Wilkins.

Specific Studies

Beedie, C., et al. 2007. Positive and negative placebo effects resulting from the deceptive administration of an ergogenic aid. *International Journal of Sport Nutrition & Exercise Metabolism* 17:259–69.

Bouchard, C., et al. 2000. Genomic scan for maximal oxygen uptake and its response to training in the HERITAGE family study. *Journal of Applied Physiology* 88:551–59.

Dascombe, B., et al. 2010. Nutritional supplementation habits and perceptions of elite athletes within a state-based sporting institute. *Journal of Science and Medicine in Sport* 13:274–80.

Erdman, K. 2006. Influence of performance level on dietary supplementation in elite Canadian athletes. *Medicine & Science in Sports & Exercise* 38:348–56.

Hinton, P., et al. 2004. Nutrient intakes and dietary behaviors of male and female collegiate athletes. *International Journal of Sport Nutrition and Exercise Metabolism* 14:389–405.

Ioannidis, J. 2005. Contradicted and initially stronger effects in highly cited clinical research. *JAMA* 294:218–28.

Jacobson, B., et al. 2001. Nutrition practices and knowledge of college varsity athletes: A follow-up. *Journal of Strength and Conditioning Research* 15:63–68.

Jonnalagadda, S., et al. 2000. Assessment of under-reporting of energy intake of elite female gymnasts. *International Journal of Sport Nutrition and Exercise Metabolism* 10:315–25.

King, D., et al. 2009. Adherence to healthy lifestyle habits in US adults, 1988–2006. *American Journal of Medicine* 122:528–34.

Krebs-Smith, S., et al. 2010. Americans do not meet federal dietary recommendations. *Journal of Nutrition* 140:1832–8.

Kristiansen, M., et al. 2005. Dietary supplement use by varsity athletes at a Canadian University. *International Journal of Sport Nutrition and Exercise Metabolism* 15:195–210.

Kvaavik, E., et al. 2010. Influence of individual and combined health behaviors on total and cause-specific mortality in men and women: the United Kingdom health and lifestyle survey. *Archives of Internal Medicine* 170:711–8.

Lun, V., et al. 2009. Evaluation of nutritional intake in Canadian high-performance athletes. *Clinical Journal of Sport Medicine* 19:405–11.

Maruti, S., et al. 2008. A prospective study of age-specific physical activity and premenopausal breast cancer. *Journal of the National Cancer Institute* 100:728–37.

Morrison, L., et al. 2004. Prevalent use of dietary supplements among people who exercise at a commercial gym. *International Journal of Sport Nutrition & Exercise Metabolism* 14:481–92.

Morrow, J., et al. 2011. Long-term tracking of physical activity behaviors in women: The WIN study. *Medicine & Science in Sports & Exercise* 43:165–70.

Mullins, V., et al. 2001. Nutritional status of U.S. elite female heptathletes during training. *International Journal of Sport Nutrition and Exercise Metabolism* 11:299–314.

Peplonska, B., et al. 2008. Adulthood lifetime physical activity and breast cancer. *Epidemiology* 19:226–36.

Rosenbloom, C. 2002. Nutrition knowledge of collegiate athletes in a Division I National Collegiate Athletic Association institution. *Journal of the American Dietetic Association* 102:418–20.

Stewart, L., et al. 2007. The influence of exercise training on inflammatory cytokines and C-reactive protein. *Medicine & Science in Sports & Exercise* 39:1714–19.

Tully, M., et al. 2007. Randomised controlled trial of home-based walking program at and below current recommended levels of exercise in sedentary adults. *Journal of Epidemiology & Community Health* 61:778–83.

Ziegler, P., et al. 1999. Nutritional and physiological status of U.S. national figure skaters. *International Journal of Sport Nutrition* 9:345–60.

Zinn, C., et al. 2006. Evaluation of sports nutrition knowledge of New Zealand premier club rugby coaches. *International Journal of Sport Nutrition and Exercise Metabolism* 16:214–25.

Healthful Nutrition for Fitness and Sport: The Consumer Athlete

CHAPTER TWO

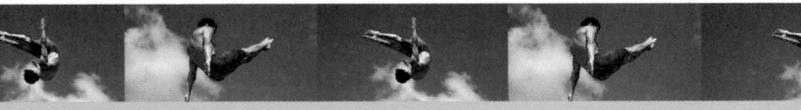

LEARNING OBJECTIVES

After studying this chapter, you should be able to:

1. List the six major classes of nutrients that are essential for human nutrition and identify specific nutrients within each class.

2. Explain the development of the DRI and explain the meaning of its various components, including the RDA, AI, AMDR, UL, EER, and EAR.

3. Discuss the concept of the balanced diet as applied to the MyPlate food guide.

4. Explain the concept of nutrient density and provide an example.

5. Outline the 12 guidelines for healthy eating and provide several examples for each as to how food might be selected or prepared in order to adhere to these guidelines.

6. Describe the various classes of vegetarians, what foods they may consume in their diets, and the potential health benefits.

7. List the nutrients that must be included on a food label and explain how reading food labels may help one consume a healthier diet.

8. Identify the various types of dietary supplements and discuss, in general, the potential benefits and risks associated with taking dietary supplements.

9. Describe how commercial and home food processing may enhance or impair the quality of food we eat.

10. Differentiate among food intolerance, food allergy, and food poisoning regarding causes and consequences of each.

11. Understand how dietary practices as related to training and competition may help optimize sport performance.

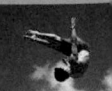

What you eat can have a significant effect on your health. Hippocrates, the Greek physician known as the father of medicine, recognized the value of nutrition and the power of food to enhance health when he declared that you should let food be your medicine and medicine be your food. As noted in chapter 1, the foods we eat contain various nutrients to sustain life by providing energy, promoting growth and development, and regulating metabolic processes. Basically, healthful nutrition is designed to optimize these life-sustaining properties of nutrients and other substances found in food.

As the human race evolved over the aeons, a natural diet of plant and animal foods provided the nutrients necessary to sustain the lives of our hunter/gatherer ancestors. As human civilization developed, however, human food consumption patterns gradually changed as the emerging food industry developed newer and increasingly more technological methods to plant, grow, process, and prepare foods. Overall, modern developments in the food industry have improved food quality and safety, but there are still some practices that are cause for consumer concern. For example, provision of a wide variety of foods has helped to eradicate most nutrient-deficiency diseases in industrialized nations. Conversely, provision of a wide variety of high-fat, high-sugar, high-Calorie, low-fiber foods appears to have increased the possibility of the development of various chronic diseases.

The three keys to a healthful diet are balance, variety, and moderation. In general, a healthful diet is simply one that provides a balanced proportion of foods from different food groups, a variety of foods from within the different food groups, and moderation in the consumption of any food. Such a diet should provide us with the nutrients we need to sustain life. In this regard, several governmental and professional health organizations have developed dietary guidelines to help us obtain the nutrients we need.

Additionally, the current major focus of nutrition research, both epidemiological and experimental, is how our diets—and even specific foods or nutrients in our diets—affect our health, primarily as related to the development of chronic diseases. Again, specific dietary guidelines have been recommended as a means to enhance one's health status, and these recommendations underlie the Prudent Healthy Diet. In essence, the basic premise of the Prudent Healthy Diet is to consume foods in as natural a state as possible, primarily relying on plant foods and a movement toward a vegetarian or semivegetarian diet.

Although the basic guidelines underlying the Prudent Healthy Diet are rather simple, selecting the appropriate foods in modern society may be somewhat confusing. Fortunately, nutrition labels should provide the knowledgeable consumer with sufficient information to make intelligent choices and select high-quality foods. Food safety is also another consumer concern, and appropriate food selection and preparation practices may help minimize most of the health risks associated with certain foods.

Another problem underlying healthy eating is the cost. A Tufts University report noted that the cost of more nutritious foods is climbing. They report that low-Calorie, nutrient-rich fruits and vegetables were far more expensive, Calorie for Calorie, than sweets and snack foods. One researcher noted that fruits and vegetables are rapidly becoming luxury goods. In one survey they reported that energy-dense foods rich in sugar and fat cost an average $1.76 for 1,000 Calories, whereas nutrient-dense foods cost $18.16 per 1,000 Calories, more than 10 times as much. However, you can reduce the cost of nutrient-dense foods with a little planning, such as the following.

- Choose seasonal fruits and vegetables.
- Capitalize on store specials on fresh chicken, fish, and low-fat meat. Buy quantities, repackage into smaller portions, and freeze for future use.
- Purchase whole grain cereals, rice, and similar products in bulk at warehouse stores.
- Buy bags of frozen vegetables, which are cheaper and do not spoil.

The Prudent Healthy Diet also serves as the basic diet for those interested in optimal physical performance, although it may be modified somewhat for specific types of athletic endeavors, as shall be noted as appropriate throughout the book.

Essential Nutrients and Recommended Nutrient Intakes

"You are what you eat" is a popular phrase that contains some truth, particularly in its implications for both health and athletic performance. The foods you eat contain a wide variety of nutrients, both essential and nonessential, as well as other substances that may affect your body functions. These nutrients are synthesized by plants from water, carbon dioxide, and various elements in the soil, and they also become concentrated in animals that consume plant foods. Various nutrients may also be added to foods in the manufacturing process. Careful selection of wholesome, natural foods will provide you with the proper amounts of nutrients to optimize energy sources, to build and repair tissues, and to regulate body processes. However, as we shall see in later chapters, poor food selection with an unbalanced intake of some nutrients may contribute to the development of significant health problems and impair sport performance.

What are essential nutrients?

As noted in chapter 1, six classes of nutrients are considered necessary in human nutrition: carbohydrates, fats, proteins, vitamins, minerals, and water. Within most of these general classes (notably protein, vitamins, and minerals) are a number of specific nutrients necessary for life. For example, more than a dozen vitamins are needed for optimal physiological functioning.

In relation to nutrition, the term **essential nutrients** describes nutrients that the body needs but cannot produce at all or cannot produce in adequate quantities. Thus, in general, essential nutrients must be obtained from the food we eat. Essential nutrients also are known as *indispensable nutrients*.

Table 2.1 lists the specific nutrients currently known to be essential or probably essential to humans. Some of the nutrients listed have been shown to be essential for various animals and are theorized to be essential for humans. Curing a nutrient-deficiency disease by a specific nutrient has been the key factor underlying the determination of nutrient essentiality. However, the concept of nutrient essentiality has evolved to include substances that may help prevent the development of chronic diseases. Most recently, the essentiality of choline was included with the B vitamin group, and the list is likely to expand in the future as research reveals health benefits of various plant substances.

Some foods, such as whole wheat bread, may contain all six general classes of nutrients, whereas others, such as table sugar, contain only one nutrient class. However, whole wheat bread cannot be considered a complete food because it does not contain a proper balance of all essential nutrients.

The human body requires substantial amounts of some nutrients, particularly those that may provide energy and support growth and development of the body tissues, namely carbohydrate, fat, protein, water, and several minerals and electrolytes. These nutrients are referred to as **macronutrients** because the daily requirement usually is greater than a few grams. Most nutrients that help to regulate metabolic processes, particularly

vitamins and minerals, are needed in much smaller amounts (usually measured in milligrams or micrograms) and are referred to as **micronutrients,** although as noted in chapter 8, minerals may be classified by other terminology according to the daily requirement.

Essential nutrients are necessary for human life. An inadequate intake may lead to disturbed body metabolism, certain disease states, or death. Conversely, an excess of certain nutrients may also disrupt normal metabolism and may even be lethal (see figure 2.1).

TABLE 2.1	Nutrients essential or probably essential to humans

Carbohydrates

Fiber
Sugars and starches

Fats (essential fatty acids)

Linoleic fatty acid
Alpha linolenic fatty acid

Protein (essential amino acids)

Histidine	Phenylalanine and tyrosine
Isoleucine	Threonine
Leucine	Tryptophan
Lysine	Valine
Methionine and cysteine	

Vitamins

Water soluble	*Fat soluble*
B_1 (thiamin)	A (retinol)
B_2 (riboflavin)	D (calciferol)
Niacin	E (tocopherol)
B_6 (pyridoxine)	K
Pantothenic acid	
Folacin	
B_{12} (cyanocobalamin)	
Biotin	
Choline*	
C (ascorbic acid)	

Minerals

Major	*Trace/Ultratrace*	
Calcium	Boron	Manganese
Chloride	Chromium	Molybdenum
Magnesium	Cobalt	Nickel
Phosphorus	Copper	Selenium
Potassium	Fluorine	Silicon
Sodium	Iodine	Vanadium
Sulfur	Iron	Zinc

Water

*Technically not classified as a vitamin (see chapter 7).

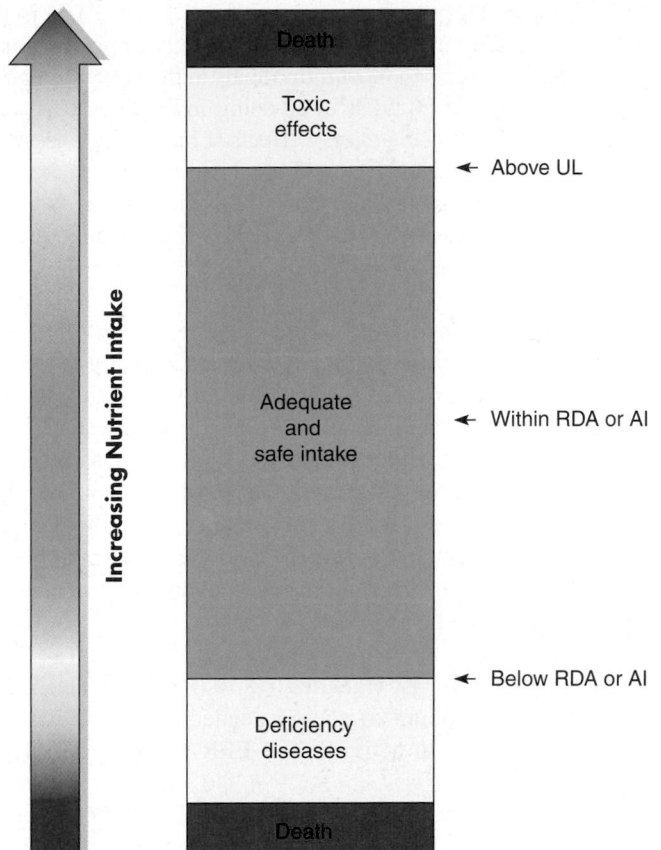

FIGURE 2.1 One model of the possible relationship between nutrient intake and health status. An inadequate intake may lead to nutrient-deficiency diseases, while excessive amounts may cause various toxic reactions. Both deficiencies and excesses may be fatal if carried to extremes. Nutrient intakes within the Recommended Dietary Allowance (RDA) or Adequate Intake (AI) levels are normally adequate and safe, while those below these levels may lead to deficiency diseases. Nutrient intakes above the Tolerable Upper Intake Level (UL) may lead to toxic reactions.

What are nonessential nutrients?

Those nutrients found in food but that also may be formed in the body are known as **nonessential nutrients,** or dispensable nutrients. A good example of a nonessential nutrient is creatine. Although we may obtain creatine from food, the body can also manufacture creatine from several amino acids when necessary. Thus, we need not consume creatine *per se,* but must consume adequate amounts of the amino acids from which creatine is made. As we shall see later, creatine combined with phosphate is a very important nutrient for energy production during very high intensity exercise.

Other than nonessential nutrients, foods contain other nonessential substances that may be involved in various metabolic processes in the body. These substances, sometimes referred to as *non-nutrients,* include those found naturally in foods and those added either intentionally or inadvertently during the various phases of food production and preparation. Classes of these substances include drugs, phytochemicals, extracts, herbals, food additives, and even antinutrients (substances that may adversely

TABLE 2.2 Examples of nonessential nutrients and other substances found in foods

Nonessential nutrients
Carnitine
Creatine
Glycerol

Drugs
Caffeine
Ephedrine

Phytochemicals
Phenols
Plant sterols
Terpenes

Extracts
Bee pollen
Ginseng
Yohimbe

Antinutrients
Phytates
Tannins

affect nutrient status). Many of these nonessential nutrients and other substances are marketed as a means to enhance health or sports performance. Table 2.2 provides some examples that will be covered later in this text.

How are recommended dietary intakes determined?

As noted in table 2.1, humans have an essential requirement for more than 40 specific nutrients. A number of countries, as well as the Food and Agriculture and World Health Organizations (FAO/WHO), have estimated the amount of each nutrient that individuals should consume in their diets. In the United States, the recommended amounts of certain of these nutrients have been established by the Food and Nutrition Board, Institute of Medicine, of the National Academy of Sciences. The first set of recommendations, **Recommended Dietary Allowances (RDA),** was published in 1941 and revised periodically over the years. In general, scientists with considerable knowledge of a specific nutrient would meet to evaluate the totality of scientific data concerning the need for that nutrient in the diet. Based on their analysis, specific dietary intake recommendations were made.

In the past the Recommended Dietary Allowances were developed to prevent deficiency diseases. For example, the RDA for vitamin C was set to prevent scurvy. However, more recently scientists have discovered that higher amounts of some nutrients may confer some health benefits in specific population groups, such as prevention of birth defects by adequate folic acid intake in the early stages of pregnancy and the prevention of various chronic diseases by sufficient intake of nutrients found in fruits and vegetables. Conversely, scientists have also noted that overconsumption of some nutrients may increase health risks.

Expert scientists still meet to evaluate the available scientific data that serve as the basis for dietary recommendations, but the basis for such recommendations has been expanded beyond the objective of simply preventing deficiency diseases. The current philosophy relative to the development of recommendations for dietary intake focuses on a continuum of nutrient intake. Several points along this continuum for a specific nutrient may be (1) the amount that prevents a nutrient-deficiency disease, (2) the amount that may reduce the risk of a specific health problem or chronic diseases, and (3) the amount that may increase health risks.

Based on this concept, the Food and Nutrition Board, working with Health Canada, is involved in a multiyear project to develop new standards for nutrient intake, the **Dietary Reference Intakes (DRI),** for Americans and Canadians. The DRI is an umbrella term, consisting of various reference intakes, that replaces and expands on the Recommended Dietary Allowances. The DRI consists of:

EARs
RDAs
AIs
DRIs
AMDRs
EERs
ULs

The Recommended Dietary Allowance (RDA) The RDA represents the average daily dietary intake that is sufficient to meet the nutrient requirement of nearly all (97 percent to 98 percent) healthy individuals in a group. The RDA is to be used as a goal for the individual. You may use the RDA to evaluate your intake of a specific nutrient. The *RDA* term is used throughout this book as the means to express nutritional adequacy.

The Adequate Intake (AI) The AI is a recommended daily intake level based on observed or experimentally determined approximations of nutrient intake by a group of healthy people. When a RDA cannot be set because extensive scientific data are not available, an AI may be established because the limited data available may provide grounds for a reasonable judgment. You may also use the AI to evaluate your intake of a specific nutrient, but remember that it is not as well established as the RDA. The *AI* term is used throughout this book as appropriate.

The Acceptable Macronutrient Distribution Range (AMDR) The AMDR is defined as a range of intakes for a particular energy source that is associated with reduced risk of chronic disease while providing adequate intakes of essential nutrients. The AMDR is expressed as a percentage of total energy intake and has both an upper and lower level. Individuals consuming below or above this range are at more risk for inappropriate intake of essential nutrients and development of chronic diseases. AMDRs have been set for carbohydrate, fat, and protein.

The Tolerable Upper Intake Level (UL) The UL is the highest level of daily nutrient intake that is likely to pose no risks of adverse health effects to most individuals in the general population. The UL is given to assist in advising individuals what levels of intake may result in adverse effects if habitually exceeded. The UL is not intended to be a recommended dietary intake; you should consider it as a maximum for your daily intake of a specific nutrient on a long-term basis. The UL is cited throughout this book when data are available.

The Estimated Average Requirement (EAR) The EAR represents a nutrient intake value that is estimated to meet the requirement of half the healthy individuals in a group. Conversely, half of the individuals consuming the EAR will not meet their nutrient needs. The EAR is used to establish the RDA. Depending on the data available, the RDA is some multiple of the EAR, mathematically calculated to provide adequate amounts to 97 percent to 98 percent of the general population. When sufficient scientific data are not available to calculate an EAR, then an AI may be provided.

The Estimated Energy Requirement (EER) The EER is an estimate of the amount of energy needed to sustain requirements for daily physical activity. The EER is covered in detail in chapter 3.

Figure 2.1 highlights several of these terms in relation to nutritional deficiency, adequacy, and excess. These terms, and others, are described in detail in the National Academy of Sciences series on Dietary Reference Intakes.

Currently, DRI have been established for all classes of essential nutrients, including carbohydrate, fat, protein and amino acids, vitamins, minerals, and water. The new DRI also, for the first time, provide recommendations for those 70 years and older. Tables containing the current DRI may be found on the inside of the front and back covers of this text. The current DRI will be updated, with inclusion of additional substances like phytochemicals, as future research data merits.

www.nap.edu   You may access the full version of the DRI for specific nutrients free of charge. Click on Special Collections and Dietary Reference Intakes.

The DRI have been developed for several purposes, one of the most important being the assessment of dietary intake and planning diets for individuals and groups. In this context, the DRI for specific nutrients will be provided in the appropriate chapter. However, another term, Daily Value (DV), is used with food labels and may be useful in helping you plan your dietary intake. The DV is discussed later in this chapter.

These new standards are designed to ensure adequate nutrition for most individuals in the population. They may also be used to plan diets for individuals with special needs. If individuals in a population consume foods in amounts adequate to meet these standards, there will be very little likelihood of nutritional inadequacy or impairment of health. An individual does not necessarily have a deficient diet if the recommendation for a given nutrient is not received daily. The daily recommendation for any nutrient should average over a five- to eight-day period, so that one may be deficient in iron consumption one day but compensate for this one-day deficiency during the remainder of the week. Thus, comparison of our nutrient intake to these standards over a sufficient period may be useful in estimating our risk for deficiency. However, one should realize that only a clinical and biochemical evaluation can reveal an individual's nutritional status in regard to any specific nutrient.

Although the RDA are useful because they state approximately how much of all the essential nutrients we need, they are not designed to inform us as to which specific foods we may need to consume to obtain these nutrients. Other dietary guidelines have been developed to help us select foods that will provide us with the RDA for all essential nutrients.

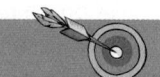

Key Concepts

▶ Balance, variety, and moderation are the three keys to a healthful diet.

▶ The principal purposes of the nutrients we eat are to provide energy, build and repair body tissues, and regulate metabolic processes in the body.

▶ More than 40 specific nutrients are essential to life processes. They may be obtained in the diet through consumption of the six major nutrient classes: carbohydrates, fats, proteins, vitamins, minerals, and water.

▶ The Dietary Reference Intakes (DRI) provide us with a set of standards for our nutritional needs and are being developed with the goal of promoting optimal health.

Check for Yourself

▶ Using the tables on the inside of the front and back covers of the text, list the DRI for yourself, including the RDA, AI, and UL.

The Balanced Diet and Nutrient Density

One of the major concepts advanced by nutritionists over the years to teach proper nutrition is that of the balanced diet, stressing variety and moderation. To help us obtain the nutrients that we need, guides to food selection have been developed, establishing various food groups with key nutrients, and in more recent years focusing on the concept of nutrient density.

What is a balanced diet?

As noted previously, the human body needs more than 40 different nutrients to function properly. The concept of the balanced diet is that by eating a wide variety of foods in moderation you will obtain all the nutrients you need to support growth and development of all tissues, regulate metabolic processes, and provide adequate energy for proper weight control (see figure 2.2). You should obtain the RDA or AI for all essential nutrients and adequate food energy to achieve a healthy body weight.

Although everyone's diet requires the essential nutrients and adequate energy, the proportions differ at different stages of the life cycle. The infant has needs differing from those of his grandfather, and the pregnant or lactating woman has needs differing from those of her adolescent daughter. There also are differences between the needs of males and females, particularly in regard to the iron content of the diet. Moreover, individual variations in lifestyle may impose different nutrient requirements. A long-distance runner in training for a marathon has some distinct nutritional needs compared to a sedentary colleague. The individual trying to lose weight needs to balance Calorie losses with nutrient adequacy. The diabetic individual needs strict nutritional counseling for a balanced diet. Thus, there are a number of different conditions that may influence nutrient needs and the concept of a balanced diet.

The food supply in the United States is extremely varied, and most individuals who consume a wide variety of foods do receive an adequate supply of nutrients. However, there appears to be some concern that many Americans are not receiving optimal nutrition because they consume excessive amounts of highly processed foods. This may be true, as improper food processing may lead to depletion of key nutrients and the addition of high-Calorie and low-nutrient ingredients, such as fat and sugar. More than half of the Calories that the average American eats are derived from fat and sugar.

An unbalanced diet is due not to the unavailability of proper foods but rather to our choice of foods. To improve our nutritional habits we need to learn to select our foods more wisely.

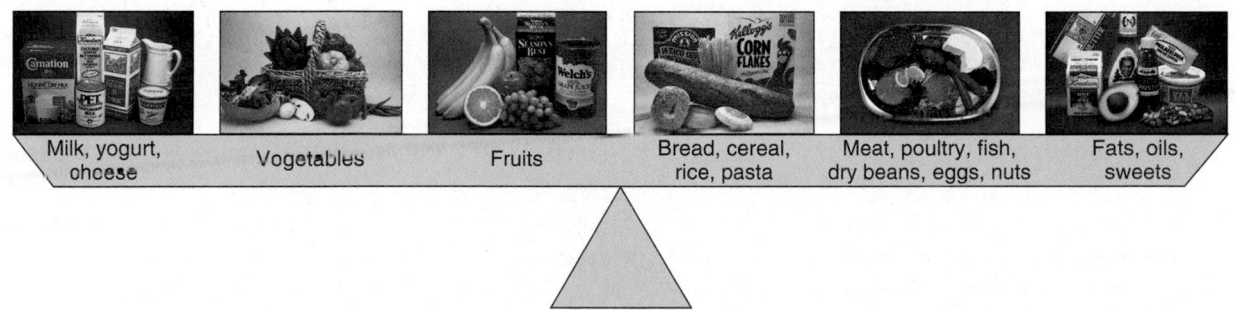

FIGURE 2.2 The key to sound nutrition is a balanced diet that is high in nutrients and low in Calories. For balance, select a wide variety of foods from among and within the food groups in the MyPlate food guide or the Exchange Lists (Appendix E).

What foods should I eat to obtain the nutrients I need?

Although the RDA, AI, and AMDR provide us with information relative to the nutrients we need, they don't guide us in appropriate food selection. Thus, over the years a number of different educational approaches have been used to convey the concept of a balanced diet to help individuals select foods that will provide sufficient amounts of all essential nutrients. In essence, foods with similar nutrient content were grouped into categories.

In the past, foods were grouped into the Basic Seven or the Basic Four Food Groups, but today there is some consensus that six general categories of foods may be used to represent the grouping of various nutrients. Although different terminology may be used with various food guides, the six categories are: (1) dairy, (2) protein foods, (3) grains, (4) vegetables, (5) fruits, and (6) oils and empty Calories. Table 2.3 lists some of the major nutrients found in each of these six food categories.

One concept of balance focuses on the macronutrients, from which we derive our food energy. Although a RDA for protein had previously been established, the National Academy of Sciences has since released DRI for carbohydrate, fat, and protein as a guide to provide adequate energy but also to help minimize the risk of chronic disease. For adults, the AMDR should be composed of approximately 45–65 percent of carbohydrate, 20–35 percent of fat, and 10–35 percent of protein. Similar percentages are recommended for children, except that younger children need a slightly higher percentage of fat. Carbohydrates are found primarily in the Grains group, the vegetable category, and the fruit category, but also in beans and sweets listed in other categories. Protein and fats are both found primarily in the Protein foods group and the Dairy group while solid fats and added sugars are major components of the Oils and empty Calories group.

Two contemporary food guides using a six-level classification system are the MyPlate and the Food Exchange System.

What is the MyPlate Food Guide?

The most recent government food guide designed to provide sound nutritional advice for daily food selection is MyPlate (figure 2.3), developed by the United States Department of Agriculture (USDA). The USDA originally published guidance on healthy eating in the early 1900s. In the 1940s, the Basic Seven food guide program was published, which was changed to the Four Food Groups program in 1956. The 1979 Hassle-Free daily food guide featured the basic four food groups, but also suggested moderate intake of a fifth group consisting of fats, sweets, and alcohol. In 1984, the Food Wheel was published, which featured the five groups that formed the basis of the Food Guide Pyramid. The Food Guide Pyramid existed from 1992 to 2011. In addition to the food groups included, the food guide pyramid graphically illustrated how variety, moderation, and proportion were important for healthy eating. The pyramid evolved into the MyPyramid Food Guidance System in 2005, which was based on the 2005 Dietary Guidelines for Americans and included physical activity and the slogan "steps to a healthier you." MyPyramid featured an interactive website which allowed consumers to personalize their nutritional and physical activity programs. MyPlate represents the 2010 Dietary Guidelines for Americans. Health Canada has developed a similar program, Eating Well with Canada's Food Guide, as have many other countries. MyPlate replaces the Food Guide Pyramid program formerly found on MyPyramid.gov.

http://www.choosemyplate.gov/ Use to access the MyPlate food guide.
http://health.gov/dietaryguidelines/ Use to access the full documentation of the development of the 2010 Dietary Guidelines for Americans.

MyPlate helps people focus on healthy behaviors and includes messages such as: enjoy your food, but eat less; avoid oversized portions; make half of your plate fruits and vegetables; switch to fat-free or low-fat (1%) milk; make at least half of your grains whole grains; compare sodium in foods like soup, bread, and frozen meals– and choose foods with lower numbers; and drink water instead of sugary drinks.

The features of the ChooseMyPlate website can be found under the menus on the top and bottom of the page on your computer screen. These features include sections to educate about nutrition basics, information for specific audiences, and resources for health professionals. By selecting Food Groups, one can access information about the five groups: grains, vegetables, fruits,

TABLE 2.3 Major nutrients found in the five food groups and the oils and empty Calories categories described in the MyPlate food guide

Dairy group	Protein foods group	Grains group	Vegetable group	Fruit group	Oils and empty Calories*
Calcium	Protein	B Vitamins	Vitamin A (carotene)	Vitamin A (carotene)	Vitamin A
Protein	B vitamins	Iron	Vitamin C	Vitamin C	Vitamin D
Riboflavin	Iron	Fiber	Iron	Fiber	Vitamin E
Vitamins A, D	Zinc		Fiber		

*Mainly contains Calories. Fat-soluble vitamins found in some foods.

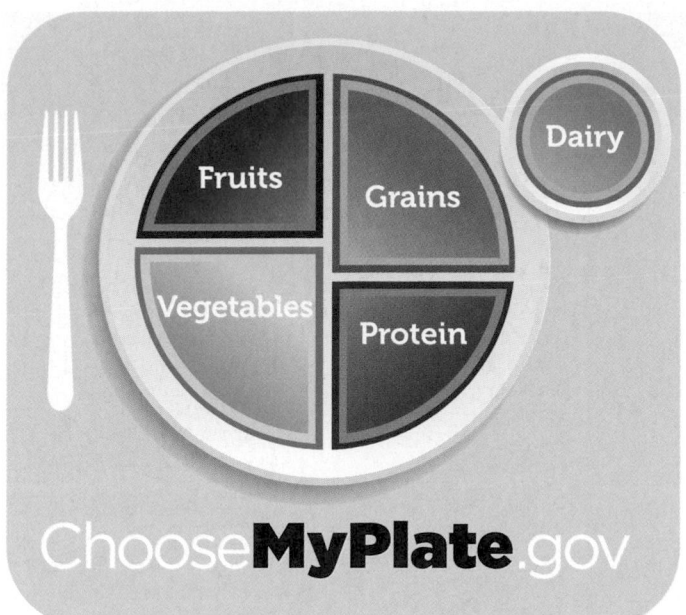

FIGURE 2.3 The new food guide for the *2010 Dietary Guidelines for Americans* is MyPlate. The guide consists of five food groups, plus oils and empty Calories, and offers tips on how to balance Calories, which foods to increase in the diet, and which foods to reduce. Physical activity is an important part of the MyPlate program. Personalized diet and physical activity programs are available through the ChooseMyPlate.gov Website.

Source: U.S. Department of Agriculture, U.S. Department of Health and Human Services.

dairy, proteins, and the additional related topics on oils and empty calories. Each food group features a brief tip, such as "make at least half your grains whole," "or go lean with protein," which encourages a healthy eating behavior. Upon selection of any of the food groups, a detailed web page that includes suggested food choices and access to a digital food gallery appears. The Ten Tips Nutrition Education Series is a collection of printable handouts consisting of ten practical tips for each of fourteen different areas of nutrition, including: Got Your Dairy Today?; Healthy Eating for Vegetarians; Salt and Sodium; and many more. The new Super-Tracker feature offers programs to: help identify personal recommendations for dietary intake and physical activity; create daily food plans; track food intake and physical activity; compare personal dietary intake and physical activity with the 2010 Dietary Guidelines for Americans and the 2008 Physical Activity Guidelines for Americans; develop customized to achieve personal goals; and monitor and measure progress. Advice for specific populations such as pregnant or breastfeeding women, preschoolers, kids, and those attempting to lose weight is also available. A complementary program can be found at www.myfoodapedia.gov. The MyFood-a-pedia program is a convenient searchable web-based database that can be used to find the Calories of a food, the food group, and to compare the Calorie content of two foods.

MyPlate is designed to be simple, yet motivational, with the intent to help individuals make healthier lifestyle choices relative to diet and exercise. Serving sizes for each food group are presented in table 2.4, while key points for healthful eating and physical activity are presented in figure 2.4. One of the key points of MyPlate is to make changes in your diet and physical activity levels gradually, or in small steps one at a time. A list of 120 small steps to improve your diet and physical activity is presented in appendix H.

The beauty of the new MyPlate, as the name implies, is its design to individualize dietary recommendations. Here is what you can do when you access the MyPlate Website.

- You are asked to input your age, gender, and activity level. You will be provided with one of 12 dietary patterns, ranging from 1,000 to 3,200 Calories, based on your individual nutrition needs.
- You can develop an individualized food plan of the types and amount of foods to suit your dietary preferences and daily caloric needs, including dietary plans for a healthier body weight.
- You can print a personalized pyramid to use as a guide for one day or a week, and a worksheet to help you track your progress and choose goals for tomorrow and the future. An example of a 7-day meal plan for 2,000 Calories is presented in appendix I.
- You may use *SuperTracker* and other tools to provide a detailed assessment and analysis of your current eating and physical activity habits, which may be compared to the 2010 Dietary Guidelines for Americans and the 2008 Physical Activity Guidelines for Americans.

TABLE 2.4 Serving sizes for the MyPlate food guide

MyPlate food group	Serving size
Dairy	1 cup of milk or yogurt 1 1/2 ounces natural cheese 2 ounces of processed cheese
Protein	1 ounce of cooked lean meat, poultry, or fish 1/4 cup of cooked dry beans 1 egg 1 tablespoon peanut butter
Grains	1 slice of bread 1 ounce of ready-to-eat cereal 1/2 cup of cooked cereal, rice, or pasta
Vegetable	1 cup of raw, leafy vegetables 1/2 cup of other vegetables, cooked or chopped raw 1 cup vegetable juice
Fruit	1 medium apple, banana, or orange 1 cup of chopped, cooked, or canned fruit 1 cup of fruit juice 1/2 cup dried fruit
Oils (Not an official food group)	1 teaspoon

GRAINS Make half your grains whole	VEGETABLES Vary your veggies	FRUITS Focus on fruits	DAIRY Get your calcium-rich foods	PROTEIN Go lean with protein
Eat at least 3 oz. of whole-grain cereals, breads, crackers, rice, or pasta every day 1 oz. is about 1 slice of bread, about 1 cup of breakfast cereal, or ½ cup of cooked rice, cereal, or pasta	Eat more dark-green veggies like broccoli, spinach, and other dark leafy greens Eat more orange vegetables like carrots and sweet potatoes Eat more dry beans and peas like pinto beans, kidney beans, and lentils	Eat a variety of fruit Choose fresh, frozen, canned, or dried fruit Go easy on fruit juices	Go low-fat or fat-free when you choose milk, yogurt, and other milk products If you don't or can't consume milk, choose lactose-free products or other calcium sources such as fortified foods and beverages	Choose low-fat or lean meats and poultry Bake it, broil it, or grill it Vary your protein routine — choose more fish, beans, peas, nuts, and seeds

For a 2,000-Calorie diet, you need the amounts below from each food group. To find the amounts that are right for you, go to ChooseMyPlate.gov.

Eat 6 oz. every day	Eat 2½ cups every day	Eat 2 cups every day	Get 3 cups every day; for kids aged 2 to 8, it's 2	Eat 5½ oz. every day

Find your balance between food and physical activity
- Be sure to stay within your daily Calorie needs.
- Be physically active for at least 30 minutes most days of the week.
- About 60 minutes a day of physical activity may be needed to prevent weight gain.
- For sustaining weight loss, at least 60 to 90 minutes a day of physical activity may be required.
- Children and teenagers should be physically active for 60 minutes every day, or most days.

Know the limits on fats, sugars, and salt (sodium)
- Make most of your fat sources from fish, nuts, and vegetable oils.
- Limit solid fats like butter, stick margarine, shortening, and lard, as well as foods that contain these.
- Check the Nutrition Facts label to keep saturated fats, *trans* fats, and sodium low.
- Choose food and beverages low in added sugars. Added sugars contribute Calories with few, if any, nutrients.

Source: United States Department of Agriculture; ChooseMyPlate.gov

FIGURE 2.4 MyPlate provides guidelines for healthful eating and physical activity.

- You may use *SuperTracker* to track your diet and physical activity history for up to one year.
- You may obtain detailed information about each food group and physical activity. For example, for each food group information is provided relative to the foods in that group, and appropriate serving size (accompanied by a food photo gallery to illustrate serving sizes), associated nutrients, and health benefits.
- You may obtain information for special populations, such as pregnant women, children ages 6 to 11, overweight children and adults, and the elderly. For kids, computer games are designed to promote healthy eating and daily exercise as a means of preventing childhood obesity.
- If you are a health professional, you may access materials for educational purposes.

Although the MyPlate figure representing the new dietary guidelines provides a very broad overview of a healthy diet, the Website contains an impressive amount of very specific useful information. You may also find some helpful information in *The Pocket Idiot's Guide to the New Food Pyramids* by Ward.

www.ChooseMyPlate.gov Provides an impressive amount of valuable information regarding diet and exercise, personalized for you with the *SuperTracker* program.

www.healthcanada.org Click on Food and Nutrition to access *EatingWell with Canada's Food Guide.*

What is the food exchange system?

A food guide similar to MyPlate is the **Food Exchange System**, a grouping of foods developed by the American Dietetic Association, American Diabetes Association, and other professional and governmental health organizations. Foods in each of the six exchanges contain similar amounts of Calories, carbohydrate, fat, and protein. As with the MyPlate food guide, eating a wide variety of foods from the various food exchanges will help guarantee that you receive the RDA for essential nutrients. The basic content of the six primary food exchanges is presented in table 2.5. There are several differences between the food groups in MyPlate and the Food Exchange Lists. First, the milk exchange list has three levels based on fat content. Second, cheese is found in the meat and meat substitutes exchange list. Third, the meat and meat substitutes exchange list has four levels based on fat content. Fourth, the starch exchange list includes starchy vegetables. Fifth, nuts and seeds are found in the fat exchange list. A detailed list of common foods in the various exchanges may be found in appendix E. The Food Exchange System was developed for diabetics and for weight control. Because it may be an effective means to judge the caloric content of foods during a weight management program, it will be covered in greater detail in chapter 11.

TABLE 2.5 Carbohydrate, fat, protein, and Calories in the six food exchanges (typical serving sizes)

Food exchange	Carbohydrate	Fat	Protein	Calories
Milk (1 cup)				
Skim/very low fat	12	0–3	8	90
Low fat	12	5	8	120
Whole	12	8	8	150
Meat and meat substitutes (1 ounce)				
Very lean*	0	0–1	7	35
Lean	0	3	7	55
Medium fat	0	5	7	75
High fat	0	8	7	100
Starch (1 ounce; 1/2 cup)	15	0–1	3	80
Fruit (1 medium; 1/2 cup)	15	0	0	60
Vegetable (1/2 cup)	5	0	2	25
Fat (1 teaspoon)	0	5	0	45

Carbohydrate, fat, and protein in grams (g)
  1 g carbohydrate = 4 Calories
      1 g fat = 9 Calories
     1 g protein = 4 Calories

*Legumes (beans) are meat substitutes, but per ounce have more carbohydrate (~7 grams) and less protein (~2 grams) than very lean meat, fish, or poultry.

What is the key-nutrient concept for obtaining a balanced diet?

As already noted, humans require many diverse nutrients, including 20 amino acids, 13 vitamins, and more than 15 minerals. To plan our daily diet to include all of these nutrients would be mind-boggling, so simplified approaches to diet planning have been developed.

The nutritional composition of foods varies tremendously. If you wish, you may evaluate the nutrient content of your favorite foods on the MyPlate Website, or for a more detailed evaluation go to the USDA Website.

http://www.nal.usda.gov/fnic/foodcomp/search Provides a detailed analysis of the nutrient content, over 60 individual nutrients, of various foods.

This site analyzes for nearly 120 nutrients and food components. If you examine a food-composition table, you will quickly see that no two foods are exactly alike in nutrient composition. However, certain foods are similar enough in nutrient content to be grouped accordingly. This fact is the basis for approaching nutrition education by way of the MyPlate food guide and the Food Exchange Lists. In essence, foods are grouped or listed according to approximate caloric content and nutrients in which they are rich.

Eight nutrients are central to human nutrition: protein, thiamin, riboflavin, niacin, vitamins A and C, iron, and calcium (figure 2.5). When found naturally in plant and animal sources, these nutrients are usually accompanied by other essential nutrients. The central theme of the **key-nutrient concept** is simply that if these eight key nutrients are adequate in your diet, you will probably receive an ample supply of *all* nutrients essential to humans. It is important to

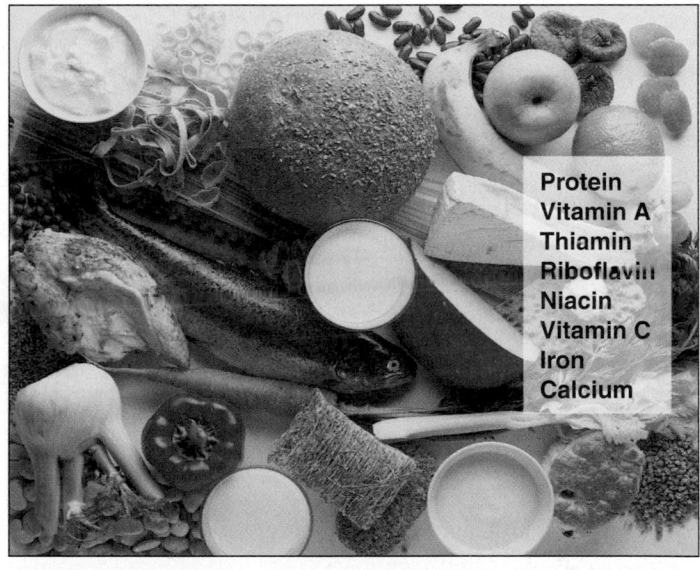

Protein
Vitamin A
Thiamin
Riboflavin
Niacin
Vitamin C
Iron
Calcium

FIGURE 2.5 The key-nutrient concept. Obtaining the RDA or AI for these eight key nutrients from a balanced diet of wholesome, natural foods among the six food exchanges will most likely support your daily needs for all other essential nutrients.

note that for the key-nutrient concept to work, you must obtain the nutrients from a wide variety of minimally processed whole foods. For example, highly processed foods to which some vitamins have been added will not contain all of the trace elements, such as chromium, that were removed during processing.

Table 2.6 presents the eight key nutrients and some significant plant and animal sources. You can see that the food groups and

TABLE 2.6 Eight key nutrients and significant food sources from plants and animals

Nutrient	RDA or AI		Plant source	Animal source	Food group/ Food exchange
	M	F			
Protein	58 g	46 g	Dried beans and peas, nuts	Meat, poultry, fish, cheese, milk	Meat, milk
Vitamin A	0.9 mg	0.7 mg	Dark-green leafy vegetables, orange-yellow vegetables, margarine	Butter, fortified milk, liver	Vegetable, fat, meat
Vitamin C	90 mg	75 mg	Citrus fruits, broccoli, potatoes, strawberries, tomatoes, cabbage, dark-green leafy vegetables	Liver	Fruit, vegetable
Thiamin (vitamin B_1)	1.2 mg	1.1 mg	Breads, cereals, pasta, nuts	Pork, ham	Grain (starch), meat
Riboflavin (vitamin B_2)	1.3 mg	1.1 mg	Breads, cereals, pasta	Milk, cheese, liver	Grain (starch), milk
Niacin	16 mg	14 mg	Breads, cereals, pasta, nuts	Meat, fish, poultry	Grain (starch), meat
Iron	8 mg	18 mg	Dried peas and beans, spinach, asparagus, dried fruits	Meat, liver	Meat, grain (starch)
Calcium	1,000 mg	1,000 mg	Turnip greens, okra, broccoli, spinach, kale	Milk, cheese, sardines, salmon	Milk, meat (fish), vegetable

Recommended Dietary Allowance (RDA) or Adequate Intake (AI) for males (M) and females (F) age 19–50. See inside of text cover for other age groups.

food exchanges can be a useful guide to securing these eight key nutrients. Keep in mind, however, that there is some variation in the proportion of the nutrients, not only between the food groups but also within each food group. For example, the grain food group does contain some protein, but it is not as good a source as the meat or milk group. Within the fruit group, oranges are an excellent source of vitamin C, but peaches are not, although peaches are high in vitamin A. If you select a wide range of foods within each group, the nutrient intake should be balanced over time. Table 2.7 presents a daily diet based upon the food exchanges. An example of a low-Calorie diet plan based upon the food exchanges is presented in chapter 11, together with methods for planning a diet based upon a specific number of Calories.

What is the concept of nutrient density?

As mentioned before, the nutrient content of foods varies considerably, and the differences between food groups are more distinct than the differences between foods in the same group. **Nutrient density** is an important concept relative to the proportions of essential nutrients such as protein, vitamins, and minerals that are found in specific foods. In essence, a food with high nutrient density possesses a significant amount of a specific nutrient or nutrients per serving compared to its caloric content. We refer to these as *quality Calories*.

Let's look at an extreme example between two different food groups. Consider the nutrient differences between six ounces of

baked yellowfin tuna (meat and meat substitute exchange) and six strips of fried bacon (fat exchange), each containing about 220 Calories. The tuna fish would provide a young adult female with 100 percent of her requirement for two key nutrients (protein and niacin) along with substantial amounts of several other vitamins, and minerals, but very little fat. The bacon would contain less than 25 percent of the protein requirement and about 10 percent of the niacin requirement, with greater amounts of total and saturated fat. Hence, the tuna fish has greater nutrient density and considerably greater nutritional value. Another example is presented in figure 2.6, which compares the nutrient density of milk and sweetened cola.

Let's also look at a comparison of two foods within the same group, the meat and meat substitute exchange. Consider the following nutritional data for three ounces of tuna fish and three ounces of clams:

	Calories	Protein	Iron
3 oz. tuna:	118	24 g	0.8 mg
3 oz. clams:	126	22 g	24 mg

The protein density is similar in the two foods. However, clams contain more than 30 times the amount of iron per serving. Both foods are excellent sources of protein for the amount of Calories consumed, and although tuna fish is also a good source of iron, clams are a much superior source. These examples illustrate the need to consume a wide variety of foods

TABLE 2.7   Example of a daily menu based on the food exchanges

Exchange	Food selections	Exchange	Food selections
Breakfast		*Dinner*	
Meat	Canadian bacon	Meat substitute	Baked beans
Starch	English muffin, whole wheat	Starch	Rice or pasta
Milk	Skim milk		Bagel
Fruit	Orange juice	Milk	Yogurt
Fat	Low-fat margarine, *trans* fat free	Fruit	Sliced peaches (in yogurt)
		Vegetable	Mixed salad
Lunch		Fat	Low-fat salad dressing
Meat	Tuna fish (water pack)	*Snacks*	
Starch	Whole wheat bread		
Milk	Skim milk	Fruit	Banana
Fruit	Apple		
Vegetable	Lettuce and tomato		
Fat	Low-fat mayonnaise		

Note: This table presents some common examples of foods within each of the six food exchanges. As discussed in the text, however, you should select food wisely among exchanges and within each exchange. For example, to avoid excessive amounts of Calories, cholesterol, and saturated fats, you should select skim milk, lean meats such as skinless turkey and chicken, water-packed tuna fish, low-fat yogurt, and low-fat, soft tub margarine.

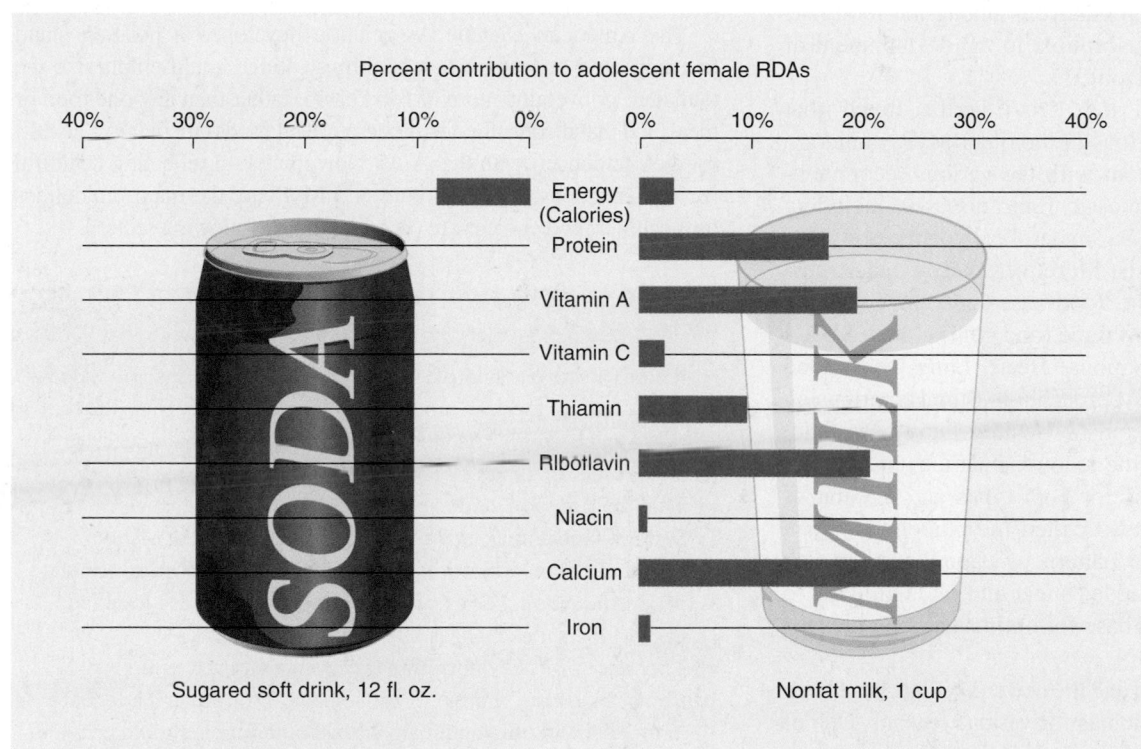

Sugared soft drink, 12 fl. oz.   Nonfat milk, 1 cup

FIGURE 2.6
Comparison of the nutrient density of a sugared soft drink with that of nonfat milk. Both contribute fluid to the diet. However, choosing a glass of nonfat milk makes a significantly greater contribution to nutrient intake in comparison with a sugared soft drink. An easy way to determine nutrient density is to see how many of the nutrient bars in the graph are longer than the Energy (Calories) bar. The soft drink has no longer nutrient bars. Nonfat milk has longer nutrient bars for protein, vitamin A, thiamin, riboflavin, and calcium. Including many nutrient-dense foods in your diet aids in meeting nutrient needs.

among food groups and within each food group to satisfy your nutrient needs.

Several groups offer tools to help increase dietary nutrient density. Yale University's Griffin Prevention Research Center developed an Overall Nutritional Quality Index (ONQI), which rates individual foods on a scale from 1 to 100 based on nutrient content and effects on health concerns. For example, broccoli scores 100 while soda scores 1. This ONQI will serve as the basis for the NuVal™ Nutritional Scoring System to rate foods in supermarkets.

The Nutrient Rich Foods Coalition is a group of researchers, health professionals, communications experts, and 21 agricultural commodity organizations that represent the five basic food groups. This coalition has created a Website to help people increase the nutrient density of their diets. The Website includes handouts on how to make smart choices when dining out, a nutrient-rich shopping checklist, a portion size guide, a nutrient-rich recipe database, and advice on how to shop to help achieve the goals of the USDA's MyPlate.

Will use of the MyPlate food guide or the food exchange system guarantee me optimal nutrition?

If you use the key-nutrient and nutrient density concepts, MyPlate or the Food Exchange System may be an effective means to obtain optimal nutrition and help sustain a healthful body weight. However, although the MyPlate Food Guide and the Food Exchange System represent a significant improvement over previous food guides to help ensure proper nutrition, both have some flaws if foods are not selected carefully. For example, the Food Exchange System does provide some classification for high-fat and low-fat foods in the milk and meat exchanges, but individuals who predominantly choose the high-fat and high-sugar foods from among the food lists may be more susceptible to the development of chronic health problems.

Krebs-Smith and Kris-Etherton noted that the recommendations in the older MyPyramid are remarkably consistent with the various recommendations to control most chronic diseases, including diabetes, heart disease and stroke, hypertension, cancer, and osteoporosis. Moreover, Reedy and Krebs-Smith compared the food-based recommendations and nutrient values of three food guides: the USDA's MyPyramid; the National Heart, Lung, and Blood Institute's Dietary Approaches to Stop Hypertension Eating Plan, and Harvard University's Healthy Eating Pyramid. In essence, they concluded that the recommendations are similar regarding almost all food groups for both types and amount of foods people should eat. They also called the guidelines *future proof*, suggesting that the basic pattern of eating nutrient-rich foods and limited calories from added sugar and fat is unlikely to change even though the research base for optimal eating practices continues to evolve.

Nevertheless, both MyPyramid and the newer MyPlate have been criticized by some health professionals for various reasons. One of the main criticisms is MyPyramid by itself lacked clarity because it did not indicate what specific foods may be more healthful and which foods may be less healthful. Another criticism indicates the basic diet plan does not use height and weight to help determine caloric requirement. Still another is that you need to be computer literate and have access to a computer with an Internet connection to access the Website. These, as well as others, may be legitimate criticisms, but are not insurmountable. Although neither the MyPyramid nor the MyPlate figure by itself indicates which foods are healthful or unhealthful, the accompanying guidelines do. For example, the seven key guidelines presented in figure 2.4 provide individuals with suggestions for selecting healthier foods and limiting less healthful foods. More detailed information concerning healthful food selection is presented on the Website. Although the basic diet plan does not use your height and weight to calculate caloric needs, the *SuperTracker* Daily Food Plan program does. Those without Internet access may find assistance available in local libraries.

Prior to the development of the MyPyramid and MyPlate food guidelines, the previous Food Guide Pyramid received considerable criticism, so much so that other, more healthful models were proposed, such as the Mediteranean Food Guide Pyramid, the California Cuisine Food Pyramid, the Harvard Pyramid, and the Vegetarian Food Guide Pyramid. Basically, all proposed healthy modifications to the former Food Guide Pyramid attempt to reduce the consumption of or modify the type of fat, to increase the consumption of whole-grain products, and to increase the consumption of plant products, particularly beans and other legumes, fruits, and vegetables.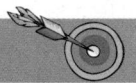

The American Dietetic Association developed a position stand focusing on the message that healthful eating should emphasize the total diet, or overall pattern of food eaten, rather than any one food or meal, and that if consumed in moderation all foods can fit into a healthful diet. In concert with this ADA viewpoint, and reflecting healthful recommendations in MyPyramid and MyPlate, the major guidelines for healthier food choices are presented in the following section.

Key Concepts

▶ If most healthy individuals in a given population consume wholesome, natural foods in amounts adequate to meet their RDA, there will be very little likelihood of nutritional inadequacy or impairment of health.

▶ The MyPlate food guide and the related Food Exchange System—meat, milk, starch, fruit, vegetable, and fat—should be viewed as an educational approach to help individuals obtain proper nutrition. Foods of similar nutrient value are found in each of the six exchanges.

▶ There are eight key nutrients (protein, vitamin A, thiamin, riboflavin, niacin, vitamin C, calcium, and iron) that, if adequate in the diet and obtained from wholesome foods, should provide an ample supply of all nutrients essential to human nutrition.

▶ Some foods contain a greater proportion of these key essential nutrients than other foods and thus have a greater nutrient density or nutritional value.

Check for Yourself

▶ Using the record of all the food you consumed in one day, as recommended in chapter 1, try to categorize the food you have eaten by the Food Exchange System.

Healthful Dietary Guidelines

In the past most morbidity and mortality in industrialized nations were caused by nutrient-deficiency diseases and infectious diseases, but advances in nutritional and medical science have almost eliminated most of the adverse health consequences associated with these diseases. Today, most morbidity and mortality are associated with various chronic diseases (e.g., coronary heart disease, stroke, cancer, diabetes, osteoporosis, obesity), and most dietary guidelines for healthful nutrition are targeted to prevent these chronic diseases.

Nutrition scientists are using both epidemiological and experimental research in attempts to determine what types of diet, specific foods, and specific nutrients or food constituents may either cause or prevent the development of chronic diseases. Such research, coupled with the application of nutrigenomics, may provide each of us with individualized diets for optimal health.

What is the basis underlying the development of healthful dietary guidelines?

In general, healthful dietary guidelines are based on appropriate research. Over the years, epidemiologists have attempted to determine the relationship between diet and the development of chronic diseases. In early research, the focus was simply on the overall diet and its relationship to disease, such as comparing the typical American diet to the Mediterranean (Greece, Italy, Spain) or Japanese diet. If a significant relationship was found between the diets of two nations, say more heart disease among Americans compared to those consuming the Mediterranean diet, scientists then attempted to determine what specific foods, particularly which macronutrients (carbohydrate, fat, and protein) in those foods, may have been related to either an increased or decreased risk for heart disease. In more recent years, scientists have been investigating the roles of specific nutrients or food constituents and their potential to prevent or deter chronic diseases.

Based on the evaluation of current research findings, nutritional scientists believe that the development of most chronic diseases may be associated with either deficiencies or excesses of various nutrients or food constituents in the diet. As mentioned previously, most Americans eat more food than they need and eat less of the food they need more.

In general, many Americans eat too many Calories, consume too much fat, saturated fat, cholesterol, refined sugars and starches, and salt and sodium, and drink too much alcohol. Such dietary practices may predispose one to several chronic diseases, including obesity, heart disease, hypertension, and cancer.

Conversely, possibly because they rely more on highly processed foods, many Americans do not consume a diet rich in whole grain products, legumes, fruits, and vegetables, foods that are rich in dietary fiber and other healthful nutrients such as antioxidant vitamins. Some may not obtain adequate amounts of calcium and iron. These dietary practices may lead to such chronic diseases as cancer, osteoporosis, and anemia.

To help prevent chronic diseases, over the years numerous governmental and professional health organizations have developed general dietary guidelines for good health. Some of these guidelines have been criticized, possibly because they were not based on the best science, as recently noted in the book *Good Calories, Bad Calories: Challenging the Conventional Wisdom on Diet, Weight Control, and Disease* by Gary Taubes. Most of the early research relating diet to disease was epidemiological in nature, which may have led to some erroneous dietary recommendations. However, experimental studies involving randomized controlled trials (RCTs) have predominated in recent years and, as noted by Woolf, rigorous procedures involving evidence-based approaches are currently used to develop dietary guidelines to promote health. For example, a recent RCT by Appel and others provided some evidence that modifying the type of carbohydrate, fat, and protein intake, referred to as the OmniHeart diet, could have favorable effects on several risk factors for heart disease.

Although there is no absolute proof that dietary changes will enhance the health status of every member of the population, scientists involved in the development of healthful dietary guidelines believe that they are *prudent* recommendations for most individuals and are based on the available scientific evidence.

> www.omniheart.org   Provides general and specific tips to improve the quality of your diet.
>
> www.hsph.harvard.edu/nutritionsource   Excellent Website for nutrition information from the Harvard School of Public Health.

What are the recommended dietary guidelines for reducing the risk of chronic disease?

These prudent dietary recommendations represent a synthesis of various recent reports from governmental, educational, and professional health organizations, including the following:

- American Cancer Society
- American Diabetes Association
- American Dietetic Association
- American Heart Association
- American Institute of Cancer Research
- Harvard School of Public Health
- United States Department of Agriculture
- United States Department of Health and Human Services

These recommendations are also in accord with *Dietary Guidelines for Americans,* 2010. The guidelines are not considered to be static, and may be modified somewhat as we gain more knowledge through research. In particular, healthful dietary recommendations may be individualized in the future when the full impact of nutrigenomics is realized.

Taken together, these recommendations may be helpful in preventing most chronic diseases, including cardiovascular diseases and cancer. The rationale as to how these dozen healthful dietary recommendations may promote good health is presented in later chapters where appropriate. These guidelines do, however, come with several caveats.

Remember, diet is only one factor that may influence the development of chronic diseases. As noted by the American

Heart Association Nutrition Committee, other positive lifestyle behaviors, such as exercise and avoiding tobacco use, are also important.

Most dietary guidelines have been developed for Americans over age 2, but some organizations, such as the American Heart Association, have developed separate dietary guidelines for children. Children and adolescents need energy to support growth and development, so it is important that adequate Calories be provided if dietary fat is restricted. Several of the guidelines presented in this section have special implications for children.

Although research shows that some foods, such as fruits and vegetables, may be protective against the development of chronic diseases, it is the total diet that is important. The benefits that may accrue from adhering to only a few healthful eating recommendations may be negated if most dietary guidelines are ignored. You can maximize your health benefits by adopting as many of these healthful dietary guidelines as possible. In general, your diet should focus on *good* carbohydrates, *good* fats, and *good* protein, some of which are highlighted in table 2.8.

1. *Balance the food you eat with physical activity to maintain or achieve a healthy body weight.* Consume only moderate food portions. Be physically active every day. Preventing obesity helps to reduce the risk of numerous chronic diseases, such as heart disease and cancer. To avoid becoming overweight, you should consume only as many Calories as you expend daily. Methods of regulating your body weight are presented in detail in chapter 11. An appropriate exercise program and adherence to the concept of nutrient density, which includes a number of the following recommendations, could serve as the basis for a sound weight-control program.

2. *Eat a nutritionally adequate diet consisting of a wide variety of nutrient-rich foods.* Build a healthy base. Eating a wide variety of natural foods from within (and among) the MyPlate food groups or the Food Exchange Lists will assure you of obtaining a balanced and adequate intake of all essential nutrients. Stress foods that are nutrient dense, particularly those that are rich in the key nutrients.

TABLE 2.8 Examples of healthy, or so-called *good* carbohydrates, *good* fats, and *good* proteins that should constitute the majority of the daily caloric intake.

Good carbohydrates	Good fats	Good proteins
Whole wheat or grain	Plant oils	Very lean meat,
Bread	Olive oil	fish, poultry
Cereal	Canola oil	Egg whites or
Rice	Unsalted nuts	substitutes
Pasta	and seeds	Legumes, beans
Fruits	Pecans, walnuts,	Vegetables
Vegetables	almonds	Meat substitutes
	Fish and seafood oil	Unsalted nuts
	Avocados and olives	and seeds
		Pecans, walnuts,
		almonds

However, keep the concept of variety in perspective. Research has shown that the more food choices we have, the more likely we are to eat more. Our supermarket society, with more than 50,000 food products in the typical store, provides us with so many choices that it is very easy to overeat and become overweight. Thus, although consuming a wide variety of foods is a good strategy to get the nutrients we need, we must keep in mind the first point, to maintain or achieve a healthy body weight. An excellent book by Marion Nestle, a renowned professor of nutrition at New York University, entitled *What to Eat: An Aisle-to-Aisle Guide to Savvy Food Choices and Good Eating* provides some excellent advice about supermarket shopping.

3. *Choose a diet moderate in total fat, but low in saturated and trans fats and cholesterol.* There is no specific requirement for fat in the diet. However, a need exists for essential fatty acids (linoleic and alpha-linolenic fatty acids) and vitamins that are components of fat. Since almost all foods contain some fat, sufficient amounts of the essential fatty acids and related vitamins are found in the average diet. Even on a vegetarian diet of fruits, vegetables, legumes, and grain products, about 5 to 10 percent of the Calories are derived from fat, thus supplying enough of these essential nutrients. The following are some healthful recommendations for daily fat and cholesterol intake:

   • 20–35 percent of Calories from fat, which is consistent with the AMDR
   • 10 percent or less of Calories from saturated fat
   • Less than 1 percent of Calories from *trans* fat
   • 300 milligrams or less of cholesterol

However, some health groups specifically recommend lower amounts. The Consumers Union suggests that females with a personal or family history of breast cancer cut back on fat to 15 percent. The American Heart Association suggests limiting saturated fat to less than 7 percent of Calories.

The following practical suggestions will help you meet the recommended dietary goal.

   a. Choose plant oils or other healthy fats. In general, most dietary fat should come from sources of monounsaturated and polyunsaturated fatty acids, such as fish, nuts, seeds, and vegetable oils, particularly olive and canola oil.
   b. Eat less meat with a high-fat content. Avoid hot dogs, luncheon meats, sausage, and bacon. Trim off excess fat before cooking. Eat only limited amounts of meat, mostly lean red meat and white meat, such as turkey and chicken, which have less fat. Remove the skin from poultry. Eat no more than 3–6 ounces of animal meat per day.
   c. Eat more fish. Many fish, such as sardines, salmon, tuna, and mackerel, are rich in omega-3 fatty acids. White fish, such as flounder, is very low in fat Calories. However, as noted in chapter 5, children and some women should avoid fish that may be polluted with mercury.
   d. Eat only several eggs per week. One egg yolk contains about 220–250 milligrams of cholesterol, close to the limit

of 300 milligrams per day. Egg whites have no cholesterol and are an excellent source of high-quality protein. You may use commercially prepared egg substitutes, particularly those that are low in fat.

e. Eat fewer dairy products that are high in fat. Switch from whole milk to low-fat or skim milk. Eat other dairy products made from skim or nonfat milk, such as yogurt and cottage cheese. Most cheeses, except low-fat cottage cheese, are high in fat and Calories, but some fat-free cheeses are now available.

f. Eat less butter, which is high in saturated fats, by substituting soft margarine made from liquid oils that are monounsaturated or polyunsaturated, such as corn oil. Avoid hard margarine made from hydrogenated or partially hydrogenated oils that produce *trans* fatty acids, which basically are metabolized like saturated fats. Eat butter and margarine sparingly. Some fat-free and other healthier margarines are also available.

g. Eat fewer commercially prepared baked goods made with eggs and saturated or hydrogenated fats. Many of these foods may also contain significant amounts of *trans* fatty acids.

h. Limit your consumption of fast foods. Although fast-food chains generally serve grade A foods, many of their products are high in fat. The average fast-food sandwich contains approximately 50 percent of its Calories in fat. Appendix F provides a breakdown of the fat Calories and milligrams of cholesterol in products served by popular fast-food restaurants. Some fast-food restaurants do serve nutrient-dense foods. Wise choices, such as baked fish, grilled skinless chicken, lean meat, baked potatoes, and salads, can provide healthy nutrition. But, avoid high-fat sauces. For example, the mayonnaise serving on a Burger King TENDERGRILL® chicken sandwich adds 110 Calories, or 12 grams of fat, which accounts for 21 percent of the total Calories of the sandwich.

i. Use food labels to help you select foods low in total fat, saturated fat, *trans* fat, and fat Calories, all of which are listed on the food label for most products. In the ingredients list, look for the terms presented in figure 2.7, all of which contain fat.

j. Broil, bake, or microwave your foods. Limit frying. If you must use oil in your cooking or food preparation, try to use monounsaturated oils such as olive, canola, or peanut oil. For other health reasons, as noted later, avoid charring foods when grilling or broiling.

4. *Choose a plant-rich diet with plenty of fruits and vegetables, whole-grain products, and legumes, foods that are rich in complex carbohydrates, phytochemicals, and fiber* (see figure 2.8). In general, about 45–65 percent or more of your daily Calories should come from carbohydrates, about 35–55 percent from complex carbohydrates, and the other 10 percent from simple, naturally occurring carbohydrates. To accomplish this, you need to eat more whole-grain breads, cereal, rice, and pasta; more legumes such as beans and peas;

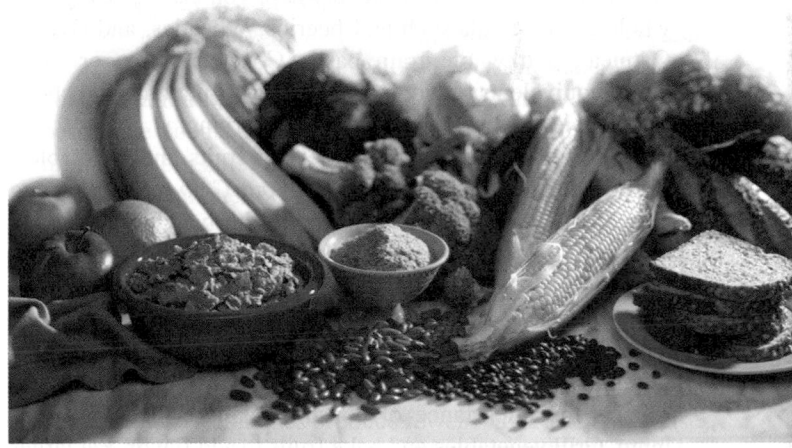

FIGURE 2.8 Include in your diet foods high in plant starch and fiber. Eat more fruits, vegetables, and whole-grain products.

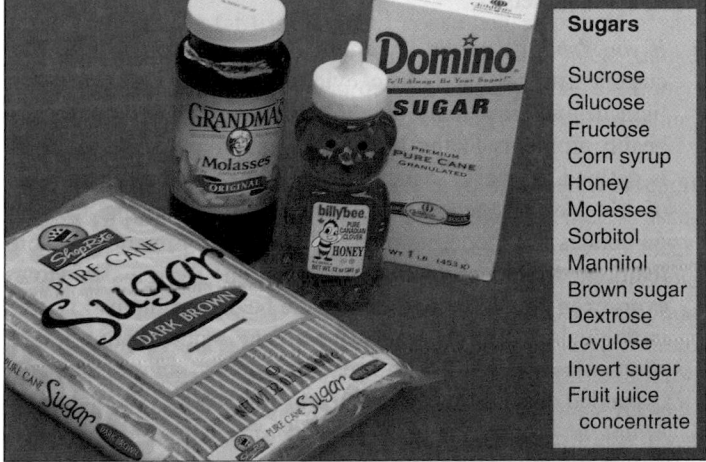

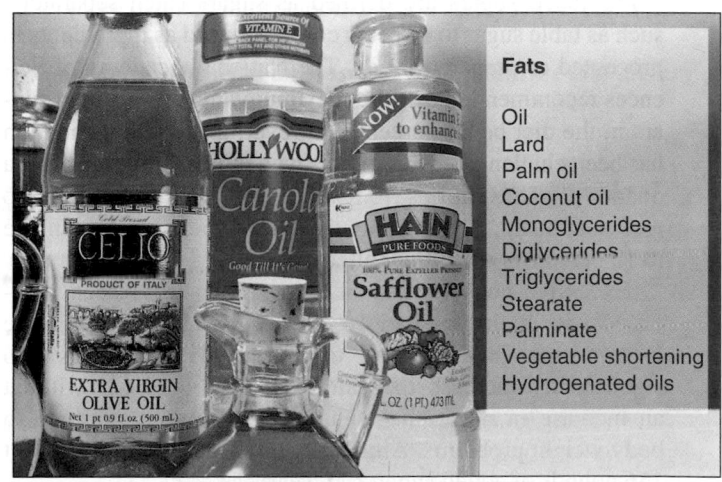

FIGURE 2.7 Nutritional labeling as a guide to sugar and fat in processed foods. Refined sugar and fats may appear in processed foods in a variety of forms. Check for these terms on nutrition labels.

TABLE 2.10 Daily food guidelines for a vegetarian (vegan) diet

Grains and starchy vegetables

Servings: 8–11 or more daily

Note: Use whole wheat or other whole grains. Products made of oats, rice, rye, corn, and whole wheat are good sources of protein, B vitamins, and iron, more so if they are fortified products. Fortified cereals may provide adequate vitamin B_{12}.

Food examples:

Barley	Macaroni, enriched
Bran flakes	Oatmeal
Bread, whole wheat	Potatoes
Buckwheat pancakes	Rice, brown
Corn	Rye wafers
Corn muffins	Spaghetti, enriched
Farina, cooked	Sweet potatoes
Fortified cereals	Wheat, shredded

Legumes

Servings: 3 or more daily

Note: Good sources of protein, niacin, iron, and Calories.

Food examples:

Great northern beans	Soybeans
Navy beans	Tofu
Red kidney beans	Split peas
Pinto beans	Chickpeas
Lima beans	Lentils

Nuts and seeds

Servings: 3 or more daily

Note: Good sources of Calories, protein, niacin, and iron. May be excellent snack foods.

Food examples:

Almonds	Pecans
Brazil nuts	Walnuts
Cashew nuts	Sesame seeds
Peanuts	Sunflower seeds
Peanut butter	Pumpkin seeds

Fruits

Servings: 4 or more daily

Note: Fruits are generally good sources of vitamins and minerals. At least one fruit should come from the citrus group and one from the high-iron group. Select fruits of different colors.

Food examples:

Regular	Citrus	High iron
Apples	Oranges	Dried apricots
Bananas	Orange juice	Dried prunes
Grapes	Grapefruit	Dried dates
Peaches	Grapefruit juice	Dried figs
Pears	Lemon juice	Dried peaches
Pineapple		Raisins
		Prune juice

Vegetables

Servings: 4–6 or more daily

Note: Vegetables are good sources of vitamins and minerals. At least one serving should come from the dark-green or deep-yellow vegetables. Select other color vegetables as well.

Food examples:

Regular	Dark-green or deep-yellow
Artichokes	Beet greens
Asparagus	Broccoli
Beans, green	Carrots
Cabbage	Collard greens
Cauliflower	Lettuce
Cucumbers	Spinach
Eggplant	Squash
Radishes	
Tomatoes	

Milk products (calcium-rich foods)

Servings: 3 or more daily

Note: Good source of protein and calcium, if fortified.

Food examples:

Non-dairy soy milk
Non-dairy rice milk

Sweets and vegetable oils may be added to increase caloric intake.

---

should have no problem getting the required amounts. A vegan will need a source of B_{12}, such as fortified soy milk, fortified breakfast cereal, or a B_{12} supplement. If not exposed to sunlight, vegans will also need dietary supplements of vitamin D, which is not found in plant foods.

Minerals Mineral deficiencies of iron, calcium, and zinc may occur. During the digestion process, some plant foods form compounds known as phytates and oxalates that can bind these minerals so that they cannot be absorbed into the body. Avoidance of unleavened bread helps reduce this effect, as does thorough cooking of legumes such as beans. In general, research has revealed that a balanced intake of grains, legumes, and vegetables will not significantly impair mineral absorption. Foods rich in iron, calcium, and zinc should also be included in the vegetarian diet.

Iron-rich plant foods include nuts, beans, split peas, dates, prune juice, raisins, green leafy vegetables, and many iron-enriched grain products. Special attention should be given to dietary practices that promote absorption of iron and zinc from plant foods. For example, consuming foods rich in vitamin C will increase the absorption of dietary iron from plant sources. Semivegetarians may obtain high-quality iron in fish and poultry.

Calcium-rich plant foods include many green vegetables like broccoli, cabbage, mustard greens, and spinach. Dairy products added to the diet supply very significant amounts of calcium, as do calcium-fortified soy milk or fruit juices. According to the American Dietetic Association, the calcium intake of some vegan vegetarians is below recommended levels, while calcium intake in ovolacto vegetarians is similar to that of nonvegetarians. Craig notes that increased bone fracture risk in vegans may be a consequence of low calcium intake.

Zinc-rich plant foods include whole wheat bread, peas, corn, and carrots. Egg yolk and seafood also add substantial zinc to the diet.

Iodine deficiency may occur with strict vegetarian diets, particularly when plant foods grown in iodine-depleted soils are ingested. In such cases, use of iodized salt will prevent iodine deficiency.

Protein　The major concern of the vegetarian is to obtain adequate amounts of the right type of protein, particularly in the case of young children. Generally speaking, consuming enough Calories to maintain an optimal body weight will provide adequate amounts of protein.

As will be noted in chapter 6, proteins are classified as either complete or incomplete. A protein is complete if it contains all of the essential amino acids that the human body cannot manufacture. Animal products generally contain complete proteins, whereas plant proteins are incomplete. However, certain vegetable products may also provide good sources of protein. Grain products such as wheat, rice, and corn, as well as beans (particularly soybeans), peas, and nuts, have a substantial protein content. However, most vegetable products lack one or more essential amino acids in sufficient quantity. They are incomplete proteins and, eaten individually, are generally not adequate for maintaining proper human nutrition. But, if certain plant foods are eaten together, they may supply all the essential amino acids necessary for human nutrition and may be as good as animal protein (see figure 2.9).

The strict vegetarian must receive nutrients from breads and cereals, nuts and seeds, legumes, fruits, and vegetables. To receive a balanced distribution of the essential amino acids, the vegan must eat plant foods that possess **complementary proteins.** In essence, a vegetable product that is low in a particular amino acid is eaten with a food that is high in that same amino acid. For example, grains and cereals, which are low in lysine, are complemented by legumes, which have adequate amounts of lysine. The low level of methionine in the legumes is offset by its high concentration in the grain products. These types of food combinations are practiced throughout the world. Traditionally, many Hispanic peoples have eaten beans and corn; many Asians, soybeans and rice. Through the proper selection of foods that contain complementary proteins, the vegan can get an adequate intake of the essential amino acids. Because all amino acids must be present for tissue formation, a deficiency of one or two essential amino acids will limit the proper development of protein structures in the body.

In their position statement regarding vegetarian diets, the American Dietetic Association and Dietitians of Canada stated that complementary proteins should be consumed over the course of the day. The ADA noted that because endogenous sources of amino acids are available, it is not necessary that complementation of amino acids occur at the same meal.

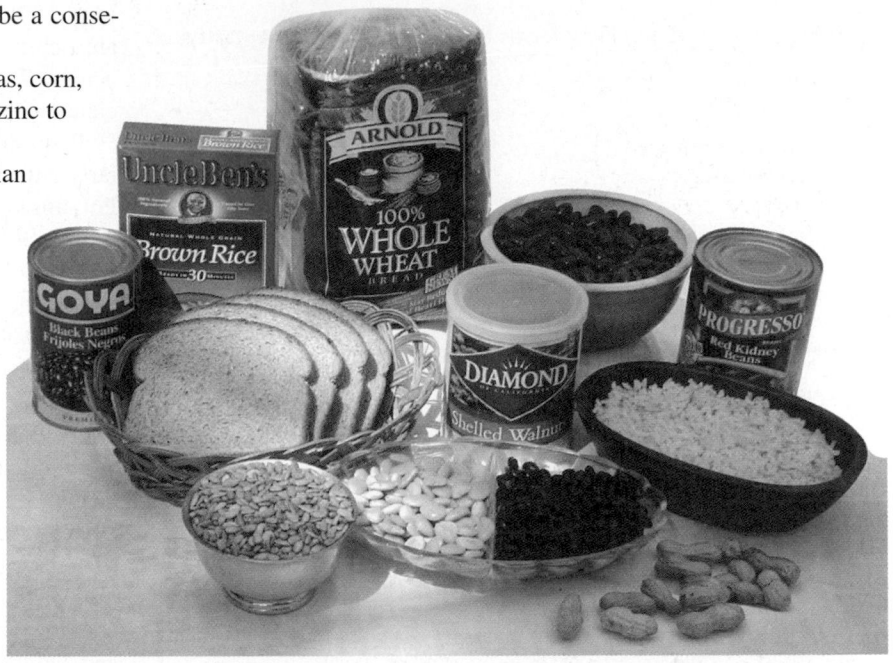

FIGURE 2.9　It is important for the vegetarian to eat protein foods that complement each other (e.g., nuts and bread, rice and beans) so that all the essential amino acids are obtained in the diet.

Table 2.11 provides some examples of food combinations that achieve protein complementarity. Milk is included because it is a common means of enhancing the quality of plant protein for lactovegetarians, but eggs could also be substituted by ovovegetarians where appropriate. The two most common plant foods that vegans combine to achieve protein complementarity are grains and legumes. Grains such as wheat, corn, rice, and oats are combined with legumes such as soybeans, peanuts, navy beans, kidney beans, lima beans, black-eyed peas, and chickpeas.

Is a vegetarian diet more healthful than a nonvegetarian diet?

Numerous epidemiological studies have suggested that a vegetarian diet, when compared to the typical nonvegetarian Western diet, is associated with reduced risk for numerous chronic diseases and health problems, including obesity, hypertension, blood sugar and lipid control, heart disease, stroke, and some types of cancer. For example, Bazzano and others reported that an increased intake of fruits and vegetables was associated with a decreased risk of strokes, cardiovascular disease, and all-cause mortality in nearly 10,000 Americans over a 19-year period. The vegetarian diet is based on nutritional concepts that may reduce health risks, including the following.

Nutrient Density　Vegetarian diets contain substantial amounts of nutrient-dense foods, particularly vegetables. For example, one 54-Calorie cup of cooked broccoli contains the following:

- 4 grams of protein
- 5 grams of dietary fiber
- 10 or more vitamins and minerals
- 170 percent of the Daily Value for vitamin C

TABLE 2.11 Combining foods for protein complementarity

Milk and grains

Pasta with milk or cheese
Rice and milk pudding
Cereal with milk
Macaroni and cheese
Cheese sandwich
Cheese on nachos*

Milk and legumes

Creamed bean soups*
Cheese on refried beans*

Grains and legumes

Rice and bean casserole
Wheat bread and baked beans
Corn tortillas and refried beans*
Pea soup and toast
Peanut-butter sandwich

*Low-fat, low-sodium versions should be selected to minimize excessive saturated fat and sodium intake.

- 50 percent of the Daily Value for vitamin A, as carotenoids
- 42 percent of the Daily Value for folate
- 30 percent of the Daily Value for potassium
- 6 percent of the Daily Value for calcium and iron

Low Fat and Cholesterol The total fat and saturated fat content in a vegetarian diet is usually low because the small amounts of fats found in plant foods are generally polyunsaturated. Plants also do not contain cholesterol; this compound is found only in animal products. These two factors account for the finding that vegetarians generally have lower blood triglycerides and cholesterol than meat eaters, and these lower levels may be important to the prevention of coronary heart disease.

High Fiber Plant foods possess a high content of fiber, which may help reduce levels of serum cholesterol and help in the prevention of heart disease. Diets rich in fiber may also prevent certain disorders in the gastrointestinal tract. Moreover, increased fiber intake may help maintain normal blood glucose levels and a healthy body weight, two factors involved in the prevention of diabetes. More details on the health benefits of fiber are presented in chapter 4.

Low Calorie If the proper foods are selected, the vegetarian diet supplies more than an adequate amount of nutrients and is rather low in caloric content. Plant foods can be high in nutrient density, providing bulk in the diet without the added Calories of fat. Hence, the vegetarian diet can be an effective dietary regimen for losing excess body weight. However, vegetarians who consume dairy products need to select low-fat versions instead of high-fat cheeses and whole milk.

High Vitamin and Phytochemical Content Plant foods are rich in various vitamins, including folic acid. As discussed in chapter 7, diets containing good sources of folic acid may be associated with lower risks of cardiovascular disease.

Plant foods are also rich in antioxidant vitamins, particularly vitamin C and beta-carotene, a precursor to vitamin A. Polyunsaturated plant oils provide substantial amounts of vitamin E. Selenium, an antioxidant mineral, is found in other plant foods.

Other than nutrients, plants also contain numerous **phytochemicals** (plant chemicals), compounds, such as phenols, plant sterols, and terpenes, which are not considered essential nutrients but may still influence various metabolic processes in the body. Collectively, these antioxidant nutrients and phytochemicals are referred to as **nutraceuticals,** parts of food that may provide a medical or health benefit, as suggested in a position stand of the American Dietetic Association on phytochemicals. Table 2.12 provides a list of some antioxidant nutrients and phytochemicals and their common plant sources.

Although the exact mechanisms whereby antioxidant nutrients and phytochemicals may help prevent chronic diseases such as cancer or heart disease have not been identified, several hypotheses are being studied. Potential health benefits of antioxidants and phytochemicals may be related to one or more of their possible roles in human metabolism:

- affect enzyme activity
- detoxify carcinogenic compounds
- block cell receptors for natural hormones
- prevent formation of excess oxygen-free radicals
- alter cell membrane structure and integrity
- suppress DNA and protein synthesis

Some of these actions may favorably affect health, as in the following two examples. Antioxidants, such as carotenoids, may block the oxidation of certain forms of serum cholesterol, reducing their potential to cause atherosclerosis and possible heart disease. Also, phytochemicals known as phytoestrogens may compete with natural forms of estrogen in the body for estrogen receptors in various tissues, blocking estrogen's natural proliferative activity and possibly suppressing cancer development.

Considerable epidemiological research has suggested that foods rich in antioxidants and phytochemicals may possess therapeutic value. Conversely, a few studies have suggested that excess of some phytochemicals may be harmful. For example, Halliwell notes that excess flavonoid intake may be mutagenic or pro-oxidant, generating free radicals. Experimental research in this area is limited. Studies involving supplementation with soy protein, which contains numerous phytochemicals, have reported beneficial health effects. However, Mares-Perlman and others noted that although certain phytochemicals in foods, such as the carotenoids lutein and zeaxanthin, may protect against the development of several chronic diseases, research is needed to evaluate the effect of their consumption independent of other nutrients in fruits and vegetables.

TABLE 2.12 Some antioxidant nutrients and phytochemicals with common food sources

Antioxidant nutrients	Common plant sources
Vitamin C	Citrus fruits
	Potatoes
	Strawberries
Vitamin E	Dark-green leafy vegetables
	Margarine
	Vegetable oils
	Wheat germ
	Whole grains

Phytochemicals	Common plant sources
Allium sulfides	Garlic
	Onions
Anthocyanins	Blueberries
Capsaicin	Hot peppers
Carotenoids	Carrots
Beta-carotene	Dark-green leafy vegetables
Lycopene	Sweet potatoes
Lutein	Tomatoes
Flavonoids	Citrus fruits
Quercetin	Apples
Catechin	Tea
Indoles	Cruciferous vegetables
	Broccoli
	Brussels sprouts
	Cabbage
	Cauliflower
	Kale
Isoflavones	Soybeans
Phytoestrogens	Peanuts
Genistein	Soy milk
Isothiocyanates	Cruciferous vegetables
Sulforaphane	Brocoli
	Brussels sprouts
	Cabbage
	Cauliflower
	Kale
Phenolic acids	Carrots
	Citrus fruits
	Tomatoes
	Whole grains
Polyphenols	Grapes
Resveratrol	Red wines
	Grapes
Saponins	Beans
	Legumes
Terpenes	Cherries
Limonene	Citrus fruits

www.ars-grin.gov/duke/plants.html   Obtain a list of all the vitamins and other phytochemicals found in your favorite food or plant, like strawberries.

Most nutrition scientists indicate that many of these nutrients and phytochemicals share the same food sources, so the protective health effect associated with a plant-rich diet may not be attributed to a single food constituent, but may be due to the collective effect of multiple nutraceuticals. Thus, health professionals currently recommend that consuming natural plant foods, rather than supplements, is the best way to obtain these purported nutraceuticals.

To help ensure that you obtain a wide variety of healthful phytochemicals in your diet, eating foods of many different colors is one strategy recommended by health professionals. Details are provided in several books, including *The Color Code: A Revolutionary Eating Plan for Optimal Health* by Joseph and Nadeau. Fruits and vegetables may contain numerous vitamins and phytochemicals, each of which may have some beneficial health effect. Table 2.13 lists the key colors and some examples of foods found within each color group. In brief, the following highlights one of the main health effects for one food of each color:

Red—Tomatoes and tomato products contain lycopene, which may help prevent prostate cancer.
Blue/purple—Blueberries contain anthocyanins, which may help lower blood pressure and risk of heart disease.
Yellow/orange—Carrots contain carotenoids, which may reduce risk of heart disease.
Green—Broccoli contains sulforaphane, which may help prevent cancer.
White/brown—Onions contain allicin, which may help lower cholesterol and risk of heart disease.

In summary, although a vegetarian diet is more healthful than a typical high-fat diet, it should be emphasized that the nonvegetarian who carefully selects foods from the meat and milk group, including limited amounts of lean red meat, may attain the same health benefits as the vegetarian. The major nutritional difference between a vegetarian and a nonvegetarian diet appears to be the higher content of saturated fats and cholesterol and lower amounts of fruits and vegetables in the latter. Selection of animal products with a low-fat and low-cholesterol content helps avoid one of these problems and also assures consumption of very high-quality proteins. In two reviews, Mann and Truswell noted that lean meat may not be as detrimental to health as once assumed, although adverse health effects may be associated with high-fat meats and unsafe methods of preparation. The National Research Council, in *Diet and Health: Implications for Reducing Chronic Disease Risk,* did not recommend against eating meat, but advised eating leaner meat in smaller and fewer portions than is customary in the United States.

How can I become a vegetarian?

People become vegetarians for a number of reasons, including weight control, improved health, religion, love for all animals, protecting the environment, and taste preferences. Choosing to adopt a vegetarian diet is up to the individual and represents a significant change in dietary habits. Anyone desiring to make an abrupt change to a vegetarian diet should do some serious reading on the matter beforehand. Once you have done some reading

TABLE 2.13 Food colors of various fruits and vegetables

Red	Yellow/orange	Green	Blue/purple	White/brown
Cherries	Apricots	Artichokes	Blackberries	Bananas
Cranberries	Cantaloupe	Avocados	Blueberries	Cauliflower
Raspberries	Corn	Collards	Dried plums	Garlic
Red cabbage	Carrots	Cucumbers	Eggplant	Jicama
Red grapes	Lemons	Green grapes	Plums	Onions
Strawberries	Mangos	Kiwi fruit	Purple cabbage	Pears
Tomatoes	Oranges	Lettuce	Purple grapes	Potatoes
Watermelon	Pineapple	Spinach	Raisins	Turnips

on vegetarianism, there may be several ways to gradually phase yourself into a vegetarian diet.

- You may become a part-time vegetarian simply by eating less red meat. For example, you may have several meatless meals each day by skipping the ham or sausage at breakfast and having a big salad for lunch. Eventually, you may move toward having several meatless days per week, possibly incorporating vegetarian "meats" such as meatless chicken, meatless smoked turkey, or tasty veggie burgers in your meals.
- You may become a semivegetarian, substituting white meat such as chicken and turkey breast, with its generally lower fat content, for red meat. You may become a pescovegetarian, eating fish as your main animal food.
- You may wish to become an ovolactovegetarian, eating eggs and dairy products. These excellent sources of complete protein can be blended with many vegetable products or eaten separately.
- You may use the above methods as forerunners to a strict vegan diet, gradually phasing out animal products altogether as you learn to select and prepare vegetable foods to obtain protein complementarity and adequate intake of essential nutrients.

The following simple suggestions may help you incorporate more fruits, vegetables, and whole grains in your diet.

- Keep 100-percent fruit juices available, but limit those which provide few nutrients, such as apple and white grape juice.
- Buy only bread products that list whole wheat as the first ingredient on the food label.
- Keep a variety of raw fruits handy for snacks, such as bananas, grapes, apples, and oranges.
- Keep a bowl of raw vegetables in the refrigerator, such as small carrots, cut-up celery, broccoli, cauliflower, and radishes, along with a tasty dip, for handy snacks.
- Use frozen vegetables for quick stir-fry meals.
- Add vegetables, such as onions, tomatoes, lettuce, spinach, and peppers, to your sandwiches.
- Load up on fresh vegetables at the supermarket salad bar, putting meal-sized portions in small containers to take for lunch during the week.

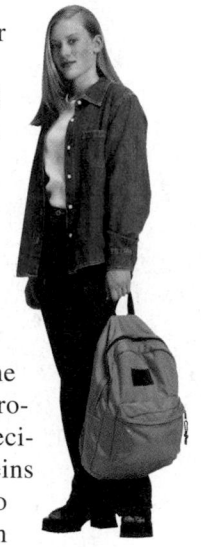

- Add cut-up vegetables to canned beans, soups, or omelets to increase their nutrient value.
- Use your microwave to cook sweet potatoes and baked potatoes, and to steam vegetables with a little water.
- Bake fruits for dessert.

The scope of this book does not permit a discussion of food preparation. A number of excellent cookbooks for vegetarian meals are available at local bookstores, the titles of which may be obtained from a local dietitian or local branch of the American Heart Association. These cookbooks provide the vegetarian with a variety of appetizing recipes that not only incorporate complementary proteins with a balance of vitamins and minerals, but also make vegetarianism a gastronomical delight. An excellent example is the *Vegetarian Times Complete Cookbook.*

www.thevegetariansite.com

www.vegan.com   Learn how to become a vegetarian with useful guidelines.

Will a vegetarian diet affect physical performance potential?

As noted previously, a diet that follows vegetarian principles is considered to be more healthful than the typical American diet today. But will such a diet have any significant impact upon physical performance? In a review of nutritional considerations for vegetarian athletes, Barr and Rideout noted that well-controlled long-term studies assessing the effects of vegetarian diets on athletes have not been conducted. Nevertheless, based on their review and the reviews of Venderley and Campbell and Fuhrman and Ferrari, the following observations can be made.

- Well-planned, appropriately supplemented vegetarian diets appear to effectively support athletic performance. Including fortified foods, such as soy milk and whole-grain cereals, may help provide adequate amounts of some vitamins and minerals that may be low in vegetarian diets.

- Plant and animal protein sources appear to provide equivalent support to athletic training and performance provided protein intakes are adequate to meet needs for total nitrogen and the essential amino acids.
- Vegetarian athletes (particularly women) are at increased risk for non-anemic iron deficiency, which may limit endurance performance.
- Vegetarian diets are low in creatine, and thus vegetarian athletes may have lower muscle creatine concentrations than meat-eating athletes. Lower creatine levels may impair very high intensity exercise. Details are presented in chapter 6.
- Vegetarian diets may be high in healthful carbohydrates and be effective for weight control, which could be to the advantage of some athletes, particularly endurance runners. However, if used improperly as a strategy for weight control, vegetarian diets could lead to eating disorders and impaired performance and health, a topic discussed in chapter 10.

Some world-class athletes have been vegetarians, and on occasion their diets have been cited as a reason for their success. On the other hand, there are a far greater number of world-class athletes who eat a balanced diet including animal products. Both types of diet may supply the nutrients necessary for the physically active individual if foods are selected properly.

However, as noted previously, if you want to shift toward a vegetarian diet, you would need to do some careful reading beforehand and then initiate the process gradually. During the process, you should listen to your body—a common phrase among many athletes today. If you are active, how do you feel during your workouts? Do you have more or less stamina? Are you gaining or losing weight? Is your physical performance getting better or worse? The answers to these questions, together with other body reactions, may offer you some feedback as to whether the dietary change is beneficial.

Remember, there is nothing magical about a vegetarian diet that will increase your physical performance capacity. It can be a healthful way to obtain the nutrients your physically active body needs, but so too is a well-balanced diet containing animal products.

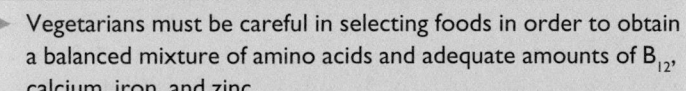

Key Concepts

▶ Vegetarians must be careful in selecting foods in order to obtain a balanced mixture of amino acids and adequate amounts of B_{12}, calcium, iron, and zinc.

▶ Vegetarian diets are based on healthful nutritional concepts that may help reduce chronic disease, particularly cardiovascular disease, but nonvegetarian diets may confer similar health and performance benefits if limited animal foods are carefully chosen.

Check for Yourself

▶ If you are not a vegetarian, eat a vegetarian diet for a day or two to see if it may fit into your lifestyle.

Consumer Nutrition— Food Labels and Health Claims

Guidelines for a healthful diet will not be effective unless people change their behavior to buy and eat healthier foods. A model often used to explain the development of a set of behaviors involves a sequence of (1) acquisition of knowledge, (2) formation of an attitude or set of values, and (3) development of a particular behavior. In this sequence, knowledge is the first step that may enhance the development of proper health behaviors. Knowing how to interpret food labels may guide you in developing a nutritious, safe, and healthful diet.

What nutrition information do food labels provide?

Food manufacturers view labels as a device for persuading you to buy their product instead of a competitor's product. Just walk down the cereal aisle next time you visit the supermarket and notice the bewildering number of choices. As manufactured food products multiplied over the years, and as competition for your food dollar intensified, food companies began to manipulate their labels to enhance sales. Unfortunately, many of these practices were deceptive, and the consumer had a difficult time determining the nutritional quality of many processed foods. Thus, Congress passed a law designed to establish a set of standards to help Americans base their food choices on sound nutritional information.

This set of standards resulted in **nutritional labeling,** whereby major nutrients found in a food product must be listed on the label. It is not the total solution to the problem of poor food selection existing among many Americans, but combined with an educational program to increase nutritional awareness, it may effectively improve the nutritional health of our nation.

Initial food labeling legislation was passed in 1973, but it contained numerous flaws. Because of pressure from a variety of consumer interest groups, a major overhaul of the nutritional labeling program was signed into law as the Nutrition Labeling and Education Act in 1990, and it was in full effect in 1994. Under this law, nutrition labeling is mandatory for almost all foods regulated by the Food and Drug Administration (FDA). However, there are some exceptions. Food produced by very small businesses; food served in restaurants, hospital cafeterias, and airplanes; ready-to-eat food prepared primarily on site; and several other categories are exempt from these regulations. Other modifications may be used for children under the age of 2, and others for children under the age of 4. Additionally, providing nutrition information is currently voluntary for many raw foods such as fresh fruits, vegetables, meat, and fish, but may become mandatory in the future.

The food label illustrated in figure 2.10 is called *Nutrition Facts,* and it is designed to provide information on the nutrients

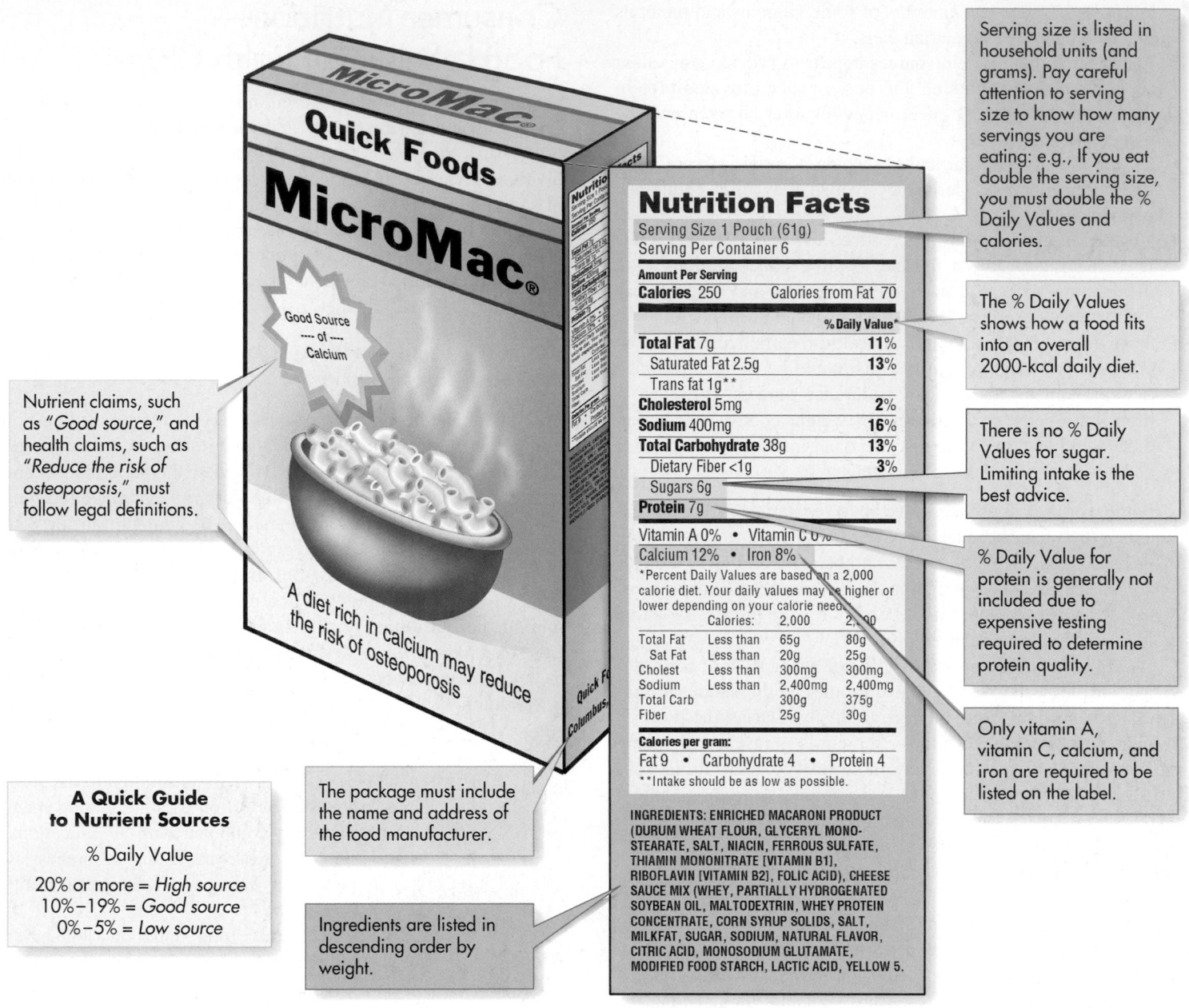

Nutrition Facts

Serving Size 1 Pouch (61g)
Serving Per Container 6

Amount Per Serving

Calories 250   Calories from Fat 70

	% Daily Value*
Total Fat 7g	**11**%
Saturated Fat 2.5g	**13**%
Trans fat 1g**	
Cholesterol 5mg	**2**%
Sodium 400mg	**16**%
Total Carbohydrate 38g	**13**%
Dietary Fiber <1g	**3**%
Sugars 6g	
Protein 7g	

Vitamin A 0% • Vitamin C 0%
Calcium 12% • Iron 8%

*Percent Daily Values are based on a 2,000 calorie diet. Your daily values may be higher or lower depending on your calorie needs:

		Calories:	2,000	2,500
Total Fat	Less than		65g	80g
Sat Fat	Less than		20g	25g
Cholest	Less than		300mg	300mg
Sodium	Less than		2,400mg	2,400mg
Total Carb			300g	375g
Fiber			25g	30g

Calories per gram:
Fat 9 • Carbohydrate 4 • Protein 4

**Intake should be as low as possible.

INGREDIENTS: ENRICHED MACARONI PRODUCT (DURUM WHEAT FLOUR, GLYCERYL MONO-STEARATE, SALT, NIACIN, FERROUS SULFATE, THIAMIN MONONITRATE [VITAMIN B1], RIBOFLAVIN [VITAMIN B2], FOLIC ACID), CHEESE SAUCE MIX (WHEY, PARTIALLY HYDROGENATED SOYBEAN OIL, MALTODEXTRIN, WHEY PROTEIN CONCENTRATE, CORN SYRUP SOLIDS, SALT, MILKFAT, SUGAR, SODIUM, NATURAL FLAVOR, CITRIC ACID, MONOSODIUM GLUTAMATE, MODIFIED FOOD STARCH, LACTIC ACID, YELLOW 5.

Quick Foods

MicroMac®

Good Source of Calcium

A diet rich in calcium may reduce the risk of osteoporosis

Serving size is listed in household units (and grams). Pay careful attention to serving size to know how many servings you are eating: e.g., If you eat double the serving size, you must double the % Daily Values and calories.

The % Daily Values shows how a food fits into an overall 2000-kcal daily diet.

There is no % Daily Values for sugar. Limiting intake is the best advice.

% Daily Value for protein is generally not included due to expensive testing required to determine protein quality.

Only vitamin A, vitamin C, calcium, and iron are required to be listed on the label.

Nutrient claims, such as "Good source," and health claims, such as "Reduce the risk of osteoporosis," must follow legal definitions.

A Quick Guide to Nutrient Sources

% Daily Value

20% or more = *High source*
10%–19% = *Good source*
0%–5% = *Low source*

The package must include the name and address of the food manufacturer.

Ingredients are listed in descending order by weight.

FIGURE 2.10 The Nutrition Facts panel on a current food label. This nutrition information is required on virtually all processed food products. The % Daily Value listed on the label is the percentage of the generally accepted amount of a nutrient needed daily that is present in one serving of the product. See text for additional discussion.

that are of major concern for consumers. Food labels must contain the following information:

List of ingredients
    Ingredients will be listed in descending order by weight.
    Serving size
        Serving size has been standardized.
    Servings per container
    Amount per serving of the following:
        Total Calories
            Calories from fat

Total fat
    Saturated fat
    Trans fat
Cholesterol
Sodium
Total carbohydrate
    Dietary fiber
    Sugars
Protein
Vitamin A
Vitamin C

Calcium
Iron

The following are optional:

Calories from saturated fat	Phosphorus
Polyunsaturated fat	Magnesium
Monounsaturated fat	Zinc
Potassium	Selenium
Soluble fiber	Copper
Insoluble fiber	Manganese
Sugar alcohols	Molybdenum
Other carbohydrates	Iodine
Vitamins D, E, K	Potassium
All B vitamins	Chloride

How can I use this information to select a healthier diet?

The **Daily Value (DV),** which is based on dietary standards discussed earlier in this chapter, represents how much of a specific nutrient you should obtain in your daily diet. DVs have been established for macronutrients and micronutrients that may affect our health. In essence, a food label indicates how much of a given nutrient is present in that product, and for some nutrients, what percentage of the DV is provided by one serving.

The DVs cover the macronutrients that are sources of energy, consisting of carbohydrate (including fiber), fat, and protein, as well as cholesterol, sodium, and potassium, which contain no Calories. The DVs for the energy-producing nutrients are based on the number of Calories consumed daily. On the food label, the percent of the DV that a single serving of a food contains is based on a 2,000-Calorie diet, which has been selected because it is believed to have the greatest public health benefit for the nation. However, the DV may be higher or lower depending on your Caloric needs. Values for some of the macronutrients are also provided for a 2,500-Calorie diet on the food label.

The DVs are based on certain minimum and maximum allowances, including the following for a 2,000-Calorie diet:

Total fat: Maximum of 30 percent of Calories, or less than 65 grams.
Saturated fat: Maximum of 10 percent of Calories, or less than 20 grams.
Carbohydrate: Minimum of 60 percent of Calories, or more than 300 grams.
Protein: Based on 10 percent of Calories. Applicable only to adults and children over age 4; 50 grams for a 2,000-Calorie diet.
Fiber: Based on 12.5 grams of fiber per 1,000 Calories.
Cholesterol: Less than 300 milligrams.
Sodium: Less than 2,400 milligrams.

The DVs for vitamins and minerals, based on previously established RDA, are presented in table 2.14. The list includes those whose listing is mandatory and some selected others. Although the RDA for several nutrients has changed with recent DRI updates, the DVs are still based on 1968 standards of the RDA. However, the

TABLE 2.14 DVs for protein, dietary fiber, and some vitamins and minerals on food labels

Mandatory listing	
Protein	56 grams
Vitamin A	5,000 IU; 1 milligram
Vitamin C	60 milligrams
Calcium	1,000 milligrams
Iron	18 milligrams
Dietary Fiber	25 grams

Optional listing	
Thiamin	1.5 milligrams
Riboflavin	1.7 milligrams
Niacin	20 milligrams
Vitamin D	400 IU
Vitamin E	30 IU
Vitamin B_6	2 milligrams
Folic acid	400 micrograms
Vitamin B_{12}	6 micrograms
Zinc	15 milligrams
Copper	2 milligrams
Magnesium	400 milligrams

Food and Drug Administration, along with Health Canada, is collaborating with the Institute of Medicine in the process of revamping current food labels, changing the DV for various nutrients and focusing on caloric content. For example, one proposal is to reduce the DV for iron from 18 to 8 milligrams and another is to develop a DV for Calories and to list caloric content on the front of the label.

Some important points to consider in reading a food label are as follows:

1. The DV for a nutrient represents the percentage contribution one serving of the food makes to the daily diet for that nutrient based on current recommendations for healthful diets. A lower DV is desirable for total fat, saturated fat, cholesterol, and sodium; a DV of 5 percent or less is a good indicator. There is no DV for *trans* fat; only the number of grams is listed, and intake should be as low as possible, preferably 0 grams. A higher DV is desirable for total carbohydrates, dietary fiber, iron, calcium, vitamins A and C, and other vitamins and minerals that may be listed, with 10 percent or more representing a good source.
2. To calculate the percentage of fat Calories in one serving, divide the value for Calories from fat by the total Calories and multiply by 100. For example, if one serving contains 70 Calories from fat and the total number of Calories is 120, the food consists of 58 percent fat Calories (70/120 × 100). It should be noted that this percentage is not the same as the DV percentage for fat, which is based on your total daily diet, not an individual serving of the food product.
3. Related to carbohydrates, sugars include both natural and added sugars. Dietary fiber is the total amount of fiber per serving. Other carbohydrates represent total carbohydrates minus sugars and dietary fiber.

4. Be aware of serving size tricks. A serving size for a cola drink may be 8 ounces (100 Calories), so a 20-ounce bottle of soda is 2.5 servings (250 Calories). However, most people drink it all at one time, thinking it is only one serving and may consume more than twice the Calories as expected. Recommended changes are to provide nutrition information for a single serving as well as for the entire package; so for a 20-ounce bottle of soda, you will get the nutrition breakdown for 8 ounces as well as for the entire 20 ounces.

Labels also must disclose certain ingredients, such as sulfites, certain food dyes, and eight food allergens, so food-sensitive consumers may avoid foods that may cause allergic responses. Others may be added as deemed necessary. Food allergies are discussed later in this chapter.

In the past, many terms used on food labels, such as "lean" and "light," had no definite meaning. However, under the new regulations, most terms used have specific definitions. A summary of these terms is presented in table 2.15. Additionally, new milk labels are based on fat content, expressed as percent or grams of fat, as follows: fat-free, skim, or nonfat milk (0 grams); low-fat or light milk (1% or 2.5 grams); reduced fat milk (2% or 5 grams); and whole milk (3.5% or 8 grams).

In a survey, Rothman and others reported that many Americans, even well-educated individuals with good literacy and math skills, do not know how to interpret food labels. However, other studies have shown that reading food labels carefully helps individuals to limit their fat intake, one of the most significant changes we can make in our diet. Individuals with high blood pressure have also used food labels to reduce their consumption of sodium, a dietary risk factor for some. Take time to learn to read food labels; it's a smart thing to do.

http://www.fda.gov/Food/LabelingNutrition/ConsumerInformation/ ucm114022.htm The FDA provides a program, *Make Your Calories Count,* featuring the animated character *Labelman,* to help people read food labels to plan a healthy diet while balancing caloric intake.

What health claims are allowed on food products?

Food manufacturers want your business. Given the public's growing awareness of the relationship between nutrition and health, many food labels now list various health claims that may entice you to buy that product. And consumers do view a food product as healthier if it carries a health claim.

The FDA permits food manufacturers to make specific health claims on food labels only if the food meets certain minimum standards. These health claims are permitted because the FDA believes there may be significant scientific agreement supporting a relationship between consumption of a specific nutrient and possible prevention of a certain chronic disease. However, there are several requirements, such as not stating the degree of risk reduction, using only terms such as "may" or "might" in reference to reducing health risks, and indicating that other foods may provide similar benefits. Figure 2.11 provides an example.

The FDA ranks health claims for food labels based on the quality of the underlying scientific evidence. In brief, the following system is used:

A—Significant scientific evidence supports the claim.
B—Scientific evidence supports the claim, but the evidence is not conclusive.
C—Some scientific evidence supports the claim, but the evidence is limited and not conclusive.
D—Little scientific evidence supports the claim.

The current FDA-approved model for A-level health claims, or qualified health claims, is presented in table 2.16. The FDA also may approve a "qualified health claim" for food products that evidence suggests, but does not prove, may reduce disease risk. One example is omega-3 fatty acids and reduced risk of coronary heart disease.

www.fda.gov In the search box, type in "Qualified Health Claims" to obtain details on currently approved health claims for food labels. Also, several letters of denial for petitions to obtain an approved qualified health claim are available on the FDA Website. Among the denials for qualified approved health claims are green tea and reduced risk of cardiovascular disease and lycopene and various cancers.

Although food labeling in the United States continues to improve to help us select healthier foods, many still find it is too complex. Some countries, such as Sweden and Great Britain, have a national system that uses traffic light symbols (Red = High; Yellow = Medium; Green = Low) to instantly highlight the contents of less healthy ingredients, such as fat, saturated fat, sugars, and sodium. Consumer groups in the United States have petitioned the FDA to develop a similar national system for supermarkets. The FDA is currently considering major changes to the current Nutrition Facts label, including more realistic serving sizes, an emphasis on Calories, and possibly removing the DV, but has not set any timetable. In the meantime, the FDA has a Website to help consumers use the food label to select healthier foods. Some food companies have already developed healthy food logos for their products, such as Kraft's *Sensible Solution,* that help to identify healthier foods.

www.cfsan.fda.gov/~dms/foodlab.html Consult for a detailed description on how to use the current Nutrition Facts food label to improve your dietary choices.

What are functional foods?

In 1994, the FDA permitted dietary supplement manufacturers to make structure and function claims on their products. Basically, a structure and function claim simply means that the food product may affect body physiology in some way, usually in some way beneficial to health or performance. These claims may not be as authoritative as the FDA-approved claims cited above (such as reducing the risk of heart disease or cancer), but these claims may use such terminology as "helps to maintain healthy cholesterol levels" or "supports your immune system" that the consumer may interpret as

Sugar
- **Sugar free:** less than 0.5 g per serving
- **No added sugar; without added sugar; no sugar added:**
  - No sugars were added during processing or packing, including ingredients that contain sugars (for example, fruit juices, applesauce, or jam).
  - Processing does not increase the sugar content above the amount naturally present in the ingredients. (A functionally insignificant increase in sugars is acceptable for processes used for purposes other than increasing sugar content.)
  - The food that it resembles and for which it substitutes normally contains added sugars.
  - If the food doesn't meet the requirements for a low- or reduced-Calorie food, the product bears a statement that the food is not low Calorie or Calorie reduced and directs consumers' attention to the Nutrition Facts panel for further information on sugars and Calorie content.
- **Reduced sugar:** at least 25% less sugar per serving than reference food

Calories
- **Calorie free:** fewer than 5 kcal per serving
- **Low Calorie:** 40 kcal or less per serving and, if the serving is 30 g or less or 2 tbsp or less, per 50 g of the food
- **Reduced or fewer Calories:** least 25% fewer kcal per serving than reference food

Fiber
- **High fiber:** 5 g or more per serving. (Foods making high-fiber claims must meet the definition for low fat, or the level of total fat must appear next to the high-fiber claim.)
- **Good source of fiber:** 2.5 to 4.9 g per serving
- **More or added fiber:** at least 2.5 g more per serving than reference food

Fat
- **Fat free:** less than 0.5 g of fat per serving
- **Saturated fat free:** less than 0.5 g per serving, and the level of *trans* fatty acids does not exceed 0.5 g per serving
- **Low fat:** 3 g or less per serving and, if the serving is 30 g or less or 2 tbsp or less, per 50 g of the food. 2% milk can no longer be labeled low-fat, as it exceeds 3 g per serving. *Reduced fat* is the term used instead.
- **Low saturated fat:** 1 g or less per serving and not more than 15% of kcal from saturated fatty acids

- **Reduced or less fat:** at least 25% less per serving than reference food
- **Reduced or less saturated fat:** at least 25% less per serving than reference food

Cholesterol
- **Cholesterol free:** less than 2 mg of cholesterol and 2 g or less of saturated fat per serving
- **Low cholesterol:** 20 mg or less cholesterol and 2 g or less of saturated fat per serving and, if the serving is 30 g or less or 2 tbsp or less, per 50 g of the food
- **Reduced or less cholesterol:** at least 25% less cholesterol and 2 g or less of saturated fat per serving than reference food

Sodium
- **Sodium free:** less than 5 mg per serving
- **Very low sodium:** 35 mg or less per serving and, if the serving is 30 g or less or 2 tbsp or less, per 50 g of the food
- **Low sodium:** 140 mg or less per serving and, if the serving is 30 g or less or 2 tbsp or less, per 50 g of the food
- **Light in sodium:** at least 50% less per serving than reference food
- **Reduced or less sodium:** at least 25% less per serving than reference food

Other Terms
- **Fortified or enriched:** Vitamins and/or minerals have been added to the product in amounts in excess of at least 10% of that normally present in the usual product. *Enriched* generally refers to replacing nutrients lost in processing, whereas *fortified* refers to adding nutrients not originally present in the specific food.
- **Healthy:** An individual food that is low fat and low saturated fat and has no more than 360 to 480 mg of sodium or 60 mg of cholesterol per serving can be labeled "healthy" if it provides at least 10% of the Daily Value for vitamin A, vitamin C, protein, calcium, iron, or fiber.
- **Light or lite:** The descriptor *light* or *lite* can mean two things: first, that a nutritionally altered product contains one-third fewer kcal or half the fat of reference food (if the food derives 50% or more of its kcal from fat, the reduction must be 50% of the fat) and, second, that the sodium content of a low-calorie, low-fat food has been reduced by 50%. In addition, "light in sodium" may be used for foods in which the sodium content has been reduced by at least 50%. The term *light* may still be used to describe such prop-

erties as texture and color, as long as the label explains the intent—for example, "light brown sugar" and "light and fluffy."
- **Diet:** A food may be labeled with terms such as *diet, dietetic, artificially sweetened,* or *sweetened with nonnutritive sweetener* only if the claim is not false or misleading. The food can also be labeled *low calorie* or *reduced calorie.*
- **Good source:** *Good source* means that a serving of the food contains 10 to 19% of the Daily Value for a particular nutrient. If 5% or less, it is a **low source.**
- **High:** *High* means that a serving of the food contains 20% or more of the Daily Value for a particular nutrient.
- **Organic:** Federal standards for organic

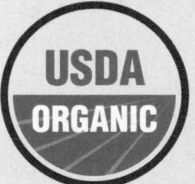

foods allow claims when much of the ingredients do not use chemical fertilizers or pesticides, genetic engineering, sewage sludge, antibiotics, or irradiation in their production. At least 95% of ingredients (by weight) must meet these guidelines to be labeled "organic" on the front of the package. If the front label instead says "made with organic ingredients," only 70% of the ingredients must be organic. For livestock, the animals need to be allowed to graze outdoors and be fed organic feed as well. They also cannot be exposed to large amounts of antibiotics or growth hormones.
- **Natural:** The food must be free of food colors, synthetic flavors, or any other synthetic substance.

Milk
- **Fat-free, skim, or nonfat:** Contains 0 grams of fat
- **Low-fat or light:** Contains 1% or 2.5 grams of fat
- **Reduced fat:** Contains 2% or 5 grams of fat
- **Whole:** Contains 3.5% or 8 grams of fat

The following terms apply only to meat and poultry products regulated by USDA.
- **Extra lean:** less than 5 g of fat, 2 g of saturated fat, and 95 mg of cholesterol per serving (or 100 g of an individual food)
- **Lean:** less than 10 g of fat, 4.5 g of saturated fat, and 95 mg of cholesterol per serving (or 100 g of an individual food)

Many definitions are from FDA's *Dictionary of Terms,* as established in conjunction with the 1990 Nutrition Education and Labeling Act (NELA).

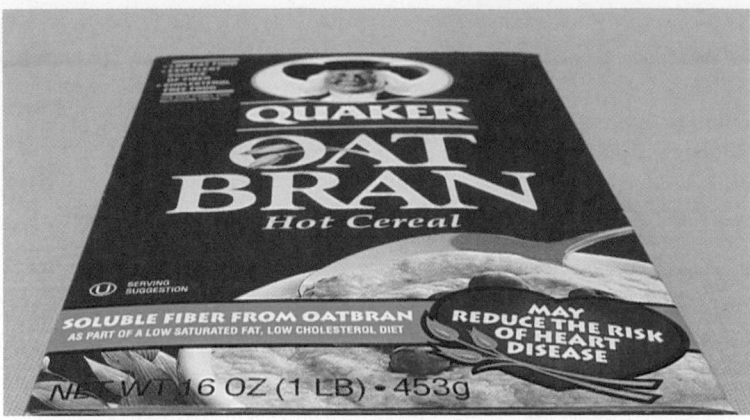

FIGURE 2.11 An example of a Nutrition Fact food label with an approved health claim.

preventing heart disease or cancer. Technically, these health claims must be correct, but they need not have as much supportive scientific evidence, nor do they have to have approval from the FDA.

Dietary supplements sales have skyrocketed in the past 15 years, and the food industry jumped on the bandwagon. In recent years, numerous food manufacturers, including some giants such as Kellogg, Tropicana, and Procter & Gamble, have marketed products that have been referred to as functional foods.

Functional foods are food products designed to provide health benefits beyond basic nutrition, the benefits being attributed mostly to vitamins, minerals, phytochemicals, and herbals. Some refer to them as *medical foods*. Many natural foods have been modified in attempts to make them more healthful. For example, meat animals have been bred for lower fat content and plant fatty acid content has been altered to achieve desired ratios of beneficial fatty acids in the extracted oil. In its position stand, the American Dietetic Association indicated that functional foods, including whole foods and fortified, enriched, or enhanced foods, have a potentially beneficial effect on health when consumed as part of a varied diet on a regular basis. Indeed, some contend that in the

TABLE 2.16 Qualified health claims. FDA-approved model health claims for foods that have significant scientific evidence supporting the claim

Calcium and osteoporosis: Regular exercise and a healthy diet with enough calcium helps teen and young adult white and Asian women maintain good bone health and may reduce their high risk of osteoporosis later in life.

Dietary fat and cancer: Development of cancer depends on many factors. A diet low in total fat may reduce the risk of some cancers.

Dietary saturated fat and cholesterol and risk of coronary heart disease: Development of heart disease depends upon many factors, but its risk may be reduced by diets low in saturated fat and cholesterol and healthy lifestyles.

Dietary sugar alcohols and dental caries: Frequent eating of foods high in sugars and starches as between-meal snacks can promote tooth decay. The sugar alcohol used to sweeten this food may reduce the risk of dental caries.

Fiber-containing grain products, fruits, and vegetables and cancer: Low fat diets rich in fiber-containing grain products, fruits, and vegetables may reduce the risk of some types of cancer, a disease associated with many factors.

Folate and neural-tube defects (spina bifida): Healthful diets with adequate folate may reduce a woman's risk of having a child with a brain or spinal cord birth defect.

Fruits and vegetables and cancer: Low-fat diets rich in fruits and vegetables (foods that are low in fat and may contain dietary fiber, vitamin A, and vitamin C) may reduce the risk of some types of cancer, a disease associated with many factors.

Fruits, vegetables, and grain products that contain fiber, particularly soluble fiber, and risk of coronary heart disease: Diets low in saturated fat and cholesterol and rich in fruits, vegetables, and grain products that contain some types of dietary fiber, particularly soluble fiber, may reduce the risk of heart disease, a disease associated with many factors.

Sodium and hypertension: Diets low in sodium may reduce the risk of high blood pressure, a disease associated with many factors.

Soluble fiber from certain foods and risk of coronary heart disease: Soluble fiber from foods such as oats and barley, as part of a diet low in saturated fat and cholesterol, may reduce the risk of heart disease. A serving of this food supplies 0.75 gram of the soluble fiber from oats necessary per day to have this effect.

Soy protein and risk of coronary heart disease: Diets low in saturated fat and cholesterol that include 25 grams of soy protein a day may reduce the risk of heart disease. One serving of this food provides 8 grams of soy protein.

Plant sterol/stanol esters and risk of coronary heart disease: Foods containing at least 0.65 g per serving of *plant sterol* esters eaten twice a day with meals for a daily total intake of at least 1.3 g (or 1.7 g per serving of *plant stanol* esters for a total daily intake of at least 3.4 g) as part of a diet low in saturated fat and cholesterol may reduce the risk of heart disease. A serving of this food supplies 0.75 gram of vegetable oil sterol (stanol) esters.

Source: U. S. Food and Drug Administration. Health Claims that Meet Significant Scientific Agreement.

future it may be possible to design foods and diets to help regulate gene expression that may enhance health.

Fortification with nutrients or nutraceuticals is a current technique to make functional foods. In a sense, functional foods have been around for nearly a century, as salt was fortified with iodine, and milk was fortified with vitamins A and D, to help prevent nutrient deficiencies. More recently, calcium-fortified juices and multivitamin/mineral-fortified cereals are breakfast mainstays designed, in part, to help us obtain adequate amounts of specific nutrients. Some of these products may be worthwhile, for they may be in accord with the principles underlying FDA approval of food health claims. For example, the Consumers Union notes that calcium-fortified orange juice may be an excellent source of calcium for someone who does not drink milk. Cereals fortified with psyllium may be an excellent source of soluble dietary fiber. On the other hand, a sugar drink with added vitamins is a different story, as it is simply a vitamin pill with added sugar.

Some functional foods are designed to satisfy the criteria for qualified health claims on food labels. Many other products marketed as functional foods are simply dietary supplements in disguise, and use structure and function claims to suggest health benefits. Such products include soups with St. John's wort, snack foods with kava kava, cereals with ginkgo biloba, and energy drinks with caffeine.

In the next section we discuss dietary supplements and health claims. However, in the meantime, remember that fruits, vegetables, whole grains, and other plant foods are the optimal functional foods. Their health benefits have been well established.

Key Concepts

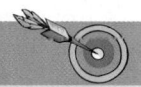

▶ Information provided through nutritional labeling on most food products may serve as a useful guide in finding foods that have a high nutrient density and are healthy choices.

▶ The Daily Value (DV) for a single serving on a food label represents the percentage of a nutrient, such as saturated fat or carbohydrate, that is recommended for an individual who consumes 2,000 Calories daily.

▶ Terms used on food labels, such as fat free, must meet specific standards. In this case, use of *fat free* indicates that a serving of the food contains less than 0.5 grams of fat.

▶ Health claims may be placed on food labels only if they are supported by adequate scientific data and have been approved by the Food and Drug Administration (FDA).

▶ Some functional foods may provide some health benefits, adhering to qualified health claims. Other products marketed as functional foods may use structure and function claims, which do not have the scientific support of qualified health claims.

Check for Yourself

▶ Go to a supermarket and compare food labels for various products. In particular, compare the caloric content of some fat-free products with their non–fat-free counterparts to see the Calorie reduction, if there is any.

Consumer Nutrition—Dietary Supplements and Health

Nutrition scientists indicate that foods, particularly fruits and vegetables, contain numerous nutrients or other food substances that may have pharmaceutical properties when taken in appropriate dosages. The potential health benefits of specific nutrients will be covered in appropriate chapters. The purpose of this section is to provide a broad overview of possible health effects of dietary supplements.

What are dietary supplements?

The dietary supplement industry is a multibillion-dollar business. According to Blendon and colleagues, about 48 percent of adults use dietary supplements. Cohen and others estimate that this is about 64 percent in older adults (65 years of age or older) (figure 2.12). In the United States, the Dietary Supplements Health and Education Act (DSHEA) defines a **dietary supplement** as a food product, added to the total diet, that contains at least one of the following ingredients:

- vitamin
- mineral
- herb or botanical
- amino acid
- metabolite
- constituent

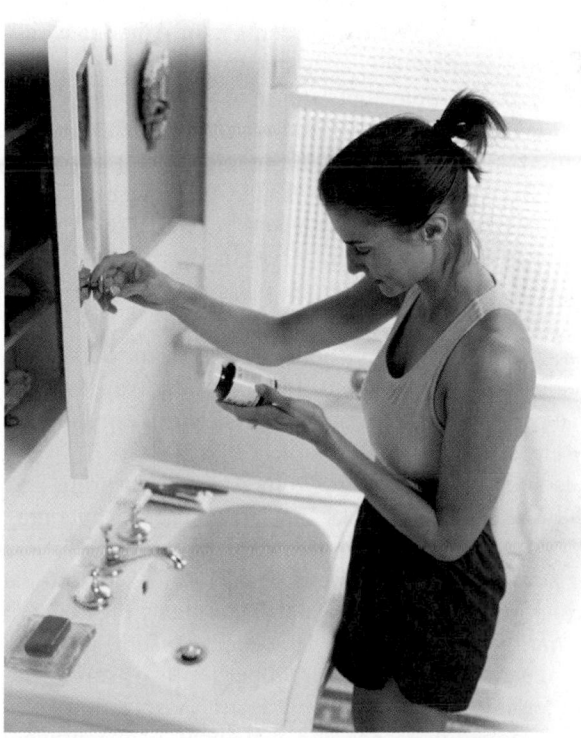

FIGURE 2.12 Dietary supplements are marketed as a means of enhancing both health and physical performance.

- extract
- combination of any of these ingredients

It is important to note that the DSHEA stipulates that a dietary supplement cannot be represented as a conventional food or as the sole item of a meal or diet.

As noted by this definition, dietary supplements may contain essential nutrients such as essential vitamins, minerals, and amino acids, but also other nonessential substances such as ginseng, ginkgo, yohimbe, ma huang, and other herbal products. The technical definition of a supplement is something added, particularly to correct a deficiency. Theoretically then, dietary supplements should be used to correct a deficiency of a specific nutrient, such as vitamin C. However, numerous dietary supplements contain substances other than essential nutrients and are marketed not to correct a deficiency, but rather to increase the total dietary intake of some food or plant substance that allegedly may enhance one's health status. Like foods, dietary supplements must carry labels, or *supplement facts;* an example is presented in figure 7.5.

Will dietary supplements improve my health?

Dietary supplements are usually advertised to the general public as a means to improve some facet of their health, and are usually under governmental regulation. In the United States, dietary supplements are regulated under food law by the Food and Drug Administration, and thus are eligible for FDA-authorized health claims, as discussed previously. Dietary supplement health claims in Canada are governed by Health Canada's Natural Health Products Directorate. In some countries, such as Germany, a medical prescription is needed to obtain some dietary supplements containing strong herbal products. Blendon and others noted that a substantial percentage of Americans regularly take dietary supplements as a part of their routine health regimen. Can dietary supplements improve your health? Possibly, but there are several caveats.

In its position statement on dietary supplements, the American Dietetic Association (ADA) indicated that the best nutritional strategy for promoting health and reducing the risk of chronic disease is to wisely choose a wide variety of foods. Essential nutrients and phytochemicals found in most dietary supplements are readily available for us in fruits, vegetables, legumes, fish, and other healthy foods. However, the ADA also notes that additional vitamins and minerals from supplements can help some people meet their nutritional needs as specified by the Dietary Reference Intakes.

Individuals such as the elderly, women of childbearing age, vegans, and those on weight-loss diets may not be obtaining adequate amounts of various vitamins and minerals. Fairfield and Fletcher note that most people do not consume an optimal amount of vitamins by diet alone. Such individuals may benefit from a daily multivitamin/mineral. However, consumers should be aware of exceeding recommended upper limits of some vitamins and minerals. The American Dietetic Association reinforces this viewpoint in its position statement. Some prudent recommendations for vitamin and mineral supplementation will be presented in chapters 7 and 8.

In general, as shall be noted in chapter 6, individual amino acid supplements may not enhance health if adequate protein is consumed in the diet. However, research is ongoing with several amino acids.

Of the other classes of nonvitamin, nonmineral dietary supplements (herb or botanical, metabolite, constituent, extract, or combinations), numerous products are marketed for their purported health benefits. In a survey of college students by Newberry and others, nearly 50 percent had used such supplements within the past year. Although we have no specific requirement for these substances, as they are not essential for normal physiological function, some may affect physiological functions in the body associated with health benefits. Using a broad interpretation of the FDA health claim regulations for dietary supplements, some supplement companies advertise their supplements as "miracle products" that can produce "magical results" in a short period of time.

The Consumers Union notes that, under current federal law, any dietary supplement can be marketed without advance testing. The only restriction is that the label cannot claim that the product will treat, prevent, or cure a disease. However, as noted previously, the label may make vague claims, referred to as structure/function claims, like "enhances energy" or "supports testosterone production." Unfortunately, as Nesheim notes, for most of these dietary supplements there are few research data to support their claims. Most advertisements are based on theory alone, testimonials or anecdotal information, or on the exaggeration or misinterpretation of research findings relative to the health effects of specific nutrients or other food constituents. Many labels carry a notice stating that *This statement has not been evaluated by the FDA,* a disclaimer regarding the health claim. Moreover, although advertisers may not make unsubstantiated health claims, the 1994 DSHEA stipulates that the burden of proving the claims false rests with the government. Currently, under the DSHEA, the FDA must show in court that an unreasonable risk is posed by consumption of a dietary supplement. Thus, numerous unsupported health claims are being made in advertisements and even on dietary supplement labels.

Help is on the way. The Center for Food Safety and Applied Nutrition of the FDA recently launched a ten-year plan to develop a science-based regulatory program that will provide consumers with a high level of confidence in the safety, composition, and labeling of dietary supplement products. The FDA has established current good manufacturing practice requirements, noting that manufacturers are required to evaluate the identity, purity, quality, strength, and composition of dietary supplements. The Federal Trade Commission has indicated that marketers of dietary supplements must have above-board scientific evidence to support any health claims. Additionally, U.S. Pharmacopeia, a respected nonprofit medical agency, launched a certification program for dietary supplements. If the dietary supplement contains what the label indicates, then it may carry the USP seal of approval. However, the USP seal does not mean the product is effective or even that it is safe to use, just that it contains what the label promises.

It should be noted that some of these types of dietary supplements, such as herbals and food extracts, have been the subject of research to evaluate their health effects. Such effects will be discussed in later chapters as appropriate.

Again, to reiterate the point, dietary supplements may exert some beneficial healthful effects in certain cases, but as Thomas points out, for most of us the substances found in most dietary supplements are readily available in familiar and attractive packages called fruits, vegetables, legumes, fish, and other healthy foods. Although the Prudent Healthy Diet is the optimal means to obtain the nutrients we need, dietary supplements may be recommended under certain circumstances. When deemed to be prudent behavior, such recommendations will be provided at specific points in this text.

Can dietary supplements harm my health?

In his review of dietary supplements, Thomas noted that although they may be beneficial to some individuals, their use may be harmful in some ways. Some of his key points, and others, are:

1. Nutrition is only one factor that influences health, well-being, and resistance to disease. Individuals who rely on dietary supplements to guarantee their health may disregard other very important lifestyle behaviors, such as appropriate exercise and a healthy diet.
2. Dietary supplements may provide a false sense of security to some individuals who may use them as substitutes for a healthful diet, believing they are eating healthfully and not attempting to eat right.
3. Taking supplements of single nutrients in large doses may have detrimental effects on nutritional status and health. Although large doses of some vitamins or minerals may be taken to prevent some conditions, excesses may lead to other health problems.
4. Individuals who use dietary supplements as an alternative form of medicine may avoid seeking effective medical treatment.
5. Dietary supplements vary tremendously in quality. Numerous independent analyses of specific dietary supplements, such as those by ConsumerLab.com, reveal that some may contain less than that listed, sometimes even none of the main ingredient. Some products often contain substances not listed on the label. This may pose a health risk.
6. Numerous case studies have shown that the use of various dietary supplements may impair health, and may even be fatal. Use of ephedrine-containing dietary supplements for weight loss have resulted in deaths.

www.ConsumerLab.com Check the content analysis of various brands of popular dietary supplements. Fee charged for some reports.

www.ods.od.nih.gov/factsheets Provides detailed information on specific dietary supplements.

http://dietarysupplements.nlm.nih.gov Check dietary supplements by specific brands or active ingredient. Indicates uses for the product. Provides list of research studies regarding effectiveness.

Nonetheless, some research suggests that use of several herbal products may have some healthful effects. In some countries,

such as Germany, herbs are approved for medical use by agencies comparable to the U.S. FDA.

In contrast, a Consumers Union report noted that various herbal preparations were associated with stomach disorders, nonviral hepatitis (rapid liver damage), obstructed blood flow to the liver and possible cirrhosis, and even death.

Where appropriate, the effectiveness and safety of various dietary supplements will be discussed in later sections of this book, but some general safeguards recommended by the Consumers Union to protect your health represent sound advice.

- Before trying a dietary supplement to treat a health problem, try changing your diet or lifestyle first.
- Check with your doctor before taking any dietary supplement, particularly herbal preparations. This is especially important for pregnant and nursing women, children, and individuals taking prescribed drugs whose effects may be impaired by herbal interactions.
- Buy standardized products. Most dietary supplements in the United States should be standardized according to federal regulations. Supplement Facts labels should provide information comparable to the Nutrition Facts food label.
- Use only single-ingredient dietary supplements. Use of combination supplements may make it difficult to determine the cause of any side effects.
- Be alert to both the positive and negative effects of the supplement. Try to keep an objective record of the effects.
- Stop taking the supplement immediately if you experience any health-related problems. Contact your physician and local health authorities to report the problem. This may help establish a database for the safety of dietary supplements.

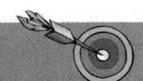

Key Concepts

▶ As defined by the Dietary Supplement Health and Education Act (DSHEA), a dietary supplement is a food product, added to the total diet, that may contain vitamins, minerals, herbs or botanicals, amino acids, metabolites, constituents, extracts, or any combination of the above.

▶ Although some people may need dietary supplements for various reasons, particularly vitamins and minerals, the use of supplements should not be routine practice for most individuals. Obtain nutrients through natural foods.

Consumer Nutrition— Food Quality and Safety

We Americans and Canadians have the basic assumption that the food we eat is safe and of high quality. Several federal agencies, such as the FDA's Center for Food Safety and Applied Nutrition, effectively regulate food quality and safety, so in general this assumption is correct. However, foods are not necessarily risk free or high quality. Many factors may influence food quality and safety in the development of a food product. For example,

pesticides in your diet, you might consider choosing organic alternatives for the *dirty* dozen.

www.foodnews.org Provides a complete list of 45 fruits and vegetables ranked on level of pesticides from highest to lowest amount.

Are organic foods safer and healthier choices?

The USDA has established rules regarding certified **organic foods.** One stipulation is prohibition of certain synthetic pesticides and fertilizers in plant production. Additionally, the use of antibiotics and growth hormones in animal production is prohibited, as is the use of irradiation and genetically modified organisms.

Foods that are 95–100 percent organic can carry the USDA organic label (see table 2.15), while foods with the notation "Made With Organic Ingredients" must contain at least 70 percent organic ingredients, but cannot use the organic label. Are such foods safer or healthier? Let's look at several proposed differences between organic and conventional food products.

Pesticides Baker and others, analyzing data drawn from more than 94,000 food samples, concluded that organically grown foods have fewer and generally lower pesticide residues than conventionally grown foods. However, Magkos and others note that although organic foods may contain less pesticide residues than conventionally grown foods, the significance of this difference is questionable, inasmuch as actual levels of contamination in both types of food are generally well below acceptable limits. This is especially so with the *clean* dozen fruits and vegetables. Most health professionals agree that you should not cut back on fruits and vegetables, because the associated health benefits discussed previously far outweigh potential risks from pesticides.

Bacteria Bacteria levels in organic foods are comparable to those in conventional foods. The Center for Science in the Public Interest indicated that organic fruits or vegetables are no less likely to be contaminated with bacteria, such as *E. coli,* than conventional ones. The Consumers Union also notes that chickens labeled as *organic* were more likely to harbor salmonella bacteria than were conventionally produced broilers. Magkos and others indicate that what should be made clear is that *organic* does not automatically equal *safe.* However, the Centers for Disease Control and Prevention indicated that there is no evidence that foodborne diseases, such as food poisoning, are a greater or lesser risk with organic foods. As discussed later in this chapter, food poisoning may have serious health consequences.

Nutritional Value The British Nutrition Foundation indicates that there is no strong scientific evidence to show that crops grown organically have a better nutrient content than those produced nonorganically. Conversely, Worthington noted that there appear to be genuine differences in the nutrient content of organic and conventional foods, with higher amounts of vitamin C, iron, and magnesium in organic foods. Moreover, organic meat may have

a different fatty acid profile because of the differences in the diet provided for the animals.

The Consumers Union notes that as more companies enter the organic market, government standards come under attack. Today we have numerous organic products in the marketplace, some of which have been termed *organic junk foods,* such as peanut butter cookies, sweetened cereals, potato chips, and soda, which may contain significant amounts of sugar and fat; although organic, such foods may not be healthful.

In a systematic review, Dangour and others determined that evidence is lacking for health effects resulting from the consumption of organic foods. However, Dangour and Williams note that we need higher quality research than that currently available.

Beyond health considerations, many promote buying organic as a means to help protect the environment. Organic farming practices may reduce pollution of our waters, while organic animal farming may be more humane.

Does commercial food processing affect food quality and safety?

Ideally, commercial food processing would make food more healthy, safe, delicious, attractive, and stable. In many cases it does, but certain commercial food-processing practices may be detrimental to our health in several ways. Potential health risks of several food-processing practices, such as the intentional inclusion of food additives and the unintentional inclusion of bacteria, are discussed later in this chapter. The major problem with some forms of commercial food-processing techniques is adding the wrong stuff and taking away the good stuff.

One potential health risk of commercial food processing is the conversion of a healthful food into a potentially harmful one. The major feature of the Prudent Healthy Diet is the consumption of wholesome, natural, low-fat foods. But most of us do consume a wide variety of packaged foods, some of which may be highly processed and may be of questionable nutritional value. There has been increasing concern over the years that the nutritional quality of our food has been declining because many of our foods are overprocessed. They contain too much refined sugar, extracted oils, or white flour, all products of a refinement process. Refined sugar is pure carbohydrate with no nutritional value except Calories. The same can be said for extracted oils, which are pure fat. In the bleaching and processing of wheat to white flour, at least 22 known essential nutrients are removed, including the B vitamins, vitamin E, calcium, phosphorus, potassium, and magnesium. In addition, many fruits and vegetables are artificially ripened before they have reached maturity and contain smaller quantities of vitamins and minerals than naturally ripened ones do. We also consume many totally synthetic products such as artificial orange juice, nondairy creamers, and imitation ice cream, which do not possess the same nutrient value as their natural counterparts. Concern about the declining nutritional value of our food supply appears to be legitimate. Much of the blame is assigned to the processing of food, rightfully so but not necessarily so.

In the mind of the public, processed foods more and more are thought to be inferior foods as compared with natural sources—for example, frozen peas versus fresh peas. The major purpose of food processing is to prevent waste through deterioration or spoilage. There are a variety of ways to do this, including heat, irradiation, dehydration, refrigeration, freezing, and the use of chemicals. Commercial food processing results in the loss of some nutrients, but preservation techniques in common use today do not cause major nutrient losses in the foods we eat. Commercial food processing may actually cause less nutrient loss than home processing. For example, some frozen foods may have higher concentrations of nutrients than their fresh counterparts because they are usually "flash-frozen" soon after picking. Processed tomatoes may increase the bioavailability of phytochemicals, such as lycopene, by breaking cell walls. In addition, food companies may enrich or fortify certain products before marketing. Examples include the addition of some B vitamins and iron to grain products, vitamins A and D to milk, vitamin A to margarine, and iodine to table salt. In some cases not all of the nutrients that were removed in processing are returned, but in some products a greater amount is returned or added.

Nevertheless, a few nutrients may be susceptible to loss through processing. Finley and others indicated that heat is particularly destructive to nutrients, especially vitamins. However, processing at optimal temperature and time may minimize nutrient loss.

The key point is that commercial processing of food does not necessarily lead to a nutritionally inferior product. Even if commercial food processing does cause a slight decrease in nutritional quality, it helps provide a greater and more varied food supply with adequate amounts of dietary nutrients.

The major problem with food processing is the excessive use of highly refined products like sugar, oils, fats, unenriched white flour, and salt. Additionally, some foods are fortified with vitamins and minerals up to 100 percent of the RDA. Consumption of multiple servings of such products may exceed the UL for several nutrients. Wise food selection can help avoid these problems, though this may be somewhat tricky in today's food marketplace. It requires careful reading of food labels.

Another potential health problem with commercial food processing is the inadvertent inclusion of bacteria. Although bacteria may be added unintentionally during commercial processing, improper food preparation at home also may contribute to the development of health problems, as discussed below.

Does home food processing affect food quality and safety?

Somewhat like commercial food processing, you process food at home. You may wash, cut, blend, freeze, and cook a variety of foods at home in preparation for a meal, and home food processing, like commercial food processing, may lead to loss of some nutrients, particularly several water-soluble vitamins. You can minimize nutrient losses and preserve the healthful quality of foods by following these procedures at home:

- Keep most fruits and vegetables chilled in the refrigerator to prevent enzymic destruction of nutrients. For similar reasons, keep frozen foods in the freezer until ready for preparation to eat.

- After cutting, wrap most fruits and vegetables tightly to prevent exposure to air, which may accelerate oxidation and spoiling, and store them in the refrigerator.
- Buy milk in cardboard or opaque plastic containers to prevent light from destroying riboflavin, a B vitamin. For similar reasons, keep most grain products stored in opaque containers or dark cupboards.
- Steam or microwave vegetables in very little water to prevent the loss of water-soluble vitamins and some minerals. Microwaving is very effective in preserving the nutrient value of food. Use microwave-safe dishes or glass cookware. Do not use plastic wrap, plastic containers, or Styrofoam because chemicals can leach into the food when heated. Cover food with a paper towel instead.
- Avoid cooking with high temperatures and prolonged cooking of foods, particularly in hot water, which may increase nutrient losses such as of water-soluble vitamins.
- Avoid excess cooking of foods, which may produce several carcinogens. Recent research indicates prolonged, high-temperature cooking, such as when French fries and other starchy foods are fried or baked at high temperatures (over 250°F), may produce acrylamide, a cancer-causing agent. In particular, avoid grilling or broiling foods, especially meats, over open flames on a daily basis as charring may lead to the formation of heterocyclic amines, a known carcinogen. Frying foods may also produce HCAs, but steaming, boiling, stir-frying, poaching, or microwaving meat are probably the healthiest cooking methods.

Using these techniques, nutrient losses incurred with home food processing are minimal, and an adequate nutrient intake will be obtained if you consume a wide variety of foods.

What is food poisoning?

The major health problem associated with home food processing is the presence of foodborne bacteria. Food bacteria are of two types. One type causes food spoilage, which probably won't make you sick, while the other type doesn't spoil food, but can make you sick.

Food poisoning is caused primarily by consuming foods contaminated with certain bacteria, particularly Salmonella, Escherichia, Staphylococcus, Clostridium, Campylobacter, and Listeria. *Campylobacter jejuni* and Salmonella are the most commonly reported bacterial causes of food poisoning in the United States. With increasing globalization of food distribution, foodborne illness is likely to become a major public health focus worldwide.

Bacteria that cause food poisoning are found mainly in animal foods. The Consumers Union reported that 83 percent of whole chicken broilers bought nationwide, even premium and organic broilers, harbored Campylobacter or Salmonella. Bacteria are also common in produce. The contamination of fresh spinach with the bacterium *Escherichia coli (E. coli)* led to one of the largest and deadliest outbreaks of foodborne illness in recent years. There were 31 cases of kidney failure, with 3 deaths. The most common sources of food poisoning are

- Raw and undercooked meat and poultry
- Raw or undercooked eggs
- Raw or undercooked shellfish
- Contaminated produce
- Improperly canned foods

The most common symptoms of food poisoning include nausea, vomiting, or diarrhea, which normally clear up in a day or two. However, individuals should seek medical help in cases involving headache, stiff neck, and fever occurring together; bloody diarrhea; diarrhea lasting longer than three days; fever that lasts more than 24 hours; or sensations of weakness, numbness, and tingling in the arms and legs. Some cases of food poisoning may lead to lifelong health problems and may be fatal if not treated properly.

Most cases of food poisoning occur at home, and may be associated with inappropriate commercial food processing. Although governmental health agencies attempt to control the spread of bacteria to food through appropriate regulations governing the food industry, the Consumers Union noted that occasional outbreaks do occur because of food contamination during industrial processing, such as ground meat contamination with *Escherichia coli* (*E. coli*). *E. coli* can lead to kidney failure. Millions of Americans experience a significant foodborne illness each year, with several thousand fatalities.

Food poisoning may be prevented by improving both commercial and home food processing. The Consumers Union notes that government action within recent years has reduced bacterial contamination of the food supply. New processes to eradicate bacteria are being used, such as pulsed electrical fields and ultrasound. One procedure is **irradiation,** a process whereby food products are subjected to powerful gamma rays from ionizing radiation, such as radioactive cobalt-60. Parnes and Lichtenstein indicate that irradiating food can greatly reduce illness from foodborne pathogens and extend food shelf life by delaying ripening, inhibiting spoilage, and minimizing contamination, and may do so without affecting nutritional or taste qualities. Irradiation may also reduce the need for many food preservatives. The FDA has approved irradiation for poultry, beef, pork, and lamb. Irradiated food products must have a label containing a statement that they have been treated and the international symbol of irradiation known as a *radura*, which is depicted in figure 2.13. The position of the

American Dietetic Association, developed by Wood and Bruhn, is that food irradiation enhances the safety and quality of the food supply and helps protect consumers from foodborne illness.

If you prefer to not purchase irradiated meats, at the minimum the following guidelines should be helpful in preventing the spread of bacteria in food prepared at home. Even if you buy irradiated foods, which may reduce the possibility of bacterial contamination, these guidelines are still recommended.

1. Wash hands thoroughly and often before and during food preparations.
2. Treat all raw meat, poultry, fish, seafood, and eggs as if they were contaminated. When shopping, place meat in separate bags, and store them that way in the refrigerator. Rinsing raw meat is more likely to contaminate the kitchen than decontaminate the food. Handle raw meat in just one part of the kitchen, on a cutting board used only for such food. Prevent juices from getting on other foods.
3. Eating raw fruits and vegetables is healthy. However, produce is often coated with wax, which can trap potentially dangerous pesticides. Wash all fruits and vegetables thoroughly with running water, even if you are going to peel them with a knife. The knife can transfer bacteria to the fruit as you recut it.
4. Thoroughly clean with hot soapy water all utensils used in food preparation. Microwaving your sponges and other food preparation utensils for about 30 to 60 seconds may help kill bacteria.
5. Use a clean preparation surface. After preparing poultry or other animal foods, clean the preparation surface thoroughly before using it to prepare other foods. When using the same surface, prepare animal foods last.
6. Do not use canned foods that are extensively dented or bulging.
7. Cook all meat, poultry, seafood, and eggs thoroughly according to directions. Use a meat thermometer inserted deep into the meat, especially with ground meat, because bacteria may get from the surface to the interior. Heat meat to the desired temperature, usually noted on the meat package. Guidelines include heating beef, pork, lamb, and veal to 160° and poultry to 170°–180°. However, do not overcook or char meats, as this process may produce carcinogens.
8. Do not eat raw shellfish.
9. Store heated foods promptly in the refrigerator or freezer. Reheat foods thoroughly.
10. Use leftovers within a few days. When in doubt, throw it out.

Are food additives safe?

Do you ever read the list of ingredients on the labels of highly processed food products? If not, check one out soon. My guess is you will not know what half the ingredients are or why they are there (unless the reason is listed). A recently purchased box of Long Grain & Wild Rice with Herb Seasoning, thought to be totally natural, had the main ingredients of enriched parboiled long grain rice, wild rice, and dehydrated vegetables (onion, parsley, spinach, garlic, celery) as the herb seasoning—along with hydrolyzed

FIGURE 2.13 The radura, the international symbol of irradiation.

vegetable protein, salt, sugar, monosodium glutamate, autolyzed yeast, sodium silicoaluminate, disodium inosinate, disodium guanylate, and sodium sulfite. The rice was delicious, but were all the additives necessary?

The Food and Drug Administration classifies a **food additive** as any substance added directly to food. There are more than 40 different purposes for the additives in the foods we eat, but the four most common are to add flavor, to enhance color, to improve texture, and to preserve the food. For example, vanilla extract may be added to ice cream to impart a vanilla flavor, vitamin C (ascorbic acid) may be added to fruits and vegetables to prevent discoloration, emulsifiers may be added to help blend oil evenly throughout a product, and sodium propionate may be used to prolong shelf life. Nutrients may also be added to increase the quality of the product, a process called *fortification*.

To earn FDA approval, additives must be **generally recognized as safe (GRAS).** The Office of Food Additive Safety of the FDA has determined an acceptable daily intake (ADI) for some, but not all, food additives. The ADI represents the amount of food additive that an individual may consume daily without any adverse effect, and includes a 100-fold safety factor. Additives may be added only to specific foods for specific purposes, and in general must improve the quality of the food without posing any hazards to humans. Only the minimum amount necessary to achieve the desired purpose may be added.

Although we realize that absolute safety does not exist in anything we do, including eating, we do have a right to expect that the food we purchase is generally safe for consumption. The government and food manufacturers must take utmost care to ensure that food additives do not create any appreciable health risks. On the other hand, we as consumers also have a responsibility to select foods necessary for good nutrition. Food product labeling has helped us in this regard, for we now can tell what ingredients we are eating, although we may not always know why they are there.

In the past, the major concern with most additives was the possibility that they could cause cancer. The Delaney Clause to the Food, Drug, and Cosmetic Act prohibits the addition of any additive to foods if it has been shown to cause cancer in animals or humans at any dose. Saccharin, which has been shown to cause cancer in laboratory animals when given in high doses, was exempted from the Delaney Clause by an act of Congress. More recently, in its position statement on food and water safety, the American Dietetic Association cited a National Research Council report indicating that people should worry less about the risk of cancer from food additives and be more concerned about the carcinogenic effects of excess macronutrients (sugar and fat), evidenced by the linkage of obesity to various cancers.

In general, the additives in today's food are regarded safe. Nevertheless, in a review of more than 70 food additives, the Center for Science in the Public Interest noted that although most were safe, others could pose some health problems. The CSPI recommended that individuals cut back on some additives because, although not toxic, large amounts may be unsafe or unhealthy. Included in this list are corn syrup, partially hydrogenated vegetable oil, and sugar, all products with high caloric content.

Some additives were recommended to be treated with caution, as they may pose a risk and should be better tested, such as some artificial colorings and aspartame. The CSPI noted that certain people should avoid other additives, such as caffeine and sulfites. Finally, the CSPI recommended that everyone avoid several products because they are unsafe or very poorly tested and not worth the risk, such as ephedrine and the fat-substitute olestra. The health aspects of many of these food additives will be discussed in later chapters where appropriate.

www.cspinet.org/reports/chemcuisine.html   The Center for Science in the Public Interest has developed a guide to safety of food additives, including the following five categories: Safe; Cut Back; Caution; Certain People Should Avoid; Everyone Should Avoid.

Why do some people experience adverse reactions to some foods?

Although most food we eat is safe and causes no acute health problems, some individuals may experience mild to severe reactions, or possibly death, from eating certain foods. These reactions may be attributed to food intolerance or food allergy.

Food intolerance, the most common problem, is a general term for any adverse reaction to a food or food component that does not involve the immune system. The body cannot properly digest a portion of the food because it lacks the appropriate enzyme, resulting in gastrointestinal distress such as bloating, abdominal pain, nausea, and diarrhea. For example, many African Americans lack lactase, the enzyme needed to digest lactose (milk sugar), and thus suffer from lactose intolerance, a topic that is covered in chapter 4. Other common culprits in food intolerance are fructose, as found in fruit juice and high-fructose corn syrup, and gluten, a protein found in wheat, rye, and barley.

Food allergy, also known as food hypersensitivity, involves an adverse immune response to an otherwise harmless food substance. Many foods contain allergens, usually proteins, that may stimulate the immune system to manufacture antibodies (immunoglobulin E, or IgE) specific to that food. When individuals who have inherited a food allergy are first exposed to that food, their immune system produces millions of IgE antibodies. These antibodies reside in some white blood cells and mast cells in the body, particularly in the skin, respiratory tract, and gastrointestinal tract, the parts of the body that come into contact with air and the food we eat. These cells also contain substances, such as histamine, that are released when the antibodies are exposed again to the offending food allergen.

Histamine and other chemicals cause the allergic reaction, which may involve the skin (swelling, hives, itchy skin and eyes), gastrointestinal tract (nausea, vomiting, abdominal cramps, diarrhea), or respiratory tract (runny nose, sneezing, coughing). In severe cases, an allergic response may involve anaphylactic shock and death by respiratory failure. Food allergies affect approximately 2–4 percent of adults and 6–8 percent of children in the United States, or more than 6 million individuals. Keet and Wood note that some allergies are mostly outgrown, whereas others are lifelong.

More than 700 food allergens have been identified. Although allergens may be found in many foods, 90 percent of the offenders are proteins found in several common foods. The FDA mandates clear labeling and source of ingredients derived from commonly allergenic sources. Labels are required to state clearly whether the food contains one of the eight "major food allergens" listed:

- Milk
- Fish
- Tree nuts
- Wheat
- Eggs
- Crustacean shellfish
- Peanuts
- Soybeans

Some additives also may cause allergic responses, particularly sulfites used as preservatives.

For individuals who know which food substances may trigger an allergic response, food labels may be helpful in determining the allergen's presence. Food manufacturers are placing notices on food labels for "Food Allergic Consumers" to check the ingredient list, and also note that the product may have been manufactured in a factory that makes other products containing allergenic foods.

If you experience problems when you consume certain foods, you may be able to make a self-diagnosis by simply avoiding that food and noting whether or not you experience a recurrence. But, because there may be many causes of food-related illness, you should consult an allergist or other appropriate physician to determine whether you have either food intolerance or food allergy. Once the offending food is determined, you may need to eliminate that food from your diet or reduce the amount you consume. In some cases this is relatively simple. For example, if you develop a reaction to clams, a common problem, you should have no difficulty finding other sources of high-quality protein. However, if you react to milk, it may be more difficult to obtain an adequate dietary intake of calcium. A dietitian will be able to assist you in planning a diet that compensates for the reduced intake of calcium. Some suggestions are presented in chapter 8.

If you want to complain to the FDA about food-related illnesses, adverse events after taking dietary supplements, products not labeled for allergens, or other problems with food products, you may use the Consumer Complaint System.

www.fda.gov/opacom/backgrounders/complain.htm **To complain** to the FDA about various food-related health problems, this site provides a contact phone number for your state and information to include in your report.

Key Concepts

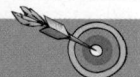

▶ In general, current food biotechnology techniques, such as genetically modified (GM) food, help provide a food supply that is high quality and safe. However, preventing the introduction of allergy-causing ingredients in GM foods is a concern.

▶ Pesticide residues in most foods are minimal, but some foods may contain more than others. The major concern is reducing pesticide intake in children, as some scientists believe neurological development may be impaired.

▶ Although organic foods may contain lesser amounts of pesticides than conventional foods, they may not contain fewer bacteria or higher nutrient density. The available research is insufficient to determine whether consumption of organic foods confers any health benefits.

▶ Commercial food processing can provide safe and healthful foods. However, excess sugar and fat added during commercial food processing may dilute health benefits.

▶ Proper food preparation practices may help preserve the nutrient quality and safety of foods prepared at home.

▶ Certain individuals may be intolerant to various foods or experience allergic responses to others and thus should take precautions to avoid such foods.

Check for Yourself

▶ Check the food label for several commercial food products you love most. Check the list of ingredients. Do you recognize any of the additives?

Healthful Nutrition: Recommendations for Better Physical Performance

Sports nutrition for the physically active person may be viewed from two aspects: nutrition for training and nutrition for competition. Of the three basic purposes of food—to provide energy, to regulate metabolic processes, and to support growth and development—the first two are of prime importance during athletic competition, while all three must be considered during the training period in preparation for competition.

Articles about nutrition for athletes in popular sports magazines, and food supplements advertised therein, give the impression that athletes have special nutritional requirements above those of nonathletes. In general, however, the diet that is optimal for health is also optimal for physical or sport performance. The Prudent Healthy Diet will provide adequate food energy and nutrients to meet the need of almost all athletes in training and competition.

Nevertheless, modifications to the Prudent Healthy Diet may help enhance performance for certain athletic endeavors, and subsequent chapters will focus on specific recommendations relative to the use of various nutrients and dietary supplements to enhance physical performance. The purpose of this section is to provide some general recommendations regarding use of the Prudent Healthy Diet by the athlete for training and competition.

However, it is very important for athletes to individualize their dietary practices. All athletes should keep track of what, how much, and when they eat and drink during training and competition, and experiment with dietary strategies to find those that are optimal. The United States Anti-Doping Agency has developed a pamphlet, *Optimal Dietary Intake for Sport, for Life* with a focus on a healthy diet and appropriate modifications for sport performance.

www.usada.org Click on Substances and then on Effects of Substances to access the 32-page pamphlet *Optimal Dietary Intake for Sport, for Life.*

What should I eat during training?

Sport scientists and coaches both stress the importance of proper nutrition during training. Ron Maughan, an expert in exercise metabolism and sports nutrition, notes that the main role of nutrition for the athlete may be to support consistent intensive training, while Chris Carmichael, former coach and nutritionist for seven-time Tour de France champion Lance Armstrong, indicates that athletes need to match their nutritional intake to the demands of their training. As noted in chapter 1, optimal training is the most important factor contributing to improved sport performance.

Because energy expenditure increases during a training period, the caloric intake needed to maintain body weight may increase considerably—an additional 500–1,000 Calories or more per day in certain activities. By selecting these additional Calories wisely from a wide variety of foods, you should obtain an adequate amount of all nutrients essential for the formation of new body tissues and proper functioning of the energy systems that work harder during exercise. A balanced intake of carbohydrate, fat, protein, vitamins, minerals, and water is all that is necessary. For endurance athletes, dietary carbohydrates should receive even greater emphasis.

However, there may be some circumstances during sport training that make particular attention to the diet important. For example, during the early phases of training, the body will begin to make adjustments in the energy systems so that they become more efficient. This is the so-called **chronic training effect,** and many of the body's adjustments incorporate specific nutrients. For example, one of the chronic effects of long-distance running is an increased hemoglobin content in the blood and increased myoglobin and cytochromes in the muscle cells; all three compounds require iron in order to be formed. Hence, the daily diet would have to contain adequate amounts of iron not only to meet normal needs, but also to make effective body adjustments due to the chronic effects of training.

Timing of nutrient intake during training may also be very important. In a review, John Hawley, a renowned sports scientist from Australia, noted that the beneficial effects of exercise training are believed to occur during recovery from each exercise bout, and evidence is accumulating that nutrient supplementation can serve as a potent modulator of many of the acute responses to both endurance and resistance training. Consuming a carbohydrate/protein combination shortly after strenuous exercise may be a recommended procedure.

Breakfast may be especially important during training. A balanced breakfast provides a significant amount of Calories and other nutrients in the daily diet of the physically active person. A breakfast of skim milk, a poached egg, whole-grain toast, fortified high-fiber cereal, and orange juice will help provide a substantial part of the RDA for protein, calcium, iron, fiber, vitamin C, and other nutrients and is also relatively high in complex carbohydrates. A balanced breakfast high in fiber with an average amount of protein also will help prevent the onset of mid-morning hunger. The fiber and protein may help maintain a feeling of satiety throughout the morning, whereas a breakfast of refined carbohydrates, like doughnuts, may trigger an insulin response and produce hypoglycemia (low blood sugar) in the middle of the morning. The resultant hunger is typically satisfied by eating other refined carbohydrates, which will satisfy the hunger urge only until about lunchtime. A balanced breakfast having a high nutrient density is therefore preferable to a breakfast based on refined carbohydrate products. Nontraditional breakfast foods, such as pizza, may also provide a balanced meal for breakfast.

Skipping breakfast would be comparable to a small fast, as the individual might not eat for 12 to 14 hours. Although some believe that exercising after a small fast increases fat burning and weight loss, this is not the case. Paoli and others recently reported that a light meal prior to physical activity increased oxygen consumption and lipid use for 24 hours relative to a fasting condition. Moreover, for young athletes, Nicklas and others have noted that breakfast consumption is an important factor in their nutritional well-being, enhancing their academic performance, an important consideration for those aspiring to college scholarships. Although individual preferences should be taken into account, a balanced breakfast could provide a good source of some major nutrients to the individual who is involved in a physical conditioning program. For those on a tight time schedule, a bowl of ready-to-eat, fortified high-fiber cereal with skim milk and fruit may be an ideal choice. Nancy Clark, a nationally acclaimed sports nutritionist, notes that this breakfast is not only quick, easy, and convenient but also rich in carbohydrate, fiber, iron, calcium, and vitamins.

Proper nutrition should enhance the physiological responses to training, and thus enhance competitive sports performance. The nutrient needs of athletes in training will be highlighted throughout the remainder of this text where relevant.

When and what should I eat just prior to competition?

In competition an athlete will utilize specific body energy sources and systems, depending upon the intensity and duration of the exercise. The three human energy systems will be discussed in detail in chapter 3. Briefly, however, high-energy compounds stored in the muscle are utilized during very short, high-intensity exercise; carbohydrate stored in the muscle as glycogen may be used without oxygen for intense exercise lasting about 1 to 3 minutes; and the oxidation of glycogen and fats becomes increasingly important in endurance activities lasting longer than 5 minutes. The release of energy in each of these three systems may require certain vitamins and minerals for optimal efficiency.

If an individual is well nourished, athletic competition normally will not impose any special demands for any of the six major classes of nutrients. Body energy stores of carbohydrate and fat are adequate to satisfy the energy demands of most activities lasting less than 1 hour. Protein is not generally considered a significant energy source during exercise. The vitamin and mineral content of the body will be sufficient to help regulate the increased levels of metabolic activity, and body-water supply will be adequate under normal environmental conditions.

However, content and timing of the precompetition intake may be critical. It is a well-established fact that the ingestion of food just prior to competition will not benefit physical performance in most athletic events, yet the pregame meal, so to speak, is one of the major topics of discussion among athletes. A number of special meals have been utilized throughout the years because of their alleged benefits to physical performance, and special products have been marketed as pre-event nutritional supplements. Although research has not substantiated the value of any one particular precompetition meal, some general guidelines have been developed from practical experience over the years.

There are several major goals of the precompetition meal that may be achieved through proper timing and composition. In general, the precompetition meal should do the following:

1. *Allow the stomach to be relatively empty at the start of competition.* In general, a solid meal should be eaten about 3 to 4 hours prior to competition. This should allow ample time for digestion to occur so that the stomach is relatively empty, and yet hunger sensations are minimized. However, pre-event emotional tension or anxiety may delay digestive time, as will a meal with a high-fat or high-protein content. Hence, the composition of the meal is critical. It should be high in carbohydrate, low in fat, and low to moderate in protein, providing for easy digestibility.
2. *Help to prevent or minimize gastrointestinal distress.* The composition of the precompetition meal should not contribute to any gastrointestinal distress, such as flatulence, increased acidity in the stomach, heartburn, or increased bulk that may stimulate the need for a bowel movement during competition. In general, foods to be avoided include gas formers like beans, spicy foods that may elicit heartburn, and bulk foods like bran products. High-sugar compounds may delay gastric emptying or create a reverse osmotic effect, possibly increasing the fluid content of the stomach, which may lead to a feeling of distress, cramps, or nausea. High-sugar loads, particularly fructose, may also lead to other forms of gastrointestinal distress, such as diarrhea. Individuals with known food intolerances, such as lactose intolerance, should use due caution. Through experience, you should learn what foods

disagree with you during performance, and of course, you should avoid these prior to competition.
3. *Help avoid sensations of hunger, lightheadedness, or fatigue.* A small amount of protein in a carbohydrate meal will help delay the onset of hunger. Large amounts of concentrated sugars can cause a reactive drop in blood sugar in susceptible individuals, which may cause lightheadedness and fatigue.
4. *Provide adequate energy supplies, primarily carbohydrate, in the blood and muscles.* A wide variety of foods may be selected for the precompetition meal. The meal should consist of foods that are high in complex carbohydrates with moderate to low amounts of protein. Examples of such foods are presented in later chapters and also may be found in appendix E, particularly those in the starch list. The foods should be agreeable to you. You should eat what you like within the guidelines presented above.
5. *Provide an adequate amount of body water.* Adequate fluid intake should be assured prior to an event, particularly if the event will be of long duration or conducted under hot environmental conditions. Diuretics such as alcohol, which increase the excretion of body water, should be avoided. Large amounts of protein increase the water output of the kidneys and thus should be avoided. Fluids may be taken up to 15 to 30 minutes prior to competition to help ensure adequate hydration.

Two examples of precompetition meals, each containing about 500–600 Calories with substantial amounts of carbohydrate, are presented in table 2.18. Bloch and Wheeler presented an excellent overview of practical approaches to feeding athletes. A similar approach, based on the Food Exchange System, is presented in chapter 11 as a means of designing comprehensive diet plans for physically active individuals.

One important last point. Meals other than the precompetition meal eaten on the same day should not be skipped. They should adhere to the basic principles set forth earlier in this chapter. Follow these general recommendations.

1. For events in the morning, eat a precompetition meal similar to breakfast; for example, meal A in table 2.18.
2. For events in early to mid-afternoon, eat breakfast and lunch. You might consume a more substantial breakfast, along with meal B in table 2.18 as a precompetition meal for lunch.
3. For events in the late afternoon, eat breakfast, lunch, and a snack. Again, eat a substantial breakfast and lunch and

TABLE 2.18 Two examples of precompetition meals containing 500–600 Calories

Meal A	Meal B
Glass of orange juice	One cup low-fat yogurt
One bowl of oatmeal	One banana
Two pieces of toast with jelly	One toasted bagel
Sliced peaches with skim milk	One ounce of turkey breast
	One-half cup of raisins

consume snacks that appeal to you, such as fruit, bagels with jelly, or other easily digestible foods.

4. For events in the evening, eat breakfast, lunch, and a precompetition meal for dinner.

Pre-event nutritional strategies will vary somewhat for athletes involved in prolonged exercise tasks, such as running a marathon. As noted by prominent Australian exercise scientist Mark Hargreaves, body stores of both carbohydrate and fluids should be optimized. To achieve this goal, athletes may engage in practices such as carbohydrate loading and water hyperhydration, which will be detailed in chapters 4 and 9.

What should I eat during competition?

There is no need to consume anything during most types of athletic competition with the possible exception of carbohydrate and water. Carbohydrate may provide additional supplies of the preferred energy source during high-intensity intermittent and prolonged exercise, while water intake may be critical for regulation of body temperature when exercising in warm environments. In ultradistance competition, a hypotonic salt solution also may be recommended. Appropriate details are presented in chapters 4 and 9.

What should I eat after competition?

In general, a balanced diet is all that is necessary to meet your nutrient needs and restore your nutritional status to normal following competition or daily, hard physical training. Carbohydrate and fat are the main nutrients used during exercise and can be replaced easily from foods among the food exchange lists. The increased caloric intake that is needed to replace your energy expenditure also will help provide you with the additional small amounts of protein, vitamins, minerals, and electrolytes that may be necessary for effective recovery. Thirst will normally help replace water losses on a day-to-day basis; you can check this by recording your body weight each morning to see if it is back to normal.

As noted previously, timing of food intake may be an important consideration. Simple sugars eaten immediately after a hard workout may help restore muscle glycogen fairly rapidly. Consuming a small amount of high-quality protein may also be prudent. Specific guidelines are presented in chapters 4 and 6.

For those who must compete several times daily and eat between competitions, such as in tennis tournaments or swim meets, the principles relative to pregame meals may be relevant, with a focus on carbohydrate-rich foods or fluids and moderate protein intake.

Should athletes use commercial sports foods?

The sports nutrition industry is booming. Numerous products are marketed to athletes, including meal replacement powders, sports drinks, sports bars, sports gels, sports candy, and sports supplements. It is important to note that although many of these products may be convenient and appropriate for a pregame, post-training, or post-competition meal, they do not contain all the healthful nutrients found in natural foods and thus should not be used on a long-term basis to replace the Prudent Healthy Diet.

Liquid Sports Meals **Liquid meals,** many of them designed specifically for athletes, usually contain high-quality sources of carbohydrate and protein, a low-to-moderate fat content, vitamins and minerals, and various other supplements. The food label will provide the amounts of each. They are very convenient for precompetition meals as well as for recovery nutrition after training or competition.

Liquid meals available include Nutrament, Ensure, Slim-Fast, Boost, Gatorade Nutrition Shake, and PowerBar ProteinPlus. Some liquid meals come premixed, while others come as powders. You can make your own liquid sports meal, or *smoothie,* from high-quality carbohydrate/protein powders, such as nonfat dry milk powder, and/or other healthful sources of carbohydrate and protein, such as yogurt and fruits. The following formula will provide one quart of a tasty liquid meal:

½ cup water/ice cubes
½ cup of nonfat dry milk powder
¼ cup of a glucose polymer
1 frozen banana
3 cups of cold skim milk
1 teaspoon of flavoring for palatability (cherry, vanilla)

A liquid meal may be assimilated more readily than a solid meal, and thus may be useful as a precompetition meal because it may be taken closer to competition, say 2 to 3 hours before. Research has shown that there is no difference between a liquid and a solid meal relative to subsequent hunger, nausea, diarrhea, or physical performance.

Sports Bars Sports bars have become increasingly popular in recent years, and several dozen products are targeted to physically active individuals. **Sports bars** vary in composition. Some are high carbohydrate, some high protein, and some have nearly equal mixtures of carbohydrate, protein, and fat. Many are vitamin and mineral fortified, and some are designed to serve as a meal replacement. Others contain drugs, such as caffeine. As with liquid meals, the food label on the sports bar will describe its contents. When compared to comparable energy sources from ordinary food, sports bars do not possess any magical qualities to enhance physical performance, but they possess some advantages similar to liquid meals, such as convenience. Because the major ingredient in many sports bars is carbohydrate, an expanded discussion is presented in chapter 4.

Sports Drinks Sports drinks are generally referred to as carbohydrate and electrolyte replacement fluids, and may be consumed by athletes before, during, and after training and competition. Examples include Gatorade and PowerAde. They are designed to provide carbohydrate, water, and electrolytes, and their role in sport is discussed in chapters 4 and 9.

Sports Gels and Candy Sports gels and candy normally provide carbohydrate, but may contain other substances such as vitamins, minerals, and caffeine. Their primary purpose is to provide a source of easily digested carbohydrates for energy during exercise.

Sports Supplements   As noted in chapter 1, numerous sports supplements are marketed to athletes, including various forms of carbohydrates, fats, and protein, many vitamins and minerals, several food drugs, and selected herbal or botanical products. Based on the available scientific data, the use of most sports supplements does not appear to be necessary for the well-nourished athlete during training. However, nutrient supplementation may be warranted in some cases. For example, in activities where excess body weight may serve to handicap performance, a loss of some body fat may be helpful. During weight loss, vitamin-mineral supplements may be recommended to prevent a nutrient deficiency. Furthermore, use of several sport supplements has been supported by research because they may enhance physical performance, may not pose any health risks, and may be legal. Research evaluating the effectiveness of purported sport ergogenics is presented throughout the book. Pertinent discussion topics include the following.

Chapter 4: Carbohydrate ergogenics
Chapter 5: Ergogenics that affect fat metabolism
Chapter 6: Amino acids, creatine, and other protein-related ergogenics
Chapter 7: Vitamins and other vitamin-related ergogenics
Chapter 8: Mineral ergogenics
Chapter 9: Glycerol
Chapter 13: Alcohol, caffeine, and other food–drug and herbal ergogenics

How can I eat more nutritiously while traveling for competition?

Athletes who must travel to compete are often faced with the problem of obtaining proper pre-event and postevent nutrition. After reading this chapter, you should be aware of how to select foods that are high in carbohydrate, low in fat, and moderate in protein. More guidelines are presented in chapters 4 through 6. One possible solution is to pack your own food and fluids in a traveling bag or cooler. Foods from each of the Food Exchange Lists can be easily packed or kept on ice, such as skim milk; precooked low-fat meats; bagels and cereal; fruits, juices, and vegetables; sports drinks; and high-carbohydrate snacks including whole wheat crackers and pretzels, and low-fat cookies such as Fig Newtons and vanilla wafers. Small containers of condiments can also be easily transported in the cooler, along with proper eating utensils. Taking your own food means you can eat your pre-event or post event meal as planned, and you may save money as well. Such an approach may be very effective for short, one-day trips and may also be used to complement other meals on longer journeys. Some easily packed snack foods are presented in table 2.19.

While traveling, you have a variety of eating places from which to select your food, including full-service restaurants, restaurants with all-you-can-eat buffets, steakhouses and fishhouses, fast-food restaurants, pizza parlors, sub shops, supermarkets, convenience stores, and even vending machines. With a solid background on the nutritional principles presented in this chapter, you should be able to select healthful, high-carbohydrate and low-fat foods at any of these establishments, but of course the variety of food choices will vary depending on the place you choose. Keep in

TABLE 2.19   Easily packed snacks for traveling or brown bag lunches

Grains	Meats	Vegetables
Bagels	Small can of baked beans	Sliced carrots
Pita bread	Cooked chicken or turkey, small 2-ounce commercial	Broccoli stalks
Muffins	packages, packed in airtight plastic bags	Cauliflower pieces
Fig Newtons	Small can of tuna fish, salmon, or sardines	Tomatoes
Vanilla wafers	Peanut butter	Canned vegetable juices
Whole wheat crackers	Reduced-fat cheese slices	
Graham crackers	String cheese	
Dry cereals		
Wheat Chex		
Grapenuts		
Plain popcorn		

Fruits	Milk	Nuts
Small cans of fruit in own juice	Small containers of skim or low-fat milk; chocolate	Almonds
Small containers of fruit juice, aseptic	milk; aseptic packaging if available	Walnuts
packages	Dried skim milk powder, to be reconstituted	
Oranges	Packaged yogurt	
Apples		
Other raw fruits		
Dried fruits		

mind that you can always ask to see if they will create a meal for you. For example, order a salad and ask to have extra vegetables and fish or chicken breast added, with the dressing on the side.

Although all fast foods can be part of a healthy diet when consumed in moderation, many are relatively high in fat content, and their intake should be restricted. However, many restaurants do provide a few healthier choices with individual sandwiches containing less than 30 percent of their Calories from fat, including grilled or broiled chicken, lean roast beef, and veggie burgers. In some cases, particularly with grilled, skinless chicken sandwiches, much of the fat content is in the sauce added to the sandwich, so ordering the sauce on the side allows you to control the amount added. Other sandwich shops, such as Au Bon Pain and Subway, may serve healthful sandwiches, but unwise selections in these stores may also contain substantial amounts of fat.

You can eat fast food and stay within the recommended nutrition guidelines for a healthy diet, but obtaining a healthful diet requires careful selection of foods. Fast-food restaurants provide materials detailing the nutrient content of each of their products. In some cases the materials may be obtained in the restaurant, and all have Websites detailing nutrient analysis of their products. See appendix F for the fat percentages of specific fast-food products and appropriate Websites.

The following suggestions may be helpful if you are dining in a fast-food or budget-type restaurant, such as McDonald's, Wendy's, Arby's, Pizza Hut, Baja Fresh, Applebee's, or Ruby Tuesday. Many supermarkets also have takeout departments or salad bars from which to select lunch or dinner.

Breakfast selections
   English muffins, unbuttered, with jelly
   English muffins with Canadian bacon
   Whole wheat pancakes with syrup
   French toast
   Bran muffins, fat-free or low-fat
   Hot whole-grain cereal, oatmeal
   Ready-to-eat fortified, high-fiber cereal
   Skim or low fat milk
   Orange juice
   Hot cocoa

Lunch or dinner selections
   Any low-fat sandwiches, no mayonnaise or high-fat sauces
   Grilled chicken breast sandwich, on whole-grain bun
   Baked or broiled fish sandwich
   Lean roast beef sandwich, on whole-grain bun
   Single, plain hamburger, on whole-grain bun
   Baked potato, with toppings on the side (add sparingly)
   Pasta dishes, spaghetti, and macaroni, with low-fat sauces
   Rice dishes
   Lo mein noodles, not chow mein (fried noodles)
   Soups, rice and noodle
   Salsas, made with tomatoes
   Chicken or seafood tostadas, made with cornmeal tortillas
   Bean and rice dishes
   All whole-grain and other breads
   Salads, low-fat dressing

Salad bar, focus on vegetables and high-carbohydrate foods; avoid high-fat items
Pizza, thick crust, vegetable type with minimum cheese topping
Skim or low-fat milk; chocolate milk
Orange juice
Frozen yogurt, fat-free or low-fat
Sherbet

With any of these selections, it is always a good idea to order toppings, for example, mayonnaise, salad dressing, and so on, on the side so that you can control portions. When selecting sandwiches, ask for those that are either baked, broiled, or grilled.

For the most part, research supports the general finding that the diet that is optimal for your health is also the optimal diet for your performance. Eating right, both for health and performance, does not mean you need to eat bland foods, because all foods, some in moderation, can be tastefully prepared and blended into the Prudent Healthy Diet.

How do gender and age influence nutritional recommendations for enhanced physical performance?

The diet that is optimal for health is the optimal diet for physical performance. This is the key principle of sports nutrition and it applies to physically active males and females of all ages. However, as shall be noted at certain points in this text, specific nutrient needs may vary by gender and age, and various forms of exercise training may influence nutrient requirements as well.

Gender   Seiler and others note that exercise performance is, in general, about 10 percent greater in males than females, mainly because males have greater levels of muscle mass and strength, anaerobic power and capacity, and maximal aerobic capacity, as well as lower levels of body fat. Nevertheless, most physiological adaptations to exercise are similar for males and females. Moreover, Maughan and Shirreffs, discussing nutrition and hydration needs of football (soccer) players, noted that the differences between males and females are smaller than differences between individuals, so that principles developed for male players also apply to women. However, several metabolic differences between males and females could influence nutritional requirements. For example, as shall be noted in chapter 5, female endurance athletes oxidize more fat and less carbohydrate during exercise as compared to males, which may influence various dietary strategies such as carbohydrate loading.

Adolescent and adult premenopausal females need more dietary iron than males. Female athletes, especially those participating in aerobic endurance sports such as distance running, must include iron-rich foods in their diet or risk incurring iron-deficiency anemia and impaired running ability. Being smaller in size, women need fewer Calories than men, yet many may not consume adequate energy and may develop disordered eating practices as they attempt to lose body mass for competition purposes. Disordered eating is more prevalent in female athletes and may contribute to the development of premature osteoporosis, prompting the American College of Sports Medicine to develop a position stand on the Female Athlete Triad, an important issue discussed in chapters 8 and 10. Such athletes may need more dietary calcium. Because of gender differences, some sports nutrition products have been designed for women only.

Age Youth sports competition is worldwide, ranging from community-based games to Olympic competition, and proper nutrition is important for these young athletes. Petrie and others have noted that child and adolescent athletes typically consume more food to meet their energy expenditure and thus are more likely to obtain an adequate supply of nutrients. However, Oded Bar-Or noted that while nutritional considerations are similar for all athletes irrespective of age, children have several physiological characteristics that may require specific nutritional considerations. For example, their relative protein needs may be greater to support growth, and their relative calcium needs may be greater for optimal bone development. Young athletes may experience greater thermal stress during exercise. Roberts indicates it may be unwise to allow children to exercise hard in high heat and humidity conditions, but also notes that there are few data to support this concern. Those who participate in weight-control sports involving excessive exercise and inadequate energy intake may be at risk for nutrient deficiencies and impaired growth and development. The American Academy of Pediatrics has developed a policy stand on promotion of healthy weight-control practices in young athletes.

Sport participation is also very popular at the other end of the age spectrum, and older athletes may also have special nutrient needs. In general, resting metabolism declines in older age, so caloric need may decrease. Older people also eat less, so they need to make wiser food choices, that is, foods with high nutrient density. Campbell and Geik recently noted that nutrition is a tool that the older athlete should use to enhance exercise performance and health. In particular, they noted that older athletes may need to focus on obtaining sufficient micronutrients, such as the B vitamins and

vitamin D. Supplements may be recommended to obtain adequate vitamin B_{12} and calcium if not obtained from the diet, such as from fortified foods. Female athletes over age 50, because of decreased estrogen levels associated with menopause, need to focus on obtaining adequate calcium. However, they may need less dietary iron compared to their younger counterparts. Older individuals also need to ensure adequate fluid intake because of increased susceptibility to dehydration.

The special nutrient requirements of females, the young, and the elderly, as they relate to physical activity, will be incorporated in the text where relevant. However, most of the nutritional principles underlying exercise and sport performance that are presented in this text apply to most physically active individuals.

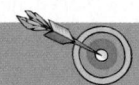

Key Concepts

▶ The precompetition meal should be easily digestible, high in carbohydrates, moderate in protein, and low in fat, and it should be consumed about 3–4 hours prior to competition. Athletes should determine what types of foods are compatible with their sport.

▶ Liquid meals and sports bars may be convenient as an occasional meal replacement, including use as a precompetition meal, but should be used only occasionally and not serve as a substitute for healthful whole foods.

▶ A healthful diet is the key to nutrition for male and female athletes at all age levels. However, female, young, and older athletes may have some specific nutritional needs in certain circumstances.

Check for Yourself

▶ Interview a coach or some athletes at your school about their meal strategies prior to competition. How do their strategies compare with general recommendations?

APPLICATION EXERCISE

In chapter 1 we recommended that you consume your normal daily diet, record the foods you have eaten, and then rate your diet using the quiz on pp. 00–00. Do the same but switch to a vegetarian diet, as close to a vegan diet as possible, for the day and compare the two rating scores.

1. The guide to eating from the United States Department of Agriculture, MyPlate, has five food groups. Which of the following is *not* considered a food group by the USDA?

   a. grains
   b. protein
   c. oils
   d. fruit
   e. dairy
   f. vegetables

2. Which of the following is not an acceptable definition for food labels with the listing "free"?

   a. fat free—less than 0.5 grams of total fat per serving
   b. cholesterol free—less than 2 milligrams per serving
   c. sugar free—less than 0.5 grams per serving
   d. Calorie free—less than 40 Calories per serving
   e. sodium free—less than 5 milligrams per serving

3. Approximately how many Calories are in a meal with two starch/bread exchanges, four lean meat exchanges, one fruit exchange, two vegetable exchanges, three fat exchanges, and one skim milk exchange?

   a. 450
   b. 540
   c. 670
   d. 715
   e. 780

4. Which of the following statements regarding consumer nutrition is false?

   a. Dietary supplements include vitamins, minerals, amino acids, herbals and botanicals, and various extracts and metabolites.
   b. Genetically modified foods may be designed to increase the content of a specific nutrient.
   c. Organic foods are healthier than conventional foods because they contain fewer bacteria and substantially more healthful nutrients.
   d. Various products in foods may cause food intolerance or food allergies in susceptible individuals.
   e. Food poisoning may be fatal.

5. Which of the following is not a key (indicator) nutrient as defined by the key-nutrient concept?

   a. iron
   b. calcium
   c. vitamin A
   d. protein
   e. vitamin D
   f. riboflavin
   g. niacin
   h. all are key nutrients

6. The recommended dietary goals for healthy Americans suggest that the intake of saturated fat, as a percentage of daily Calories, be less than what percent?

   a. 10
   b. 20
   c. 30
   d. 40
   e. 50

7. Which key nutrient is not usually found in substantial amounts in the meat group?

   a. vitamin C
   b. iron
   c. protein
   d. niacin
   e. thiamin

8. A food label lists the amount of complex carbohydrates as 5 grams, the amount of simple sugars as 10 grams, the amount of protein as 5 grams, and the amount of fat as 10 grams. Which of the following is true?

   a. Simple sugars make up the majority of the Calories.
   b. Carbohydrate makes up the majority of the Calories.
   c. The amount of Calories from protein and carbohydrate is equal.
   d. The majority of the Calories is derived from fat.
   e. None of the above statements is true.

9. A vegetarian-type diet may be more healthful than the current typical American diet for all of the following reasons *except* which?

   a. higher in iron
   b. higher in fiber
   c. lower in saturated fats
   d. a higher polyunsaturated to saturated fat ratio
   e. lower in cholesterol

10. Which of the following is a recommendation for the precompetition meal for an endurance athlete who will be competing in warm environmental conditions?

    a. water
    b. sports drinks
    c. high carbohydrate content
    d. moderate protein content
    e. moderate salt content
    f. all of the above

Answers to multiple-choice questions: 1. c; 2. d; 3. d; 4. c; 5. e; 6. a; 7. a; 8. d; 9. a; 10. f.

1. Name the eight key nutrients and identify a food source that is particularly rich in each nutrient. For example, lean meat is a rich source of iron.

2. Discuss the five categories of foods depicted in the MyPlate design in respect to the concepts of variety, proportionality, and moderation.

3. Compare and contrast the MyPlate food guide with the Food Exchange System. What similarities and differences do you note?

4. List and explain the potential health benefits of a vegan diet as compared to the typical American diet today.

5. Identify the nutrients that must be listed on food labels, how the DV is determined for each, and why you may want to have a high percent of the DV for some and a low percent for others.

References

Books

American Dietetic Association and American Diabetes Association. 1995. *Exchange Lists for Meal Planning.* Chicago: American Dietetic Association.

American Institute for Cancer Research. 2007. *Food, Nutrition, Physical Activity, and the Prevention of Cancer: A Global Perspective.* Washington, DC: AICR.

Bratman, S. 2000. *Health Food Junkies: Overcoming the Obsession with Healthful Eating.* New York: Bantam Doubleday.

Carmichael, C. 2004. *Food for Fitness: Eat Right to Train Right.* New York: G.P. Putnam's Sons.

Joseph, J., and Nadeau, D. 2002. *The Color Code: A Revolutionary Eating Plan for Optimal Health.* New York: Hyperion.

Larson-Meyer, D. 2007. *Vegetarian Sports Nutrition.* Champaign, IL: Human Kinetics.

National Academy of Sciences. Institute of Medicine, Food and Nutrition Board. 2010. *Dietary Reference Intakes for Calcium and Vitamin D.* Washington, DC: National Academy Press.

National Academy of Sciences. Institute of Medicine, Food and Nutrition Board. 2004. *Dietary Reference Intakes for Water, Potassium, Sodium, Chloride, and Sulfate.* Washington, DC: National Academy Press.

National Academy of Sciences. Institute of Medicine. Food and Nutrition Board. 2003. *Dietary Reference Intakes: Guiding Principles for Nutrition Labeling and Fortification.* Washington, DC: National Academy Press.

National Academy of Sciences. Institute of Medicine, Food and Nutrition Board. 2002. *Dietary Reference Intakes for Vitamin A, Vitamin K, Arsenic, Boron, Chromium, Copper, Iodine, Iron, Manganese, Molybdenum, Nickel, Silicon, Vanadium, and Zinc.* Washington, DC: National Academy Press.

National Academy of Sciences. Institute of Medicine, Food and Nutrition Board. 2002. *Dietary Reference Intakes for Energy, Carbohydrates, Fiber, Fat, Protein and Amino Acids (Macronutrients).* Washington, DC: National Academy Press.

National Academy of Sciences. Institute of Medicine, Food and Nutrition Board. 2000. *Dietary Reference Intakes for Thiamin, Riboflavin, Niacin, Vitamin B_6, Folate, Vitamin B_{12}, Pantothenic Acid, Biotin, and Choline.* Washington, DC: National Academy Press.

National Academy of Sciences. Institute of Medicine, Food and Nutrition Board. 2000. *Dietary Reference Intakes for Vitamin C, Vitamin E, Selenium, and Carotenoids.* Washington, DC: National Academy Press.

National Academy of Sciences. Institute of Medicine, Food and Nutrition Board. 1999. *Dietary Reference Intakes for Calcium, Phosphorus, Magnesium, Vitamin D, and Fluoride.* Washington, DC: National Academy Press.

National Research Council. 1989. *Diet and Health: Implications for Reducing Chronic Disease Risk.* Washington, DC: National Academy Press.

Nestle, M. 2006. *What to Eat: An Aisle-to-Aisle Guide to Savvy Food Choices and Good Eating.* New York: North Point Press.

Otten, J., et al. 2000. *Dietary Reference Intakes: The Essential Guide to Nutrient Requirements.* Washington, DC: National Academies Press.

Shils, M., et al. (Eds.). 2006. *Modern Nutrition in Health and Disease.* Philadelphia: Lippincott Williams & Wilkins.

Taubes, G. 2007. *Good Calories, Bad Calories: Challenging the Conventional Wisdom on Diet, Weight Control, and Disease.* New York: Alfred A. Knopf.

United States Anti-Doping Agency. 2005. *Optimal Dietary Intake.* Colorado Springs, CO.

U.S. Department of Agriculture and U.S. Department of Health and Human Services. 2005. *Nutrition and Your Health: Dietary Guidelines for Americans.* Washington, DC: U.S. Government Printing Office.

U.S. Department of Health and Human Services. 2000. *Healthy People 2010: National Health Promotion and Disease Prevention Objectives.* Washington, DC: U.S. Government Printing Office.

Ward, M. S. 2006. *The Pocket Idiot's Guide to the New Food Pyramids.* Indianapolis: Alpha Books/Penguin.

Review Articles

Ackerman, J. 2002. *Food: How safe; How altered? National Geographic* 201 (5):2–51.

Allen, K., et al. 2006. Food allergy in childhood. *Medical Journal of Australia* 185:394–400.

American Academy of Pediatrics. 2005. Promotion of healthy weight-control practices in young athletes. *Pediatrics* 116:1557–64.

American Academy of Pediatrics. 2003. Oral health risk assessment timing and establishment of dental home. *Pediatrics* 111:1113–16.

American Cancer Society 2001 Nutrition and Physical Activity Guidelines Advisory Committee. 2002. American Cancer Society guidelines on nutrition and physical activity for cancer prevention: Reducing the risk of cancer with healthy food choices and physical activity. *CA: A Cancer Journal for Clinicians* 52:92–119.

American Diabetes Association. 2003. Evidence-based nutrition principles and recommendations for the treatment and prevention of diabetes and related complications. *Diabetes Care* 26:S51–61.

American Dietetic Association. 2009. Position of the American Dietetic Association: Functional foods. *Journal of the American Dietetic Association* 109:735–46.

American Dietetic Association. 2009. Position of the American Dietetic Association: Vegetarian diets. *Journal of the American Dietetic Association* 109:1266–82.

American Dietetic Association. 2009. Position of the American Dietetic Association: Nutrient supplementation. *Journal of the American Dietetic Association* 109: 2073–85.

American Dietetic Association. 2002. Position of the American Dietetic Association: Total diet approach to communicating food and nutrition information. *Journal of the American Dietetic Association* 102:100–108.

American Dietetic Association. 2000. *10 tips to healthy eating.* Chicago: The American Dietetic Association.

American Heart Association. 2006. Diet and lifestyle recommendations revision 2006: A scientific statement from the American Heart Association Nutrition Committee. *Circulation* 114:82–96.

American Heart Association. 2002. *Dietary Guidelines for Healthy Children.* Dallas: AHA.

Ames, B. N., and Gold, L. S. 1998. The causes and prevention of cancer: The role of environment. *Biotherapy* 11:205–20.

Aoi, W., et al. 2006. Exercise and functional foods. *Nutrition Journal* 5:15.

Bar-Or, O. 2001. Nutritional considerations for the child athlete. *Canadian Journal of Applied Physiology* 26:S186–91.

Barr, S., and Rideout, C. 2004. Nutritional considerations for vegetarian athletes. *Nutrition* 20:696–703.

Bidlack, W., and Wang, W. 1999. Designing functional foods. In *Modern Nutrition in Health and Disease,* eds. M. Shils et al. Baltimore: Williams & Wilkins.

Blendon, R., et al. 2001. America's view on the use and regulation of dietary supplements. *Archives of Internal Medicine* 161:805–10.

Bloch, T., and Wheeler, K. 1999. Dietary examples: A practical approach to feeding athletes. *Clinics in Sports Medicine* 18:703–11.

Bren, L. 2003. Turning up the heat on acrylamide. *FDA Consumer* 37 (1):10–11.

Burks, W. 2002. Current understanding of food allergy. *Annals of the New York Academy of Sciences* 964:1–12.

Byers, T., et al. 2002. American Cancer Society guidelines on nutrition and physical activity for cancer prevention: Reducing the risk of cancer with healthy food choices and physical activity. *CA: A Cancer Journal for Clinicians* 52:92–119.

Campbell, W., and Geik, R. 2004. Nutritional considerations for the older athlete. *Nutrition* 20:603–8.

Center for Science in the Public Interest. 2008. Chemical cuisine: A guide to food additives. *Nutrition Action Health Letter* 35 (4):1–8.

Center for Science in the Public Interest. 2006. Eating green: The case for a plant-based diet. *Nutrition Action Health Letter* 33 (7):3–7.

Center for Science in the Public Interest. 2006. Fear of fresh. *Nutrition Action Health Letter* 33 (10):3–6.

Center for Science in the Public Interest. 2002. Genetically engineered foods: Are they safe? *Nutrition Action Health Letter* 28 (9):1–8.

Center for Science in the Public Interest. 1999. Chemical cuisine. *Nutrition Action Health Letter* 26 (2):4–9.

Clark, N. 1987. Breakfast of champions. *Physician and Sportsmedicine* 15(January):209–12.

Consumers Union. 2007. Dirty birds. *Consumer Reports* 72 (1):20–23.

Consumers Union. 2007. Functional—or dysfunctional—foods. *Consumer Reports on Health* 19 (2):8–9.

Consumers Union. 2007. Eat right, at any age. *Consumer Reports on Health* 19 (8):1, 4–5.

Consumers Union. 2006. Buy quality organic foods and save. *Consumer Reports* 71 (2):12–17.

Consumers Union. 2006. Diet and cancer: Can one size fit all? *Consumer Reports on Health* 18 (11):8–9.

Consumers Union. 2005. 'Super' foods: Do you really need them. *Consumer Reports on Health* 17 (6):1, 4–6.

Consumers Union. 2005. The new do's and dont's for protecting your heart. *Consumer Reports on Health* 17 (7):1, 4–6.

Consumers Union. 2005. You are what they eat. *Consumer Reports* 70 (1):26–31.

Consumers Union. 2004. Dangerous supplements: Still at large. *Consumer Reports* 69 (5):12–17.

Consumers Union. 2003. The truth about irradiated meat. *Consumer Reports* 68 (8):34–37.

Consumers Union. 2002. How safe is that burger? *Consumer Reports* 67 (11):29–35.

Consumers Union. 2000. Debate over genetically engineered food heats up. *Consumer Reports* 65 (6):48.

Corliss, R. 2002. Should we all be vegetarians? Would we be healthier? Would the planet? The risks and benefits of a meat-free life. *Time* 160 (3):48–56.

Craig, W. 2009. Health effects of vegan diets. *American Journal of Clinical Nutrition* 89:1627S–1633S.

Dangour, A., et al. 2010. Nutrition-related health effects of organic foods: A systematic review. *American Journal of Clinical Nutrition* 92:203–10.

Ding, E., and Mozaffarian, D. 2006. Optimal dietary habits for prevention of stroke. *Seminars in Neurology* 26:11–23.

Fairfield, K., and Fletcher, R. 2002. Vitamins for chronic disease prevention in adults. *Journal of the American Medical Association* 287:3116–26.

Feldeisen, S., and Tucker, K. 2007. Nutritional strategies in the prevention and treatment of metabolic syndrome. *Applied Physiology, Nutrition & Metabolism* 32:46–60.

Felton, J., et al. 2002. Human exposure to heterocyclic amine food mutagens/carcinogens: Relevance to breast cancer. *Environmental Molecular Mutagenesis* 39:112–18.

Finley, J., et al. 2006. Food processing: Nutrition, safety, and quality. In *Modern Nutrition in Health and Disease,* eds. M. Shils et al. Philadelphia: Lippincott Williams & Wilkins.

Fletcher, R., and Fairfield, K. 2002. Vitamins for chronic disease prevention in adults: Clinical applications. *Journal of the American Medical Association* 287:3127–29.

Fuhrman, J., and Ferreri, D. 2010. Fueling the vegetarian (vegan) athlete. *Current Sports Medicine Reports* 9:233–41.

Giugliano, D., et al. 2006. The effects of diet on inflammation: Emphasis on metabolic syndrome. *Journal of the American College of Cardiology* 48:677–85.

Halliwell, B. 2007. Dietary polyphenols: Good, bad, or indifferent for your health? *Cardiovascular Research* 73:341–347.

Hargreaves, M. 2001. Pre-exercise nutritional strategies: Effects on metabolism and performance. *Canadian Journal of Applied Physiology* 26:S64–70.

Hawley, J., et al. 2006. Promoting training adaptations through nutritional interventions. *Journal of Sports Sciences* 24:709–21.

Heber, D. 2004. Vegetables, fruits and phytoestrogens in the prevention of diseases. *Journal of Postgraduate Medicine* 50:145–49.

Hefle, S., and Taylor, S. 2004. Food allergy and the food industry. *Current Allergy & Asthma Reports* 4:55–59.

Hsieh, Y., and Ofori, J. 2007. Innovations in food technology for health. *Asia Pacific Journal of Clinical Nutrition* 16 (Supplement 1):65–73.

Hunt, J. 2002. Moving toward a plant-based diet: Are iron and zinc at risk? *Nutrition Reviews* 60:127–34.

Hurley, J., and Liebman, B. 2005. Fast food in '05. *Nutrition Action Health Letter* 32 (2):12–15.

International Food Information Council Foundation. 1999. Myths and facts about food biotechnology. *Food Insight* September/October:2–3.

Johnston, P., and Sabate, J. 2006. Nutritional implications of vegetarian diets. In *Modern Nutrition in Health and Disease,* eds. M. Shils et al. Philadelphia: Lippincott Williams & Wilkins.

Katsilambros, N., et al. 2006. Critical review of the international guidelines: What is agreed upon—what is not? *Nestle Nutrition Workshop Series: Clinical & Performance Programme* 11:207–18.

Kavanaugh, C., et al. 2007. The U.S. Food and Drug Administration's evidence-based review for qualified health claims: Tomatoes, lycopene, and cancer. *Journal of the*

National Cancer Institute 99: 1074–85.

Keet, C., and Wood, R. 2007. Food allergy and anaphylaxis. *Immunology & Allergy Clinics of North America* 27:193–212.

Kennedy, D. 2004. Dietary diversity, diet quality, and body weight regulation. *Nutrition Reviews* 62:S78–S81.

Kennedy, E. 2006. Evidence for nutritional benefits in prolonging wellness. *American Journal of Clinical Nutrition* 83: 410S–14S.

King, J. 2002. Biotechnology: A solution for improving nutrient bioavailability. *International Journal of Vitamin & Nutrition Research* 72:7–12.

Krebs-Smith, S., and Kris-Etherton, P. 2007. How does MyPyramid compare to other population-based recommendations for controlling chronic disease? *Journal of the American Dietetic Association* 107:830–37.

Lichtenstein, A., and Russell, R. 2005. Essential nutrients: Food or supplements? Where should the emphasis be? *Journal of the American Medical Association* 294:351–58.

Liu, R. 2004. Potential synergy of phytochemicals in cancer prevention: Mechanism of action. *Journal of Nutrition* 134:3479S–85S.

Lynn, A., et al. 2006. Cruciferous vegetables and colorectal cancer. *Proceedings of the Nutrition Society* 65:135–44.

Magkos, F., et al. 2006. Organic food: Buying more safety or just peace of mind? A critical review of the literature. *Critical Reviews in Food Science & Nutrition* 46:23–56.

Mann, N. 2000. Dietary lean meat and human evolution. *European Journal of Nutrition* 39:71–79.

Mares-Perlman, J., et al. 2002. The body of evidence to support a protective role for lutein and zeaxanthin in delaying chronic disease: Overview. *Journal of Nutrition* 132:518S–24S.

Massey, B. 2002. Dietary supplements. *Medical Clinics of North America* 86:127–47.

Maughan, R. 2002. The athlete's diet: Nutritional goals and dietary strategies. *Proceedings of the Nutrition Society* 6:87–96.

Maughan, R., and Shirreffs, S. 2007. Nutrition and hydration concerns of the female football player. *British Journal of Sports Medicine* 41 (Supplement 1):60–63.

Meadows, M. 2007. How the FDA works to keep produce safe. *FDA Consumer* 41 (2):13–19.

Meadows, M. 2002. Plastics and the microwave. *FDA Consumer* 36 (6):30.

Michels, K., et al. 2007. Diet and breast cancer: A review of the prospective observational studies. *Cancer* 109:2712–49.

Mozaffarian, D., and Rimm, E. 2006. Fish intake, contaminants, and human health: Evaluating the risks and the benefits. *Journal of the American Medical Association* 296:1885–99.

Needham, L., et al. 2005. Concentrations of environmental chemicals associated with neurodevelopmental effects in U.S. population. *Neurotoxicology* 26:531–45.

Nesheim, M. 1999. What is the research base for the use of dietary supplements? *Public Health Nutrition* 2:35–38.

Neuhouser, M. 2004. Dietary flavonoids and cancer risk: Evidence from human population studies. *Nutrition & Cancer* 50:1–7.

Nicklas, T., et al. 1998. Nutrient contribution of breakfast, secular trends, and the role of ready-to-eat cereals: A review of data from the Bogalusa Heart Study. *American Journal of Clinical Nutrition* 67:757S–763S.

Ortega, R. 2006. Importance of functional foods in the Mediterranean diet. *Public Health Nutrition* 9:1136–40.

Parnes, R., and Lichtenstein, A. 2004. Food irradiation: A safe and useful technology. *Nutrition in Clinical Care* 7:149–55.

Petrie, H., et al. 2004. Nutritional concerns for the child and adolescent competitor. *Nutrition* 20:620–31.

Reedy, J., and Krebs-Smith, S. 2008. A comparison of food-based recommendations and nutrient values of three food guides: USDA's MyPyramid, NHLBI's Dietary Approaches to Stop Hypertension Eating Plan, and Harvard's Healthy Eating Pyramid. *Journal of the American Dietetic Association* 108:522–28.

Roberts, W. O. 2007. Can children and adolescents run marathons? *Sports Medicine* 37:299–301.

Rock, C. 2007. Multivitamin-multimineral supplements: Who uses them? *American Journal of Clinical Nutrition* 85: 277S–79S.

Rosenbloom, C., et al. 2006. Special populations: The female player and the youth player. *Journal of Sports Sciences* 24: 783–93.

Schardt, D. 2007. Organic foods: Worth the price? *Nutrition Action Health Letter* 34 (6):3–8.

Seal, C. 2006. Whole grains and CVD risk. *Proceedings of the Nutrition Society* 65:24–34.

Seiler, S., et al. 2007. The fall and rise of the gender difference in elite anaerobic performance 1952–2006. *Medicine and Science in Sports & Exercise* 39:534–40.

Skibola, C., and Smith, M. 2000. Potential health impacts of excessive flavonoid intake. *Free Radicals in Biology & Medicine* 29:375–83.

Thomas, P. 1996. Food for thought about dietary supplements: Scientific review. *Nutrition Today* 31 (March/April):46–54.

Thompson, L. 2000. Are bioengineered foods safe? *FDA Consumer* 34 (1):18–23.

Truswell, A. 2002. Meat consumption and cancer of the large bowel. *European Journal of Clinical Nutrition* 56:S19–24.

Tufts University. 2008. Can you afford to eat right? *Health & Nutrition Letter* 26 (3):4–5.

Tufts University. 2007. Eating to beat cancer. *Health and Nutrition Letter* 25 (3): Special.

Tufts University. 2007. Five new reasons to get whole grains. *Health & Nutrition Letter* 25 (6):1–2.

Tufts University. 2005. Beef: Is it still what's for dinner? *Tufts University Health and Nutrition Letter* 23 (8): Supplement, 1–4.

Van Duyn, M., and Pivonka, E. 2000. Overview of the health benefits of fruit and vegetable consumption for the dietetics professional: Selected literature. *Journal of the American Dietetic Association* 100:1511–21.

Van Maele-Fabry, G., et al. 2006. Review and meta-analysis of risk estimates for prostate cancer in pesticide manufacturing workers. *Cancer Causes & Control* 17:353–73.

Venderley, A., and Campbell, W. 2006. Vegetarian diets: Nutritional considerations for athletes. *Sports Medicine* 36:293–305.

Volek, J., et al. 2006. Nutritional aspects of women strength athletes. *British Journal of Sports Medicine* 40:742–48.

Weiss, B., et al. 2004. Pesticides. *Pediatrics* 113:1030–36.

Willett, W. 2006. The Mediterranean diet: Science and practice. *Public Health & Nutrition* 9:105–10.

Williams, C. 2006. Nutrition to promote recovery from exercise. *Sports Science Exchange* 19 (1):1–6.

Williams, C. 2002. Nutritional quality of organic food: Shades of grey or shades of green? *Proceedings of the Nutrition Society* 61:19–24.

Williams, M. 2008. Nutrition for the school aged child athlete. In *The Young Athlete,* eds. H. Hebestreit and O. Bar-Or. Oxford: Blackwell Publishing.

Wilson, B., and Bahna, S. 2005. Adverse reactions to food additives. *Annals* of Allergy, Asthma & Immunology 95:499–507.

Wood, O., and Bruhn, C. 2000. Position of the American Dietetic Association: Food irradiation. *Journal of the American Dietetic Association* 100:246–53.

Woolf, S. 2006. Weighing the evidence to formulate dietary guidelines. *Journal of the American College of Nutrition* 25:277S–84S.

Worthington, V. 2001. Nutritional quality of organic versus conventional fruits, vegetables, and grains. *Journal of Alternative & Complementary Medicine* 7:161–73.

Yates, A., et al. 1998. Dietary Reference Intakes: The new basis for recommendations for calcium and related nutrients, B vitamins, and choline. *Journal of the American Dietetic Association* 98:699–706.

Specific Studies

Appel, L., et al. 2005. Effects of protein, monounsaturated fat, and carbohydrate intake on blood pressure and serum lipids: Results of the OmniHeart randomized trial. *Journal of the American Medical Association* 294:2455–64.

Baker, B., et al. 2002. Pesticide residues in conventional, integrated pest management (IPM)-grown and organic foods: Insights from three US data sets. *Food Additives & Contaminants* 19:427–46.

Bazzano, L., et al. 2002. Fruit and vegetable intake and risk of cardiovascular disease in US adults: The first National Health and Nutrition Examination Survey Epidemiologic Follow-up Study. *American Journal of Clinical Nutrition* 76:93–99.

Bray, G., et al. 2007. Hormonal responses to a fast-food meal compared with nutritionally comparable meals of different composition. *Annals of Nutrition and Metabolism* 51:163–71.

Chao, A., et al. 2005. Meat consumption and risk of colorectal cancer. *JAMA* 293:172–82.

Cho, E., et al. 2006. Red meat intake and risk of breast cancer among premenopausal women. *Archives of Internal Medicine* 166:2253–59.

Cohen, R., et al. 2002. Complementary and alternative medicine (CAM) use by older adults: A comparison of self-report and physician chart documentation. *Journal of Gerontology Medical Sciences* 57:M223–7.

Dragsted, L., et al. 2006. Biological effects of fruits and vegetables. *Proceedings of the Nutrition Society* 65:61–67.

Jensen, M., et al. 2004. Intakes of whole grains, bran, and germ and the risk of coronary heart disease in men. *American Journal of Clinical Nutrition* 80:1492–99.

Maffucci, D., and McMurray, R. 2000. Towards optimizing the timing of the pre-exercise meal. *International Journal of Sport Nutrition & Exercise Metabolism* 10:103–13.

Martins, Y., et al. 1999. Restrained eating among vegetarians: Does a vegetarian eating style mask concerns about weight? *Appetite* 32:145–54.

McCann, D., et al. 2007. Food additives and hyperactive behaviour in 3-year-old and 8/9-year-old children in the community: A randomised, double-blinded, placebo-controlled trial. *Lancet* 370:1560–67.

Neuhouser, M., et al. 1999. Use of food nutrition labels is associated with lower fat intake. *Journal of the American Dietetic Association* 99:45–53.

Newberry, H., et al. 2001. Use of nonvitamin, nonmineral dietary supplements among college students. *Journal of the American College of Health* 50:123–29.

Nicholls, S., et al. 2006. Consumption of saturated fat impairs the anti-inflammatory properties of high-density lipoproteins and endothelial function. *Journal of the American College of Cardiology* 48:715–20.

O'Neil, C., et al. 2010. Whole-grain consumption is associated with diet quality and nutrient intake in adults: The National Health and Nutrition Examination Survey, 1999–2004. *Journal of the American Dietetic Association* 110:1461–8.

Paoli, A., et al. 2011. Exercising fasting or fed to enhance fat loss? Influence of food intake on respiratory ratio and excess postexercise oxygen consumption after a bout of endurance training. *International Journal of Sport Nutrition & Exercise Metabolism* 21:48–54.

Pereira, M., et al. 2005. Fast-food habits, weight gain, and insulin resistance (the CARDIA study): 15-year prospective analysis. *The Lancet* 365:36–42.

Rothman, R., et al. 2006. Patient understanding of food labels: The role of literacy and numeracy. *American Journal of Preventive Medicine* 31:391–98.

Sinha, R., et al. 2009. Meat intake and mortality: A prospective study of over half a million people. *Archives of Internal Medicine* 169:562–71.

Steck, S., et al. 2007. Cooked meat and risk of breast cancer—lifetime versus recent dietary intake. *Epidemiology* 18:373–82.

Taylor, E., et al. 2007. Meat consumption and risk of breast cancer in the UK Women's cohort study. *British Journal of Cancer* 96:1139–46.

CHAPTER THREE

Human Energy

L E A R N I N G   O B J E C T I V E S

After studying this chapter, you should be able to:

1. Understand the interrelationships among the various forms of chemical, thermal, and mechanical energy, and be able to perform mathematical conversions from one form of energy to another.

2. Identify the three major human energy systems, their major energy sources as stored in the body, and various nutrients needed to sustain them.

3. List the components of total daily energy expenditure (TDEE) and how each contributes to the total amount of caloric energy expended over a 24-hour period.

4. Describe the various factors that may influence resting energy expenditure (REE).

5. List and explain the various means whereby energy expenditure during exercise, or the thermic effect of exercise (TEE), may be measured, and be able to calculate conversions among the various methods.

6. Describe the three different muscle fiber types and the major characteristics of each in relation to energy production during exercise.

7. Explain the relationship between exercise intensity, particularly walking and running, and energy expenditure, and relate walking and running intensity to other types of physical activities.

8. Understand the concept of the physical activity level (PAL) and how it relates to estimated energy expenditure (EER). Calculate your EER based on an estimate of your PAL and the physical activity coefficient (PA).

9. Describe the role of the three energy systems during exercise.

10. Explain the various causes of fatigue during exercise and discuss nutritional interventions that may help delay the onset of fatigue.

As noted in chapter 1, the body uses the food we eat to provide energy, to build and repair tissues, and to regulate metabolism. Of these three functions, the human body ranks energy production first and will use food for this purpose at the expense of the other two functions in time of need. Energy is the essence of life.

Through technological processes, humans have harnessed a variety of energy sources, such as wind, waterfalls, the sun, wood, and oil, to operate the machines invented to make life easier. However, humans cannot use any of these energy sources for their own metabolism, but must rely on food sources found in nature. The food we eat must be converted into energy forms that the body can use. Thus, the human body is equipped with a number of metabolic systems to produce and regulate energy for its diverse needs, such as synthesis of tissues, movement of substances between tissues, and muscular contraction.

Sport energy! The underlying basis for the control of movement in all sports is human energy, and successful performance depends upon the ability of the athlete to produce the right amount of energy and to control its application to the specific demands of the sport. Sports differ in their energy demands. In some events, such as the 100-meter dash, success is dependent primarily upon the ability to produce energy very rapidly. In others, such as the 26.2-mile marathon, energy need not be produced so rapidly, but must be sustained at an optimal rate for a much longer period. In still other sports, such as golf, the athlete need not only produce energy at varying rates (compare the drive with the putt) but must carefully control the application of that energy. Thus, each sport imposes specific energy demands upon the athlete.

A discussion of the role of nutrition as a means to help provide and control human energy is important from several standpoints. First, inadequate supplies of necessary energy nutrients, such as muscle glycogen or blood glucose, may cause fatigue. Fatigue also may be caused by the inability of the energy systems to function optimally because of a deficiency of other nutrients, such as selected vitamins and minerals. In addition, the human body is capable of storing energy reserves in a variety of body forms, including body fat and muscle tissue. Excess body weight in the form of fat or decreased body weight due to losses of muscle tissue may adversely affect some types of athletic performance.

One purpose of this chapter is to review briefly the major human energy systems and how they are used in the body under conditions of exercise and rest. Following this, chapters 4 through 9 discuss the role of each of the major classes of nutrients as they relate to energy production in the human body, with the primary focus on prevention of fatigue caused by impaired energy production; chapter 13 details the effects of various food drugs and supplements on human energy systems. Another purpose of this chapter is to discuss the means by which humans store and expend energy. Chapters 10 through 12 focus on weight control methods and expand on some of the concepts presented in this chapter.

Measures of Energy

What is energy?

For our purposes, **energy** represents the capacity to do work. **Work** is one form of energy, often called *mechanical* or *kinetic energy*. When we throw a ball or run a mile, we have done work; we have produced mechanical energy.

Energy exists in a variety of other forms in nature, such as the light energy of the sun, nuclear energy in uranium, electrical energy in lightning storms, heat energy in fires, and chemical energy in oil. The six forms of energy—mechanical, chemical, heat, electrical, light, and nuclear—are interchangeable according to various laws of thermodynamics. We take advantage of these laws every day. One such example is the use of the chemical energy in gasoline to produce mechanical energy—the movement of our cars.

In the human body, four of these types of energy are important. Our bodies possess stores of *chemical energy* that can be used to produce *electrical energy* for creation of electrical nerve impulses, to produce *heat energy* to help keep our body temperature at 37°C (98.6°F) even on cold days, and to produce *mechanical energy* through muscle shortening so that we may move about.

The sun is the ultimate source of energy. Solar energy is harnessed by plants, through photosynthesis, to produce either plant carbohydrates, fats, or proteins, all forms of stored chemical energy. When humans consume plant and animal foods, the carbohydrates, fats, and proteins undergo a series of metabolic changes and are utilized to develop body structure, to regulate body processes, or to provide a storage form of chemical energy (figure 3.1).

The optimal intake and output of energy is important to all individuals, but especially for the physically active person. To perform to capacity, body energy stores must be used in the most efficient manner possible.

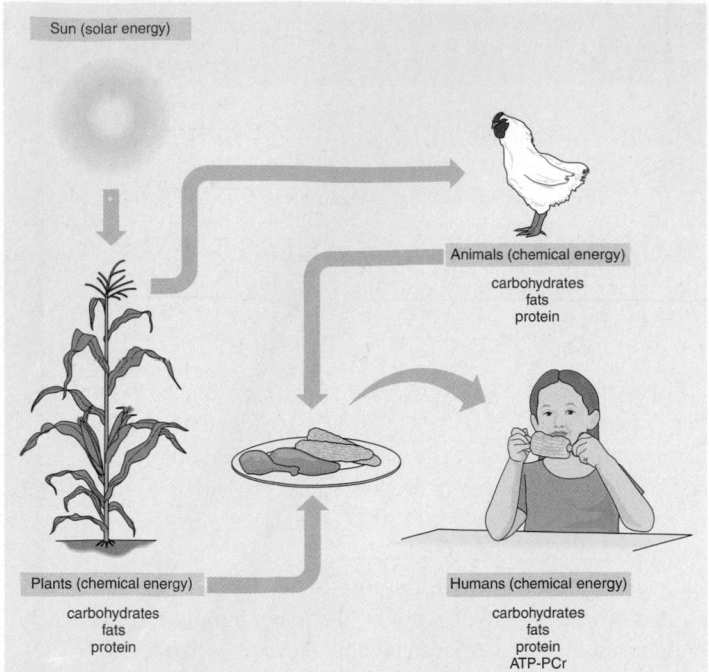

FIGURE 3.1 Through photosynthesis, plants utilize solar energy and convert it to chemical energy in the form of carbohydrates, fats, or proteins. Animals eat plants and convert the chemical energy into their own stores of chemical energy—primarily fat and protein. Humans ingest food from both plant and animal sources and convert the chemical energy for their own stores and use.

How do we measure work, physical activity, and energy expenditure?

Energy has been defined as the ability to do work. According to the physicist's definition, work is simply the product of force times vertical distance, or in formula format, Work = Force × Distance. When we speak of how fast work is done, the term **power** is used. Power is simply work divided by time, or Power = Work/Time.

Two major measurement systems have been used in the past to express energy in terms of either work or power. The metric system has been in use by most of the world, while England, its colonies, and the United States have used the English system. In an attempt to provide some uniformity in measurement systems around the world, the International Unit System (*Systeme International d'Unites,* or SI) has been developed. Most of the world has adopted the SI. Although legislation has been passed by Congress to convert the United States to the SI, and terms such as *gram, kilogram, milliliter, liter,* and *kilometer* are becoming more prevalent, it appears that it will take some time before this system becomes part of our everyday language.

The SI is used in most scientific journals today, but the other two systems appear in older journals. Terms that are used in each system are presented in table 3.1. For our purposes in this text, we shall use several English terms that are still in common usage in the United States, but if you read scientific literature, you should be able to convert values among the various systems if necessary. For example, work may be expressed as either foot-pounds, kilogram-meters (kgm), joules, or watts. If you weigh 150 pounds and climb a 20-foot flight

TABLE 3.1 Terms in the English, metric, and international systems

Unit	English system	Metric system	International system
Mass	slug	kilogram (kg)	kilogram (kg)
Distance	foot (ft)	meter (m)	meter (m)
Time	second (s)	second (s)	second (s)
Force	pound (lb)	newton (N)	newton (N)
Work	foot-pound (ft-lb)	kilogram-meter (kgm)	joule (J)
Power	horsepower (hp)	watt (W)	watt (W)

of stairs in one minute, you have done 3,000 foot-pounds of work. One kgm is equal to 7.23 foot-pounds, so you would do about 415 kgm. One **joule** is equal to about 0.102 kgm, so you have done about 4,062 joules of work. One watt is equal to one joule per second, so you have generated about 68 watts of power. Some basic interrelationships among the measurement systems are noted in table 3.2. Other equivalents may be found in appendix A.

In general, exercise and nutrition scientists are interested in measuring work output and energy expenditure under two conditions. One condition involves specific techniques in controlled laboratory research, whereas the other condition involves normal daily activities, including actual sports performance.

To measure work we need to know the weight of an object and the vertical distance through which it is moved. This is fine according to the formal definition of work, but are you doing work while holding a stationary weight out in front of your body? According to the formal definition, the answer is no, because the distance the weight moved is zero. How about when you come down stairs as compared to going up? It is much easier to descend the stairs, and yet according to the formula you have done the same amount of work. Also, how about when you run a mile? You know you have worked, but most of the distance you covered was horizontal, not vertical.

To accurately measure work output under laboratory conditions, scientists use devices known as ergometers. An **ergometer,** such as a cycle or arm ergometer, is designed to provide accurate measurements of work, including measures of power and total work output over specific periods of time.

Research on physical activity and energy expenditure assessment has increased dramatically during the past several years, and activity monitors such as pedometers and accelerometers are now widely used by the general public and researchers. Pedometers, which measure step counts but do not provide exercise intensity, can be used to measure or alter physical activity behaviors. Tudor-Locke and Lutes report that when self-monitoring of step counts is combined with recording of daily values, motivation to engage in physical activity may increase.

Accelerometers, which measure changes in acceleration in one to three planes, can be used to assess physical activity and energy expenditure, and can estimate exercise intensity. The newest accelerometers are smaller and lighter, contain long-lasting batteries, have increased memory capacity, and use advanced signal processing techniques to

TABLE 3.2 Some interrelationships between work measurement systems

Weight	Distance	Work	Power
1 kilogram = 2.2 pounds	1 meter = 3.28 feet	1 kgm = 7.23 foot-pounds	1 watt = 1 joule per second
1 kilogram = 1,000 grams	1 meter = 1.09 yards	1 kgm = 9.8 joules	1 watt = 6.12 kgm per minute 1 watt = 0.0013 horsepower
454 grams = 1 pound	1 foot = 0.30 meter	1 foot-pound = 0.138 kgm	1 horsepower = 550 foot-pounds per second
1 pound = 16 ounces	1,000 meters = 1 kilometer	1 foot-pound = 1.35 joules	1 horsepower = 33,000 foot-pounds per minute
1 ounce = 28.4 grams	1 kilometer = 0.6215 mile	1 newton = 0.102 kg	1 horsepower = 745.8 watts
3.5 ounces = 100 grams	1 mile = 1.61 kilometers 1 inch = 2.54 centimeters 1 centimeter = 0.39 inch	1 joule = 1 newton meter 1 kilojoule = 1,000 joules 1 megajoule = 1,000,000 joules 1 joule = 0.102 kgm 1 joule = 0.736 foot-pound 1 kilojoule = 102 kgm	

determine activity intensity, duration, and type. Pober and Staudenmayer, researchers in Patty Freedson's Physical Activity Laboratory in the Department of Kinesiology at the University of Massachusetts, are using sophisticated mathematical principles such as Hidden Markov Models and neural networks that allow the monitor to recognize what the wearer is doing. For instance, accelerometers can determine whether a person is performing household chores or playing a sport. Another advancement in the assessment of physical activity and energy expenditure is the characterization and measurement of sedentary behavior, which is a low level of physical activity that is below light intensity activity, but above resting levels. Matthews and others have shown, in a study of more than 6,000 participants (from children to older adults), that almost 55 percent of daily time is spent sedentary. The authors noted that Americans spend most of their time expending very little energy, which is critical, as Katzmarzyk and colleagues have shown a relationship between sitting time and all-cause and cardiovascular disease mortality. Thus, in addition to the recommendation to increase moderate- to vigorous-intensity physical activity, a reduction in sitting time and time spent in sedentary activities should also be encouraged. Improvements in physical activity and energy expenditure assessment will continue to improve with the combination of accelerometer signals and other factors such as location (using global positioning systems [GPS]) and biological variables such as galvanic skin temperature response.

Several methods are available to measure energy expenditure in humans. One is **calorimetry,** which measures heat energy. Figure 3.2 illustrates a bomb calorimeter, which may be used to measure the energy content of a given substance. For example, a gram of fat contains a certain amount of chemical energy. When placed in the calorimeter and oxidized completely, the heat it gives off can be recorded. We then know the heat energy of one gram of fat and can equate it to chemical or work units of energy if needed. Large, expensive whole-room calorimeters (metabolic chambers) are available that can accommodate human beings and measure their heat production under normal home activities and some conditions of exercise. This technique is known as *direct calorimetry.*

A second, more commonly used method of measuring energy expenditure is to determine the amount of oxygen an individual consumes, an *indirect calorimetry* technique. This procedure is normally done under laboratory conditions (see figure 3.3), but lightweight portable oxygen analyzers are also available to record energy expenditure in freely moving individuals. The volume of oxygen one uses is usually expressed in liters (L) or milliliters (ml); one L is equal to 1,000 ml. One liter is slightly larger than a quart. In general, humans need oxygen, which helps metabolize the various nutrients in the body to produce energy. It is known that when

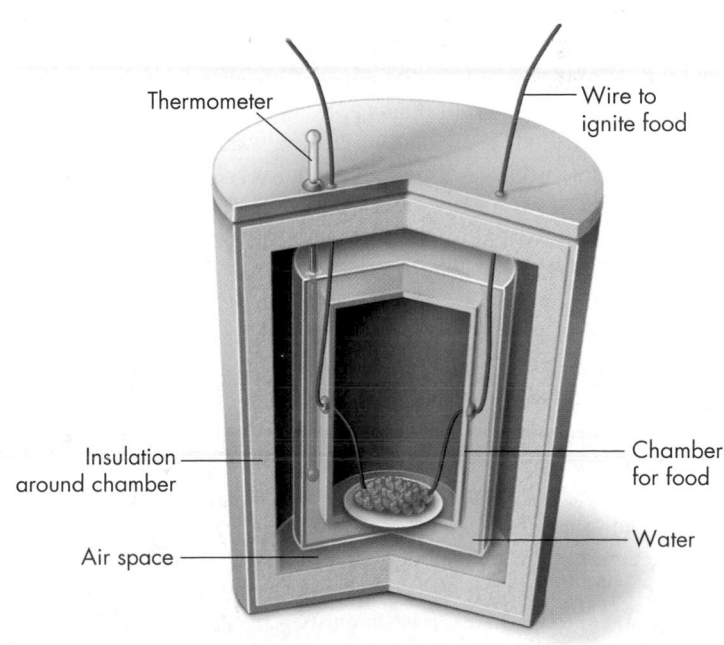

FIGURE 3.2 A bomb calorimeter. The food in the calorimeter is combusted via electrical ignition. The heat (Calories) given off by the food raises the temperature of the water, thereby providing data about the caloric content of specific foodstuffs.

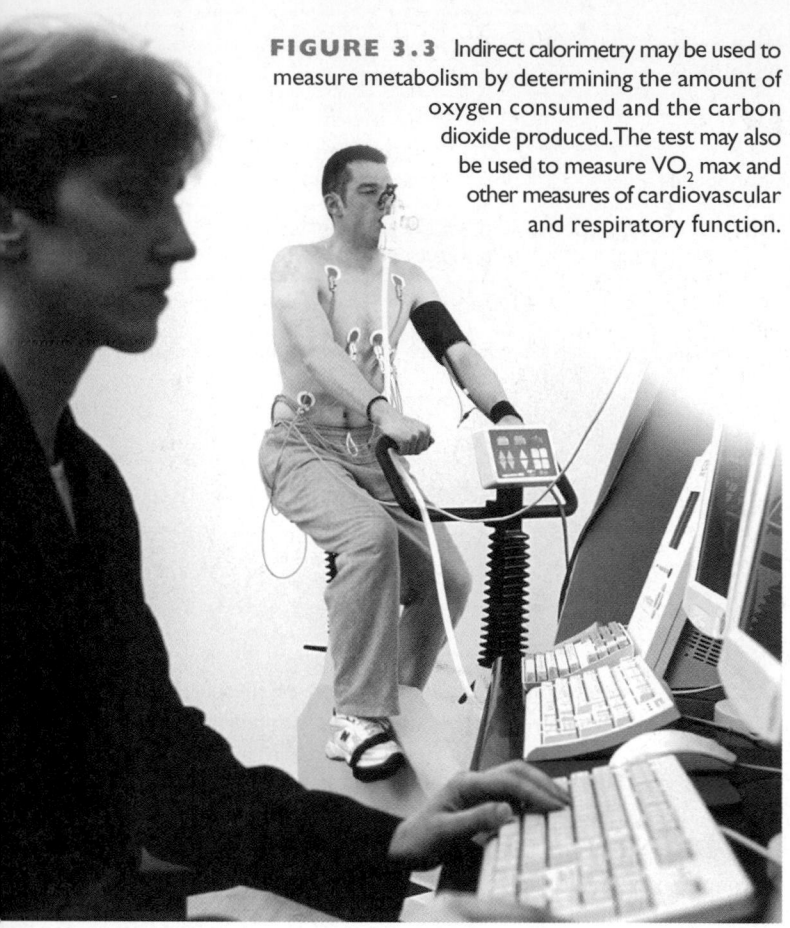

FIGURE 3.3 Indirect calorimetry may be used to measure metabolism by determining the amount of oxygen consumed and the carbon dioxide produced. The test may also be used to measure VO$_2$ max and other measures of cardiovascular and respiratory function.

oxygen combines with a gram of carbohydrate, fat, or protein, a certain amount of energy is released. If we can accurately measure the oxygen consumption (and carbon dioxide production) of an individual, we can get a pretty good measure of energy expenditure. The amount of oxygen used can be equated to other forms of energy, such as work done in foot-pounds or heat produced in Calories.

Another method is the doubly labeled water (DLW) technique in which stable isotopes of hydrogen and oxygen in water (^{2}H$_2$^{18}O) are ingested. This is a safe procedure, as the isotopes are stable and emit no radiation. Analysis of urine and blood samples provides data on ^{2}H and ^{18}O excretion. The labeled oxygen is eliminated from the body as water and carbon dioxide, whereas the hydrogen is eliminated only as water. Subtracting the hydrogen losses from the oxygen losses provides a measure of carbon dioxide fluctuation, which may be converted to energy expenditure. Although expensive, the advantage of this technique is that it may be used with individuals while they perform their normal daily activities, and they need not be confined to a metabolic chamber or be attached to equipment to measure oxygen consumption. Despite the advantages of the doubly labeled water technique, this method does not provide an estimate of exercise intensity. Whereas energy expended may be useful in energy balance or weight management, exercise intensity is needed to prescribe exercise programs that reduce disease risk or improve fitness according to the guidelines set by the American College of Sports Medicine.

Although all of these techniques to measure work and energy expenditure have limitations, they do provide useful data relative to the approximate energy cost of exercise and normal daily activities.

What is the most commonly used measure of energy?

Although there are a number of different ways to express energy, the most common term used in the past and still most prevalent and understood in the United States by most people is **Calorie.**

A calorie is a measure of heat. One gram calorie represents the amount of heat needed to raise the temperature of one gram of water one degree Celsius. A kilocalorie is equal to 1,000 small calories. It is the amount of heat needed to raise 1 kg of water (1 L) one degree Celsius. In human nutrition, because the gram calorie is so small, the kilocalorie is the main expression of energy. It is usually abbreviated as kcal, kc, or C, or capitalized as Calorie. Throughout this book, *Calorie* or *C* will refer to the kilocalorie.

According to the principles underlying the first law of thermodynamics, energy may be equated from one form to another. Thus, the Calorie, which represents thermal or heat energy, may be equated to other forms of energy. Relative to our discussion concerning physical work such as exercise and its interrelationships with nutrition, it is important to equate the Calorie with mechanical work and the chemical energy stored in the body. As will be explained later, most stored chemical energy must undergo some form of oxidation in order to release its energy content as work.

The following represents some equivalent energy values for the Calorie in terms of mechanical work and oxygen utilization. Some examples illustrating several of the interrelationships will be used in later chapters.

$$1\ C = 3,086\ \text{foot-pounds}$$
$$1\ C = 427\ \text{kgm}$$
$$1\ C = 4.2\ \text{kilojoules (kJ) or 4,200 joules}$$
$$1\ C = 200\ \text{ml oxygen (approximately)}$$

Although the Calorie is the most commonly used expression in the United States for energy, work, and heat, the **kilojoule** is the proper term in the SI and is used by the rest of the world. It is important for you to be able to convert from Calories to kilojoules, and vice versa. To convert Calories to kilojoules, multiply the number of Calories by 4.2 (4.186 to be exact); to convert kilojoules to Calories, divide the number of kilojoules by 4.2. Simply multiplying or dividing by 4 for each respective conversion will provide a ballpark estimate. In some cases megajoules (MJ), a million joules, are used to express energy. One MJ equals about 240 Calories, or 4.2 MJ is the equivalent of about 1,000 Calories.

Through the use of a calorimeter, the energy contents of the basic nutrients have been determined. Energy may be derived from the three major foodstuffs—carbohydrate, fat, and protein—plus alcohol. The caloric value of each of these three nutrients may vary somewhat, depending on the particular structure of the different forms. For example, carbohydrate may exist in several forms—as glucose, sucrose, or starch—and the caloric value of each will differ slightly. In general, one gram of each of the three nutrients and alcohol, measured in a calorimeter, yields the following Calories:

$$1\ \text{gram carbohydrate} = 4.30\ C$$
$$1\ \text{gram fat} = 9.45\ C$$

1 gram protein = 5.65 C

1 gram alcohol = 7.00 C

Unfortunately, or fortunately if one is trying to lose weight, humans do not extract all of this energy from the food they eat. The human body is not as efficient as the calorimeter. For one, the body cannot completely absorb all the food eaten. Only about 97 percent of ingested carbohydrate, 95 percent of fat, and 92 percent of protein are absorbed. In addition, a good percentage of the protein is not completely oxidized in the body, with some of the nitrogen waste products being excreted in the urine. In summary, then, the caloric value of food is reduced somewhat in relation to the values given previously. Although the following values are not exactly precise, they are approximate enough to be used effectively in determining the caloric values of the foods we eat. Thus, the following caloric values are used throughout this text as a practical guide:

Carbohydrate
4 kcal per gram

Protein
4 kcal per gram

Energy sources for body functions

Alcohol
7 kcal per gram

Fat
9 kcal per gram

1 gram carbohydrate = 4 C

1 gram fat = 9 C

1 gram protein = 4 C

1 gram alcohol = 7 C

For our purposes, the Calories in food represent a form of potential energy to be used by our bodies to produce heat and work (figure 3.4). However, the fact that fat has about twice the amount of energy per gram as carbohydrate (figure 3.5) does not mean that it is a better energy source for the active individual, as we shall see in later chapters when we talk of the efficient utilization of body fuels.

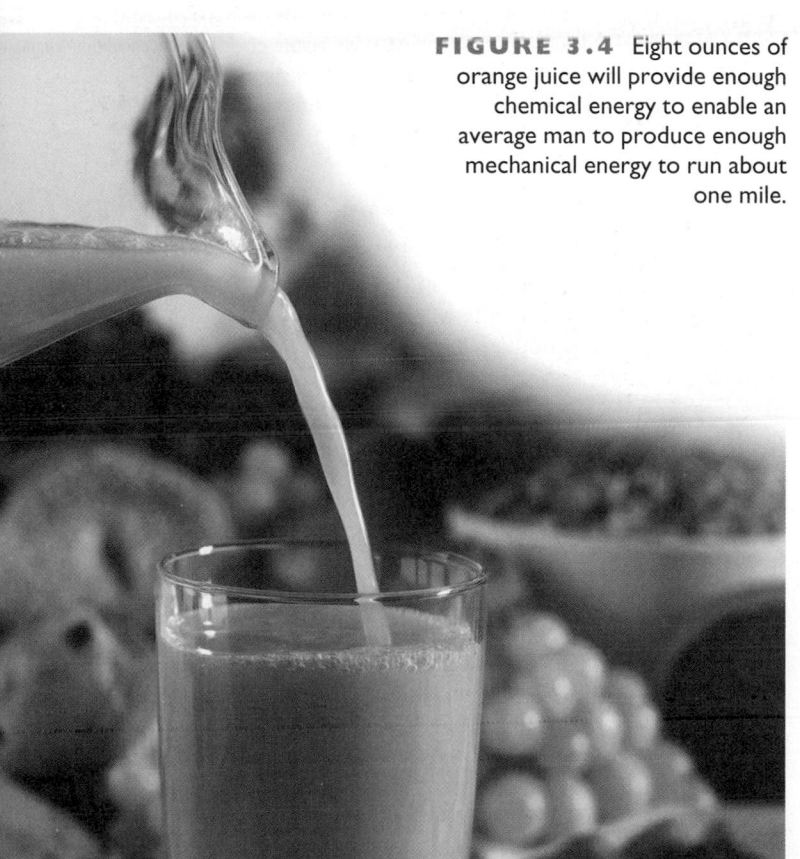

FIGURE 3.4 Eight ounces of orange juice will provide enough chemical energy to enable an average man to produce enough mechanical energy to run about one mile.

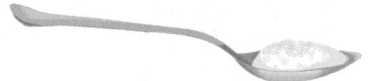

1 teaspoon sugar = 5 grams carbohydrate = 20 Calories

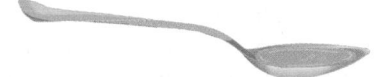

1 teaspoon salad oil = 5 grams fat = 45 Calories

FIGURE 3.5 The Calorie as a measure of energy.

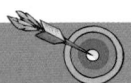

Key Concepts

- Energy represents the capacity to do work, and food is the source of energy for humans.
- Energy expenditure in humans may be estimated in a variety of different ways, including both direct and indirect calorimetry, doubly labeled water, accelerometers, and pedometers. Each of these techniques has advantages and disadvantages.
- The Calorie, or kilocalorie, is a measure of chemical energy stored in foods; this chemical energy can be transformed into heat and mechanical work energy in the body. A related measure is the kilojoule. One Calorie is equal to 4.2 kilojoules.
- Carbohydrates and fats are the primary energy nutrients, but protein may also be an energy source during rest and exercise. In the human body 1 gram of carbohydrate = 4 Calories, 1 gram of fat = 9 Calories, and 1 gram of protein = 4 Calories. Alcohol is also a source of energy; 1 gram = 7 Calories.

Check for Yourself

- Measure the height of a step on a flight of stairs or bleachers and convert it to feet (9 inches = 0.75 foot). Stepping in place, count the total number of steps you do in one minute. Multiply your count by the step height to determine the number of feet you have climbed. Next, multiply this value by your body weight in pounds to determine the number of foot-pounds of work you have done. Then, convert this number of foot-pounds to the equivalent amount of kilogram-meters (kgm), kilojoules (kJ), and Calories.

Human Energy Systems

How is energy stored in the body?

The ultimate source of all energy on earth is the sun. Solar energy is harnessed by plants, which take carbon, hydrogen, oxygen, and nitrogen from their environment and manufacture either carbohydrate, fat, or protein. These foods possess stored energy. When we consume these foods, our digestive processes break them down into simple compounds that are absorbed into the body and transported to various cells. One of the basic purposes of body cells is to transform the chemical energy of these simple compounds into forms that may be available for immediate use or other forms that may be available for future use.

Energy in the body is available for immediate use in the form of **adenosine triphosphate (ATP).** It is a complex molecule constructed with high-energy bonds, which, when split by enzyme action, can release energy rapidly for a number of body processes, including muscle contraction. ATP is classified as a high-energy compound and is stored in the tissues in small amounts. It is important to note that ATP is the immediate source of energy for all body functions, and the other energy stores are used to replenish ATP at varying rates. Myburgh notes that muscle contraction is totally dependent on ATP, so the body has developed an intricate system to help replenish ATP as rapidly as needed.

Another related high-energy phosphate compound, **phosphocreatine (PCr),** is also found in the tissues in small amounts. Although it cannot be used as an immediate source of energy, it can rapidly replenish ATP.

ATP may be formed from either carbohydrate, fat, or protein after those nutrients have undergone some complex biochemical changes in the body. Figure 3.6 represents a basic schematic of how ATP is formed from each of these three nutrients.

Because ATP and PCr are found in very small amounts in the body and can be used up in a matter of seconds, it is important to have adequate energy stores as a backup system. Your body stores of carbohydrate, fat, and protein can provide you with ample amounts of ATP, enough to last for many weeks even on a starvation diet. The digestion and metabolism of carbohydrate, fat, and protein are discussed in their respective chapters, so it is unnecessary to present that full discussion here. However, you may wish to preview figure 3.12 to visualize the metabolic interrelationships among the three nutrients in the body. For those who desire more detailed schematics of energy pathways, appendix G provides some of the major metabolic pathways for carbohydrate, fat, and protein.

It is important to note that parts of each energy nutrient may be converted to the other two nutrients in the body under certain circumstances. For example, protein may be converted into carbohydrate during prolonged exercise, whereas excess dietary carbohydrate may be converted to fat in the body during rest.

Table 3.3 summarizes how much energy is stored in the human body as ATP, PCr, and various forms of carbohydrate, fat, and protein. The total amount of energy, represented by Calories, is approximate and may vary considerably between individuals. Carbohydrate is stored in limited amounts as blood (serum) glucose, liver glycogen, and muscle glycogen. The largest amount of energy is stored in the body as fats. Fats are stored as triglycerides in both muscle tissue and adipose (fat) tissue; triglycerides and free fatty acids (FFA) in the blood are a limited supply. The protein of the body tissues, particularly muscle tissue, is a large reservoir of energy but is not used to any great extent under normal circumstances. Table 3.3 also depicts how far an individual could run using the total of each of these energy sources as the sole supply. The role of each of these macronutrient energy stores during exercise is an important consideration that is discussed briefly in this chapter and more extensively in their respective chapters.

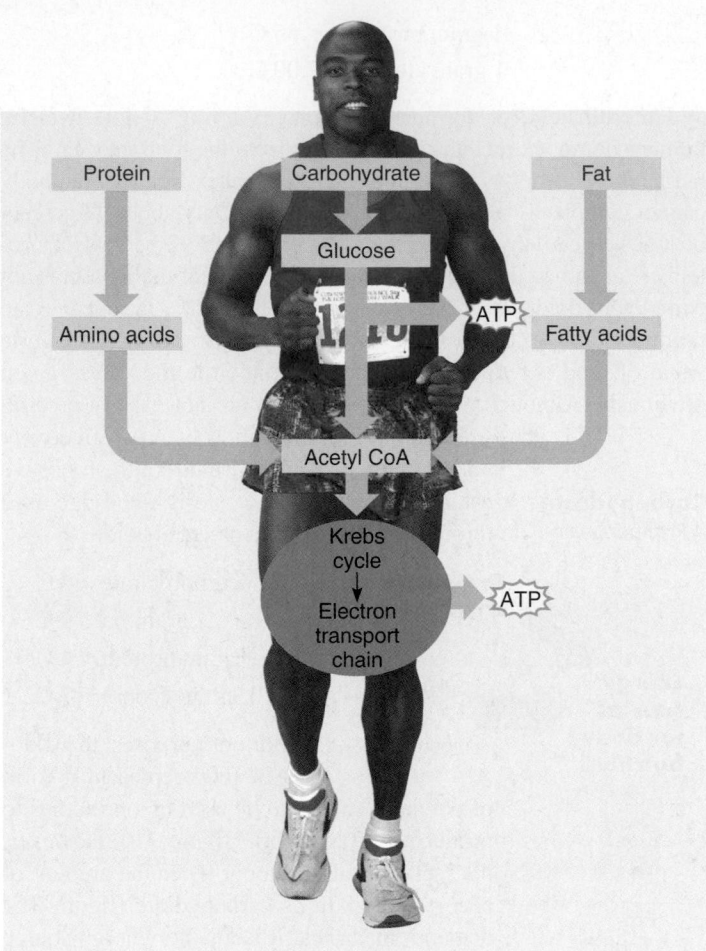

FIGURE 3.6 Simplified schematic of ATP formation from carbohydrate, fat, and protein. All three nutrients may be used to form ATP, but carbohydrate and fat are the major sources via the aerobic metabolism of the Krebs cycle. Carbohydrate may be used to produce small amounts of ATP under anaerobic conditions, thus providing humans with the ability to produce energy rapidly without oxygen for relatively short periods. For more details, see appendix G.

What are the human energy systems?

Why does the human body store chemical energy in a variety of different forms? If we look at human energy needs from an historical perspective, the answer becomes obvious. Sometimes humans needed to produce energy at a rapid rate, such as when sprinting to safety to avoid dangerous animals. Thus, a fast rate of energy production was an important human energy feature that helped ensure survival. At other times, our ancient ancestors may have been deprived of adequate food for long periods, and thus needed a storage capacity for chemical energy that would sustain life throughout these times of deprivation. Hence, the ability to store large amounts of energy was also important for survival. These two factors—rate of energy production and energy capacity—appear to be determining factors in the development of human energy systems.

One need only watch weekend television programming for several weeks to realize the diversity of sports popular throughout

TABLE 3.3   Major energy stores in the human body with approximate total caloric value*

Energy source	Major storage form	Total body Calories	Total body kilojoules	Distance covered**
ATP	Tissues	1	4.2	17.5 yards
PCr	Tissues	4	16.8	70 yards
Carbohydrate	Serum glucose	20	88	350 yards
	Liver glycogen	400	1,680	4 miles
	Muscle glycogen	1,500	6,300	15 miles
Fat	Serum-free fatty acids	7	29.2	123 yards
	Serum triglycerides	75	315	0.75 mile
	Muscle triglycerides	2,500	10,500	25 miles
	Adipose tissue triglycerides	80,000	336,000	800 miles
Protein	Muscle protein	30,000	126,000	300 miles

See text for discussion.
*These values may have extreme variations depending on the size of the individual, amount of body fat, physical fitness level, and diet.
**Running at an energy cost of 100 Calories per mile (1.6 kilometers).

the world. Each of these sports imposes certain requirements on humans who want to be successful competitors. For some sports, such as weight lifting, the main requirement is brute strength, while for others such as tennis, quick reactions and hand/eye coordination are important. A major consideration in most sports is the rate of energy production, which can range from the explosive power needed by a shot-putter to the tremendous endurance capacity of an ultramarathoner. The physical performance demands of different sports require specific sources of energy.

As noted previously, the body stores energy in a variety of ways—in ATP, PCr, muscle glycogen, and so on. In order for this energy to be used to produce muscular contractions and movement, it must undergo certain biochemical reactions in the muscle. These biochemical reactions serve as a basis for classifying human energy expenditure by several energy, or power, systems.

In the text *Sports Physiology,* one of the first to discuss the application of human energy systems to sport, Edward L. Fox named three human energy systems—the ATP-PCr system, the lactic acid system, and the oxygen system. As noted below, other terminology may be used to describe the metabolic relationships to these three energy systems, but the original classification is still useful when discussing the application of human energy to sport performance.

The **ATP-PCr system** is also known as the *phosphagen system* because both adenosine triphosphate and phosphocreatine contain phosphates. ATP is the immediate source of energy for almost all body processes, including muscle contraction. This high-energy compound, stored in the muscles, rapidly releases energy when an electrical impulse arrives in the muscle. See figure 3.7 for a graphical representation of ATP breakdown. No matter what you do, scratch your nose or lift 100 pounds, ATP breakdown

makes the movement possible. ATP must be present for the muscles to contract. The body has a limited supply of ATP and must replace it rapidly if muscular work is to continue. The main purpose of every other energy system, including PCr, is to help regenerate ATP to enable muscle contraction to continue at the optimal desired rate.

PCr, which is also a high-energy compound found in the muscle, can help form ATP rapidly as ATP is used. Energy released when PCr splits is used to form ATP from ADP and P. PCr is also in short supply (but more than ATP) and has to be replenished if used. PCr breakdown to help resynthesize ATP is illustrated in figure 3.8.

The ATP-PCr system is critical to energy production. Because these phosphagens are in short supply, any all-out exercise for 5 to 10 seconds could deplete the supply, particularly PCr, in a given muscle. Hence, the phosphagens must be replaced, and this is the function of the other energy sources. Increasing the level of PCr in the muscle would provide a greater fuel reserve and possibly enhance the performance of brief high-intensity exercise. Creatine supplementation, discussed in later chapters, is one way athletes

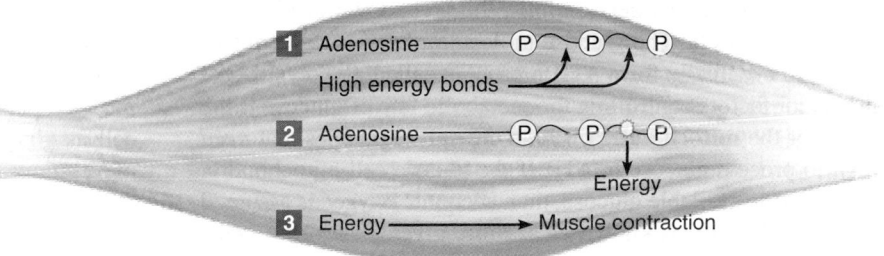

FIGURE 3.7 ATP, adenosine triphosphate. *(1)* ATP is stored in the muscle in limited amounts. *(2)* Splitting of a high-energy bond releases adenosine diphosphate (ADP), inorganic phosphate (P), and energy, which *(3)* can be used for many body processes, including muscular contraction. The ATP stores may be used maximally for fast, all-out bursts of power that last about one second. ATP must be replenished from other sources for muscle contraction to continue.

Granata and Brandon analyzed 50 studies and noted many discrepant findings. Nonetheless, small changes in energy intake or expenditure can cause weight gain or weight loss over time. This topic is discussed in chapters 10 and 11 concerning diets for weight control.

How can I estimate my daily resting energy expenditure (REE)?

There are several ways to estimate your REE, but whichever method is used, the value obtained is an estimate and will have some error associated with it. To get a truly accurate value you would need a clinical evaluation, such as a standard BMR test. Accurate determination of REE is important for clinicians dealing with obesity patients, for such testing is needed to rule out hypometabolism. However, a number of formula estimates may give you an approximation of your daily REE.

Table 3.4 provides a simple method for calculating the REE of males and females of varying ages. Examples are provided

TABLE 3.4	Estimation of the daily resting energy expenditure (REE)
Age (years)	**Equation**
Males	
3–9	(22.7 × body weight*) + 495
10–17	(17.5 × body weight) + 651
18–29	(15.3 × body weight) + 679
30–60	(11.6 × body weight) + 879
>60	(13.5 × body weight) + 487
Example	
154-lb male, age 20	
154 lbs/2.2 = 70 kg	
(15.3 × 70) + 679 = 1,750	
Females	
3–9	(22.5 × body weight*) + 499
10–17	(12.2 × body weight) + 746
18–29	(14.7 × body weight) + 496
30–60	(8.7 × body weight) + 829
>60	(10.5 × body weight) + 596
Example	
121-lb female, age 20	
121 lbs/2.2 = 55 kg	
(14.7 × 55) + 496 = 1,304	

To get a range of values, simply add or subtract a normal 10-percent variation to the RMR estimate.

Male example: 10 percent of 1,750 = 175 Calories
Normal range = 1,575–1,925 Calories/day
Female example: 10 percent of 1,304 = 130 Calories
Normal range = 1,174–1,434 Calories/day

*Body weight is expressed in kilograms (kg).

in the table along with calculation of a 10-percent variability. Keep in mind that this is only an estimate of the daily REE, and additional energy would be expended during the day through the TEF effect and the effect of physical activity, as noted later.

A very simple, rough estimate of your REE is one Calorie per kilogram body weight per hour. Using this procedure, the estimated value for the male in table 3.4 is 1,680 Calories per day (1 × 70 kg × 24 hours) and for the female is 1,320 Calories (1 × 55 kg × 24 hours), values that are not substantially different from those calculated by the table procedure.

What genetic factors affect my REE?

Your REE is directly related to the amount of metabolically active tissue you possess. At rest, tissues such as the heart, liver, kidneys, and other internal organs are more metabolically active than muscle tissue, but muscle tissue is more metabolically active than fat. Changes in the proportion of these tissues in your body will therefore cause changes in your REE.

Many factors influencing the REE, such as age, sex, natural hormonal activity, body size and surface area, and to a degree, body composition, are genetically determined. The effect of some of these factors on the REE is generally well known. Because infants have a large proportion of metabolically active tissue and are growing rapidly, their REE is extremely high. The REE declines through childhood, adolescence, and adulthood as full growth and maturation are achieved. Individuals with naturally greater muscle mass in comparison to body fat have a higher REE; the REE of women is about 10–15 percent lower than that of men, mainly because women have a higher proportion of fat to muscle tissue. Genetically lean individuals have a higher REE than do stocky individuals because their body surface area ratio is larger in proportion to their weight (body volume) and they lose more body heat through radiation.

How does body composition affect my REE?

Body composition may be changed so as to alter REE. Losing body weight, including both body fat and muscle tissue, generally lowers the total daily REE. The REE may be decreased significantly in obese individuals who go on a very low-Calorie diet of less than 800 Calories per day. The decrease in the REE, which is greater than would be due to weight loss alone, may be caused by lowered levels of thyroid hormones. In one study, the REE of obese subjects dropped 9.4 percent on a diet containing only 472 Calories per day. This topic is covered in more detail in chapters 10 and 11. The possibility of decreased REE in some athletes who maintain low body weight through exercise, such as female distance runners and male wrestlers, has been the subject of recent debate and will be covered in chapter 10 when we discuss body composition.

In contrast, maintaining normal body weight while reducing body fat and increasing muscle mass may raise the REE slightly because muscle tissue has a somewhat higher metabolic level than fat tissue or because the ratio of body surface area to body weight is increased. The decline in the REE that occurs with aging may be attributed partially to physical inactivity with a consequent loss of the more metabolically active muscle tissue and an accumulation of body fat. Methods to lose body fat and increase muscle mass are covered in chapters 11 and 12.

What environmental factors may also influence the REE?

Several lifestyle and environmental factors may influence our metabolism. For example, although caffeine is not a food, it is a common ingredient in some of the foods we may eat or drink. Caffeine is a stimulant and may elicit a significant rise in the REE. One study reported that the caffeine in 2–3 cups of regular coffee increased the REE 10–12 percent.

Smoking cigarettes also raises the REE. Apparently the nicotine in tobacco stimulates the metabolism similarly to caffeine. This may be one of the reasons why some individuals gain weight when they stop smoking.

Climatic conditions, especially temperature changes, may also raise the REE. Exposure to the cold may stimulate the secretion of several hormones and muscular shivering, which may stimulate heat production up to 400 percent. Exposure to warm or hot environments will increase energy expenditure through greater cardiovascular demands and the sweating response. Altitude exposure will also increase REE due to increased ventilation.

Many of these factors influencing the REE are important in themselves, but may also be important considerations relative to weight control programs and body temperature regulation. Thus, they are discussed further in later chapters.

As we shall see in the next section, the most important factor that can increase the metabolic rate is exercise.

What energy sources are used during rest?

The vast majority of the energy consumed during a resting situation is used to drive the automatic physiological processes in the body. Because the muscles expend little energy during rest, there is no need to produce ATP rapidly. Hence, the oxygen system is able to provide the necessary ATP for resting physiological processes.

The oxygen system can use carbohydrates, fats, and protein as energy sources. However, as noted in chapter 6, protein is not used as a major energy source under normal dietary conditions. Carbohydrates and fats, when combined with oxygen in the cells, are the major energy substrates during rest. Several factors may influence which of the two nutrients is predominantly used. In general, though, on a mixed diet of carbohydrate, protein, and fat, about 40 percent of the REE is derived from carbohydrate and about 60 percent comes from fat. However, eating a diet rich in carbohydrate or fat will increase the percent of the REE derived, respectively, from carbohydrate and fat. Also, when carbohydrate levels are low, such as after an overnight fast, the percentage of the REE derived from fat increases.

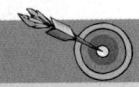

Key Concepts

- Human metabolism represents the sum total of all physiological processes in the body, and the metabolic rate reflects the speed at which the body utilizes energy.
- The basal metabolic rate (BMR) represents the energy requirements necessary to maintain physiological processes in a resting, postabsorptive state, while the resting metabolic rate (RMR) is a little higher due to the effects of prior eating and physical activity. The terms BEE and REE represent basal energy expenditure and resting energy expenditure, respectively, totaled over a 24-hour period.
- Eating a meal increases the metabolic rate as the digestive system absorbs, metabolizes, and stores the energy nutrients, a process termed the thermic effect of food (TEF). A meal will increase the RMR by about 5–10 percent, and some meals will elevate the RMR more than others.
- Various methods may be used to estimate daily resting energy expenditure (REE), but one simple means is to use the value of one (1) Calorie per kilogram body weight per hour. For a 60-kilogram (132-pound) individual, this would represent 1,440 Calories over the course of 24 hours ($60 \times 1.0 \times 24$).
- A number of different factors may affect the REE, including body composition, drugs, climatic conditions, and prior exercise.
- Fats stored in the body serve as the main source of energy during rest.

Check for Yourself

- Using the formula in table 3.4, estimate your daily resting energy expenditure (REE) in Calories. Keep this record for later comparisons.

Human Energy Metabolism during Exercise

Exercise is a stressor to the body, and almost all body systems respond. If the exercise is continued daily, the body systems begin to adapt to the stress of exercise. As noted previously and as we shall see in later chapters, these adaptations may have significant health benefits. The two body systems most involved in exercise are the nervous system and the muscular system. The nervous system is needed to activate muscle contraction, but it is in the muscle cell itself that the energetics of exercise occur. Most other body systems are simply designed to serve the needs of the muscle cell during exercise.

How do my muscles influence the amount of energy I can produce during exercise?

Muscles comprise a significant percentage of our body weight, approximating 45 percent in the typical adult male and 35 percent in the typical adult female. However, in any given individual these percentages may vary tremendously depending on level and type of physical activity. We shall discuss the potential health and sports performance benefits associated with modifying muscle mass in later chapters, but our focus here is on energy production for exercise.

The muscle cell, or muscle fiber, is a rather simple machine in design but extremely complex in function. It is a tube-like structure containing filaments that can slide by one another to shorten the total muscle. The shortening of the muscle moves bones, and hence work is accomplished, be it simply the raising of a barbell as in weight training or moving the whole body as in running. Like most other machines, the muscle cell has the capability of producing work at different rates, ranging from very low levels of energy expenditure during sleep to nearly a 90-fold increase during maximal, short-term anaerobic exercise.

The human body possesses several different types of muscle fibers, and their primary differences are in the ability to produce energy. Various types of proteins are found in muscle cells, and the production of energy is dependent on the specific type of proteins present. In general, three different types of muscle fiber types have been differentiated based on their rate of energy production, and table 3.5 presents various characteristics associated with each.

Type I muscle fiber is also known as the *slow twitch red fiber,* and as this name implies is used for slow muscle contractions, such as during rest and light aerobic physical activity. It is often referred to as the *slow-oxidative (SO) fiber.* The characteristics associated with it, such as high mitochondria and myoglobin content, support its high oxidative capacity and resistance to fatigue. Use of the type I fiber is important during events associated with aerobic capacity and aerobic power.

The type IIa muscle fiber, also known as the *fast twitch red fiber,* also possesses good aerobic capacity, but not as high as the type I fiber. However, it may also produce energy anaerobically via the lactic acid energy system. Hence, it is often referred to as the fast-oxidative glycolytic (FOG) fiber. It also has high ATP-PCr capacity. Use of the type IIa fiber is important during events associated with aerobic power and anaerobic capacity, but it fatigues sooner than the type I muscle fiber.

The type IIb muscle fiber, also known as the fast *twitch white fiber,* possesses poor aerobic capacity and is used primarily for anaerobic energy production. It is often referred to as the fast glycolytic (FG) fiber. Like the type IIa fiber, it also has high ATP-PCr capacity. Use of the type IIb muscle fiber is important during events associated with anaerobic power and anaerobic capacity, but it fatigues very rapidly.

Most muscles contain all three types of muscle fibers, and all fibers are used during exercise tasks of varying intensity. However, the use of one fiber type will usually predominate, dependent on the intensity of the exercise task and the associated human energy system. Physical training can improve the efficacy of each muscle fiber type, and the benefits that accrue to each depend on the type and extent of exercise training. Moreover, the distribution of muscle fiber types will vary among different individuals due to genetic predisposition, and such differences may influence the level of success in certain sport endeavors.

What effect does muscular exercise have on the metabolic rate?

As noted in the previous section, the REE is measured with the subject at rest in a reclining position. Any physical activity will raise metabolic activity above the REE and thus increase energy expenditure. Accounting for changes in physical activity over the day may provide a reasonable, although imprecise, estimate of the total daily energy expenditure. Very light activities such as sitting, standing, playing cards, cooking, and typing all increase energy output above the REE, but we normally do not think of them as exercise, as noted later in this chapter. For purposes of this discussion, the **exercise metabolic rate (EMR),** represents the increase in metabolism brought about by moderate or strenuous physical activity such as brisk walking, climbing stairs, cycling, dancing, running, and other such planned exercise activities. The EMR is known more appropriately as the **thermic effect of exercise (TEE).**

The most important factor affecting the metabolic rate is the intensity or speed of the exercise. To move faster, your muscles must contract more rapidly, consuming proportionately more energy. Use of type I muscle fibers predominates during low-intensity exercise, and type II fibers are increasingly recruited with more intense exercise. The following represents approximate energy expenditure in Calories per minute for increasing levels of exercise intensity for an average-sized

TABLE 3.5 Characteristics associated with the three types of muscle fibers

Type	I	IIa	IIb (IIx)
Twitch speed	Slow	Faster	Fastest
Color	Red	Red	White
Size (diameter)	Small	Medium	Large
Fatigability	Slow	Moderate	Fast
Force production	Low	High	Highest
Oxidative processes	Highest	Moderate	Lowest
Mitochondria	Highest	Moderate	Low
Myoglobin	Highest	Moderate	Low
Blood flow	Highest	Moderate	Lowest
Triglyceride use	Highest	Moderate	Lowest
Glycogen use	Lowest	Moderate	Highest
Phosphocreatine levels	Lowest	Higher	Higher
Energy for sports	Aerobic capacity; aerobic power	Aerobic power; anaerobic capacity	Anaerobic power; anaerobic capacity

adult male. However, for most of us it would be impossible to sustain the higher levels of energy expenditure for a minute, and the highest level could be sustained for only a second or so.

Level of intensity	Caloric expenditure per minute
Resting metabolic rate	1.0
Sitting and writing	2.0
Walking at 2 mph	3.3
Walking at 3 mph	4.2
Running at 5 mph	9.4
Running at 10 mph	18.8
Running at 15 mph	29.3
Running at 20 mph	38.7
Maximal power weightlift	>90.0

Although the intensity of the exercise is the most important factor affecting the magnitude of the metabolic rate, there are some other important considerations. In some activities the increase in energy expenditure is not directly proportional to speed, for the efficiency of movement will affect caloric expenditure. Very fast walking becomes more inefficient, so the individual burns more Calories per mile walking briskly compared to more leisurely walking. A beginning swimmer wastes a lot of energy, whereas one who is more accomplished may swim with less effort, saving Calories when swimming a given distance. Swimming and cycling at very high speeds exponentially increase water or air resistance, so caloric expenditure also increases exponentially. Moreover, the individual with a greater body weight will burn more Calories for any given amount of work in which the body has to be moved, as in walking, jogging, or running. It simply costs more total energy to move a heavier load.

How is exercise intensity measured?

The intensity of a given exercise may be measured in two general ways. One way is to measure the actual work output or power of the activity, such as foot-pounds per second, kilojoules per second, or watts. In some cases this is rather easy to do because some machines, such as bicycle ergometers, are designed to provide an accurate measure of work output. However, the actual work output of a basketball player during a game is more difficult to measure, although use of accelerometers and other motion-detection devices help. The majority of accelerometer research focuses on walking, running, and activities of daily living, and few studies are available to quantify work during sports activties. In an analysis of the ability of accelerometers to predict energy expenditure, Lyden and others reported that current accelerometer prediction equations often misclassify vigorous intensity activities. Although promising, more research must be conducted before accelerometers can be widely used to quantify work during sports activities.

A second way is to measure the physiological cost of the activity by monitoring the activity of the three human energy systems. Ward-Smith noted that due to accurate measurements of oxygen uptake and carbon dioxide output, the energy contributions from aerobic metabolism are readily quantifiable, whereas the energy contribution from anaerobic metabolism is far more difficult to determine.

Energy production from the ATP-PCr energy system has been measured by several procedures. One procedure involves a muscle biopsy with subsequent analysis for ATP and PCr levels to determine use following exercise, but the small muscle biopsy may not represent ATP-PCr use in other muscles. ATP and PCr levels may also be determined by computerized imaging procedures, a noninvasive procedure, but the exercise task must be confined to specific movements due to the nature of the imaging equipment. Thus, Lange and Bury indicate that it is difficult to obtain precise physiological or biochemical data during common explosive-type exercise tests, such as short sprints.

Laboratory techniques are also available to measure the role of the lactic acid system in exercise, primarily by measuring the concentration of lactic acid in the blood or in muscle tissues. One measure of exercise intensity is the so-called anaerobic threshold, or that point where the metabolism is believed to shift to a greater use of the lactic acid system. This point is often termed the **onset of blood lactic acid (OBLA),** or *lactate threshold*. The anaerobic threshold may also be referred to as the **steady-state threshold,** indicating that endurance exercise may continue for prolonged periods if you exercise below this threshold value. Exercise physiologists disagree about which is the better term, but all terms may be found in scientific literature. Some sport scientists also use specific measurements to define these terms, such as a certain level of blood lactic acid.

Laboratory tests also are necessary to measure the contribution of the oxygen system during exercise, and this is the most commonly used technique for measuring exercise intensity (see figure 3.3). The most commonly used measurement is the **maximal oxygen uptake,** which represents the highest amount of oxygen that an individual may consume under exercise situations. In essence, the technique consists of monitoring the oxygen uptake of the individual while the exercise intensity is increased in stages. When oxygen uptake does not increase with an increase in workload, the maximal oxygen uptake has been reached. Maximal oxygen uptake is usually expressed as VO_2 **max,** which may be stated as liters per minute or milliliters per kilogram body weight per minute. An example is provided in figure 3.13. A commonly used technique to indicate exercise intensity is to report it as a certain percentage of an individual's VO_2 max, such as 50 or 75 percent. If blood samples are taken periodically to measure serum levels of lactic acid, the percent of VO_2 max at which the steady-state threshold occurs may be determined. Additionally, measurement of oxygen during recovery from exercise may be used to calculate the maximal accumulated oxygen deficit (MAOD), an indirect marker for anaerobic contributions to energy expenditure during exercise. Proper training may increase both VO_2 max and the steady-state threshold, as illustrated in figure 3.14.

In summary, measurement of the three energy systems during exercise provides us with a measure of the energy cost of the physical activity.

How is the energy expenditure of exercise metabolism expressed?

A number of research studies have been conducted to determine the energy expenditure of a wide variety of sports and other physical activities.

FIGURE 3.13

Maximal oxygen uptake (VO_2 max). The best way to express VO_2 max is in milliliters of oxygen per kilogram (kg) of body weight per minute (ml O_2/kg/min). As noted in the figure, the smaller individual has a lower VO_2 max in liters but a higher VO_2 max when expressed relative to weight. In this case, the smaller individual has a higher degree of aerobic fitness, at least as measured by VO_2 max per unit body weight.

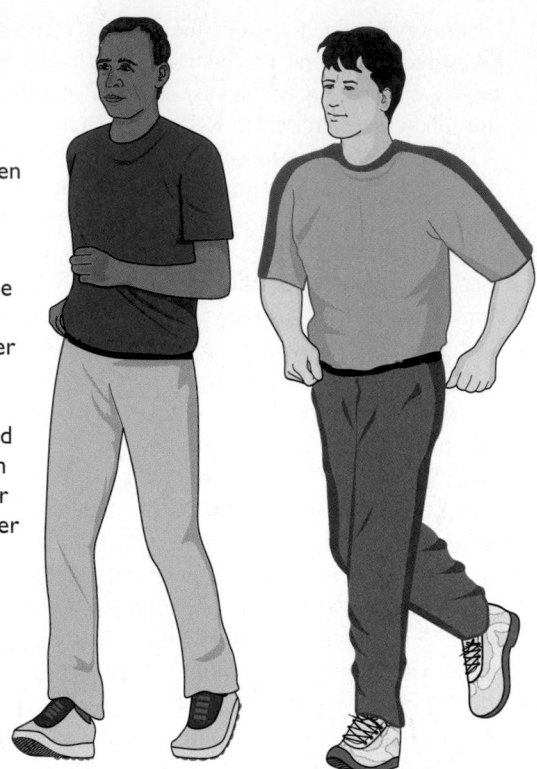

VO_2 max: liters/minute	3.6 L (3600 ml)	4.0 L (4000 ml)
kg body weight	60	80
VO_2 max: ml O_2/kg/minute	60	50

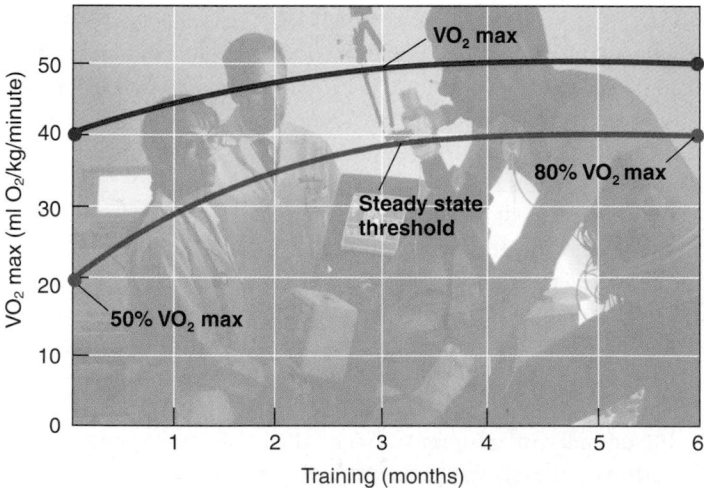

FIGURE 3.14 The effect of training upon VO_2 max and the steady-state threshold. Training increases both your VO_2 max and your steady-state threshold, which is the ability to work at a greater percentage of your VO_2 max without producing excessive lactic acid—a causative factor in fatigue. For example, before training the VO_2 max may be 40 ml while the steady-state threshold is only 20 ml (50% of VO_2 max). After training, VO_2 max may rise to 50 ml, but the steady-state threshold may rise to 40 ml (80% of the VO_2 max).

The energy costs have been reported in a variety of ways, including Calories, kilojoules (kJ), oxygen uptake, and **METS.** The MET is a unit that represents multiples of the resting metabolic rate (see figure 3.15). These concepts are, of course, all interrelated, so an exercise can be expressed in any one of the four terms and converted into the others. For our purposes, we will express energy cost in Calories per minute based upon body weight, as that appears to be the most practical method for this book. However, just in case you see the other values in another book or magazine, here is how you may simplify the conversion. We know the following approximate values:

$$1 \text{ C} = 4 \text{ kJ}$$
$$1 \text{ L } O_2 = 5 \text{ C}$$
$$1 \text{ MET} = 3.5 \text{ ml } O_2/\text{kg body weight/min}$$
(amount of oxygen consumed during rest)

These values are needed for the following calculations:
Example: Exercise cost = 20 kJ/minute
To get Calorie cost, divide kJ by the equivalent value for Calories.

$$20 \text{ kJ/min}/4 = 5 \text{ C/min}$$

Example: Exercise cost = 3 L of O_2/min
To get Calorie cost, multiply liters of O_2 × Calories per liter.

$$\text{Caloric cost} = 3 \times 5 = 15 \text{ C/min}$$

Example: Exercise cost = 25 ml O_2/kg body weight/min
You need body weight in kg, which is weight in pounds divided by 2.2. For this example 154 lbs = 70 kg. Determine total O_2 cost/min by multiplying body weight times O_2 cost/kg/min.

$$70 \times 25 = 1,750 \text{ ml } O_2$$

Convert ml to L: 1,750 ml = 1.75 L
Multiply liters O_2 × Calories per liter
Caloric cost = 1.75 × 5 = 8.75 C/min

Example: Exercise cost = 12 METS
You need body weight in kg—for this example, 70 kg.
Multiply total METS times O_2 equivalent of 1 MET.

$$12 \times 3.5 \text{ ml } O_2/\text{kg/min} = 42.0 \text{ ml } O_2/\text{kg/min}$$

Multiply body weight times this result
70 × 42 ml O_2/kg/min = 2,940 ml O_2/min
Convert ml to L: 2,940 ml O_2/min = 2.94 L O_2/min
Multiply liters O_2 × Calories per liter
Caloric cost = 2.94 × 5 = 14.70 C/min

How can I tell what my metabolic rate is during exercise?

The human body is basically a muscle machine designed for movement. Almost all of the other body systems serve the muscular system. The nervous system causes the muscles to contract. The digestive system supplies nutrients. The cardiovascular system delivers these nutrients along with oxygen in cooperation with the respiratory system. The endocrine system secretes hormones that affect muscle nutrition. The excretory system removes

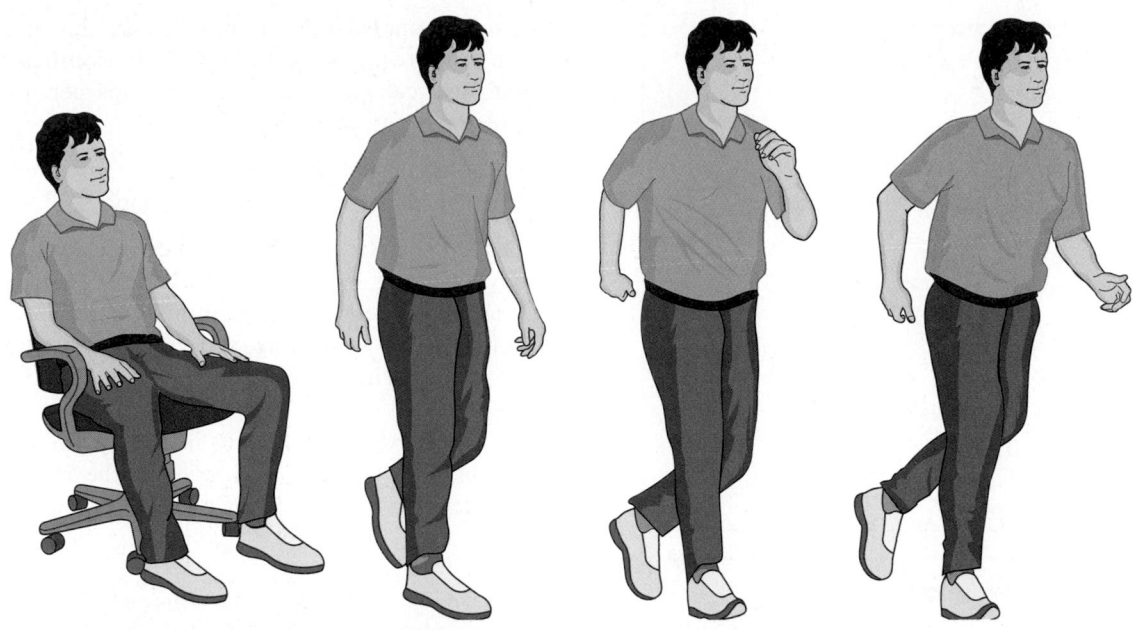

	Rest	Slow walk (2 mph)	Fast walk (5 mph)	Run (8 mph)
Liters of oxygen/minute	.25	.5–.75	1.5–1.75	2.5–3.0
Calories/minute	1.25	2.5–3.75	7.5–8.75	12.5–15.0
Kilojoules/minute	5	10–15	30–35	50–60
METS	1	2–3	6–7	10–12

FIGURE 3.15 Energy equivalents in oxygen consumption, Calories, Kilojoules, and METS. This figure depicts four means of expressing energy expenditure during four levels of activity. These approximate values are for an average male of 154 pounds (70 kg). If you weigh more or less, the values will increase or decrease accordingly.

waste products. When humans exercise, almost all body systems increase their activity to accommodate the increased energy demands of the muscle cell. In most types of sustained exercises, however, the major demand of the muscle cells is for oxygen.

As noted previously, the major technique for evaluating metabolic rate is to measure the oxygen consumption of an individual during exercise. Athletes may benefit from such physiological testing. Measurements of VO_2 max, maximal heart rate, and the anaerobic threshold may help in planning an optimal training program, and subsequent testing may illustrate training effects. Such testing is becoming increasingly available at various universities and comprehensive fitness/wellness centers.

Unfortunately, this may not be practical for most of us. However, because of some interesting relationships among exercise intensity, oxygen consumption, and heart rate, the average individual may be able to get a relative approximation of the metabolic rate during exercise. A more or less linear relationship exists between exercise intensity and oxygen uptake. As the

intensity level of work increases, so does the amount of oxygen consumed. The two systems primarily responsible for delivering the oxygen to the muscles are the cardiovascular and respiratory systems. There is also a fairly linear relationship between their responses and oxygen consumption. In general, maximal heart rate (HRmax) and VO_2 max coincide at the same exercise intensity level. A simplified schematic is presented in figure 3.16.

Because the heart rate (HR) generally is linearly related to oxygen consumption (the main expression of metabolic rate), and because it is easy to measure this physiological response during exercise either at the wrist or neck pulse, it may prove to be a practical guide to your metabolic rate. The higher your heart rate, the greater your metabolic rate. However, a number of factors may influence your specific heart rate response to exercise, such as the type of exercise (running vs. swimming), your level of physical fitness, sex, age, skill efficiency, percentage of body fat, and a number of environmental conditions. Thus, it is difficult to predict your exact metabolic rate from your exercise HR. As we shall see in chapter 11, however, the HR data during exercise may be used as a basis for establishing a personal fitness program for health and weight control, either directly by measuring the heart rate or indirectly by how intense we perceive the exercise to be, or our *rating of perceived exertion.*

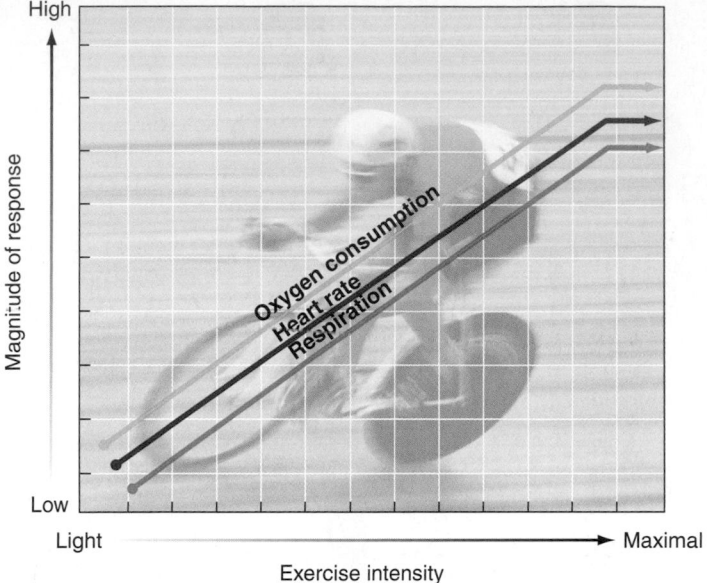

FIGURE 3.16 Relationships between oxygen consumption, heart rate, and respiration responses to increasing exercise rates. In general, as the intensity of exercise continues, there is a rise in oxygen consumption, which is accompanied by proportional increases in heart rate and respiration. VO_2 max and HRmax usually occur at the same exercise intensity.

How can I determine the energy cost of exercise?

To facilitate the determination of the energy cost of a wide variety of physical activities, appendix B has been developed. This is a composite table of a wide variety of individual reports in the literature. When using this appendix, keep the following points in mind.

1. The figures include the REE. Thus, the total cost of the exercise includes not only the energy expended by the exercise itself, but also the amount you would have used anyway during that same period. Suppose you ran for 1 hour and the calculated energy cost was 800 Calories. During that same time at rest you may have expended 75 Calories as your REE. The net cost of the exercise is only 725 Calories.
2. The figures in the table are only for the time you are doing the activity. For example, in an hour of basketball you may exercise strenuously for only 35–40 minutes, as you may take timeouts and rest during foul shots. In general, record only the amount of time that you are actually moving during the activity.
3. The figures may give you some guidelines to total energy expenditure, but actual caloric cost might vary somewhat because of such factors as your skill level, running against the wind or uphill, and so forth.
4. Not all body weights could be listed, but you may approximate by going to the closest weight listed.
5. There may be small differences between men and women, but not enough to make a marked difference in the total caloric value for most exercises.

As one example, suppose we calculate the energy expenditure of a 154-pound individual who ran 5 miles in 30 minutes. You must calculate either the minutes per mile or miles per hour (mph).

1. 30 minutes/5 miles = 6 min/mile
2. 60 minutes/6 minutes/mile = 10 mph

Consult appendix B and find the caloric value per minute for a body weight of 155 lbs and a running speed of 10 mph, a value of 18.8 Calories/minute. Multiply this value times the number of minutes of running, and you get the total caloric cost of that exercise. In this example, 30 × 18.8 = 564 total Calories expended.

If the activity you do does not appear in appendix B, try to find one you think closely matches the movements found in your activity. Then check the caloric expenditure for the related activity.

http://sites.google.com/site/compendiumofphysicalactivities/ **Presents** a complete compendium of the metabolic cost, in MET values, for hundreds of different activities of daily living, specific exercises, and sports. The compendium was developed by Barbara Ainsworth, from Arizona State University, and other health professionals.

What are the best types of activities to increase energy expenditure?

Activities that use the large muscle groups of the body and are performed continuously usually will expend the greatest amount of Calories. Intensity and duration are the two key determinants of total energy expenditure. Activities in which you may be able to exercise continuously at a fairly high intensity for a prolonged period will maximize your total caloric loss. Although this may encompass a wide variety of different physical activities, those that have become increasingly popular include walking, running, swimming, bicycling, and aerobic dance. A few general comments about these common modes of exercising would appear to be in order.

Walking and Running Walking and running are popular exercises because they are so practical to do. All you need is a good pair of shoes.

Walking Walking is more economical than running. Kuo and others note that walking is a pendular motion, with the stance leg behaving like an inverted pendulum and the swing leg like a regular pendulum. Thus, walking appears to be optimized with respect to metabolic cost. A good rule of thumb is that you expend about 1 Calorie per kilogram/body weight per mile walking at a speed of 2–4 miles per hour, and the following represents the number of Calories expended walking a kilometer or mile for an average adult male and female.

Walking		
	Male (165 lbs, 75 kg)	Female (132 lbs, 60 kg)
Kilometer	47	37
Mile	75	60

Running		
	Male (165 lbs, 75 kg)	Female (132 lbs, 60 kg)
Kilometer	75	60
Mile	120	96

However, walking faster may increase energy expenditure exponentially. A study by Thomas and Londeree has shown that the caloric cost of walking at 4.7 mph is only about 5 percent less than jogging at the same speed. At high walking speeds (above 5 mph), you may possibly expend more energy than if you jogged at the same speed. Fast, vigorous walking, known as aerobic walking, can be an effective means to expend Calories. However, as with other exercise activities, it takes practice to become a fast walker.

Walking intensity can be increased in other ways. Climbing stairs, at home, at work, in an athletic stadium, or on step machines, is one means to make walking more vigorous.

Many individuals use small weights in conjunction with their walking or running programs either by carrying them or strapping them to the ankles or wrists. The most popular technique is to carry small weights of 1–3 pounds. A number of research studies have reported that this technique, particularly if the arms are swung vigorously through a wide range of motion during walking, may increase the energy expenditure about 5–10 percent or higher above unweighted walking at the same speed. Use of walking poles, similar to ski poles, may increase caloric expenditure by 15 percent. Increases in energy expenditure greater than 30 percent have been reported with vigorous pumping of 1-pound hand weights as compared with just running at the same speed. The heart rate response also increases, and using hand weights with fast walking is an adequate stimulus to promote a training effect on the cardiovascular system. However, use of hand weights exaggerates the blood pressure response, and thus should be used with caution by individuals with blood pressure problems. Since some researchers have noted that simply walking a little faster without weights will have the same effect on energy cost and heart rate response, this may be a good alternative. Nevertheless, at any given walking speed, hand weights will increase energy expenditure. Addition of weights to the ankle also will increase energy expenditure, but it may also change the normal walking style and may predispose one to injury.

Running Running a given distance expends more energy than walking the same distance. As a general rule, the caloric cost of running a given distance does not depend on the speed. It will take you a longer time to cover the distance at a slower running speed, but the total caloric cost will be similar to that expended at a faster speed. A good rule of thumb is that you expend about 1 Calorie per kilogram/body weight per kilometer, which approximates about 0.73 Calorie per pound/body weight per mile. The following represents the number of Calories expended running a kilometer or mile for an average adult male and female. In general, research indicates that running expends approximately 30–40 percent more energy per mile or kilometer compared to walking the same distance.

Swimming Because of water resistance, swimming takes more energy to cover a given distance than does either walking or running. Although the amount of energy expended depends somewhat on the type of swimming stroke used and the ability of the swimmer, swimming a given distance takes about four times as much energy as running. For example, swimming a quarter-mile is the energy equivalent of running a mile. Water aerobics and water running (doing aerobics or running in waist-deep, chest-deep, or deep water) may be effective exercise regimens that help prevent injuries due to impact.

Cycling Bicycling takes less energy to cover a given distance in comparison to running on a level surface. The energy cost of bicycling depends on a number of factors such as body weight, the type of bicycle, hills, and body position on the bike (assuming a streamlined position to reduce air resistance). Owing to rapidly increasing air resistance at higher speeds such as 20 mph, the energy cost of bicycling increases at a much faster rate at such speeds. A detailed method for calculating energy expenditure during bicycling is presented in the article by Hagberg and Pena. In general, cycling 1 mile is approximately the energy equivalent of running one third the distance.

Group Exercise Various types of group exercise classes have been popular for more than 30 years. These classes can include high- and low-impact aerobic dance, step aerobics, spin classes, and cardio-kickboxing. All of these classes vary in intensity based on participant effort, but have been shown to burn up to about 10 Calories per minute. Though the energy expenditure of group exercise can be comparable to individual exercise tasks such as running or cycling, the greatest benefit of group exercise might be improved exercise adherence. Burke and colleagues examined 44 studies and showed that when exercisers are given the opportunity to interact with others, as when exercising in a group, adherence was better and the exercise program was more effective.

Home Aerobic Exercise Equipment Home exercise equipment may also provide a strenuous aerobic workout. Recent research suggests that for any given level of perceived effort, treadmill running burned the most Calories. Exercising on elliptical trainers, cross-country ski machines, rowing ergometers, and stair-climbing apparatus also expended significant amounts of Calories, more so than bicycling apparatus. Many modern pieces of exercise equipment are electronically equipped with small computers to calculate approximate energy cost as Calories per minute and total caloric cost of the exercise. However, research shows that exercise adherence is better when there is contact with fellow exercisers, as in group exercise settings.

Resistance or Weight Training Resistance training, or weight training, may be an effective way to expend energy, but it is not as effective as aerobic types of exercise. For example, Bloomer compared energy expenditure during resistance training (free-weight squatting at 70% maximal) to aerobic training (cycling at 70 percent VO_2 max) for 30 minutes. Although the heart rates were the same for both types of exercise, the cycling protocol expended 441 Calories while the squatting protocol expended only 269 Calories, a 64 percent difference. Although this is a significant difference, Bloomer noted that the resistance exercise, if performed 4–5 days a week, would meet the recommendations for energy expenditure as suggested by the ACSM.

Passive and Occupational Energy Expenditure Advances in technology have changed the way people accomplish their jobs. Specifically, people are spending more time sitting than ever, which has been implicated in decreased daily energy expenditure and as a contributing factor to the obesity epidemic. One way people are increasing energy expenditure at work is to sit on a Physioball instead of a desk chair, or to abandon sitting entirely and simply do their job while standing. Beers and others noted that sitting on a Physioball or standing while performing clerical work burns 6 percent more Calories than sitting in a desk chair. Now that sitting itself has been identified as an independent risk factor for mortality, researchers are focusing on how to increase passive energy expenditure to combat the decrease in occupational energy expenditure and to supplement daily energy expenditure to help maintain a healthy body weight.

Table 3.6 provides a classification of some common physical activities based upon rate of energy expenditure. The implications of these types of exercises for weight control programs are discussed in later chapters.

www.ChooseMyPlate.gov Click on Interactive Tools, then Food Tracker to assess your physical activity.

www.internetfitness.com Click on Calorie Burning Calculator for the energy cost of various physical activities.

Does exercise affect my resting energy expenditure (REE)?

Exercise not only raises the metabolic rate during exercise, but also, depending on the intensity and duration of the activity, will keep the REE elevated during the recovery period. The increase in body temperature and in the amounts of circulating hormones such as adrenaline (epinephrine) will continue to influence some cellular activity, and some other metabolic processes, such as circulation and respiration, will remain elevated for a limited time. This effect, which has been labeled the **metabolic aftereffects of exercise,** is calculated by monitoring the oxygen consumption for several hours during the recovery period after the exercise task. The amount of oxygen in excess of the preexercise REE, often called excess postexercise oxygen consumption (EPOC), reflects the additional caloric cost of the exercise above and beyond that expended during the exercise task itself.

Some older research noted that the average number of additional Calories expended after each exercise session would be about 45–50. However, in a series of more recent studies with more appropriate controls, although most investigators did report an increased REE following exercise of varying durations and intensities, the magnitude of the response was generally lower. Depending on the intensity and duration of the exercise bout in these studies, the REE during the recovery period ranged from 4–16 percent higher than the preexercise

TABLE 3.6 Classification of physical activities based upon rate of energy expenditure*

Light, mild aerobic exercise (<5 Calories/min)

Archery	Bowling	Horseback riding (walk)
Badminton, social	Dancing, waltz	Swimming (20–25 yards/min)
Baseball	Golf (using cart)	Walking (2–3 mph)
Bicycling (5 mph)		

Moderate aerobic exercise (5–10 Calories/min)

Badminton, competitive	Golf (carrying clubs)	Swimming (30–40 yards/min)
Basketball, recreational	Rope skipping (60 rpm)	Tennis, recreational
Bicycling (10 mph)	Running (5 mph)	Walking (3–4.5 mph)
Dancing, aerobic	Skiing, cross-country (2.5 mph)	Weight training

Moderately heavy to heavy aerobic exercise (>10 Calories/min)

Bicycling (15–20 mph)	Rope skipping (120–140 rpm)	Swimming (50–70 yards/min)
Calisthenics, vigorous	Running (6–9 mph)	Tennis, competitive
In-line skating (10–15 mph)	Skiing, cross-country (5–6 mph)	Walking (5.0–6.0 mph)

*Calories per minute based upon a body weight of 70 kg, or 154 pounds. Those weighing more or less will expend more or fewer Calories, respectively, but the intensity level of the exercise will be the same. The actual amount of Calories expended may also depend on a number of other factors, depending on the activity. For example, bicycling into or with the wind will increase or decrease, respectively, the energy cost. See appendix B for more details.

Source: Modified from M.H. Williams, *Nutritional Aspects of Human Physical and Athletic Performance,* 1985, Charles C Thomas Publishers, Springfield, IL.

REE, and it remained elevated for only 15–20 minutes in some studies but up to 4–5 hours in others. Both aerobic and resistance-type exercises increase EPOC, with greater increases associated with high-intensity, long-duration exercise. Burleson and others reported that when matched for oxygen consumption during exercise, weight training exhibited a greater postexercise oxygen consumption, but the amount was rather small. Using the oxygen consumption values presented in these studies, the additional energy expenditure ranged from 3–30 Calories. For example, Haddock and Wilkin found that although a bout of resistance training increased the resting metabolic rate for 120 minutes afterwards, subjects expended only about 23 more Calories above the normal resting level for that time frame.

Although the metabolic aftereffects of exercise would not appear to make a significant contribution to weight loss, exercise may help mitigate the decrease in the REE often seen in individuals on very low-Calorie diets. This point is explored further in chapter 11.

Does exercise affect the thermic effect of food (TEF)?

Many studies have been conducted to investigate the effect of exercise on the thermic effect of food. Unfortunately, no clear answer has been found. Some studies have reported an increase in TEF when subjects exercise either before or after the meal, whereas others revealed little or no effects. Some research even suggests that exercise training decreases the TEF. Other studies have investigated differences between exercise-trained and untrained individuals relative to TEF, and although some preliminary research noted a decreased TEF in endurance-trained athletes, Tremblay and others also noted that it is still unclear if training causes any significant alterations in TEF. In any case, the increases or decreases noted in the TEF due to either exercise or exercise training were minor, averaging about 5–9 Calories for several hours.

How much energy do I need to consume daily?

The National Academy of Sciences, through the Institute of Medicine, has released its DRI for energy in conjunction with DRI for carbohydrate, fat, and protein, as noted in chapter 2. Because of possible problems in developing obesity, no RDA or UL were developed for energy. Instead, the Institute of Medicine uses the term **Estimated Energy Requirement (EER),** which it defines as the dietary intake that is predicted to maintain energy balance in a healthy adult of a defined age, gender, weight, height, and level of physical activity consistent with good health. In essence, the EER estimates your REE based on age, gender, weight, and height, and then modifies this value depending on your daily level of physical activity, which we refer to in this book as TEE.

Your total daily energy expenditure (TDEE) is the sum of your BEE, your TEF, and your TEE. Figure 3.17 provides some approximate values for the typical active individual, indicating that BEE accounts for 60–75 percent of the total daily energy expenditure, TEF represents 5–10 percent, and TEE explains 15–30 percent. These values are approximate and may vary tremendously, particularly TEE, which may range from near 0 percent in the totally sedentary individual to 50 percent or more in ultraendurance athletes.

To illustrate the effect that physical activity, or TEE, may have on your TDEE, the Institute of Medicine developed four **physical**

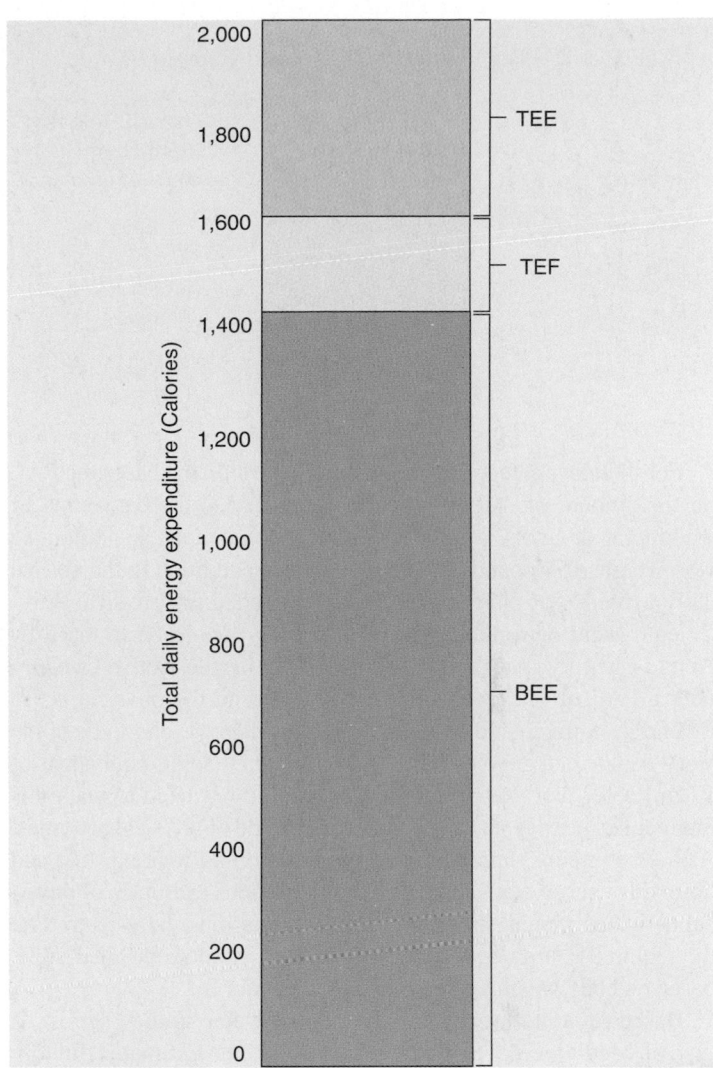

FIGURE 3.17 Total daily energy expenditure. Three major factors account for the total daily energy expenditure. Basal energy expenditure (BEE) accounts for 60–75 percent, the thermic effect of food (TEF) accounts for 5–10 percent, and 15–30 percent is accounted for by the thermic effect of exercise (TEE). However, all of these percentages are variable in different individuals, with exercise being the most modifiable component. In the figure, the BEE is 70 percent, the TEF is 10 percent, and the TEE is 20 percent.

activity level (PAL) categories, which are presented in table 3.7. The PAL describes the ratio of the TDEE divided by the BEE over a 24-hour period. The PAL in figure 3.17 is 1.43, or low active. The higher the ratio, the greater the amount of daily physical activity.

The energy expenditure in individuals in the Sedentary category represents their REE, including the TEF, plus various physical activities associated with independent living, such as walking from the house or work to the car, typing, and other forms of very light activity. Levine has coined the term **nonexercise activity thermogenesis (NEAT)** for these very light activities, which represent all the energy we expend daily that is not sleeping, eating, or sports-related exercise. NEAT includes such activities as playing the piano, dancing, housework, washing the car, and similar daily physical activities. We shall discuss the role of NEAT in weight control in chapter 10.

TABLE 3.7 The Physical Activity Level Categories

Category	Physical Activity Level (PAL)	Physical Activity Coefficient (PA) Males/Females
Sedentary	≥ 1.0 – < 1.4	1.00/1.00
Low Active	≥ 1.4 – < 1.6	1.11/1.12
Active	≥1.6 – < 1.9	1.25/1.27
Very Active	≥1.9 – < 2.5	1.48/1.45

For the other categories, the Institute of Medicine bases the PAL on the amount of daily physical activity that is the equivalent of walking at a rate of 3–4 miles per hour. For example, an adult male who weighs 154 pounds (70 kg) and who, in addition to the normal daily activities of independent living, expended the physical activity equivalent of walking 2.2 miles per day would be in the Low Active category, with a PAL of 1.5. To be in the Active category with a PAL of 1.75, he would need to expend the physical activity energy equivalent of walking 7.0 miles per day, and to be in the Very Active category with a PAL of 2.2, the energy equivalent of 17 miles per day. Keep in mind that you do not need to walk this many miles per day, but simply do a multitude of physical activities, such as climbing stairs, golfing, swimming, and jogging, that add up to this energy equivalent. Table 3.6 provides examples of physical activities ranging from light to heavy that may be used to total the required energy equivalents of walking. A more detailed table, based on body weight, is presented in appendix B.

Based on a number of doubly labeled water studies, the Institute of Medicine developed equations for the Estimated Energy Requirement (EER). Here are two:

Males, 19 years and older:

$$EER = 662 - 9.53 \times age + [PA \times (15.91 \times Weight + 539.6 \times Height)]$$

Females, 19 years and older:

$$EER = 354 - 6.91 \times age + [PA \times (9.361 \times Weight + 726 \times Height)]$$

Age: In years.

Weight: In kilograms (kg). To convert weight in pounds to kilograms, multiply by 0.454.

Height: In meters (m). To convert height in inches to meters, multiply by 0.0254.

PA: PA is the physical activity coefficient, which is based on the PAL. Based on mathematical consideration to equate energy expenditure between the various PAL categories, the PA coefficient for the Sedentary category was set at 1.0 and the PA for the other categories adjusted accordingly. The PAs for the four PAL categories are presented for adult males and females in table 3.7.

Although there may be variances in this estimate of your EER, the estimate may provide you with a ballpark figure of your daily energy needs. Let's look at an example, as depicted in figure 3.18, of the difference that physical activity may have on the daily energy needs of a sedentary and very active adult female. Both are 20 years old, weigh 132 pounds (60 kg), and are 55 inches (1.4 m) tall.

Sedentary:

$$EER = 354 - 6.91 \times 20 + [1.0 \times (9.361 \times 60 + 726 \times 1.4)]$$
$$EER = 354 - 138.2 + [1.0 \times (561.66 + 1,016.4)]$$
$$EER = 215.8 + [1,578.06] = 1,794 \text{ Calories}$$

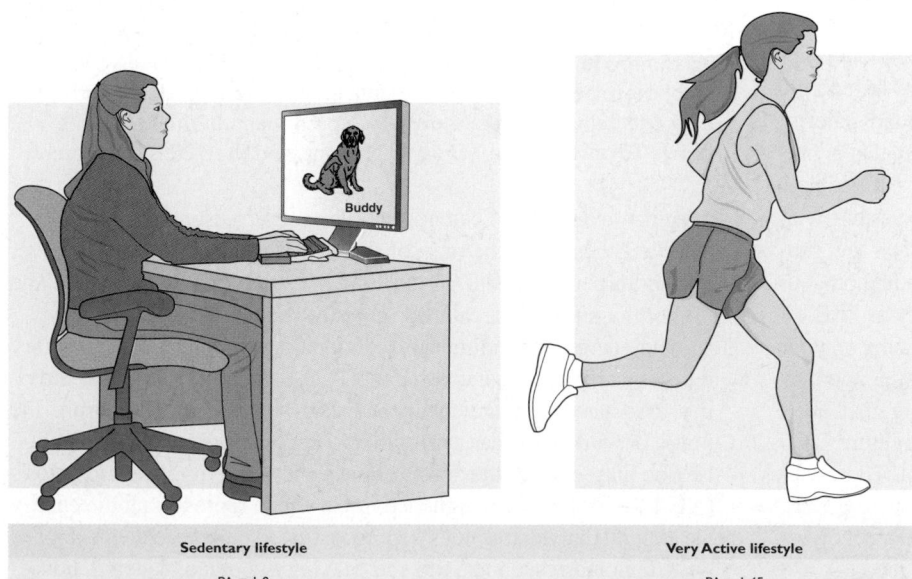

Sedentary lifestyle
PA = 1.0
EER = 1,794 Calories

Very Active lifestyle
PA = 1.45
EER = 2,504 Calories

FIGURE 3.18 Estimated Energy Requirement (EER) for two 20-year-old females. Both weigh 132 pounds (60 kg) and are 55 inches (1.4 m) tall. The sedentary female has a Physical Activity Coefficient (PA) of 1.0, whereas the very active female has a PA of 1.45. Compared to her sedentary counterpart, the very active female needs about 700 additional Calories to sustain her physically active lifestyle.

Very active:

$$EER = 354 - 6.91 \times 20 + [1.45 \times (9.361 \times 60 + 726 \times 1.4)]$$
$$EER = 354 - 138.2 + [1.45 \times (561.66 + 1,016.4)]$$
$$EER = 2,15.8 + [2,288.19] = 2,504 \text{ Calories}$$

The total caloric difference between the sedentary and very active women approximates 700 Calories per day, which may be important in several ways for the very active female. First, as noted in chapter 1, increased physical activity is an important aspect of a healthy lifestyle to prevent a variety of chronic diseases. Second, this additional 700 Calories of energy expenditure daily could have a significant impact on her body weight over time, approximating a loss of more than a pound per week if not compensated for by increased food intake. Third, if she is at an optimal body weight, she may consume an additional 700 Calories per day without gaining weight.

If you are interested in increasing your PAL, then your best bet is to incorporate more light, moderate, and moderately heavy to heavy physical activities into your daily lifestyle. Some additional guidelines for estimating your daily TDEE and EER, particularly in the design of a proper weight control program, are presented in chapter 11.

www.nap.edu Full details concerning the EER and PAL are provided by the National Academies Press. Type in *Dietary Reference Intake for Energy* in the search box. Review chapters 5 and 12, which focus on energy and physical activity.

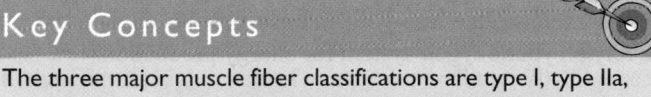

Key Concepts

▶ The three major muscle fiber classifications are type I, type IIa, and type IIb. Type I, known as a slow-oxidative fiber, produces ATP aerobically. Type IIa, also known as a fast-oxidative glycolytic fiber, produces ATP both aerobically and anaerobically. Type IIb, also known as a fast glycolytic fiber, produces ATP anaerobically.

▶ The thermic effect of exercise (TEE), or exercise metabolic rate (EMR) provides us with the most practical means to increase energy expenditure.

▶ The metabolic rate during exercise is directly proportional to the intensity of the exercise, and the exercise heart rate may serve as a general indicator of the metabolic rate.

▶ Activities that use the large muscle groups of the body, such as running, swimming, bicycling, and aerobic dance, facilitate energy expenditure. Resistance training of sufficient intensity and duration may also help expend enough energy to satisfy exercise recommendations for caloric expenditure.

▶ The total daily energy expenditure (TDEE) is accounted for by BEE (60–75 percent), TEF (5–10 percent), and TEE (15–30 percent), although these percentages may vary considerably among individuals.

▶ The Estimated Energy Requirement (EER) is defined as the dietary intake that is predicted to maintain energy balance in a healthy adult of a defined age, gender, height, weight, and level of physical activity consistent with good health. Changing from a sedentary Physical Activity Level (PAL) to a very active PAL is a very effective means to increase TDEE and EER.

Check for Yourself

▶ Record the types and amounts (in minutes) of your daily physical activity (or use the record from Chapter 1) and consult appendix B to determine your total amount of daily energy expenditure through physical activity and exercise. The application exercise on page 113 may be useful.

Human Energy Systems and Fatigue during Exercise

What energy systems are used during exercise?

In sport, energy expenditure can vary tremendously. For example, Asker Jeukendrup and his associates noted that in one sport, World Class Cycling, events may range in duration from 10 seconds to 3 weeks, involving race distances between 200 meters to 4,000 kilometers. Exercise intensity in a 200-meter event would be extremely high, and much lower during the prolonged event.

The most important factor determining which energy system will be used is the intensity of the exercise, which is the rate, speed, or tempo at which you pursue a given activity. In general, the faster you do something, the higher your rate of energy expenditure and the more rapidly you must produce ATP for muscular contraction. Very rapid muscular movements are characterized by high rates of power production. If you were asked to run 100 meters as fast as you could, you would exert maximal speed for a short time. On the other hand, if you were asked to run 5 miles, you certainly would not run at the same speed as you would for the 100 meters. In the 100-meter run your energy expenditure would be very rapid, characterized by a high-power production. The 5-mile run would be characterized by low-power production, or endurance.

The requirement of energy for exercise is related to a power-endurance continuum. On the power end, we have extremely high rates of energy expenditure that a sprinter might use; on the endurance end, we see lower rates that might be characteristic of a marathon runner. The closer we are to the power end of the continuum, the more rapidly we must produce ATP. As we move toward the endurance end, our rate of ATP production does not have to be as great, but we need the capacity to produce ATP for a longer time.

It should be noted from the outset that all three energy systems—ATP-PCr, lactic acid, and oxygen—are used in one way or another during most athletic activities. (Gastin provides an excellent overview.) However, one system may predominate, depending primarily on the intensity level of the activity. In this regard, the three human energy systems may be ranked according to several characteristics, which are displayed in table 3.8.

Both the ATP-PCr and the lactic acid systems are able to produce ATP rapidly and are used in events characterized by high intensity levels that occur for short periods, because their capacity for total ATP production is limited. Because both of these systems may function without oxygen, they are called anaerobic. Relative to running performance, the ATP-PCr system predominates in short,

the 400-meter dash may involve depletion of PCr and muscle glycogen, but may also be associated with increases in hydrogen ion concentration.

How can I delay the onset of fatigue?

The most important factor in the prevention of premature fatigue is proper training, including physiological, psychological, and biomechanical training.

Physiologically, athletes must train specifically on the energy system or systems that are inherent to their event. Under the guidance of sport physiologists and coaches, appropriate physiological training for each specific energy system may increase its energy stores, enzymatic activity, and metabolic efficiency, thus enhancing energy production. Physiological training enhances physical power.

Psychologically, athletes must train the mind to tolerate the stresses associated with their specific event. Sport psychologists may help provide the athlete with various mental strategies, such as inducing either a state of relaxation or arousal, whichever may be appropriate for their sport. Physiological training may also confer some psychological advantages, such as tolerating higher levels of pain associated with intense exercise. Psychological training enhances mental strength.

Biomechanically, athletes must maximize the mechanical skills associated with their sport. For any sport, sport biomechanists can analyze the athlete's skill level and recommend modifications in movement patterns or equipment to improve energy production or efficiency. In many cases, modification of the amount of body fat and muscle mass may provide the athlete with a biomechanical advantage. Biomechanical training helps provide a mechanical edge.

Proper physiological, psychological, and biomechanical training represents the best means to help deter premature fatigue. However, what you eat may affect physiological, psychological,

and biomechanical aspects of sport performance. Thus, nutrition is an important consideration in delaying the onset of fatigue during sport training and competition.

How is nutrition related to fatigue processes?

As noted in our discussion of the power-endurance continuum, we can exercise at different intensities, but the duration of our exercise is inversely related to the intensity. We can exercise at a high intensity for a short time or at a low intensity for a long time. The importance of nutrition to fatigue is determined by this intensity-duration interrelationship.

In very mild aerobic activities, such as distance walking or low-speed running in a trained ultramarathoner, the body can sustain energy production by using fat as the primary fuel when carbohydrate levels diminish. Because the body has large stores of fat, energy supply is not a problem. However, low blood sugar levels, dehydration, and excessive loss of minerals may lead to the development of both mental and physical fatigue in very prolonged activities.

In moderate to heavy aerobic exercise, the body needs to use more carbohydrate as an energy source and thus will run out of muscle glycogen faster. As we shall see later, carbohydrate is a more efficient fuel than fat, so the athlete will have to reduce the pace of the activity when liver and muscle carbohydrate stores are depleted, such as during endurance-type activities lasting more than 90 minutes. Thus, energy supply may be critical. Low blood sugar, changes in blood constituents such as certain amino acids, and dehydration also may be important factors contributing to the development of mental or physical fatigue in this type of endeavor.

In very high-intensity exercise lasting only 1 or 2 minutes, the probable cause of fatigue is the disruption of cellular metabolism caused by the accumulation of hydrogen ions resulting from

TABLE 3.11 Examples of some nutritional ergogenic aids and, theoretically, how they may influence physiological, psychological, or biomechanical processes to delay fatigue

Provide energy substrate	**Attenuate fatigue-related metabolic by-products**
Carbohydrate: Energy substrate for aerobic glycolysis	Beta-alanine: Amino acid that acts as an intracellular buffer and attenuates acidosis
Creatine: Substrate for formation of phosphocreatine (PCr)	Sodium bicarbonate: Buffer to reduce effects of lactic acid
Enhance energy-generating metabolic pathways	**Prevent catabolism of energy-generating cells**
B vitamins: Coenzymes in aerobic and anaerobic glycolysis	Antioxidants: Vitamins to prevent unwanted oxidation of cell membranes
Carnitine: Enzyme substrate to facilitate fat metabolism	HMB: By-product of amino acid metabolism to prevent protein degradation
Increase cardiovascular-respiratory function	**Ameliorate psychological function**
Iron: Substrate for hemoglobin formation and oxygen transport	BCAA: Amino acids that favorably modify neurotransmitter production
Glycerol: Substance to increase blood volume	Choline: Substrate for formation of acetylcholine, a neurotransmitter
Increase size or number of energy-generating cells	**Improve mechanical efficiency**
Arginine and ornithine: Amino acids that stimulate production of human growth hormone, an anabolic hormone	Ma huang: Stimulant to increase metabolism for fat loss
Chromium: Mineral to potentiate activity of insulin, an anabolic hormone	Hydroxycitrate (HCA): Supplement to increase fat oxidation for fat loss

Note: These examples as to how nutritional aids may delay fatigue are based on theoretical considerations. As shall be shown in respective chapters, supplementation with most of these nutritional ergogenic aids has not been shown to enhance exercise or sport performance.

excess lactic acid production. There is some evidence to suggest that sodium bicarbonate and beta alanine (discussed in chapter 13), which promote intracellular buffering, may help reduce the disruptive effect of lactic acid to some extent. Furthermore, a very low supply of muscle glycogen in fast-twitch muscle fibers may impair this type of performance.

In extremely intense exercise lasting only 5–10 seconds, a depletion of phosphocreatine (PCr) may be related to the inability to maintain a high force production. Although some nutritional practices, such as phosphate loading or gelatin supplements, have been used in attempts to increase PCr, they have not been regarded as effective. However, recent research involving creatine supplements has shown some beneficial effects, which are discussed in chapter 6.

In summary, a deficiency of almost every nutrient may be a causative factor in the development of fatigue. A poor diet can hasten the onset of fatigue. Proper nutrition is essential to assure the athlete that an adequate supply of nutrients is available in the diet, not only to provide the necessary energy, such as through carbohydrate and fat, but also to ensure optimal metabolism of the energy substrate via protein, vitamins, minerals, and water. The role of specific nutrients or dietary supplements relative to fatigue processes will be discussed in later sections of the book where appropriate. Table 3.11 provides some examples of how some nutrients or dietary supplements are thought to delay fatigue.

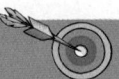

Key Concepts

► The ATP-PCr and lactic acid energy systems are used primarily during fast, anaerobic, power-type events, while the oxygen system is used primarily during aerobic, endurance-type events.
► Fats serve as the primary source of fuel during mild levels of aerobic exercise intensity, but carbohydrates begin to be the preferred fuel as exercise intensity increases.
► Fatigue may be classified as central (neural) or peripheral (muscular) fatigue. Fatigue may also be caused by a variety of factors, including the depletion of energy substrate or the accumulation of fatigue-causing metabolites.
► A sound training program and proper nutrition are important factors in the prevention of fatigue during exercise.

Check for Yourself

► Check the world records in running for 100 meters, 400 meters, 1,500 meters, and the marathon (42,200 meters). Calculate the average speed for each distance. Can you relate your findings to the human energy systems and their relationship to fatigue?

APPLICATION EXERCISE

Borrow, rent, or buy a pedometer or an accelerometer and keep a record of your daily movement (recording the amount every 2 hours). This will provide you with an estimate of your daily physical activity involving movement and will be useful in determining your estimated energy requirement (EER) and maintaining an optimal body weight as discussed in chapter 11.

	Distance logged Sunday	Distance logged Monday	Distance logged Tuesday	Distance logged Wednesday	Distance logged Thursday	Distance logged Friday	Distance logged Saturday
12:00–2:00 A.M.							
2:00–4:00 A.M.							
4:00–6:00 A.M.							
6:00–8:00 A.M.							
8:00–10:00 A.M.							
10:00–12:00 A.M.							
12:00–2:00 P.M.							
2:00–4:00 P.M.							
4:00–6:00 P.M.							
6:00–8:00 P.M.							
8:00–10:00 P.M.							
10:00–12:00 P.M.							

1. Which energy system would predominate in an all-out, high-intensity, 400-meter dash in track?

   a. ATP-PCr
   b. lactic acid
   c. oxygen–carbohydrate
   d. oxygen–fat
   e. oxygen–protein

2. If a 50-kilogram body-weight athlete was exercising at an oxygen consumption level of 2.45 liters (2,450 ml) per minute, approximately how many METS would she be attaining?

   a. 8
   b. 10
   c. 11
   d. 12
   e. 14
   f. insufficient data to calculate the answer

3. Which of the following classifications of physical activity is rated as light, mild aerobic exercise—because it is likely to burn less than 7 Calories per minute?

   a. competitive racquetball
   b. running at a speed of 7 miles per hour
   c. walking at a speed of 2.0 miles per hour
   d. competitive singles tennis
   e. bicycling at a speed of 12 miles per hour

4. Which of the following statements relative to the basal metabolic rate or resting metabolic rate is false?

   a. The BMR is high in infancy but declines throughout adolescence and adulthood.
   b. The BMR is higher in women than in men due to the generally higher levels of body fat in women.

   c. The resting metabolic rate is the equivalent of one MET.
   d. The resting metabolic rate is higher than the BMR.
   e. Dietary-induced thermogenesis raises the resting metabolic rate.

5. Which of the following is not likely to be a cause of fatigue?

   a. depletion of PCr in fast-twitch fibers in a 200-meter dash
   b. depletion of muscle glycogen in fast-twitch fibers in a 400-meter dash
   c. depletion of adipose cell fatty acids in a marathon
   d. depletion of muscle glycogen in a marathon
   e. accumulation of hydrogen ions in a 400-meter dash

6. Of the following statements concerning the interrelationships between various forms of energy, which one is false?

   a. A kilojoule is greater than a kilocalorie.
   b. A kilogram-meter is equal to 7.23 foot-pounds.
   c. A gram of fat has more Calories than a gram of carbohydrate.
   d. A gram of fat has more Calories than a gram of protein.
   e. A liter of oxygen can release more than one kilocalorie when metabolizing carbohydrate.

7. Approximately how many Calories will a 200-pound individual use while jogging a mile?

   a. 70   d. 255
   b. 145   e. 440
   c. 200

8. Which of the following statements relative to exercise and metabolic rate is false?

   a. The intensity of the exercise is the most important factor to increase the metabolic rate.
   b. Increased efficiency for swimming a set distance will decrease the energy cost.
   c. The heavier person will burn more Calories running a mile than a lighter person.
   d. Oxygen consumption and heart rate are two ways to monitor the metabolic rate.
   e. Walking a mile slowly or jogging a mile cost the same amount of Calories.

9. Which energy system has the greatest capacity for energy production, (i.e., endurance?)

   a. ATP-PCr
   b. lactic acid
   c. anaerobic glycolysis
   d. oxygen
   e. phosphagens

10. Which of the following is *not* needed to calculate the estimated energy requirement (EER)?

   a. body fat percentage
   b. age
   c. height
   d. weight
   e. physical activity level (PAL)

1. b; 2. e; 3. c; 4. b; 5. c; 6. a; 7. b; 8. e; 9. d; 10. a.

1. If an individual performed 5,000 foot-pounds of work in one minute, how many kilojoules of work were accomplished?

2. Name the sources of energy stored in the human body and discuss their role in the three human energy systems.

3. Differentiate between BMR, RMR, BEE, REE, TEF, TEE, EER, and TDEE as defined in this text.

4. Explain the role of the three energy systems during exercise and provide an example using track running events. Which muscle fiber types are the major source

of energy production during these track events?

5. List the major causes of fatigue during exercise and indicate how various nutritional interventions may help prevent premature fatigue.

Books

Fox, E. L. 1979. *Sports Physiology.* Dubuque, IA: Wm. C. Brown.

Houston, M. 2006. *Biochemistry Primer for Exercise Science.* Champaign, IL: Human Kinetics.

Lee, R., and Nieman, D. 2003. *Nutritional Assessment.* Boston: McGraw-Hill.

Mooren, F., and Völker, K. 2005. *Molecular and Cellular Exercise Physiology.* Champaign, IL: Human Kinetics.

National Academy of Sciences. 2005. *Dietary Reference Intakes for Energy, Carbohydrates, Fiber, Fat, Protein, and Amino Acids (Macronutrients).* Washington, DC: National Academy Press.

Welk, G. 2002. *Physical Activity Assessments for Health-Related Research.* Champaign, IL: Human Kinetics.

Review Articles

Ainsworth, B., et al. 2011. 2011 Compendium of Physical Activities: A second update of codes and MET values. *Medicine and Science in Sports and Exercise* 43:1575–81.

Baker, L., and Kenney, W. 2007. Exercising in the heat and sun. *President's Council on Physical Fitness and Sports Research Digest* 8 (2):1–8.

Brooks, G. 1998. Mammalian fuel utilization during sustained exercise. *Comparative Biochemistry & Physiology: Part B. Biochemistry Molecular & Biology* 120:89–107.

Budgett, R. 1998. Fatigue and underperformance in athletes: The overtraining syndrome. *British Journal of Sports Medicine* 32:107–10.

Burke, S., et al. 2006. Group versus individual approach? A meta-analysis of the effectiveness of interventions to promote physical activity. *Sport & Exercise Psychology Review* 2:19–35.

Cairns, S., et al. 2005. Evaluation of models used to study neuromuscular fatigue. *Exercise & Sports Sciences Reviews* 33:9–16.

Conley, K., et al. 2001. Limits to sustainable muscle performance: Interaction between glycolysis and oxidative phosphorylation. *Journal of Experimental Biology* 204:3189–94.

Coyle, E. 2007. Physiological regulation of marathon performance. *Sports Medicine* 37:306–11.

Davis, J., et al. 2000. Serotonin and central nervous system fatigue: Nutritional considerations. *American Journal of Clinical Nutrition* 72:573S–78S.

de Jonge, L., and Bray, G. 1997. The thermic effect of food and obesity. *Obesity Research* 5:622–31.

Dempsey, J., et al. 2008. Respiratory system determinants of peripheral fatigue and endurance performance. *Medicine & Science in Sports & Exercise* 40:457–61.

Edgerton, V., and Roy, R. 2006. The nervous system and movement. In *ACSM's Advanced Exercise Physiology,* ed. C. M. Tipton. Philadelphia: Lippincott Williams & Wilkins.

Evans, W., and Lambert, C. 2007. Physiological basis of fatigue. *American Journal of Physical Medicine & Rehabilitation* 86:S29–S46.

Fitts, R. 2008. The cross-bridge cycle and skeletal muscle fatigue. *Journal of Applied Physiology* 104:551–58.

Fitts, R. 2006. The muscular system: Fatigue processes. In *ACSM's Advanced Exercise Physiology,* ed. C. M. Tipton. Philadelphia: Lippincott Williams & Wilkins.

Garber, C., et al. 2011. American College of Sports Medicine Position Stand: Quantity and quality of exercise for developing and maintaining cardiorespiratory, musculoskeletal, and neuromotor fitness in apparently healthy adults: Guidance for prescribing exercise. *Medicine & Science in Sports & Exercise* 43:1334–59.

Gastin, P. 2001. Energy system interaction and relative contribution during maximal exercise. *Sports Medicine* 31:725–41.

Goran, M. 1997. Genetic influence on human energy expenditure and substrate utilization. *Behavior Genetics* 27:389–99.

Granata, G., and Brandon, L. 2002. The thermic effect of food and obesity: Discrepant results and methodological variations. *Nutrition Reviews* 60:223–33.

Green, H. 2004. Mechanisms and management of fatigue in health and disease: Symposium introduction. *Canadian Journal of Applied Physiology* 29:264–73.

Hagberg, J., and Pena, N. 1989. Bicycling's exclusive calorie counter. *Bicycling* 30:100–103.

Halson, S., and Jeukendrup, A. 2004. Does overtraining exist? An analysis of overreaching and overtraining research. *Sports Medicine* 34:967–81.

Hargreaves, M. 2005. Metabolic factors in fatigue. *Sports Science Exchange* 18 (3):1–6.

Hargreaves, M. 2000. Skeletal muscle metabolism during exercise in humans. *Clinical & Experimental Pharmacology & Physiology* 27:225–28.

Hawley, J., and Hopkins, W. 1995. Aerobic glycolytic and aerobic lipolytic power systems. *Sports Medicine* 19:240–50.

Holloszy, J., et al. 1998. The regulation of carbohydrate and fat metabolism during and after exercise. *Frontiers in Bioscience* 3:D1011–27.

Hoppeler, H., and Weibel, E. 2000. Structural and functional limits for oxygen supply to muscle. *Acta Physiologica Scandinavica* 168:445–56.

International Life Sciences Institute. 2000. Measurement of moderate physical activity: Advances in assessment techniques. *Medicine and Science in Sports and Exercise* 32: S438–516.

Jeukendrup, A., et al. 2000. The bioenergetics of World Class Cycling. *Journal of Science & Medicine in Sport* 3:414–33.

Kearney, J., et al. 2000. Measurement of work and power in sport. In *Exercise and Sport Sciences,* eds. W. E. Garrett and D. T. Kirkendall. Philadelphia: Lippincott Williams & Wilkins.

Knuttgen, H. 1995. Force, work, and power in athletic training. *Sports Science Exchange* 8(4):1–6.

Kovacs, M. 2007. Tennis physiology: Training the competitive athlete. *Sports Medicine* 37:189–98.

Kuo, A., et al. 2005. Energetic consequences of walking like an inverted pendulum: Step-to-step transitions. *Exercise & Sports Sciences Reviews* 33:88–97.

Lambert, C., and Flynn, M. 2002. Fatigue during high-intensity intermittent exercise: Application to bodybuilding. *Sports Medicine* 32:511–22.

Lambert, E., et al. 2005. Complex systems model of fatigue: Integrative homeostatic control of peripheral physiological systems during exercise in humans. *British Journal of Sports Medicine* 39:52–62.

Lange, B., and Bury, T. 2001. Physiologic evaluation of explosive force in sports. *Revue Medicale de Liege* 56:233–38.

Levine, J. 2005. Measurement of energy expenditure. *Public Health Nutrition* 8:1123–32.

Levine, J. 2004. Non-exercise activity thermogenesis. *Nutrition Reviews* 62:S82–S97.

Melanson, E., et al. 2009. Exercise improves fat metabolism in muscle but does not increase 24-h fat oxidation. *Exercise & Sports Science Reviews* 37:93–101.

McMahon, S., and Jenkins, D. 2002. Factors affecting the rate of phosphocreatine resynthesis following intense exercise. *Sports Medicine* 32:761–84.

Meeusen, R., et al. 2006. The brain and fatigue: New opportunities for nutritional interventions? *Journal of Sports Sciences* 24:773–82.

Mooren, F., et al. 2005. Inter- and intracellular signaling. In *Molecular and Cellular Exercise Physiology,* eds. F. Mooren and K. Völker. Champaign, IL: Human Kinetics.

Myburgh, K. 2004. Protecting muscle ATP: Positive roles for peripheral defense mechanisms. *Medicine & Science in Sports & Exercise* 37:16–19.

Neiss, A. 2005. Generation and disposal of reactive oxygen and nitrogen species. In *Molecular and Cellular Exercise Physiology,* eds. F. Mooren and K. Völker. Champaign, IL: Human Kinetics.

Newsholme, E. 1993. Application of knowledge of metabolic integration to the problem of metabolic limitations in sprints, middle distance and marathon running. In *Principles of Exercise Biochemistry,* ed. J. Poortmans. Basel, Switzerland: Karger.

Noakes, T. 2011. Time to move beyond a brainless exercise physiology: The evidence for complex regulation of human exercise performance. *Applied Physiology Nutrition and Metabolism* 36:23–35.

Noakes, T. 2007. The central governor model of exercise regulation applies to the marathon. *Sports Medicine* 37:374–77.

Nybo, L., and Rasmussen, P. 2007. Inadequate cerebral oxygen delivery and central fatigue during strenuous exercise. *Exercise and Sport Sciences Reviews* 35:110–118.

O'Connor, P., Puetz, T. 2005. Chronic physical activity and feelings of energy and fatigue. *Medicine & Science in Sports and Exercise* 37:299–305.

Peters, A., et al. 2004. The selfish brain: Competition for energy resources. *Neuroscience and Biobehavior Reviews* 28:143–80.

Sale, C., et al. 2010. Effect of beta-alanine supplementation on muscle carnosine concentrations exercise performance. *Amino Acids* 39:321–33.

Shephard, R. 2001. Chronic fatigue syndrome: An update. *Sports Medicine* 31:167–94.

Skinner, J. 2004. Chronic fatigue syndrome. *Physician and Sportsmedicine* 32 (2):28–32.

Stager, J., et al. 1995. The use of doubly labelled water in quantifying energy expenditure during prolonged activity. *Sports Medicine* 19:166–72.

Thompson, J., et al. 1996. Effects of diet and diet-plus-exercise programs on resting metabolic rate: A meta-analysis. *International Journal of Sport Nutrition* 6:41–61.

Tremblay, A., et al. 1985. The effects of exercise-training on energy balance and adipose tissue morphology and metabolism. *Sports Medicine* 2:223–33.

Tudor-Locke, C. and Lutes, L. 2009. Why do pedometers work?: A reflection upon the factors related to successfully increasing physical activity. *Sports Medicine* 39:981–93.

Vaz, M., et al. 2005. A compilation of energy costs of physical activities. *Public Health Nutrition* I8:1153–83.

Ward, D., et al. 2005. Accelerometer use in physical activity: Best practices and research recommendations. *Medicine & Science in Sports & Exercise* 37:S582–S588.

Weir, J., et al. 2006. Is fatigue all in your head? A critical review of the central governor model. *British Journal of Sports Medicine* 40:573–86.

Wyller, V. 2007. The chronic fatigue syndrome—an update. *Acta Neurologica Scandinavica Supplementum* 187:7–14.

Specific Studies

Beers, E., et al. 2008. Increasing passive energy expenditure during clerical work. *European Journal of Applied Physiology* 103:353–60.

Biewener, A., et al. 2004. Muscle mechanical advantage of human walking and running: Implications for energy cost. *Journal of Applied Physiology* 97:2266–74.

Bloomer, R. 2005. Energy cost of moderate-duration resistance and aerobic exercise. *Journal of Strength and Conditioning Research* 19:878–82.

Burleson, M., et al. 1998. Effect of weight training exercise and treadmill exercise on post-exercise oxygen consumption. *Medicine & Science in Sports Exercise* 30:518–22.

Coutts, A., et al. 2007. Monitoring for overreaching in rugby league players. *European Journal of Applied Physiology* 99:313–24.

Crovetti, R., et al. 1998. The influence of thermic effect of food on satiety. *European Journal of Clinical Nutrition* 52:482–88.

Esliger, D., and Tremblay, M. 2006. Technical reliability assessment of three accelerometer models in a mechanical setup. *Medicine & Science in Sports & Exercise* 38:2173–81.

Gillette, C., et al. 1994. Postexercise energy expenditure in response to acute aerobic or resistive exercise. *International Journal of Sport Nutrition* 4:347–60.

Graves, J., et al. 1987. The effect of hand-held weights on the physiological responses to walking exercise. *Medicine & Science in Sports & Exercise* 19:260–65.

Haddock, B., and Wilkin, L. 2006. Resistance training volume and post-exercise energy expenditure. *International Journal of Sports Medicine* 27:143–48.

Hall, C., et al. 2004. Energy expenditure of walking and running: Comparison of prediction equations. *Medicine & Science in Sports & Exercise* 36:2128–34.

Katzmarzyk, P., et al. 2009. Sitting time and mortality from all causes, cardiovascular disease, and cancer. *Medicine & Science in Sports & Exercise* 41:998–1005.

Leblanc, J. 1992. Mechanisms of adaptation to cold. *International Journal of Sports Medicine* 13 (Supplement 1): S169–78.

Lyden, K., et al. 2011. A comprehensive evaluation of commonly used accelerometer energy expenditure and MET prediction equations. *European Journal of Applied Physiology* 111:187–201.

Matthews, C., et al. 2008. Amount of time spent in sedentary behaviors in the United States, 2003–2004. *American Journal of Epidemiology* 167:875–81.

Nijs, J., et al. 2005. Chronic fatigue syndrome: Exercise performance related to immune dysfunction. *Medicine & Science in Sports & Exercise* 37:1647–54.

Paoli, A., et al. 2011. Exercising fasting or fed to enhance fat loss? Influence of food intake on respiratory ratio and excess postexercise oxygen consumption after a bout of endurance training. *International Journal of Sports Nutrition & Exercise Metabolism* 21:48–54.

Pober, D., et al. 2006. Development of novel techniques to classify physical activity mode using accelerometers. *Medicine & Science in Sports & Exercise* 38:1626–34.

Reed, G., and Hill, J. 1996. Measuring the thermic effect of food. *American Journal of Clinical Nutrition* 63:164–69.

Schoeller, D., and Hnilicka, J. 1996. Reliability of the doubly labeled water method for the measurement of total daily energy expenditure in free-living subjects. *Journal of Nutrition* 126:348S–354S.

Sjodin, A., et al. 1996. The influence of physical activity on BMR. *Medicine & Science in Sports & Exercise* 28:85–91.

Spencer, M., and Gastin, P. 2001. Energy system contribution during 200- to 1500-m running in highly trained athletes. *Medicine & Science in Sports & Exercise* 33:157–62.

Staudenmayer, J., et al. 2009. An artificial neural network to estimate physical activity energy expenditure and identify physical activity type from an accelerometer. *Journal of Applied Physiology* 107:1300–7.

Thomas, T., and Londeree, B. 1989. Energy cost during prolonged walking vs jogging exercise. *Physician and Sportsmedicine* 17 (5):93–102.

Tremblay, A., et al. 1990. Long-term exercise training with constant energy intake. 2: effect of glucose metabolism and resting energy expenditure. *International Journal of Obesity* 14:75–81.

Ward-Smith, A. J. 1999. Aerobic and anaerobic energy conversion during high-intensity exercise. *Medicine & Science in Sports Exercise* 31:1855–60.

Wilmore, J. H., et al. 1998. Alterations in resting metabolic rate as a consequence of 20 wk of endurance training: The HERITAGE Family Study. *American Journal of Clinical Nutrition* 68:66–71.

Carbohydrates: The Main Energy Food

CHAPTER FOUR

LEARNING OBJECTIVES

After studying this chapter, you should be able to:

1. List the different types of dietary carbohydrates and identify foods typically rich in the different types.

2. Calculate the approximate number of Calories from carbohydrate that should be included in your daily diet.

3. Describe how dietary carbohydrate is absorbed, how it is distributed in the body, and what its major functions are in human metabolism.

4. Explain the role of carbohydrate in human energy systems during exercise.

5. Describe the various mechanisms whereby inadequate amounts of dietary carbohydrate may contribute to fatigue during exercise.

6. Understand the mechanisms whereby various dietary strategies involving carbohydrate intake (amount, type, and timing) before, during, and after exercise may help to optimize training for and competition in sport.

7. Identify athletes for whom carbohydrate loading may be appropriate, and describe the full carbohydrate loading protocol, highlighting dietary intake and exercise training considerations.

8. Evaluate the efficacy of metabolic by-products of carbohydrate metabolism as ergogenic aids.

9. Identify carbohydrate-containing foods that are considered to be more healthful and explain why.

10. Describe the effects of chronic endurance exercise training on the subsequent use of carbohydrate as an energy source during exercise, including underlying mechanisms and potential health benefits.

One of the most important nutrients in your diet, from the standpoint of both health and athletic performance, is dietary carbohydrate.

Over the years the reputation of carbohydrate, particularly as a component of a weight control diet, has seesawed between friend and foe. Most recently, some have dubbed carbohydrate as foe, alleging that high-carbohydrate diets are contributing to the epidemic of obesity within industrialized nations. However, most dietitians and nutrition scientists consider consumption of carbohydrate-rich foods to be one of the most important components of a healthful diet, not only for its potential in preventing certain chronic diseases but also as an integral part of a proper diet to lose excess body fat. However, as noted in the OmniHeart study, choosing *good* carbohydrates is the key. The possible health benefits of a diet high in complex carbohydrates and fiber and low in added sugars were introduced in chapter 2 and are explained further in this chapter. The role of carbohydrate foods in a weight control plan will be addressed in chapter 11 and, as we shall see, carbohydrates *per se* do not cause obesity, but excess Calories do.

As noted in chapter 3, the major role of carbohydrate in human nutrition is to provide energy, and scientists have long known that carbohydrate is one of the prime sources of energy during exercise. Of all the nutrients we consume, carbohydrate has received the most research attention in regard to a potential influence upon athletic performance, particularly in exercise tasks characterized by endurance, such as long-distance running, cycling, and triathloning. Such research is important to athletes who are concerned about optimal carbohydrate nutrition during training and competition. Indeed, continued research over the past quarter century has enabled sports nutritionists to provide more specific and useful responses to athletes' questions. For example, compared to the first edition of this book published in 1983, readers of this edition will note several

significant differences concerning dietary carbohydrate recommendations to athletes.

In this chapter, we explore the nature of dietary carbohydrates, their metabolic fates and interactions in the human body, their possible influence upon health status, and their potential application to physical performance, including the following: the adverse effects of low-carbohydrate diets; the value of carbohydrate intake before, during, and after exercise; the efficacy of different types of carbohydrates; the role of carbohydrate loading; and carbohydrate foods or compounds with alleged ergogenic properties. Although the role of sports drinks containing carbohydrate, such as Gatorade and PowerAde, is introduced in this chapter, additional detailed coverage of these beverages and their effect upon performance is presented in chapter 9: Water, Electrolytes, and Temperature Regulation.

Dietary Carbohydrates

What are the different types of dietary carbohydrates?

Carbohydrates represent one of the least expensive forms of Calories and hence are one of the major food supplies for the vast majority of the world's peoples. They are one of the three basic energy nutrients formed when the energy from the sun is harnessed in plants through the process of photosynthesis. Although the energy content of the various forms of carbohydrate varies slightly, each gram of carbohydrate contains approximately 4 Calories.

Carbohydrates are organic compounds that contain carbon, hydrogen, and oxygen in various combinations. A wide variety of different forms exist in nature and in the human body, and novel manufactured carbohydrates, including sports drinks, have been

developed for the food industry. In general terms, the major categories of importance to our discussion are simple carbohydrates, complex carbohydrates, and dietary fiber.

Simple carbohydrates, which are usually known as sugars, can be subdivided into two categories: disaccharides and monosaccharides. *Saccharide* means "sugar" or "sweet." Think of saccharin, a noncaloric sweetener. The three major **monosaccharides** (single sugars) are **glucose, fructose,** and **galactose.** Glucose and fructose occur widely in nature, primarily in fruits, as free monosaccharides. Glucose is often called *dextrose* or *grape sugar,* while fructose is known as *levulose* or *fruit sugar.* Galactose is found in milk as part of lactose. Figure 4.1 presents two configurations illustrating the structure of monosaccharides.

The combination of two monosaccharides yields a **disaccharide.** The disaccharides (double sugars) include maltose (malt sugar), lactose (milk sugar), and sucrose (cane sugar or table sugar). Upon digestion these disaccharides yield the monosaccharides as follows:

to foods durir
with the total
and grams o
percentage of
drate and fibe

As carboh,
several produc
drinks, sports
and PowerAd
or about 14–1
bohydrate sou
of one of the
polymers. Mo
Sports gels, su
tain forms of
but in a more
ers (usually a
carbohydrate.
athletes. They
2.3–8 grams o
carbohydrate,
amount and ty
ally ranging b
may contain s
or more gram
sports and "e
information o
carbohydrate,
as caffeine, ar
reading and pr
on some prod
so purchasing
value may pro

Foods high
foods in the s
beans and pea
sources of insc
vegetables are
ported health
new products
lium, rich in bc
breakfast cerea
common foods
Currently food
future labels m

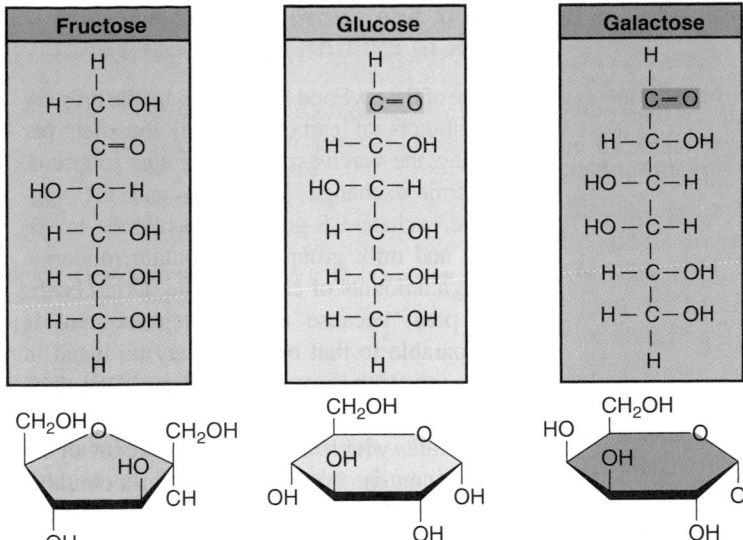

FIGURE 4.1 Chemical structure of the three monosaccharides is depicted in both the linear and ring configurations. Each corner in the ring structure contains a carbon atom, for a total of six carbons for each monosaccharide.

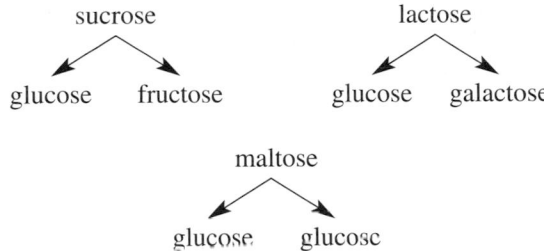

Monosaccharides and disaccharides, such as glucose and sucrose, may be isolated from foods in purified forms known as *refined sugars.* Trisaccharides and higher saccharides also exist, and may be found in commonly used sweeteners such as corn syrup. For example, high-fructose corn syrup, a common food additive, is a manufactured carbohydrate derived from the conversion of glucose in corn starch to fructose. Other food additives that are primarily sugar include honey, brown sugar, maple syrup, molasses, and fruit juice concentrate.

Complex carbohydrates, commonly known as *starches,* are generally formed when three or more glucose molecules combine. This combination is known as a **polysaccharide** when more than ten glucose molecules are combined, and may contain thousands of linked glucose molecules. Starches, which exist in a variety of forms such as amylose, amylopectin, and resistant starch, are the storage form of carbohydrates. The vast majority of carbohydrates that exist in the plant world are in polysaccharide form. Of prime interest to us are the plant starches, through which we obtain a good proportion of our daily Calories along with a wide variety of nutrients, and the animal starch, glycogen, about which we shall hear more later in relation to energy for exercise. Additionally, **glucose polymers** are polysaccharides prepared commercially by controlled hydrolysis of starch. Maltodextrins are common glucose polymers used in sports drinks, which are discussed later.

Unfortunately, because of disagreements over the classification of various forms of carbohydrate, the term "complex carbohydrate" does not appear on the Nutrition Facts food label. You may obtain a rough estimate of the complex carbohydrate content by subtracting the grams of sugar from the grams of total carbohydrate. In some cases, the term "other carbohydrates" is used, which could include complex carbohydrates and other forms of carbohydrate as well.

Fiber is a complex carbohydrate. In its recent report on Dietary Reference Intakes, the National Academy of Sciences settled on three terms to define fiber. **Dietary fiber** consists of nondigestible carbohydrates and lignin that are intrinsic and intact in plants; this would include resistant starch. **Functional fiber** consists of isolated, nondigestible carbohydrates that have beneficial physiological effects in humans. **Total fiber** is the sum of dietary fiber and functional fiber. These nondigestible substances, which means that they are not digested and absorbed in the human small intestine, are usually a mixture of polysaccharides found in the plant wall or intracellular structures.

The National Academy of Sciences carefully defines both dietary and functional fiber, particularly as they may affect health. In essence, dietary fiber is consumed as part of intact foods (even if mechanically altered) containing other macronutrients, such as digestible carbohydrate and protein. For example, cereal brans derived from whole grains contain carbohydrate and protein, along with nondigestible fiber. Some examples of dietary fiber are cellulose, hemicellulose, lignin, pectin, and gums. When studying the health effects of dietary fiber, it is difficult to determine if health benefits are attributed to dietary fiber or to other potential healthful substances, such as certain phytochemicals, found in the food. The definition of dietary fiber includes the phytochemicals that come with it.

Functional fibers, in contrast, may be isolated or extracted from foods by chemical or other means, and may be manufactured synthetically. For example, various gums may be extracted from seeds and used as food ingredients for various purposes. Some examples of functional fiber are pectin, gums, and resistant starch. The specific fiber has to demonstrate a physiological effect in the body to be classified as a functional fiber, and this effect may be associated with a specific health benefit.

Total fiber is the sum of dietary fiber and functional fiber. A specific fiber may be classified as both dietary fiber and functional fiber. For example, cellulose can be classified as dietary fiber as a natural ingredient of an intact food, or it may be considered to be a functional fiber if extracted from a natural source and added to another food.

Previously, the various components of dietary and functional fiber have been classified on the basis of their solubility in water. Some fibers have been referred to as water soluble because they have been found to dissolve or swell in water and may be metabolized by bacteria in the large intestine. Others that do not possess these characteristics have been referred to as water-insoluble fibers. Common water-soluble fibers include gums, beta-glucans, and pectins. Common water-insoluble fibers include cellulose, hemicellulose, and lignin. Each of these types of fibers may confer specific health benefits, which will be discussed later in this chapter.

Sugar substitutes are designed to provide the sweetness of sugars, but with no or fewer Calories. Two of the most commonly used sugar substitutes include aspartame, a derivative of two

TABLE 4.1

Monosacchari

Glucose
Fructose
Galactose

Dietary fiber

Hemicellulose
Resistant starch

*Certain forms
**Dietary fiber if four
***See text for food

amino acids, a
sugar substitute
   A summary
in table 4.1, an
physical perfor

TABLE 4.2

**Starch
exchange
(15 grams)**

Whole grain
   Brown rice
   Corn tortillas
   Granola
   Oatmeal
   Ready-to-eat
   cereal*
   Rye crackers
   Whole wheat
   bread
Enriched
   Bagels
   English muffins
   Pasta
   Ready-to-eat
   cereal*
   White bread
   White rice
Starchy vegetable
   Corn
   Green peas
   Potatoes

*May be whole wheat
†Typical serving sizes a
exchange (½ cup). Che

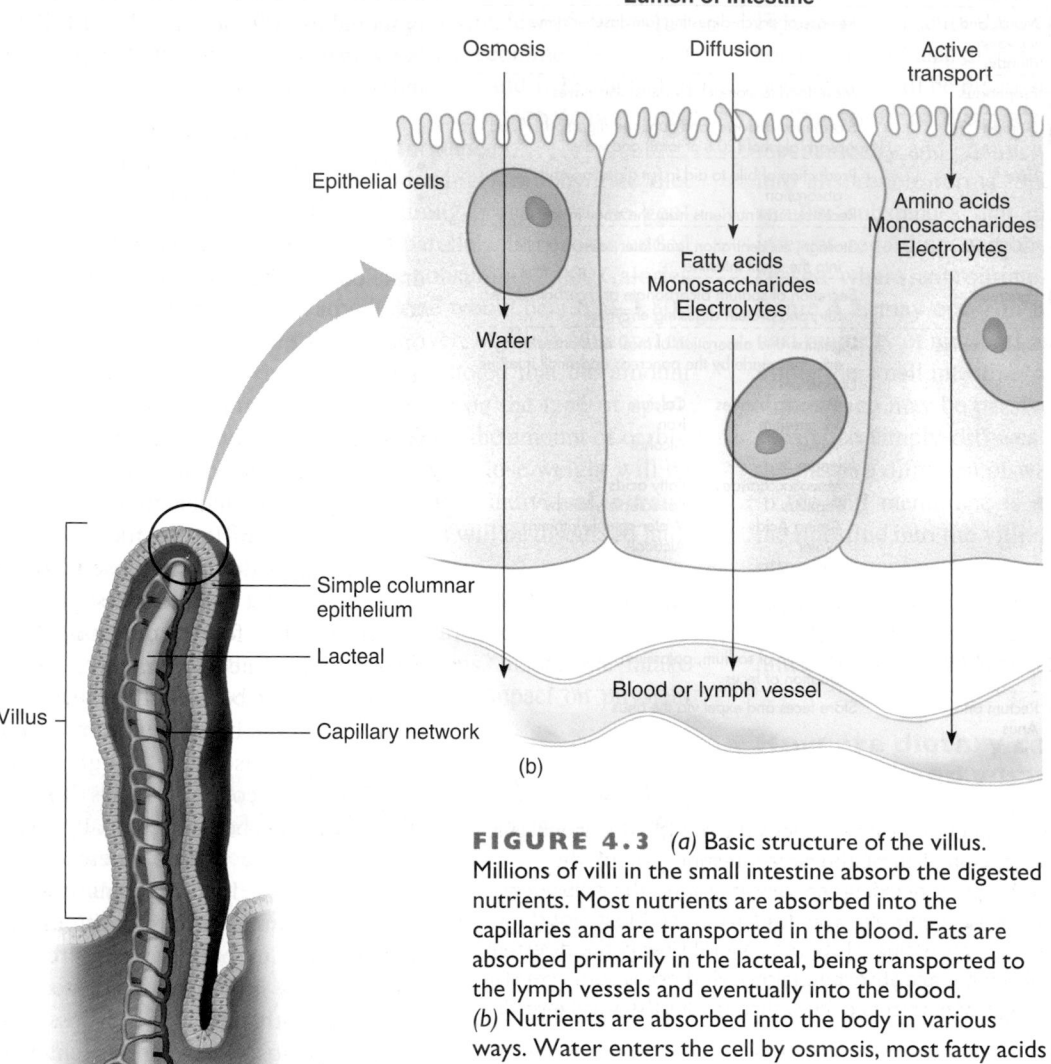

Lumen of Intestine

(a)

(b)

FIGURE 4.3 (a) Basic structure of the villus. Millions of villi in the small intestine absorb the digested nutrients. Most nutrients are absorbed into the capillaries and are transported in the blood. Fats are absorbed primarily in the lacteal, being transported to the lymph vessels and eventually into the blood. (b) Nutrients are absorbed into the body in various ways. Water enters the cell by osmosis, most fatty acids by diffusion, and amino acids enter via active transport, a process that requires energy. Monosaccharides and electrolytes may use two pathways, (i.e., diffusion and active transport).

from someone else's response. Moreover, individuals do not normally consume carbohydrate foods by themselves, but usually with other foods containing fat and protein such as a hamburger on a bun. The addition of fat and protein will usually reduce the glycemic index and glycemic load. Nevertheless, Keegan indicates that the glycemic index and glycemic load have been used to help select more healthful carbohydrates. In general, the lower the glycemic index or glycemic load, the more healthful the source of carbohydrate, as discussed later in this chapter.

www.mendosa.com/gilists.htm   Check the glycemic index and the glycemic load for a wide variety of carbohydrate-containing foods.

What is the metabolic fate of blood glucose?

Normal blood glucose levels (normoglycemia) range between 80–100 milligrams per deciliter of blood (80–100 mg/ml, or 80–100 milligram percent). The maintenance of a normal blood glucose level is very important for proper metabolism. Thus, the human body possesses a variety of mechanisms, primarily hormones, to help keep blood glucose levels under precise control. The rise in blood glucose, also known as *serum glucose,* stimulates the pancreas to secrete insulin into the blood. **Insulin** is a hormone that facilitates the uptake and utilization of glucose (facilitated diffusion) by various tissues in the body, most notably the muscles and adipose (fat) tissue. Cell membranes contain receptors to transport glucose into the cell. The primary receptors in muscle and fat cell membranes are known as GLUT-4 receptors, which are directly activated by insulin (see figure 4.5). Exercise also activates these receptors to transport blood glucose into the muscle cell, independently of the effect of insulin. Other hormones, discussed later in this chapter, are also involved in regulating blood glucose. With normal amounts of carbohydrate intake in a mixed meal, blood glucose levels remain normal.

   However, foods with a high glycemic index may lead rapidly to high blood glucose levels, possibly **hyperglycemia** (>140 mg percent), which will cause an enhanced secretion of insulin from the pancreas. High serum levels of insulin will then lead to a rapid, and possibly excessive, transport of blood glucose into the tissues. This may lead in turn to **hypoglycemia** (<40–50 mg percent), or low blood glucose level. This insulin response and **reactive hypoglycemia** following carbohydrate intake may be an important consideration for some athletes and is discussed later.

   Foods with a low glycemic index, particularly soluble fiber forms, lead to a slower insulin response and a more stable blood glucose level. Consuming a diet based on the glycemic index has been studied as a possible means to enhance health, as well as sports performance, as noted later in this chapter.

   The fate of blood glucose is dependent upon a multitude of factors, and exercise is one of the most important. The following

Carbohydrates

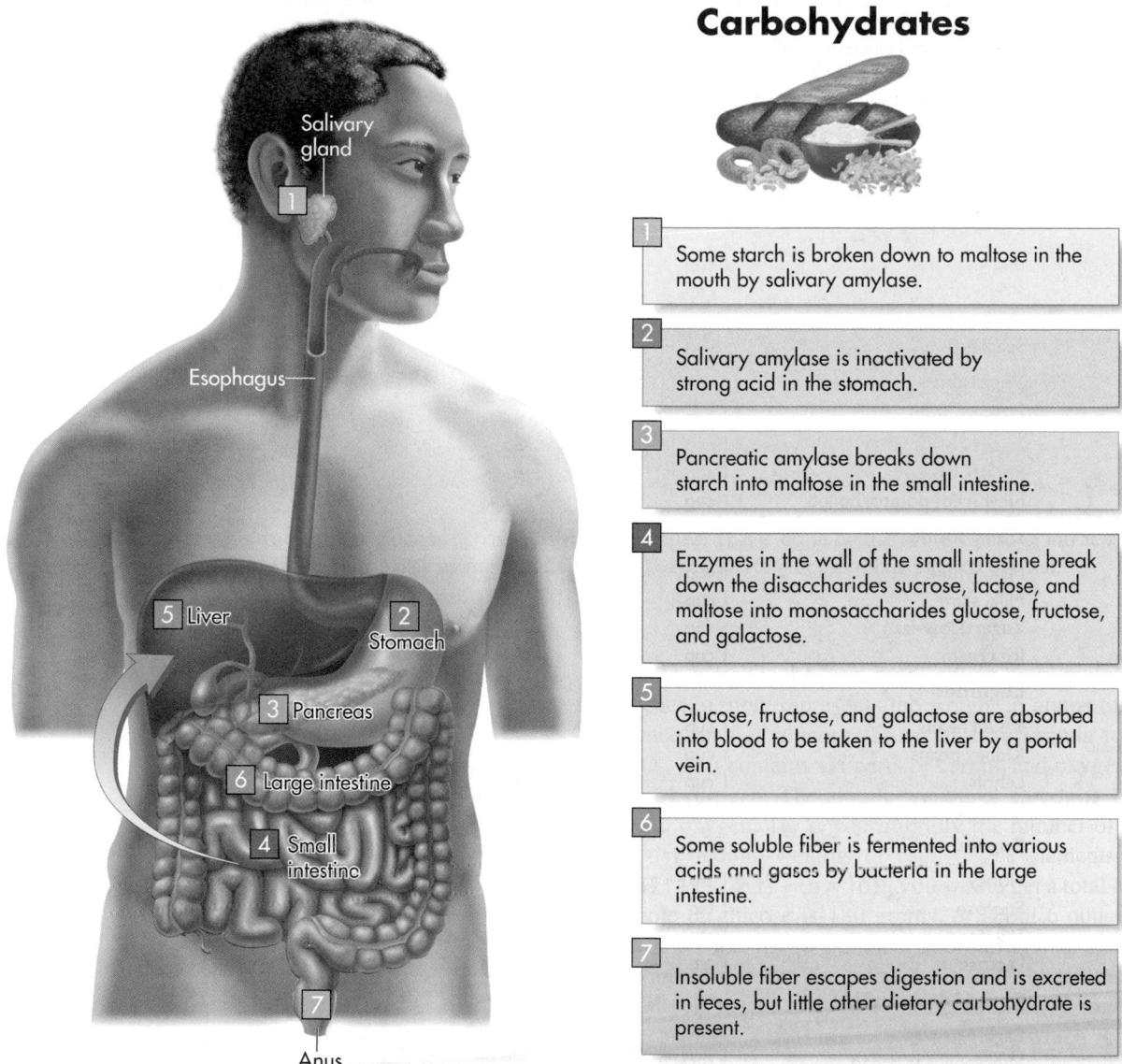

1. Some starch is broken down to maltose in the mouth by salivary amylase.

2. Salivary amylase is inactivated by strong acid in the stomach.

3. Pancreatic amylase breaks down starch into maltose in the small intestine.

4. Enzymes in the wall of the small intestine break down the disaccharides sucrose, lactose, and maltose into monosaccharides glucose, fructose, and galactose.

5. Glucose, fructose, and galactose are absorbed into blood to be taken to the liver by a portal vein.

6. Some soluble fiber is fermented into various acids and gases by bacteria in the large intestine.

7. Insoluble fiber escapes digestion and is excreted in feces, but little other dietary carbohydrate is present.

FIGURE 4.4 Carbohydrate digestion and absorption. Enzymes made by the mouth, pancreas, and small intestine participate in the process of digestion. Most carbohydrate digestion and absorption take place in the small intestine.

points represent the major fates of blood glucose. Figure 4.6 schematically represents these fates.

1. Blood glucose may be used for energy, particularly by the brain and other parts of the nervous system that rely primarily on glucose for their metabolism. Hypoglycemia can impair the normal function of the brain. Although hypoglycemia as a clinical condition is quite rare in the general population, transitory hypoglycemia may occur in very prolonged endurance exercise.

2. Blood glucose may be converted to either liver or muscle glycogen. It is important to note that liver glycogen may later be reconverted to blood glucose. However, this does not occur to any appreciable extent with muscle glycogen. In essence, glucose is locked in the muscle once it enters, owing to the lack of a specific enzyme needed to change its form so it can cross the cell membrane back into the bloodstream. Most of the muscle glycogen is converted to this locked form of glucose

during the production of energy. Researchers discovered two forms of muscle glycogen, proglycogen and macroglycogen. Hargreaves indicates that the functional significance of these glycogen forms remains to be fully elucidated. Houston indicates that proglycogen seems to be preferentially used during muscle activity, while the macroglycogen may be more of a reserve supply of carbohydrate for prolonged exercise. In this text we shall use the term *glycogen* to represent both forms.

3. Blood glucose may be converted to and stored as fat in the adipose tissue. This situation occurs when the dietary carbohydrate, in combination with caloric intake of other nutrients, exceeds the energy demands of the body and the storage capacity of the liver and muscles for glycogen.

4. Some blood glucose also may be excreted in the urine if an excessive amount occurs in the blood because of rapid ingestion of simple sugars.

shown some glycogen remaining even though subjects were exhausted. Several mechanisms have been postulated to explain the development of fatigue even with some muscle glycogen remaining.

- Location of glycogen. Costill has indicated that performance would be adversely affected only when muscle glycogen levels went below 40 mmol/kg of muscle tissue. It may be that complete depletion of muscle glycogen is not necessary for performance to suffer, for glycolysis may be impaired with lower glycogen levels or the glycogen in the muscle fiber may be located where it is not readily available for glycolysis.

- Rate of energy production. Shulman and Rothman propose a model in which energy is supplied in milliseconds via glycogenolysis, and indicate that one possible mechanism for muscle fatigue is that at low, but nonzero glycogen concentrations, there is not enough glycogen to supply millisecond energy needs. In a related vein, Fitts notes that low levels of muscle glycogen may interfere with maintenance of optimal levels of Krebs cycle intermediates, which can reduce the rate of aerobic ATP production, and further notes that the metabolism of blood-borne substrates (blood glucose and FFA) is simply too slow to maintain heavy exercise intensities.

- Muscle fiber type. The fatigue that develops may be related to the depletion of muscle glycogen from specific muscle fiber types. In prolonged exercise at 60–75 percent of VO_2 max, type I fibers (red, oxidative slow twitch) and type IIa fibers (red, oxidative-glycolytic fast twitch) are recruited during the early stages of the task, but as muscle glycogen is depleted, the athlete must recruit type IIb fibers (white, glycolytic fast twitch) to maintain the same pace. However, it takes more mental effort to recruit the type IIb fibers, which will be more stressful to the athlete. Type IIb fibers also are more likely to produce lactic acid, increasing the acidity, which may increase the perceived stress of the exercise. In a study, Krustrup and others reported that glycogen depletion of the slow-twitch muscle fibers, necessitating recruitment of fast-twitch muscle fibers and increased energy demands, is a factor that may predispose to fatigue.

- Use of fat for energy. As muscle glycogen becomes depleted in the slow-twitch muscle fibers, the muscle cell will rely more on fat as the primary energy source. Because fat is a less efficient fuel than carbohydrate, the pace will slow down.

- Role of the brain. Signals sent from peripheral tissues to the brain may regulate energy metabolism. A low glycogen level in exercising muscle may be such a signal, and may invoke neural responses causing fatigue.

Low Muscle Glycogen and Anaerobic Exercise
Fatigue in very high-intensity, anaerobic-type exercise generally is attributed to the detrimental effects of the acidity in the muscle cell associated with lactic acid production. Research has now shown that maximal high-intensity exercise, lasting only about 60 seconds, is not impaired by a very low muscle glycogen concentration, approximately 30 mmol/kg muscle. However, it is possible that performance in such very high-intensity, short-term exercise tasks may be impaired with extremely low muscle glycogen in the fast-twitch muscle fibers. Moreover, with somewhat longer anaerobic tasks, approximating 3 minutes, one laboratory study reported a reduced performance in the time to exhaustion test after 4 days of a low-carbohydrate, high-fat diet when compared to a normal, mixed diet and a high-carbohydrate diet. Although muscle glycogen levels were not measured, a logical assumption is that they were lower on the low-carbohydrate diet.

In addition, field research has suggested that slower overall sprint speed, such as in the latter parts of prolonged athletic contests like soccer and ice hockey, may be due to muscle glycogen depletion. Muscle biopsies of these athletes revealed very low glycogen levels, which were attributed not only to the strenuous exercise in the contest but also to the fact that these athletes were consuming diets low in carbohydrates. In support of these field studies, Balsom and others reported that low muscle glycogen levels impaired laboratory exercise performance in repeated bouts of very high-intensity intermittent exercise, 6-second cycle ergometer performance followed by 30 seconds of rest. Krustrup and others reported that almost 50 percent of muscle fibers were completely or almost empty of glycogen following a soccer game, and suggested that slower sprint performance in the latter part of a game may be explained by low glycogen levels in individual muscle fibers. Also, low muscle glycogen stores may lead to a decrease in exercise intensity during training.

Low muscle glycogen levels, because they are associated with premature fatigue, have been theorized to be a major cause of the overtraining syndrome in endurance athletes. However, in her review, Ann Snyder noted that cyclists who met the criteria of short-term overtraining maintained their muscle glycogen levels. Thus, she concluded that some other mechanism than reduced muscle glycogen levels must be responsible for the development of the overtraining syndrome.

In summary, low levels of glycogen in the white, fast-twitch IIb muscle fibers may limit performance in intermittent, anaerobic-type exercise tasks. Both hypoglycemia and low glycogen in the red muscle fiber types, most likely a combination of the two, may be contributing factors to fatigue in prolonged endurance exercise.

How are low endogenous carbohydrate levels related to the central fatigue hypothesis?

As noted previously, hypoglycemia and low muscle glycogen levels may impair exercise performance, and one mechanism for each involves adverse effects on brain function. Collectively, they may contribute to central fatigue in a different way.

In the latter stages of prolonged exercise bouts, low muscle glycogen, in combination with decreased blood glucose levels, will stimulate gluconeogenesis from muscle protein. In particular, branched-chain amino acids (BCAAs) in the muscle will be catabolized to provide energy. Because BCAA release from the liver may be decreased, or uptake by the muscle may increase, blood levels of BCAA decline. The *central fatigue hypothesis* during prolonged exercise suggests that this decline in blood BCAA may contribute to fatigue. In general, fatigue is hypothesized to occur when BCAA levels drop and the concentration of another amino acid—tryptophan—increases in its free form, or free tryptophan (fTRP). BCAA compete with fTRP for similar receptors that facilitate their entry into the brain, so high BCAA levels prevent brain uptake of fTRP. With an increased fTRP:BCAA ratio, entry of fTRP into the brain cells will be facilitated. Increased brain levels of tryptophan may stimulate the formation of serotonin, a neurotransmitter in the brain that may be related to fatigue sensations (see figure 4.11). Preventing the increase in the fTRP:BCAA ratio is theorized to prevent the premature development of fatigue, and the use of BCAA supplements in this regard will be covered in chapter 6. However, carbohydrate intake during exercise may also be helpful, as discussed later in this section.

Will eating carbohydrate immediately before or during an event improve physical performance?

Because hypoglycemia or muscle glycogen depletion may be causes of fatigue during endurance exercise, supplementation with glucose or other forms of carbohydrate before or during exercise may be theorized to delay the onset of fatigue and improve performance. Thousands of studies have been conducted on this topic ever since carbohydrates were identified as the most efficient energy source for exercise (more than 80 years ago), and researchers' interest in this topic remains unabated today. In

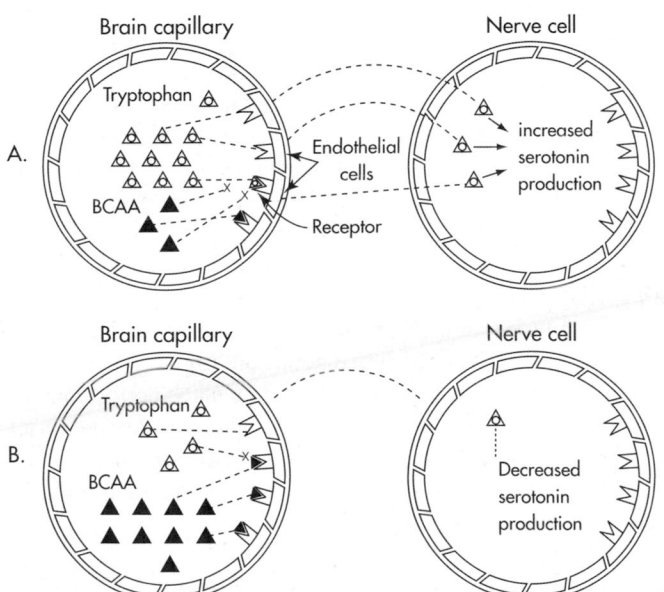

FIGURE 4.11 BCAA and the central fatigue hypothesis. (A) An increased level of serum free-tryptophan (fTRP ▲) resulting in a high fTRP:BCAA ratio will bind to receptors in the capillary for transport to nerve cells and increased serotonin formation, which may be associated with central fatigue. (B) An increased level of BCAAs (▲) will compete with the fTRP for receptors, blocking them from entering the nerve cell and decreasing production of serotonin, helping to prevent central fatigue.

recent years, the research designs have usually been highly sophisticated as investigators have attempted to provide specific answers relative to the type, amount, and timing of carbohydrate ingestion before and during performance. Although some problems remain in providing quantitative data, the use of stable isotopes of ingested carbohydrates (referred to as *exogenous* carbohydrates in comparison to *endogenous* stores in the body), as detailed by Wolfe and George, has enhanced our understanding of their metabolic fate when ingested prior to or during exercise.

However, the reviewer attempting to synthesize the available research is confronted with a difficult task, as the experimental designs varied considerably. The amount and type of carbohydrate ingested, the use of liquid or solid forms, the method of administration (oral ingestion or venous infusion), the time prior to or during the exercise that it was taken, the diet of the subject several days prior to the study, the amount of glycogen in the muscle and liver, the intensity and duration of the exercise, the type of exercise task (running, swimming, cycling, etc.), the fitness level of the subjects, the environmental temperature, and the method used to evaluate blood glucose and muscle glycogen utilization are some of the important differences between studies.

Although the results from all of these studies were not similar, some general consistencies have evolved. The role of carbohydrate supplementation on exercise performance has been the subject of numerous reviews, and a number of contemporary reviews may be found in the reference list at the end of this chapter. Based on these reviews and an overall review of specific studies, the following generalizations appear to be logical. More specific information relative to practical recommendations is provided following this discussion.

Use of the Ingested Carbohydrate Using labeled carbohydrate sources and analyzing the expired carbon dioxide for radioactivity, investigators have shown that some of the ingested, or exogenous, carbohydrate may be used as an energy source within 5–10 minutes, indicating that it may empty rapidly from the stomach, be absorbed from the small intestine into the blood, and enter into metabolic pathways. Peak use of exogenous carbohydrate appears to occur 75 to 90 minutes after ingestion. A number of studies have shown that the ingested carbohydrate may contribute a significant percentage of the carbohydrate energy source during exercise, ranging from 20–40 percent in some studies, but as much as 60–70 percent during the latter stages of exercise, when endogenous liver and muscle glycogen stores become depleted.

Possible Fatigue-Delaying Mechanisms The precise mechanism whereby glucose ingestion helps delay the onset of fatigue during moderate- to high-intensity exercise (i.e., > 65 percent VO_2 max) has not been totally elucidated, but several theories have been studied.

Maintenance of blood glucose levels The available data suggest that the ability of carbohydrate intake to delay fatigue may be related to the maintenance of higher blood glucose levels, possibly by sparing liver glycogen until late in the exercise, and the prevention of hypoglycemia in susceptible individuals; blood glucose would be available to enter the muscle and provide a source of energy for aerobic glycolysis, and may also provide glucose to the brain to prevent premature central fatigue. As noted, exogenous glucose is used increasingly as the exercise task becomes prolonged.

Reduction of psychological effort   Some research has shown that glucose ingestion could make an endurance task psychologically easier and suggested that the physiological effects of the glucose, either in the brain or in the muscles, reduced the stressful effects of exercise. Several studies by Utter and others found that carbohydrate ingestion reduced the ratings of perceived exertion during prolonged running and cycling. For example, they reported that marathoners ingesting carbohydrate compared to placebo beverages were able to run at a higher intensity during a competitive marathon, and yet the ratings of perceived exertion (RPE) were similar in both groups of runners, suggesting that the carbohydrate may have permitted them to run at a faster rate with similar psychological effort. However, it has not been determined whether these ergogenic effects may be attributed to the effect of glucose as a source of energy in the muscle or to its effect on the central nervous system, either as a direct energy source for brain metabolism or through its effect on BCAA levels.

In several studies, carbohydrate supplementation during exercise has been reported to prevent the decrease in serum BCAA during the later stages of prolonged exercise, possibly by mitigating secretion of cortisol. According to the central fatigue hypothesis, preventing an increase in the fTRP:BCAA ratio would deter the onset of mental fatigue.

Sparing of muscle glycogen   Although sparing of muscle glycogen could be another benefit of carbohydrate ingestion before or during moderate- to high-intensity exercise, research findings are equivocal.

In a unique experiment from the University of Texas, subjects received venous glucose infusions to maintain a hyperglycemic state during 2 hours of exercise at 73 percent of VO_2 max, but the net rate of muscle glycogen utilization was not affected compared to control conditions. Arkinstall and Chryssanthopoulos and their colleagues also noted no muscle glycogen sparing effect with carbohydrate supplementation during the exercise task.

In contrast, Yaspelkis and others, also from the University of Texas, noted that during low-intensity exercise (i.e., <50 percent VO_2 max) or during low- to moderate-intensity exercise tasks, carbohydrate supplementation during exercise could spare use of muscle glycogen in slow-twitch muscle fibers and enhance performance. They noted that during low-intensity exercise the serum levels of both glucose and insulin were elevated, which could promote muscle use of serum glucose and sparing of muscle glycogen. Bosch and others, as well as Tsintzas and others, reported that carbohydrate intake during prolonged exercise at about 70 percent VO_2 max did spare muscle glycogen use, and the Tsintzas group reported that the sparing effect occurred in the type I, slow-twitch muscle fibers, but not in the type II fast-twitch fibers. Williams noted that although other reviewers concluded that consuming carbohydrate during exercise did not spare use of muscle glycogen in cyclists, research findings from his laboratory did find glycogen sparing in runners who consumed carbohydrate drinks throughout prolonged exercise, and the glycogen sparing occurred early in the exercise task. Hargreaves noted also that the breakdown of muscle glycogen may be slowed because the supply of blood glucose is improved when carbohydrate is consumed.

Limitations to Prevent Fatigue   Although glucose ingestion may help delay fatigue during moderately high-intensity exercise, it cannot totally prevent the onset of fatigue. It appears that a maximum of about 1.5 to 1.7 grams of the ingested carbohydrate may be available each minute, which is much lower than the required energy needs at 65–85 percent of VO_2 max. Jeukendrup and Jentjens indicate that the intestines and liver may be limiting factors, the intestines being unable to absorb the ingested carbohydrate at a faster rate, while the liver may limit the amount of glucose released into the blood. When blood glucose, BCAA, and/or muscle glycogen levels are eventually reduced to a critical level, fatigue occurs.

Initial Endogenous Stores   If the individual has normal liver and muscle glycogen stores, glucose feedings are unnecessary for continuous moderately high-intensity exercise bouts lasting 60–90 minutes or less, but may be beneficial for high-intensity exercise tasks of similar duration, as noted below. Because the body can store carbohydrate in the muscles and liver, the usefulness of glucose or other carbohydrate intake before or during exercise depends on the adequacy of those supplies already in the muscle and liver to meet energy needs. For competition, the muscle and liver glycogen stores should be adequate to meet carbohydrate energy needs. The critical point is to consume substantial amounts of carbohydrates a day or two prior to the event and to decrease the duration and intensity of training to assure ample endogenous glycogen supplies.

The available research has shown that the consumption of glucose, fructose, sucrose, maltodextrin (a glucose polymer), or other carbohydrate combinations immediately prior to events of short or moderate duration has a negligible effect upon performance. Adding a gallon of gas to a full tank will not make a car go faster during a short ride. The same is true of sugar to a muscle already filled with glycogen. If, however, muscle glycogen levels are low and the exercise task is somewhat prolonged, then ingestion of carbohydrate just prior to the exercise bout may improve performance. It is important to note, however, that to enhance performance, the exogenous carbohydrate source must be able to delay the onset of fatigue that might otherwise occur as a result of premature depletion of endogenous carbohydrate sources, a viewpoint also proposed by Tsintzas and Williams.

Exercise Intensity and Duration   The potential beneficial effects of carbohydrate supplementation depend on the interaction of exercise intensity and duration, which of course are interrelated. The shorter the duration, the greater the exercise intensity can be. The following time frames are representative of those that have been studied to evaluate the effects of carbohydrate supplementation. A summary of the science-based recommendations for carbohydrate intake before, during, and after exercise or sport performance is presented in table 4.7.

TABLE 4.7 Some recommended guidelines for carbohydrate intake as a means to help optimize exercise/sport performance. Carbohydrate intake before and during exercise may help optimize performance, whereas carbohydrate intake after exercise may facilitate recovery for subsequent training or competition. In general, the lower the intensity and the shorter the duration of exercise, the less the need for additional carbohydrate. Recommendations are based on scientific studies. Physically active individuals should consume various types and amounts of carbohydrate before and during exercise and sport training to determine personal optimal dietary strategies. See the text for additional information and guidelines.

Exercise intensity/sport	Duration	Before exercise*	During exercise**	After exercise***
Very high intensity aerobic (5K run)	<30 minutes	None needed	None needed	None needed
High-intensity aerobic (10K run)	30–90 minutes	20–25 grams	30–60 grams	60–80 grams/hour for 3–4 hours
Intermittent high-intensity (Team sports, such as soccer)	60–90 minutes	20–25 grams	30–60 grams	60–80 grams/hour for 3–4 hours
Moderate- to high-intensity aerobic (half-marathon; marathon)	>90 minutes	20–50 grams Carbohydrate loading	60–80 grams/hour	60 grams/hour for 3–4 hours
Moderate-intensity aerobic (Ironman-distance triathlon; 140 miles; 226 kilometers)	>6 hour	20–50 grams Carbohydrate loading	60–80 grams/hour	60–80 grams/hour for 3–4 hours
High-intensity resistance training (Lifting weights)	1–2 hours	None needed	None needed	60–80 grams/hour for 3–4 hours

*Within 10–15 minutes of the start of exercise. All individuals should consume a pregame meal sometime between 1–4 hours prior to exercise in order to ensure normal muscle glycogen and blood glucose levels. Carbohydrate intake 3–4 hours before should average about 3–4 grams per kilogram body weight, but only 1–2 grams per kilogram body weight if consumed within 1–2 hours exercise.

**Fluids such as sports drinks are recommended. Drinking about 8 ounces (240 milliliters) of a typical sport drink every 15 minutes will provide about 60 grams of carbohydrate per hour.

***For most athletes, consuming a diet with substantial amounts of healthful carbohydrates over the course of 24 hours will replace muscle glycogen levels to normal. For those who want a speedy recovery of muscle glycogen for subsequent intense training or competition the same or following day, using this rapid muscle glycogen replacement protocol may be recommended. Athletes may also benefit by consuming some protein with the carbohydrate, about 1 gram of protein for every 4 grams of carbohydrate.

Very high intensity exercise for less than 30 minutes   Research suggests that carbohydrate supplementation will not enhance performance in high-intensity exercise bouts less than 30 minutes in length. For example, Palmer and others noted that consuming carbohydrate 10 minutes before competing in a 20-kilometer cycle time trial did not enhance performance in well-trained cyclists. Nevertheless, if carbohydrate supplements could ameliorate a muscle or liver glycogen deficiency, performance might improve. For example, Walberg-Rankin reported that carbohydrate supplementation improved high-intensity anaerobic exercise performance in wrestlers following a drastic weight reduction program with very limited carbohydrate intake. Presumably, the carbohydrate supplement, consumed in a 5-hour period before testing, increased muscle glycogen levels, particularly in fast-twitch fibers, enhancing carbohydrate utilization and subsequent performance.

Very high intensity resistance exercise training   In a review, Conley and Stone noted that resistance, or strength, training, may use considerable amounts of muscle glycogen, which can lead to fatigue and strength loss. However, they noted that there are inadequate data to determine whether carbohydrate supplements increase performance if consumed before or during training. Kulik and colleagues reported that carbohydrate consumed before and between sets does not enhance performance of squats performed with 85 percent 1-RM to volitional failure. Moreover, Utter and others reported no significant effects of carbohydrate supplementation (sports drink) on ratings of perceived exertion during a 2-hour resistance training workout.

High-intensity exercise for 30 to 90 minutes   Within this time frame, the potential benefit of carbohydrate consumption may depend on the duration of the exercise, intensity of exercise, and training level of the athlete. For example, two studies found that neither consumption of a 6 percent carbohydrate solution nor infusing glucose at the rate of 1 gram per minute improved performance in a one-hour maximal cycling protocol. Additionally, Burke and others reported no effect of a commercial gel supplying about 1.1 grams of carbohydrate per kilogram body weight on half-marathon performance compared to the placebo. However, in a review, Karelis and colleagues examined studies with exercise times ranging between 30 and 60 minutes. They noted a beneficial effect of carbohydrate ingestion with exercise lasting at least 40–50 minutes. Moreover, supplementation may benefit well-trained athletes who may be able to exercise at high intensity for about an hour. For example, Jeukendrup and el-Sayed, with their associates, reported that cyclists exercising for about an hour at high intensity significantly improved their performance following ingestion of a carbohydrate supplement, as compared to a placebo. Also, Ball and others reported that carbohydrate intake during a simulated time trial improved performance in a sprint at the end of 50 minutes of high-intensity cycling. In such cases, it is possible that the ingested carbohydrates may help provide glucose to the fast-twitch muscle fibers or prevent premature depletion in the slow-twitch fibers.

Jeukendrup hypothesizes that carbohydrate intake seems to positively affect the central nervous system during more intense exercise. Research from his laboratory, by Carter and others, found that simply swishing a carbohydrate (maltodextrin) solution in the mouth periodically during exercise enhanced performance in a 1-hour cycle time trial, an effect suggested to be due to increased central nervous system drive or motivation from carbohydrate receptors in the mouth.

Intermittent high-intensity exercise for 60 to 90 minutes

Research has shown that individuals engaged in endurance-type contests with intermittent bouts of sprinting, such as soccer, ice hockey, or tennis, may benefit from carbohydrate supplements taken before and during the game. In a controlled laboratory protocol representative of a 60-minute intermittent, high-intensity competitive sport such as soccer or field hockey, Welsh and colleagues, from Mark Davis's laboratory, reported that carbohydrate intake before and during the exercise task resulted in significant improvements in various tests of physical and mental functions performed throughout the experimental trial. Toward the end of the 60-minute period, the carbohydrate trial resulted in faster 20-meter sprint time, longer time to fatigue in a shuttle run, enhanced whole body motor skills, and decreased self-reported perceptions of fatigue. The results suggested a beneficial role of carbohydrate-electrolyte ingestion on physical and mental functions during intermittent exercise similar to that of many competitive team sports. Similar findings were reported by Winnick and others. Other field research studies, although not universally supportive, have shown similar benefits of carbohydrate intake under game conditions. Several reviewers, such as Kirkendall and Kovacs, indicate that carbohydrate intake before and during prolonged, intermittent high-intensity exercise sports may enhance performance.

High- to moderate-intensity exercise greater than 90 minutes

Research generally supports a beneficial effect of carbohydrate intake on exercise performance tasks greater than 90 minutes (if the exercise intensity is high enough), particularly so when the task is more prolonged, such as 2 hours or more. For example, Kimber and others reported a significant inverse correlation between the amount of carbohydrate consumed and the finishing time of male triathletes in an Ironman triathlon, suggesting that increasing carbohydrate consumption during such a prolonged event may enhance performance. Jeukendrup indicates that the performance benefits of carbohydrate ingestion are likely achieved by maintaining or raising plasma glucose concentrations to help sustain high rates of carbohydrate oxidation.

When, how much, and in what form should carbohydrates be consumed before or during exercise?

The most common athletic events or physical performance activities that may benefit from carbohydrate feedings are those associated with long duration (90–120 minutes or more) at moderate- to high-intensity levels. Marathon running, cross-country skiing, and endurance cycling are common sports of this kind. Other sports that require intermittent bouts of intensive activity over a prolonged period, such as soccer, may also benefit. However, the individual participating in these activities, particularly under warm or hot environmental conditions, also needs to replenish fluid losses incurred through sweating. In such cases, fluid replenishment is more critical than carbohydrate. The topic of fluid replacement during exercise is covered in more detail in chapter 9, but because carbohydrate is one of the contents in the majority of the sport drinks developed as fluid replacements for athletes, its role is discussed briefly here.

Many studies have been conducted to determine the best carbohydrate feeding regimen to prevent fatigue during prolonged exercise. A number of different variables have been studied, such as the timing of the feeding and the type, amount, and concentration of carbohydrate.

Again, based on current reviews by the primary investigators regarding carbohydrate supplementation for exercise performance and a careful analysis of individual studies, the following points represent the general conclusions and recommendations for individuals who may be exercising at 60–80 percent of their VO_2 max or greater for 1–2 hours or longer. These points may also be applicable to athletes engaged in intermittent high-intensity exercise sports that last an hour or more. But remember, individuals may have varied reactions to carbohydrate intake, so athletes should experiment in training before using these recommendations in actual competition.

Pre-Exercise: When and How Much?

Four hours or less before exercise   Carbohydrate intake 60–240 minutes prior to prolonged exercise tasks (longer than 90 minutes) may enhance performance. Research has demonstrated improved performance when adequate carbohydrate was consumed either 1, 3, or 4 hours prior to a prolonged exercise task involving simulated racing conditions during the latter stage. Other research revealed no significant differences in 30-kilometer run performance when equal amounts of carbohydrate were supplemented either 4 hours before or during the run, suggesting the ingested carbohydrate was available for energy production using either strategy.

The amount of carbohydrate ingested 4 hours prior to performance should be based upon body weight. Several studies have used 4–5 grams/kg (1.8–2.3 grams/pound) with good results. For an athlete who weighs 60 kg (132 pounds), the recommended amount would be 240–300 grams. The carbohydrates could be consumed in any of several forms, including fluids such as juices or glucose polymer solutions, or solid carbohydrates such as fruits or starches. The fiber content should be minimized to prevent possible intestinal problems during exercise. Keep in mind that 300 grams of carbohydrate is about 1,200 Calories, a somewhat substantial meal. You may consult appendix E for an expanded list of foods high in carbohydrate. Table 4.8 presents a quick estimate of carbohydrates in the various food exchanges and sports products.

The guidelines presented on pages 76–77 relative to precompetition meals provide appropriate guidelines.

Less than I hour before exercise Jeukendrup and Killer reviewed the myths surrounding pre-exercise carbohydrate feedings. They found that the ingestion of carbohydrates in the hour before exercise either improved performance or had no impact on performance. Based on these findings, there is little evidence to abstain from carbohydrate ingestion in the hour prior to exercise, for those who do not experience symptoms of hypoglycemia. Prudence suggests that individuals who may be prone to reactive hypoglycemia should avoid carbohydrate intake, particularly high-glycemic-index foods, 15–60 minutes prior to performance. Simple sugars ingested within this time frame may actually impair physical performance in such individuals because of the adverse effects of reactive hypoglycemia, such as muscular weakness. Moreover, this same insulin response may speed up muscle glycogen utilization. This may be a disadvantage to the marathoner, whose glycogen levels may be depleted too early in the race. Several earlier studies showed that run time to exhaustion was shorter by about 20–25 percent after athletes consumed 2–3 ounces of glucose within an hour before the endurance test.

The guidelines presented on pages 76–77

TABLE 4.8 Grams of carbohydrate in selected food exchanges and sports products

I fruit exchange = 15 grams carbohydrate
  I apple
  I orange
  1/2 banana
  4 ounces orange juice
I starch exchange = 15 grams carbohydrate
  I slice bread
  1/2 cup cereal
  1/4 large bagel
  1/2 cup cooked pasta
  I small baked potato
Sports drinks: 7–8 ounces = 15 grams carbohydrate
  Gatorade
  PowerAde
  SportAde
Sports bars = 20–50 grams carbohydrate
  I PR Bar
  I Power Bar
Sports gels = 20–30 grams carbohydrate
  I Power Gel packet
  I ReLode packet
Energy Drinks: 8 ounces = 25–50 grams carbohydrate
  Gatorade Energy Drink
  SoBe Energy

However, not all individuals experience reactive hypoglycemia. Kuipers and others noted that about one-third of well-trained subjects experienced hypoglycemia following the ingestion of 50 grams of glucose after a 4-hour fast. However, the hypoglycemia was transient, as blood glucose levels returned to normal after 20 minutes of exercise at 60 percent VO_2 max. No performance data were measured. In a study by Seifert and others, subjects were given various carbohydrate solutions to raise their insulin levels; when their insulin levels peaked, they undertook an exercise task at 60 percent of VO_2 max for 50 minutes. No hypoglycemia developed, nor were there any adverse sensory or psychological responses.

If carbohydrate is consumed approximately 1 hour prior to performance, about 1–2 grams/kg (60–120 grams for a 60-kg athlete) may be recommended, for these levels have been shown to enhance performance in several studies. One study using only 12 grams 1 hour prior to performance showed no beneficial effect. Both glucose polymers and foods with a low glycemic index have been used successfully.

Immediately before exercise As noted previously, consuming carbohydrate immediately before exercise of short duration, and even exercise tasks of less than 90 minutes or so, normally will not enhance performance. For example, Marjerrison and others found that the ingestion of a carbohydrate solution 30 minutes before undertaking four 30-second anaerobic Wingate tests had no effect on power output; Smith and others reported no significant effect on swim time performance of ingesting a 10-percent glucose solution 5 minutes before a 4-kilometer swim of approximately 70 minutes. However, carbohydrate intake immediately prior to (within 5–10 minutes) prolonged endurance exercise tasks of 2 hours or more may help delay the development of fatigue and improve performance if the athlete is exercising at a level greater than 50 percent VO_2 max, such as 60–75 percent. The majority of the studies, including controlled laboratory investigations and field research involving different types of endurance athletes, support this point of view. At this level of exercise intensity, the insulin response to glucose ingestion is suppressed; in addition, the secretion of epinephrine is increased. These two hormonal responses interact to help maintain or elevate the blood glucose level and prevent the hypoglycemic response that typically may occur in reactive individuals if more time elapses between the ingestion of the carbohydrate and the initiation of exercise.

If carbohydrates are consumed immediately before exercise, that is, within 10 minutes of the start, about 50–60 grams of a glucose polymer in a 40–50 percent solution has been used effectively in some studies. Dry glucose polymers are available commercially. One tablespoon is about 15 grams. To make a 50 percent solution containing 50 grams of the polymer, put about 3 level tablespoons of the polymer into 100 milliliters (about 3–4 ounces) of water. To make a 7.5 percent solution containing 15 grams, put 1 tablespoon of the polymer into 200 milliliters (about 7 ounces) of water. Several commercial "energy" drinks contain 25–50 grams of carbohydrate per 8 fluid ounces, which are about 10–20 percent solutions.

During exercise Carbohydrate ingested during prolonged exercise can help maintain blood glucose levels and reduce the psychological perception of effort, as measured by the ratings of perceived exertion, during the latter stages of an endurance task. As the exercise task continues and the muscle glycogen level falls, the amount of energy derived from the ingested carbohydrates increases. Most research supports the benefits of consuming carbohydrates early in and throughout the exercise task, but even a single carbohydrate feeding late in a prolonged exercise bout may help replenish blood glucose levels, increase carbohydrate oxidation, and delay fatigue.

All major investigators who have published extensive reviews, notably Mark Hargreaves and Asker Jeukendrup, conclude that carbohydrate intake during prolonged exercise, when contrasted with placebo conditions, will enhance performance. This general finding is supported by both laboratory and field studies and applies to both females and males.

During Exercise: When and How Much?

During exercise, feedings every 15–20 minutes appear to be a reasonable schedule, but possibly more frequently when attempting to maximize carbohydrate intake or to obtain fluids when exercising under warm or hot environmental conditions. Although you may consume considerable quantities of carbohydrate during exercise, your ability to use this exogenous source for energy is limited. The reason is not known, but as noted previously, may be related to insufficient intestinal absorption or impaired delivery from the liver.

In the past, reasonable evidence-based estimates suggested that athletes could use approximately 0.5–1 gram of ingested carbohydrate per minute, or about 30–60 grams of carbohydrate per hour. In general, research indicates that equally trained males and females can oxidize equivalent amounts of ingested carbohydrate. More recently, studies have shown that ingesting various combinations of carbohydrates could increase this amount to 1.2–1.7 grams per minute, or about 72–102 grams per hour. The rationale is presented in the next section.

Sports drinks averaging 6–10 percent carbohydrate have been found to enhance prolonged endurance performance. A typical serving of a sport drink (8 ounces) would contain about 14–24 grams of carbohydrate, so depending on the concentration, an athlete who wanted to maximize utilizable carbohydrate intake would need to drink about 32–56 ounces to obtain about 100 grams of carbohydrate per hour. Drinking 8 ounces every 15 minutes would provide 32 ounces (1 quart) over the course of an hour, but consumption would have to be more frequent to obtain 56 ounces. Consuming 56 ounces of fluid over the course of an hour might be difficult, and may pose a potential health risk for some individuals. Although the fluids could provide the desired amount of carbohydrate, excessive fluid consumption could lead to overhydration and a serious medical condition known as hyponatremia, as shall be discussed in chapter 9.

Several other protocols have been effective. One involved consumption of a high concentration (about 1 gram carbohydrate/kg body weight) immediately before or during the first 20 minutes of the exercise, and then use of lower concentrations such as found in commercial sports drinks at regular intervals. Other investigators have noted that taking a single more concentrated dose of carbohydrate, such as 100–200 grams total, in the latter stages of prolonged exercise may be beneficial. Additionally, because of the nature of their sport, soccer players and other such athletes may need to consume a high concentration before the game and during halftime, or breaks in the game as they occur.

It should be noted that consumption of carbohydrate solutions above 10 percent during exercise may cause gastrointestinal distress, as may other high concentrations of simple carbohydrates. However, some athletes may learn to tolerate larger concentrations, such as 15–20 percent. Ultradistance athletes, who exercise at a lower intensity, may tolerate even higher concentrations ranging from 20–50 percent.

Although athletes may learn to tolerate higher amounts of carbohydrate intake during exercise, Asker Jeukendrup, an authority on carbohydrate use during exercise, has recommended the following, which are less likely to cause gastrointestinal disturbances:

• Maximal exercise lasting less than 45 minutes	None required
• Maximal exercise lasting about 45–60 minutes	Less than 30 grams/hour
• Team sports lasting about 90 minutes	Up to 50 grams/hour
• Submaximal exercise lasting more than 2 hours	Up to 60 grams/hour
• Near-maximal and maximal exercise lasting more than 2 hours	Up to 50–70 grams/hour
• Ultraendurance events	60–90 grams/hour

Optimal Supplementation Protocol Several studies have indicated that although the intake of carbohydrate either before or during exercise may separately enhance performance, the best effect was observed when carbohydrate was consumed both before and during exercise. For example, Chryssanthopoulos and others had subjects run to exhaustion at 70 percent VO_2 max and found that although a high-carbohydrate meal 3 hours prior to performance improved endurance time, the combination of the meal and a carbohydrate-electrolyte solution during exercise further improved endurance running capacity.

Type of Carbohydrate A number of different types of carbohydrates have been studied, including glucose, fructose, galactose, sucrose, maltose, glucose polymers such as maltodextrins, both individually and in various combinations, as well as soluble starch (a very long polymer), high-glycemic-index foods like potatoes, and low-glycemic-index foods such as legumes. In general, there appears to be no difference between these different types of carbohydrates as a means to enhance endurance performance when used appropriately. However, there may be some important considerations relative to the use of various carbohydrate combinations, fructose, solid carbohydrates, and low-glycemic-index foods.

Carbohydrate combinations Jeukendrup noted studies showing that a single carbohydrate ingested during exercise will be oxidized at rates up to about 1 gram/minute, even when large amounts of carbohydrate are ingested. However, combinations of carbohydrate, particularly glucose and fructose, that use different intestinal transporters for absorption have been shown to result in higher oxidation rates (see figure 4.12). This seems to be the way to increase exogenous carbohydrate oxidation rates, up to 1.7 grams/minute. Combinations of carbohydrates are recommended to increase glucose oxidation at a rate of more than 60 grams per hour. Currell and Jeukendrup reported that ingestion of a drink containing multiple carbohydrates (glucose and fructose), as compared to either a glucose drink or water, improved performance by 8 and 19 percent, respectively, in time-trial performance following a 2-hour bout of cycling. Power output was greater throughout the approximate one-hour time trial with the glucose/fructose drink. Single sources of carbohydrate, such as glucose, appear to be adequate when less is needed. As noted later in this chapter, lactate has also been incorporated into a sports drink and preliminary research suggests a potential ergogenic effect. Thus, check food labels for ingredients to ensure that the chosen sports drink contains such combinations.

Fructose   Fructose has been theorized to be a better source of carbohydrate than glucose because it is absorbed more slowly from the intestine and hence will not create an insulin response and the potential reactive hypoglycemia. Indeed, research has shown that fructose, compared to glucose, may lead to a more stable blood sugar during the early stages of prolonged exercise when ingested 45 minutes prior to the activity, for most ingested fructose is eventually converted to glucose in the liver. However, when fructose is ingested immediately before or during exercise, its effect on the blood sugar and carbohydrate metabolism appears to be little different from that of glucose.

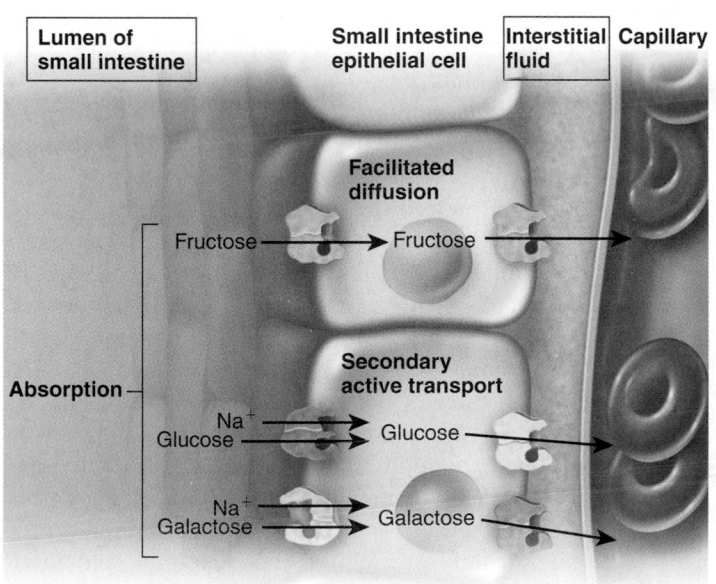

FIGURE 4.12 The villi in the intestines contain different receptors for the monosaccharides, which may increase carbohydrate absorption when multiple sources of carbohydrate are ingested.

Most people can tolerate small amounts of fructose. It is found naturally in fruits, and is an ingredient in some sports drinks. However, consuming larger amounts may pose problems. Because fructose is absorbed slowly from the intestinal tract, it can create a significant osmotic effect in the intestines, leading to diarrhea and gastrointestinal distress in some individuals. Research has indicated that a 6 percent solution of fructose, when compared to similar solutions of glucose and sucrose, caused significant gastrointestinal distress and an impairment in exercise performance. The athlete should be cautious in using fructose as the sole source of carbohydrate before or during exercise. Sports drinks containing fructose include it in small concentrations.

Additionally, high-fructose corn syrup, although rich in fructose, is treated as an added sugar. The health risks of added sugars are covered later in this chapter.

Solid and liquid carbohydrates   In her review, Coleman noted that solid and liquid forms of carbohydrate were equally effective in maintaining blood glucose levels and enhancing exercise performance. Pfeiffer and others confirmed this viewpoint, finding that delivery and oxidation of carbohydrate in the form of a glucose-fructose blend during exercise were as effective when ingested as a semisolid gel compared with a drink. However, Peters and others noted that triathletes who consumed a liquid form of carbohydrates performed better on a 3-hour cycling-running exercise task when compared to both a placebo trial and a trial in which the triathletes consumed isocaloric semisolid carbohydrate foods (orange juice, white bread, marmalade, and bananas). The authors did note that the athletes may have had a negative perception of eating solid foods during performance, which could have adversely affected their performance in that trial. Still, concentrated forms of carbohydrate, as found in products marketed to endurance athletes, appear to provide similar benefits. Campbell and others studied the effect of different forms of carbohydrate (liquid, gel, and jellybeans) on endurance exercise performance and found that all carbohydrate-supplement forms were equally effective in maintaining blood glucose levels during exercise and improving exercise performance compared to water only.

Although the effects of consuming equivalent amounts of carbohydrate in either liquid or solid form would appear to be minimal (providing adequate fluid intake in each case), more research is desirable to explore this issue, particularly with ultraendurance performance events where many athletes may consume both liquid and solid carbohydrate sources.

Low-glycemic-index foods   Although research has been conducted on glycemic index and performance for 20 years, Donaldson and colleagues concluded in a review that there is still a lack of agreement on the benefits of consuming high- and low-GI diets on performance. In examining feedings 1–3 hours prior to exercise, they found that only 5 of the 13 studies included a measure of performance. Of these five, only two demonstrated enhanced performance following consumption of a low-GI diet. The underlying mechanism might be a slower rate of absorption, resulting in a blunted insulin response and maintenance of higher blood glucose levels during prolonged exercise, an effect associated with soluble fiber. Febbraio and Stewart provided either a low-glycemic-index meal, a high-glycemic-index meal, or a control meal to trained individuals before cycling at 70 percent VO_2 max for 2 hours, followed by a 15-minute performance ride. Although the high-glycemic-index food increased blood glucose levels and depressed free fatty acid levels during the early stages, there were no differences later in the exercise task and no effects on the rate of muscle glycogen use or exercise performance. Several other well-controlled studies from Febbraio's laboratory, using similar glycemic-index meal and exercise protocols, reported no significant differences between the meals and performance. Other studies support this viewpoint. Erith and others reported no significant differences between diets of different glycemic indices on performance following overnight recovery. Semiprofessional soccer players performed a fatiguing intermittent high-intensity shuttle run test, and during the succeeding day interval consumed either a high-glycemic-index diet (GI = 70) or a low-glycemic-index diet (GI = 35). No differences were noted between trials for performance or rate of fatigue as measured by the test. Earnest and others also found no differences between a high-GI and low-GI diet on performance in a 64-kilometer cycling time trial. Chen and others compared the effects of pre-exercise meals with different glycemic indices and glycemic loads on performance in an exercise test involving running for 60 minutes at 70 percent VO_2 max, followed by a 10-kilometer performance run. Although the high- and low-glycemic meals modified carbohydrate and fat oxidation somewhat, there was no effect on 10-kilometer time.

Conversely, recent preliminary research from Clyde Williams's laboratory at the University of Loughborough has suggested some beneficial effects of a low-GI diet on endurance exercise performance. Several well-controlled studies by Stevenson and others compared the effects of a high- and low-GI diet on substrate utilization during exercise at 65 to 70 percent of VO_2 max, and reported a higher rate of fat oxidation following the low-GI meal. In one of these studies, run time to exhaustion at 70 percent of VO_2 max was greater following the low-GI diet. Wong and colleagues found that consumption of a low-GI meal resulted in a 2.8 percent improvement in a 21-km performance run compared with consumption of an isocaloric high-GI meal. They found carbohydrate oxidation to be 9.5 percent lower and fat oxidation to be 17.9 percent higher during exercise in the low-GI meal compared with the high-GI meal. In another study, Wu and Williams also reported higher rates of fat oxidation and a greater run to exhaustion at 70 percent of VO_2 max following a low-GI meal (GI = 37), as compared to a high-GI meal (GI = 77). They speculated that the enhanced oxidation of fats may have optimized carbohydrate metabolism in some way to enhance performance.

Given the conflicting data, additional research is needed to evaluate the effect of a low-GI diet on endurance exercise performance.

Carbohydrate with protein Studies have been conducted to determine the impact on performance of consuming protein with carbohydrate during exercise. McCleave and others found time to exhaustion to be 15.2 percent longer for female competitive cyclists and triathletes when a 3 percent carbohydrate/1.2 percent protein supplement was consumed every 20 minutes, compared to a 6 percent carbohydrate supplement. Using similar supplementation, Ferguson-Stegall found that total time to exhaustion was greater for cyclists and triathletes for intensities at or below the ventilatory threshold. Subjects cycling to exhaustion above the ventilatory threshold demonstrated no difference in performance with the supplements. However, it is unclear whether adding protein to carbohydrate during recovery will enhance subsequent endurance performance.

Several studies have compared the effects of carbohydrate supplementation alone to carbohydrate/protein supplementation on performance following recovery from previous exercise. Betts and others had subjects complete a 90-minute run at 70 percent of VO_2 max, followed by a 4-hour recovery period during which they consumed either a carbohydrate or a carbohydrate/protein mixture. The subjects then ran to exhaustion at 85 percent of VO_2 max, but there was no difference between treatments. Romano-Ely and others investigated the effect of a carbohydrate-protein-antioxidant drink, as compared to an isocaloric carbohydrate drink, on cycling time to exhaustion at 70 percent VO_2 max and, 24 hours later, at 80 percent VO_2 max. The drinks were consumed every 15 minutes during exercise and immediately afterward. There were no significant differences between the treatments on performance time during either of the cycling tests. Conversely, Bernardi and others had subjects complete a 60-minute time trial followed by a 6-hour recovery period during which the subjects consumed either carbohydrate or carbohydrate/protein. The subjects then repeated the 60 minute time-trial ride. Ingestion of carbohydrate/protein increased fat oxidation, increased recovery, and improved performance relative to isoenergetic carbohydrate ingestion. In a meta-analysis, Stearns and colleagues demonstrated an average 9 percent improvement in subsequent endurance performance with co-ingestion of protein and carbohydrate compared to carbohydrate alone. They also found an ergogenic effect when supplements were matched for carbohydrate content.

The use of chocolate milk has been reviewed by Roy and others as a more economical alternative to sports drinks during recovery from exercise. Benefits to this beverage include a ratio of carbohydrates to protein in the range recommended by the International Society of Sports Nutrition and its naturally high concentrations of electrolytes; it also affords a greater feeling of fullness compared to water or carbohydrate beverages. Karp and colleagues had highly trained cyclists perform an interval workout followed by 4 hours of recovery and then an endurance trial to exhaustion at 70 percent VO_2 max. During recovery, subjects consumed the same volume of chocolate milk, fluid replacement drink, or carbohydrate replacement drink. The carbohydrate content was equivalent for the chocolate milk and the carbohydrate replacement drink. Total time to exhaustion and total work were significantly greater for chocolate-milk and fluid-replacement subject compared to the carbohydrate replacement drink group. These results are supported by research done by Pritchett, Thomas, and Gilson who also found at least as effective muscle recovery responses with chocolate milk and carbohydrate recovery drinks.

Individuality Probably the most important recommendation is for the athlete to experiment with different types and amounts of carbohydrate during training before using them in competition. Just as it is important for you to know your optimal race pace for an endurance event, so too must you know how well you can tolerate different amounts and concentrations and types of carbohydrates. Williams noted that the type of event may influence the amount of carbohydrate ingested, as runners may be more prone to gastrointestinal distress than cyclists. "Runner's trots" is a form of diarrhea, that may be associated with excess consumption of highly concentrated sugar solutions, such as "energy" drinks.

Just as you train your muscles to learn their capacity, you may also be able to train your digestive system to know its limits. During training, experiment with various types and concentrations of carbohydrate, both before and during exercise. Ron Maughan, an internationally respected authority in sport nutrition, indicated that the optimal strategy relative to carbohydrate utilization is to use your own subjective experience, which you can gain during training.

What is the importance of carbohydrate replenishment after prolonged exercise?

There are several possible applications of this question. One is the athlete who may be involved in a prolonged exercise bout, have a rest period of 1–4 hours, and then must exercise again, such as athletes who train two or three times daily. Benefits may accrue to anaerobic endurance-, aerobic endurance-, and resistance-trained individuals. A second application is the athlete who trains intensely every day and must have an adequate recovery in the one-day rest interval. A third application, covered in the next section, is the technique of carbohydrate loading.

After prolonged exercise, increased levels of GLUT-4 receptors in the muscle cell membrane help move available blood glucose into the muscle for resynthesis to muscle glycogen. Several studies have shown that ingesting carbohydrate during the rest interval between two prolonged exercise bouts improves performance in the second bout. This finding is comparable to the beneficial effects of carbohydrate intake during prolonged exercise bouts. The carbohydrate can help restore blood glucose levels but may also be used to resynthesize muscle glycogen. In cases such as this, where the rate of muscle glycogen resynthesis is important, high-glycemic-index foods, such as potatoes, bread, glucose, or glucose polymers, would be the preferred source of carbohydrate, for they apparently lead to a faster restoration of muscle glycogen than does a meal rich in low-glycemic-index foods. For repeat prolonged exercise tasks with about a 4-hour interval, a general recommendation is to consume 1 gram of carbohydrate per kilogram body weight immediately after the first event and again 2 hours prior to the second event. Additional carbohydrate may also be consumed immediately before and during the second event.

Carbohydrate with protein Carbohydrate has been combined with other nutrients, particularly protein, in attempts to enhance muscle glycogen resynthesis. Protein and some amino acids, such as arginine, may stimulate the release of insulin which, if added to the effects of carbohydrate-mediated insulin release, could increase the rate at which glucose is transported into the muscle cell. In a review, Beelen and colleagues concluded that the inclusion of protein or amino acids with carbohydrates does not further enhance post-exercise muscle glycogen synthesis when an adequate amount of carbohydrate (1.2 g/kg/hr) is ingested at frequent intervals (every 15–30 minutes). They added that this combination may accelerate postexercise muscle glycogen synthesis rates when less carbohydrate is provided (<1.0 g/kg/hr). Kerksick and others recently published the International Society of Sports Nutrition position stand on nutrient timing. It states that adding protein to carbohydrate (ratio of 1: 3–4) may increase endurance performance and maximally promotes glycogen synthesis during acute and subsequent endurance exercise. Several studies, such as those by Baty and Romano-Ely and their colleagues, have shown that carbohydrate/protein supplementation may also reduce the incidence of muscle soreness following exercise, including lower levels of serum enzymes used as markers of muscle tissue damage. Moreover, as shall be noted in chapter 6, consuming some additional protein following strenuous exercise may have some beneficial effects, such as improved muscle protein balance.

If rapid resynthesis of muscle glycogen is not important, it is good to note that studies have shown that consumption of adequate amounts of carbohydrate over a 24-hour period will restore muscle glycogen levels to normal. For athletes who train intensely on a daily basis with either resistive or aerobic exercise that leads to muscle glycogen depletion, sport nutritionists normally recommend that approximately 8–10 grams of carbohydrate per kilogram body weight should be consumed daily to restore muscle glycogen levels to normal. For an individual who weighs 70 kilograms, this approximates 560–700 grams of carbohydrate, or 2,240–2,800 carbohydrate Calories. This amount of carbohydrate would represent about 65–80 percent of the daily caloric intake of an athlete consuming 3,500 Calories. Over the 24-hour period, the rate of muscle glycogen recovery is approximately 5–7 percent per hour. Sports drinks may be a convenient means to consume carbohydrate immediately after exercise. The remaining carbohydrate should be derived from other natural sources in the diet, including both simple carbohydrates in fruits and complex carbohydrates in grains, potatoes, and other foods with adequate dietary fiber and other nutrients. The inclusion of high-glycemic-index foods in the daily diet will help speed resynthesis of muscle glycogen over the 24-hour period, and may be very compatible with the Prudent Healthy Diet. Regular meals consumed during the 24-hour recovery period should include healthful low-glycemic-index foods with adequate amounts of protein.

Following prolonged, high-intensity competitive exercise performance, such as running a marathon, the resulting muscle damage will limit muscle glycogen replenishment for several days. Rest is important during this time, and muscle glycogen levels may return to normal following seven or more days of high-carbohydrate meals.

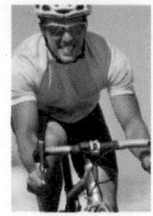

Will a high-carbohydrate diet enhance my daily exercise training?

Most scientists and sport nutritionists who study carbohydrate metabolism in athletes recommend a high-carbohydrate diet for most athletes, particularly endurance athletes, because success in athletic competition is contingent upon optimal training, and for the endurance athlete, optimal training may be contingent upon adequate nutrition, primarily the ingestion of sufficient carbohydrate every day. Louise Burke, a prominent sports nutritionist, and her associates recommended that athletes in general training should consume daily approximately 5–7 grams of carbohydrate per kilogram body weight, but endurance athletes should consume about 7–10 grams per kilogram. These recommendations are comparable to those of Melinda Manore, another sport nutrition expert. Burke and others noted that most male athletes may be meeting these needs, but many female endurance athletes, particularly those attempting to lose weight for competition, may not. Older athletes may need to ensure adequate carbohydrate intake during training. According to Mittendorfer and Klein, aging causes a shift in energy substrate use during exercise with an increased oxidation of glucose and less fat, presumably caused by age-related changes in skeletal muscle.

There are some limited data supporting the concept of enhanced training following a high-carbohydrate diet. A number of field and laboratory studies with athletes have attempted to mimic actual sport conditions. For example, one group of soccer players improved performance on an intermittent exercise task designed to mimic physical activity in a game, while another group improved performance in a standardized intermittent running task and a run to exhaustion. In other studies, runners were able to endure longer on a treadmill run to exhaustion; swimmers were better able to maintain 400-meter swim velocity; and triathletes experienced a significant improvement in treadmill endurance following 30 minutes of swimming, cycling, and running. Based on the available data, Edward Coyle, an international authority in carbohydrate metabolism during exercise, indicated that physical performance seems better maintained with a high- versus moderate-carbohydrate diet. In general, the normal carbohydrate intake of athletes in training studies was increased from approximately 40–45 percent to 55–70 percent of the daily Calories for varying periods, but usually a week or more. This level of carbohydrate approximates the upper levels of the AMDR for carbohydrate.

Not all athletes, including endurance athletes, need high-carbohydrate diets all the time. In a meta-analysis, Erlenbusch and others indicated that subjects following a high-carbohydrate diet could exercise longer until exhaustion, but this finding applied more to untrained individuals than trained individuals. As you may recall, aerobic exercise training improves the ability of the muscles to use fat as an energy source, so they may be somewhat less dependent on carbohydrate for a given training protocol. Thus, a moderate-carbohydrate diet may be adequate for trained athletes. For example, obtaining 45 percent of daily energy needs from carbohydrate might be considered moderate, as it is at the lower end of the AMDR. On such a diet, an endurance athlete who consumes 3,000 Calories per day during training would derive 1,350 Calories from carbohydrate ($0.45 \times 3,000$), which is about 340 grams of carbohydrate. For a 60-kilogram athlete, this is about 5.6 grams of carbohydrate per kilogram body weight. Although this is slightly less than that recommended for endurance athletes, research has shown that such amounts may be sufficient to maintain training on a daily basis.

However, training may appear more stressful psychologically. In several studies, the psychological status of athletes, as measured by the vigor and fatigue components of the Profile of Mood States (POMS) questionnaire and their rating of perceived exertion (RPE) during exercise, was improved when they switched from moderate- to higher-carbohydrate diets. In his review, Coyle concluded that mood state seems better maintained with a high- rather than moderate-carbohydrate diet. Utter and others reported reduced ratings of perceived exertion in subjects involved in prolonged (2.6 hours), intermittent cycling following ingestion of carbohydrate before and during the exercise bout.

Coyle also indicates that a high-carbohydrate diet may help reduce symptoms of overreaching and, possibly, overtraining. Gleeson and others note that heavy prolonged exertion is associated with numerous hormonal and biochemical changes in the body, many of which may have detrimental effects on immune function. A well-balanced diet helps promote optimal immune function, and reviews by Gleeson and Nieman indicate that consuming carbohydrate during exercise attenuates rises in stress hormones such as cortisol and appears to limit the degree of exercise-induced immunosuppression. An impaired immune response is one possible factor associated with the overtraining syndrome. Carbohydrate intake following exercise also promotes protein synthesis via the insulin effect, which may enhance muscle and overall recovery.

Some nutritionists indicate that many athletes do not eat high carbohydrate diets because it may be impractical for them to do so. Selecting foods high in carbohydrate content, highlighted earlier in this chapter, provides a sound guide to increase the carbohydrate content of the diet, as do some of the recommendations in the following section regarding carbohydrate loading. Chapter 11 will provide additional information specific to daily caloric intake for planning a diet.

In summary, as Coyle notes, athletes do not train hard every day, so they do not require a high intake of carbohydrate every day of training. Nevertheless, a diet rich in healthful carbohydrates not only may have several major health benefits, but may also help guarantee optimal energy sources for daily exercise training. Moreover, as Louise Burke points out, experts in the field of energy metabolism indicate that there is no evidence that diets which are restricted in carbohydrate, such as the "zone" diet discussed in chapters 5 and 6, enhance training. Carbohydrate is the major fuel for most athletes in training. The slogan *Train high and compete high* refers to the concept of training and competing with high carbohydrate intake.

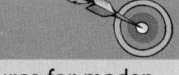

Carbohydrate Loading

What is carbohydrate, or glycogen, loading?

Because carbohydrate becomes increasingly important as a fuel for muscular exercise as the intensity of the exercise increases, and because the amount of carbohydrate stored in the body is limited, muscle and liver glycogen depletion could be factors that may limit performance capacity in distance events characterized by high levels of energy expenditure for prolonged periods. **Carbohydrate loading,** also called *glycogen loading* and *glycogen supercompensation,* is a dietary technique designed to promote a significant increase in the glycogen content in both the liver and the muscles in an attempt to delay the onset of fatigue. It is generally used for 3–7 days in preparation for major athletic competitions.

What type of athlete would benefit from carbohydrate loading?

In general, carbohydrate loading is primarily suited for individuals who will sustain high levels of continuous energy expenditure for prolonged periods, such as long-distance runners, swimmers, bicyclists, triathletes, cross-country skiers, and similar athletes. In addition, athletes who are involved in prolonged stop-and-go activities, such as soccer, lacrosse, and tournament-play sports like tennis and handball, may benefit. For example, Rico-Sanz and others concluded that exhaustion during soccer-specific performance is related to the capacity to use muscle glycogen, underlying the importance of glycogen loading. In essence, carbohydrate loading may be effective for athletes engaged in events that use muscle glycogen as the major energy source and that may lead to a depletion of glycogen in the muscle fibers. Athletes who compete in sports involving high-intensity, short-duration energy expenditure will not benefit from carbohydrate loading. For example, Hatfield and others reported no effects of carbohydrate loading on performance in resistance training involving multiple sets of maximal jump squats. However, bodybuilders have been reported to carbohydrate load in attempts to appear more muscular owing to increased muscle glycogen levels and associated water retention.

Recall from chapter 3 that humans have several different types of skeletal muscle fibers. In general, the slow-twitch red and fast-twitch red fibers are used mainly during long, continuous activities and are aerobic in nature, whereas the fast-twitch white fibers are used for short, fast activities and are anaerobic in nature. Consider the differences between a distance runner and a soccer player. The former may run at a steady pace for hours, whereas the latter will constantly be changing speeds, with many bouts of full speed interspersed with recovery periods of slower running. Research has shown that glycogen depletion patterns of the two different muscle fiber types are related to the type of exercise. Long, continuous exercise depletes glycogen principally in the slow-twitch red and fast-twitch red fibers, whereas fast, intermittent bouts of exercise with periods of rest—actually a form of interval training—primarily deplete glycogen in the fast-twitch white fibers. However, it should be noted that glycogen depletion may occur in all types of fibers in either prolonged continuous or intermittent exercise and may be quite appreciable, depending upon intensity and duration of the exercise bouts. If carbohydrate loading works for the specific muscle fiber involved, then both types of athletes may benefit. Both should have greater glycogen stores in the latter stages of their respective athletic contests.

How do you carbohydrate load?

As you might suspect, the key to carbohydrate loading is to switch from the normal, balanced diet to one very high in carbohydrate content. The original, classic carbohydrate loading technique, emanating from earlier Scandinavian research, involved a glycogen depletion stage induced by prolonged exercise and a restricted diet. For example, a runner might go for an 18- to 20-mile run to use as much stored glycogen as possible, and then ingest very little carbohydrate in the following 2- to 3-day period. Exercise is continued during this 2- to 3-day period to keep glycogen stores low. Following the depletion stage, the loading stage began. During this phase, carbohydrate may contribute 70 or more percent of the caloric intake. The intensity and duration of exercise during this phase were reduced considerably. The usual case was to rest fully for 2 to 3 days. Thus, the classic carbohydrate loading pattern involved three stages: depletion, carbohydrate deprivation (high-fat/protein diet), and carbohydrate loading. However, this original method may be particularly difficult to tolerate, especially if one tries to exercise at high levels during the depletion phase. The lack of carbohydrate in the diet combined with the exercise bouts may elicit symptoms of hypoglycemia (weakness, lethargy, irritability). Moreover, prolonged exhaustive exercise may lead to muscle trauma, which may actually impair the storage of extra glycogen. This classic, original method is presented in table 4.9.

Although some early research supported this technique, more recent data suggest that this strict routine may be unnecessary, particularly the total program of depletion. For example, in trained runners, research has shown that simply changing to a very high-carbohydrate diet, combined with 1 or 2 days of rest or reduced activity levels (tapering), will effectively increase muscle and liver glycogen. Well-controlled research has revealed that exhaustive running is not necessary to achieve muscle glycogen supercompensation. It appears to be important to continue endurance training, or other high-intensity training specific to the sport, during the 7–14 days prior to competition. Such training will serve to maintain adequate levels of GLUT-4 receptors to transfer blood glucose into the muscle cell and of glycogen synthase, the enzyme in the muscle that synthesizes glycogen from glucose. Evidence also suggests that if the total carbohydrate content is consumed over the entire week, in contrast to concentrating it in 2–3 days, there will be little difference in the muscle glycogen content between the two techniques.

Although there may be a number of variations in the carbohydrate loading protocol, a generally recommended format is also presented in table 4.9. The interested athlete may want to experiment with both techniques, and also make adjustments through experience.

Sports scientists have generally recommended that carbohydrate intake during carbohydrate loading should be about 8–10 grams per kilogram body weight, and Louise Burke, from the Australian Institute of Sport, recommended that marathon runners should consume about 10–12 grams per kilogram body weight over the 36–48 hours prior to the race. These recommendations could total about 400–800 grams per day, depending on the size of the individual, which is not too different from the generally recommended dietary content of carbohydrate for the endurance athlete in regular training; Burke recommends that marathoners consume 7–12 grams of carbohydrate per kilogram body mass during training. It is important to note that the athlete should not change his or her diet drastically prior to competition. Consuming a high-carbohydrate diet during training will condition the body to metabolize carbohydrate properly during this loading phase. Table 4.10 represents a general dietary plan for carbohydrate loading. The total caloric value and grams of carbohydrate should be adjusted to individual needs. They are dependent upon the size of the individual and daily energy expenditure in exercise. It is important not to consume excess

---

TABLE 4.9 Different methods for carbohydrate loading

A recommended method		Original, classic method	
1st day:	tapering exercise	1st day:	depletion exercise
2nd day:	mixed diet, moderate carbohydrate; tapering exercise	2nd day:	high-protein/fat diet; low carbohydrate; tapering exercise
3rd day:	mixed diet, moderate carbohydrate; tapering exercise	3rd day:	high-protein/fat diet; low carbohydrate; tapering exercise
4th day:	mixed diet, moderate carbohydrate; tapering exercise	4th day:	high-protein/fat diet; low carbohydrate; tapering exercise
5th day:	high-carbohydrate diet; tapering exercise	5th day:	high-carbohydrate diet; tapering exercise
6th day:	high-carbohydrate diet; tapering exercise or rest	6th day:	high-carbohydrate diet; tapering exercise or rest
7th day:	high-carbohydrate diet; tapering exercise or rest	7th day:	high-carbohydrate diet; tapering exercise or rest
8th day:	competition	8th day:	competition

High-carbohydrate diet: 400–800 g per day depending on body weight; about 70–80 percent of dietary Calories should be carbohydrate.

TABLE 4.10 Daily food plan for carbohydrate loading

Dietary sources of fats, proteins, and carbohydrates	Amount and calories	Grams of carbohydrate, protein, and fat
Meat, fish, poultry, eggs, cheese, select low-fat items	6–8 oz Calories: 330–440	0 grams carbohydrate* 42–56 grams protein 18–24 grams fat
Breads, cereals, and grain products	10–20 servings Calories: 800–1,600	150–300 grams carbohydrate 24–60 grams protein
Vegetables, high Calorie (such as corn)	4 servings Calories: 280	60 grams carbohydrate 8 grams protein
Fruits	4 servings Calories: 240	60 grams carbohydrate
Fats and oils	2–4 teaspoons Calories: 90–180	10–20 grams fat
Milk, skim	2 servings Calories: 180	24 grams carbohydrate 16 grams protein
Desserts, like pie	2 servings Calories: 700	102 grams carbohydrate 6 grams protein 30 grams fat
Beverages, naturally sweetened	8–24 ounces Calories: 80–240	20–60 grams carbohydrate
Water	8 or more servings Calories: 0	
TOTAL KCAL	2,700–3,860	

TOTAL GRAMS AND APPROXIMATE % OF DIETARY CALORIES

Carbohydrate	416–606	65%
Protein	96–146	15%
Fat	58–74	20%

Consult table 4.2 for specific high-carbohydrate foods in each of the food sources.

*Beans are listed in the meat group because of their high protein content; however, they are also low in fat and high in carbohydrates, so they are an excellent selection from this food group. Substitution of beans for meat will increase the total grams of carbohydrate and the percentage of dietary Calories from carbohydrate.

Including high-carbohydrate drinks, such as glucose polymers, can add significant amounts of carbohydrate to the diet and may substitute for other foods, such as desserts.

Source: Adapted from M. Forgac, "Carbohydrate Loading: A Review" in *Journal of the American Dietetic Association* 75:42–5, 1979.

Moreover, the diet should also include the daily requirements for protein and fat.

If, for some reason, the athlete cannot carbohydrate load over the 3–7 day period, a rapid protocol may be effective. Fairchild and others found that one day of a high-carbohydrate intake, approximately 10 grams of high-glycemic-index carbohydrate per kilogram body mass, nearly doubled the muscle glycogen concentration, from 109 to 198 mmol/kg wet weight muscle. The carbohydrate feeding was preceded by a short bout of near maximal-intensity exercise for 3 minutes. They reported that these muscle glycogen levels were comparable to those achieved over a 2–6 day regimen.

Most prolonged endurance events begin in the morning. The last large meal should be about 15 hours prior to race time, possibly topped off with a simple carbohydrate snack before retiring for the night. Some athletes drink a glucose polymer for the last major meal to avoid the presence of intestinal residue the morning of competition. A carbohydrate breakfast such as orange juice, toast, jelly, or other carbohydrates along with some protein may be eaten 3 to 4 hours prior to competition. Review the discussion of precompetition meals in chapter 2. This overall dietary regimen should help maximize muscle and liver glycogen stores. The athlete should then follow the guidelines presented previously relative to carbohydrate intake before and during performance.

Calories, for they may be converted into body fat if in excess of the maximal storage capacity of the muscle and liver for glycogen.

Some guidelines for replenishment of glycogen were presented earlier. Because glycogen loading for long-distance events occurs over two to three days, it would be wise to stress complex carbohydrates in the diet because of their higher nutrient content. However, simple carbohydrates may also be used effectively to increase muscle glycogen stores, as can high-carbohydrate sports drinks such as Gatorade Energy Drink.

Will carbohydrate loading increase muscle glycogen concentration?

Most, but not all, studies show that an appropriate carbohydrate loading protocol, compared to normal or low dietary carbohydrate intake, will substantially increase muscle glycogen levels. Although some previous research found that muscle glycogen levels in the early phases of loading did not increase as much in females as in males, more recent, better controlled research by James, Paul, and Tarnopolsky, with their associates, revealed that carbohydrate loading increased muscle glycogen

Based on the current data, it would appear that lactate preparations may provide additional energy, somewhat comparable to carbohydrate sources. The preliminary research findings showing a more ergogenic effect of Cytomax™ over other sports drinks need confirmation from other research laboratories.

Ribose Ribose is a 5-carbon monosaccharide found throughout body cells as part of various compounds, such as RNA (ribonucleic acid) in the cell nucleus. Ribose also comprises the sugar portion of adenosine, the nucleotide found in ATP (adenosine triphosphate). ATP, as you recall, is the immediate source of energy for muscle contraction both in the heart and skeletal muscles.

Although found in nature, very little ribose is consumed in a natural diet. Instead, a specific metabolic pathway (pentose phosphate pathway) produces ribose from glucose to meet our body needs. Recently, ribose supplements (made from corn sugar) have been marketed to physically active individuals as a means to promote faster recovery in heart and skeletal muscles, presumably by facilitating the formation of adenosine, one of the major components of ATP.

Research indicates that strenuous exercise may necessitate rapid recovery of adenosine within muscle cells, which might benefit from adequate ribose. Pliml and others found that ribose ingestion (60 grams daily for 3 days) improved exercise performance time in patients with severe coronary artery disease, while other studies have suggested that ribose, when supplemented, could serve as an energy source and promote adenosine synthesis in various patient groups.

The effect of ribose supplementation has been evaluated using healthy, physically active individuals and athletes. Several studies used an acute supplementation protocol. Kerksick and others reported that 3 grams of ribose, provided to moderately trained male cyclists about 25 minutes prior to exercise, had no effect on 5 maximal 30-second anaerobic capacity cycling tests with a 3-minute recovery. In a crossover study, Peveler and others also found no effect of an acute 625-milligram dose of ribose on peak power, mean power, or rate of fatigue in 3 intermittent 30-second Wingate tests of anaerobic capacity in healthy males.

Research using chronic supplementation of ribose also does not support an ergogenic effect. Berardi and Ziegenfuss studied the effect of oral ribose supplementation (32 grams over a 36-hour period) on high-intensity, intermittent, anaerobic cycle ergometer performance; the exercise task consisted of six 10-second sprints with a 60-second recovery. They concluded that ribose supplementation does not have a consistent or substantial effect on anaerobic cycle sprinting as evaluated by peak and mean power output. Hellsten and others reported that 3 days of ribose supplementation (based on body weight, approximately 45 grams daily) elicited a greater resynthesis of ATP compared to the placebo. However, the slight increase in ATP availability did not enhance performance, as there were no differences between the placebo and ribose supplement for mean and peak power outputs. The authors note that a small reduction in muscle ATP does not appear to limit high-intensity exercise performance. In a well-designed study, Op 'T Eijnde and others evaluated the effect of oral ribose supplementation (16 grams/day for 6 days) on two maximal knee-extension exercise protocols and ATP recovery. The exercise bouts were separated by a 60-minute rest period. They concluded that oral ribose supplementation had no effect on maximal intermittent exercise performance or ATP recovery. In the longest supplementation protocol, Dunne and others compared the effects of ribose or dextrose (10 grams each before and after practice) supplementation for 8 weeks on 2,000-meter rowing performance in female collegiate rowers. Over the course of the 8 weeks, performance in both groups improved, but the dextrose group (about 10 seconds faster) showed significantly more improvement at 8 weeks than the ribose group. The investigators thought that the ribose did not impair performance, but the dextrose simply may have elicited a greater improvement. In their review, Dhanoa and Housner note that although ribose manufacturers claim it provides an ergogenic benefit, scientific research does not support this claim.

Current data do not support an ergogenic effect of ribose supplementation.

Multiple Carbohydrate By-Products Sports supplements manufacturers often combine multiple nutrients in a single supplement on the theory that each may exhibit an ergogenic effect, but the effect will be amplified with multiple components. Limited research is available with multiple by-products of carbohydrate metabolism, but Brown and others investigated the ergogenic potential of a multinutrient supplement composed primarily of intermediates of the Krebs cycle, which may be derived from carbohydrate, fat, or protein. Three weeks of supplementation did not improve cycling time to exhaustion at approximately 70–75 percent VO_2 max, nor did it improve the rate of recovery.

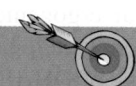

Key Concept

▶ Metabolic by-products of carbohydrate metabolism have been tested as ergogenics. Most have been found to be ineffective, although research with physically trained individuals is limited with several purported ergogenic products.

Check for Yourself

▶ Go to a health food store that sells sports supplements and ask the clerk for carbohydrate products, including metabolites, that may help you train or compete more effectively. Evaluate the supplement fact labels for content and performance claims. What is your judgment?

Dietary Carbohydrates: Health Implications

Although improving somewhat, the diet of the typical American and Canadian still appears to be unbalanced. In general, we consume too many Calories for the level of physical activity we do, and we eat too much of the unhealthy fats and carbohydrates. Such a diet may pose several health problems. As we shall see in chapter 5, excessive consumption of total and saturated fat appears to be of major concern relative to the development of several chronic diseases. In this section, we discuss the health aspects of dietary carbohydrates. In general, the health effects associated with various sugars and starches is not in the substances themselves, but rather in the nutrients that accompany them in the foods we eat. For example, sugar in orange juice is little different from sugar in a soda, but the orange juice contains substantial amounts of vitamin C, potassium, and other nutrients, whereas the soda has none unless fortified. Whole grains contain more fiber and more of some micronutrients than refined grains.

In the recent past, low-carbohydrate diets have been all the rage. As shall be noted in chapter 10, research has indicated that such diets may have some health benefits, but these health benefits appear to be attributed more to decreased caloric intake than to diet composition. The pendulum, rightfully so, has shifted toward a diet rich in carbohydrate, specifically healthier carbohydrate choices.

Nutritional objectives in *Healthy People 2020* and in the *2010 Dietary Guidelines for Americans* recommend that we should consume more grains, making whole grains half of all grains consumed. We should also reduce the consumption of refined carbohydrates and added sugars, often referred to as *bad carbs*. Although no foods, or carbohydrates, are inherently good or bad, following these two general guidelines may produce some significant health benefits. Additionally, an appropriate exercise program may have a healthful influence on carbohydrate metabolism.

How do refined sugars and starches affect my health?

As noted previously, sugars may be found naturally in foods, or they may be manufactured from starches, such as high-fructose corn syrup, and added to foods. Refined starches are predominant in many foods, such as white bread, pasta, and rice. Consumption of refined sugars and starches in excess may be associated with various health risks, attributed mainly to their high glycemic index.

Dental Caries   One of the most common health problems that has been associated with dietary sugar is tooth decay, or dental caries. However, the National Institutes of Health, in its consensus statement on management of dental caries throughout life, noted that effective preventive practice involves a number of factors, including proper oral hygiene (brushing, flossing, use of fluoride) and dietary modifications (use of sugarless products). Tooth decay is not necessarily a matter of how much sugar one eats, but in what form and how often. Dental erosion is increasing and is associated with dietary acids, a major source of which is soft drinks. Sticky, chewy, sugary foods eaten often between meals increase the risk of developing dental caries. Starchy foods that adhere to teeth, like bread, are also cariogenic. Such foods may increase the presence of dental plaque, which may lead to periodontal infection. Seymour and others cite epidemiological research supporting a relationship between periodontal infection and various systemic diseases, such as coronary heart disease, stroke, and diabetes. The infection may lead to systemic inflammation, which may induce adverse effects, such as atherosclerosis. Seymour and others indicate that the control of oral disease is essential in the prevention and management of these systemic conditions.

Of particular interest to athletes, von Fraunhofer and Rogers reported far greater enamel dissolution in flavored and energy (sports) drinks than previously noted for water. They noted that sipping sports drinks over long periods of time may erode tooth enamel; therefore, drink quickly. In contrast, Mathew and others reported no relationship between consumption of sports drinks and dental erosion in university athletes. Nevertheless, scientists have developed a prototype sports drink, containing substantial amounts of calcium and maltodextrins, which is alleged to cause less dental enamel erosion than the typical commercial sports drink.

Chronic Diseases   Over the years, dietary intake of refined sugar has been alleged to contribute to a wide variety of health problems, including obesity, diabetes, heart disease, and cancer, as well as various psychological afflictions such as hyperactivity in children, premenstrual syndrome (PMS), and seasonal affective disorder (SAD). Such allegations have been based mainly on theoretical considerations, but with support from some recent epidemiological studies. An habitual diet rich in high-glycemic-index foods theoretically may lead to insulin resistance and high serum triglyceride levels, risk factors for diabetes and heart disease, respectively. This may be especially so in individuals who are obese, and will be discussed in detail in chapter 10. Bantle also indicated that fructose, which is a low-glycemic-index sugar, may increase serum triglycerides and may be a contributing factor to obesity. Individuals should avoid high-fructose corn syrup, but eating fruits with naturally occurring fructose is not a cause for concern. Added sugars can increase caloric intake and predispose to obesity.

As a part of the National Health and Nutrition Examination Survey (NHANES 2003–2006) of 4,258 healthy adults, fructose intake was calculated and blood pressure was directly measured. Jalal and colleagues determined a median fructose intake of 74 g/d (equivalent to 2.5 sugary soft drinks per day). They also found this fructose intake to be associated with a 26, 30, and 77 percent higher risk for blood pressure values of $\geq 135/85$, $\geq 140/90$, and $> 160/100$ mmHg, respectively. Fung and others conducted a 24-year follow-up with the Nurses' Health Study cohort and identified a significant positive association between sugar-sweetened beverage intake and coronary heart disease risk.

High-sugar intake has been associated with development of cancer. Two large epidemiological studies by Larsson and Stattin and their associates found that increased consumption of sugar and high-sugar foods, particularly sugar-sweetened sodas, increases the risk of pancreatic cancer. The increased sugar intake may cause the pancreas to produce more insulin, which may cause hyperinsulinemia and increased insulin-like growth factor, factors that may stimulate cell division in the pancreas and lead to cancer.

Additionally, as discussed previously, a high-carbohydrate diet can affect the fTRP:BCAA ratio and formation of the neurotransmitter serotonin. Serotonin may influence mood and behavior associated with PMS and SAD or other psychological states.

The National Academy of Sciences, in its DRI recommendations for carbohydrate, noted that given the currently available scientific evidence relative to the effect of dietary sugar on dental caries, psychological behavior, cancer, risk of obesity, and risk of hyperlipidemia, there is insufficient evidence to set a UL for total or added sugar in the diet. Nevertheless, the Academy noted that the theory linking a high glycemic index to certain health problems, such as diabetes and CHD, appears to be valid and supported by some studies, but the evidence at this time appears to be insufficient to substantiate the theory. Furthermore, the Academy noted that individuals who consume excess amounts of added sugars may not obtain sufficient amounts of various micronutrients, and that this may lead to adverse health effects. Johnson and others, in the American Heart Association scientific statement on dietary sugars intake and cardiovascular health, recommend an upper limit of half the discretionary calorie allowance from added sugars. For most American women, this is no more than 100 Calories per day, and for most American men it is no more than 150 Calories per day from added sugars.

Given these considerations, and the fact that many health organizations recommend a reduced intake of refined sugars to about 10 percent or less of the daily caloric intake, it appears to be prudent to moderate your consumption of refined sugars and starches.

Suggestions to decrease intake of refined starches and sugars were presented in chapter 2.

Are artificial sweeteners safe?

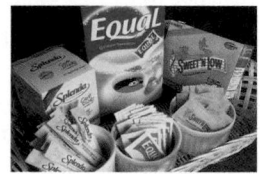

Artificial sweeteners are products designed to provide sweetness, but fewer or no Calories, as a means for individuals to reduce refined sugar consumption. However, Liebman noted that although dietary intake of artificial sweeteners has increased over the past ten years, so too has the consumption of refined sugars. As these products have been used as food additives, their safety has been evaluated.

A number of artificial sweeteners have been produced over the years, and currently several are approved for use by the FDA in the United States (see table 4.11). Saccharin is a noncaloric derivative of coal tar. Aspartame is derived from two amino acids (aspartic acid and phenylalanine) and contains 4 Calories per gram. Neotame is derived from the same amino acids as aspartame. Acesulfame-K is a naturally occurring potassium salt. Sucralose is produced by altering the sugar molecule. Sugar alcohols, such as sorbitol, erythritol, mannitol, and lactitol, are not absorbed, so they are low glycemic and provide no Calories.

Years ago, saccharin in extremely large doses had been shown to cause urinary bladder cancer in laboratory animals, and according to the Delaney clause, it should be banned as an additive to food products. However, the United States Congress passed a law exempting saccharin from the Delaney clause. Nevertheless, a warning relative to the association between saccharine and cancer was required on food labels for products containing saccharin. Epidemiological data with humans have not shown any relationship between urinary bladder cancer and saccharin at levels normally consumed by the general population, so it is assumed to be safe and has been removed from the government's list of carcinogens. The food label warning is no longer required in the United States. However, Canada still prohibits the use of saccharin in foods, and some consumer protection groups, such as the Center for Science in the Public Interest, recommend avoidance of saccharin-containing products.

The safety of aspartame, also known as Equal or NutraSweet, has been questioned because some reports have associated it with headaches, dizziness, or fatigue in some individuals, which may have been allergic reactions. Previous studies also have associated aspartame use with brain tumors. More recently, an Italian study, with rats, found that aspartame use was linked to leukemia and lymphoma (cancers of the blood cells and lymphatic system); however, in a review the FDA noted that the European Food Safety Authority indicated that the conclusions were not supported by the data.

TABLE 4.11 Artificial sweeteners approved for use in the United States

Name	Brand name	Times sweeter than sugar	Calories per typical serving
Acesulfame-K (potassium)	Sunett Sweet One	200	0
Aspartame	Equal NutraSweet	200	0
Neotame	*	7,000–13,000	0
Saccharin	Necta Sweet Sweet'n Low Sweet Twin	200–700	0
Sucralose	Splenda	600	0

*No brand name yet

In a major review, Magnuson and others noted that current use levels of aspartame, even by high users in special subgroups, remain well below the U.S. FDA established acceptable daily intake levels. Moreover, they conducted a critical review of all carcinogenicity studies conducted on aspartame and found no credible evidence that aspartame is carcinogenic. The data from the extensive investigations into the possibility of neurotoxic effects of aspartame, in general, do not support the hypothesis that aspartame in the human diet will affect nervous system function, learning, or behavior. They concluded that the weight of existing evidence is that aspartame is safe at current levels of consumption as a nonnutritive sweetener. Other research by Lim and Gallus and their colleagues support this conclusion. Additionally, the Food and Drug Administration and other federal health agencies consider aspartame to confer no significant health risks, with the exception of individuals who have phenylketonuria (PKU), a rare genetic disease that limits the ability to metabolize phenylalanine. Such individuals are aware of their condition, and products containing aspartame must carry a warning on the label that the product contains phenylalanine.

In a review, the Consumers Union concluded that all artificial sweeteners appear to be safe in small amounts. In particular, studies have raised no safety concerns at all about sucralose. Grotz and Munro reviewed the safety of sucralose and concluded that sucralose and sucralose-mixed products are safe for use in food. However, the Consumers Union states several caveats. For one, high intakes of sugar alcohols, because they are not absorbed, may cause gastrointestinal distress. For another, individuals who may suffer from headaches or other symptoms from aspartame should avoid it.

Some contend that use of sugar substitutes perpetuates cravings for sweet foods, and does nothing to promote good health. However, artificial sweeteners may be effective in weight control programs, and their role will be discussed in chapter 11. Nevertheless, one should keep in mind that *sugar free* does not mean low-Calorie; check the food label for Calories per serving.

Why are complex carbohydrates thought to be beneficial to my health?

To increase consumption of total carbohydrate in the diet while reducing the consumption of refined sugars, one must increase the consumption of complex carbohydrates. Some diet plans developed for health, such as the Pritikin program, recommend that 80 percent of the dietary Calories be supplied by carbohydrates, mostly complex and unrefined. More recently, the OmniHeart diet focused on healthy carbohydrates, fats, and proteins. The OmniHeart diet plan includes the following tips for increasing consumption of healthier carbohydrates:

- Eat 1–2 servings of fruit at every meal and have an extra fruit at breakfast.
- Have 2–3 servings of vegetables at lunch and dinner.
- Create a fruit and nut trail mix for snacks: ¼ cup dried fruit with 1 oz unsalted nuts.
- Use whole grains rather than refined grains as often as possible.
- Select legumes for a carbohydrate and protein source several times a week.

A diet rich in complex carbohydrates may reduce the percentage contribution from fats if excessive, which may confer significant health benefits, as noted in chapter 5. Complex carbohydrates are found primarily in starchy vegetables, whole grains, and legumes, but small amounts are also found in fruits.

Whole-grain products are one of the best sources of healthy carbohydrates. As defined by the FDA, whole grains contain all three ingredients of a cereal grain, namely the outer bran and the inner germ and endosperm, and in the same proportion as found in nature (see figure 4.13). Seal noted that an increasing body of evidence from both epidemiological and prospective studies supports an inverse relationship between consumption of whole-grain foods and risk of coronary heart disease. For example, Djoussé and Gaziano found that those who ate the most whole-grain cereals over the course of the week had the greatest reduction in risk of heart failure. Over the course of approximately 20 years, those who consumed no whole-grain cereals weekly had a relative risk (RR) of heart failure of 1.0; those who consumed 2–6 servings weekly had a RR of 0.79, and those who consumed 7 or more servings had a RR of 0.71, which represents about a 22–28 percent lower risk of heart failure.

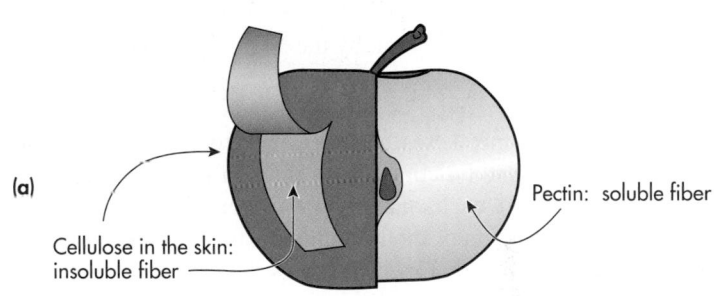

(a)

Cellulose in the skin: insoluble fiber

Pectin: soluble fiber

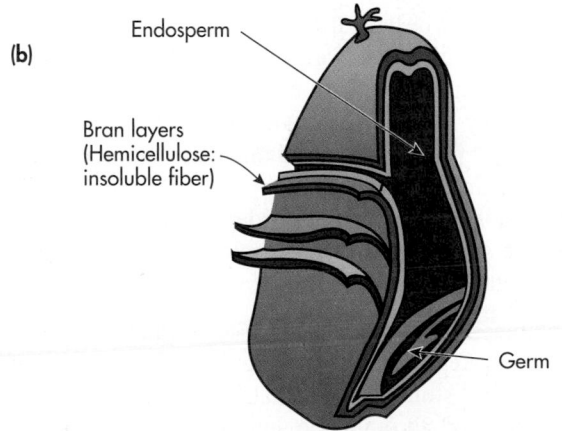

(b)

Endosperm

Bran layers (Hemicellulose: insoluble fiber)

Germ

FIGURE 4.13 Various forms of fiber. *(a)* The skin of an apple consists of the insoluble fiber cellulose, which provides structure for the fruit. The soluble fiber pectin "glues" the fruit cells together. *(b)* The outside layer of a wheat kernel is made of layers of bran—insoluble fiber—making this grain a good source of fiber. Fruits, vegetables, whole grains, and legumes such as beans are rich in fiber.

When shopping, look for products labeled 100% Whole Wheat or 100% Whole Grains. Products labeled 100% wheat, multigrain, or stone ground may be made primarily from refined grains. The first ingredient listed should be whole oats, whole rye, whole wheat, or other whole grains such as brown rice, bulgur, or oatmeal. Many vitamins, minerals, phytonutrients, antioxidants, and fiber may be lost in processing of whole grain to refined grain. Some, but not all, may be replaced during processing, so you may not get the synergistic health effects of the multiple nutrients. In your efforts to increase fiber intake, look at the 10 Tips To Help You Eat Whole Grains on the www.ChooseMyPlate.gov site.

Current thinking supports the concept that the beneficial health effects of a diet rich in complex carbohydrates, which may be considered to be a low-glycemic-index diet, may be linked to several important attributes of such a diet, including the collective presence of various phytochemicals, vitamins, minerals, and dietary fiber. The health benefits of phytochemicals were discussed in chapter 2, while the benefits of vitamins and minerals will be covered in chapters 7 and 8. Most research relative to the healthful benefits of complex carbohydrates has focused on dietary fiber.

Why should I eat foods rich in fiber?

The current AI recommendation by the National Academy of Sciences for total fiber has been set at 14 grams per 1,000 Calories, or 38 grams for men and 25 grams for women up to age 50 and slightly lesser amounts thereafter. Recall that total fiber consists of both dietary fiber and functional fiber, and various specific forms of fiber are found in each category; some specific forms of fiber may be classified as both dietary and functional fiber. Although the Academy indicates that specific forms of fibers have properties that result in different physiological effects that may impact health, it did not feel that the evidence was sufficient to establish separate recommendations for each type of fiber. Nevertheless, some feel that the use of the water-solubility classifications system, as discussed previously, might be useful conceptually to illustrate the potential health benefits of certain forms of fiber. As noted earlier, dietary fiber is found naturally in various plant foods.

Exactly how dietary fiber may be protective is not known, but several mechanisms have been proposed that may help in the prevention of certain forms of cancer, coronary heart disease, obesity, diabetes, hypertension, and various disorders of the gastrointestinal tract. Here are some of the theories relative to the potential health benefits of total fiber:

1. Water-insoluble fibers are considered to be those with the greatest effect on fecal bulk. Adding bulk to the contents of the large intestine stimulates peristalsis and speeds up the transit time of food through the intestines. The increased bulk has been shown to dilute any possible cancer-causing (carcinogens) that might attack cell walls, while faster transit diminishes the time carcinogens may have to act. Increased bulk—and peristalsis—also decreases the incidence rate of diverticulosis, an inflammatory disorder in the large intestine that may cause rupture, leading to serious complications.

2. Fiber-rich foods are low-glycemic-index foods, and may increase insulin sensitivity and prevention of weight gain. Fiber slows down gastric (stomach) emptying and thereby slows glucose absorption in the small intestine. The high viscosity of soluble fiber also decreases intestinal absorption. These effects may lead to better control of blood sugar and may also lengthen the sensation of fullness or satiety, which may be important to individuals on weight-loss diets. Fiber-rich diets are frequently lower in fat and added sugars, and thus contain fewer Calories. So, high-fiber diets may be useful in the prevention or treatment of obesity and obesity-related chronic diseases such as diabetes and hypertension.

3. Fiber, particularly gummy forms of water-soluble fiber like beta-glucans in oats, may bind with various substances in the gastrointestinal tract. Soluble fiber may bind with carcinogens so that they are excreted by the bowel. Soluble fibers may also bind with and lead to the excretion of bile salts, which contain cholesterol; normally bile salts are reabsorbed into the body, but excretion of bile salts, along with their cholesterol content, may help reduce serum cholesterol levels. This effect may decrease the risk of coronary heart disease. (Lower serum cholesterol levels decrease the risk of atherosclerosis, a major cause of heart disease.)

4. Some water-soluble fibers may be fermented in the large intestine to form short-chain fatty acids (SCFAs). Wong and others noted that several of these SCFAs are theorized to help prevent gastrointestinal disorders, cancer, and cardiovascular disease. Some act in the colon; others are absorbed into the blood, delivered to the liver, and may help decrease synthesis of cholesterol.

Although it may be illustrative to view the health benefits of fiber based on its water solubility, Joanne Slavin, a scholar on the health effects of dietary fiber, notes that it is difficult to generalize as to the physiological effects of fiber based on this classification system. For example, she notes that rice bran, which is devoid of soluble fiber, has been shown to reduce serum cholesterol, while recent research has also supported the effect of insoluble fiber to reduce the risk of heart disease. Thus, health benefits may be attributable to total fiber.

Numerous studies, including major epidemiological studies and clinical trials, have investigated the effect of total fiber on reducing the risk or incidence of chronic diseases. Based on these studies, the National Academy of Sciences established the AI for total fiber because it may reduce the risk of coronary heart disease, and more recent research supports this concept.

The Academy cited studies showing a beneficial effect of total fiber and a low-glycemic-index diet on other health problems, particularly in individuals with diabetes or hyperlipidemia, but the evidence was not as convincing as that for prevention of heart disease.

Scientists have expressed different opinions regarding the use of the glycemic index, which is associated with fiber intake, as a means to design a diet for enhanced health. For example, in a meta-analysis of 45 studies, Livesey and others concluded that consumption of reduced glycemic response diets are followed by favorable changes in various health markers. Kendall and others also note that sufficient positive research findings have emerged to suggest that the glycemic index is an aspect of diet of potential importance in the treatment and prevention of chronic diseases, such as diabetes and cardiovascular disease. In contrast, Howlett and Ashwell, summarizing a workshop on the glycemic index and health, reported that although lower GI and GL diets are beneficial for health in persons with impaired glucose metabolism, it is as yet unclear what they mean for healthy persons.

Even though there may be debate over the usefulness of the glycemic index as a means to design a healthful diet for chronic diseases other than heart disease, consuming a fiber-rich diet is certainly prudent dietary behavior given that coronary heart disease is the number one cause of death in Western societies. And, although the National Academy of Sciences indicates that the relationship of fiber intake to other health problems is the subject of ongoing investigation and currently unresolved, there appear to be no adverse health effects associated with a fiber-rich or low-glycemic-index diet. Indeed, a fiber-rich diet may be useful for other possible health benefits.

Prevention of colon cancer has been one of the main theories underlying the promotion of a high-fiber diet. Rock has indicated that the relationship between dietary fiber intake and colorectal cancer has been inconsistent. However, she noted that no significant relationship between fiber intake (or major food sources of fiber) and risk for colorectal cancer was observed in a recently reported, large pooled analysis of several studies. Nevertheless, she notes limitations in epidemiological studies and indicates that the effect of increased dietary fiber intake on risk for colorectal cancer has not been adequately addressed in studies conducted to date. More research, including longer-term trials and higher levels of fiber intake, is needed to increase knowledge in this area.

As the different types of fiber appear to convey health benefits in different ways, a balanced intake of total fiber appears to be the best approach. The Academy notes that although the AI are based on total fiber, the greatest health benefits may come from the ingestion of cereal fibers and various viscous fibers, including gums and pectins, which are found in fruits and vegetables. Obtaining 25–38 grams of fiber daily is not difficult, but you have to eat more whole grains, fruits, vegetables, and legumes. Total fiber is listed on food labels. In particular, check food labels on breads and cereals, staples of the daily diet. According to the *2010 Dietary Guidelines for Americans,* although Americans eat adequate amounts of total grains, most of these come from refined sources rather than whole grains. Additionally, on average Americans eat less than 1 ounce-equivalent of whole grains per day, and less than 5 percent consume the minimum amount of whole grains. Refined grains contain little or no fiber, whereas whole grains are usually rich in fiber. Some brands of bread contain 3 grams of fiber per slice, and only 50 Calories. Breakfast cereals may also be very high in fiber, some containing 10 or more grams per serving.

Here are some suggestions from *Consumer Reports on Health* for ten easy ways to eat more fiber:

- Look for "good sources" of fiber (~3 grams per serving)
- Choose whole grains (100 percent whole wheat or 100 percent whole grain)
- Start the day right (oatmeal or a high-fiber cereal)
- Choose fiber-filled snacks (raw carrots or celery, popcorn, or fiber-rich crackers)
- Drink it up (blend chunks of fruit or vegetables with yogurt, juice, or soy milk)
- Look for fiber-fortified pastas
- Don't forget legumes (add beans or lentils)
- Keep the skin on (wash, but don't peel skins of fruits and vegetables)
- Bake it in (add crushed bran cereal or flax or sesame seeds to baked items)
- Consider a supplement (if foods are not enough)

According to one physician, a good way to see if you are eating enough fiber is to observe the buoyancy of your stool in the toilet. It should float, or at least appear flaky and break apart. If it sinks or does not break apart, you are not eating enough fiber.

There appear to be few or no health disadvantages to a high-fiber diet. As we shall see in chapter 8, there has been some concern that high-fiber diets could lead to increased losses of certain minerals, such as iron and zinc, but research has shown that such concerns are generally unwarranted if one follows the recommendations just given.

Schneeman, discussing development of a scientific consensus on the importance of dietary fiber, notes that fiber serves as a marker for diets rich in plant foods, which provide additional benefits for maintaining health. Liebman notes that it is important to recognize that the health benefits attributed to dietary fiber may be associated with the form in which the fiber is consumed—as part of a whole, natural food containing other potential health-promoting nutrients such as vitamins and phytochemicals, rather than by consumption of a purified supplement form. This is in accord with the position stand of the American Dietetic Association, written by Marlett and others, on dietary fiber. Get more plant foods in your diet!

Do some carbohydrate foods cause food intolerance?

About one in nine Americans may develop gastrointestinal distress when they consume dairy products containing substantial amounts of lactose, particularly milk. African-Americans are more likely to suffer lactose intolerance. Such individuals lack the enzyme lactase and hence cannot metabolize lactose in the digestive tract. The most common symptoms of **lactose intolerance** are gas, bloating, abdominal pain, and diarrhea, although headache and fatigue may also occur. Levey has noted that lactose intolerance may be the cause of runner's diarrhea that often occurs during exercise.

Individuals may be diagnosed as being lactose intolerant through a lactose tolerance test administered by a physician. One physician suggests, however, that a self-detection technique may be an effective approach. If you experience problems such as gas and diarrhea after consuming milk, abstain from all dairy products for 2 weeks and then evaluate the results. If the symptoms resolve, and then reoccur when you resume dairy food consumption, you may need to reduce the amount of lactose in your diet. Unfortunately, usually this means a reduced intake of dairy foods, which are considered to be the main dietary source of not only lactose, but calcium as well. Di Stefano and others indicated that lactose intolerance may prevent the achievement of adequate peak bone mass in young adults and may, therefore, predispose to severe osteoporosis.

Calcium will be discussed in detail in chapter 8, but here are several strategies lactose-intolerant individuals may use to obtain adequate calcium intake. In a meta-analysis of well-designed studies, Savaiano and others indicated that symptoms of lactose intolerance may be minimal with small amounts of dairy foods, such as one cup or less. Consuming small amounts of milk over the course of the day may provide significant amounts of calcium. Reduced-lactose milk is available, as are enzyme supplements, such as Lactaid, to help prevent indigestion. Other dairy products which have been fermented, such as yogurt, may be tolerated and provide a good calcium source. Cheese may also be a good source of calcium, although it is high in fat. Dark-green leafy vegetables, tofu, sardines, and salmon are all nondairy sources of calcium. Additionally, calcium supplements may be useful either in tablet form or as added to various foods, such as soy milk, rice milk, or orange juice.

Wheat products may produce gastrointestinal symptoms comparable to lactose intolerance. The problem is not the wheat itself, but rather a protein called gluten. Gluten is found in wheat, rye, and barley, which are the main constituents in most of the grain-based products we eat, such as cereals, breads, and pasta. **Gluten intolerance** represents a sensitivity to gluten; the immune system recognizes gluten as a foreign substance, but does not induce an allergic response. Some sports nutritionists note that simple gluten intolerance can be uncomfortable, but the symptoms are fleeting. Symptoms may vary from none to severe. Simple gluten intolerance could be problematic for endurance athletes. Alternate sources of carbohydrate, such as corn, potatoes, rice, soybeans, and similar foods, will be needed to replace grain-based foods. Gluten-free products are currently available in the marketplace.

Gluten intolerance is also known as *celiac (coeliac) disease,* and in severe cases the gluten damages the lining of the small intestine. This leads to impaired nutrient absorption and a variety of nutrient-deficiency diseases, including weight loss, anemia, and osteoporosis. Celiac disease necessitates medical treatment and a lifelong gluten-free diet.

Does exercise exert any beneficial health effects related to carbohydrate metabolism?

As noted in chapter 1, an appropriate exercise program may provide a variety of health benefits. In subsequent chapters, we shall detail the preventive health effects of exercise as related to several major health problems, such as obesity, diabetes, hypertension, and coronary heart disease. Some of these beneficial effects may be attributed to the effect of exercise on carbohydrate metabolism.

Aging is normally associated with impaired glucose tolerance, which is associated with decreased insulin sensitivity. As shall be noted in chapter 10, such effects may contribute to metabolic aberrations associated with the development of coronary heart disease. However, Holloszy and Greiwe noted that these deleterious changes are not inevitable, but are most likely related to a sedentary lifestyle and increased body weight. They found that athletic individuals 60 years and older had glucose tolerance and insulin action as good as young athletes nearly half their age.

Exercise may enhance glucose tolerance and insulin sensitivity in several ways. In their review, Borghouts and Keizer noted that both acute and chronic exercise may affect blood glucose and insulin activity favorably. Up to two hours after an acute bout of exercise, glucose uptake is in part elevated due to insulin-independent mechanisms, probably involving an increase in GLUT-4 receptors in the cell membrane induced by exercise. Additionally, an exercise bout can increase insulin sensitivity for up to 16 hours afterwards. Chronic exercise training potentiates the effect of exercise on insulin sensitivity through multiple adaptations in glucose transport and metabolism. Frøsig and others suggested that improved insulin-stimulated glucose uptake associated with endurance training may result from hemodynamic adaptations, such as greater blood flow to the muscle, as well as increased cellular protein content of individual insulin signaling components and molecules involved in glucose transport and metabolism. Borghouts and Keizer conclude that exercise plays an important, if not essential, role in the prevention and treatment of impaired insulin sensitivity.

Given the epidemic of obesity and type 2 diabetes in the United States and other industrialized nations, these beneficial effects of exercise on carbohydrate metabolism underscore its importance as preventive medicine. More details are presented in chapter 10.

Key Concepts

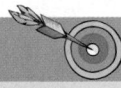

▶ Added sugars should be limited in the diet. The maximal recommended amount is 25 percent of daily energy intake, but some health professionals recommend lower amounts of about 10 percent. Intake of refined starches should also be limited.

▶ An increase in the amount of total fiber to about 25–38 grams per day may be helpful as a protective measure against the development of heart disease, and possibly other chronic diseases. Consuming more whole grains, more fresh fruits, more nonstarchy vegetables, and more legumes, which are low-GI foods, will help ensure adequate fiber intake.

Check for Yourself

▶ Check the food labels of various breads for fiber content. Do some brands have significantly more than others? What impact could switching breads have on meeting the recommended daily fiber intake of 25 grams for females and 38 grams for males?

If you are not currently eating enough fiber, try this experiment. Keep a record of your appetite and your bowel movements for a week or so, and then switch to a high-fiber diet, consuming fruits and vegetables, whole wheat and whole-grain breads, and other high-fiber foods as documented by food labels.

Record approximate grams of total fiber consumed daily. Also record an increase (↑), decrease (↓), or no change (NC) for appetite, and record the number of daily bowel movements. Compare your appetite and bowel movements to the previous week. Did the high-fiber diet influence either?

Week 1 (Normal diet)

	Sunday	Monday	Tuesday	Wednesday	Thursday	Friday	Saturday
Breakfast							
Lunch							
Dinner							
Snacks							
Appetite							
Bowel Movement(s)							

Week 2 (High-fiber diet)

	Sunday	Monday	Tuesday	Wednesday	Thursday	Friday	Saturday
Breakfast							
Lunch							
Dinner							
Snacks							
Appetite							
Bowel Movement(s)							

Review Questions—Multiple Choice

1. Which of the following statements relative to carbohydrate loading is false?

   a. It is beneficial primarily for athletes involved in prolonged endurance events, such as the typical marathon (26.2 miles).

   b. It involves the intake of about 500–600 grams of carbohydrate each day for several days prior to competition.

   c. Research generally supports its effectiveness as a means of improving performance by helping to delay the onset of fatigue in the latter stages of prolonged exercise tasks.

   d. The major advantage of carbohydrate loading is the increased storage of glycogen in the adipose cells for use during exercise.

   e. The increase in carbohydrate stores in the body may be detected by the increased body weight attributed to the water-binding effect of stored glycogen.

2. If you were to recommend to a runner a fluid replacement protocol, including carbohydrate content, for use during a marathon, which of the following would you *not* recommend?

   a. Use a 50–60 percent solution of galactose.

   b. Provide approximately 10–15 grams of carbohydrate per feeding.

   c. Provide feedings about every 15–20 minutes.

   d. Limit the amount of fructose in the solution.

   e. Choose a combination of carbohydrates.

3. Which of the following statements relative to the intake of carbohydrates and physical performance is false?
   a. If an individual has normal glycogen levels in the muscle and liver, carbohydrate feedings are usually not necessary if the exercise task is only about 60–90 minutes.
   b. The intake of concentrated sugar solutions may actually impair performance if they lead to osmosis of fluids into the stomach and precipitate the feeling of gastric distress.
   c. Carbohydrate intake may help delay the onset of fatigue in prolonged exercise by either preventing the early onset of hypoglycemia or delaying the depletion of muscle glycogen levels.
   d. Carbohydrate intake prior to and during endurance exercise tasks lasting more than 2 hours may be helpful as a means of enhancing performance.
   e. If consumed during exercise, it takes approximately 60–90 minutes for the carbohydrate to find its way into the muscle and be used as an energy source.

4. Following a meal high in simple carbohydrate, which of the following is most likely to occur in the next 1–2 hours?
   a. suppression of insulin with a resultant hyperglycemia
   b. hyperglycemia, which stimulates insulin secretion followed by possible hypoglycemia
   c. hypoglycemia, which stimulates insulin secretion and a return to normal blood glucose levels
   d. hyperglycemia with a suppression of insulin and movement of blood glucose into the liver and muscle tissues
   e. no change in blood glucose level

5. Which of the following is *not* one of the potential health benefits of dietary fiber?
   a. It may increase the bulk in the large intestine and dilute possible carcinogens.
   b. It may increase the bulk in the large intestine and help speed up intestinal transit.
   c. It may bind with carcinogens and help to excrete them.
   d. It may help excrete bile salts and reduce serum cholesterol levels.
   e. It may bind with certain minerals such as zinc and help to excrete them.

6. Which of the following food exchanges is least likely to be high in dietary fiber?
   a. vegetable
   b. starch/bread
   c. milk
   d. fruit
   e. legumes (meat exchange)

7. What two tissues in the body store the most carbohydrate?
   a. adipose and kidney
   b. kidney and liver
   c. liver and muscles
   d. muscles and kidney
   e. adipose and muscles

8. Common table sugar is:
   a. glucose.
   b. dextrose.
   c. fructose.
   d. sucrose.
   e. maltose.

9. The total amount of carbohydrate, as a percentage of the daily calories, that represents the Acceptable Macronutrient Distribution Range (AMDR) for Americans and Canadians is:
   a. 12–15.
   b. 20–30.
   c. 30–45.
   d. 45–65.
   e. 85–90.

10. The glycemic index represents:
    a. the degree to which an athlete suffers from hypoglycemia.
    b. the amount of glucose released into the blood in response to exercise.
    c. the effect a particular food has on the rate and amount of increase in the blood glucose level.
    d. the amount of stored glycogen in the muscle and liver.
    e. the total amount of insulin released in response to food intake.

Answers to multiple-choice questions:
1. d; 2. a; 3. e; 4. b; 5. e; 6. c; 7. c; 8. d; 9. d; 10. c.

Review Questions—Essay

1. Differentiate between dietary fiber and functional fiber, and contrast the new AI for total fiber with the current Daily Value (DV) used on food labels.
2. You have eaten a high-carbohydrate meal for lunch. Explain the digestion and metabolic fate of this carbohydrate over the next five hours, including an hour of running at the end of this time frame.
3. Explain three possible mechanisms of fatigue due to inadequate carbohydrate intake prior to and during the running of a 26.2 mile marathon.
4. Identify athletes who might benefit from carbohydrate loading and present details of the dietary and exercise training protocol.
5. Discuss the possible health benefits associated with a diet rich in complex carbohydrates and low to moderate in refined carbohydrates.

Books

American Institute of Cancer Research. 2007. *Food, Nutrition, Physical Activity and the Prevention of Cancer: A Global Perspective.* Washington, DC: American Institute of Cancer Research.

Houston, M. 2006. *Biochemistry Primer for Exercise Science.* Champaign, IL: Human Kinetics.

Maughan, R., and Murray, R. 2001. *Sports Drinks.* Boca Raton, FL: CRC Press.

National Academy of Sciences. 2005. *Dietary Reference Intakes for Energy, Carbohydrates, Fiber, Fat, Fatty Acids, Cholesterol, Protein and Amino Acids.* Washington, DC: National Academy Press.

U.S. Department of Health and Human Services Public Health Service. 2010. *Healthy People 2020.* Washington, DC: Government Printing Office.

Reviews

Bangsbo, J., et al. 2006. Physical and metabolic demands of training and match-play in the elite football player. *Journal of Sports Sciences* 24:665–74.

Bantle, J. 2006. Is fructose the optimal glycemic index sweetener? *Nestle Nutrition Workshop Series: Clinical & Performance Programme* 11:83–91.

Beelen, M., et al. 2010. Nutritional strategies to promote postexercise recovery. *International Journal of Sport Nutrition & Exercise Metabolism* 20:515–32.

Borghouts, L., and Keizer, H. 2000. Exercise and insulin sensitivity: A review. *International Journal of Sports Medicine* 21:1–12.

Braun, B. 2008. Effects of high altitude on substrate use and metabolic economy: Cause and effect? *Medicine & Science in Sports & Exercise* 40:1495–1500.

Brooks, G. 2007. Lactate: Link between glycolytic and oxidative metabolism. *Sports Medicine* 37:341–43.

Brown, L., et al. 1999. Cholesterol-lowering effects of dietary fiber: A meta-analysis. *American Journal of Clinical Nutrition* 69:30–42.

Burke, L. 2007. Nutrition strategies for the marathon. *Sports Medicine* 37:344–47.

Burke, L. 2001. Nutritional practices of male and female endurance cyclists. *Sports Medicine* 31:521–32.

Burke, L., et al. 2006. Energy and carbohydrate for training and recovery. *Journal of Sports Sciences* 24:675–85.

Burke, L., et al. 2004. Carbohydrates and fat for training and recovery. *Journal of Sports Sciences* 22:15–30.

Burke, L., et al. 2001. Guidelines for daily carbohydrate intake: Do athletes achieve them? *Sports Medicine* 31:267–99.

Coleman, E. 1994. Update on carbohydrate: Solid versus liquid. *International Journal of Sport Nutrition* 4:80–88.

Conley, M., and Stone, M. 1996. Carbohydrate ingestion/supplementation for resistance exercise and training. *Sports Medicine* 21:7–17.

Consumers Union. 2009. 10 easy ways to eat more fiber. *Consumer Reports on Health* 21 (12):7.

Consumers Union. 2005. Sweeteners can sour your health. *Consumer Reports on Health* 17 (1):8–9.

Costill, D. 1988. Carbohydrates for exercise: Dietary demands for optimal performance. *International Journal of Sports Medicine* 9:1–18.

Coyle, E. 2007. Physiological regulation of marathon performance. *Sports Medicine* 37:306–11.

Coyle, E. 2004. Highs and lows of carbohydrate diets. *Sports Science Exchange* 17 (2):1–6.

Coyle, E. 2000. Physical activity as a metabolic stressor. *American Journal of Clinical Nutrition* 72:512S–20S.

Coyle, E. 1995. Substrate utilization during exercise in active people. *American Journal of Clinical Nutrition* 61 (Supplement): 968S–979S.

Davis, J. 1996. Carbohydrates, branched-chain amino acids and endurance: The central fatigue hypothesis. *Sports Science Exchange* 9 (2): 1–6.

Dhanoa, T., and Housner, J. 2007. Ribose: More than a simple sugar? *Current Sports Medicine Reports* 6:254–57.

Donaldson, C., et al. 2010. Glycemic index and exercise endurance. *International Journal of Sport Nutrition & Exercise Metabolism* 20:154–65.

Edgerton, V., and Roy, R. 2006. The nervous system and movement. In *ACSM's Advanced Exercise Physiology,* ed. C. M. Tipton. Philadelphia: Lippincott Williams & Wilkins.

Erlenbusch, M., et al. 2005. Effect of high-fat or high-carbohydrate diets on endurance exercise: A meta-analysis. *International Journal of Sport Nutrition and Exercise Metabolism* 15:1–14.

Febbraio, M. 2001. Alterations in energy metabolism during exercise and heat stress. *Sports Medicine* 31:47–59.

Fehm, H., et al. 2006. The selfish brain: Competition for energy resources. *Progress in Brain Research* 153:129–40.

Fitts, R. 2006. The muscular system: Fatigue processes. In *ACSM's Advanced Exercise Physiology,* ed. C. M. Tipton. Philadelphia: Lippincott Williams & Wilkins.

Food and Drug Administration. 2006. Artificial sweeteners: No calories … Sweet! *FDA Consumer* 40 (4):27–28.

Gallus, S., et al. 2007. Artificial sweeteners and cancer risk in a network of case-control studies. *Annals of Oncology* 18:40–44.

Gleeson, M. 2006. Can nutrition limit exercise-induced immunodepression? *Nutrition Reviews* 64:119–31.

Gleeson, M., et al. 2004. Exercise, nutrition and immune function. *Journal of Sports Sciences* 22:115–25.

Grotz, V., and Munro, I. 2009. An overview of the safety of sucralose. *Regulatory Toxicology & Pharmacology* 55:1–5.

Hargreaves, M. 2006. The metabolic systems: Carbohydrate metabolism. In *ACSM's Advanced Exercise Physiology,* ed. C. M. Tipton. Philadelphia: Lippincott Williams & Wilkins.

Hargreaves, M. 2005. Metabolic factors in fatigue. *Sports Science Exchange* 18 (3):1–6.

Hargreaves, M. 2000. Carbohydrate metabolism and exercise. In *Exercise and Sport Science,* eds. W. E. Garrett and D. T. Kirkendall. Philadelphia: Lippincott Williams & Wilkins.

Hargreaves, M. 2000. Carbohydrate replacement during exercise. In *Nutrition in Sport,* ed. R. J. Maughan. Oxford: Blackwell Science.

Hargreaves, M., et al. 2004. Pre-exercise carbohydrate and fat ingestion: Effects on metabolism and performance. *Journal of Sports Sciences* 22:31–38.

Hashimoto, T., and Brooks, G. 2008. Mitochondrial lactate oxidation complex and an adaptive role for lactate production. *Medicine & Science in Sports & Exercise* 40:486–94.

Hawley, J., et al. 1997. Carbohydrate-loading and exercise performance: An update. *Sports Medicine* 24:73–81.

Holloszy, J. 2005. Exercise-induced increase in muscle insulin sensitivity. *Journal of Applied Physiology* 99:338–43.

Holloszy, J., and Greiwe, J. 2001. Overview of glucose metabolism and aging. *International Journal of Sport Nutrition & Exercise Metabolism* S58–63.

Holloszy, J., et al. 1998. The regulation of carbohydrate and fat metabolism during and after exercise. *Frontiers in Science* 3:D1011–27.

Howlett, J., and Ashwell, M. 2008. Glycemic response and health: Summary of a workshop. *American Journal of Clinical Nutrition* 212S–16S.

Jeukendrup, A. 2007. Carbohydrate supplementation during exercise: Does it help? How much is too much? *Sports Science Exchange* 20 (3):1–6.

Jeukendrup, A. 2004. Carbohydrate intake during exercise and performance. *Nutrition* 20:669–77.

Jeukendrup, A., and Jentjens, R. 2000. Oxidation of carbohydrate feedings during prolonged exercise: Current thoughts, guidelines and directions for future research. *Sports Medicine* 29:407–24.

Jeukendrup, A., and Killer, S. 2010. The myths surrounding pre-exercise carbohydrate feeding. *Annals of Nutrition & Metabolism* 57 (suppl. 2):18–25.

Johnson, R., et al. 2009. Dietary sugars intake and cardiovascular health: A scientific statement from the American Heart Association. *Circulation* 120:1011–20.

Karelis, A., et al. 2010. Carbohydrate administration and exercise performance: What are the mechanisms involved? *Sports Medicine* 40 (9):747–63.

Keegan, A. 2007. The glycemic index debate. *Diabetes Forecast* 60 (11):16, 19.

Keim, N., et al. 2006. Carbohydrates. In *Modern Nutrition in Health and Disease,* eds. M. Shils, et al. Philadelphia: Lippincott Williams & Wilkins.

Kendall, C., et al. 2006. The glycemic index: Methodology and use. *Nestle Nutrition Workshop Series: Clinical & Performance Programme* 11:43–53.

Kerksick, C., et al. 2008. International Society of Sports Nutrition position stand: Nutrient timing. *Journal of the International Society of Sports Nutrition* 5:17.

Kirkendall, D. 2004. Creatine, carbs, and fluids: How important in soccer nutrition? *Sports Science Exchange* 17 (3):1–6.

Kjaer, M. 1998. Hepatic glucose production during exercise. *Advances in Experimental Medicine & Biology* 441:117–27.

Kovacs, M. 2006. Carbohydrate intake and tennis: Are there benefits? *British Journal of Sports Medicine* 40 (5):e13.

Kreider, R., et al. 2010. International Society of Sports Nutrition exercise and sport nutrition review: Research and recommendations. *Journal of the International Society of Sports Nutrition* 7:7.

Kreitzman, S., et al. 1992. Glycogen storage: Illusions of easy weight loss, excessive weight regain, and distortions in estimates of body composition. *American Journal of Clinical Nutrition* 56:292S–293S.

Levey, J. 2000. Runner's diarrhea. *AMAA Quarterly* 14 (1): 6–7.

Liebman, B. 2008. Fiber free-for-all: Not all fibers are equal. *Nutrition Action Health Letter* 35 (6):1–7.

Liebman, B. 1998. Sugar: The sweetening of the American diet. *Nutrition Action Health Letter* 25 (9):1–8.

Livesey, G., et al. 2008. Glycemic response and health: A systematic review and meta-analysis: Relations between dietary glycemic properties and health outcomes. *American Journal of Clinical Nutrition* 258S–68S.

Lupton, J., and Trumbo, P. 2006. Dietary fiber. In *Modern Nutrition in Health and Disease,* eds. M. Shils, et al. Philadelphia: Lippincott Williams & Wilkins.

Ma, Y., et al. 2005. Association between dietary carbohydrates and body weight. *American Journal of Epidemiology* 161:359–67.

Magnuson, B., et al. 2007. Aspartame: A safety evaluation based on current use levels, regulations, and toxicological and epidemiological studies. *Critical Reviews in Toxicology* 37:629–727.

Manore, M. 2002. Carbohydrate: Friend or foe? *ACSM's Health & Fitness Journal* 6 (5): 25–27.

Marlett, J., et al. 2002. Position of the American Dietetic Association: Health implications of dietary fiber. *Journal of the American Dietetic Association* 102:993–1010.

Maughan, R., et al. 1997. Diet composition and the performance of high-intensity exercise. *Journal of Sports Sciences* 15:265–75.

Mazzeo, R., and Fulco, C. 2006. Physiological systems and their responses to conditions of hypoxia. In *ACSM's Advanced Exercise Physiology,* ed. C. M. Tipton. Philadelphia: Lippincott Williams & Wilkins.

Mittendorfer, B., and Klein, S. 2001. Effect of aging on glucose and lipid metabolism during endurance exercise. *International Journal of Sport Nutrition & Exercise Metabolism* 11:S86–91.

National Institutes of Health. 2001. Diagnosis and management of dental caries throughout life. *NIH Consensus Statement* 18 (1): 1–23.

Nieman, D. 2007. Marathon training and immune function. *Sports Medicine* 37:412–15.

Nieman, D., and Bishop, N. 2006. Nutritional strategies to counter stress to the immune system in athletes, with special reference to football. *Journal of Sports Sciences* 24:763–72.

Peters, E. 2003. Nutritional aspects in ultra-endurance exercise. *Current Opinions in Clinical Nutrition & Metabolic Care* 6:427–34.

Pi-Sunyer, F. 2002. Glycemic index and disease. *American Journal of Clinical Nutrition* 76:290S–98S.

Rauch, H., et al. 2005. A signalling role for muscle glycogen in the regulation of pace during prolonged exercise. *British Journal of Sports Medicine* 39:34–38.

Richter, E., et al. 2001. Regulation of muscle glucose transport during exercise. *International Journal of Sport Nutrition & Exercise Metabolism* 11:S71–77.

Rock, C. 2007. Primary dietary prevention: Is the fiber story over? *Recent Results in Cancer Research* 173:171–77.

Roy, B. 2008. Milk: The new sports drink? A review. *Journal of the International Society of Sports Nutrition* 5:15.

Savaiano, D., et al. 2006. Lactose intolerance symptoms assessed by meta-analysis: A grain of truth that leads to exaggeration. *Journal of Nutrition* 136:1107–13.

Sawka, M., and Young, A. 2006. Physiological systems and their responses to conditions of heat and cold. In *ACSM's Advanced Exercise Physiology,* ed. C. M. Tipton. Philadelphia: Lippincott Williams & Wilkins.

Schneeman, B. 1999. Building scientific consensus: The importance of dietary fiber. *American Journal of Clinical Nutrition* 69:30–42.

Seal, C. 2006. Whole grains and CVD risk. *Proceedings of the Nutrition Society* 65:24–34.

Seymour, G., et al. 2007. Relationship between periodontal infections and systemic disease. *Clinical Microbiology & Infection* 13 (Supplement 4):3–10.

Short, S. 1993. Surveys of dietary intake and nutrition knowledge of athletes and their coaches. In *Nutrition in Exercise and Sport,* eds. I. Wolinsky and J. Hickson. Boca Raton, FL: CRC Press.

Shulman, R., and Rothman, D. 2001. The "glycogen shunt" in exercising muscle: A role of glycogen in muscle energetics and fatigue. *Proceedings of the National Academy of Sciences* 98:457–61.

Slavin, J., et al. 2001. The role of whole grains in disease prevention. *Journal of the American Dietetic Association* 101:780–85.

Snyder, A. 1998. Overtraining and glycogen depletion hypothesis. *Medicine & Science in Sports & Exercise* 30:1146–50.

Spriet, L. 2007. Regulation of substrate use during the marathon. *Sports Medicine* 37:332–36.

Stearns, R., et al. 2010. Effects of ingesting protein in combination with carbohydrate during exercise on endurance performance: A systematic review with meta-analysis. *Journal of Strength & Conditioning Research* 24 (8):2192–202.

Tarnopolsky, M. 2008. Sex differences in exercise metabolism and the role of 17-beta estradiol. *Medicine & Science in Sports & Exercise* 40:648–54.

Tarnopolsky, M. 2000. Gender differences in substrate metabolism during endurance exercise. *Canadian Journal of Applied Physiology* 25:312–27.

Tufts University. 2007. Five new reasons to get whole grains. *Health & Nutrition Letter* 25 (6):1–2.

Tsintzas, K., and Williams, C. 1998. Human muscle glycogen metabolism during exercise: Effect of carbohydrate supplementation. *Sports Medicine* 25:7–23.

Van Hall, G. 2000. Lactate as fuel for mitochondrial regeneration. *Acta Physiologica Scandinavica* 168:643–56.

Walberg-Rankin, J. 2000. Dietary carbohydrate and performance of brief, intense exercise. *Sports Science Exchange* 13 (4):1–4.

Williams, C. 2006. Nutrition to promote recovery from exercise. *Medicine & Science in Sports & Exercise* 19:1–6.

Williams, C. 1998. Diet and sports performance. In *Oxford Textbook of Sports Medicine.* eds. M. Harries, et al. Oxford: Oxford University Press.

Williams, C., and Lamb, D. 2008. Do high-carbohydrate diets improve exercise performance? *Sports Science Exchange* 21 (1):1–6.

Wolfe, R., and George, S. 1993. Stable isotopic tracers as metabolic probes in exercise. *Exercise & Sports Science Reviews* 21:1–31.

Zierler, K. 1999. Whole body glucose metabolism. *American Journal of Physiology* 276:E409–26.

Specific Studies

Achten, J., et al. 2004. Higher dietary carbohydrate content during intensified running training results in better maintenance of performance and mood state. *Journal of Applied Physiology* 96:1331–40.

Akermark, C., et al. 1996. Diet and muscle glycogen concentration in relation to physical performance in Swedish elite ice hockey players. *International Journal of Sport Nutrition* 6:272–84.

Appel, L., et al. 2005. Effects of protein, monounsaturated fat, and carbohydrate intake on blood pressure and serum lipids: Results of the OmniHeart randomized trial. *JAMA* 294:2455–64.

Arkinstall, M., et al. 2001. Effect of carbohydrate ingestion on metabolism during running and cycling. *Journal of Applied Physiology* 91:2125–34.

Azevedo, J., et al. 2007. Lactate, fructose and glucose oxidation profiles in sports drinks and the effect on exercise performance. *PLoS ONE* 26;2(9):e927.

Ball, T., et al. 1995. Periodic carbohydrate replacement during 50 min of high intensity cycling improves subsequent sprint performance. *International Journal of Sport Nutrition* 5:151–58.

Balsom, P., et al. 1999. High-intensity exercise and muscle glycogen availability in humans. *Acta Physiologica Scandinavica* 165:337–45.

Baty, J. 2007. The effect of a carbohydrate and protein supplement on resistance exercise performance, hormonal response, and muscle damage. *Journal of Strength & Conditioning Research* 21 (2): 321–29.

Berardi, J., and Ziegenfuss, T. 2003. Effects of ribose supplementation on repeated sprint performance in men. *Journal of Strength Conditioning Research* 17:47–52.

Berardi, J., et al. 2008. Recovery from a cycling time trial is enhanced with carbohydrate-protein supplementation vs. isoenergetic carbohydrate supplementation. *Journal of the International Society of Sports Nutrition* 5:24.

Betts, J., et al. 2005. Recovery of endurance running capacity: Effect of carbohydrate-protein mixture. *International Journal of Sport Nutrition* 590–609.

Blair, S., et al. 1980. Blood lipid and ECG response to carbohydrate loading. *Physician & Sports Medicine* 8:69–75.

Bosch, A., et al. 1994. Influence of carbohydrate ingestion on fuel substrate turnover and oxidation during prolonged exercise. *Journal of Applied Physiology* 76:2364–72.

Brouns, F., et al. 1995. Chronic oral lactate supplementation does not affect lactate disappearance from blood after exercise. *International Journal of Sport Nutrition* 5:117–24.

Brown, A., et al. 2004. Tricarboxylic-acid-cycle intermediates and cycle endurance capacity. *International Journal of Sport Nutrition & Exercise Metabolism* 14:720–29.

Bryner, R., et al. 1998. Effect of lactate consumption on exercise performance. *Journal of Sports Medicine & Physical Fitness* 38:116–23.

Burke, L., et al. 2005. Effect of carbohydrate intake on half-marathon performance of well-trained runners. *International Journal of Sport Nutrition & Exercise Metabolism* 5:573–89.

Burke, L., et al. 2000. Carbohydrate loading failed to improve 100-km cycling performance in a placebo-controlled trial. *Journal of Applied Physiology* 88:1284–90.

Campbell, C., et al. 2008. Carbohydrate-supplement form and exercise performance. *International Journal of Sport Nutrition & Exercise Metabolism* 18:179–90.

Carter, J., et al. 2004. The effect of carbohydrate mouth rinse on 1-h cycle time trial performance. *Medicine & Science in Sports & Exercise* 36:2107–11.

Carter, J., et al. 2004. The effect of glucose infusion on glucose kinetics during a 1-h time trial. *Medicine & Science in Sports & Exercise* 36:1543–50.

Chen, Y., et al. 2008. Effect of preexercise meals with different glycemic indices and loads on metabolic responses and endurance running. *International Journal of Sport Nutrition & Exercise Metabolism* 18:281–300.

Chryssanthopoulos, C., et al. 2002. Influence of a carbohydrate-electrolyte solution ingested during running on muscle glycogen utilization in fed humans. *International Journal of Sports Medicine* 23:279–84.

Chryssanthopoulos, C., et al. 2002. The effect of a high carbohydrate meal on endurance running capacity. *International Journal of Sport Nutrition & Exercise Metabolism* 12:157–71.

Currell, K., and Jeukendrup, A. 2008. Superior endurance performance with ingestion of multiple transportable carbohydrates. *Medicine & Science in Sports & Exercise* 40:275–81.

Desbrow, B., et al. 2004. Carbohydrate-electrolyte feedings and 1 h time trial cycling performance. *International Journal of Sport Nutrition & Exercise Metabolism* 14:541–49.

Di Stefano, M., et al. 2002. Lactose malabsorption and intolerance and peak bone mass. *Gastroenterology* 122:1793–99.

Djoussé, L., and Gaziano, J. 2007. Breakfast cereals and risk of heart failure in the physicians' health study I. *Archives of Internal Medicine* 167:2080–85.

Dunne, L., et al. 2006. Ribose versus dextrose supplementation, association with rowing performance: A double-blind study. *Clinical Journal of Sport Medicine* 16:68–71.

Earnest, C., et al. 2004. Low vs. high glycemic index carbohydrate gel ingestion during simulated 64-km cycling time trial performance. *Journal of Strength Conditioning Research* 18:466–72.

el-Sayed, M., et al. 1997. Carbohydrate ingestion improves performance during a 1 h simulated cycling trial. *Journal of Sports Sciences* 15:223–30.

Erith, S., et al. 2006. The effect of high carbohydrate meals with different glycemic indices on recovery of performance during prolonged intermittent high-intensity shuttle running. *International Journal of Sport Nutrition & Exercise Metabolism* 16:393–404.

Fahey, T., et al. 1991. The effects of ingesting polylactate or glucose polymer drinks during prolonged exercise. *International Journal of Sport Nutrition* 1:249–56.

Fairchild, T., et al. 2002. Rapid carbohydrate loading after a short bout of near maximal-intensity exercise. *Medicine & Science in Sports & Exercise* 34:980–86.

Febbraio, M., and Stewart, K. 1996. CHO feeding before prolonged exercise: Effect of glycemic index on muscle glycogenolysis and exercise performance. *Journal of Applied Physiology* 81:1115–20.

Febbraio, M., et al. 2000. Effects of carbohydrate ingestion before and during exercise on glucose kinetics and performance. *Journal of Applied Physiology* 89:2220–26.

Febbraio, M., et al. 2000. Pre-exercise carbohydrate ingestion, glucose kinetics, and muscle glycogen use: Effect of the glycemic index. *Journal of Applied Physiology* 89:1845–51.

Ferguson-Stegall, L., et al. 2010. The effect of a low carbohydrate beverage with added protein on cycling endurance performance in trained athletes. *Journal of Strength & Conditioning Research* 24 (10): 2577–86.

Fogelholm, M., et al. 1991. Carbohydrate loading in practice: High muscle glycogen concentration is not certain. *British Journal of Sports Medicine* 25:41–44.

Frøsig, C., et al. 2007. Effects of endurance exercise training on insulin signaling in human skeletal muscle: Interactions at the level of phosphatidylinositol 3-kinase, Akt, and AS160. *Diabetes* 56:2093–102.

Fung, T., et al. 2009. Sweetened beverage consumption and risk of coronary heart disease in women. *American Journal of Clinical Nutrition* 89:1037–42.

Gilson, S., et al. 2010. Effects of chocolate milk consumption on markers of muscle recovery following soccer training: A randomized cross-over study. *Journal of the International Society of Sports Nutrition* 7:19.

Hargreaves, M., et al. 1995. Influence of muscle glycogen on glycogenolysis and glucose uptake during exercise in humans. *Journal of Applied Physiology* 78:288–92.

Hatfield, D., et al. 2006. The effects of carbohydrate loading on repetitive jump squat power performance. *Journal of Strength Conditioning & Research* 20:167–71.

Hellsten, Y., et al. 2004. Effect of ribose supplementation on resynthesis of adenine nucleotides after intense intermittent training in humans. *American Journal of Physiology. Regulatory, Integrative, & Comparative Physiology* 286:R182–88.

Jalal, D., et al. Increased fructose associates with elevated blood pressure. *Journal of the American Society of Nephrology* 21:1543–49.

James, A., et al. 2001. Muscle glycogen supercompensation: Absence of a gender-related difference. *European Journal of Applied Physiology* 85:533–58.

Jentjens, R., et al. 2006. Exogenous carbohydrate oxidation rates are elevated after combined ingestion of glucose and fructose during exercise in the heat. *Journal of Applied Physiology* 100:807–16.

Jeukendrup, A., et al. 2006. Exogenous carbohydrate oxidation during ultraendurance exercise. *Journal of Applied Physiology* 100:1134–41.

Jeukendrup, A., et al. 1997. Carbohydrate-electrolyte feedings improve 1-h time trial cycling performance. *International Journal of Sports Medicine* 18:125–29.

Kalman, D., et al. 1999. The effects of pyruvate supplementation on body composition in overweight individuals. *Nutrition* 15:337–40.

Kang, J., et al. 1995. Effect of carbohydrate ingestion subsequent to carbohydrate supercompensation on endurance performance. *International Journal of Sport Nutrition* 5:329–43.

Karp, J., et al. 2006. Chocolate milk as a post-exercise recovery aid. *International Journal of Sport Nutrition & Exercise Metabolism* 16:78–91.

Kavouras, S., et al. 2004. The influence of low versus high carbohydrate diet on a 45-min strenuous cycling exercise. *International Journal of Sport Nutrition & Exercise Metabolism* 14:62–72.

Kerksick, C., et al. 2005. Effects of ribose supplementation prior to and during intense exercise on anaerobic capacity and metabolic markers. *International Journal of Sport Nutrition & Exercise Metabolism* 15:653–64.

Kimber, N., et al. 2002. Energy balance during an Ironman triathlon in male and female triathletes. *International Journal of Sport Nutrition & Exercise Metabolism* 12:47–62.

Koh-Banerjee, P., et al. 2005. Effects of calcium pyruvate supplementation during training on body composition, exercise capacity, and metabolic responses to exercise. *Nutrition* 21:312–19.

Krustrup, P., et al. 2006. Muscle and blood metabolites during a soccer game: Implications for sprint performance. *Medicine & Science in Sports & Exercise* 38:1165–74.

Krustrup, P., et al. 2004. Slow-twitch fiber glycogen depletion elevates moderate-exercise fast-twitch fiber activity and O_2 uptake. *Medicine & Science in Sports & Exercise* 36:973–82.

Kuipers, H., et al. 1999. Pre-exercise ingestion of carbohydrate and transient hypoglycemia during exercise. *International Journal of Sports Medicine* 20:227–31.

Kulik, J., et al. 2008. Supplemental carbohydrate ingestion does not improve performance of high-intensity resistance exercise. *Journal of Strength and Conditioning Research* 22:1101–7.

Larsson, S., et al. 2006. Consumption of sugar and sugar-sweetened foods and the risk of pancreatic cancer in a prospective study. *American Journal of Clinical Nutrition* 184:1171–76.

Lim, U., et al. 2006. Consumption of aspartame-containing beverages and incidence of hematopoietic and brain malignancies. *Cancer Epidemiology, Biomarkers & Prevention* 15:1654–59.

Marjerrison, A., et al. 2007. Preexercise carbohydrate consumption and repeated anaerobic performance in pre- and early-pubertal boys. *International Journal of Sport Nutrition & Exercise Metabolism* 17:140–51.

Mathew, T., et al. 2002. Relationship between sports drinks and dental erosion in 304 university athletes. *Caries Research* 36:281–87.

McCleave, E., et al. 2011. A low carbohydrate-protein supplement improves endurance performance in female athletes. *Journal of Strength & Conditioning Research* 25 (4):879–88.

McInerney, P., et al. 2005. Failure to repeatedly supercompensate muscle glycogen stores in highly trained men. *Medicine & Science in Sports & Exercise* 37:404–11.

McLay, R., et al. 2007. Carbohydrate loading and female endurance athletes: Effect of menstrual-cycle phase. *International Journal of Sport Nutrition & Exercise Metabolism* 17:189–205.

Morrison, M., et al. 2000. Pyruvate ingestion for 7 days does not improve aerobic performance in well-trained individuals. *Journal of Applied Physiology* 89:549–56.

Murray, R., et al. 1989. The effects of glucose, fructose, and sucrose ingestion during exercise. *Medicine & Science in Sports & Exercise* 21:275–82.

Op 'T Eijnde, B., et al. 2001. No effects of oral ribose supplementation on repeated maximal exercise and de novo ATP resynthesis. *Journal of Applied Physiology* 91:2275–81.

Ostojic, S., and Ahmetovic, Z. 2009. The effect of 4 weeks treatment with a 2-gram daily dose of pyruvate on body composition in healthy trained men. *International Journal for Vitamin & Nutrition Research* 79 (3):173–79.

Palmer, G., et al. 1998. Carbohydrate ingestion immediately before exercise does not improve 20 km time trial performance in well trained cyclists. *International Journal of Sports Medicine* 19:415–18.

Paul, D., et al. 2001. Carbohydrate during the follicular phase of the menstrual cycle: Effects on muscle glycogen and exercise performance. *International Journal of Sport Nutrition & Exercise Metabolism* 11:430–31.

Peters, H., et al. 1995. Exercise performance as a function of semi-solid and liquid carbohydrate feedings during prolonged exercise. *International Journal of Sports Medicine* 16:105–13.

Peveler, W., et al. 2006. Effects of ribose as an ergogenic aid. *Journal of Strength & Conditioning Research* 20:519–22.

Pfeiffer, B., et al. 2010. CHO oxidation from a CHO gel compared with a drink during exercise. *Medicine & Science in Sports & Exercise* 42 (11):2038–45.

Pizza, F., et al. 1995. A carbohydrate loading regimen improves high intensity, short duration exercise performance. *International Journal of Sport Nutrition* 5:110–16.

Pliml, W., et al. 1992. Effects of ribose on exercise-induced ischaemia in stable coronary artery disease. *Lancet* 340:507–10.

Pritchett, K., et al. 2009. Acute effects of chocolate milk and a commercial recovery beverage on postexercise recovery indices and endurance cycling performance. *Applied Physiology, Nutrition, & Metabolism* 34:1017–22.

Rico-Sanz, J., et al. 1999. Muscle glycogen degradation during simulation of a fatiguing soccer match in elite soccer players examined noninvasively by 13C-MRS. *Medicine & Science in Sports & Exercise* 31:1587–93.

Romano-Ely, B., et al. 2006. Effect of an isocaloric carbohydrate-protein-antioxidant drink on cycling performance. *Medicine & Science in Sports & Exercise* 38:1608–16.

Saris, W. 1989. Study of food intake and energy expenditure during extreme sustained exercise: The Tour de France. *International Journal of Sports Medicine* 10:S26–S31.

Seifert, J., et al. 1994. Glycemic and insulinemic response to preexercise carbohydrate feedings. *International Journal of Sport Nutrition* 4:46–53.

Smith, G., et al. 2002. The effect of pre-exercise glucose ingestion on performance during prolonged swimming. *International Journal of Sport Nutrition & Exercise Metabolism* 12:136–44.

Stanko, R., et al. 1990. Enhanced leg exercise endurance with a high-carbohydrate diet and dihydroxyacetone and pyruvate. *Journal of Applied Physiology* 69:1651–56.

Stanko, R., et al. 1990. Enhancement of arm exercise endurance capacity with dihydroxyacetone and pyruvate. *Journal of Applied Physiology* 68:119–24.

Stattin, P., et al. 2007. Prospective study of hyperglycemia and cancer risk. *Diabetes Care* 30:561–67.

Stevenson, E., et al. 2006. Influence of high-carbohydrate mixed meals with different glycemic indexes on substrate utilization during subsequent exercise in women. *American Journal of Clinical Nutrition* 84:354–60.

Stevenson, E., et al. 2005. Improved recovery from prolonged exercise following the consumption of low glycemic index carbohydrate meals. *International Journal of Sport Nutrition & Exercise Metabolism* 15:350–65.

Tarnopolsky, M., et al. 2001. Gender differences in carbohydrate loading are related to energy intake. *Journal of Applied Physiology* 91:225–30.

Thomas, K., et al. 2009. Improved endurance capacity following chocolate milk consumption compared with 2 commercially available sport drinks. *Applied Physiology, Nutrition, & Metabolism* 34:78–82.

Tsintzas, K., et al. 2001. Phosphocreatine degradation in type I and type II muscle fibers during submaximal exercise in man: Effect of carbohydrate ingestion. *Journal of Physiology* 537:305–11.

Utter, A., et al. 2007. Carbohydrate attenuates perceived exertion during intermittent exercise and recovery. *Medicine & Science in Sports & Exercise* 39:880–85.

Utter, A., et al. 2005. Carbohydrate supplementation and perceived exertion during resistance training. *Journal of Strength & Conditioning Research* 19:939–43.

Utter, A., et al. 2004. Carbohydrate supplementation and perceived exertion during prolonged running. *Medicine & Science in Sports & Exercise* 36:1036–41.

Utter, A., et al. 2002. Effect of carbohydrate ingestion on ratings of perceived exertion during a marathon. *Medicine & Science in Sports & Exercise* 34:1779–84.

Vandenberghe, K., et al. 1995. No effect of glycogen level on glycogen metabolism during high intensity exercise. *Medicine & Science in Sports & Exercise* 27:1278–83.

van Loon, L., et al. 2001. The effects of increasing exercise intensity on muscle fuel utilisation in humans. *Journal of Physiology* 536:295–304.

Venables, M., et al. 2005. Erosive effect of a new sports drink on dental enamel during exercise. *Medicine & Science in Sports & Exercise* 37:39–44.

von Fraunhofer, J., and Rogers, M. 2005. Effects of sports drinks and other beverages on dental enamel. *General Dentistry* 53:28–31.

Walker, J., et al. 2000. Dietary carbohydrate, muscle glycogen content, and endurance performance in well-trained women. *Journal of Applied Physiology* 88:2151–58.

Wallis, G., et al. 2007. Dose-response effects of ingested carbohydrate on exercise metabolism in women. *Medicine & Science in Sports & Exercise* 39:131–38.

Welsh, R., et al. 2002. Carbohydrates and physical/mental performance during intermittent exercise to fatigue. *Medicine & Science in Sports & Exercise* 34:723–31.

Weltan, S., et al. 1998. Influence of muscle glycogen content on metabolic regulation. *American Journal of Physiology* 274: E72–E82.

Weltan, S., et al. 1998. Preexercise muscle glycogen content affects metabolism during exercise despite maintenance of hyperglycemia. *American Journal of Physiology* 274:E83–E88.

Williams, C., et al. 1992. The effect of a high carbohydrate diet on running performance during a 30-km treadmill time trial. *European Journal of Applied Physiology* 65:18–24.

Winnick, J., et al. 2005. Carbohydrate feedings during team sport exercise preserve physical and CNS function. *Medicine & Science in Sports & Exercise* 37:306–15.

Wong, J., et al. 2006. Colonic health: Fermentation and short chain fatty acids. *Journal of Clinical Gastroenterology* 40:235–43.

Wong, S., et al. 2009. Effect of preexercise glycemic-index meal on running when CHO-electrolyte solution is consumed during exercise. *International Journal of Sport Nutrition & Exercise Metabolism* 19 (3):222–42.

Wu, C., and Williams, C. 2006. A low glycemic index meal before exercise improves endurance running capacity in men. *International Journal of Sport Nutrition & Exercise Metabolism* 16:510–27.

Yaspelkis, B., et al. 1993. Carbohydrate supplementation spares muscle glycogen during variable-intensity exercise. *Journal of Applied Physiology* 75:1477–85.

Fat: An Important Energy Source During Exercise

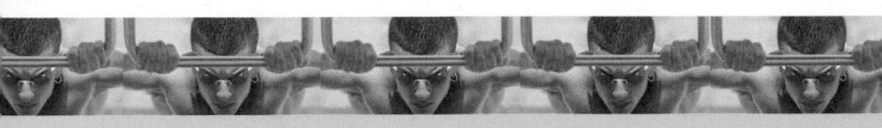

CHAPTER FIVE

LEARNING OBJECTIVES

After studying this chapter, you should be able to:

1. List the different types of dietary fatty acids and identify general types of foods in which they are found.

2. Calculate the approximate amount, in grams or milligrams, of total fat, saturated fat, and cholesterol that should be included in your daily diet.

3. Describe how dietary fat is absorbed, how it is distributed in the body, and what its major functions are in human metabolism.

4. Explain the role of fat in human energy systems during exercise and how endurance exercise training affects exercise fat metabolism.

5. Explain the theory underlying the role of increased fat oxidation to enhance prolonged aerobic endurance performance.

6. List the various dietary fat strategies and dietary supplements that have been investigated as a means of enhancing exercise performance, and highlight the major findings.

7. Describe the proposed process underlying the development of atherosclerosis and cardiovascular disease, including the role that dietary fat and cholesterol may play in its etiology.

8. List and describe at least eight of the ten dietary strategies that are proposed to help treat or prevent the development of atherosclerosis and cardiovascular disease.

9. Explain the role of exercise as a means of helping prevent the development of atherosclerosis and cardiovascular disease.

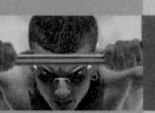

From a health standpoint, dietary fat is the nutrient of greatest concern to the American Heart Association because excessive consumption of certain types of fat has been associated with the development of coronary heart disease. Excessive consumption of dietary fat may also contribute to the development of obesity, a risk factor for several other chronic diseases, such as diabetes. Thus, one of the major recommendations advocated in Healthy People 2020 *for a healthier diet is to reduce the amount of dietary fat intake to a reasonable level. Part of the rationale for this recommendation and some general guidelines for implementing it are presented in this chapter, but additional information may also be found in chapters 2 and 11.*

We need some fat in our diet. Despite its potential health hazards when consumed in excess, dietary fat contains several essential nutrients that serve a variety of important functions in human nutrition. The National Academy of Sciences has set an Acceptable Macronutrient Distribution Range (AMDR) for total fat of 20–35 percent of daily energy intake. Because some types of fat may confer various health benefits, the Academy also set Adequate Intakes (AI) for several fatty acids. Moreover, in its position statement regarding nutrition and athletic performance, the American Dietetic Association, Dietitians of Canada, and the American College of Sports Medicine noted that, overall, diets should provide moderate amounts of energy from fat (20 to 35 percent of energy) and that there is no health or performance benefit to consuming a diet containing less than 20 percent energy from fat. For the endurance athlete, one of the most important functions of fat is to provide energy during exercise, and researchers have explored a variety of techniques in attempts to improve endurance performance by increasing the ability of the muscle to use fat as a fuel.

To clarify the role of dietary fat in health and its possible relevance to sports, this chapter presents information on the basic nature of dietary fats and associated lipids, the metabolic fate and physiological functions of fats and cholesterol in the body, the role of fat as an energy source during exercise, the use of various dietary practices or ergogenic aids in attempts to improve fat metabolism and endurance performance, and possible health problems associated with excessive dietary fat.

Dietary Fats

What are the different types of dietary fats?

What we commonly call fat in our diet actually consists of several substances classified as lipids. **Lipids** represent a class of organic substances that are insoluble in water but soluble in certain solvents like alcohol or ether. The three major dietary lipids of importance to humans are triglycerides, cholesterol, and phospholipids. All three have major functions in the body.

What are triglycerides?

The **triglycerides,** also known as the true fats or the neutral fats, are the principal form in which fats are eaten and stored in the human body. Triglycerides are composed of two different compounds—fatty acids and glycerol. When an acid (fatty acid) and an alcohol (glycerol) combine, an **ester** is formed, the process being known as *esterification.* (Three fatty acids are attached to each glycerol molecule.) Figure 5.1 is a diagram of a triglyceride.

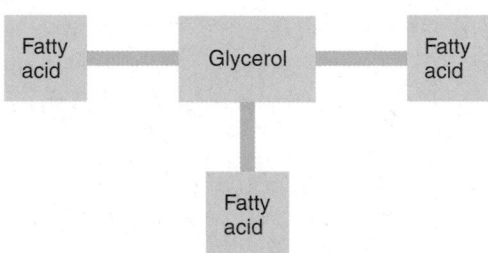

FIGURE 5.1 Structure of a triglyceride. Three fatty acids combine with glycerol to form a triglyceride.

Another term used for triglyceride is *triacylglycerol.* Some triglycerides may be modified commercially to contain only two fatty acids, known as diglycerides, or diacylglycerols.

Fatty acids, one of the components of fat, are chains of carbon, oxygen, and hydrogen atoms that vary in length and in the degree of saturation of carbon with hydrogen. Short-chain fatty acids (SCFAs) contain fewer than 6 carbons, medium-chain fatty acids (MCFAs) have 6 to 12 carbons, and long-chain fatty acids (LCFAs) have 14 or more carbons.

Fatty acids may be saturated or unsaturated. A **saturated fatty acid** contains a full quota of hydrogenated ions so that all of its carbon bonds are full; saturated fats such as butter are solid at room temperature. Carbon molecules in unsaturated fatty acids may incorporate more hydrogen because they have some unfilled bonds, or double bonds. These unsaturated fatty acids may be classified as **monounsaturated,** having a single double bond and capable of incorporating two hydrogen ions, and **polyunsaturated,** having two or more double bonds and capable of incorporating four or more hydrogen ions; monounsaturated and polyunsaturated fats as oils are liquid at room temperature.

Polyunsaturated fatty acids are further identified according to the location of the first carbon double bond from the last, or omega, carbon. **Omega-3** and **omega-6 fatty acids** are the two major types, and the numeric represents the location of the first double bond. Other terminology to identify these two fatty acids are ω-3 and n-3, and ω-6 and n-6. Adequate amounts of omega-3 and omega-6 fatty acids may confer health benefits, as noted later in the chapter. At room temperature, saturated fats are usually solid, while unsaturated fats are usually liquid. **Partially hydrogenated fats** or oils have been treated by a process that adds hydrogen to some of the unfilled bonds, thereby hardening the fat or oil. In essence, the fat becomes more saturated. During the hydrogenation process, the normal position of hydrogen ions at the double bond is on the "same side" (*cis*). This is known as a *cis* **fatty acid,** but if partially hydrogenated so that hydrogen ions are on opposite sides of the double bond, it results in a *trans* **fatty acid.** Figure 5.2 represents the structural difference between a saturated, a monounsaturated, a polyunsaturated (*cis* and *trans*), and an omega-3 polyunsaturated fatty acid. The health implications of these different types of fats are discussed later in this chapter. In general though, excess intake of saturated and *trans* fatty acids is associated with increased health risks, whereas adequate intake of monounsaturated, polyunsaturated, and omega-3 fatty acids may be associated with neutral or some beneficial health effects. Bell and others noted that food technology is evolving to create structured triglycerides that may possess health benefits.

Glycerol is an alcohol, a clear, colorless syrupy liquid. It is obtained in the diet as part of triglycerides, but it also may be produced in the body as a by-product of carbohydrate metabolism. On the other hand, glycerol can be converted back to carbohydrate in the process of gluconeogenesis in the liver.

What are some common foods high in fat content?

The fat content in foods can vary from 100 percent, as found in most cooking oils, to minor trace amounts, less than 5–10 percent, as found in most fruits and vegetables. Some foods obviously have a high-fat content: butter, oils, shortening, mayonnaise, margarine, and the visible fat on meat. However, in other foods the fat content may be high but not as obvious. This is known as **hidden fat.** Whole milk, cheese, nuts, desserts, crackers, potato chips, and a wide variety of commercially prepared foods may contain considerable amounts of hidden fat. For example, a

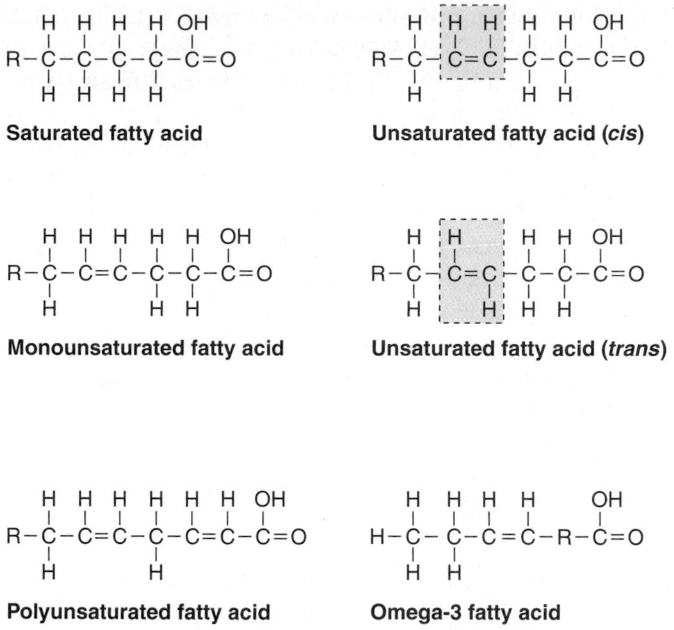

FIGURE 5.2 Structural differences between saturated, monounsaturated, and polyunsaturated fatty acids (including the *cis* and *trans* forms) and the omega-3 fatty acid. Note there is a single double bond between carbon atoms in the monounsaturated fatty acid and two or more in the polyunsaturated fatty acid. In the omega-3 fatty acid, the double bond is located three carbons from the last, or omega, carbon. The R represents the radical, or the presence of many more C–H bonds. In the *trans* configuration, one of the hydrogen ions is moved to the opposite side.

5-ounce baked potato contains 145 Calories with about 3 percent fat, while a 5-ounce serving of potato chips contains 795 Calories, more than 60 percent of them from fat.

In general, animal foods found in the meat and milk groups are high in fat, particularly saturated fat. Hamburger meat contributes the most saturated fat to the typical American diet. However, careful selection and preparation of foods in these groups will considerably reduce fat content. The percentage of fat in meat and milk products may vary considerably; beef, pork, and cheese products usually contain considerable amounts of fat, up to 70 percent or more fat Calories. The meat and dairy industries are responding to dietary modifications by many Americans and are making low-fat red meats and low-fat cheeses available to consumers. For example, 3 ounces of beef eye of round or pork tenderloin contain about 140 Calories, 4 grams of total fat, and 1.5 grams of saturated fat; both cuts of meat contain fewer than 30 percent of their Calories as fat. Lean cuts of poultry and fish have much lower levels of fat. Trimming the fat from meats or removing the skin from poultry drastically reduces the fat content. Some fish, such as flounder and tuna, are remarkably low in fat, whereas others, such as salmon and mackerel, are higher in total fat content but contain greater amounts of omega-3 fatty acids. Look for foods in the very lean meat exchange list in appendix E. In the milk group, whole milk contains about 8 grams of fat per cup; skim milk contains about 0.5–1.0 grams, which is much less than whole milk. Low-fat cheese alternatives containing soy or rice are available.

Small amounts of *trans* fatty acids are found naturally in beef, butter, and milk, but deep-fried foods and commercially prepared products, particularly stick margarine and snack foods such as chips, cakes, and cookies, may contain substantial amounts. The health risks associated with *trans* fatty acids are discussed later in this chapter.

Most plant foods, such as vegetables, fruits, beans, and natural whole-grain products, generally are low in fat content, and the fat they do contain is mostly unsaturated. On the other hand, some plant foods, such as nuts, seeds, and avocados, are very high in fat, but again primarily unsaturated fats. However, coconuts and palm kernels are extremely high in both total and saturated fats.

All fats contain a mixture of saturated, monounsaturated, and polyunsaturated fatty acids. Later in this chapter we discuss some health implications relating to the types of fats we eat; figure 5.3 presents an approximate percentage of the amount of saturated, monounsaturated, and polyunsaturated fatty acids found in some common oils and fats. Several high-content sources for each of the various types of fatty acids are noted.

How do I calculate the percentage of fat Calories in a food?

It is important to realize that a product advertised as 95 percent fat free (or only 5 percent fat) may contain a considerably higher percentage of its Calories as fat: The advertised percentage refers to the *weight of the product, not its caloric content*. The product may contain a considerable amount of water, which contains no Calories. Thus, luncheon meat advertised as 95 percent fat free may actually contain more than 40 percent of its Calories from fat depending on the water weight. Foods with a high water content contain even higher percentages of fat Calories. A striking example is whole milk, which is only 3.5 percent fat by weight; however, one glass of milk contains about 150 Calories and 8 grams of fat, which accounts for 48 percent of the caloric content ($8 \times 9 = 72; 72/150 = 48$). Even low-fat milk (2 percent fat) contains about 37 percent fat Calories.

If you want to calculate the percentage of fat calories in most foods you eat, you can get the information you need from the food label, which will include the total Calories and the Calories from

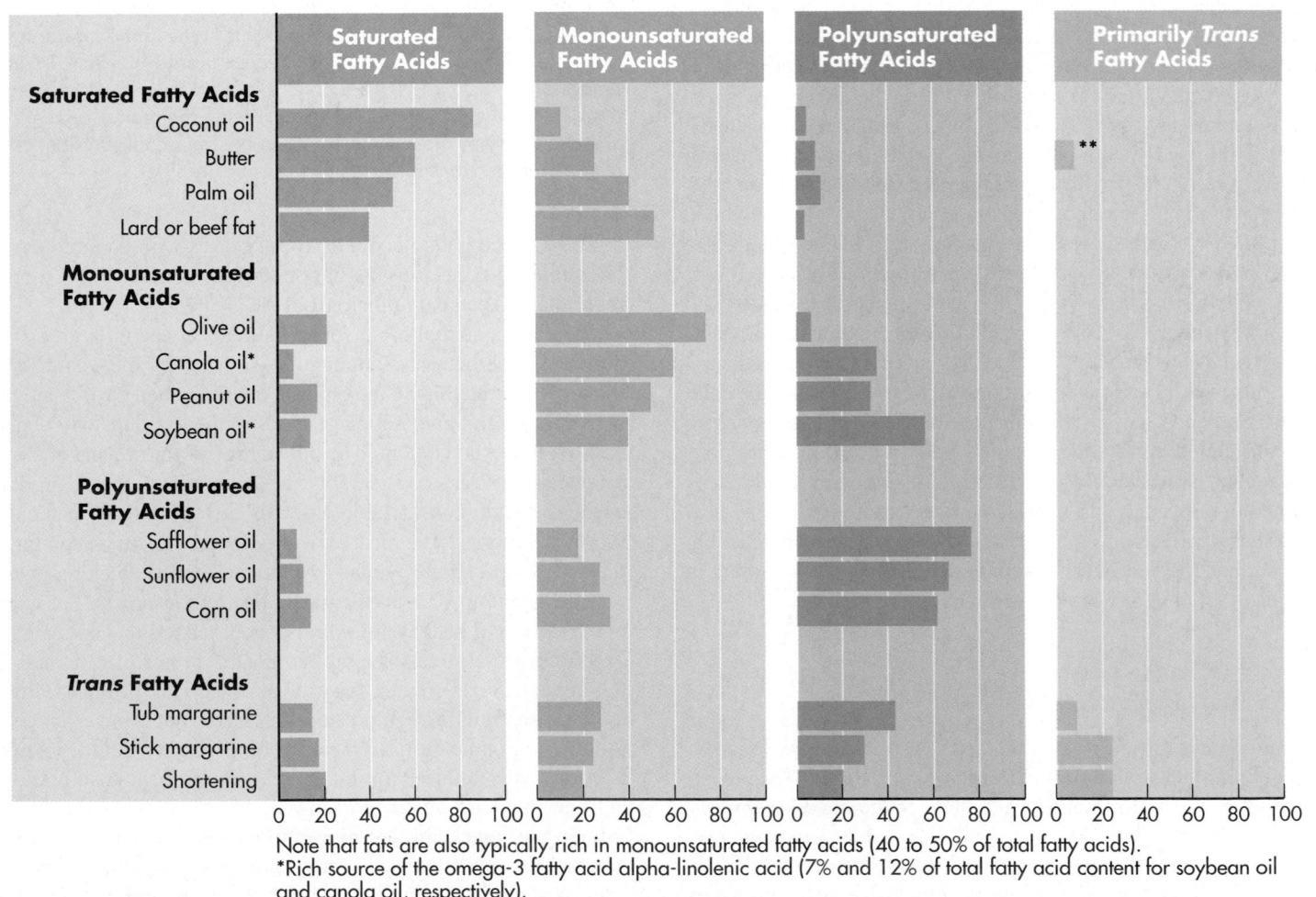

Note that fats are also typically rich in monounsaturated fatty acids (40 to 50% of total fatty acids).
*Rich source of the omega-3 fatty acid alpha-linolenic acid (7% and 12% of total fatty acid content for soybean oil and canola oil, respectively).
**Natural *trans* fatty acids in butter are not harmful.

FIGURE 5.3 Saturated, monounsaturated, polyunsaturated, and *trans* fatty acid composition of common fats and oils (expressed as % of all fatty acids in the product.

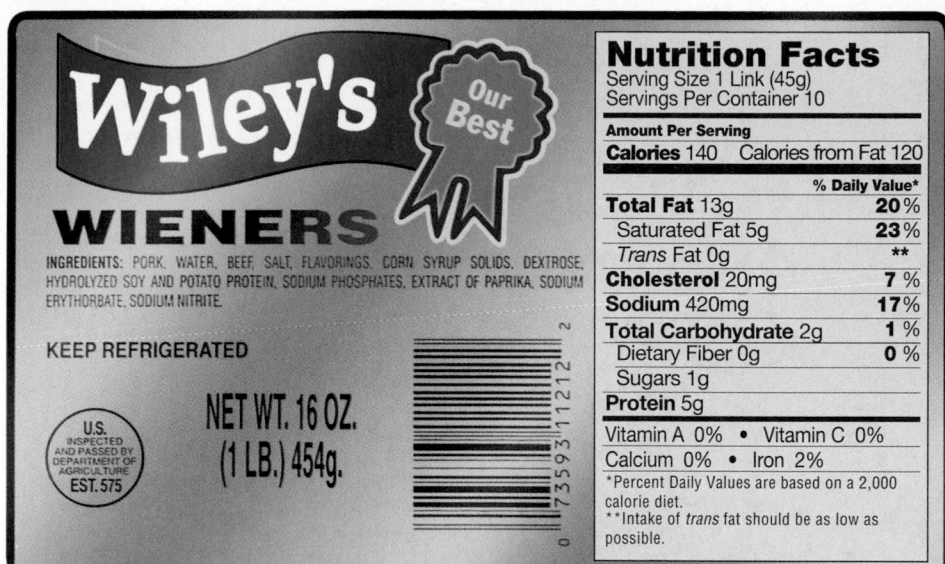

FIGURE 5.4 Reading labels helps locate hidden fat. Who would think that wieners (hot dogs) can contain about 85 percent of energy content as fat? Looking at the hot dog itself does not suggest that almost all its energy content comes from fat, but the label shows otherwise. Do the math: 120/140 Calories = 0.85 or 85 percent.

fat; additional mandatory information is the total fat, saturated fat, and *trans* fatty acid content. The label optionally may list the Calories from saturated fat and the amounts of polyunsaturated and monounsaturated fat. Figure 5.4 presents a food label to help illustrate the hidden fat in a hot dog (wiener). If you do not have a food label, then you will need to know the Calories and grams of fat for the food. Both of these values can be obtained from a food composition table found in most basic nutrition texts or online. Table 5.1 presents the methods for calculating the percent of fat Calories and percent of saturated fat Calories from either a food label or food composition table. Table 5.2 represents the percentage of food energy that is derived from fat in some common foods; the percentages are indicated for both total fat and saturated fat. Additional information is presented in chapter 11, where the focus is on reducing high-fat foods in the diet as a means to Calorie control.

www.ars.usda.gov/ba/bhnrc/ndl   To obtain the total Calories and grams of fat for a given food, click on search and enter the name of the food. The amounts of all types of fats and cholesterol, as well as numerous other nutrients, are also provided.

What are fat substitutes?

Fat substitutes, or fat replacers, are supposedly designed to provide the taste and texture of fats, but without the Calories (9 Calories per gram), saturated fat, or cholesterol. They are found in many normally high-fat products, such as ice cream, that are marketed as fat free. Fat substitutes may be manufactured from carbohydrate, protein, or fats. Although a number of fat substitutes are under development, the following are commonly used.

Some carbohydrates, such as starches and gums, provide thickness and structure and are useful as fat substitutes. Guar gum, gum arabic, and cellulose gel are examples. Oatrim, made from oats, is being used to replace fat in milk. Depending on the form used, the caloric content may range from 0–4 Calories

TABLE 5.1 Calculation of the percentage of Calories in foods that are derived from fat

Method A. Data from food label

Amount per serving

Calories = 90
Calories from fat = 30
To calculate percentage of food Calories that consists of fat, simply divide the Calories from fat by the Calories per serving and multiply by 100 to express as a percent.
     30/90 = 0.33   0.33 × 100 = 33 percent fat Calories

Method B. Data from food composition table

Amount per serving

Calories = 90
Total fat, grams = 8
Saturated fat, grams = 3
To calculate percentage of food Calories that consists of total fat or saturated fat, use the caloric value for fat of 1 gram = 9 Calories.
Total fat = 8 grams
Total fat Calories = 8 grams × 9 Calories/gram = 72 Calories
Use the same procedure as in Method A.
     72/90 = 0.80   0.80 × 100 = 80 percent fat Calories
Saturated fat = 3 grams
Saturated fat Calories = 3 grams × 9 Calories/gram = 27 Calories
     27/90 = 0.30   0.30 × 100 = 30 percent saturated fat Calories

per gram. Simplesse is manufactured from milk or egg protein by a microparticulation process so that it has the taste and texture of fat. The caloric value of Simplesse is only 1.3 Calories per gram. The use of Simplesse has been approved by the FDA. Salatrim, which is an acronym for short- and long-chain fatty acid triglyceride molecule, is a modified fat containing only

TABLE 5.2 Percentage of total fat Calories and saturated fat Calories in some common foods*

Food	% Calories total fat	% Calories saturated fat	Food	% Calories total fat	% Calories saturated fat
Meat group			*Vegetables*		
Bacon	80	30	Asparagus	8	2
Beef, lean and fat (untrimmed)	70	32	Beans, green	7	1.5
			Broccoli	12	1.5
Beef, lean only (trimmed)	35	15	Carrots	4	< 1
			Potatoes	1	< 1
Hamburger, regular	62	29	*Fruits*		
Chicken, breast (with skin)	35	11			
Chicken, breast (without skin)	19	5	Apples	5	< 1
			Bananas	5	2
Luncheon meat (bologna)	82	35	Oranges	4	< 1
Salmon	37	7	*Starches/Breads/Cereals*		
Flounder, tuna	8	2			
Egg, white and yolk	67	22	Bread		
Egg, white	0	0	White	12	2
Milk group			Whole wheat	12	2
			Crackers	30	12
Milk, whole	45	28	Doughnuts	43	7
Milk, skim	5	2.5	Macaroni	5	< 1
Cheese, cheddar	74	47	Macaroni and cheese	46	20
Cheese, mozzarella, part skim	56	35	Oatmeal	13	2
			Pancakes, wheat	30	7
Ice cream	49	28	Spaghetti	5	< 1
Ice milk	31	18	*Fats and oils*		
Yogurt, partially skim milk	29	14			
Dried beans and nuts			Butter	99	62
			Lard	99	40
Beans, dry, navy	4	< 1	Margarine	99	21
Beans, navy, canned with pork	28	12	Oil, corn	100	13
Peanuts	77	17	Oil, coconut	100	87
Peanut butter	76	19	Salad dressings		
			French	95	15
			French, special dietary low fat	14	< 1

< 1 = less than 1 percent

*Percentages may vary. See food labels for specific information when available.

5 Calories per gram. Olestra is an ester of sucrose with long-chain fatty acids, a structure that cannot be hydrolyzed by digestive enzymes or absorbed by the gastrointestinal tract and therefore supplies no Calories to the body.

The effect of fat substitutes on health is covered later in this chapter, and their use in weight control programs is detailed in chapter 11.

What is cholesterol?

Cholesterol is one of the lipids known as *sterols*. It is not a fat, but it is a fat-like pearly substance found in animal tissues. Cholesterol is not an essential nutrient for humans because it is manufactured naturally in the liver from fatty acids and from the breakdown products of carbohydrate and protein—glucose and amino acids.

What foods contain cholesterol?

Cholesterol is found only in animal products and is not found in fruits, vegetables, nuts, grains, or other nonanimal foods. Table 5.3 presents some foods from the meat and milk groups with the cholesterol content in milligrams. Several foods from the bread/cereal group are also included, indicating that the preparation of some bread/cereal products may add cholesterol by including some animal product containing cholesterol, mainly eggs.

TABLE 5.3	Cholesterol content, in milligrams, for some common foods		
		Amount	Cholesterol
Meat group			
Beef, pork, ham		1 oz	25
Poultry		1 oz	23
Fish		1 oz	21
Shrimp		1 oz	45
Lobster		1 oz	25
Eggs		1	220
Liver		1 oz	120
Milk group			
Milk, whole		1 cup	27
Milk, 2%		1 cup	15
Milk, skim		1 cup	7
Butter		1 tsp	12
Margarine		1 tsp	0
Cream cheese		1 tbsp	18
Ice milk		1 cup	10
Ice cream		1 cup	85
Bread/Cereal group			
Bread		1 slice	0
Biscuit		1	17
Pancake		1	40
Sweet roll		1	25
French toast		1 slice	130
Doughnut		1	28
Cereal, cooked		1 cup	0

Fruits, vegetables, grains, and nuts have no cholesterol.

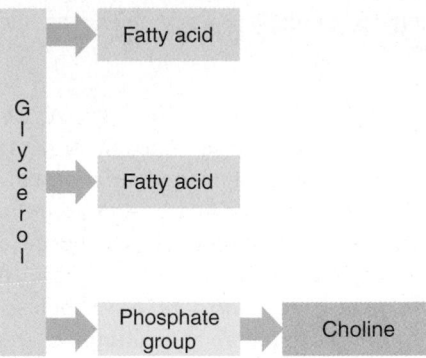

FIGURE 5.5 Simplified diagram of the phospholipid lecithin.

Some plants contain various products that resemble cholesterol. Plant sterols and stanols may possess some health benefits, as noted later in this chapter.

What are phospholipids?

Chemically, **phospholipids** are somewhat comparable to triglycerides. They have a glycerol base, one or two attached fatty acids, and an additional structure that contains a phosphate group. One of the most common phospholipids is **lecithin,** whose structure is depicted as a simple diagram in figure 5.5. Phospholipids are not essential nutrients, as the body can make them from triglycerides. As discussed later in this chapter, some phospholipids have been studied as a potential ergogenic aid.

What foods contain phospholipids?

Egg yolks provide substantial amounts of lecithin, and other good sources include liver, wheat germ, and peanuts. However, lecithin may be degraded in the digestive tract to smaller constituents. Your body can make all of the phospholipids it needs. Because

dietary phospholipids are not associated with any health risks, there is little concern with dietary intake.

How much fat and cholesterol do we need in the diet?

In a review, Jequier indicated that we need dietary fat for three reasons: to meet energy needs; to provide essential fatty acids; and to provide essential fat-soluble vitamins.

Dietary fats are a concentrated source of energy, and adequate dietary intake is very important during the growth and development years. Dietary fats also provide several essential fatty acids, without which various health problems would develop. Dietary fats also provide the fat-soluble vitamins A, D, E, and K.

These factors, along with possible implications for health, were taken into consideration in the development of Dietary Reference Intakes for dietary fats, which may be found in the DRI table for macronutrients in the front inside cover. For the purpose of developing its DRI, the National Academy of Sciences classified fat into the following categories:

Total fat
Saturated fatty acids (SFAs)
Cis monounsaturated fatty acids (MUFAs)
Cis polyunsaturated fatty acids (PUFAs)
   n-6 fatty acids (omega-6)
   n-3 fatty acids (omega-3)
Trans fatty acids

The abbreviations for the various fatty acids, as well as the omega classification, will be used interchangeably with the respective fat or fatty acids.

Total Fat The Academy developed an AMDR of 20–35 percent of daily energy intake from total fat, which is an estimate based on adverse effects that may occur from consuming either a low-fat or high-fat diet. Individuals should obtain sufficient but not excessive amounts of dietary fat within this range of energy intake. No RDA, AI, or UL have been developed for total fat because of insufficient evidence, but diets higher than 35 percent dietary fat are not recommended because saturated fat intake may be increased beyond this level. Other health professional groups have recommended 30 percent of daily energy intake as the maximal from fat.

Saturated Fatty Acids and *Trans* Fatty Acids   The Academy did not develop an RDA, AI, or UL for saturated fat or *trans* fat. However, increased intake of both of these fats is associated with increased risk of coronary heart disease. Although the Academy notes that because most diets contain fats, and because most fats contain a mixture of fatty acids, it is not possible to consume a diet devoid of saturated and *trans* fats. Nevertheless, the prevailing undertone in this DRI report is to minimize the dietary intake of these two types of fat. Other health organizations suggest a maximum of 7–10 percent of the daily energy intake be derived from the combination of saturated and *trans* fats. In the popular media, saturated and *trans* fats are often referred to as *bad* fats.

Cis Monounsaturated Fatty Acids   The Academy did not develop an RDA, AI, or UL for monounsaturated fats, indicating that they are not essential fatty acids because they may be synthesized by the body. About 20–40 percent of the fat we consume is monounsaturated, and primarily olive oil. Although no DRI have been set for monounsaturated fat, the Academy notes that they may have some benefit in the prevention of chronic disease. Olive oil is a staple in the Mediterranean diet and its alleged health benefits will be discussed later in this chapter. In the popular media, monounsaturated fats are often referred to as *good* fats.

Cis Polyunsaturated Fatty Acids   The Academy developed an AI for polyunsaturated fatty acids because there may be some health benefits associated with such dietary intakes. AI were set for both omega-6 and omega-3 fatty acids. In the popular media, some polyunsaturated fats, particularly omega-3 fatty acids, are often referred to as *good* fats.

Omega-6 fatty acids   Linoleic acid, an essential omega-6 polyunsaturated fatty acid, must be supplied in the diet because the body cannot produce it from other fatty acids. The AI for adult males age 19–50 is 17 grams of linoleic acid daily, and 12 grams per day for females. For males and females age 51 and over the AI is 14 and 11 grams daily, respectively. Somewhat smaller AIs have been developed for children and adolescents age 9–18. Linoleic acid is found in vegetable and nut oils—such as corn, sunflower, peanut, and soy oils—that constitute food products such as margarine, salad dressings, and cooking oils. **Conjugated linoleic acid (CLA),** an isomer of linoleic acid, has been suggested to be ergogenic and possess health benefits, which will be discussed in later sections of this chapter.

Omega-3 fatty acids   Alpha-linolenic acid, an omega-3 polyunsaturated fatty acid, is also considered to be an essential fatty acid. The AI for adult males age 19 and older is 1.6 grams of alpha-linolenic acid daily, and 1.1 grams per day for females. Somewhat smaller AIs have been developed for children and adolescents age 9–18. Alpha-linolenic acid is found in green leafy vegetables, canola oil, flaxseed oil, soy products, some nuts,

and fish. The potential health benefits of omega-3 fatty acids, including several derived from fish oils (eicosapentaenoic acid, EPA; docosahexaenoic acid, DHA), are discussed later in this chapter.

Cholesterol   Cholesterol is vital to human physiology in a variety of ways, so the body needs an adequate supply. Because cholesterol may be manufactured in the body from either fats, carbohydrate, or protein, however, there is apparently little need for us to obtain large amounts, if any, in the foods we eat. Also, because a positive relationship has been established between high blood cholesterol levels and coronary heart disease, reduction of dietary cholesterol has been advocated by a number of health-related associations. The American Heart Association, in its set of dietary guidelines, recommends that cholesterol intake be less than 300 milligrams per day, or about 100 milligrams of cholesterol for every 1,000 Calories you eat.

Table 5.4 indicates the grams of fat and saturated fat and milligrams of cholesterol that may be consumed daily on a diet containing 30 percent of the Calories as fat and less than 300 milligrams of cholesterol. For the 30 percent recommendation, a very simple method to determine the grams of total fat you may consume on a given caloric diet is to simply drop the zero from the daily caloric total and divide by 3. For example,

$$2{,}100 \text{ Calorie diet}$$
$$2{,}100 = 210$$
$$210/3 = 70 \text{ grams total fat}$$

For lower percentages of fat Calories, say 20 percent, simply multiply the daily caloric intake by the percentage desired and divide by 9 to get the grams of fat allowed per day. For example, 20 percent of 2,500 Calories would permit 500 Calories from fat, or about 55 grams per day.

As we shall see later in this chapter and in chapter 10, excessive consumption of dietary fat and cholesterol may be linked to a variety of chronic diseases, including heart disease and obesity. In certain individuals with blood lipid abnormalities, the recommended reduction in dietary fats and cholesterol is even greater than the Prudent Healthy Diet, with the total dietary Calories

TABLE 5.4 Daily allowance for grams of fat and saturated fat, and milligrams of cholesterol*

Total Calories	Fat Calories	Grams of fat	Grams of saturated fat	mg of cholesterol
1,000	300	33	11	100
1,500	450	50	16	150
2,000	600	66	22	200
2,500	750	83	27	250
3,000	900	100	33	300

*Based upon a diet containing 30 percent of Calories as fat with 100 milligrams of cholesterol per 1,000 Calories.

from fat being 20 percent or lower in some diet plans, as in the Ornish diet plan.

Theoretically, high-fat diets may be deleterious to physical performance in several ways. The fat may displace carbohydrate in the diet, may lead to excessive caloric intake and body weight, and may cause gastrointestinal distress if consumed as part of a pregame meal. All of these factors could possibly impair physical performance. On the other hand, some investigators have contended that high-fat diets may enhance exercise performance. These issues will be discussed later in this chapter.

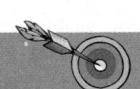

Key Concepts

▶ The three major lipids in human nutrition are triglycerides, cholesterol, and phospholipids.

▶ Triglycerides, which consist of fatty acids and glycerol, account for about 98 percent of the lipids we eat. Fatty acids may be saturated or unsaturated. Unsaturated fatty acids may be monounsaturated and polyunsaturated. Polyunsaturated fatty acids may exist in two forms, *cis* and *trans*. Omega-3 fatty acids are also polyunsaturated.

▶ The fat content of foods varies considerably, but generally the fruit, vegetable, and starch food exchanges are good sources of unsaturated fats and are low in total fat, whereas the meat and milk food exchanges contain foods that may have a high total fat and saturated fat content.

▶ Cholesterol is a nonfat substance vital to human metabolism, and although it may be obtained in the diet only from animal foods, the body can produce its own supply from other dietary nutrients such as saturated fats.

▶ The AMDR for dietary fat is 20–35 percent of daily caloric intake. Although some fat is essential in the diet as a source of essential fatty acids (linoleic and alpha-linolenic) and the fat-soluble vitamins (A, D, E, K), these nutrients may be obtained from polyunsaturated fats. The total amount of saturated and *trans* fats in the diet should be less than 10 percent, preferably 7 percent of daily caloric intake, while monounsaturated and polyunsaturated fats should constitute the majority of the AMDR.

Check for Yourself

▶ Peruse food labels of some of your favorite foods and check the fat content. Pay particular attention to percent of daily value for total fat, saturated fat, and cholesterol. Check also for *trans* fat content.

Metabolism and Function

In this section we briefly cover the digestion of dietary lipids, their metabolic disposal in the body, interactions with carbohydrate and protein, the major functions of fats in the body, and energy stores of fat.

How does dietary fat get into the body?

The major dietary sources of lipids are the triglycerides, comprising about 98 percent, while the other 2 percent consists mainly of sterols and phospholipids. Most of the dietary triglycerides contain long-chain fatty acids (14 or more carbons). Lipids are insoluble in water, and therefore their digestion and absorption is somewhat more complicated than that of carbohydrates; a broad overview is presented in figure 5.6. As lipids enter the small intestine, they stimulate hormonal secretion by the intestines that culminates in the secretion of bile from the gallbladder and lipases from the pancreas into the intestinal lumen. The bile salts serve as emulsifiers, breaking up the lipid droplets into smaller segments that may be hydrolyzed by the lipid enzymes, pancreatic lipases, and cholesterases. In essence, lipids are hydrolyzed into free fatty acids (FFA), glycerol, cholesterol, and phospholipids, which through an intricate process are then absorbed into the cells of the intestinal mucosa. Here they are combined into a fat droplet called a **chylomicron,** which contains a large amount of triglyceride and smaller amounts of cholesterol, phospholipids, and protein. The chylomicron is one form of a **lipoprotein,** which, by its name, you can see is composed of lipids and protein. A diagram of a lipoprotein is presented in figure 5.7. The chylomicron then leaves the intestinal cell and is absorbed by the lacteal in the villi, where it is eventually transported in the lymphatic system to the blood. A schematic of the absorption process is presented in figure 5.8.

Medium-chain triglycerides (MCTs) release medium-chain fatty acids (MCFAs) with shorter carbon chain lengths (6–12 carbons), enabling them to be absorbed directly into the blood without being converted into chylomicrons. They are transported directly to the liver. Because of this rapid processing, MCTs have been theorized to possess ergogenic potential, and their efficacy in this regard will be discussed in a later section. Short-chain fatty acids (SCFAs) derived from triglycerides are also absorbed like MCFAs.

What happens to the lipid once it gets in the body?

The digestion of lipids into chylomicrons is slow, and the absorption after a high-fat meal can last several hours. As the chylomicron circulates in the blood, it reacts with various cells in the body, particularly cells in the muscle and adipose tissues. Specific proteins in the outer coat of lipoproteins are known as apolipoproteins. **Apolipoproteins,** or *apoproteins,* increase lipid solubility and enable the various lipoproteins to react with specific receptors in cells throughout the body. The apolipoproteins in the chylomicron interact with an enzyme, lipoprotein lipase, which is produced in the muscle and adipose cells and released to the capillary blood vessels surrounding the cells. The lipoprotein lipase releases fatty acids and glycerol from the chylomicron. The fatty acids are absorbed into the cells by simple diffusion and receptors for some LCFAs, while the glycerol is transported primarily to the liver for conversion to glucose. The remains of the chylomicron, the chylomicron remnant, are transported to the liver for disposal.

FIGURE 5.6 A summary of fat digestion and absorption.

Fats

1 Very minor fat digestion in stomach

2 Fat digested mainly into monoglycerides and free fatty acids by a lipase enzyme released from the pancreas

3 Bile made by the liver aids fat digestion and absorption

4 Fat absorbed is mostly made into chylomicrons and transferred into the lymph

5 Less than 5% of fat normally excreted in feces

3 Liver   **1** Stomach

2 Pancreas

4 Small intestine

5

Anus

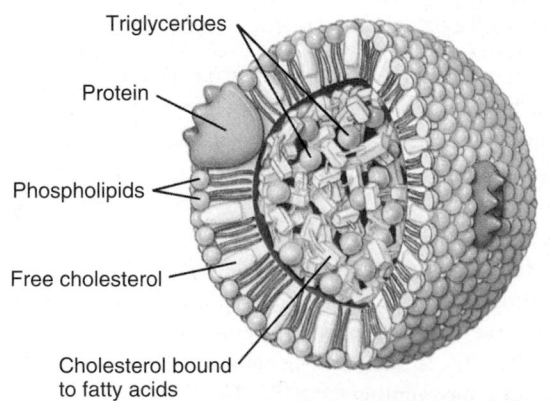

Triglycerides

Protein

Phospholipids

Free cholesterol

Cholesterol bound to fatty acids

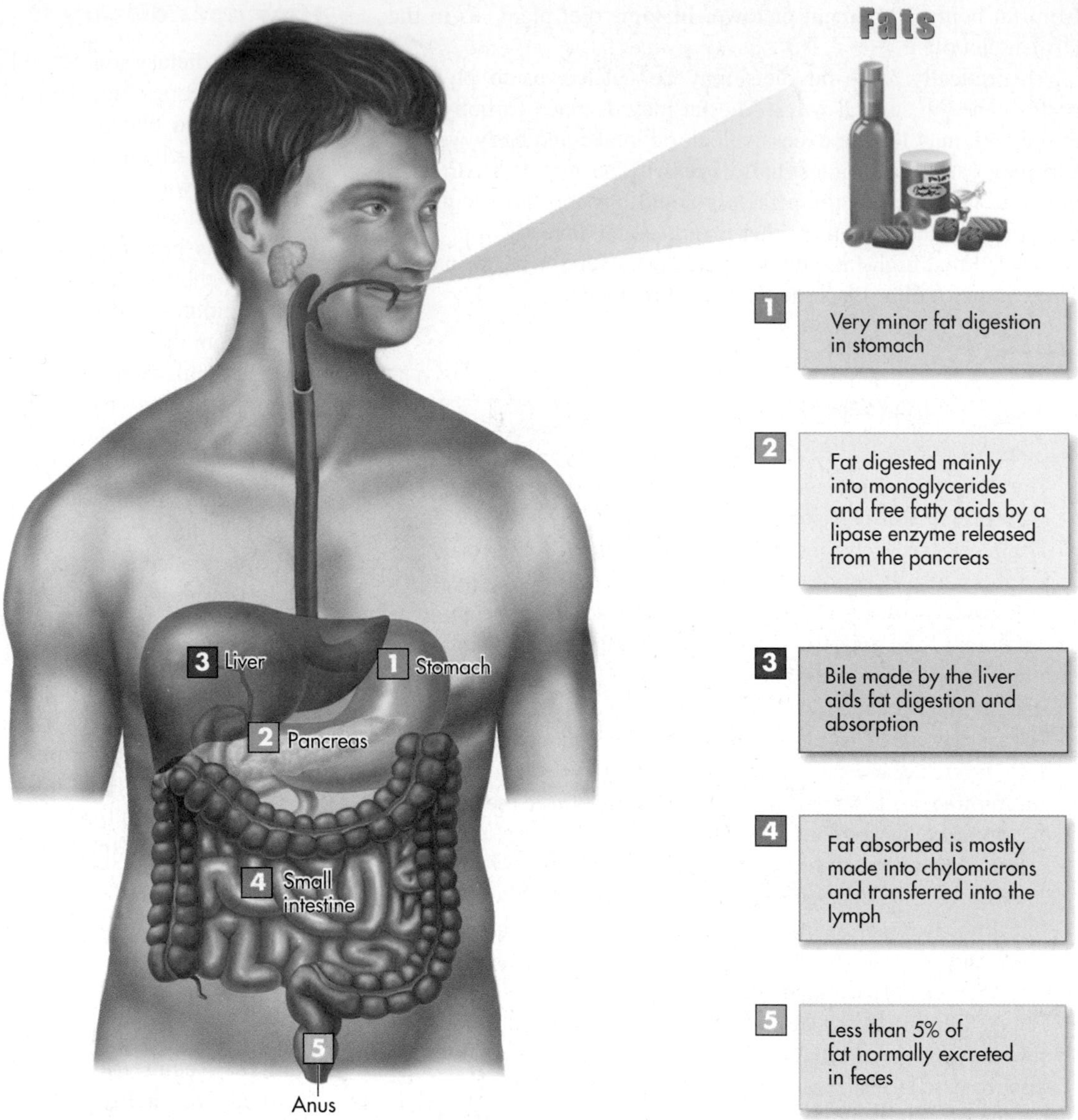

FIGURE 5.7 Schematic of a lipoprotein. Lipoproteins contain a core of triglycerides and cholesterol esters surrounded by a coat of apoproteins, cholesterol, and phospholipids. The proportion of protein, cholesterol, triglycerides, and phospholipids varies between the different types of lipoproteins.

In the muscle, the fatty acids may either be used as a source of energy or may combine with newly generated glycerol, which is derived as a metabolic by-product of glycolysis, leading to the formation and storage of muscle triglycerides. In exercise science literature, intramuscular triglycerides are often referred to as *intramyocellular triacylglycerol (IMTG)*. In the adipose cell, most of the fatty acids combine with glycerol and are stored as adipose cell triglycerides.

The key organ in the body for the metabolism of most nutrients is the liver. It is a clearinghouse in human metabolism. As blood passes through the liver, its cells take the basic nutrients and convert them into other forms. As mentioned in chapter 4, the liver is able to manufacture glucose from a variety of other nutrients, including glycerol. Pertinent to our discussion here is its role in lipid metabolism. As noted previously, glycerol and chylomicron remnants, including phospholipids, are transported to the liver, as are the MCFAs and SCFAs directly from the intestinal tract. Adipose cells are metabolically active in the sense that they are constantly releasing fatty acids for use by the body, including the

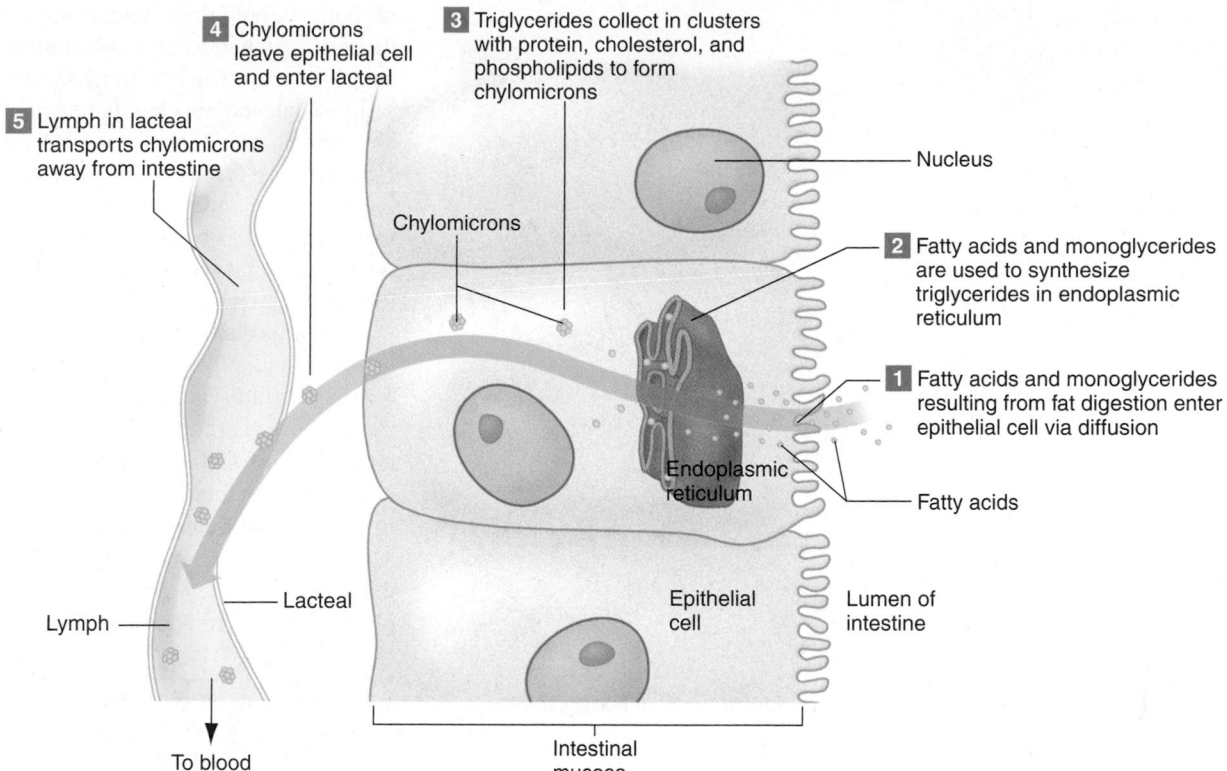

FIGURE 5.8 The absorption of lipids. In the lumen of the intestine, several lipases, assisted by bile salts, digest lipids to various forms of fatty acids, phospholipids, cholesterol, and glycerol, which are absorbed by an intricate process into the epithelial cells of the intestinal mucosa. Here they are combined with protein to form chylomicrons, a form of lipoprotein, which are transported out of the cell and into the lacteal, where the lymph eventually carries them to the blood. Medium chain triglycerides (MCTs) may be absorbed directly into the blood (not depicted).

liver. The major role of the liver is to combine these various components (fatty acids, glycerol, cholesterol, and phospholipids), along with protein, into various forms of lipoproteins.

What are the different types of lipoproteins?

After the chylomicrons have been cleared from the blood, which may take several hours, other lipoproteins constitute approximately 95 percent of the serum lipids. The metabolism of lipoproteins is complex, for they are constantly being synthesized and catabolized by the liver and other body tissues. As a result, there is an exchange of protein and lipid components among the different classes of lipoproteins, which can lead to the conversion of one form into another.

The classification of lipoproteins may be determined by several methods. One of the methods is by the type of apolipoprotein present and its functions. Lipoproteins have a number of different apoproteins, which enable them to react with different tissues. The letters *A, B, C, D,* and *E,* including subdivisions such as *A-I* and *A-II,* are common designations. The second method, most popularly known, is based on the density of the lipoprotein particle. Designations range from high to very low density.

The chylomicron is one form of lipoprotein, but it is relatively short-lived because it is derived from dietary fat intake. For our purposes in this book, the major classifications of

lipoproteins along with their suggested composition and function are listed next; a graphical depiction is presented in figure 5.9. However, it should be noted that a wide variety of lipoproteins exists, based upon their specific lipid and protein content. Additionally, their metabolism and complete functions have not been totally elucidated.

VLDL (very low-density lipoproteins). **VLDL** consist primarily of triglycerides formed in the liver from endogenous sources, whereas chylomicrons contain triglycerides from exogenous sources, that is, the diet. Like chylomicrons, VLDL are transported to the tissues to provide fatty acids and glycerol. The loss of some triglycerides to the liver or tissues produces VLDL remnants, referred to as IDL (intermediate-density lipoprotein) or TRL (triglyceride-rich lipoprotein). These remnants are either taken up by the liver or converted to LDL. Apoprotein B is the major apoprotein associated with both VLDL and IDL.

LDL (low-density lipoproteins). **LDL** contain a high proportion of cholesterol and phospholipids, but little triglycerides. LDL are formed after the VLDL and IDL release most of their stores of triglycerides. LDL size may be important. One form of LDL, a small, dense LDL, with important health implications has been identified. LDL, interacting with cell membrane receptors, deliver cholesterol into body cells. Apolipoprotein B is the major apolipoprotein associated with LDL.

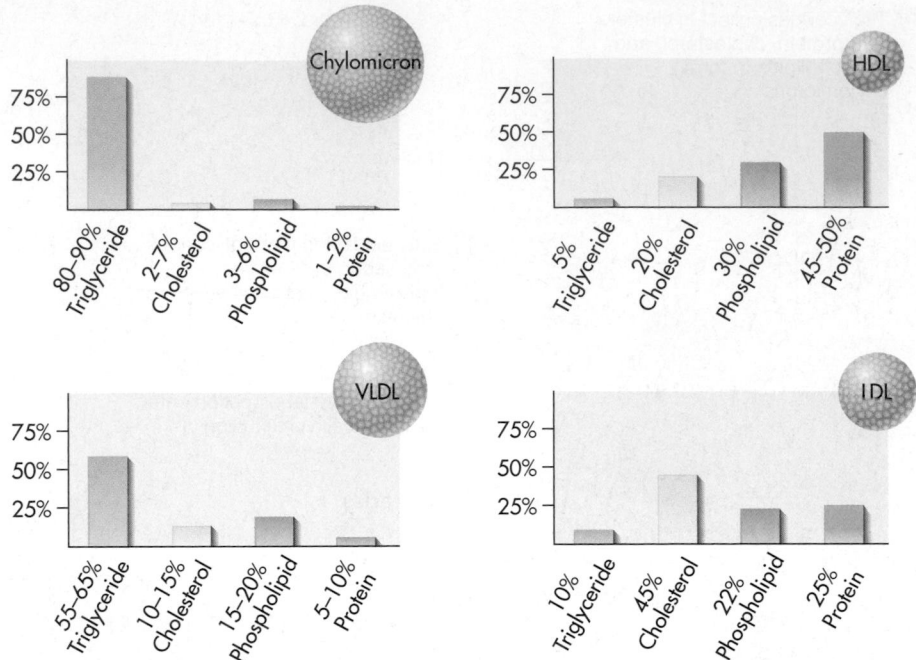

FIGURE 5.9 The approximate content of four different types of lipoproteins.

of both carbohydrate and protein and convert them to fat when caloric expenditure is less than caloric intake. Thus, in general, it is not necessarily what you eat, but rather how much, that determines whether or not you gain body fat. However, as discussed in chapters 10 and 11, there is some evidence to suggest that dietary fat may be stored as body fat more readily than carbohydrate or protein, and thus may be a factor in the development of obesity.

It is important to note that although carbohydrates and protein may be converted to fat (primarily fatty acids), fatty acids cannot be converted to carbohydrate or protein. If excess nitrogen is available from protein, it may combine with metabolic by-products of fatty acids to form nonessential amino acids—but fatty acids cannot be converted into protein without this excess nitrogen. Although keep in mind that glycerol can be converted into carbohydrate.

What are the major functions of the body lipids?

The body lipids are derived from the dietary lipids and other carbon sources, namely carbohydrate and protein, but with the exception of linoleic fatty acid and alpha-linolenic fatty acid, all lipids essential to human metabolism may be produced by the liver. The body lipids serve a variety of functions, including all three purposes of food: they form body structures, help regulate metabolism, and provide a source of energy.

Structure The structure of virtually all cell membranes, including the nerve membranes, consists partly of lipids, notably cholesterol and phospholipids. Lipids form myelin, an important component in the sheath covering nerve fibers. The structural fat deposits in the adipose tissues are used as insulators to conserve body heat and shock absorbers to protect various organs.

Metabolic Regulation Various fatty acids interact with proteins, the major metabolic regulators in the body. Essential fatty acids are found in cell membranes and are involved in various intracellular metabolic pathways, including regulation of gene expression. Cholesterol is a component of several hormones, such as testosterone and estrogen, which have diverse effects in the regulation of human metabolism. The majority of cholesterol in the body is used by the liver to produce bile salts, essential for the digestion of fats. Phospholipids are also instrumental for blood clotting.

Adipose cells produce various substances called **adipokines** (adipocytokines) and release them into the bloodstream. These adipokines may function as hormones, affecting tissues in other parts of the body. Leptin is one such adipokine that we will discuss in chapter 10.

Some derivatives of the omega-6 and omega-3 fatty acids formed by oxidation have some potent biologic functions in the body. These derivatives—prostaglandins, prostacyclins, thromboxanes,

HDL (high-density lipoproteins). **HDL** contain a high proportion of protein (about 45–50 percent), moderate amounts of cholesterol and phospholipids, and very little triglycerides. Various HDL are produced in the liver and intestinal tract. Several subclasses of HDL have been identified, most notably HDL_2 and HDL_3. HDL transport cholesterol from peripheral cells to the liver, known as *reverse cholesterol transport.* Apolipoprotein A is the major apolipoprotein associated with HDL.

Lipoprotein (a). **Lipoprotein (a)** is very similar to the LDL, being in the upper LDL density range. The principal apolipoprotein associated with lipoprotein (a) is apolipoprotein (a).

Other apolipoproteins comprise the structure of lipoproteins. For example, apolipoprotein E is formed in the liver and present in all lipoproteins. These lipoproteins are needed to bind with cell membrane receptors.

A simplified schematic of fat metabolism is presented in figure 5.10. A more detailed diagram of lipoprotein interactions is presented in appendix G.4B.

Can the body make fat from protein and carbohydrate?

You may recall that glycogen is made up of many individual glucose molecules and is a glucose polymer. In essence, fatty acids are polymers of acetyl CoA, the primary substrate for the Krebs cycle.

As noted in figure 4.9, the amino acids of protein may be converted to acetyl CoA, which can then be converted into fat. Carbohydrates also may be converted to fat via acetyl CoA. It is important to understand that the body will take excess amounts

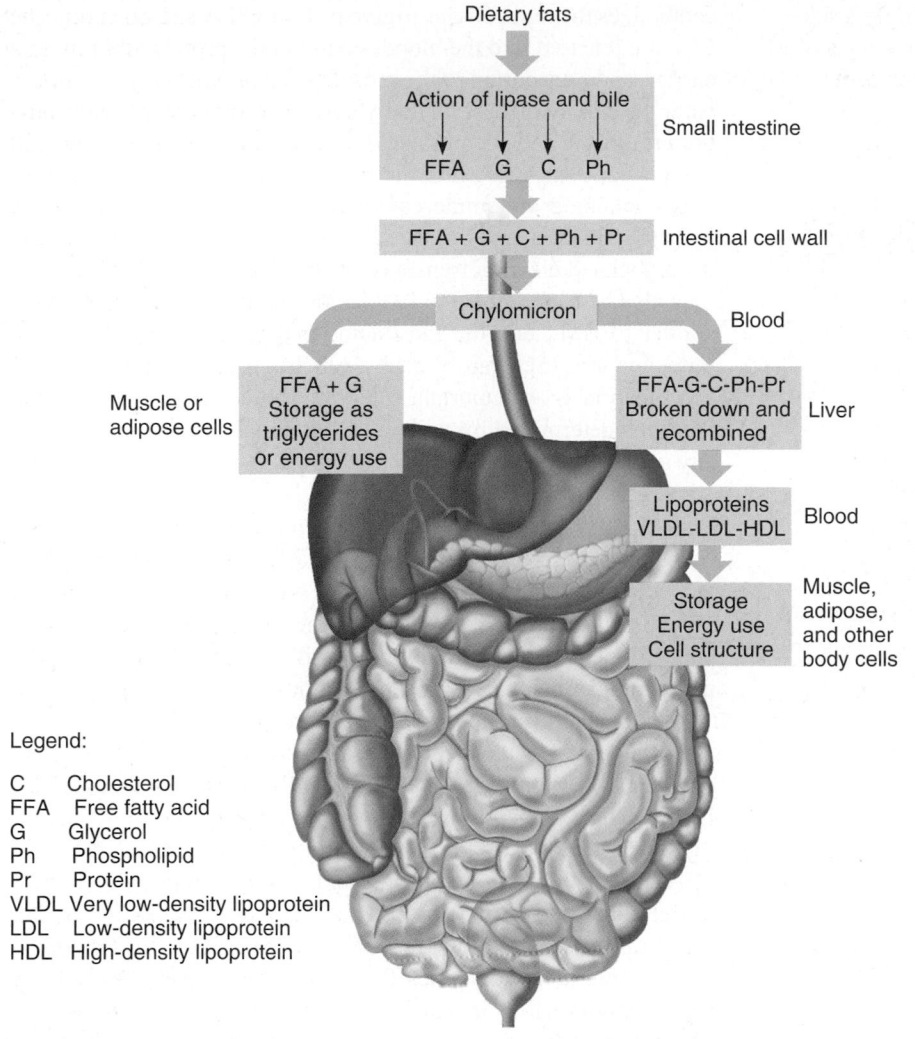

Dietary fats

Action of lipase and bile — Small intestine

FFA   G   C   Ph

FFA + G + C + Ph + Pr — Intestinal cell wall

Chylomicron

Blood

Muscle or adipose cells

FFA + G
Storage as triglycerides or energy use

FFA-G-C-Ph-Pr
Broken down and recombined — Liver

Lipoproteins
VLDL-LDL-HDL — Blood

Storage
Energy use
Cell structure

Muscle, adipose, and other body cells

Legend:

C   Cholesterol
FFA   Free fatty acid
G   Glycerol
Ph   Phospholipid
Pr   Protein
VLDL Very low-density lipoprotein
LDL   Low-density lipoprotein
HDL   High-density lipoprotein

FIGURE 5.10 Simplified diagram of fat metabolism. After digestion, most of the fats are carried in the blood as chylomicrons. Through the metabolic processes in the body, fat may be utilized as a major source of energy, used to help develop cell structure, or stored as a future energy source.

During rest, nearly 60 percent of the energy supply is provided by the metabolism of fats when the individual consumes a mixed diet, but may be higher when blood glucose is low, as after an overnight fast. Most of the energy provided is presented to cells as fatty acids, either FFA delivered via the blood or fatty acids from stored intracellular triglycerides. Inside the cell, the metabolism of fatty acids into acetyl CoA (a 2-carbon molecule) is known as **beta-oxidation,** for the beta carbon is the second carbon on the fatty acid chain. The acetyl-CoA is then processed through the citric acid (Krebs) cycle and associated electron transport system for production of energy as ATP. At rest, a high-fat meal will increase the proportion of energy derived from fat. In general, the greater the amount of fatty acids available in the plasma, the greater their use as a source of energy. For example, the heart muscle may derive 100 percent of its energy needs from fatty acids after a lipid-rich meal.

Ketones, ketoacids that are metabolic by-products of excess fatty acid metabolism, may also serve as an energy source for body cells. Ketones diffuse from the liver into the blood, and are transported to the body tissues where they can eventually be used as a source of energy. The major ketones are acetoacetic acid, beta-hydroxybutyric acid, and acetone. These ketones usually are produced in small amounts, but when the use of fatty acids as an energy source is high (such as with fasting, high-fat diets, and diabetes) ketone levels in the blood will increase. Ketones are an important energy source during fasting or starvation. However, excessive accumulation may lead to acidosis (ketosis) in the blood, a condition which may cause coma and death, such as in uncontrolled diabetes.

and leukotrienes—are collectively known as **eicosanoids.** These eicosanoids possess local hormone-like properties that influence a number of physiological functions, including several that may have implications for health or physical performance. Several important eicosanoids are derived from omega-3 fatty acids, and the theorized health and performance implications will be discussed in later sections of this chapter.

Energy Source In general, the function of the majority of the body lipids, the triglycerides, is to provide energy to drive metabolic processes. The majority of the triglycerides in the body are stored in the adipose tissue. They break down to free fatty acids (FFA) and glycerol, which are released into the blood, with the FFA being transported to the tissues and the glycerol going to the liver. In the tissues, the FFA are reduced to acetyl CoA and enter the Krebs cycle to produce energy via the oxygen system. The glycerol is used by the liver to form other lipids or glucose. This energy-yielding process is illustrated in appendix G, figure G.4A.

How much total energy is stored in the body as fat?

The greatest amount of energy stored in the body is fat in the form of triglycerides. Fat is a very efficient, compact means to store energy, for several reasons. First, fat has 9 Calories per gram, more than twice the value of carbohydrate and protein. Also, there is very little water in body fat compared to the 3–4 grams of water stored with each gram of carbohydrate or protein. In essence, based on weight, body fat may be about 5–6 times as efficient an energy store as carbohydrate and protein. If the average 154-pound man had to carry all the potential energy of his fat stores as carbohydrate, he would weigh nearly 300 pounds.

Most of the triglycerides are stored in the adipose tissues, approximately 80,000–100,000 Calories of energy in the average adult male with normal body fat. The triglycerides within and between the muscle cells may provide approximately 2,500–2,800 Calories, while those in the blood provide only about 70–80 Calories. The free fatty acids (FFA) in the blood total about 7–8 Calories.

The liver also contains an appreciable store of triglycerides. Thus, you can see that the human body contains a huge reservoir of energy Calories in the form of fat. A summary is presented in chapter 3, table 3.3.

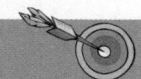

Key Concepts

▶ Fats are transported in the blood primarily as lipoproteins. Lipoproteins may be classified by their density and have various functions. In general, VLDL transport fats to the tissues, LDL transport cholesterol to the tissues, and HDL transport cholesterol from the tissues.

▶ Dietary lipids may serve the three major functions of nutrients. They may be utilized as an energy source, used as part of body-cell structure, and by-products of fat metabolism, known as eicosanoids, may act as local hormones and affect a variety of metabolic functions.

▶ The vast majority of dietary fats are stored as triglycerides in the adipose cells, but significant amounts may also be stored in the muscles as intramuscular triglycerides, also known as intramyocellular triacylglycerols.

Fats and Exercise

Are fats used as an energy source during exercise?

The two major energy sources for the production of ATP during exercise are carbohydrates in the form of muscle glycogen and fats in the form of fatty acids, mainly LCFA. In steady-state exercise, both can be converted to acetyl CoA for subsequent oxidation in the citric acid cycle. In general, a mixture of both fuel sources is used during exercise, although the quantitative values may vary depending on a variety of factors, including the intensity and duration of the exercise bout, the diet, and the training status of the individual. The use of fat as an energy source during endurance exercise, including the marathon, has been the subject of several recent symposia and reviews, including those by Hawley, Jeukendrup, Roepstorff, Spriet, and Spriet and Hargreaves, and several key studies, such as those by Romijn and associates. The following discussion represents some of the key findings from these reviews and studies.

Fat Energy Sources   The fatty acids used by the muscle cells during exercise may be derived from a variety of sources, including the plasma triglycerides in the chylomicrons and VLDL, but these sources are considered to be minor, providing less than 10 percent of fat energy.

The two major energy sources are the plasma FFA and the fatty acids derived from intramuscular triglycerides (IMTGs). The plasma FFA are in very short supply, so they must be replenished by the vast stores of triglycerides in the adipose tissue. An enzyme in the adipose cells, known as hormone-sensitive lipase (HSL),

catabolizes the intracellular triglycerides to FFA and glycerol. The FFA are released into the blood, bound to the protein albumin as a carrier, and transported to the muscle cells or other cells. The FFA enter the cell by diffusion and by specific protein receptors (transporters) in the cell membrane. The FFA are activated in the cell cytoplasm, transported into the mitochondria by an enzyme complex containing the amine **carnitine,** metabolized to acetyl CoA by beta-oxidation, and produce energy via the citric acid cycle and the associated electron transport system. The muscle triglycerides may also be metabolized to fatty acids and glycerol by an enzyme similar to HSL, and the fatty acids may be transported into the mitochondria. (See figure 5.11.) van Loon indicated that IMTG can function as an important substrate source during exercise and its use is determined by various factors, including exercise intensity and training status.

Use During Exercise   During rest, most of the fat energy needs of the body are met by the supply of plasma FFA to the cells. Fatty acids are constantly being mobilized from the adipose tissues to replenish the plasma FFA. Most of the FFA released during rest, about 70 percent, are actually re-esterified back into triglycerides, the remainder being delivered to the body cells for energy.

During exercise, only about 25 percent of these FFA are re-esterified, so this alone provides a substantial increase in FFA delivery to the muscle cells. Additionally, hormones that activate HSL, such as epinephrine, are secreted during exercise, stimulating the breakdown of adipose cell triglycerides and the release of FFA into the blood for transport and entrance to the muscle cell. Spriet noted that fatty acid proteins may be important in regulating the FFA transport into cells, and as Glatz and others reported, muscle contraction activates the fatty transporters in the muscle cell membrane, thus increasing FFA uptake into the muscle cell. Epinephrine also stimulates intramuscular lipases to catabolize muscle triglycerides into FFA. These fatty acids then enter the mitochondria and are degraded to acetyl CoA.

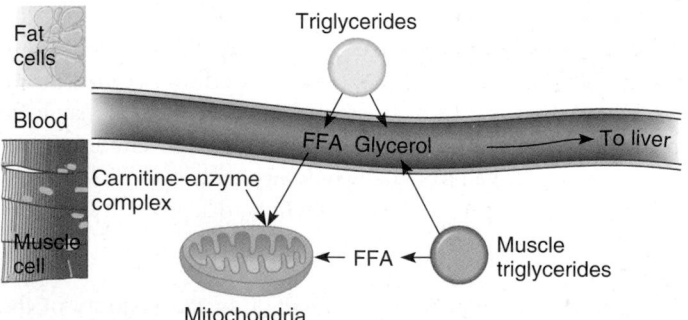

FIGURE 5.11 Fat as an energy source during exercise. Free fatty acids (FFA) are an important energy source during endurance exercise. They may be released by the adipose tissue triglycerides and travel by the blood to the muscle cells, and also may be derived from the muscle cell triglycerides. A carnitine-enzyme complex is needed to transport the FFA into the mitochondria. The glycerol that is released from the triglycerides may be transported to the liver for gluconeogenesis. (See appendix G, figure G.4A, for more details.)

During mild exercise at about 25 percent of VO_2 max, 20 percent or less of the total energy cost is derived from carbohydrate while the other 80 percent or more comes from fat. Wolfe indicates that exercise-induced lipolysis normally provides FFA at a rate in excess of that needed during exercise. Thus, the plasma FFA provided by the adipose tissue appear to be the major source of fat energy during mild exercise, but their percentage use decreases and that of muscle triglycerides increases as the exercise intensity increases up to about 65 percent VO_2 max. At this point, fats and carbohydrates appear to contribute equally to the energy expenditure, and the plasma FFA and muscle triglycerides contribute equally to the energy derived from fats. Carbohydrate increasingly becomes the predominant fuel as exercise exceeds 65 percent of VO_2 max. At high-intensity exercise levels, about 85 percent VO_2 max, the percentage contribution from fats (mostly muscle triglycerides) diminishes to 25 percent or less as muscle glycogen becomes the preferential energy source. These percentages are relevant to trained athletes, and will be somewhat lower in untrained individuals. A summary of fat utilization during exercise is presented in table 5.5.

Limiting Factors In a review, Lange stated that the human being is far from optimally designed for fat oxidation during exercise, noting that fat oxidation alone can sustain a metabolic rate corresponding to only 50–60 percent of VO_2 max. Although reviewers contend that factors limiting fatty acid utilization during high-intensity exercise are largely unknown, several have been suggested. First, inadequate FFA mobilization from adipose tissue may limit FFA delivery to the muscle. Wolfe indicates that fat oxidation is increased significantly at exercise intensities of 85 percent VO_2 max when lipid is infused, but carbohydrate still remains the most significant source of energy. Second, suboptimal intramuscular processes may also limit fat oxidation. For example, Wolfe indicated that the high rate of carbohydrate oxidation during high-intensity exercise may inhibit fatty acid oxidation by limiting transport into the mitochondria, possibly by inhibition of the carnitine-enzyme complex.

In his review, Spriet noted that these two factors may limit fat utilization during high-intensity exercise, but other regulatory factors may be involved as well, such as limited transport of fatty acids into the muscle cell and the optimal muscle triglyceride lipase activity. Frayn, in a review, concluded that there is a problem with delivery of sufficient fatty acids to muscle from adipose tissue only during high-intensity exercise. This limitation may be due to feedback inhibition of lipolysis, possibly due to lactate or catecholamine concentrations. As noted by Spriet, research is needed to determine what down-regulates fat use during exercise intensity above 85 percent of VO_2 max.

Dietary Effects As noted in previous chapters, the amount of energy that may be obtained from muscle and liver glycogen is rather limited. Feeding carbohydrate before and during exercise may reduce fat utilization. Spriet and Hargreaves indicated that the reduction in fat metabolism following glucose ingestion appears to be the result of increased plasma insulin levels. Insulin may decrease adipose tissue lipolysis, thus decreasing FFA availability in the plasma. Also, insulin may reduce fatty acid oxidation in the muscle, possibly by inhibiting fatty acid transport into the mitochondria. Although fat oxidation may possibly be reduced, the available carbohydrate would provide a more efficient energy source. In one study, Larson-Meyer and others found that reducing intramuscular lipid levels with a low-fat diet over the course of 3 days had no effect on endurance running performance, as measured by a 2-hour run at 62 percent of VO_2 max followed by a 10-kilometer time trial.

Carbohydrate intake before and during prolonged exercise helps, but within 90–120 minutes or more of high-intensity aerobic exercise, glycogen stores approach very low levels and the body shifts to an increasing usage of FFA, leading to a decrease in the intensity of the exercise. In cases such as prolonged endurance tasks like ultramarathons, FFA may provide nearly 90 percent of the energy in the latter stages of the event when muscle glycogen and blood glucose levels are inadequate to sustain higher-intensity exercise.

Use of Ketones Although ketones may be utilized by the muscle, they do not appear to contribute significantly to energy production during exercise.

TABLE 5.5 Fat energy sources during exercise

Plasma chylomicrons	Not a major source
Plasma VLDL	Not a major source
Plasma FFA	Major source; Replenished by adipose cell release of FFA; Used in exercise at low to moderate intensity, i.e., 25–65 percent VO_2 max; Use decreases as exercise intensity increases toward 65 percent VO_2 max
Muscle FFA	Major source; Released from intramuscular triglycerides; Low use during mild exercise; Used increasingly as exercise intensity increases toward 65 percent VO_2 max

Note: With high-intensity exercise, 65 percent VO_2 max or higher, total fat oxidation falls.

Does gender or age influence the use of fats as an energy source during exercise?

Gender Women possess a greater percentage of body fat than men, and several writers for popular runners' magazines have suggested that women could process this fat more efficiently and thus be more effective in ultramarathon events. Tarnopolsky indicated some theoretical rationale supports this viewpoint, as both the muscle lipid content and the maximal activity of a key enzyme in fat metabolism are higher in females. The greater fat oxidation for women during submaximal endurance exercise compared with men seems to occur partly through a sex hormone-mediated enhancement of lipid-oxidation pathways. In several studies Tarnopolsky and his associates, using the respiratory exchange ratio to evaluate energy substrate utilization following carbohydrate loading, reported that women oxidized significantly more fat and less carbohydrate than men when exercising at 65 or 75 percent VO_2 max. Similar findings were presented in studies headed by Knechtle and Venables. Roepstorff noted that some sport scientists think women may use more IMTG during exercise than men, possibly attributed to gender differences in skeletal muscle HSL regulation.

However, other studies have shown that the utilization of fat as an energy source by men and women during exercise is similar, particularly when matched for their aerobic capacity. Replicating their previous study with males, Romijn and others studied substrate metabolism in well-trained females at 25, 65, and 85 percent of VO_2 max. As with the men, carbohydrate oxidation in women increased progressively with exercise intensity, whereas the highest rate of fat oxidation was during exercise at 65 percent of VO_2 max. They concluded that the patterns of use of carbohydrate and fat during moderate- and high-intensity exercise are similar in trained men and women.

Whether or not women oxidize fat more efficiently than men appears to be debatable, and whether or not it improves ultraendurance performance is also questionable. For example, in one of their studies cited previously, Tarnopolsky and others found that although the women oxidized more fat and less carbohydrate than the men, the men improved their performance in the exercise task following carbohydrate loading but the women did not.

Age Young children may use more fat for energy during exercise compared to older postpubertal children and adults. Aucouturier and others suggested that a low activity of glycolytic enzymes in children may lead to greater use of lipid for energy during submaximal exercise. In a 60-minute cycling task at 70 percent VO_2 max, Timmons and others reported a higher utilization of fat in 12-year-old preadolescent girls as compared to adolescent 14-year-old girls. In another comparably designed study, they reported similar findings between 12-year-old boys in various stages of puberty and 14-year-old pubertal boys. Stephens and others also found that young males in the early and middle stages of puberty, as compared to males in late puberty and early adulthood, used more fat and less carbohydrate during exercise at intensities ranging from 30–70 percent of VO_2 peak. However, they indicated that the conversion to an adult-like metabolic profile of fuel utilization during exercise appears to be complete by the end of puberty in males.

What effect does exercise training have on fat metabolism during exercise?

A single bout of exercise influences fat utilization during exercise. Tunstall and others found that a single endurance exercise session led to an increased expression of genes in the skeletal muscle that increase the capacity for fat oxidation, and 9 days of training augmented this effect.

In general, reviewers indicate that trained athletes use more fat than untrained athletes during a standardized exercise task.

TABLE 5.6 Possible mechanisms associated with the increased use of fat as an energy source during aerobic endurance exercise following exercise training

- Increased blood flow and capillarization to the muscle, delivering more plasma FFA.
- Increased muscle triglyceride content, possibly associated with increased insulin sensitivity. Insulin regulates movement of FFA into muscle cells. Exercise training may also increase the activity of lipoprotein lipase or fatty acid transporters at the muscle cell membrane.
- Increased sensitivity of both adipose and muscle cells to epinephrine, resulting in increased FFA release to the plasma and within the muscle from triglycerides.
- Increased number of fatty acid transporters in the muscle cell membrane to move fatty acids from the plasma into the muscle cell.
- Improved ability to use ketones as an energy source.
- Increased number and size of mitochondria, and associated oxidative enzymes for processing of activated FFA.
- Increased activation of FFA and transport across the mitochondrial membrane.
- Increased activity of oxidative enzymes.

For example, if you ran an 8-minute mile both before and after a 2-month endurance training program, you would use the same amount of caloric energy each time. However, after training, more of that energy would be derived from fat. Hence, training helps you become a better fat burner, so to speak, which may help spare some of the glycogen in your muscles. Although the exact mechanisms have not been identified, the reviews by Horowitz and Klein and Jeukendrup and his colleagues document multiple factors, as presented in table 5.6.

Overall, according to Martin, the increased content and use of muscle triglycerides may be the primary mechanism underlying the greater capacity of trained muscle to oxidize fatty acids during exercise. Increased utilization of fat during exercise is one of the major effects of training experienced by the endurance athlete.

Although carbohydrate becomes more important as an energy source during high-intensity exercise, Coggan and others found highly trained endurance athletes may be able to use fats more efficiently at exercise intensity levels of 75–80 percent VO_2 max, and in a review Spriet noted that IMTG is an important energy source during prolonged, moderate dynamic exercise up to about 85 percent of VO_2 max in well-trained athletes. The ability to derive a substantial proportion of the energy demands of intensive exercise from fatty acids is extremely important for athletes such as marathoners who may be able to save some of their muscle glycogen for utilization in the latter stages of the race. An optimal mixture of fatty acids and glycogen for energy will enable them to sustain their pace, whereas the total depletion of muscle glycogen and subsequent reliance on fatty acids as the sole energy supply would force them to slow down. Thus, it is important for the endurance athlete to become a better "fat burner," and a variety of ergogenic aids have been proposed to enhance this effect.

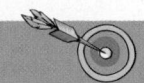
Fats: Ergogenic Aspects

Because exercise training leads to an increased utilization of fatty acids as an energy source and improved performance in prolonged endurance events (theoretically by sparing muscle glycogen), a variety of dietary practices, dietary supplements, and pharmacological agents have been employed in attempts to facilitate this metabolic process during exercise. In a review of the proposed mechanism, Jeukendrup noted that the increased availability and oxidation of fatty acids would generate more acetyl CoA, which in turn would inhibit a cascade of events that would essentially decrease the activity of enzymes involved in carbohydrate breakdown. Such an effect could spare the use of muscle glycogen and enhance endurance performance. As noted in chapter 4, preliminary studies from Clyde Williams's laboratory at Loughborough suggest that an increased fat metabolism may be the mechanism underlying enhanced endurance performance following a low-glycemic-index diet.

Both acute and chronic dietary strategies have been used to increase the concentration of muscle triglycerides or serum level of FFA. Such strategies include high-fat diets, fasting, and even infusion of lipids into the bloodstream. Dietary supplements and drugs have been used to either increase the supply of oxidizable fats or the rate of fat metabolism. Dietary supplements include medium-chain triglycerides, lecithin, glycerol, omega-3 fatty acids, carnitine, hydroxycitrate, conjugated linoleic acid, and phosphatidylserine. Caffeine also has been theorized to enhance fat oxidation, and its role as an ergogenic aid is covered in chapter 13.

What is fat loading?

Dietary strategies designed to increase the supply or metabolism of fat as an energy source during exercise may be referred to as **fat loading.** Fat loading may be done on an acute or chronic basis.

Acute fat loading involves dietary strategies immediately before exercise. Hargreaves notes that elevated plasma FFA levels are associated with reduced muscle glycogenolysis, which could help spare muscle glycogen. Because the rate at which FFA are oxidized in the muscle is dependent in part upon their concentration in the blood plasma, several different acute dietary techniques have been tried in attempts to increase plasma FFA levels.

Chronic fat loading involves dietary strategies about a week or so prior to endurance exercise. These strategies are designed to increase lipid metabolism and gene expression in skeletal muscle, resulting in an increased ability of the skeletal muscle to use fat as an energy source during exercise. In a review, Roepstorff and others indicated that ingestion of a fat-rich diet induces an increase in intramuscular triglyceride (IMTG) content, primarily in the type I muscle fibers used for oxidative energy production. Spriet and Hargreaves reported that IMTG levels can be increased by 50 to 80 percent following the consumption of a high-fat diet. Thus, chronic high-fat diets are designed primarily to increase IMTG. Some investigators have also evaluated the effect of chronic fat loading prior to 1–2 days of carbohydrate loading to see if there were any additional benefits associated with this dietary protocol. This latter dietary protocol is similar to the classic carbohydrate-loading protocol discussed in chapter 4.

Acute High-fat Diets Lipid digestion and absorption are slow, so one strategy is to infuse a lipid solution (such as Intralipid) directly into the blood along with heparin, a substance that stimulates lipoprotein lipase activity and increases plasma FFA levels. Such a strategy increases fat oxidation and reduces carbohydrate oxidation, which may enhance endurance exercise performance. However, after a lipid solution was used by a national team in the Tour de France, the entire team withdrew from the race allegedly due to adverse reactions. No research has been uncovered that supports this ergogenic technique.

A second strategy is to ingest a high-fat meal prior to exercise performance. For example, in two studies Okano and others reported no significant differences between a high-fat meal (61 percent fat content) and a control or low-fat meal on performance in a cycling test to exhaustion at 78–80 percent VO_2 max following 2 hours of riding at 60–67 percent VO_2 max. Additionally, Rowlands and Hopkins investigated the effect of a high-fat (85 percent fat energy) meal, as compared to a high-carbohydrate (85 percent carbohydrate energy) meal and high-protein (30 percent protein energy) meal consumed 90 minutes before an endurance cycling test, which involved a 1-hour preload at 55 percent VO_2 max, five 10-minute incremental loads from 55–82 percent of peak power, and a 50-kilometer time trial that included several 1-km and 4-km sprints. Subjects consumed a carbohydrate supplement during the cycling protocol. The meal composition had no clear effect on sprint or 50-kilometer cycle performance.

An acute high-fat dietary strategy does not appear to enhance performance, and, in fact, may actually impair performance if it contributes to gastrointestinal distress because of the delayed gastric emptying associated with fats. Research has shown that consuming a high-fat diet for 1 or 2 days, another acute approach, may actually impair performance in high-intensity exercise tasks.

Chronic High-fat Diets   Several investigators have challenged the dogma that endurance athletes need high-carbohydrate diets and suggest that endurance performance may benefit from diets containing about 50 percent or more energy from fat. Brown and Cox note that athletes can adapt to such a diet and maintain physical endurance capacity, will increase their muscle triglyceride levels, and may increase the use of fat and decrease use of carbohydrate during exercise. Stellingwerff and others recently reported that 5 days of a high-fat diet while training increases rates of whole body fat oxidation and decreases carbohydrate oxidation during aerobic cycling. In general, research has shown that when an individual is placed on a chronic low-carbohydrate and high-fat diet for about a week or more, the body adjusts its metabolism to use fats more efficiently. According to Yeo and others, it appears that there are responders and nonresponders to this practice. Thus, preliminary screening may be helpful to determine which athletes may benefit from this dietary intervention. But do such changes lead to enhanced endurance exercise performance?

Studies showing ergogenic effect   Several studies support an ergogenic effect of chronic fat loading. Pendergast and Horvath, along with their associates, conducted several of the first contemporary studies. Although two studies from their laboratory have shown that adapting to a high-fat diet (38–41 percent fat content) over a 1–4 week period improved treadmill running time to exhaustion, both studies had problems with the experimental design, such as no random assignment of the diet conditions and no counterbalancing of diet order. Moreover, the diets were not exceptionally high in fat content. Muoio and others acknowledged the limitations to experimental design in their prototype study, and the interested reader is referred to the other study by Venkatraman and Pendergast.

More recently, Horvath and others had male and female runners consume diets of 16 and 31 percent fat for 4 weeks, and then about half the subjects increased their dietary fat intake to 44 percent. All diets were designed to be isocaloric, but the runners actually consumed about 19 percent fewer Calories on the low-fat (16 percent) diet. There were no differences among the diets for VO_2 max, anaerobic power, or body mass, but the endurance run after the low-fat diet was reduced compared to the medium- and high-fat diets. However, it is possible that decreased energy intake may have contributed to this decrease in performance.

Lambert and her colleagues also found some ergogenic effects in several studies. In one study, they placed athletes on a high-fat (70 percent fat Calories) diet or low-fat (12 percent fat Calories) diet for 2 weeks, testing the effects on three performance tests done in consecutive order with 30 minutes rest between each. The three exercise tests included a Wingate high-power test, a high-intensity test to exhaustion at 90 percent VO_2 max, and a moderate-intensity test to exhaustion at 60 percent VO_2 max. Although there were no significant effects between the two diets for performance in the first two exercise tests, the cyclists rode significantly longer on the moderate-intensity test following adaptation to the high-fat diet. The investigators noted that adaptation to the high-fat diet decreased the reliance on carbohydrate as an energy source during exercise, and thus suggested the improved performance was due to muscle-glycogen sparing.

In a subsequent study, Lambert and others evaluated the effect of a 10-day high-fat diet, prior to 3 days of a carbohydrate-loading regimen, on cycling performance in a trial consisting of 150 minutes at 70 percent VO_2 max followed by a 20-kilometer time trial. Compared to their habitual diet with carbohydrate loading, the high-fat diet enabled the endurance cyclists to increase total fat oxidation and reduce carbohydrate oxidation, and significantly improve time trial performance by 1.4 minutes.

Studies showing no ergogenic effect   Conversely, other well-controlled research suggests that chronic high-fat diets do not benefit endurance performance. Using well-trained cyclists as subjects, Havemann and others reported no significant differences in 100-kilometer time-trial performance when consuming either a high-fat (68 percent fat) or high-carbohydrate (68 percent carbohydrate) diet for 6 days, followed by 1 day of carbohydrate loading, but the high-fat diet impaired 1-kilometer sprint power. The authors noted that although the high-fat diet increased fat oxidation, it compromised high-intensity sprint performance.

Several recent studies have shown no effect of chronic fat loading on endurance performance in trained individuals. Brown and Cox, in a randomized study using 32 endurance-trained cyclists, reported no difference in 20-km road time performance over a period of 12 weeks when subjects consumed either a high-fat (47 percent of energy) versus a high-carbohydrate (69 percent of energy) diet. Burke and her associates found no beneficial effects in two studies. In the first study they investigated the effects of a high-fat diet for 5 days, followed by a 1-day high-carbohydrate diet, on an endurance cycling protocol involving cycling at 70 percent VO_2 max for 2 hours followed by an intense time trial. Compared to a high-carbohydrate diet, the high-fat diet induced greater utilization of fat with an associated muscle glycogen sparing, but there was no significant improvement in the cycling time trial, even though performance following the high-fat phase was about 3.4 minutes faster. In a subsequent study using a similar protocol, Burke and her associates reported no significant effect on endurance performance.

In a similar vein, Rowlands and Hopkins compared the effects of three different 14-day dietary regimens on 100-kilometer cycling performance. One of the diets was high-carbohydrate, one was high-fat, and one was high-fat before 2.5 days of carbohydrate loading. Both high-fat diets increased fat oxidation during the cycling trial, and although there were no significant differences between the three trials, the 100-kilometer performance was approximately 3–4 percent faster with the high-fat diets. Interestingly, power output in the last 5 kilometers of the time trial was significantly greater for the high-fat with carbohydrate-loading trial as compared to the high-carbohydrate trial. The authors noted that although the main effects of the study were not significant, there was some evidence for enhanced ultraendurance cycling with a high-fat diet compared to a high-carbohydrate diet. Carey and others compared the effects of two 6-day diets, either high-carbohydrate or high-fat, on a prolonged cycling task involving

4 hours at 65 percent VO$_2$ peak followed by a 1-hour time trial. In both diets, a high-carbohydrate diet was consumed on the day prior to testing. Similar to other studies, the high-fat diet increased total fat oxidation and reduced carbohydrate oxidation, but there was no effect on cycling performance. However, the power output was 11 percent higher during the time trial after the high-fat diet as compared to the high-carbohydrate condition, but this difference was not statistically significant.

It is interesting to note that in three of these contemporary studies, although the chronic fat-loading protocol was not shown statistically to improve performance, the investigators did note that performance was generally improved compared to the other diets.

In a crossover design study, Holloway and others recently placed healthy men on 5-day diets of high fat (70 percent fat, 4 percent carbohydrates, and 26 percent protein) and a control (24 percent fat, 50 percent carbohydrates, and 26 percent protein). Men in the study ingested one diet and following a 2-week washout period consumed the other diet. The high-fat diet impaired cognitive function in the areas of attention, speed, and mood. A decrement in any one of these areas could affect an individual's ability to train and compete, particularly in activities that require an athlete to react to an opponent or conditions.

Reviews concluding an ergogenic effect Several reviewers from the same research group have concluded that chronic high-fat diets may enhance endurance performance. Venkatraman and others have noted that short-term, high-fat diets may improve endurance exercise performance at 60–80 percent VO$_2$ max in endurance cyclists and runners. Pendergast and others cited various studies indicating high-fat diets (42–55 percent of energy) that maintained adequate carbohydrate levels have shown increased endurance capacity in both men and women when compared with low-fat diets (10–15 percent of energy).

Reviews concluding no ergogenic effect Conversely, other reviewers concluded that chronic high-fat diets are not ergogenic. In her review, Bente Kiens noted that varying periods of fat adaptation followed by a carbohydrate-rich diet, despite an increased fat oxidation and a concomitant decrease in carbohydrate oxidation during submaximal exercise, exerts no beneficial effects on subsequent time trial endurance cycling performance.

In their review, Burke and Hawley indicated that endurance athletes who consume chronic high-fat diets, as compared to isocaloric high-carbohydrate diets, may increase fat oxidation and spare use of muscle glycogen during submaximal exercise. They noted that these effects persist even under conditions in which carbohydrate availability is increased, either by consuming a high-carbohydrate meal before exercise and/or ingesting glucose solutions during exercise. Yet, despite marked changes in the patterns of fuel utilization that favor fat oxidation, they conclude that this strategy does not provide clear benefits to the performance of prolonged endurance exercise. Helge reiterates the potential beneficial ergogenic effects of chronic high-fat diets, but indicates that overall the scientific evidence suggests that endurance performance can, at best, only be maintained on such diets when compared with carbohydrate-rich diets, and therefore long-term fat diet usage cannot

be recommended as a tool to improve endurance performance, a conclusion also supported by Hargreaves and others.

Given these studies and reviews, the findings appear to be equivocal but generally support the conclusion that chronic high-fat diets for 1–2 weeks are not ergogenic for endurance athletes. Nevertheless, if this dietary regimen could spare the use of muscle glycogen during exercise as noted in several studies, and if indeed muscle glycogen stores represent a limiting factor in the premature development of fatigue, then such a dietary strategy could possibly enhance endurance performance in events that may benefit from preservation of muscle glycogen.

A high-fat diet does not appear to be recommended on a long-term basis. One reason may be possible adverse health effects associated with such diets, as discussed later in this chapter, although athletes involved in intense training may not experience such adverse effects. Another reason may be the quality of training. Helge noted that optimal competitive performance is dependent on several factors, including the quality and quantity of training. Training may be compromised on a fat-rich diet as it compromises glycogen storage in both muscle and liver. Although Stepto and others found that endurance athletes could maintain levels of high-intensity training while adapting to a high-fat diet over a 3-day period, the training sessions were associated with increased ratings of perceived exertion when compared to training with a high-carbohydrate diet. Thus, such diets may make training more psychologically stressful.

Will fasting help improve my performance?

Sherman and Leenders indicate that fasting for 24 hours may increase the plasma FFA availability. Unfortunately, endurance exercise performance is usually impaired because fasting reduces muscle glycogen stores or induces hypoglycemia. For example, in one study, Gutierrez and others evaluated the effects of a 3-day fast on exercise performance in young men during training. The researchers reported a significantly decreased aerobic endurance physical working capacity based on heart rate responses to a cycling exercise protocol. Ferguson and others examined the impact of caloric restriction and an overnight fast on physiological responses to a cycling endurance task. Trained competitive cyclists were placed on a 3-week caloric restriction (60 percent of Calories for maintenance) with no change in their training routine. At the end of the 3 weeks, there was no impact on power output, heart rate, RER, or VO$_2$ during a 2-hour cycling endurance ride. The overall weight, fat weight, and body fat percentages decreased, which aided in an improved power-to-weight ratio. Because the 2-hour cycling ride was not a performance ride, it is not possible to determine the influence of the 3-week Calorie restriction on performance. Oliver and others reported impaired performance in a 30-minute treadmill run time trial following a 2-day modified fast in which subjects consumed less than 300 Calories per day. Fasting for several days may impair carbohydrate metabolism and is not a recommended procedure for aerobic endurance athletes. The effect of fasting on physical performance when athletes attempt to lose body weight for sport competition is covered in chapter 10.

Can the use of medium-chain triglycerides improve endurance performance?

Medium-chain triglycerides (MCTs) have been suggested to be ergogenic, possibly because they are water soluble, which may confer two advantages: they can be absorbed by the portal circulation and delivered directly to the liver instead of via the chylomicron route in the lymph and they more readily enter the mitochondria in the muscle cells as they do not need carnitine. MCTs have been marketed commercially. Research has shown that MCTs do not inhibit gastric emptying as common fat does and may be absorbed rapidly in the small intestine. Also, Massicotte and his associates reported that exogenous MCTs are oxidized at a rate comparable to exogenous glucose, being oxidized within the first 30 minutes of exercise. Researchers have investigated the ergogenic effect of MCT supplementation by itself and also combined with carbohydrate. Most studies provided the supplements just before and during the exercise task, but one study involved chronic supplementation.

Some early research found that MCT supplementation alone may actually impair endurance exercise performance, whereas an MCT-carbohydrate supplement might be ergogenic. Van Zyl and others, using endurance-trained cyclists, compared the effects of three supplements on an endurance performance task consisting of a 2-hour ride at 60 percent VO_2 max followed by a 40-kilometer performance ride. The three supplements, consumed throughout the performance task, were carbohydrate only, MCTs only, and carbohydrate with MCTs; the MCT dose was about 86 grams. Compared to the carbohydrate supplement, the MCT supplement actually impaired 40-kilometer performance, whereas the combination carbohydrate-MCT supplement improved performance. These investigators suggested that the carbohydrate-MCT supplement improved performance in the 40-kilometer performance ride by decreasing oxidation of muscle glycogen during the preliminary submaximal 2-hour ride, thus sparing the glycogen for the more intense exercise task.

However, most studies have not shown any beneficial effects of MCT supplementation, either alone or combined with carbohydrate, on endurance exercise performance. One such study was conducted by Goedecke and others, from Tim Noakes' laboratory in South Africa. Nine endurance-trained cyclists cycled for 2 hours at 63 percent of VO_2 peak, and then completed a 40-kilometer time trial under three conditions: glucose, glucose and low-dose MCTs, and glucose and high-dose MCTs, all in solution. The solutions were ingested immediately before and every 10 minutes during exercise. Although MCT ingestion increased serum FFA concentration, there were no beneficial effects on performance as compared to the glucose trial. In a well-designed crossover study, Angus and others compared the effects of carbohydrate to carbohydrate plus MCT on 100-kilometer cycling time trial in eight endurance-trained males. The beverages were provided during the trial at about every 15 minutes, and consisted of a 6 percent carbohydrate solution with and without a 4.2 percent MCT solution. Compared to the placebo trial, they found that the carbohydrate enhanced 100-kilometer cycling performance, but the addition

of MCT did not provide any further performance enhancement. In a similar study with ultraendurance athletes, but with carbohydrate or MCTs provided before an ultradistance ride, Goedecke and others reported that MCT supplementation actually impaired periodic sprint performance within the event. Using muscle biopsies, Horowitz and others have also shown that a carbohydrate-MCT solution does not spare muscle glycogen during high-intensity aerobic exercise.

Using a chronic MCT feeding protocol, Misell and others had 12 trained male endurance runners consume either corn oil (LCT) or MCT (60 grams) daily for 2 weeks. The runners then performed an endurance treadmill test consisting of a 30-minute run at 85 percent VO_2 max followed by a run to exhaustion at 75 percent VO_2 max. The investigators reported that chronic MCT consumption neither enhances endurance performance nor significantly alters exercise metabolism in trained male runners. In a review, Clegg concluded that medium-chain triglyceride supplementation is ineffective in improving exercise performance. However, medium-chain triglyceride feedings increase fat oxidation and energy expenditure. Clegg stated that future work should focus more on the potential health benefits rather than on the ergogenic benefits.

Is the glycerol portion of triglycerides an effective ergogenic aid?

As you may recall, glycerol is one of the by-products of triglyceride breakdown. Burelle and others have noted that exogenous glycerol can be oxidized during prolonged exercise, presumably following conversion into glucose in the liver. Thus, researchers theorized that it could be an efficient energy source during exercise. However, in well-controlled research, glycerol feedings did not prevent either hypoglycemia or muscle glycogen depletion patterns in several prolonged exercise tasks. Apparently the rate at which the human liver converts glycerol to glucose is not rapid enough to be an effective energy source during strenuous prolonged exercise. However, as noted in chapter 9, glycerol may be used to increase body water stores, including plasma volume, prior to exercise, and has been theorized to be ergogenic for endurance athletes performing under warm environmental conditions.

Are phospholipid dietary supplements effective ergogenic aids?

Lecithin Lecithin, also known as *phosphatidylcholine,* is a phospholipid that occurs naturally in a variety of foods, such as beans, eggs, and wheat germ. Because it is an important component of many types of human body tissues, contains choline needed for the synthesis of acetylcholine (an important neurotransmitter), and contains phosphorus, it has been theorized to be ergogenic in nature. Several German studies conducted more than 50 years ago reported increases in power and strength following several days of supplementation with 22–83 milligrams of lecithin. However, these early studies have been discredited because of poor experimental design. In a study with better experimental design, Staton reported that 30 grams of lecithin supplementation daily for 2 weeks had no effect upon grip strength.

Although lecithin does not appear to be an effective ergogenic aid, several of its constituents have been theorized to enhance exercise performance. Choline, an amine associated with vitamin-like activity, has been studied independently or as part of lecithin for potential ergogenic effects on endurance performance, and is discussed in chapter 7. Phosphate salts are covered in chapter 8.

Phosphatidylserine **Phosphatidylserine,** like phosphatidylcholine, is a naturally occurring phospholipid found in cell membranes. Food products that are good sources of phosphatidylserine include green leafy vegetables, rice, fish, and soybeans. Dietary supplements, some marketed as Phosphatidyl Serine, are derived primarily from soybeans and are marketed to improve brain health, claiming to be essential for normal functioning of neuronal cell membranes.

Several recent studies have evaluated the effect of phosphatidylserine supplementation on various responses to exercise and exercise performance. Kingsley notes that phosphatidylserine may serve as an antioxidant, which may help reduce muscle tissue damage. It also may help promote optimal balance of calcium and other minerals in the cell during exercise, which might influence exercise performance, because of its role in promoting transport of substances across cell membranes. Kingsley also notes early research indicating that oral supplementation with phosphatidylserine moderated exercise-induced changes in the hypothalamic-pituitary-adrenal axis, which could affect hormonal responses to exercise that may influence performance.

In one of the first studies, Kingsley and others provided male soccer players with 750 milligrams of soy phosphatidylserine daily for 10 days. The players engaged in intermittent exercise designed to simulate soccer match play, immediately followed by an exhaustive run. The supplement had no effect on muscle soreness or markers of muscle damage and lipid peroxidation following exhaustive running; however, supplementation tended to increase running time to exhaustion, but the difference between the treatment and placebo group was not statistically significant. In another study with a similar supplementation protocol, Kingsley and others reported no significant effect of phosphatidylserine supplementation on markers of muscle tissue damage, inflammation, and oxidative stress, or on delayed onset of muscle soreness following downhill running for nearly an hour.

Although phosphatidylserine supplementation appears to have little effect on reducing markers of muscle damage or soreness after severe exercise, Kingsley and others did find improved exercise performance in one study. Using a similar supplementation protocol (750 milligrams for 10 days), phosphatidylserine supplementation significantly increased cycling time to exhaustion at 85 percent VO_2 max, and the authors suggested that phosphatidylserine supplementation might possess ergogenic potential.

These findings are interesting, but research with phosphatidylserine supplementation and exercise performance is in its preliminary stages and additional research is merited.

Why are omega-3 fatty acids suggested to be ergogenic, and do they work?

Omega-3 fatty acids are theorized to be ergogenic, not because of their energy content, but because they may elicit favorable physiological effects relative to several types of physical performance. One theory is based on the finding that omega-3 fatty acids may be incorporated into the membrane of the red blood cell (RBC), making the RBC less viscous and less resistant to flow. Another theory is based on the role of certain by-products—the eicosanoids mentioned previously—whose production in the body cells is related to omega-3 fatty acid metabolism. In particular, two specific forms of the eicosanoids, prostaglandin E_1 (PGE_1) and prostaglandin I_2 (PGI_2), may elicit a vasodilation effect on the blood vessels. Walser and others noted that 6 weeks of EPA and DHA (total 5 g/d) supplementation enhances blood flow during exercise in healthy individuals. Theoretically, the less viscous RBC and the vasodilative effect should enhance blood flow, facilitating the delivery of blood and oxygen to the muscles during exercise, benefiting the endurance athlete. These prostaglandins may also stimulate the release of human growth hormone. The increased secretion of human growth hormone might stimulate muscle growth and benefit the strength/power athlete and may also facilitate recovery from intense exercise bouts.

Unfortunately, although the ergogenic potential of omega-3 fatty acids is an interesting hypothesis, there are few supportive scientific data. Results from well-controlled, peer-reviewed scientific research indicate that omega-3 fatty acids do not affect energy metabolism during exercise. For example, Bortolotti and others recently reported that supplementation with 7.2 grams of fish oil daily, containing 1.1 g/day eicosapentaenoic acid and 0.7 g/day docosahexaenoic acid, for 14 days exerted no effect on glucose or lipid energy metabolism during 30 minutes of cycling at 50 percent VO_2 max.

Research also indicates that omega-3 fatty acid supplementation has no effect on aerobic endurance performance. Buckley and others supplemented the diets of 25 professional Australian Football League players for 5 weeks in a randomized, double-blind study. The players were matched for performance of a 2,200-meter running time trial and provided either 6 × 1 gram capsules of either sunflower oil (placebo) or DHA-rich fish oil (1.56 grams DHA and 0.36 grams of eicosapentaenoic acid). At the end of the 5 weeks of supplementation, the fish oil group had lower serum triglycerides and lower heart rate during submaximal exercise. Buckley and others did not find improvements in endurance exercise performance, as determined by time to exhaustion, or recovery. In a slightly longer study, Peoples and colleagues supplemented the diets of 16 well-trained male cyclists for 8 weeks with either 8 × 1 grams of olive oil (control) or fish oil in a doubleblind, parallel design. The fish oil supplementation lowered heart rate during VO_2 peak testing and steady-state submaximal exercise, as well as whole-body oxygen consumption and rate pressure product. Time to voluntary fatigue was not influenced by fish oil supplementation.

As noted previously, some foods are rich in omega-3 fatty acids. Certain diet plans incorporate such foods, and one plan suggests that such a diet may enhance sport performance. In his best-selling book, *The Zone,* Barry Sears describes his diet plan for health and appearance, mainly weight loss. Basically the diet consists of a set ratio of Calories from carbohydrate (40 percent), fat (30 percent), and protein (30 percent), and is often referred to as the 40:30:30 diet. It is basically a low-carbohydrate, moderate-fat, and high-protein diet.

Sears suggests that certain fats in the "zone" diet may be of value to athletes, and part of the underlying theory may be the eicosanoid-generating fatty acids, particularly the omega-3 fatty acids. Indeed, some companies manufacture food products based on the 40:30:30 ratio and target them at the sport nutrition market. Sports bars including omega-3 fatty acids are one example. However, Cheuvront recently noted that the key eicosanoid reportedly produced in the "zone" diet and responsible for improved muscle oxygenation is not found in skeletal muscle. Several reports in swimming magazines indicated that such a diet was instrumental in the success of the Stanford University swim team, but the data presented were anecdotal rather than scientific. Cheuvront also indicated that based on the best available scientific evidence, the "zone" diet should be considered more ergolytic than ergogenic to performance. As this diet is primarily a high-protein diet, it will be discussed further in the next chapter.

At the present time, there do not appear to be sufficient data to support an ergogenic effect of omega-3 fatty acids. However, Mickleborough indicates that omega-3 fatty acids from fish oils may be helpful in decreasing exercise-induced asthma (EIA), possibly functioning as an anti-inflammatory compound to help prevent bronchoconstriction. If so, athletes with EIA could possibly benefit. Tartibian and colleagues examined the impact of omega-3 supplementation on the pulmonary function of young wrestlers. In this double-blind study, the wrestlers were randomly assigned to groups and provided either 1,000-mg omega-3 fatty acids or matched placebo capsules each day for 12 weeks. Incremental training took place for the subjects during this time. At the end of the experimental period, a significant positive effect on five measures of lung function was seen for those subjects receiving the supplement. Further research is required to examine the relationship between omega-3 supplementation and pulmonary function.

Can carnitine supplements enhance fat metabolism and physical performance?

Carnitine is a water-soluble, vitamin-like compound that facilitates the transport of long-chain fatty acids into the mitochondria. There are basically two forms of carnitine, L-carnitine and D-carnitine, but other forms are available, such as L-propionylcarnitine. L-carnitine is the physiologically active form in the body, so in the following discussion, carnitine will refer mostly to L-carnitine, but in some studies L-propionylcarnitine has been used.

Dietary Sources Carnitine was discovered in 1905 and was considered to be an essential vitamin (B_T) at one time; more recently Kelly labeled it a conditionally essential amino acid. Although Rebouche has indicated that carnitine is an extremely important catalyst for metabolic reactions in the muscle, carnitine is not an essential dietary nutrient because it may be formed in the liver from other nutrients—principally two amino acids, lysine and methionine. Also, carnitine is found in substantial amounts in animal foods. Meat products, particularly beef and pork, are good sources of carnitine; much less is found in fish and poultry, and even lower amounts in dairy products. Only minimal amounts of carnitine are found in fruits, vegetables, and grains. For example, for similar weights, beef has about 300 times as much carnitine as bread; 3 ounces of beef contains about 60 mg of carnitine. There is no RDA for carnitine. Most individuals consume enough carnitine in the daily diet, and the body also has an effective conservation system. The typical nonvegetarian diet provides about 100–300 milligrams per day. Carnitine deficiencies are very rare. Rebouche indicated that there is no evidence that carnitine deficiency occurs in the general population of strict vegetarians, whose diet generally provides a very minimal amount of carnitine.

Theory as an Ergogenic Aid Carnitine supplementation has been theorized to enhance physical performance because of several of its metabolic functions in the muscle cell. Approximately 90 percent of the body supply of carnitine is located in the muscle tissues where it is part of an enzyme (carnitine palmitoyl transferase) important for transport of long-chain fatty acids into the mitochondria for oxidation. Theoretically, supplemental carnitine might facilitate the transport of LCFAs into the mitochondria for oxidation, which would be an important consideration if the oxidation of fatty acids was limited by their transport into the mitochondria. Some research has reported an increase in respiratory chain enzymes in the mitochondria of long-distance runners following carnitine supplementation. Combining these two potential effects, carnitine would theoretically be beneficial for athletes in very prolonged endurance events by increasing the utilization of fatty acids during exercise and sparing the use of muscle glycogen. This is the primary theory underlying carnitine supplementation for endurance athletes. Stephens and others provide insights on the role of carnitine in the regulation of muscle energy metabolism related to exercise performance.

Given the theory of carnitine supplementation to increase fatty acid oxidation, Villani and others have noted that manufacturers marketed it as a weight-loss supplement, either alone or combined with exercise to facilitate fat burning. Inducing a loss of excess body fat could provide a mechanical edge to some athletes.

Carnitine plays other metabolic roles that have been theorized to be ergogenic. Wagenmakers notes that carnitine may facilitate the oxidation of pyruvate, which may possibly enhance the utilization of glucose and reduce the production of lactic acid during exercise, factors that may enhance performance in short-term maximal or supramaximal exercise, such as in a 400-meter or 800-meter run. Wagenmakers also notes that carnitine may increase blood flow both at rest and during exercise, which may enhance delivery of both oxygen and energy substrate to the muscle during exercise, a theoretical ergogenic effect independent of the role of carnitine in the muscle cells.

Conversely, Wagenmakers notes that carnitine may expedite the oxidation of branched-chain amino acids (BCAAs), leading to a series of biochemical reactions that could lead to premature fatigue, an ergolytic rather than ergogenic effect.

Carnitine supplementation, particularly L-propionylcarnitine, has been used effectively to improve exercise capability in patients with serious diseases. After carnitine supplementation for several weeks, patients with peripheral vascular disease increased their walking distance before experiencing pain. Several studies have also reported improved exercise capacity in patients with heart and end-stage renal disease following carnitine supplementation. In a review, Kraemer and others indicated that improvements in exercise performance and recovery may be seen in individuals with specific disorders, such as congestive heart failure, peripheral artery disease, chronic stable angina, and chronic obstructive pulmonary disease, when taking L-carnitine.

Effects on Performance   Although these are logical theories and interesting medical applications, the available scientific evidence is somewhat equivocal, and in general does not appear to support an ergogenic effect of carnitine supplementation. Major reviews regarding the effect of carnitine supplementation on physical performance have been published, and the following are the key points regarding the ergogenic effects of carnitine supplementation emanating from these reviews and studies:

1. Supplementation will increase plasma levels of carnitine, but much of this will be excreted by the kidneys. However, although some previous research has suggested that carnitine supplementation could increase muscle carnitine levels, in his review Wagenmakers concluded that carnitine supplements do not increase muscle carnitine concentration. He based this conclusion on research using direct measurements in muscle showing no changes in muscle carnitine concentration after 14 days of supplementation with 4–6 grams of carnitine per day. Most recently, Wacher and others reported no increased muscle carnitine content following supplementation with 4 grams of L-carnitine daily for 3 months. Stephens and others note that it is doubtful that oral supplementation, or even intravenous infusion, of carnitine will increase muscle carnitine levels. However, they did note that inducing physiologically high levels of serum insulin may help increase transport of carnitine into the muscle.

2. The primary theory underlying carnitine supplementation is enhanced fat utilization. However, research by Abramowicz and Galloway, Broad, Decombaz and Vukovich, along with their colleagues, reported no effect of chronic carnitine supplementation on fat oxidation or muscle glycogen sparing under exercise conditions maximizing fatty acid oxidation.

3. Acute supplementation does not appear to enhance performance. Stuessi and others reported that supplementation with 2 grams of L-carnitine 2 hours before cycling to exhaustion at the anaerobic threshold had no effect on performance, and no effect also when the exercise test was repeated 3 hours later. Such short-term supplementation may not be adequate to increase muscle levels of carnitine.

4. Chronic supplementation, with as much as 6 grams per day for 7 days, has no effect on lactic acid accumulation during high-intensity anaerobic exercise, nor does it increase performance in such exercise tasks. For example, Trappe and others reported no effect of carnitine supplementation on performance in five repeat 100-yard swims with a 2-minute recovery.

5. Well-controlled studies, and the conclusions of most reviewers, indicated that chronic carnitine supplementation has no effect on VO_2 max or aerobic endurance. The effects of chronic carnitine supplementation on very prolonged aerobic endurance performance have not been studied extensively, but those data that are available, such as the effect on a 70-minute cycling task, cycling to exhaustion at 60 percent of maximal workload, performing a 20-kilometer cycling time trial following 90 minutes of steady-state cycling, and a 5-kilometer run, have shown no beneficial effect. There are no scientific data showing a beneficial effect of chronic carnitine supplementation on very prolonged aerobic endurance tasks, such as a marathon.

6. Preliminary data, from William Kraemer's research group at the University of Connecticut, suggest that combining carnitine with tartrate may have some beneficial effects for individuals engaged in resistance training. Tartrate, a salt, possesses antioxidant properties. Spiering and others reported that carnitine supplementation, either 1- or 2-gram doses for 3 weeks, reduced markers of metabolic stress and perceived muscle soreness following a resistance training workout. Kraemer and others noted that carnitine/tartrate supplementation may increase responses of androgenic receptors that help muscle formation, which they suggest may help promote recovery from resistance exercise. These preliminary findings are interesting and merit additional research, possibly evaluating the effects of carnitine and tartrate separately.

7. Carnitine supplementation has not been shown to reduce body fat in obese individuals, and thus would not appear to be effective in athletes either.

8. D-carnitine may be toxic, as it can deplete L-carnitine, leading to a carnitine deficiency. L-carnitine appears to be a safe supplement, but some reviewers recommend no more than 2–5 grams per day, possibly for only one month at a time.

For a detailed review of carnitine metabolism and its potential ergogenic effect, the interested reader is referred to the excellent critiques by Brass, Heinonen, Kelly, and Wagenmakers. Although interpretation of the scientific data regarding the ergogenic value of carnitine supplementation may vary somewhat, Brass indicates that there is no compelling evidence that carnitine supplementation can improve physical performance in healthy subjects. He does note, however, that additional research is needed because although the data do not allow a conclusion to be drawn that carnitine is beneficial, the negative has not been proven either. The review by Stephens and others suggests that if muscle carnitine levels are elevated, there may be some effects beneficial to exercise performance. The problem is finding a practical means by which the typical athlete may increase muscle carnitine content.

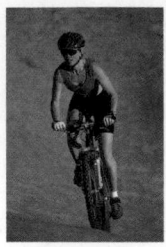

Can hydroxycitrate (HCA) enhance endurance performance?

Hydroxycitric acid is derived from a tropical fruit and marketed as a dietary supplement, hydroxycitrate (HCA). Kriketos and others noted that as a competitive inhibitor of citrate lysase, HCA has been hypothesized to modify citric acid cycle metabolism to promote fatty acid oxidation. Although some studies with mice suggest that HCA supplementation may enhance endurance performance, human studies do not support such an ergogenic effect.

Kriketos and others, in an excellent crossover study, reported no significant effect of HCA supplementation (3.0 grams/day for 3 days) on blood serum energy substrates, fat metabolism, or energy expenditure either during rest or during moderately intense exercise. However, the subjects were sedentary males. Using endurance-trained cyclists as subjects, van Loon and others evaluated the effect of HCA supplementation (3.1 ml/kilogram body mass of a 19 percent HCA solution) given twice to the cyclists before and during 2 hours of cycling at 50 percent VO_2 max. They concluded that HCA supplementation, even in large quantities, does not increase total fat oxidation in endurance-trained cyclists.

Thus, the available evidence indicates that HCA supplementation does not modify fat utilization during exercise, much less confer an ergogenic effect.

Can conjugated linoleic acid (CLA) enhance exercise performance?

Conjugated linoleic acid (CLA) has been marketed as a sports dietary supplement to resistance-trained individuals, mainly as a means to promote weight loss and to gain muscle mass. For similar and other reasons, CLA also has been marketed as a means to improve health.

Research regarding its ergogenic effect on exercise-trained individuals is very limited. Using resistance-trained athletes as subjects, Kreider and others investigated the effect of CLA supplementation (6 grams prescribed daily dose; 28 days) on body composition and muscular strength, and reported no significant effects on total body mass, fat mass, fat-free mass, or strength as measured by a single maximal repetition in the bench press and leg press. Pinkoski and others, in a crossover design, also found that CLA supplementation (5 grams daily for 7 weeks) resulted in minimal changes in body composition and no changes in the strength tests in males and females involved in resistance training. However, in the first phase of the study, which did not involve a crossover design, male subjects receiving CLA experienced significant increases in bench press strength compared to the placebo group. The crossover phase of the study, as the authors note, is a stronger experimental design.

According to Campbell and Kreider's review, very few studies have been conducted on CLA and its effect on performance. Presently, adverse reactions to CLA supplementation are mild, with gastrointestinal distress being most commonly reported. Based on limited research, CLA supplementation does not currently appear to

be an effective ergogenic aid for trained individuals, but confirming research is needed. Its role in health is discussed later in this chapter.

What's the bottom line regarding the ergogenic effects of fat burning diets or strategies?

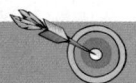

As noted in this section, numerous fat burning strategies have been employed in attempts to enhance prolonged endurance exercise performance. Theoretically, such strategies would increase the oxidation of fat, decrease the utilization of carbohydrate, and thus spare some muscle glycogen for use in the later stages of exercise. As muscle glycogen is a more efficient fuel compared to fats, performance should be enhanced.

However, John Hawley, an international sports science scholar, reviewed all such fat burning strategies and concluded that endurance exercise capacity is not systematically improved with increases in serum FFA availability, even in some studies with substantial muscle glycogen sparing. He noted that for some reason, exercise capacity is remarkably resistant to change. Other studies suggest that high-fat diets may impair performance in some events, such as high-intensity surges during a race or sprints to the finish. Moreover, individuals may find that it may be difficult to adhere to a high-fat diet.

In its booklet promoting optimal dietary intake for athletes, the U.S. Anti-Doping Agency indicates that although fat is a valuable metabolic fuel for muscles during endurance exercise and performs many important functions in the body, no attempt should be made to consume more fat. The USADA recommends that the diet of athletes should contain about 20–30 percent of Calories as fat, and note that athletes who consume high-fat diets typically consume fewer Calories from carbohydrates. As noted in chapter 4, carbohydrate replacement is important in the recovery period during intense exercise training. Although fat is used during exercise, Spriet notes that there appears to be no need for rapid fat replacement after exercise. Carbohydrate is more important; fat can be ingested in later meals.

Key Concepts

▶ Fat-loading practices, either acute or chronic, may increase utilization of fat during endurance exercise, but do not appear to enhance exercise or sport performance. Chronic high-fat diets may increase the psychological stress of exercise training.

▶ Medium-chain triglyceride (MCT) supplementation does not improve, and may impair, endurance exercise performance. Consuming an MCT-carbohydrate solution provides no additional benefits compared to a carbohydrate solution alone.

▶ Carnitine supplementation does not appear to increase muscle carnitine content, does not affect oxidation of fat during exercise, and does not enhance endurance exercise performance.

▶ In general, various dietary strategies and dietary supplements theorized to increase oxidation of fat during exercise and enhance prolonged aerobic endurance performance have not been shown to be effective ergogenic aids.

Dietary Fats and Cholesterol: Health Implications

As noted in previous chapters, the etiology of chronic diseases such as cancer and coronary heart disease is complex and involves multiple risk factors. Eliminating or reducing as many risk factors as possible is the best approach to optimize your health. Your diet is one of the most important risk factors that can be modified to promote good health, particularly the amount and composition of fat you eat. Every few years the American Dietetic Association provides a review of the evidence regarding various dietary practices and effects on cardiovascular disease, the most recent being the review by Van Horn and others. In this section we shall focus on the role of dietary fat in the etiology of coronary heart disease (CHD), and in chapter 10 we will discuss the possible role of dietary fat in obesity and related health problems, such as diabetes, high blood pressure, and various forms of cancer.

CHD is still the number one cause of death in industrialized nations. In its recommendations regarding dietary fat, the National Academy of Sciences indicated that although very-high fat diets may predispose to CHD, so too may very-low-fat diets. For example, Siri and Krauss reported that increased dietary carbohydrates, particularly simple sugars and starches with high glycemic index, can modify the serum lipid profile in ways that may also be conducive to CHD. Lipid expert Penny Kris-Etherton and her associates recently noted that the main message regarding dietary fat is very simple: Avoid diets that are *very low* and *very high* in fat. The guiding principle is that moderation in total fat is the defining benchmark for a contemporary diet that reduces risk of chronic disease. Moreover, within the range of a moderate-fat diet, it is still important to individualize the total fat prescription. Fats are not all equal. Some are better for your health than others, and, as noted, the terms *good* and *bad* fats have been popularized. Remember, however, that even some *bad* fats can fit into a healthy diet. The key is moderation.

Because the available evidence relating dietary lipids to cardiovascular disease is so compelling, we shall treat this subject in some detail. However, note that the dietary and exercise recommendations advanced later in this chapter for the prevention of cardiovascular disease may also help prevent other chronic diseases, such as obesity and certain forms of cancer.

How does cardiovascular disease develop?

Nearly one out of every two deaths in the United States is due to diseases of the heart and blood vessels. Each year, approximately one million Americans die from some form of cardiovascular disease, including coronary heart disease, stroke, hypertensive disease, rheumatic heart disease, and congenital heart disease.

Coronary heart disease is the major disease of the cardiovascular system; of the million deaths noted previously, it is responsible for more than half. Although the total percentage of deaths due to coronary heart disease has been declining in recent years, it is still an epidemic and the number one cause of death among both males and females.

Coronary heart disease (CHD) is also known as **coronary artery disease (CAD)** because obstruction of the blood flow in the coronary arteries is responsible for the pathological effects of the disease. The coronary arteries, which nourish the heart muscle, are illustrated in figure 5.12. The major manifestation of CHD is a heart attack, which results from a stoppage of blood flow to parts of the heart muscle. A decreased blood supply, known as **ischemia,** will deprive the heart of needed oxygen. In some individuals, ischemia results in **angina,** a sharp pain in the chest, jaw, or along the inside of the arm indicative of a mild heart attack. Other terms often associated with a heart attack include **coronary thrombosis,** a blockage of a blood vessel by a clot (thrombus); **coronary occlusion,** which simply means blockage; and **myocardial infarct,** death of heart cells that do not get enough oxygen due to the blocked coronary artery. The major cause of blocked arteries is atherosclerosis.

Arteriosclerosis is a term applied to a number of different pathological conditions wherein the arterial walls thicken and lose their elasticity. It is often defined as hardening of the arteries. **Atherosclerosis,** one form of arteriosclerosis, is characterized by the formation of **plaque,** an accumulation of fatty acids, oxidized LDL cholesterol, macrophages (white blood cells that oxidize LDL), foam cells (macrophages that consume cholesterol), cytokines (immune system mediators of inflammation), cellular debris, fibrin, and calcium on the inner lining of the coronary artery wall. A cap of smooth muscle cells forms around the plaque to prevent contact with the arterial wall. Figure 5.13 presents a schematic of the content of arterial plaque.

Inflammatory processes precipitated by cytokines are now recognized to play a central role in the pathogenesis of atherosclerosis by interacting with serum cholesterol and serving as an initiating factor in plaque buildup. As the plaque accumulates, the diameter of the artery is diminished, decreasing blood flow to the heart muscle. Foam cells continue to accumulate, becoming a major component of plaque. The foam cells secrete a substance that can weaken the muscle cap. If the muscle cap ruptures, plaque will leak into the bloodstream and trigger the formation of a clot, which partially or completely blocks blood flow to a section of heart muscle, leading to death of cardiac cells due to inadequate oxygen and nutrients. The process is depicted in figure 5.14.

Atherosclerosis is a slow, progressive disease that begins in childhood and usually manifests itself later in life. Because of its prevalence in industrialized society, scientists throughout the world have been conducting intensive research to identify the cause or causes of atherosclerosis and coronary heart disease. The actual cause has not yet been completely identified, but considerable evidence has identified factors that may predispose an individual.

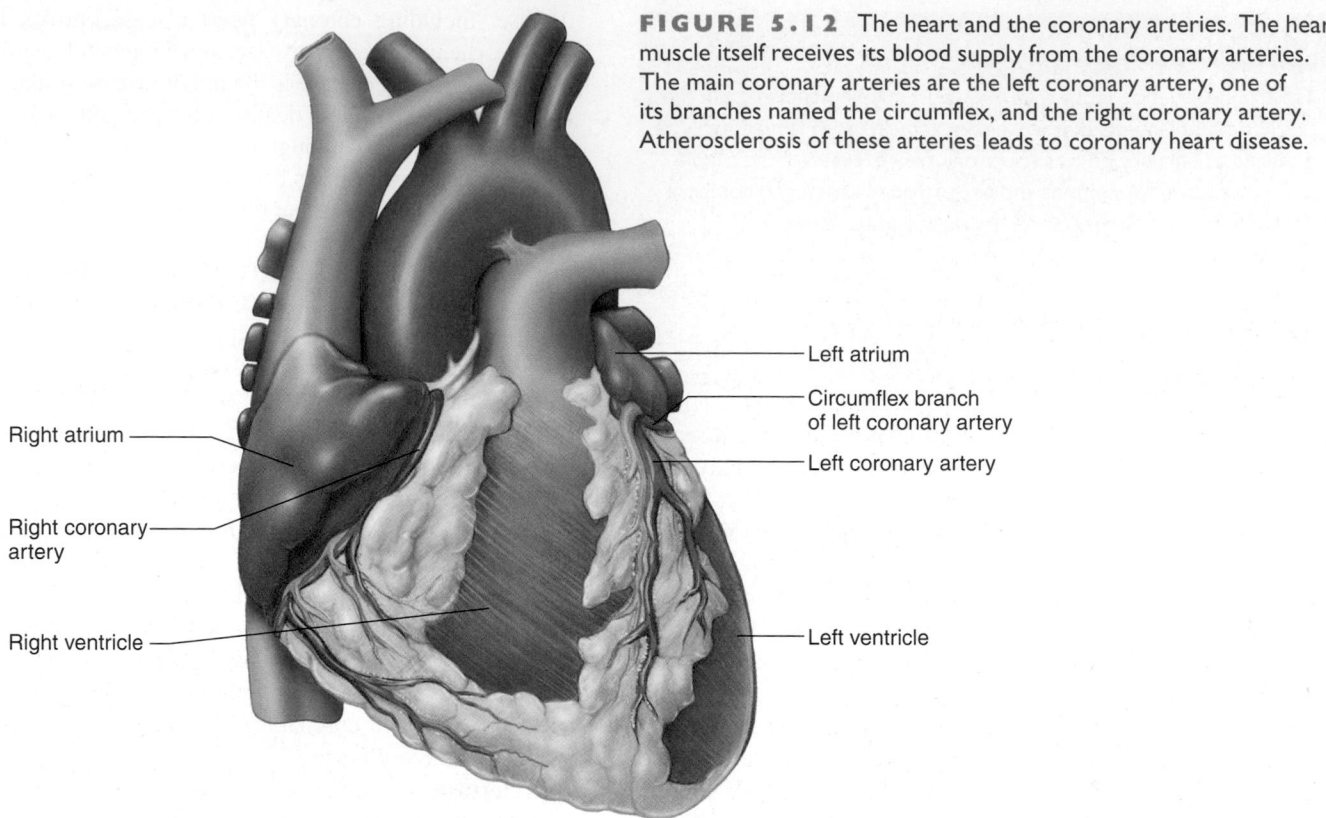

FIGURE 5.12 The heart and the coronary arteries. The heart muscle itself receives its blood supply from the coronary arteries. The main coronary arteries are the left coronary artery, one of its branches named the circumflex, and the right coronary artery. Atherosclerosis of these arteries leads to coronary heart disease.

Left atrium

Circumflex branch of left coronary artery

Left coronary artery

Right atrium

Right coronary artery

Left ventricle

Right ventricle

As noted previously, a risk factor represents a statistical relationship between two items such as high serum cholesterol and heart attack. This does not mean that a cause-and-effect relationship exists, although such a relationship is often strongly supported by the available evidence. The three principal risk factors associated with CHD are high blood pressure, high serum cholesterol levels, and cigarette smoking. Several major professional and governmental health organizations also believe that physical inactivity is a fourth principal risk factor. Other interacting risk factors are heredity, diabetes, diet, obesity, age, gender, and stress. Elevated blood levels of homocysteine and C-reactive protein (CRP) have been associated with CHD, and their role as risk factors continues to be studied. Homocysteine is discussed in chapter 7. CRP is a marker for inflammation.

www.americanheart.org/riskassessment Use this questionnaire to assess your risk of developing coronary heart disease. Knowing your cholesterol levels and blood pressure is helpful, but not required. Some information about risk factors is also presented.

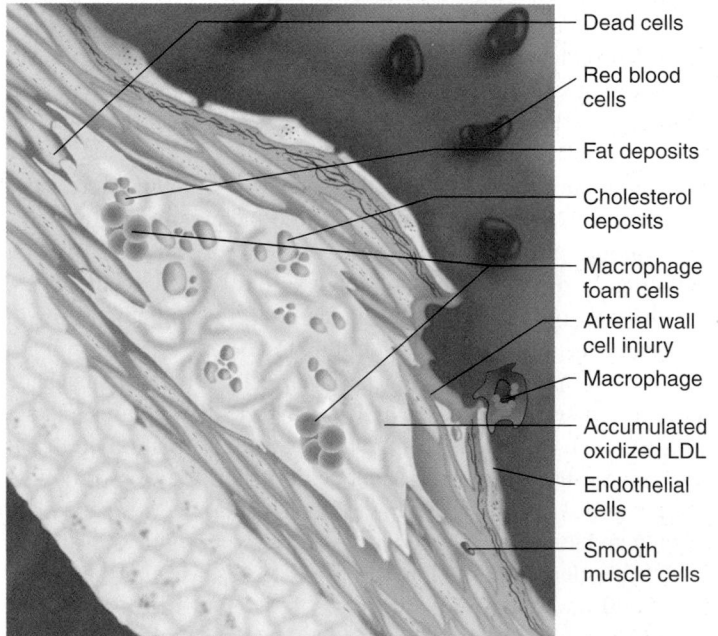

Dead cells

Red blood cells

Fat deposits

Cholesterol deposits

Macrophage foam cells

Arterial wall cell injury

Macrophage

Accumulated oxidized LDL

Endothelial cells

Smooth muscle cells

FIGURE 5.13 An enlargement of atherosclerotic plaque. Oxidized LDL cholesterol, macrophages, foam cells, fibrous material, and other debris collect beneath the endothelial cells lining the coronary artery. The site of the plaque may be initiated by some form of injury to the cell lining, possibly an ulceration as shown.

How do the different forms of serum lipids affect the development of atherosclerosis?

In atherosclerosis, the plaque that develops in the arterial walls is composed partly of fats and cholesterol. Hence, high levels of blood lipids (triglycerides and cholesterol) are associated with increased plaque formation. However, as you recall, triglycerides and cholesterol may be transported in the blood in a variety of

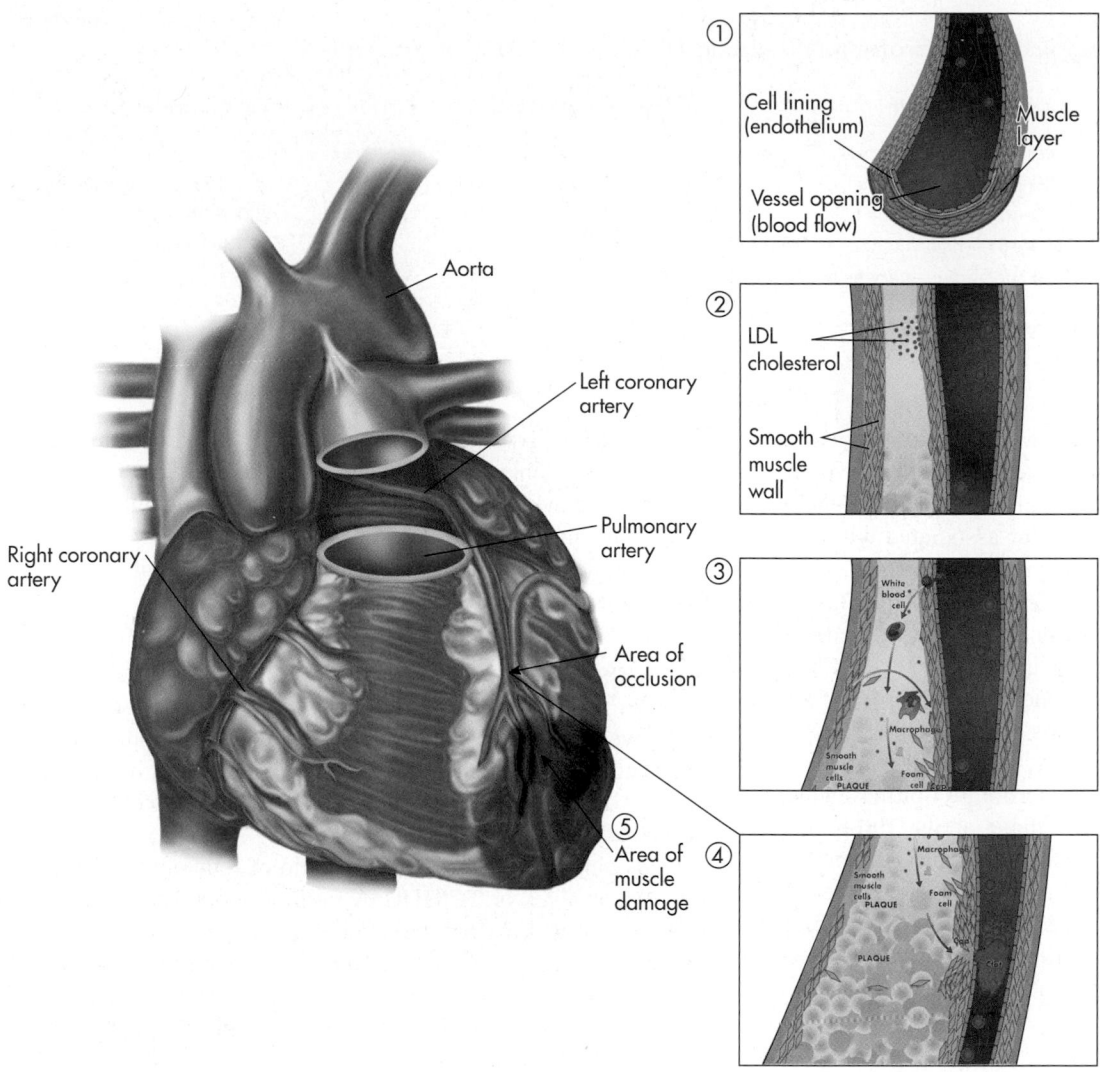

FIGURE 5.14 The developmental process of atherosclerosis and thrombosis. (1) Normal coronary artery (2) LDL-cholesterol seeps through the endothelium into the smooth muscle wall (3) Immune system responds, sending macrophages (white blood cells) to ingest the LDL-cholesterol; macrophages become foam cells, a major component of plaque; a smooth muscle cap forms to protect the endothelium (4) Foam cells accumulate secreting a substance that weakens the cap; the cap ruptures, plaque leaks into the blood stream triggering clot formation (5) Blocked artery leads to a decrease or cessation of blood flow to a section of heart tissue, leading to heart attack which may be mild or fatal depending on the severity of the blockage.

ways, but primarily as constituents of lipoproteins. Considerable research has been devoted to identifying those specific lipoproteins and other lipid components that may predispose to CHD, and although there is some debate about the meaningfulness of specific serum lipid profiles, some theories prevail.

The four main serum lipid factors associated with increased risk of atherosclerosis are total cholesterol, LDL-cholesterol, HDL-cholesterol, and triglycerides. The guidelines for the fasting blood serum level profile recommended by the National Cholesterol Education Program are presented in table 5.7.

Serum lipid levels are normally given in milligrams per deciliter (mg/dL), as shown in table 5.7. A deciliter is 100 milliliters. However, you may see cholesterol and triglyceride levels expressed as millimole per liter (mmol/L). To convert mmol/L of cholesterol to mg/dL, simply multiply mmol/L by 38.67. This applies to total cholesterol as well as LDL- and HDL-cholesterol.

Example: Total cholesterol = 7.5 mmol/L

7.5 mmol/L × 38.67 = 290 mg/dL

To convert mmol/L of triglycerides to mg/dL, simply multiply by 88.57.

Example: Serum triglycerides = 1.5 mmol/L

1.5 × 88.57 = 132.9 mg/dL

To convert in the opposite direction, from mg/dL to mmol/L, simply divide mg/dL by the appropriate numerical factor for cholesterol or triglycerides.

Total Cholesterol   The major villain appears to be serum cholesterol. Total cholesterol, expressed in milligrams per 100 milliliters of blood (mg/dL), is a significant risk factor. As noted in table 5.7, a cholesterol level below 200 is considered to be desirable, between 200 and 239 is borderline-high, and above 240 is high. However, you should be aware that there is a rather large standard error of measurement involved in some tests of cholesterol, being on the order of 30 milligrams. What this means is that if your blood cholesterol is reported as 220 (borderline-high), it may be possible that you actually have a cholesterol level of 190 (desirable) or 250 (high) if you vary, respectively, one standard error below or above your actual measurement of 220. For this reason, it may be a good idea to have a second test completed if you are concerned with your total cholesterol level.

TABLE 5.7 Recommended fasting lipoprotein profile* of the National Cholesterol Education Program

Total cholesterol	LDL-cholesterol	HDL-cholesterol	Triglycerides
Less than 200—desirable	Less than 100—optimal	Less than 40—low	Less than 150—normal
200–239—borderline high	100–129—near optimal	60 or above—protective	151–199—borderline high
240 or above—high	130–159—borderline high		200–499—high
	160–189—high		500 and above—very high
	190 and above—very high		

*Fasting levels expressed in mg/dL; testing recommended every 5 years for those over 20

LDL-Cholesterol The form by which cholesterol is transported in your blood may also be related to the development of atherosclerosis. In general, a high level of low-density lipoproteins (LDL) is the major risk factor associated with atherosclerosis. A current theory suggests various forms of LDL, such as small, dense LDL and the variant lipoprotein (a), may be more prone to oxidation by macrophages at an injured site in the arterial epithelium, leading to an influx into the cell wall and the formation of plaque. The presence of oxygen free radicals has been suggested to accelerate this process. Other mechanisms, such as increased clotting ability, may be operative. As noted in table 5.7, LDL levels less than 100 are optimal, while those above 160 pose a high risk and those above 190 a very high risk. Although not normally listed in risk factor tables, lipoprotein (a) values greater than 25–30 milligrams per deciliter of blood are associated with increased risk of CHD. A high level of IDL (which some consider a form of LDL) is also recognized as a risk factor, as is apolipoprotein B, involved in cholesterol transport to the tissues.

HDL-Cholesterol Conversely, high levels of high-density lipoproteins (HDL), particularly the subfraction HDL_2 and HDL with apolipoprotein A-I, appear to be protective against the development of atherosclerosis, although research is continuing to explore other relationships. Levels of 60 milligrams or more of HDL appear to be protective, but because HDL varies daily, several measurements over time may be required to obtain an accurate reading. Research suggests that HDL interacts with the arterial epithelium, acting as a scavenger by picking up cholesterol from the arterial wall and transporting it to the liver for removal from the body, known as *reverse cholesterol transport*. HDL may also inhibit LDL oxidation and platelet aggregation. HDL_2 levels are higher in women until menopause, and then decrease, with an associated increased risk for CHD.

Triglycerides Jacobson and others noted that elevated triglyceride levels may be a significant independent risk factor for coronary heart disease. Also, it is often associated with increased levels of LDL, particularly the small, dense LDL, and decreased levels of HDL. Current guidelines from the National Cholesterol Education Program (NCEP) indicate that triglyceride levels below 150 milligrams per deciliter are normal, whereas the risk associated

with progressively increasing levels goes from borderline high to very high (see table 5.7). Jacobson and others indicate increasing concern over the increasing rate of hypertriglyceridemia, which is associated with overweight and obesity.

A summary of serum lipid factors associated with increased risk of atherosclerosis is presented in table 5.8.

Cholesterol Ratios and Other Tests If your total blood cholesterol is borderline or high, a determination of the LDL and HDL levels may be desirable, for they provide additional information relative to your risk. Based on epidemiological data, several ratios have been developed to assess risk of CHD, with the lower the ratio, the lower the risk.

One common comparison is the ratio of total cholesterol (TC) to the HDL level, or TC/HDL. A ratio of about 4.5 is associated with an average risk for CHD. For example, an individual with a total cholesterol of 200 and an HDL of 60 would have a ratio of 3.33 (200/60), or a lower risk, while someone with the same total cholesterol but an HDL of 20 would have a much higher risk with a ratio of 10 (200/20).

Another comparison is the ratio of LDL to HDL, or LDL/HDL. An LDL to HDL ratio of about 3.5 is considered to be an average risk for CHD. Thus, a ratio of 140/60, or 2.3, would be a much lower risk than 140/20, or 7.0.

Additional tests are merited for those at high risk for CHD. Special lipoprotein tests may measure density levels of the various lipoproteins. Tests for other markers of atherosclerosis, such as homocysteine and CRP, will add to the

TABLE 5.8 Serum lipid factors associated with increased risk of atherosclerosis

High levels of total cholesterol
High levels of LDL-cholesterol
High levels of dense form of LDL-cholesterol
High levels of IDL-cholesterol
High levels of abnormal lipoprotein, lipoprotein (a)
High levels of apolipoprotein B
High levels of triglycerides
Low levels of HDL-cholesterol
Low levels of HDL_2-cholesterol
Low levels of apolipoprotein A-I

diagnosis. For example, Ridker and others noted that high CRP levels may be more effective predictors of heart attacks than high LDL-cholesterol levels, but the greatest risk is when both are high.

http://hp2010.nhlbihin.net/atpiii/calculator.asp If you know your total and HDL-cholesterol levels, as well as your systolic blood pressure, you may check your risk of having a heart attack in the next 10 years.

Can I reduce my serum lipid levels and possibly reverse atherosclerosis?

Lowering your serum cholesterol, particularly your LDL-cholesterol, is a very effective means to help prevent CHD. LaRosa indicated that for each 1 percent reduction in LDL-cholesterol, there is a corresponding 1 percent reduction in coronary heart disease risk. Several approaches may help you improve your serum lipid levels and reduce the risk of atherosclerosis. A healthy lifestyle is one, and appropriate drug therapy is another. However, even with a healthy lifestyle some individuals may have poor serum lipid profiles. Certain forms of hypercholesteremia are genetic in nature. In the future, gene therapy may be the treatment of choice for such individuals, possibly manipulating genes to decrease LDL and increase HDL.

Currently, drug therapy may be required to reduce serum lipid levels in genetically predisposed individuals, as well as in those with poor diets. Some drugs stimulate liver degradation and excretion of cholesterol, others increase lipoprotein lipase activity or LDL receptor function to decrease serum triglyceride levels, while still others may bind with bile salts in the intestines so that they are not reabsorbed; because bile salts are derived from cholesterol, it is effectively excreted from the body. Statins, drugs that inhibit an enzyme (HMG-CoA reductase) that regulates cholesterol, have been particularly effective to reduce serum LDL-cholesterol. For more detail on current and proposed medicinal means to help lower serum lipids, the interested reader is referred to the review by Jain.

The National Cholesterol Education Program indicated that individuals at high risk for cardiovascular disease might consider getting their LDL levels as low as possible and could explore with their doctor the possibility of taking lipid-lowering drugs; table 5.9 provides some guidelines. However, even if on drug therapy, individuals should not abandon a healthy lifestyle.

Adopting a healthier lifestyle is the first step in attempts to improve one's serum lipid profile. A healthy lifestyle may not only help to prevent the development of atherosclerosis, but may also lead to regression of coronary artery blockage. In their review, Greg Brown and others noted that the available data support the hypothesis that lowering of serum lipids may lead to the regression of atherosclerotic lesions and elicit improved clinical effects. For those who are interested in preventing the development of atherosclerosis or reversing its progress, an appropriate diet and exercise program, as discussed below, are two key elements of a healthy lifestyle that are recommended by health professionals. Both factors may have favorable effects not only on serum lipid levels, but on other risk factors for CHD as well, such as obesity and hypertension.

What should I eat to modify my serum lipid profile favorably?

The National Cholesterol Education Program (NCEP) was developed with the general goal of reducing the prevalence of high serum cholesterol in the United States. One of the first steps is to identify those individuals with high serum cholesterol by various simplified screening techniques, such as the measurement of total cholesterol by small samples of blood obtained through fingertip capillary blood. If this measure is borderline-high (200–239 mg/dL) or high (> 240 mg/dL), venous blood samples may be taken to determine LDL and HDL levels. If high serum cholesterol levels are detected, dietary modifications and other appropriate lifestyle changes may be recommended.

Figure 5.15 illustrates the composition of the average American diet and the Step 1 diet of the NCEP. Although the differences between the two diets appear to be small, such changes may

TABLE 5.9 National serum cholesterol guidelines

Risk category	Heart disease risk factors	Target LDL in milligrams/deciliter	Take drugs if LDL is
Low	Those with zero or one heart disease risk factor	Less than 160	190 or higher
Moderate	Those with two or more risk factors and less than a 10% to 20% risk of heart attack within 10 years	Less than 130	160 or higher
Moderately High	Those with two or more risk factors and a 10% to 20% risk of heart attack within 10 years	Less than 130 (optional goal 100)	130 or higher
High	Those who have heart disease or diabetes, or have two or more risk factors that give them greater than a 20% chance of a heart attack within 10 years	Less than 100 (optional goal 70)	100 or higher

Source: National Cholesterol Education Program Guidelines

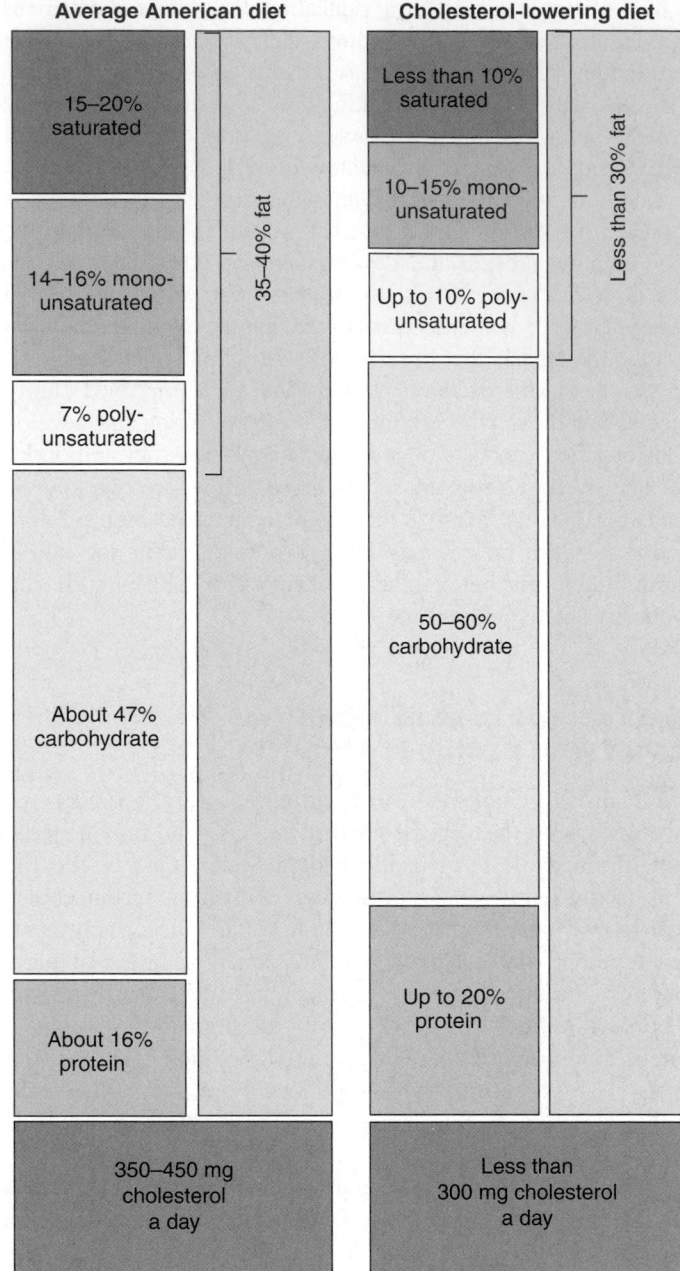

FIGURE 5.15 Comparison of the composition of the average American diet to the National Cholesterol Education Program Step 1 cholesterol-lowering diet.

Source: U.S. Department of Health and Human Services.

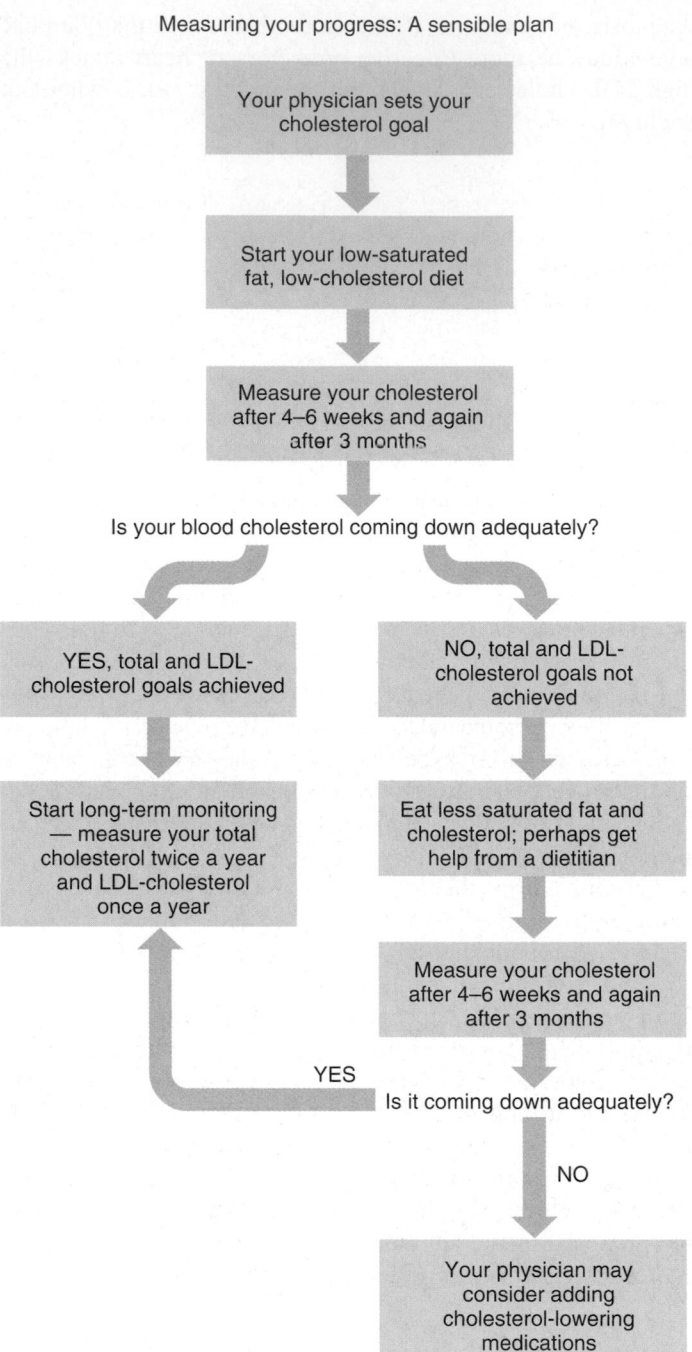

FIGURE 5.16 A sensible plan to monitor the effects of a cholesterol-lowering diet. The initial diet plan may involve the National Cholesterol Education Program Step 1 diet, but if unsuccessful, the Step 2 diet may be implemented. In individuals highly resistant to dietary modifications, drug therapy may be prescribed.

Source: U.S. Department of Health and Human Services.

reduce serum lipids. A sensible plan to reduce serum lipid levels is presented in figure 5.16, and representative results are shown in figure 5.17. If the original dietary plan is not effective after several months, the Step 2 NCEP diet may be recommended, which is essentially the same as the Step 1 diet but with less than 7 percent of the dietary Calories from saturated fat and less than 200 milligrams of cholesterol per day. Two meta-analyses revealed that the NCEP diet plan significantly decreased total blood cholesterol, and may have multiple beneficial effects on major cardiovascular risk factors.

Several health organizations, including the American Heart Association, the National Institutes of Health, and the National Heart, Lung, and Blood Institute, have recommended a number of dietary guidelines that have been shown to lower serum cholesterol or serum triglycerides. Moreover, recent studies using

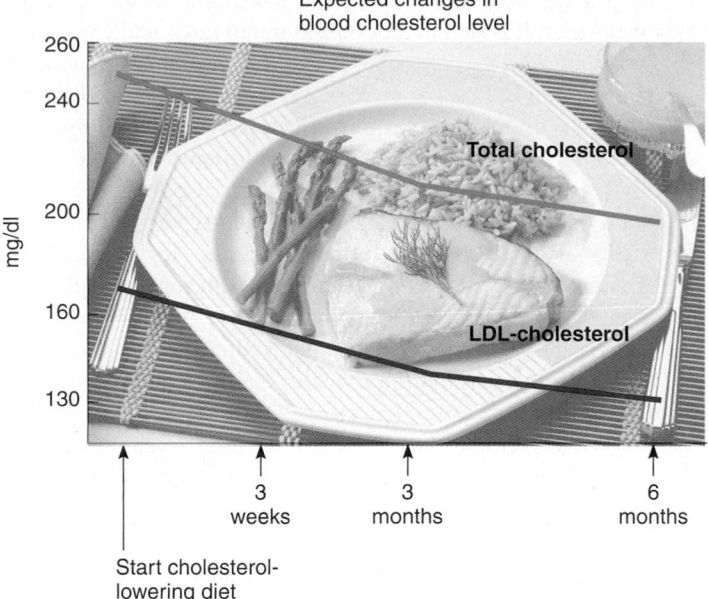

Expected changes in blood cholesterol level

260
240
200
160
130

mg/dl

Total cholesterol

LDL-cholesterol

3 weeks 3 months 6 months

Start cholesterol-lowering diet

FIGURE 5.17 Representative expected changes in total serum cholesterol and LDL-cholesterol associated with appropriate dietary modifications, such as switching from the typical American diet to the Step 1 diet of the National Cholesterol Education Program (NCEP).

Source: U.S. Department of Health and Human Services.

the DASH (Dietary Approaches to Stop Hypertension) and OmniHeart (Optimal MacroNutrient Intake for Heart Health) diet plans have also helped refine dietary recommendations for healthy eating.

Based on the available scientific evidence, the following guidelines appear to be prudent and are consistent with the National Academy of Sciences recommendations for dietary fat. Although these guidelines have been developed to help individuals reduce high serum lipid profiles, they will also help to maintain normal levels and thus may be regarded as preventive medicine. As you may note, these recommendations are extensions of some guidelines for the Prudent Healthy Diet. Each guideline may be used to select foods that appeal to personal tastes. King and Gibney noted that individuals are more likely to eat a healthful diet if it includes foods they enjoy. It should be noted that in the near future, the application of nutrigenomics may permit individualized dietary recommendations. Menus may be tailored to the genetic profile of each individual to maximize dietary effects favorable to the lipid profile and prevention of CHD, and prevention of other chronic diseases as well.

1. *Adjust caloric intake to achieve and maintain ideal body weight.* One of the most common causes of high triglyceride levels is too much body fat, particularly in the abdominal region. The health risks of obesity are detailed in chapter 10. In many cases, simply losing body weight or reducing caloric intake will reduce these levels.

2. *Reduce the total amount of fats in the diet.* The American Heart Association recently increased the upper limit of dietary fat intake from 30 percent to 35 percent. Keep in mind that is the upper limit. Reducing the total amount of fat will usually reduce the amount of Calories also, but nutrient content will actually improve. Reducing total fat intake to 20 percent or lower of total daily Calories, as recommended in some healthy diet plans, will reduce total and LDL-cholesterol even more. However, a very low-fat diet (10 percent fat Calories) may actually cause a negative lipid profile in some individuals. To help prevent this, the carbohydrate Calories that replace the fat Calories should *not* be derived from refined carbohydrates, but rather from complex carbohydrates containing dietary fiber.

The Consumers Union, summarizing a report by 50 nutrition researchers, indicated that fat intake need not be restricted drastically in the diet, as long as you watch the type of fat in your diet (discussion follows) and your total caloric intake.

3. *Reduce the amount of saturated fat to less than 7 percent of dietary Calories.* The American Heart Association decreased the upper limit of saturated fat intake from 10 percent to 7 percent. As a matter of fact, scientists recommend reducing intake of saturated fats as low as possible while consuming a nutritionally adequate diet. The National Academy of Sciences indicated that there is a positive linear trend between total saturated fatty acid intake and total and LDL cholesterol concentration and increased risk of CHD. Saturated fats may also increase blood clotting, another risk factor for CHD. In two meta-analyses, Howell and others found that consumption of saturated fatty acids was the major dietary determinant of plasma cholesterol response to diet, while Clarke and others indicated that reducing the intake of saturated fat produced the most significant benefits regarding the prevention of CHD.

Animal foods may contain significant amounts of saturated fat. The biggest contributor of saturated fat to the American diet is hamburger meat, even if it is labeled lean. However, extra lean hamburger may be low in total fat and saturated fat. Note the following comparison for one serving (4 ounces) of hamburger (ground beef) containing various percentages of fat:

Regular hamburger (25%) = 331 Calories, 28 grams of fat (10.7 grams saturated fat)
Lean hamburger (15%) = 243 Calories, 17 grams of fat (6.6 grams saturated fat)
Extra lean hamburger (5%) = 155 Calories, 5.6 grams of fat (2.5 grams saturated fat)
Extra lean hamburger (3%) = 136 Calories, 4.5 grams of fat (1.5 grams saturated fat)

Processed meats, such as most luncheon meats, are relatively high in fat. In contrast, fish, chicken, turkey, and very lean cuts of beef (eye of round) and pork (tenderloin) contain much less fat and saturated fat.

All oils contain saturated fats and unsaturated fats. Avoid the tropical oils, such as palm, palm kernel, and coconut, which may be 50–90 percent saturated fat. Use mainly monounsaturated and polyunsaturated oils that have no more than about 2 grams of saturated fat per tablespoon:

- Canola
- Safflower
- Sunflower
- Corn
- Olive
- Sesame
- Soybean
- Peanut

Food labels must list the amount of saturated fat per serving and its percentage of the Daily Value, which provides a sound means to select products with little to no saturated fat.

4. *Reduce the consumption of trans fats and, comparable to saturated fat, keep dietary intake as low as possible.* The combined total of dietary saturated and *trans* fats should not exceed 10 percent of daily caloric intake. The American Heart Association recommends much lower intake of less than 1 percent of energy from *trans* fats. In a review, Lichtenstein noted that *trans* fats elevate LDL-cholesterol, and at relatively high intakes decrease HDL-cholesterol levels. Some data suggest that *trans* fatty acids may also trigger inflammation. The National Academy of Sciences also noted that, like saturated fats, there is a positive linear trend between *trans* fat and CHD. Although some reviewers contend that the adverse effects of *trans* fatty acids are somewhat less than those associated with saturated fatty acids, Mozaffarian and others cited research indicating that they may be as bad, or even worse. They indicate that, on a per-calorie basis, *trans* fats appear to increase the risk of coronary heart disease more than any other macronutrient. An increased risk is seen with low levels of consumption corresponding to 1 to 3 percent of total energy, which for a 2,000-Calorie diet would be approximately 20–60 Calories from *trans* fat. Similarly, Remig and others found that an increase in 2 percent of total energy from *trans* fat increases cardiovascular risk by 23 percent.

To decrease *trans* fat intake, you need to know what foods contain it. Although we know that meat and dairy products contain small amounts of natural *trans* fats, the Consumers Union has referred to *trans* fat as the "stealth" fat because we may not realize it is in the foods we eat. The vast majority of *trans* fat consumed by Americans is in processed foods, particularly margarine; vegetable shortening; white bread; packaged goods such as cookies, crackers, potato chips, and cakes; and fried fast foods such as french fries. The major component of each of these foods that adds *trans* fatty acids is usually partially hydrogenated vegetable oil. *Trans* fatty acid content per serving is now listed in the Nutrition Facts food label. However, the food label may list 0 grams of *trans* fat if there is less than 0.5 gram per serving. Thus, consuming multiple servings of such products daily may accumulate, totaling several grams or more of *trans* fat.

5. *Substitute monounsaturated fats for saturated fats and simple or refined carbohydrates.* Consume about 10–15 percent of Calories from monounsaturated fats. Although no DRI have been set for monounsaturated fats, the National Academy of Sciences notes that they may have some benefit in the prevention of chronic disease.

Epidemiological research has indicated that the Mediterranean diet is associated with reduced risk of CHD. Olive oil,

the primary source of dietary fat, is a staple of the Mediterranean diet. It is rich in monounsaturated fatty acids, is a good source of various phytochemicals, and contains the antioxidant vitamin E. In separate reviews, Covas and Perez-Jimenez and others highlighted various mechanisms, such as improved serum lipoprotein profile and reduced inflammation, whereby olive oil may reduce the risk of heart disease. However, they noted that the specific mechanisms underlying the beneficial effects of olive oil need further research. Nevertheless, the FDA has approved a *qualified* health claim for olive oil, indicating that eating two tablespoons of olive oil daily may, due to its monounsaturated fat content, reduce the risk of CHD. Keep in mind that *qualified* health claims are based on limited, not conclusive, evidence.

Walter Willett, the renowned nutrition research scientist from Harvard University, reported that both epidemiologic and metabolic studies suggest that individuals can benefit greatly by adopting elements of the Mediterranean diet. Although olive oil is one of those elements, others include a diet rich in vegetables, whole grains, and seafood, all of which may confer health benefits in the prevention of CHD.

However, the Consumers Union notes that there is little, if any, scientific evidence that people who consume mostly monounsaturated fats have lower rates of heart disease or other conditions. In a review addressing the hype and truth about olive oil, the Pritikin Longevity Center made the following points:

- Olive oil, in and by itself, does not protect against CHD. When used in place of saturated fats, it may reduce the serum LDL-cholesterol level, a major risk factor for CHD. Monounsaturated fat may be considered a more *healthful* fat if it displaces the unhealthful *saturated* fat in the diet.
- Although olive oil may be a better choice than saturated fats, it still contains the same amount of Calories. Consuming large amounts of olive oil may lead to excessive energy intake and possibly contribute to weight gain.
- Olive oil may be rich in phytochemicals, such as polyphenols, but similar amounts of these phytochemicals may be obtained from fruits and vegetables with much lower caloric content.
- Olive oil may simply be a marker for the Mediterranean diet, an overall heart-healthy diet rich in whole, natural foods like vegetables, fruits, whole grains, and beans.

Other than olive oil, rich sources of MUFAs include canola oil, avocados, and nuts.

The American Heart Association provided their stamp of approval to diets rich in MUFAs, provided saturated fatty acid intake is limited to a minimum and caloric intake is in balance. These two points may be the key to the role of MUFAs, such as olive oil, in helping prevent CHD.

Additionally, the OmniHeart study by Appel and others found that substituting monounsaturated fats, mainly olive oil, canola oil, and nuts, for simple carbohydrates, primarily desserts, may help promote heart health. For example, in a pooled analysis of 25 intervention trials, Sabaté and others found that 67 grams (2.4 oz) of nuts consumed daily lowered triglyceride and LDL-cholesterol levels. These effects were dose related and more marked in those with higher LDL-cholesterol levels. Thus, consumption of nuts may lower the risk of CHD. The OmniHeart plan provides the following tips to enrich the diet with monounsaturated fats.

- Have a teaspoon per day of olive oil or canola oil-based margarine on bread at lunch.
- Have 1 or 2 tablespoons of salad dressing made with olive or canola oil and vinegar in salads each day.
- Add a teaspoon of olive or canola oil or margarine in vegetables at dinner.
- Use olive or canola oil to sauté or stir-fry vegetables and add to recipes.
- Have 1 ounce of unsalted nuts rich in monounsaturated fat, like almonds, peanuts, and pecans, as a snack or add to cereals.

6. *Consume adequate amounts of polyunsaturated fatty acids.* As indicated previously, the National Academy of Sciences developed an AI for both the omega-6 and omega-3 polyunsaturated fatty acids because there may be some health benefits associated with such dietary intakes. Both types of fatty acids help promote healthy skin and are a source of various eicosanoids that may influence health processes. When substituted for saturated fat, polyunsaturated fat may reduce total serum cholesterol, including LDL cholesterol. In their study of pooled data from 11 American and European studies, Jakobsen and others examined associations between type of fat consumed and risk of CHD. They found that when polyunsaturated fats were substituted for saturated fats, there was a reduced risk of both coronary events and coronary deaths.

Essential fatty acids Polyunsaturated fatty acids should constitute about 10 percent of the daily caloric intake, and if foods are selected wisely this should provide adequate amounts of both omega-6 and omega-3 fatty acids. The essential omega-6 linoleic fatty acid is found in various vegetable oils that constitute food products such as margarine, salad dressings, and cooking oils. Several sources are listed in table 5.10. The essential omega-3 alpha-linolenic fatty acid is found in green leafy vegetables, canola oil, flaxseed oil, soy products, some nuts, and fish. Some nuts are especially rich in both the omega-3 and omega-6 fatty acids. Although both essential fatty acids may confer separate health benefits, the omega-3 fatty acids are thought to be more important for the prevention of CHD.

Omega-3 fatty acids The three principal omega-3 fatty acids—alpha-linolenic, EPA (eicosapentaenoic acid), and DHA (docasahexaenoic acid)—are believed to reduce the risk of CHD, but EPA and DHA are believed to be more potent. EPA and DHA may be formed in the body from alpha-linolenic acid, but this process appears to be limited. However, both EPA and DHA are found in substantial quantities in various fish oils, as highlighted in table 5.11. Eggs from chickens fed a special diet may contain DHA in amounts ranging from 0.05–0.15 grams, but the eggs are still high in cholesterol. Fish oil supplements may contain 0.3–0.5 grams.

As mentioned earlier, omega-3 fatty acids have been theorized to be ergogenic in nature because of the production of specific eicosanoids. Omega-3 fatty acids are also being studied for their potential health benefits, which also may be related to specific eicosanoids that are produced. Although the health-related role of omega-3 fatty acids and eicosanoids is complex and has not been totally determined, here is a simple summarization. The cell membrane contains a variety of molecular compounds, including phospholipids and their associated fatty acids. When the diet is high in linoleic acid, one of the main fatty acids in the phospholipids is arachidonic acid, which produces one form of eicosanoids when it is metabolized. When the diet is high in fish oils, EPA and DHA become the major source of eicosanoids, which are different in nature compared to those derived from arachidonic acid. In essence, the different forms of eicosanoids function as local hormones in body cells affecting metabolism and gene expression, and the effects associated with omega-3 fatty

TABLE 5.10 Alpha-linolenic content of selected oils, nuts, and seeds

Oils, Nuts, and Seeds	Alpha-linolenic content, grams/tablespoon
Olive oil	0.1
Walnuts, English	0.7
Soybean oil	0.9
Canola oil	1.3
Walnut oil	1.4
Flaxseed	2.2
Flaxseed (linseed) oil	8.5

Source: USDA Nutrient Data Laboratory.

TABLE 5.11 Grams of EPA and DHA in fish per 3-ounce edible fish portion and in fish oils per gram of oil

> 1 gram/ 3 ounces	0.5–1.0 gram/ 3 ounces	< 0.5 gram/ 3 ounces
Herring	Halibut	Catfish
Oysters, Pacific	Omega-3 concentrate*	Cod
Salmon, Atlantic, farmed	Salmon, sockeye	Cod liver oil*
Salmon, Atlantic, wild	Trout	Crab
Salmon, chinook	Tuna, fresh	Flounder/Sole
Sardines	Tuna, white, canned in water	Haddock
		Lobster
		Oysters, Eastern
		Scallops
		Shrimp
		Tuna, light, canned in water

*Note: Omega-3 content in fish oils or supplements is per gram of oil. Check supplement labels for content.

Source: Adapted from USDA Nutrient Data Laboratory. Ranges listed are rough estimates because oil content can vary markedly with species, season, diet, and packaging and cooking methods.

acid-derived eicosanoids appear to provide some health benefits. Metcalf and others found that dietary omega-3 fatty acids are rapidly incorporated into the phospholipids of human heart muscle cells, displacing arachidonic acid.

Epidemiological research has suggested that populations consuming diets rich in fish products have a lower incidence rate of CHD, and experimental research has suggested a number of possible mechanisms underlying this relationship.

- Reduce serum triglycerides
- Increase HDL-cholesterol
- Prevent clot formation
- Decrease platelet aggregation and stickiness
- Improve vascular tone
- Decrease blood viscosity
- Optimize blood pressure
- Promote anti-inflammatory activity
- Decrease abnormal heart rhythms

Some preliminary research suggests that they may be helpful in preventing the development of type 2 diabetes, macular degeneration in the eye, arthritic pain, and the dementia (loss of intellectual functions; behavior change) associated with aging. The National Institute of Aging recently initiated a clinical trial to evaluate the effects of EPA and DHA to prevent Alzheimer's disease.

Most research has focused on the effects of fish oil or omega-3 fatty acid supplementation on CHD, and the reviews of published studies are contradictory. Robinson and Stone noted that epidemiologic studies show more consistent reductions in the incidence of nonfatal myocardial infarction and ischemic stroke than do the clinical trials of increased omega-3 fatty acid intake, which suggests important confounding factors in the observational studies. In this regard, Cundiff and others found that individuals who consumed more EPA and DHA also consumed fewer Calories, fewer Calories from total fat and saturated fat, and more dietary fiber. They suggested that the benefit of fish or omega-3 fatty acids may be due to the association of greater fish intakes with an overall healthier dietary pattern. In a recent systematic review of 48 randomized controlled trials and 41 cohort studies, which provide stronger evidence than epidemiological studies, Hooper and others concluded that there is no clear effect of omega-3 fatty acid intake on total mortality or cardiovascular events.

Nevertheless, other contemporary reviews and meta-analyses indicate that increased consumption of fish oils and omega-3 fatty acids is cardioprotective. For example, Konig and others, in a meta-analysis, concluded that consuming small quantities of fish is associated with a risk reduction for both nonfatal myocardial infarction (27 percent reduction) and CHD mortality risk (17 percent reduction). In another meta-analysis, Studer and others concluded that consumption of omega-3 fatty acids was effective as a means of preventing mortality from cardiovascular disease. Mori and Woodman also concluded that prospective studies demonstrate an inverse association between fish intake and CHD mortality.

Harris even proposed an omega-3 fatty acid index as a new marker or risk factor for CHD. The National Institutes of Health (NIH) indicate that there is significant scientific evidence supporting the claim that increased dietary omega-3 intake improves outcomes in hypertriglyceridemia, hypertension, and secondary cardiovascular disease prevention. The NIH also concluded that there is supportive, but not conclusive, evidence in the primary prevention of cardiovascular disease, which is the basis for the *qualified* health claim on food labels that consumption of conventional foods containing omega-3 fatty acids may reduce the risk of CHD.

Tufts University, one of the leading international nutrition research universities, noted that the predominance of the medical literature continues to support eating fish for cardiovascular health. Based on the available evidence, Kris-Etherton and others provided some dietary guidelines in the American Heart Association Scientific Statement: Fish Consumption, Fish Oil, Omega-3 Fatty Acids, and Cardiovascular Disease. The key points are:

- Eat fish, particularly fatty fish, at least two times a week. Fatty fish like mackerel, lake trout, herring, sardines, albacore tuna, and salmon are high in EPA and DHA.
- Eat plant foods rich in the alpha-linolenic acid, an omega-3 fatty acid that may be converted to EPA and DHA in the body.
- Individuals who have high serum triglycerides may benefit from a fish oil supplement of 2–4 grams of EPA and DHA per day. Patients with CHD may benefit but should consult with their physicians.

Although eating more fish and fish oils is a healthful recommendation, a report by the Institute of Medicine, *Seafood Choices: Balancing Benefits and Risks,* raises some some caveats. Some types of fish may contain significant amounts of mercury, as methylmercury, which if consumed in excess may harm the nervous system and impair neurodevelopment in the fetus or in young children. Sushi is generally made from large blue fin, or *ahi,* tuna, which may contain mercury. Some types of fish, particularly older, larger predatory fish like shark and farmed fish such as Atlantic salmon, may contain environmental contaminants such as dioxins and polychlorinated biphenyls.

In a major review, Mozaffarian and Rimm concluded that the benefits of fish intake exceed the potential risks. However, along with the AHA, FDA, and Consumers Union, caution is recommended depending on a person's stage in life:

- For women of childbearing age, benefits of modest fish intake, excepting a few selected species, outweigh risks. The FDA indicates that pregnant women should limit the intake of shark, swordfish, king mackerel, and tilefish, and limit consumption of other fish to no more than 12 ounces per week. The FDA indicates that shrimp, salmon, pollock, and catfish are generally low in mercury. Based on new FDA data showing that some canned light tuna may contain as much mercury as white (Albacore) tuna, the Consumers Union recommends that women who are pregnant avoid canned tuna entirely. Women of childbearing age should also limit weekly consumption of canned tuna: no more than three 6-ounce cans of light tuna or no more than one can of white tuna.

- Young children should also limit consumption of fish that may be high in mercury, including tuna. The Consumers Union recommends that young children who weigh up to 45 pounds should eat less than one can of tuna a week. Young children may also eat salmon, tilapia, shrimp, and clams daily, but should limit intake of other fish to several times a week or less.
- The health effects of low-level methylmercury in adults are not clearly established. Adults should consume a variety of seafood. Select fresh, local seafood where available. The Consumers Union recommends the following safe fish consumption for adult men and women:

Daily	Several times a week
Salmon	Flounder
Tilapia	Sole
Pollock	Herring
Sardine	Mackerel
Oyster	Croaker
Shrimp	Scallop
Clam	Crab
Crawfish	

Environmentalists recommend choosing safe, sustainable fish, such as wild Alaska salmon, canned pink or sockeye salmon, sardines, Atlantic mackerel, and farmed oysters.

www.m.edf.org/seafood The Environmental Defense Fund provides information on fish that are safe to eat and offers substitutes for overfished choices.

Although consuming fish is the recommended means to obtain EPA and DHA, fish oil supplements are also available. Weber and others noted that the possible higher mercury content of some fish may make the intake of omega-3 fatty acids as capsules the better choice. Mercury accumulates in the muscle of the fish, not the fat tissues that is the source of fish oils. Although some health professionals recommend higher amounts for individuals with high levels of serum triglycerides or heart disease, one recommendation for healthy individuals is 500 to 1,300 milligrams a day of EPA and DHA combined. This is more liberal than the recommendation from Lee and colleagues in their review. They propose at least 1 gram of long-chain omega-3 fatty acids daily for patients with known CHD, and 250–500 mg daily for those without disease. The amount of EPA and DHA in a typical fish oil capsule varies, but generally a 1,000-milligram fish oil softgel will contain about 180 mg of EPA and 120 mg of DHA, or a total of 300 mg of omega-3 fatty acids. Consuming 2–4 capsules a day would provide the recommended amount. Some capsules may contain more than 500 mg of omega-3 fatty acids. However, Brunton and Collins note that many types of omega-3 fatty acid dietary supplements are available, but the efficacy, quality, and safety of these products are open to question because they are not regulated by the same standards as pharmaceutical agents. Health professionals recommend that you discuss the benefits and risks of taking fish oil supplements with your doctor. If you do take supplements, do so with food to help absorption.

You may also see omega-3 fatty acids prominently displayed on many food labels, such as cereals, pasta, yogurt, and soy milk. However, check the ingredient list for the source. If it is soybean, canola, or flaxseed oil, the omega-3 fatty acid is alpha-linolenic, which is a good choice but not considered to be as healthful as EPA and DHA.

Conjugated linoleic acid (CLA) Conjugated linoleic acid (CLA), a polyunsaturated omega-6 fatty acid found naturally in small amounts in dairy foods and beef, has been studied for its potential to reduce body fat. Whigham and others conducted a meta-analysis of 18 human studies, and concluded that CLA supplementation in a dose of about 3.2 grams daily produces a modest loss of body fat in humans, about 0.1 pound per week. Although this may be meaningful over time, the Consumers Union reports some research suggesting that CLA supplementation may induce some effects such as impaired blood glucose regulation and inflammation, that might contribute to chronic health problems. The role of CLA in weight control will be discussed further in chapter 10, but currently those at risk for CHD might be advised not to use it.

7. *Limit the amount of dietary cholesterol.* In recent years some have contended that dietary cholesterol does not influence serum cholesterol and the development of CHD. For example, Hasler noted it is now known that there is little if any connection between dietary cholesterol and blood cholesterol levels, and consuming up to one or more eggs per day does not adversely affect blood cholesterol levels. In contrast, in a meta-analysis covering 17 studies that evaluated cholesterol intake for at least 14 days, Weggemans and others noted that the addition of 100 milligrams of dietary cholesterol per day would increase slightly the ratio of total cholesterol to HDL-cholesterol, an adverse effect on the serum cholesterol profile. They concluded that the advice to limit cholesterol intake by reducing consumption of eggs and other cholesterol-rich foods may still be valid.

Limiting cholesterol intake is particularly important for cholesterol responders, those individuals with a genetic predisposition whose body production of cholesterol does not automatically decrease when the dietary intake increases. The average U.S. daily intake is approximately 400–500 milligrams or more.

Although some countries, such as Canada and the United Kingdom, do not provide specific recommendations regarding dietary cholesterol, the United States government does, as do some health professional organizations. The amount specified in the Daily Value for food labels is 300 milligrams. The American Heart Association recommends a cholesterol intake of 300 milligrams per day or less, or 100 milligrams per 1,000 Calories consumed.

8. *If you consume foods with artificial fats, do so in moderation.* The fat substitutes discussed earlier in this chapter are generally recognized as safe and have been approved by the Food and Drug Administration (FDA). Although olestra has been approved by the FDA, some contend that its use may interfere with the absorption of several fat-soluble vitamins and beta-carotene. However, the FDA requires that products containing olestra-type fat substitutes be enriched with fat-soluble vitamins to offset potential losses.

Snack foods containing olestra, particularly when consumed in large amounts, may cause intestinal cramps and loose stools. McRorie and others reported that although olestra-containing potato chips induced a gradual stool softening effect after several days of consumption, when consumed in smaller amounts, such as 20–40 grams, there were no objective measures of diarrhea or increased gastrointestinal symptoms. Nevertheless, the Center for Science in the Public Interest noted that the FDA received more than 18,000 adverse-reaction reports from people who had eaten olestra-containing foods. Sales of such foods have dropped dramatically.

In its position statement, the American Dietetic Association (ADA) concludes that the majority of fat replacers, when used in moderation by adults, can be safe and useful adjuncts to lowering the fat content of foods and may play a role in decreasing total dietary energy and fat intake. However, the ADA notes that they are effective only if they lower the total caloric content of the food and if the consumer uses these foods as part of a balanced meal plan, such as that promoted in the 2010 *Dietary Guidelines for Americans.*

Some fat is needed in the diet to provide the essential fatty acids and fat-soluble vitamins, and this fat should be obtained easily through natural, wholesome foods such as whole grains, fruits, and vegetables. Following such appropriate guidelines, the American Diabetes Association indicated that foods with fat replacers have the potential to help people with diabetes reduce total and saturated fat intake and may help improve the serum lipid profile. Another possible health benefit of fat substitutes may be their application in weight-loss programs. This topic will be covered in chapter 11.

9. *Reduce intake of refined carbohydrates and increase consumption of plant foods high in complex carbohydrates and dietary fiber, particularly water-soluble fiber.* Refined sugar and starches provoke higher triglyceride concentrations more than complex carbohydrates with fiber do. Again, the value of complex carbohydrates in the diet is stressed, particularly high-fiber foods, as a means to help reduce serum cholesterol. Research has suggested that without adequate amounts of fiber, a diet low in saturated fats and cholesterol has only modest effects on lowering CHD risk. Thus, replace high-fat foods with high-fiber foods. Legumes, such as beans, are an excellent source of carbohydrate and water-soluble fiber. Beans also contain protein, and soy protein, as found in products such as tofu, has been shown to reduce cholesterol in men with both normal and high serum cholesterol. Oat products, such as found in oatmeal, may effectively lower serum

cholesterol. Increased consumption of fruits and vegetables is recommended as well, for they may provide substantial amounts of the antioxidant vitamins (C, E, and beta-carotene) that may help to prevent undesired oxidations in the body. Guidelines presented in the preceding chapter are helpful to increase carbohydrate intake, and the role of antioxidant vitamins will be discussed in chapter 7.

Some plant foods, such as almonds and oats, may also contain various sterols and stanols, which are known to reduce serum cholesterol. Devaraj and Jialal indicated that about 2 grams of stanols or sterols per day may lower total and LDL-cholesterol, possibly by interfering with the uptake of both dietary and biliary cholesterol from the intestinal tract. Commercial margarines such as Benecol and Take Control contain such plant stanols and sterols. In a meta-analysis of six well-designed studies, Moruisi and others concluded that fat spreads (margarines) providing about 2.5 grams of phytosterols/stanols daily over the course of 1 to 3 months reduced both total cholesterol and LDL-cholesterol. As noted in chapter 2, a diet rich in plant sterols and stanols may reduce the risk of heart disease. Plant foods also contain several phytochemicals that may reduce serum cholesterol. Many food manufacturers, such as those who produce breakfast cereals and orange juice, are fortifying their products with sterols, stanols, phytochemicals, and other nutrients, creating functional foods designed to reduce serum cholesterol and provide other health benefits as well.

10. *Nibble food throughout the day.* Interestingly, David Jenkins showed a significant reduction in serum LDL cholesterol if subjects consumed their daily Calories, actually the same food, throughout the day rather than in three concentrated meals at breakfast, lunch, and dinner. In particular, it may be wise to avoid eating a high-fat meal. Nicholls and others reported that a single meal rich in saturated fats may impair blood vessel function and reduce the anti-inflammatory potential of HDL-cholesterol. The Consumers Union noted that a single high-fat meal significantly increased serum triglycerides and decreased blood flow through the heart. Jakulj and others found that a single high-fat meal could increase the blood pressure response to a stressful situation, such as public speaking. All of these factors may increase the short-term risk of a heart attack in susceptible individuals.

In simple practical terms, what do all of these recommendations mean? You should not eliminate all fat from your diet, but simply reduce the amount of fat that you eat. In essence, eat less butter, fatty meats, organ foods such as liver and kidney, egg yolks, whole milk, cheeses, ice cream, gravies, creamed foods, high-fat desserts, and refined sugar. Eat more very lean meats, fish, poultry, egg whites, skim and low-fat milk products, fruits and vegetables, beans, and whole-grain products, or the Prudent Healthy Diet. Table 5.12 provides some specifics.

You may have noted that alcohol intake was not one of these recommendations. As detailed in chapter 13, low-risk alcohol intake may provide some protection against CHD for those who do drink. However, most health professionals do not

TABLE 5.12 General food selections to decrease total dietary fat, saturated fat, and cholesterol

	Choose	Go easy on	Decrease
Meat, poultry, fish and shellfish (up to 6 ounces a day)	Lean cuts of meat with fat trimmed, like: beef—round, sirloin, chuck, loin lamb—leg, arm, loin, rib pork—tenderloin, leg (fresh), shoulder (arm or picnic) veal—all trimmed cuts except ground poultry without skin fish, shellfish		"Prime" grade fatty cuts of meat like: beef—corned beef brisket, regular ground short ribs pork—spareribs, blade roll Goose, domestic duck Organ meats like: liver, kidney, sweetbreads, brain Highly processed meats such as sausage, bacon, frankfurters, regular luncheon meats Caviar, roe
Dairy products (2 servings a day; 3 servings for women who are pregnant or breast-feeding)	Skim milk, 1% milk, low-fat buttermilk, low-fat evaporated or nonfat milk Low-fat yogurt and low-fat frozen yogurt Low-fat soft cheeses, like: cottage, farmer, pot Cheese labeled no more than 2 to 6 grams of fat an ounce	2% milk Part-skim ricotta Part-skim or imitation hard cheeses, like: part-skim mozzarella "Light" cream cheese "Light" sour cream	Whole milk, like: regular, evaporated, condensed Cream, half-and-half, most nondairy creamers and products, real or nondairy whipped cream Cream cheese, sour cream, ice cream, custard-style yogurt Whole-milk ricotta High-fat cheeses, like: Neufchatel, Brie, Swiss, American, mozzarella, feta, cheddar, Muenster
Eggs (no more than 3 egg yolks a week)	Eggs whites Cholesterol-free egg substitutes		Egg yolks
Fats and oils (up to 6 to 8 teaspoons a day)	Unsaturated vegetable oils, like: corn, olive, peanut, rapeseed (canola oil), safflower, sesame, soybean Margarine or shortening made with unsaturated fats listed above: liquid, tub, stick Diet mayonnaise, salad dressings made with unsaturated fats listed above Low-fat dressings	Nuts and seeds Avocados and olives	Butter, coconut oil, palm kernel oil, palm oil, lard, bacon fat Margarine or shortening made with saturated fats listed above Dressings made with egg yolk
Breads, cereals, pasta, rice, dried peas and beans (6 to 11 servings a day)	Breads, like: whole wheat, pumpernickel, and rye breads; sandwich buns; dinner rolls; bagels; English muffins; rice cakes; focus on whole wheat products Low-fat crackers, like: matzo, pita, bread sticks, rye krisp, saltines, zwieback Hot cereals, most cold dry cereals Pasta, like: plain noodles, spaghetti, macaroni; all with low-fat sauces Wild rice Dried peas and beans, like: split peas, black-eyed peas, chickpeas, kidney beans, navy beans, black beans, lentils, soybeans, soybean curd (tofu)	Store-bought pancakes, waffles, biscuits, muffins, cornbread; refined grains	Croissants, butter rolls, sweet rolls, Danish pastry, doughnuts Most snack crackers, like: cheese crackers, butter crackers, those made with saturated fats Granola-type cereals made with saturated fats Pasta and rice prepared with cream, butter, or cheese sauces, egg noodles

(Continued)

207

TABLE 5.12 Continued

	Choose	Go easy on	Decrease
Fruits and vegetables (2 to 4 servings of fruit and 3 to 5 servings of vegetables)	Fresh, frozen, canned, or dried fruits and vegetables		Vegetables prepared in butter, cream, or sauce Fruits in high-sugar syrup
Sweets and snacks (avoid too many sweets)	Low-fat frozen desserts, like: sherbet, sorbet, Italian ice, frozen yogurt, popsicles Low-fat cakes, like: angel food cake Low-fat cookies, like: fig bars, gingersnaps Low-fat candy, like: jelly beans, hard candy Low-fat snacks, like: plain popcorn, pretzels Nonfat beverages, like: carbonated drinks, juices, tea, coffee	Frozen desserts, like: ice milk Homemade cakes, cookies, and pies using unsaturated oils sparingly Fruit crisps and cobblers Potato and corn chips prepared with unsaturated vegetable oil	High-fat frozen desserts, like: ice cream, frozen tofu High-fat cakes, like: most store-bought, pound, and frosted cake Store-bought pies, most store-bought cookies Most candy, like: chocolate bars Potato and corn chips prepared with saturated fat Buttered popcorn High-fat beverages, like: frappes, milkshakes, floats, eggnogs
Label ingredients (To avoid too much fat, saturated fat, or cholesterol, go easy on products that list first any fat, oil, or ingredients higher in saturated fat or cholesterol. Choose more often those products that contain ingredients lower in fat, saturated fat, and cholesterol.)	Ingredients lower in saturated fat or cholesterol: Carob, cocoa Oils, like: corn, cottonseed, olive, safflower, sesame, soybean, sunflower Nonfat dry milk, nonfat dry milk solids, skim milk		Ingredients higher in saturated fat or cholesterol: Chocolate Animal fat, like: bacon, beef, ham, lamb, meat, pork, chicken or turkey fats, butter, lard Coconut, coconut oil, palm-kernel or palm oil Cream Egg and egg-yolk solids Hardened fat or oil Hydrogenated vegetable oil Shortening or vegetable shortening, unspecified vegetable oil (could be coconut, palm-kernel, palm)

Source: Adapted from "Report of the Expert Panel of Detection, Evaluation, and Treatment of High Blood Cholesterol in Adults." National Heart, Lung, and Blood Institutes of Health.

recommend that nondrinkers begin to consume alcohol for its potential health benefits because of other health risks associated with drinking in excess.

Can exercise training also elicit favorable changes in the serum lipid profile?

Physical inactivity, or lack of exercise, has been identified as one of the primary risk factors associated with an increased incidence of atherosclerosis and cardiovascular disease. Hence, exercise programs stressing aerobic endurance-type activities have been advocated as a means of reducing the incidence levels of these conditions, possibly via direct beneficial effects on the heart or blood vessels. However, the precise mechanism whereby exercise may help reduce the morbidity and mortality of CHD has not been identified. Therefore, many authorities believe that the beneficial effect may not be due to exercise itself, but rather the possible associated effects, such as reductions in body fat and blood pressure. Although some investigators believe that endurance exercise may have a preventive function independent of these associated effects, it also exerts a significant beneficial influence on the serum lipid profile, which, like blood pressure, is one of the major risk factors.

An acute bout of exercise may reduce risk factors for CHD. For example, Thompson and others recently noted that acute exercise may reduce blood pressure and serum triglycerides, increase HDL-cholesterol, and improve insulin sensitivity and glucose homeostasis. Thus, some of the beneficial effects of exercise on risk factors for CHD, including the serum lipid profile, may be attributed to recent exercise bouts. However, some of these benefits may become long-lasting with a chronic exercise training program.

Chronic exercise training has been shown to affect favorably the serum lipid profile. Literally hundreds of epidemiological and experimental studies have been conducted over the past several decades to investigate the effects of exercise on serum lipids. Space does not permit a detailed analysis of each, but major reviews of the worldwide literature have been reported by prominent authorities such as Stefanik and Wood, Leon and Sanchez, Durstine, and Williams. Although most of these reviews involved males, similar reviews have evaluated the effects of exercise training on women, such as those by Dowling and the meta-analysis by Kelley and others. These reviews have noted a rather consistent pattern relating exercise and blood lipids, and some of the benefits have been associated with concomitant body weight control. In general, increased levels of exercise are associated with lower plasma levels of triglycerides and higher levels of HDL, as documented in several recent meta-analyses by Kelley and Kelley. However, Durstine and others note that exercise training seldom alters total and LDL cholesterol, although some studies have shown small decreases in the latter. Moreover, research has shown that exercise may not improve the lipid profile of some individuals, primarily in those with genetic defects. These individuals may receive other health benefits of exercise, but may need drug therapy to control elevated serum lipid levels.

In an attempt to quantify the serum lipid changes with the amount of exercise, Durstine and his associates conducted a meta-analysis of well-controlled studies. One of the dose-response findings from their analysis indicated that an exercise training volume of 1,200–2,200 Calories per week is often effective at elevating HDL-C levels from 2–8 mg/dL and lowering triglyceride levels by 5–38 mg/dL. Their analysis also suggests that greater increases in HDL-cholesterol can be expected with additional increases in exercise training volume. This amount of physical activity is reasonable and attainable for most individuals and is within the ACSM recommended range for healthy adults. Lifetime aerobic exercise appears to be the key, and moderately intense leisure-time activity, such as brisk walking, may elicit beneficial effects in men, women, children, and adolescents. As noted by Kelley and others, walking favorably affects the adult serum lipid profile independent of changes in body composition.

However, in women, extreme amounts of exercise combined with insufficient energy intake and leading to amenorrhea may reverse these benefits. The effects of exercise-induced amenorrhea will be discussed further in chapters 8 and 10, but it appears that the lower levels of estrogen associated with this condition may lead to lower levels of HDL-cholesterol.

As noted previously, a single high-fat meal may increase the risk of heart attack. However, Katsanos indicates that expending about 500 Calories or more through moderate-intensity exercise within 16 hours before the meal will minimize adverse changes in the lipid profile. As discussed below, this supports the finding that endurance athletes who consume diets rich in fat maintain normal serum lipid profiles.

Although the precise biochemical mechanisms underlying the beneficial effects of exercise on serum lipids have not been identified, researchers have found that in physically trained males and females, activity levels of several enzymes, such as hepatic lipase and lipoprotein lipase, are modified in such a way as to promote a more rapid catabolism of triglycerides and a greater production of HDL. The muscle cell membrane may be modified favorably to become more insulin sensitive, helping clear lipids from the blood into the muscle. Exercise may also favorably modify the serum lipid levels by helping the individual lose body fat or influencing changes in other aspects of his or her lifestyle, such as diet.

Research has revealed that the beneficial effects of exercise training are additive to a diet modified in fat content, such as one reduced in total and saturated fat. A low-fat diet will reduce total cholesterol and LDL-cholesterol but may also undesirably decrease HDL-cholesterol. Exercise may prevent or attenuate the decrease in HDL-cholesterol on such diets, but when combined with omega-3 fatty acid supplementation may actually increase serum HDL-cholesterol, as reported in a study by Thomas and others. Thus, the combination of both dietary modifications and exercise is the recommended approach to modify favorably serum lipid levels.

Research also reveals that highly trained endurance runners who increase their dietary fat to about 40 percent or more of daily caloric intake for 4 weeks do not experience any adverse effects in their blood lipid profiles. Although this type of diet is not recommended on a long-term basis, the review by Brown and Cox illustrates some of the protective effects of exercise training on serum lipid changes associated with short-term increases in dietary fat. They suggest that the strenuous physical training seems to metabolize the increased fat intake for energy and prevents adverse changes in the lipid profile.

www.americanheart.org Use this site to obtain information to help reduce the risk of heart disease and stroke. There are sections on diet and nutrition, healthy cooking, and exercise.

Key Concepts

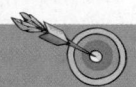

▶ Low-density forms of lipoproteins (LDL) may predispose certain individuals to coronary heart disease, whereas high-density forms (HDL) may be protective.

▶ In general, a low- to moderate-fat diet is recommended for both health and physical performance. One should consume less high-fat meat and dairy products and more fruits, vegetables, whole-grain products, dietary fiber, lean meats, and skim milk. Fish, including fatty fish like salmon, is part of a heart-healthy diet.

▶ Diets rich in saturated fats, *trans* fats, and cholesterol may increase the risk of coronary heart disease. In the United States,

in general, the recommended dietary intake of total fat is 35 percent or less of the total caloric intake, with saturated and *trans* fats at less than 7 percent of the total. The recommended cholesterol intake is less than 300 milligrams per day, or 100 milligrams per 1,000 Calories.

▶ Aerobic exercise training increases the ability of the muscles to use fat as an energy source and can be an important adjunct to diet in beneficially modifying the serum lipid profile and reducing body fat, two factors that may reduce the risk of coronary heart disease (CHD). Relative to the serum lipid profile, aerobic exercise training is most effective in reducing serum triglycerides and increasing serum HDL-cholesterol.

Check for Yourself

▶ Major professional health organizations, such as the American Heart Association, the National Cancer Society, and the American Diabetes Association, all have pamphlets or Internet sites providing dietary recommendations to help prevent related diseases. Obtain pamphlets or visit Websites for several such organizations and evaluate the findings relative to dietary fat. Compare your findings.

APPLICATION EXERCISE

The American Heart Association established its Food Certification Program in 1995 to provide consumers an easy and reliable way to identify heart-healthy foods. Foods that display the distinctive red heart with the white check mark are evaluated to meet the Program's standards.

Go to your local supermarket and look for foods with labels that display the American Heart Association *heart-check mark,* as displayed here.

Try to find foods in the different food groups, such as grains, fruits, vegetables, meats, and dairy. Make a list of foods you find in each of the food categories, and visit www.heartcheckmark.org to review the nutritional criteria these products must meet to be certified. You may notice that desserts do not have the AHA symbol. In their effort to reduce sugar intake, desserts have been taken off the list of packaged foods, according to Tufts University.

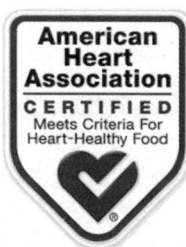

Used with permission of the American Heart Association, Inc.

Review Questions—Multiple Choice

1. If a 2,000-Calorie diet contains 100 grams of fat, the percentage of fat Calories in the diet is which of the following?
   a. 20 percent
   b. 25 percent
   c. 35 percent
   d. 45 percent
   e. 60 percent

2. Which of the following dietary supplements has been proven to increase fat utilization during exercise, store muscle glycogen, and enhance endurance exercise performance?
   a. carnitine
   b. conjugated linoleic acid
   c. omega-3 fatty acids
   d. hydroxycitrate
   e. medium-chain triglycerides
   f. a and b
   g. none of the above

3. Which of the following is most conducive to the development of atherosclerosis?
   a. a total cholesterol of 190-milligrams
   b. a low level of very low-density lipoprotein cholesterol
   c. a high-density lipoprotein cholesterol of 70 milligrams
   d. a low-density lipoprotein cholesterol of 170 milligrams

e. a total cholesterol/high-density lipoprotein cholesterol ratio of less than 3.5

4. Which lipid dietary component appears to be most likely to cause an increase in serum cholesterol and the development of atherosclerosis?
   a. saturated fats
   b. polyunsaturated fats
   c. monounsaturated fats
   d. omega-3 fatty acids
   e. phospholipids

5. What compound in the diet cannot be used to form fat if it is consumed in excess?
   a. fat
   b. complex carbohydrate
   c. simple carbohydrate
   d. protein
   e. alcohol
   f. all are capable of forming fat

6. Which essential fatty acids are needed in the diet?
   a. linoleic and alpha-linolenic
   b. oleic and linoleic
   c. stearic and alpha-linolenic
   d. palmitic and stearic
   e. palmitoleic and stearic

7. Which of the following statements relative to fats is false?
   a. Hydrogenation of fats makes them more saturated.
   b. Saturated fats are found primarily in animal foods.
   c. Vegetable fats are primarily unsaturated fats.
   d. Polyunsaturated fats are theorized to be more healthful than saturated fats.
   e. Saturated fats appear to help lower blood cholesterol levels.

8. Which of the following is not good advice in attempts to reduce *serum* cholesterol?
   a. Limit whole egg consumption to about 2–4 per week.
   b. Eat fish and white poultry meat in place of saturated fat meat.
   c. Drink skim milk instead of whole milk.
   d. Use butter instead of soft tub, non-*trans* fatty acid margarine.
   e. Eat more fruits, vegetables, and whole-grain products.

9. Fats may be a significant source of energy during exercise of low intensity and long duration. What is the main form of fats used for energy production during low-intensity exercise?
   a. phospholipids derived from the cell membrane
   b. chylomicrons from the liver
   c. free fatty acids from the adipose cells and muscle cells
   d. VLDL from the liver
   e. cholesterol from the kidney

10. Aerobic endurance exercise may have some beneficial effects on the serum lipid profile and help to prevent coronary heart disease (CHD). In particular, what aspects of the serum lipid profile are improved from exercise to help reduce risk of CHD?
    a. lower both total cholesterol and LDL-cholesterol
    b. lower total cholesterol and increase LDL-cholesterol
    c. lower both triglycerides and LDL-cholesterol
    d. lower both triglycerides and HDL-cholesterol
    e. lower triglycerides and increase HDL-cholesterol

Answers to multiple-choice questions:
1. d; 2. g; 3. d; 4. a; 5. f; 6. a; 7. e; 8. d; 9. c; 10. e.

1. List the major classes of dietary fatty acids and discuss their relative importance to cardiovascular health. Include in your discussion specific fatty acids as deemed relevant.

2. Describe the role that the blood lipoproteins play in the etiology of atherosclerosis and cardiovascular disease.

3. What is carnitine and how is it theorized to enhance endurance exercise performance? Does research support the theory?

4. Describe the process of chronic fat loading as a strategy to enhance endurance exercise performance, and provide a synthesis of research findings relative to its efficacy.

5. List at least five dietary strategies that may help reduce the risk of atherosclerosis and cardiovascular disease, including specific foods in the diet.

Books

American Institute of Cancer Research 2007. *Food, Nutrition, Physical Activity, and the Prevention of Cancer: A Global Perspective,* Washington, DC: AICR.

Houston, M. 2006. *Biochemistry Primer for Exercise Science.* Champaign, IL: Human Kinetics.

Institute of Medicine. 2006. *Seafood Choices: Balancing Benefits and Risks.* Washington, DC: National Academies Press.

Jeukendrup, A. 1997. *Aspects of Carbohydrate and Fat Metabolism During Exercise.* Haarlem the Netherlands: De Vriesborch.

Moffatt, R. and Stamford, B. 2006. *Lipid Metabolism and Health.* Boca Raton, FL: CRC Press.

National Academy of Sciences. 2005. *Dietary Reference Intakes for Energy, Carbohydrates, Fiber, Fat, Protein and Amino Acids* (Macronutrients). Washington, DC: National Academies Press.

Sears, B. 1995. The Zone. New York: Regan Books.

U.S. Anti-Doping Agency. 2005. *Optimal Dietary Intake.* Colorado Springs, CO: USADA.

U.S. Department of Health and Human Services Public Health Service. 2001. *Third Report of the National Cholesterol Education Program of the Expert Panel on Population Strategies for Blood*

Cholesterol Reduction. Bethesda, MD: National Institutes of Health.

U.S. Department of Health and Human Services Public Health Service. 2010. *Healthy People 2020: National Health Promotion and Disease Prevention Objectives.* Washington, DC: U.S. Government Printing Office.

Wardlaw, G., and Hampl, J. 2007. *Perspectives in Nutrition:* McGraw-Hill Companies.

Reviews

Achten, J., and Jeukendrup, A. 2004. Optimizing fat oxidation through exercise and diet. *Nutrition* 20:716–27.

American College of Sports Medicine, et al. 2009. Position of the American Dietetic Association, Dietitians of Canada, and the American College of Sports Medicine: Nutrition and athletic performance. *Medicine & Science in Sports & Exercise* 41:709–31.

American Diabetes Association. 2000. Role of fat replacers in diabetes medical nutrition therapy. *Diabetes Care* 23:S96–97.

American Dietetic Association: 2005. Position of the American Dietetic Association: Fat replacers. *Journal of the American Dietetic Association* 105:266–75.

American Dietetic Association, et al. 2000. Position of the American Dietetic Association, Dietitians of Canada, and the American College of Sports Medicine: Nutrition and Athletic performance. *Journal of the American Dietetic Association* 100:1543–56.

American Heart Association. 2006. Diet and lifestyle recommendations revision 2006: A scientific statement from the American Heart Association Nutrition Committee. *Circulation* 114:82–96.

American Heart Association. 1999. Monounsaturated fatty acids and risk of cardiovascular disease. *Circulation* 1253–8.

Aucouturier, J., et al. 2008. Fat and carbohydrate metabolism during submaximal exercise in children. *Sports Medicine* 38:213–38.

Bell, S., et al. 1997. The new dietary fats in health and disease. *Journal of the American Dietetic Association.* 97:280–86.

Brass, E. 2004. Carnitine and sports medicine: Use or abuse? *Annals of the New York Academy of Sciences* 1033:67–78.

Brown, G., et al. 1993. Lipid lowering and plaque regression: New insights into prevention of plaque disruption and clinical events in coronary disease. *Circulation* 87:1781–89.

Brown, R., and Cox, C. 2001. Challenging the dogma of dietary carbohydrate

requirements for endurance athletes. *American Journal of Medicine & Sports* 3:75–86.

Brunton, S., and Collins, N. 2007. Differentiating prescription omega-3-acid ethyl esters (P-OM3) from dietary-supplement omega-3 fatty acids. *Current Medical Research & Opinion* 23:1139–45.

Burke, L., and Hawley, J. 2002. Effects of short-term fat adaptation on metabolism and performance of prolonged exercise. *Medicine & Science in Sports & Exercise* 34:1492–98.

Campbell, B., and Kreider, R. 2008. Conjugated linoleic acids. *Current Sports Medicine Reports* 7:237–41.

Center for Science in the Public Interest. 1999. Olean times at P & G. *Nutrition Action Health Letter* 26 (8):2.

Cheuvront, S. 1999. The zone diet and athletic performance. *Sports Medicine* 27:213–28.

Clarke, R., et al. 1997. Dietary lipids and blood cholesterol: Quantitative meta-analysis of metabolic ward studies. *British Medical Journal* 314:112–17.

Clegg, M. 2010. Medium-chain triglycerides are advantageous in promoting weight loss although not beneficial to exercise performance. *International Journal of Food Science & Nutrition* 61:653–79.

Consumers Union. 2007. The new facts about fats. *Consumer Reports on Health* 19 (10):1, 4–5.

Consumers Union. 2006. Mercury in tuna. *Consumer Reports* 71 (7):20–21.

Consumers Union. 2002. Chest pain after eating? *Consumer Reports on Health* 14 (7):3.

Consumers Union. 1998. Finally, a consensus on fat. *Consumer Reports on Health* 10 (8):8.

Covas, M. 2007. Olive oil and the cardiovascular system. *Pharmacological Research* 55:175–86.

Cundiff, D., et al. 2007. Relation of omega-3 fatty acid intake to other dietary factors known to reduce coronary heart disease risk. *American Journal of Cardiology* 99:1230–33.

Devaraj, S., and Jialal, I. 2006. The role of dietary supplementation with plant sterols and stanols in the prevention of cardiovascular disease. *Nutrition Reviews* 64:348–54.

Dowling, E. 2001. How exercise affects lipid profiles in women. *Physician and Sportsmedicine* 29 (9):45–52.

Durstine, J., et al. 2001. Blood lipid and lipoprotein adaptations to exercise: A quantitative analysis. *Sports Medicine* 31:1033–62.

Erlenbusch, M., et al. 2004. Effect of high-fat or high-carbohydrate diets on endurance

exercise: A meta-analysis. *International Journal of Sport Nutrition & Exercise Metabolism* 15:1–14.

Frayn, K. 2010. Fat as fuel: Emerging understanding of the adipose tissue-skeletal muscle axis. *Acta Physiologica* 199:509–18.

Glatz, J., et al. 2002. Exercise and insulin increase muscle fatty acid uptake by recruiting putative fatty acid transporters to the sarcolemma. *Current Opinion in Clinical Nutrition & Metabolic Care* 5:365–70.

Grundy, S. 2006. Nutrition in the management of disorders of serum lipids and lipoproteins. In *Modern Nutrition in Health and Disease,* eds. M. Shils, et al. Philadelphia: Lippincott Williams & Wilkins.

Hargreaves, M. 2006. The metabolic systems: Carbohydrate metabolism. In *ACSM's Advanced Exercise Physiology,* ed. C. M. Tipton. Philadelphia: Lippincott Williams & Wilkins.

Hargreaves, M., et al. 2004. Pre-exercise carbohydrate and fat ingestion: Effects on metabolism and performance. *Journal of Sports Sciences* 22:31–38.

Harris, W. 2007. Omega-3 fatty acids and cardiovascular disease: A case for omega-3 index as a new risk factor. *Pharmacological Research* 55:217–23.

Harris, W. 2004. Are omega-3 fatty acids the most important nutritional modulators of coronary heart disease risk? *Current Atherosclerosis Reports* 6:447–52.

Hasler, C. 2000. The changing face of functional foods. *Journal of the American College of Nutrition* 19:499S–506S.

Hawley, J. 2002. Effect of increased fat availability on metabolism and exercise capacity. *Medicine & Science in Sports & Exercise* 34:1485–91.

Hawley, J., et al. 2000. Fat metabolism during exercise. In *Nutrition in Sport,* ed. R. Maughan. Oxford: Blackwell Scientific.

Heinonen, O. 1996. Carnitine and physical exercise. *Sports Medicine* 22:109–32.

Hooper, L., et al. 2006. Risks and benefits of omega-3 fats for mortality, cardiovascular disease, and cancer: Systematic review. *British Medical Journal* 332:752–60.

Horowitz, J., and Klein, S. 2000. Lipid metabolism during endurance exercise. *American Journal of Clinical Nutrition* 72:558S–63S.

Howell, W., et al. 1997. Plasma lipid and lipoprotein responses to dietary fat and cholesterol: A meta-analysis. *American Journal of Clinical Nutrition* 65:1747–64.

Hulbert, A. 2005. Dietary fats and membrane function: Implications for metabolism and disease. *Biological Reviews of the*

Cambridge Philosophical Society 80:155–69.

Jacobson, T., et al. 2007. Hypertriglyceridemia and cardiovascular risk reduction. *Clinical Therapy* 29:763–77.

Jain, K., et al. 2007. The biology and chemistry of hyperlipidemia. *Bioorganic & Medical Chemistry* 15:4674–99.

Jakobsen, M., et al. 2009. Major types of dietary fat and risk of coronary heart disease: A pooled analysis of 11 cohort studies. *American Journal of Clinical Nutrition* 89:1425–32.

Jequier, E. 1999. Response to and range of acceptable fat intake in adults. *European Journal of Clinical Nutrition* 53:S84–S88.

Jeukendrup, A. 2002. Regulation of fat metabolism in skeletal muscle. *Annals of the New York Academy of Sciences* 967:217–35.

Jeukendrup, A., and Aldred, S. 2004. Fat supplementation, health, and endurance performance. *Nutrition* 20:678–88.

Jeukendrup, A. E., et al. 1998. Fat metabolism during exercise: A review. Part II: Regulation of metabolism and the effects of training. *International Journal of Sports Medicine* 19:293–302.

Johnson, E., and Schaefer, E. 2006. Potential role of dietary *n*-3 fatty acids in the prevention of dementia and macular degeneration. *American Journal of Clinical Nutrition* 84:1494S–98S.

Jones, P., and Kubow, S. 2006. Lipids, sterols, and their metabolites. In *Modern Nutrition in Health & Disease,* eds. M. Shils, et al. Philadelphia: Lippincott Williams & Wilkins.

Katsanos, C. 2006. Prescribing aerobic exercise for the regulation of postprandial lipid metabolism: Current research and recommendations. *Sports Medicine* 36: 547–60.

Kelley, G., and Kelley, K. 2007. Aerobic exercise and lipids and lipoproteins in children and adolescents: A meta-analysis of randomized controlled trials. *Atherosclerosis* 191:447–53.

Kelley, G., and Kelley, K. 2006. Aerobic exercise and HDL$_2$-C: A meta-analysis of randomized controlled trials. *Atherosclerosis* 184:207–15.

Kelley, G., et al. 2004. Aerobic exercise and lipids and lipoproteins in women: A meta-analysis of randomized controlled trials. *Journal of Women's Health* 13: 1148–64.

Kelley, G., et al. 2004. Walking, lipids, and lipoproteins: A meta-analysis of randomized controlled trials. *Preventive Medicine* 38:651–61.

Kelly, G. 1998. L-carnitine: Therapeutic applications of a conditionally-essential amino acid. *Alternative Medicine Reviews* 3:345–60.

Kiens, B., and Helge, J. 2000. Adaptations to a high fat diet. In *Nutrition in Sport,* ed. R. Maughan. Oxford: Blackwell Scientific.

Kingsley, M. 2006. Effects of phosphatidylserine supplementation on exercising humans. *Sports Medicine* 36:657–69.

Kodama, S., et al. 2007. Effect of aerobic exercise training on serum levels of high-density lipoprotein cholesterol: A meta-analysis. *Archives of Internal Medicine* 167:999–1008.

Konig, A., et al. 2005. A quantitative analysis of fish consumption and coronary heart disease mortality. *American Journal of Preventive Medicine* 29:335–46.

Kraemer, W., et al. 2008. L-carnitine supplementation: Influence upon physiological function. *Current Sports Medicine Reports* 7:218–23.

Kris-Etherton, P., et al. 2002. AHA Scientific Statement: Fish, fish oils and omega-3 fatty acids. *Circulation* 106:2747–57.

Kris-Etherton, P., et al. 2002. Dietary fat: Assessing the evidence in support of a moderate-fat diet: The benchmark based on lipoprotein metabolism. *Proceedings of the Nutrition Society* 61:287–98.

Lange, K. 2004. Fat metabolism in exercise—With special reference to training and growth hormone administration. *Scandinavian Journal of Medicine & Science in Sports* 14:74–99.

LaRosa, J. 2007. Low-density lipoprotein cholesterol reduction: The end is more important than the means. *American Journal of Cardiology* 100:240–42.

Lee, J., et al. 2009. Omega-3 fatty acids: Cardiovascular benefits, sources, and sustainability. *Nature Reviews: Cardiology* 6:753–8.

Leon, A., and Sanchez, O. 2001. Response of blood lipids to exercise training alone or combined with dietary interventions. *Medicine & Science in Sports & Exercise* 33:S502–15.

Lichtenstein, A. 2000. Trans fatty acids and cardiovascular disease risk. *Current Opinion in Lipidology* 11:37–42.

Martin, W. 1997. Effect of endurance training on fatty acid metabolism during whole body exercise. *Medicine & Science in Sports & Exercise* 29:635–39.

Mickleborough, T. 2008. A nutritional approach to managing exercise-induced asthma. *Exercise & Sport Science Reviews* 36:135–44.

Mori, T., and Woodman, R. 2006. The independent effects of eicosapentaenoic acid and docosahexaenoic acid on cardiovascular risk factors in humans. *Current Opinion in Clinical Nutrition & Metabolic Care* 9:95–104.

Moruisi, K., et al. 2006. Phytosterols/stanols lower cholesterol concentrations in familial hypercholesterolemic subjects: A systematic review with meta-analysis. *Journal of the American College of Nutrition* 25:41–48.

Mozaffarian, D., et al. 2006. *Trans* fatty acids and cardiovascular disease. *New England Journal of Medicine* 354:1601–16.

Mozaffarian, D., and Rimm, E. 2006. Fish intake, contaminants, and human health: Evaluating the risks and the benefits. *Journal of the American Medical Association* 296:1885–99.

Pendergast, D., et al. 2000. A perspective on fat intake in athletes. *Journal of the American College of Nutrition* 19:345–50.

Perez-Jimenez, F., et al. 2005. International conference on the healthy effect of virgin olive oil. *European Journal of Clinical Investigation* 35:421–24.

Pritikin Longevity Center. 2006. The truth about olive oil. *Pritikin ePerspective Issue* 93: November 29.

Rebouche, C. J. 2006. Carnitine. In *Modern Nutrition in Health and Disease,* eds. M. Shils, et al. Philadelphia: Lippincott Williams & Wilkins.

Remig, V., et al. 2010. *Trans* fats in America: A review of their use, consumption, health implications, and regulation. *Journal of the American Dietetic Association* 110: 585–92.

Robinson, J., and Stone, N. 2006. Antiatherosclerotic and antithrombotic effects of omega-3 fatty acids. *American Journal of Cardiology* 98:39i–49i.

Roepstorff, C., et al. 2005. Intramuscular triacylglycerol in energy metabolism during exercise in humans. *Exercise & Sport Sciences Reviews* 33:182–88.

Sabaté, J., et al. 2010. Nut consumption and blood lipid levels. *Archives of Internal Medicine* 170:821–27.

Sherman, W., and Leenders, N. 1995. Fat loading: The next magic bullet. *International Journal of Sport Nutrition* 5:S1–S12.

Shrier, I. 2005. Mediterranean diet for reducing mortality and easing the metabolic syndrome. *Physician and Sportsmedicine* 33 (5):8–9.

Shulman, D. 2002. Fuel on fat for the long run. *Marathon & Beyond* 6 (5):128–36.

Siri, P., and Krauss, R. 2005. Influence of dietary carbohydrate and fat on LDL

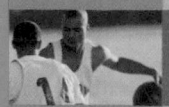

Protein is one of our most essential nutrients for optimal health. Additionally, it has a wide variety of physiological functions that are essential to optimal physical performance. For example, protein forms the structural basis of muscle tissue, is the major component of most enzymes in the muscle, and can serve as a source of energy during exercise. Because protein is so important to the development and function of muscle tissue, and because most feats of human physical performance involve strenuous muscular activity in one form or another, it is no wonder that protein has persisted throughout the years as the food of the athlete. Indeed, surveys have revealed that many high school and college athletes believe that athletic performance is improved by a high-protein diet. Protein is one of the best-selling sports supplements. A best-selling diet book suggests that protein is the key macronutrient for the athlete, and for health as well.

Companies that market nutritional supplements for athletes have capitalized on this belief. Probably the athletic groups most susceptible to the lure of protein supplements are bodybuilders and strength-type athletes, such as weight lifters and football players. Numerous high-protein products have been developed for these athletes in attempts to exploit the protein-muscle strength relationship. In recent years, specific amino acids have been theorized to maximize muscle mass and strength gains and have been advertised extensively in magazines for bodybuilders. Some advertisements even suggest that certain amino acid mixtures have an effect similar to drugs such as anabolic steroids, which have been used to stimulate muscle development.

Protein supplements are marketed for other types of athletes as well. Although protein is not regarded as a major energy source during exercise, research has suggested that endurance athletes may use some specific amino acids for energy production under certain conditions.

Protein supplements, often combined with carbohydrate, are marketed in sport drinks to endurance athletes. Additionally, specific amino acids have been theorized to delay the onset of fatigue during prolonged exercise through their effect on neurotransmitters in the brain.

There is no doubt that an adequate amount of dietary protein and related essential amino acids is required by all individuals. However, the advertisements directed toward athletes imply that additional protein, usually in the form of protein or amino acid supplements, is necessary for optimal performance. Although the National Academy of Sciences has indicated that the Recommended Daily Allowance (RDA) provides sufficient protein to athletes, some investigators recommend that athletes in training increase their protein intake. However, these investigators usually recommend that the protein be derived from natural food sources and the amount of protein recommended is well within the Acceptable Macronutrient Dietary Range (AMDR).

Other dietary supplements related to protein or amino acids, such as amines or various metabolic by-products, have become increasingly popular in recent years. One of the current hot sellers is creatine, but other supplements such as inosine and HMB are also available. In most cases these dietary supplements have been marketed to strength-trained athletes as a means to foster muscle growth and strength development, but some are intended for use by athletes involved in other sports, such as aerobic endurance events.

Does the physically active individual need more protein or related dietary supplements in the diet? The information presented in this chapter should provide a general answer to this question. Topics to be covered include dietary needs and sources of protein; metabolic fates and functions in the body; the effects of exercise on protein metabolism and dietary requirements; the ergogenic potential of protein, amino acids, or other related supplements; and health aspects of dietary protein.

Dietary Protein

What is protein?

Protein is a complex chemical structure containing carbon, hydrogen, and oxygen—just as carbohydrates and fats do. Protein has one other essential element—nitrogen, which constitutes about 16 percent of most dietary protein. These four elements are combined into a number of different structures called **amino acids,** each one possessing an amino group (NH_2) and an acid group (COOH), with the remainder being different combinations of carbon, hydrogen, oxygen, and in some cases sulfur. There are 20 amino acids, all of which can be combined in a variety of ways to form the proteins necessary for the structure and functions of the human body. The body may also modify the structure of dietary amino acids, such as converting proline to hydroxyproline, to meet its needs. Figure 6.1 depicts the formula of **alanine,** an amino acid discussed later.

Proteins are created when two amino acids link and form a peptide bond; hence, a dipeptide is formed. As more amino acids are added, a polypeptide is formed. Most proteins are polypeptides, combining up to 300 amino acids. Figure 6.2 depicts the building of a protein.

Protein is contained in both animal and plant foods. Humans obtain their supply of amino acids from these two general sources.

Is there a difference between animal and plant protein?

To answer this question, let us first look at a basic difference between two groups of amino acids. Humans can synthesize some amino acids in their bodies but cannot synthesize others. The nine amino acids that cannot be manufactured in the body are called **essential,** or **indispensable, amino acids** and must be supplied in the diet. Those that may be formed in the body are called **nonessential,** or **dispensable, amino acids.** Six of the dispensable amino acids are conditionally indispensable, which means that they must be obtained through the diet when endogenous synthesis cannot meet metabolic demands, such as in severe catabolic states. Although nutrition scientists prefer the terms *indispensable* and *dispensable,* this text uses the terms *essential* and *nonessential* because they are most commonly used.

It should be noted that all 20 amino acids are necessary for protein synthesis in the body and must be present simultaneously for optimal maintenance of body growth and function. The use of the terms *essential* and *indispensable* in relation to amino acids is to distinguish those that must be obtained in the diet. Table 6.1 presents the dietary essential, nonessential, and conditionally essential amino acids.

TABLE 6.1	The dietary amino acids
Essential amino acids	**Nonessential amino acids**
Histidine	Alanine
Isoleucine*	Arginine**
Leucine*	Asparagine
Lysine	Aspartic acid
Methionine	Cysteine**
Phenylalanine	Glutamic acid
Threonine	Glutamine**
Tryptophan	Glycine**
Valine*	Proline**
	Serine
	Tyrosine**

*Branched-chain amino acids
**Conditionally essential

The National Academy of Sciences indicates that different dietary sources of protein vary widely in their composition and nutritional value. The quality of a source of protein is an expression of its ability to provide the nitrogen and amino acid requirements for growth, maintenance, and repair. The key factors are digestibility and the ability to provide the indispensable amino acids. All natural, unprocessed animal and plant foods contain all 20 amino acids. However, the amount of each amino acid in specific foods varies. Over the years a number of different techniques have been used, usually with animals, to assess the quality of protein in selected foods. One of the most widely used is the Protein Digestibility-Corrected Amino Acid Score (PDCAAS), which incorporates real-life variables including the amino acid content and digestibility of the protein. Scores can range from 1.0 to 0.0, with 1.0 being the highest quality. We need not go into a detailed discussion of all techniques to evaluate protein quality, but essentially they focus on the concept of **nitrogen balance,** the ability of the body to retain nitrogen. In essence, nitrogen balance is protein balance. In positive nitrogen balance the body is retaining

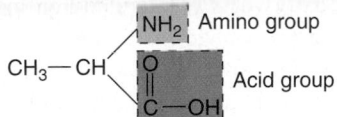

FIGURE 6.1 The chemical structure of alanine, an amino acid. The amino group (NH_2) contains nitrogen, while the acid group is represented by COOH.

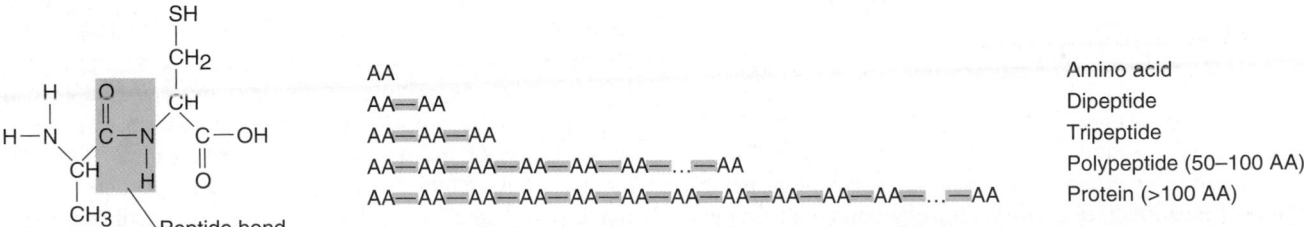

FIGURE 6.2 Formation of peptides and polypeptides from amino acids, with eventual formation of proteins.

protein to adequately support growth and development, whereas in negative nitrogen balance the body is losing protein, with possible impairment in growth and development. The quality of the protein in foods we eat may affect nitrogen balance.

In general, those foods that contain an adequate content of all nine essential amino acids to support both life and growth are known as **complete proteins,** or high-quality proteins, and will have a high PDCAAS score, while those that have a deficiency of one or more essential amino acids and are unable to support life or growth are called **incomplete proteins,** or low-quality proteins, and have a lower score. Relative to human requirements, an essential amino acid that is in limited supply in a particular food is labeled a **limiting amino acid.**

The proteins ingested as animal products are generally regarded to be of a higher quality than those found in plants. This is not to say that an amino acid found in a plant is inferior to the same amino acid found in an animal. They are the same. When we look at the distribution of all the amino acids in the two food sources, however, we can then see two major reasons why animal protein is called a high-quality protein, whereas plant protein is of lower quality. The PDCAAS for egg white and meat is, respectively, 1.0 and 0.92, while the score for kidney beans and whole wheat is, respectively, 0.68 and 0.40.

Animal protein is a complete protein because it contains each essential amino acid in the proper proportion to human requirements. As noted, all 20 amino acids must be present simultaneously for the body to synthesize them into necessary body proteins. If one amino acid is in short supply, protein construction may be blocked. Having the proper amount of animal protein in the diet is a good way to ensure receipt of a balanced supply of amino acids. Some protein supplements marketed to athletes are made from animal protein, including milk, egg, and whey protein.

Plant proteins can provide you with all the protein and amino acids you need for optimal growth and development. However, proteins usually exist in smaller concentrations in plant foods. For example, 2 ounces of fish contain about 14 grams of protein, while 2 ounces of cooked macaroni only have 2 grams; 2 ounces of beans, which are generally regarded to be good sources of protein, have only 5 grams. In addition, most plant proteins have insufficient amounts of one or more of the essential amino acids (i.e., limiting amino acids). Grain products are usually deficient in lysine, whereas legumes are low in methionine. An exception to this generality is the protein isolated from soybeans, which when processed properly is comparable to animal protein. As noted in chapter 2, vegetarians who eat plant foods in proper combinations over the course of the day will receive a balanced supply of amino acids. Some populations receive most of their protein from plant sources.

What are some common foods that are good sources of protein?

Animal Foods Animal foods in the milk and meat groups generally have substantial amounts of high-quality protein. One glass of milk or its equivalent contains about 7–8 grams of protein, as does 1 ounce of meat, fish, or poultry. One egg contains 6 grams of high-quality protein, as does one serving of Egg Beaters, but the latter has half the Calories and no fat or cholesterol.

Plant Foods and Supplements Legumes, such as dry beans (black, garbanzo, great northern, kidney, lima, navy, pinto, soybeans), lentils, and peas (black-eyed, split), are relatively good sources of protein. Legumes also are high in carbohydrate and for this reason are currently classified as a starch food exchange. However, because of their relatively high protein content, legumes may be included within the meat and meat substitutes exchange list. One-half cup contains about 7–9 grams of protein. Nuts contain fair amounts of protein but are high in fat. Fruits, vegetables, and grain products all have some protein, but the content varies; generally speaking, the protein content is low, ranging from less than 1 gram to about 3 grams of protein per serving, although some products may contain more, such as protein-enriched pasta. Some sports drinks and sports bars contain significant amounts of protein. Protein supplements targeted to strength-trained individuals may contain substantial amounts of protein, but may also be expensive.

Table 6.2 and figure 6.3 present some common foods in each of several food groups, with the number of grams of protein in each. Notice the effect combination-type foods have on protein content: for example, macaroni and cheese versus plain macaroni. Most food labels today will list the grams of protein per serving. For plant foods commonly eaten in a vegan diet, review table 2.10 in chapter 2.

How much dietary protein do I need?

Humans actually do not need protein per se, but rather an adequate amount of nitrogen and essential amino acids. However, because all nine essential amino acids and almost all dietary nitrogen are derived from dietary protein, it serves as the basis for our daily requirements. Bilsborough and Mann note that three ways of defining protein intake include absolute intake in grams per day, relative intake based on grams per unit body weight (the basis of the RDA), and as percentage of daily energy intake (the basis of the AMDR).

In the United States, the recommended dietary intake of protein is based upon the RDA. The amount of protein necessary in the diet varies in different stages of the life cycle, as may be noted in the Dietary Reference Intakes table for macronutrients in the front inside cover. During the early years of life, children manufacture protein tissue during rapid growth stages, with the rate of growth (and thus the protein needs) varying from infancy through late adolescence. In young adulthood, the protein requirement stabilizes. Throughout the life cycle, however, the protein requirement established in the RDA is based upon the body weight of the individual. As a person passes from infancy to adulthood, the protein RDA per unit body weight decreases, but the absolute amount of protein needed by the body as a whole actually increases because of increases in body weight.

Table 6.3 presents the amount of protein needed per kilogram or per pound of body weight for different age groups. A variety of scientific techniques have been used over the years to determine human protein needs, and more recent research has reaffirmed these estimates for adults and children. The values for the first year of life are AI, while the remainder are RDA. The values in this table are dependent upon adequate daily energy intake (i.e., Calories), for a low-energy diet will increase protein needs. To calculate your requirement, simply determine your body weight in kilograms or pounds and multiply by the appropriate

TABLE 6.2 Protein content in some common foods

Food	Amount	Protein (grams)	Food	Amount	Protein (grams)
Milk list			*Fruit list*		
Milk, whole	1 c	8	Banana	1	1
Milk, skim	1 c	8	Orange	1	1
Cheese, cheddar	1 oz	7	Pear	1	1
Yogurt	1 c	8			
			Starch list		
Meat list					
			Bread, wheat	1 slice	3
Beef, lean	1 oz	8	Bran flakes	1 c	4
Chicken breast	1 oz	8	Doughnuts	1	1
Luncheon meat	1 oz	5	Macaroni	1/2 c	3
Fish	1 oz	7	Macaroni and cheese	1/2 c	9
Eggs	1	6	Peas, green	1/2 c	4
Navy beans, cooked*	1/2 c	7	Potato, baked	1	3
Peanuts, roasted	1/4 c	9	Quinoa	1 c	8
Peanut butter	1 tbsp	4			
			Sports drinks and bars		
Vegetable list					
			Gatorade Nutrition Shake	11 oz	20
Broccoli	1/2 c	2	Power Bar Protein Plus	1	30
Carrots	1	1	Endurox R4 Recovery Drink	12 oz	11
			Protein sports supplements		
			GNC Pro Performance 100% Whey Protein	31 g	20

Protein (grams) may vary slightly from the food exchange lists because these data were derived from food analyses reported by the United States Department of Agriculture. Some data were obtained from company Websites.

*Found in both the meat and meat substitutes and starch lists in appendix E.

figure for your age group. Recall that 1 kilogram is equal to 2.2 pounds. As an example, compute the protein requirement for a 154-pound, or 70-kg, average 23-year-old male:

$$0.36 \text{ g protein/pound} \times \text{pounds} = 55.4 \text{ or } 56 \text{ g protein/day}$$
$$0.8 \text{ g protein/kg} \times 70 \text{ kg} = 56 \text{ g protein/day}$$

On a protein-free diet, the average individual loses approximately 0.34 g protein/kg body weight per day, which could be replaced by a similar amount of high-quality egg protein. However, allowances are made in the RDA for the fact that individual protein needs vary, that the biologic quality of all dietary protein is not as good as egg protein, and that the efficiency of utilization decreases at higher dietary protein-intake levels. Hence, the RDA is adjusted upward to account for these factors.

The RDA for protein, as noted, is based upon body weight of the individual at different ages. If you took the recommended energy intake in Calories for each age group, say 2,500 C for the average adult male, and calculated the percentage of this value that the RDA for protein supplies, the values approximate 10 percent for each age group. The National Academy of Sciences indicated that the AMDR should not be set below levels for the RDA for

protein, which is about 10 percent of energy. Mathematically, 56 grams of protein, at 4 Calories per gram, total 224 Calories, which is about 9 percent of 2,500, or near the lower limit of the AMDR.

As noted in previous chapters, the Acceptable Macronutrient Distribution Ranges (AMDRs) for individuals have been set based on evidence from interventional trials, with support of epidemiological evidence, to suggest a role in the prevention of increased risk of chronic disease and based on ensuring sufficient intakes of essential nutrients. The AMDR for protein is 10–35 percent of energy for adults and 5–20 and 10–30 percent for young and older children, respectively. The health implications of the AMDR will be discussed later in this chapter.

It is important to note, as Millward indicated in a review, that protein needs are determined by overall food energy intake. If energy intake is inadequate, such as may be the case in those on weight-loss diets or the elderly, dietary protein may be used for energy instead of its core purpose of building tissue. Thus, some individuals may need more or higher quality protein because their energy intake may be low. In particular, some exercise scientists recommend adequate protein for the elderly as a means to prevent sarcopenia (loss of muscle mass) and osteoporosis (loss of bone mass).

How much of the essential amino acids do I need?

The Academy also established RDA for the nine indispensable amino acids. The amounts for adults age 19 and over are found in table 6.4. Slightly larger amounts are recommended for children and adolescents. For the average adult, about 25 percent of the total protein requirement should consist of the essential amino acids; this amounts to about 14–15 grams. Phenylalanine is an essential amino acid, whereas tyrosine is normally listed as a nonessential amino acid. The two are of similar chemical structure so that when substantial quantities of tyrosine are contained in the diet, the need for phenylalanine will decrease somewhat. The same holds true for the essential sulfur-containing amino acid methionine and its chemically related counterpart, cysteine. Individuals who obtain the RDA for protein should have no problem obtaining these recommended values.

Fortunately, we do not need to memorize these amino acids and check our food products to see if they are present. A few general rules can help ensure that we receive a balanced supply in our diet.

What are some dietary guidelines to ensure adequate protein intake?

To answer in one sentence: Eat a wide variety of animal and plant foods. The high-quality, complete proteins are obtained primarily from animal foods. Meat, fish, eggs, poultry, milk, and cheese contain the type and amount of the essential amino

acids necessary for maintaining life and promoting growth and development. They are high-nutrient-density foods, particularly if fat content is low to moderate. Because animal protein is of high quality, you do not need as much of it to satisfy your RDA. For example, for a male who needs about 56 grams of protein per day, only 45 grams is needed if it is animal protein. One glass of milk, with 8 grams of protein, will provide almost 20 percent of his protein RDA. Two glasses of milk, one egg, and 3 ounces of lean meat, fish, or poultry will provide 100 percent of his RDA. In addition, a substantial proportion of daily vitamin and mineral needs will also be supplied in these foods. As noted in chapter 5, selection of low-fat foods will enhance the nutrient density by reducing Calories.

TABLE 6.3	Grams of protein needed per kilogram or per pound body weight during the life cycle	
Age in years	**Grams/kg body weight**	**Grams/pound body weight**
0.0–0.5	1.52	0.69
0.5–1.0	1.10	0.50
1–3	1.10	0.50
4–8	0.95	0.43
9–13	0.95	0.43
14–18	0.85	0.39
19 and up	0.8	0.36

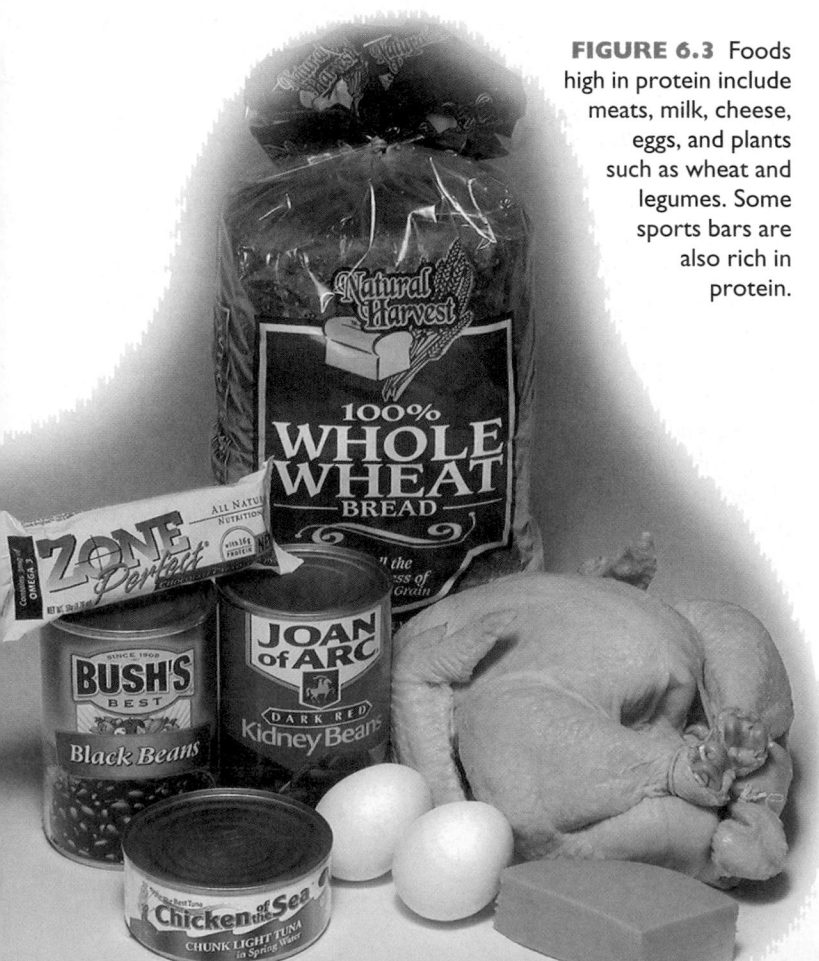

FIGURE 6.3 Foods high in protein include meats, milk, cheese, eggs, and plants such as wheat and legumes. Some sports bars are also rich in protein.

TABLE 6.4	RDA for the essential amino acids in an adult male (70 kg)	
	RDA (mg/kg)	**Total mg**
Histidine	14	980
Isoleucine	19	1,260
Leucine	42	2,940
Lysine	38	2,660
Methionine plus cysteine	19	1,260
Phenylalanine plus tyrosine	33	2,310
Threonine	20	1,400
Tryptophan	5	350
Valine	24	1,680
Total		14,840

Currently, adults in the United States consume only 3.5 ounces of fish per week. There is moderate evidence that consumption of seafood is associated with reduced risk of heart disease. Therefore, in the 2010 *Dietary Guidelines for Americans,* there is a new quantitative recommendation for seafood intake of 8 or more ounces per week from a variety of seafood. You can also go to www.ChooseMyPlate.gov. Click on Food Groups, then Protein Foods Group, to learn more about what foods are healthy choices for each of the food groups. The Food Gallery links may also help in determining serving sizes. From the www.ChooseMyPlate.gov main page, select the *10 tips Nutrition Education Series* from the right-hand side of the page. Here you will find easy-to-follow tips for consumers and professionals in a convenient format, including "With Protein Foods, Variety Is Key."

Plant foods also may provide good sources of protein. Grain products such as wheat, rice, and corn, as well as soybeans, peas, beans, and nuts, have a substantial protein content. However, most plant foods contain incomplete proteins because they lack a sufficient quantity of some essential amino acids. For this reason, the protein RDA for the adult male is 65 grams per day when plant proteins are the primary source. However, Craig and Mangels, in the position stand on vegetarian diets by the American Dietetic Association, state that if certain plant foods are eaten over the course of a day, such as grains and legumes, they may supply all the essential amino acids necessary for human nutrition and be as complete a protein as animal protein.

Some research has suggested that if the daily dietary protein is obtained through a mixture of animal and plant foods in a ratio of 30:70, that is 30 percent of the protein from animal foods and 70 from plant foods, the protein quality would be similar to the use of animal foods alone. Mixing animal and plant foods in the same meal is common, and is also healthful and nutritious. Animal foods provide excellent sources of essential minerals, such as iron, zinc, and calcium, while plant foods provide carbohydrate, dietary fiber, and various phytochemicals.

Key Concepts

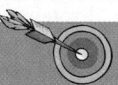

▶ Protein contains nitrogen, an element essential to the formation of 20 different amino acids, the building blocks of all body cells. All 20 amino acids are necessary for protein formation in the body.

▶ Essential, or indispensable, amino acids cannot be adequately synthesized in the body and thus must be obtained through dietary protein, whereas nonessential, or dispensable, amino acids may be synthesized in the body. Conditionally indispensable amino acids may be synthesized from other amino acids under normal conditions, but their synthesis may be limited under certain conditions when insufficient amounts of their precursors are available.

▶ The RDA for protein is based upon the body weight of the individual, and the amount needed per unit body weight is greater during childhood and adolescence than during adulthood. The

adult RDA is 0.8 gram of protein per kilogram body weight, or 0.36 gram per pound body weight.

▶ The Acceptable Macronutrient Distribution Range (AMDR) for protein indicates that dietary intake should be no less than 10 percent and no greater than 35 percent of daily energy needs.

▶ The human body needs a balanced mixture of essential amino acids, and although animal protein provides all of the essential amino acids in the proper blend, a combination of certain plant proteins, such as grains and legumes, will satisfy this dietary requirement.

▶ Although animal foods in the meat and milk groups have high protein content, they may also be high in fat. Increasing the proportion of dietary protein intake from plant sources is recommended. Combining animal and plant proteins in one meal, such as milk and cereal or stir-fry vegetables and meat, will increase the protein quality of the meal.

Check for Yourself

▶ Peruse food labels of some of your favorite foods and check the protein content. Check both animal and plant foods and compare the grams or protein provided by a serving. The percent of the Daily Value (DV) is not required, but it may be found on some labels.

Metabolism and Function

What happens to protein in the human body?

Dietary protein consists of long, complex chains of amino acids. In the digestive process, enzymes (proteases) in the stomach and small intestine break the complex protein down into polypeptides and then into individual amino acids. The amino acids are absorbed through the wall of the small intestine, pass into the blood, and then to the liver via the portal vein (see figure 6.4). The digestion of protein takes several hours, but once the amino acids enter the blood they are cleared within 5 to 10 minutes. There is a constant interchange of amino acids among the blood, the liver, and the body tissues. The liver is a critical center in amino acid metabolism. It is continually synthesizing a balanced amino acid mixture for the diverse protein requirements of the body. These amino acids are secreted into the blood and carried as free amino acids or as plasma proteins such as albumin. All these functions consume energy, and the thermic effect (TEF) is greater for protein as compared to carbohydrate and fat. Whether or not this plays an important role in weight control is discussed in chapter 10.

The most important metabolic fate of the amino acids is the formation of specific proteins, including the structural proteins such as muscle tissue and the functional proteins such as enzymes. Body cells obtain amino acids from the blood, and the genetic apparatus in the cell nucleus directs the synthesis of proteins specific to the cell needs. The body cells may also use some of the nitrogen from the amino acids to form non-protein nitrogen compounds, such as creatine. For example, the muscle cells will form

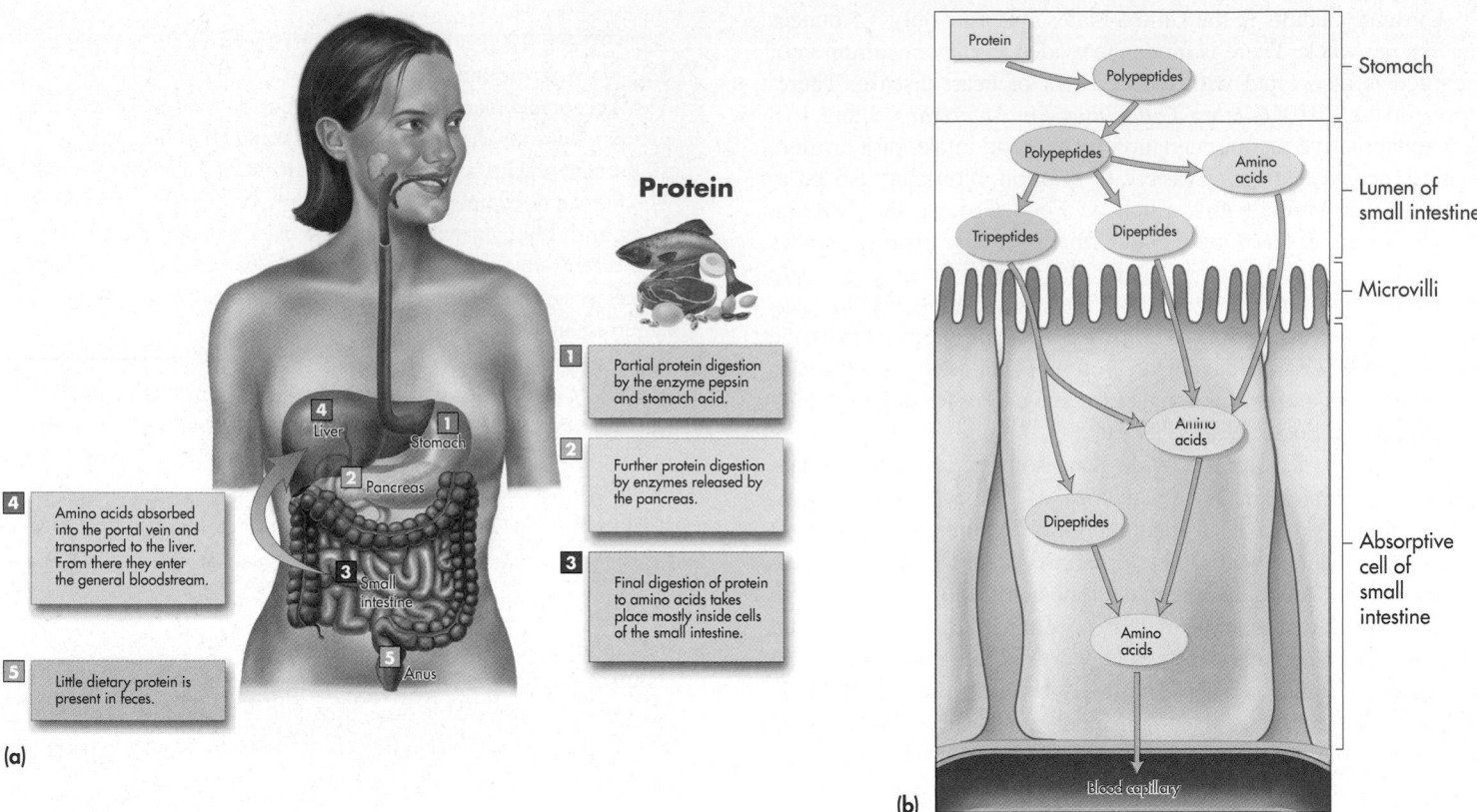

Protein

1. Partial protein digestion by the enzyme pepsin and stomach acid.
2. Further protein digestion by enzymes released by the pancreas.
3. Final digestion of protein to amino acids takes place mostly inside cells of the small intestine.
4. Amino acids absorbed into the portal vein and transported to the liver. From there they enter the general bloodstream.
5. Little dietary protein is present in feces.

(a)

(b)

FIGURE 6.4 (*a*) A summary of protein digestion and absorption. (*b*) Stomach acid and enzymes contribute to protein digestion. Enzmatic protein digestion begins in the stomach and ends in the absorptive cells of the small intestine, where the last peptides are broken down into single amino acids.

contractile proteins as well as the enzymes and creatine phosphate necessary for energy production. The body cells will use only the amount of amino acids necessary to meet their protein needs. They cannot store excess amino acids to any significant amount, although the protein formed may be catabolized to release amino acids back to the blood.

Because the human body does not have a mechanism to store excess nitrogen, it cannot store amino acids per se. Through the process of **deamination,** the amino group (NH_2) containing the nitrogen is removed from the amino acid, leaving a carbon substrate known as an **alpha-ketoacid.** The excess nitrogen must be excreted from the body. In essence, the liver forms **ammonia** (NH_3) from the excess nitrogen; the ammonia is converted into **urea,** which passes into the blood and is eventually eliminated by the kidneys into the urine.

The alpha-ketoacid that is released may have several fates. For one, this carbon substrate may be oxidized for the release of energy. For another, it may accept another amino group and be reconstituted to an amino acid. It also may be channeled into the metabolic pathways of carbohydrate and fat. The liver is the main organ where this conversion occurs. In essence, some of the amino acids are said to be **glucogenic amino acids,** that is, glucose forming. At various stages of the energy transformations within the liver, the glucogenic amino acids may be converted to glucose. As noted in chapter 4, this process is called *gluconeogenesis.* The **ketogenic amino acids**

are metabolized in the liver to acetyl CoA, which may be used for energy production via the Krebs cycle or converted to fat. The glucose and fat produced may be transported to other parts of the body to be used. Thus, although excess protein cannot be stored as amino acids in the body, the energy content is not wasted, for it is converted to either carbohydrate or fat.

Protein turnover represents the process by which all body proteins are being continuously broken down and resynthesized, and it is an ongoing process. The National Academy of Sciences indicates that about 250 grams of body protein turns over daily in an adult, or about 0.5 pound of body mass. Figure 6.5 presents a summary of the fates of protein in human metabolism. See also appendix G, figure G.5.

Can protein be formed from carbohydrates and fats?

Yes, but with some major limitations. Protein has one essential element, nitrogen, which is not possessed by either carbohydrate or fat. However, if the body has an excess of amino acids, the liver may be able to use the nitrogen-containing amino groups from these excess amino acids and combine them with alpha-ketoacids derived from either carbohydrate or fat metabolism. A key alpha-ketoacid from carbohydrate is pyruvic acid, while fat yields acetoacetic acid. The net result is the formation in the body of some of the nonessential amino acids using carbohydrates and fats as part

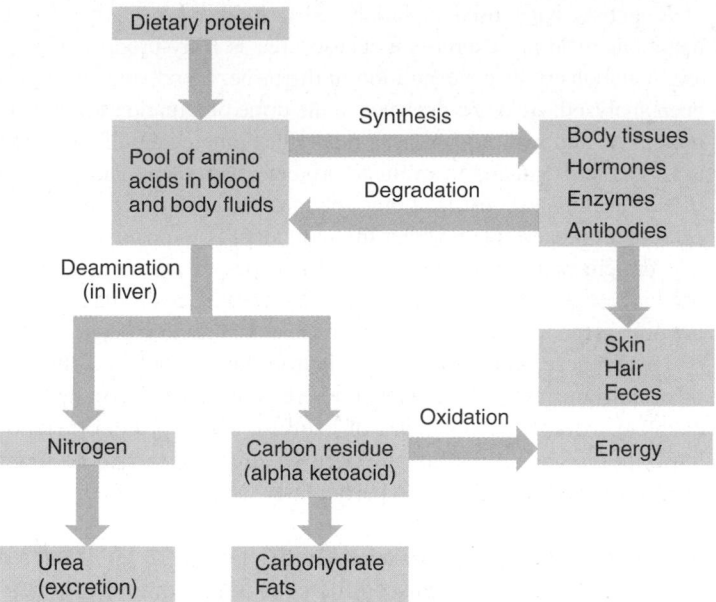

FIGURE 6.5 Simplified diagram of protein metabolism. Following the digestion of dietary proteins, one of the major functions of the amino acids is the synthesis of body tissues, enzymes, hormones, and antibodies. However, protein also is constantly being degraded by the liver. The excess nitrogen is excreted as urea while the carbon residue may be converted into carbohydrate or fat or used to produce energy.

of the building materials. Keep in mind that nitrogen must be present for this to occur, and its source is dietary protein.

What are the major functions of protein in human nutrition?

Dietary protein may be utilized to serve all three major functions of food. Through the action of the individual amino acids, protein serves as the structural basis for the vast majority of body tissues,

is essential for regulating metabolism, and can be used as an energy source. In one way or another protein is involved in almost all body functions. Its individual roles are beyond the scope of this text, so the following discussion represents just some of its major functions of importance to health and fitness. Table 6.5 highlights the major functions of protein in the body.

Protein is the main nutrient used in the formation of all body tissues. This role is extremely important in periods of rapid growth, such as childhood and adolescence. Athletes who attempt to gain muscle tissue also need an adequate dietary supply of protein to create a positive protein balance. Certain amino acids, such as the branched-chain amino acids (BCAA) leucine, isoleucine, and valine, constitute a significant amount of muscle tissue.

Protein is critical in the regulation of human metabolism. It is used in the formation of almost all enzymes, many hormones, and other compounds that control body functions. Insulin, hemoglobin, and the oxidative enzymes in the mitochondria are all proteins that have important roles in regulating metabolism during exercise. Other metabolic roles of protein include the maintenance of water balance and acid-base balance, regulation of the blood clotting process, prevention of infection, and development of immunity to disease. Proteins also serve as carriers for nutrients in the blood, such as the free fatty acids (FFA) and the lipoproteins, and help transport nutrients into the body cells.

Although protein is not a major energy source for humans at rest, it can serve such a function under several conditions. In nutritional energy balance, the priority use of dietary protein is to promote synthesis of body proteins essential for optimal structure and function. However, as noted previously, excess dietary protein may be deaminated and used for energy, or may be converted to carbohydrate or fat and then enter metabolic pathways for energy production or storage. During periods of starvation or semistarvation, adequate amounts of dietary or endogenous carbohydrates and dietary fats may not be available. Both dietary protein and the body protein stores are used for energy purposes in such a

TABLE 6.5	Summary of the functions of proteins and amino acids in human metabolism
1. Structural function	Form vital constituents of all cells in the body, such as contractile muscle proteins
2. Transport function	Transport various substances in the blood, such as the lipoproteins for conveying triglycerides
3. Enzyme function	Form almost all enzymes in the body to regulate numerous diverse physiological processes
4. Hormone and neurotransmitter function	Form various hormones, such as insulin; form various neurotransmitters, or neuropeptides, that function in the central nervous system, such as serotonin
5. Immune function	Form key components of the immune system, such as antibodies
6. Acid-base balance function	Buffer acid and alkaline substances in the blood to maintain optimal pH
7. Fluid balance function	Exert osmotic pressure to maintain optimal fluid balance in body tissues, particularly the blood
8. Energy function	Provide source of energy to the Krebs cycle when deaminated; excess protein may be converted to glucose or fat for subsequent energy production
9. Movement function	Provide movement when structural muscle proteins use energy to contract

situation, because energy production takes precedence over tissue building in metabolism. Hence, if the active individual desires to maintain lean body mass, it is essential to have not only adequate protein intake but also sufficient carbohydrate Calories in the diet to provide a **protein-sparing effect.** In other words, carbohydrate Calories will be used for energy production, thus sparing utilization of protein as an energy source and allowing it to be used for its more important structural and metabolic functions.

Although body proteins are composed of all 20 amino acids, individual amino acids may have important specific effects in the body. For example, the amino acid glycine is a neurotransmitter substance; tryptophan and tyrosine are important for the formation of several chemical transmitters in the brain; and the branched-chain amino acids (leucine, isoleucine, and valine) are major components of muscle tissue that may provide a source of energy.

Because of the diverse roles of protein and amino acids in the body, athletes have used protein supplements for years in attempts to improve performance. Amino acid supplements have also been used for this purpose. The effectiveness of such supplements is evaluated in later sections.

Key Concept

▶ The major function of dietary protein is to build and repair tissues and to synthesize hormones, enzymes, and other body compounds essential in human metabolism, but it also may be used as a significant source of energy under certain conditions.

Proteins and Exercise

Protein has always been considered one of the main staples of an athlete's diet. In this section we discuss several topics regarding protein and exercise, including its use as an energy source, possible avenues for protein loss, protein metabolism during recovery, and dietary requirements and recommendations for strength and endurance athletes.

Are proteins used for energy during exercise?

The average individual consumes about 10 percent or more of daily energy intake from protein. For individuals in protein and energy balance, this protein intake must be balanced through energy expenditure and other body losses. In general, scientists suggest that about 5 percent of daily protein intake may be used directly for energy. Protein in excess of tissue needs may be converted to carbohydrate or fat, which may also be used for energy. Protein may also be lost from the body in various ways, such as creatinine and urea excreted in the urine and sloughed body cells. In one review, Gibala noted that protein is regarded as a minor source of fuel during rest, usually accounting for less than 5 percent of total daily energy expenditure. However, given its nutritional importance, researchers have attempted to determine the effect of exercise on protein balance and needs.

Scientists have used a variety of techniques to study protein metabolism during exercise. Because urea is a by-product of protein metabolism, its concentration in the urine, blood, and sweat has been analyzed. Also, the presence in the urine of a marker for muscle protein breakdown, known as 3-methylhistidine, a modified amino acid, has been studied to evaluate protein catabolism. The nitrogen balance technique consists of precisely measuring nitrogen intake and excretion to determine whether the individual is in positive or negative protein balance. Finally, labeled isotopes of amino acids have been ingested or injected to study their metabolic fate during exercise, not only in the whole body but also in isolated muscle groups.

Using these techniques, investigators have evaluated the use of protein during both resistance exercise and aerobic endurance exercise. Although both types of exercise affect protein metabolism, the use of protein as an energy source appears to be more prevalent in aerobic exercise, particularly when prolonged.

Resistance Training In a review, Rennie and Tipton noted that resistance exercise causes little change in amino acid oxidation, but probably depresses protein synthesis and elevates breakdown acutely. In this regard, Evans suggested that the eccentric muscle contraction associated with resistance training may produce ultrastructural damage that may stimulate this protein turnover. However, Wolfe noted that factors regulating muscle protein breakdown in human subjects are complex and interactive, and proposed that muscle protein breakdown is paradoxically elevated in the anabolic state following resistance exercise. Thus, while it appears that resistance exercise does not increase protein or amino acid oxidation, it may provoke muscle tissue breakdown.

Aerobic Endurance Exercise Poortmans has noted that although protein may be used to produce significant amounts of ATP in the muscle, during aerobic endurance exercise the rate of production is much slower than with carbohydrate and fat, the preferred fuels. On the other hand, Rennie and Tipton noted that sustained dynamic exercise stimulates amino acid oxidation, mainly by activating an enzyme (BCAA dehydrogenase; BCAAD) that oxidizes BCAA and increases ammonia production in proportion to exercise intensity. If the exercise is intense enough, there is a net loss of muscle protein as a result of decreased protein synthesis, increased catabolism, or both. Some of the amino acids are oxidized as fuel, and the rest provide substrates for gluconeogenesis. In this regard, prolonged exercise may be comparable to a state of starvation. As the endurance athlete depletes the endogenous carbohydrate stores, the body catabolizes some of its protein for energy or eventual conversion to glucose. Protein catabolism has been shown to increase significantly even when muscle glycogen is depleted by only about 33–55 percent.

Mechanisms and By-Products In general, a brief session of exercise lowers the rate of protein synthesis and speeds protein breakdown. The exact mechanisms of protein metabolism during exercise have not been determined, though several mechanisms have been proposed. Parkhouse has reported that exercise, particularly exercise to exhaustion, activates specific proteolytic enzymes in the muscle that degrade the myofibrillar protein.

Fitts and Metzger found elevated levels of proteolytic enzymes in fatigued muscle. In a review, Wagenmakers indicated that six amino acids (BCAA; asparagine, aspartate, glutamate) may be metabolized in the muscle, providing the nitrogen needed for the synthesis of ammonia, alanine, and glutamine. During exercise, particularly prolonged aerobic exercise, Graham and MacLean noted significant muscle efflux of ammonia, glutamine, and alanine. These three products carry excess nitrogen from the muscle to other parts of the body, most notably the liver, for recycling or conversion to urea.

Ammonia, a nitrogen by-product of protein catabolism, is an indicator of increased muscle amino acid breakdown. Although no underlying mechanism has been identified, increasing levels of ammonia in the body have been associated with fatigue, somewhat comparable to the accumulation of lactic acid. One theory is that increased ammonia levels in the muscle may impair oxidative processes, thus decreasing energy production, while another theory suggests that increased plasma ammonia may impair brain functions and induce central fatigue. Because ammonia is formed in the muscle from the amino group, removal of the amino group by alanine or glutamine may help decrease the production of ammonia and delay the onset of fatigue.

Glutamine release from the muscle also increases during exercise, and it is an important fuel for various cells in the body, particularly those in the immune system. As we shall see later, glutamine supplementation has been studied as a means to enhance immune function in athletes.

Leucine and the Glucose-Alanine Cycle

Although a number of amino acids may be used as energy substrate during exercise, the major research effort has focused on the fate of leucine. Wagenmakers noted that the increase in BCAA oxidation during prolonged exercise seems to be specific for leucine only. In essence, the amino group of leucine catabolism eventually combines with pyruvate in the muscle cell to form alanine and leaves the residual alpha-ketoacid. The alpha-ketoacid may enter the Krebs cycle and be used for energy production. The alanine is released into the bloodstream and transported to the liver where it is converted into glucose. The glucose may then be released into the blood to be used by the central nervous system and may eventually find its way to the contracting muscle to be used as an energy source. Alanine appears to be the most important means of transporting the amino group to the liver for excretion as urea. This overall process involving gluconeogenesis, known as the glucose-alanine cycle, is depicted graphically in figure 6.6. Some investigators have noted that during the latter part of endurance exercise, the blood levels of alanine increase, presumably because more is released from the muscle. However, the estimated glucose production approximates only 4 grams per hour, which might make a limited contribution in mild-intensity exercise but is possibly insignificant during high-intensity exercise when carbohydrate use may approximate 3 grams or more per minute. Additionally, several investigators have reported an increased release of branched-chain amino acids (BCAAs) from the liver during endurance exercise, with subsequent uptake by the muscle cells.

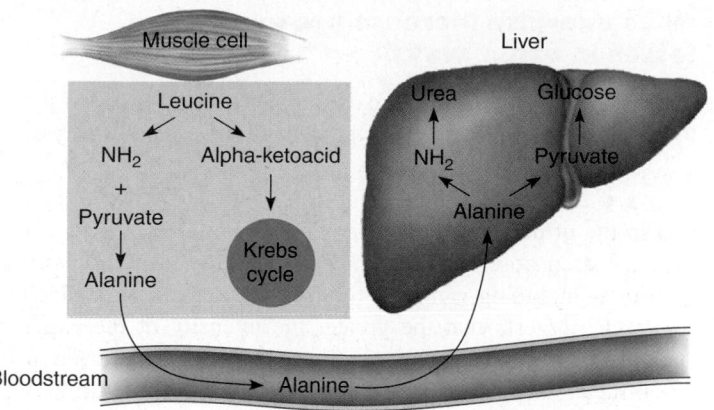

FIGURE 6.6 Glucose-alanine cycle. Alanine may be produced in the muscle tissue from the breakdown of other amino acids, most notably leucine. The alanine is then released into the blood and travels to the liver for eventual conversion to glucose through the process of gluconeogenesis. (See appendix G, figure G.5, for other amino acids that may enter energy pathways.)

Protein Use and Importance of Carbohydrate

Protein (amino acids) can be utilized during exercise to provide energy directly in the muscle and via glucose produced in the liver, particularly when the body stores of glycogen and glucose are low. In earlier research, Lemon reported that in the latter stages of prolonged endurance exercise, protein could contribute up to 15 percent of the total energy cost. However, less protein would be used for energy during the early stages of prolonged exercise when carbohydrate is adequate. Thus, Gibala suggested that the contribution of amino acid oxidation to total energy expenditure is negligible during short-term intense exercise and accounts for 3–5 percent of the total energy production during prolonged exercise. In his review, Tarnopolsky cited similar figures, indicating that protein oxidation could account for 1 to 6 percent of the energy cost of aerobic exercise. Tarnopolsky also noted that women oxidize less protein compared with men and show lower leucine oxidation during aerobic exercise.

It is important to note how dietary carbohydrate influences protein as an energy source during exercise. A low-carbohydrate diet leading to decreased muscle glycogen levels will lead to increased dependence on protein as an energy source. However, adequate carbohydrate intake before and during prolonged exercise will help reduce the use of body protein for this purpose, because the presence of adequate muscle glycogen appears to inhibit enzymes that catabolize muscle protein. Scientists from the University of Maastricht in the Netherlands noted that high-carbohydrate diets may have a protein-sparing effect for endurance athletes.

Although the available evidence suggests that metabolism of protein and its use as an energy source are increased during exercise, the magnitude of its contribution may depend on a variety of factors, such as the intensity and duration of exercise and the availability of other fuels, such as carbohydrate, either as stored muscle glycogen or consumed during exercise.

Does exercise increase protein losses in other ways?

Other than loss of protein from oxidation, exercise has been shown to increase protein losses from the body in several other ways.

Urinary Losses   Exercise may cause an elevated level of protein in the urine, a condition known as **proteinuria.** This condition has been observed following competition in a wide variety of sports, including running, football, basketball, and handball. Research suggests that the greater the intensity of the exercise, such as a high-intensity 400-meter sprint versus a lower-intensity 3,000-meter run, the greater the loss of protein in the urine. Prolonged aerobic exercise, such as the triathlon, has also increased urinary protein loss. Yaguchi and others suggested that heavy, prolonged exercise, such as a triathlon, may induce some transient kidney damage in some individuals. Such damage may explain the findings of Poortmans, who reported a decreased reabsorption of protein in the kidney tubules following intense exercise. However, the total amount of protein lost in this manner appears to be rather negligible, amounting to less than 3 grams per day.

Sweat Losses   Protein also may be lost in the sweat. Several investigators have reported the presence of both amino acids and proteins in exercise-induced sweat, with both sweat rate and sweat nitrogen losses increasing with greater exercise intensities. Again, the losses are relatively minor, on the order of 1 gram per liter of sweat in adult males. This avenue could account for 2–4 grams of protein in an endurance athlete training in a warm environment.

Gastrointestinal Losses   As shall be noted in chapter 8, prolonged intense exercise may also increase gastrointestinal losses of iron, which may be bound to blood proteins. Again, however, these protein losses would be relatively minor.

What happens to protein metabolism during recovery after exercise?

Although net protein breakdown occurs during exercise, in general protein synthesis is believed to predominate during the recovery period. In a review, Tipton and Wolfe noted that whole body protein breakdown is generally reduced following aerobic endurance exercise, while whole body protein synthesis is either increased or unchanged. However, they note that whole body protein synthesis may not represent changes in specific muscle groups. Muscle groups that have been exercised may experience protein synthesis, as they may be especially insulin sensitive after exercise. In another review, Walberg-Rankin notes that although leucine may be oxidized during moderate aerobic exercise, leucine balance returns to normal in 24 hours, indicating a reduced leucine catabolism over this time frame.

Tipton and Wolfe report that resistance exercise induces protein breakdown in the exercised muscles, which may persist in the immediate recovery period. However, over the next 24–48 hours, protein anabolism appears to predominate and the net effect is increased protein synthesis. Wolfe notes that anabolic states appear to be due more to stimulation of synthesis rather than a decrease in breakdown. This is especially so if adequate amino acids are available.

Eccentric exercise, such as lowering weights during resistance exercise or running downhill rapidly, puts tremendous stress on muscle tissue, and often induces muscle soreness in the following days. Tipton and Wolfe note that following eccentric exercise, whole body protein breakdown is increased. Microtears in muscle fibers may impair protein synthesis and delay recovery from such exercise. The muscle fiber microtears are believed to be the causative factor underlying the muscle soreness which, because its onset is usually delayed for 1–2 days, is referred to as **delayed onset of muscle soreness (DOMS).**

What effect does exercise training have upon protein metabolism?

Rennie noted that protein metabolism may also become more efficient as a result of training, noting that the response of muscle protein turnover to habitual exercise is comparable to other metabolic changes in the muscle associated with exercise training. Although an initial bout of exercise may markedly elevate protein breakdown and synthesis in an untrained individual, the effect would be much less in one who has trained habitually. Tarnopolsky indicated that training induces a decreased *activity* in BCAAD, the enzyme that oxidizes BCAAs, when exercising at a standardized workload of the same absolute intensity.

As mentioned, protein synthesis appears to predominate in the muscles during recovery. With training, or repeated bouts of exercise on a regular basis, changes in the muscle structure and function are additive. Numerous studies have found that after resistance or endurance exercise, protein balance becomes positive. Trained individuals, during rest, have been shown to experience a preferential oxidation of fat and a sparing of protein, as measured by leucine metabolism and the respiratory quotient. The specific exercise task apparently stimulates the DNA in the muscle cell nucleus to increase the synthesis of protein, and the type of protein that is synthesized is specific to the type of exercise. Aerobic exercise stimulates syntheses of mitochondria and oxidative enzymes, which are composed of protein and are necessary for energy production in the oxygen system. Resistance training promotes synthesis of the contractile muscle proteins. These adaptations are the key factors underlying improved performance (see figure 6.7).

Other than its beneficial effects in increasing structural and functional protein important to resistance or aerobic endurance exercise, training may influence protein metabolism in other ways to help prevent premature fatigue. You may recall from previous chapters that there is substantial research to support the conclusion that aerobic endurance training improves the ability of the muscle cell to use both carbohydrate and fat as energy sources during exercise. Although extensive evidence is not available, in a review, Graham and others noted that following endurance training, enzymes in the muscles appear to develop the potential

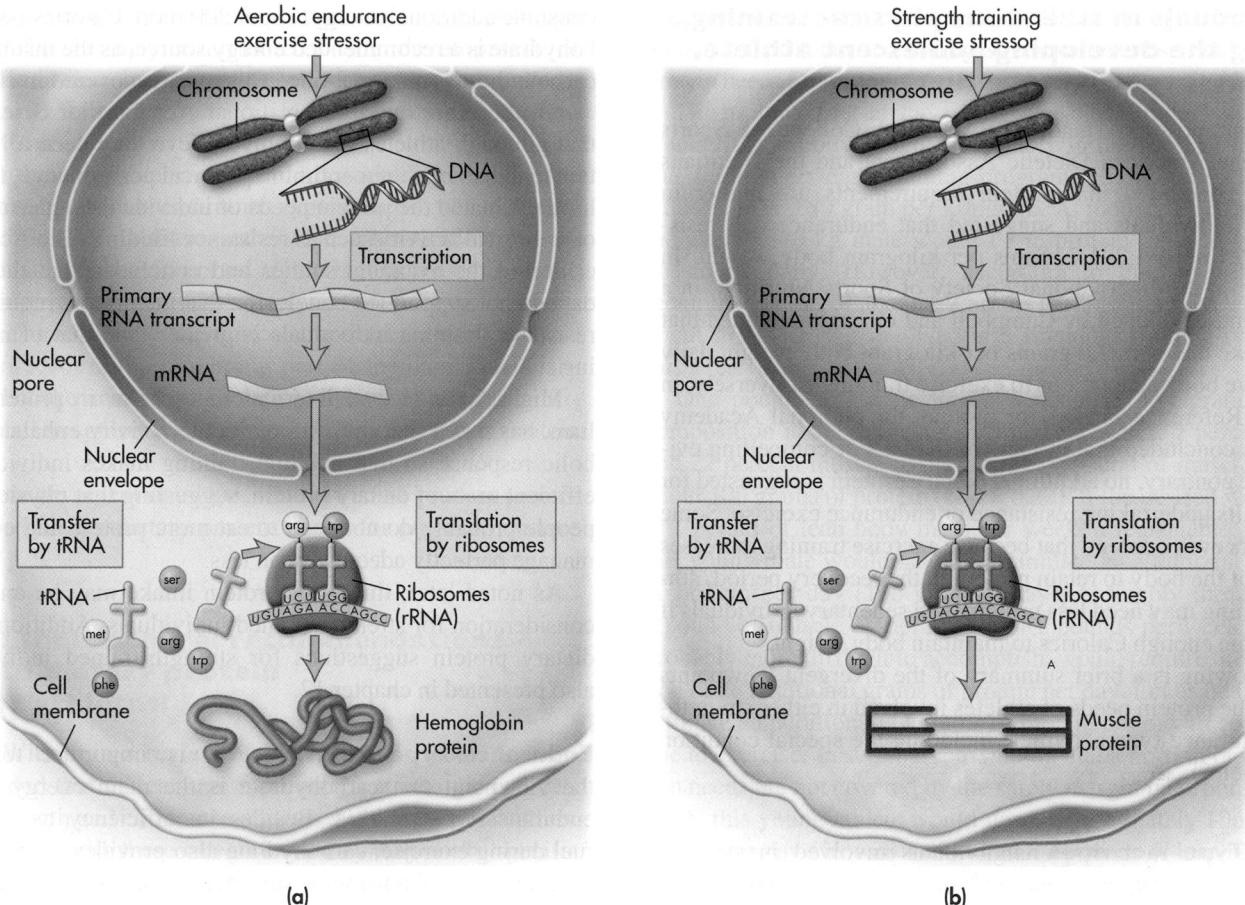

FIGURE 6.7 Adaptations in body tissues following exercise training are specific to the type of exercise. The exercise stressor influences the genes to initiate the formation of protein synthesis through the transcription, transfer, and translation process. The transcription process provides the template (messenger RNA:mRNA) for the specific protein; the transfer (transfer RNA) process moves specific amino acids to the ribosome; the translation process by the ribosomes (ribosomal RNA) forms the protein. (*a*) Aerobic exercise training will lead to an increase in serum hemoglobin levels, which transport oxygen to the muscle cells. (*b*) Resistance training will lead to an increase in skeletal muscle protein.

for increased capacity for oxidation of leucine and the other BCAAs, which are an abundant source of energy in the muscles. Thus, endurance training may increase the capacity of the muscle to derive energy from protein in a fashion similar to the increased utilization of fat, another possible means to spare the use of carbohydrates such as blood glucose, to help protect the main energy source for the brain, and muscle glycogen. Although these changes do not appear to spare the use of muscle protein, they would appear to spare the use of carbohydrate, and thus may help prevent fatigue when carbohydrate levels are decreased during exercise.

Additionally, when exercising at a standardized workload before and after training, training may also decrease the production or accumulation of ammonia. Extrapolating from animal research, some investigators theorize that instead of forming ammonia, the nitrogen is incorporated into other amino acids, such as alanine, for transportation from the muscle to the liver. Theoretically, reduced plasma ammonia levels may be associated with less fatigue.

Training properly may also help prevent muscle injury associated with eccentric exercise. Research shows that physically trained individuals, when compared to untrained individuals, do not experience as much muscle tissue damage during prolonged, eccentric exercise tasks. However, specificity of training is also important, and individuals preparing for a race with a significant downhill component, such as the Boston Marathon, should gradually incorporate increasing intensities of eccentric exercise in their training.

In general, these changes associated with appropriate training appear to represent another means whereby the body adapts to endurance training in an attempt to prevent fatigue. However, some research indicates that excessive training leading to the overtraining syndrome is associated with a persistent decrease in plasma amino acids, particularly glutamine.

The effect of training in producing a positive nitrogen balance or a positive protein balance, and possibly the effect of preventing the overtraining syndrome, depends on an adequate dietary supply of protein and Calories.

If the protein portion of the dietary Calories averaged 12 percent, a general recommended level of protein intake, then the intake of protein would approximate 1.5–1.7 grams per kilogram body weight, which parallels the amounts estimated in the examples cited previously. Currently, the protein content of the average American is 12 to 16 percent, and Walberg-Rankin noted that most athletes consume this much or more in their daily diets. Consuming a diet with a protein content of 15 percent could provide a value of 2.0 grams or more per kilogram body weight, and other surveys among strength-type athletes indicate that they obtain this amount. These values approach or exceed the higher amounts recommended by some investigators for individuals in training. The calculations are presented in table 6.6.

Some athletes may need to increase the percentage of protein in their daily caloric intake. Athletes in weight-control sports, such as wrestlers and gymnasts, may be in greater need of protein because of low caloric intake. Endurance athletes, particularly ultraendurance athletes, are susceptible to overtraining and chronic fatigue. Such athletes have been found to have depressed plasma levels of amino acids, which Kingsbury and others indicated appeared to be associated with inadequate protein intake.

Young athletes have high protein needs to support growth and development. Volek indicates that female strength athletes may require more protein than their endurance-training counterparts to attain positive nitrogen balance and promote protein synthesis. Also, some female endurance athletes may need more protein because of inadequate energy intake, and low dietary protein intake has been associated with amenorrhea, a topic discussed further in chapters 8 and 10.

Increasing the protein percentage of daily energy intake may help such athletes obtain adequate protein. For example, a young wrestler attempting to lose weight to compete in a lower weight category might be on a diet of 1,600 Calories per day. With an RDA of 0.85 gram of protein per kilogram body weight, a 60-kilogram (132 pound) wrestler would need 51 grams of protein to meet the RDA and up to 102 grams to meet the highest recommendation for strength-type athletes. To consume 51 grams of protein, the wrestler would need to obtain about 13 percent of daily energy intake from protein, but to obtain 102 grams of protein would need to obtain about 25 percent of daily energy intake from protein. These amounts are well within the AMDR for protein.

Wise selection of high-quality protein foods will provide adequate amounts through a balanced diet to meet bodily needs during the early and continued stages of training. It is not difficult to increase the protein content of the diet. For example, 8 ounces of roasted, skinless chicken breast and two glasses of skim milk, a total of less than 600 Calories, will provide more than 70 grams of high-quality protein, the RDA for our typical 70-kg adolescent and more than half of the 125 grams that may be recommended for such an athlete attempting to gain muscle mass. Perusal of table 6.2 and appendix E will help you select high-protein foods. Additional points on this subject are covered in chapter 12 under the topic of gaining weight as muscle.

2. *Consume protein, preferably with carbohydrate, before and after workouts.* Eating strategies may also be an important consideration, particularly timing of protein intake. Most research has focused on amino acid or protein ingestion following exercise, but some studies have also studied the effect of preexercise protein intake. The feedings usually occurred immediately before or within an hour of exercise. Many studies have used **protein hydrolysate,** a high-protein dietary supplement containing a solution of amino acids and peptides prepared from protein by hydrolysis. Wolfe noted that the protein supplement should contain all the essential amino acids, and many studies also added carbohydrate.

Protein intake before exercise In separate reviews, Tipton and Wolfe both noted research studies suggesting that ingestion of free amino acids plus carbohydrates before exercise results in a superior anabolic response to exercise than if ingested after exercise. Lemon indicates that the practice of consuming nutrients prior to exercise may be beneficial by providing fuel and/or minimizing catabolic processes. However, in his review Tipton noted that the difference in anabolic response between preexercise and postexercise ingestion of protein is not apparent. In 2008, the International Society of Sports Nutrition published its position stand on nutrient timing. As a part of this position stand, Kerksick and others stated that the optimal preexercise meal is dependent on several factors, including exercise duration and fitness level. General guidelines they suggest are ingestion of 1–2 grams of carbohydrate per kilogram body weight and 0.15–0.25 grams of protein per kilogram body weight in the 3–4 hours prior to competition.

Protein intake after exercise Studies from Robert Wolfe's laboratory, using both intravenous and oral administration of amino acids, have suggested that providing an ample supply to the muscle within 1–3 hours following exercise may help

TABLE 6.6	Calculation of grams protein/kilogram body weight	
Body weight: 70 kg		
One gram protein = 4 Calories		
Daily caloric intake:	3,500–4,000	3,500–4,000
Percent protein:	15	12
Calories in protein:	525–600	420–480
Grams of protein:	131–150	105–120
Grams protein/kg:	1.9–2.1	1.5–1.7

to further stimulate protein synthesis. The increased blood flow to the muscle during the immediate recovery period may permit a more effective delivery of the amino acids. In his review, Rennie indicated that muscle protein synthesis appears to be very sensitive to increased availability of amino acids in the blood and appears to be saturated by a relatively small increase in amino acid availability equivalent to about 3.5–7.0 grams of protein over an hour. Gibala indicated that consuming a drink containing about 0.1 gram of essential amino acids per kilogram of body weight (7 grams for a 70-kilogram athlete) during the first few hours of recovery from heavy resistance exercise will produce a transient, net positive increase in muscle protein balance.

This amount may be different when a complete protein is consumed. Moore and colleagues examined the impact of protein dose on muscle protein synthesis following resistance exercise. Healthy, active young men consumed, in a random order, drinks containing 0, 5, 10, 20, or 40 grams of whole egg protein after an intense bout of resistance exercise. A dose-dependent response to increasing protein intake was seen for protein synthesis after resistance exercise, with maximal stimulation after ingesting 20 grams of high-quality protein. However, according to Beelen there is still debate on the exact amount and type of protein, as well as the timing of protein intake, to maximize muscle synthesis after exercise.

Protein and carbohydrate intake after exercise Carbohydrate alone may have some effect on protein synthesis following exercise, as it may help to decrease secretion of cortisol, a hormone that promotes protein catabolism. Moreover, Lemon has noted that the insulin response to dietary carbohydrate has been shown to enhance the already elevated protein synthetic rate in muscle following a strength-training session. However, van Loon, Drummond, and others indicate that if adequate protein is available, there is no need for carbohydrates to promote muscle protein synthesis, but also noted that because resistance exercise uses muscle glycogen, the carbohydrate could help replenish muscle glycogen.

Several studies and reviews have suggested that such protein intake soon *after* exercise, possibly combined with carbohydrate, was beneficial. Anton Wagenmakers, an international authority on protein metabolism during exercise, noted that protein provides the amino acids and carbohydrate increases insulin secretion. Wagenmakers noted that the effect of amino acids and insulin on protein synthesis is substantially larger after exercise, suggesting that exercise potentiates the anabolic effect of insulin and amino acids. Levenhagen and others reported that consuming protein immediately after exercise enhanced accretion of whole body and leg protein as compared to protein consumption several hours later. These findings were supported in more recent studies by Koopman and others, who used a protein/carbohydrate solution during exercise and added leucine to a protein/carbohydrate feeding after exercise. Esmarck also

found that consumption of protein with carbohydrate soon after exercise also benefits muscle protein synthesis in the elderly as well.

Nutrient timing and performance Based on available research findings, the ratio of carbohydrates to protein requires additional investigation, as concluded by the International Society of Sports Nutrition in its position stand on nutrient timing. In this position stand, Kersick et al. conclude that the approach often used is to consume a supplement containing a ratio of 3–4 grams of carbohydrate per gram of protein within 30 minutes following exercise. Although commercial protein/carbohydrate sport drinks and supplements are available, Phillips and others recommend high-quality protein food sources, such as dairy protein, eggs, and lean meat, which provide an abundance of essential amino acids. In their review, Rennie and others note that a solution of mixed amino acids will increase human muscle protein synthesis to about the same extent as complete meals. A turkey breast sandwich on whole-wheat bread consumed with a glass of chocolate skim milk provides a good balance of protein and carbohydrate. Karp and Elliot, along with their associates, indicated that milk, including chocolate milk, may be an effective recovery drink for athletes and provides an alternative to supplements.

It should be noted that although these dietary practices may provide the nutrients necessary for an anabolic response in the muscle, Gibala indicates it remains to be determined if the acute effects of such supplementation eventually lead to greater gains in muscle mass following habitual training. In a study involving a 10-week resistance training program, Cribb and Hayes found that consuming a supplement containing protein, creatine, and glucose (1 gram/kg body weight) immediately before and after training, as compared to consuming the same supplement in the morning and evening, resulted in greater increases in lean body mass, muscle cross-section area, and muscular strength. Although this study would appear to support anabolic effects of protein and carbohydrate intake immediately before and after exercise training, the supplement also contained creatine, which as noted later in this chapter may by itself increase muscle mass and strength. Most investigators in this area indicate that more research is needed to determine the optimal combination of protein and timing for the various types of exercise training adaptations.

3. *Be prudent regarding protein intake.* Whether or not athletes in training need additional protein is not clear at this time. Two experts in protein metabolism, Kevin Tipton and Robert Wolfe, noted that given sufficient energy intake, lean body mass can be maintained within a wide range of protein intakes. They note that since a high protein intake is not likely harmful, and since there is a metabolic rationale for the efficacy of an increase in dietary protein if muscle hypertrophy is the goal, a higher protein intake within the context of an athlete's overall dietary requirements may be beneficial. However, they also note that there are few convincing data

to indicate that the ingestion of a high amount of protein (2–3 grams per kilogram body weight) is necessary. Based on current literature, they conclude that it may be too simplistic to rely on recommendations of a particular amount of protein per day, because the amount depends on energy intake, type of protein, and timing of intake.

Consuming additional protein within the AMDR is both safe and prudent. Table 6.7 presents a summary of some prudent daily protein intakes for sedentary and physically active individuals. These recommendations are in accord with those of the U.S. Anti-Doping Agency in its nutrition guide to athletes, *Optimal Dietary Intake*.

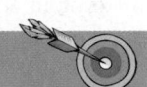

Key Concepts

▶ During aerobic endurance exercise, particularly with low carbohydrate stores in the body, muscle protein may supply nearly 5 percent of the energy Calories.

▶ Although protein catabolism may occur during exercise, protein synthesis predominates in the recovery period. The type of protein synthesized is specific to the type of exercise program, such as resistance (weight, strength) training or aerobic endurance.

▶ Several recognized authorities have recommended a protein intake of 1.6–1.7 grams per kilogram body weight per day for athletes attempting to gain weight, and about 1.2–1.4 grams per kilogram body weight per day for endurance athletes.

TABLE 6.7 Prudent protein intakes in grams per kilogram body weight for sedentary and physically active individuals	
	Grams of protein/kg body weight
Sedentary	0.8
Strength-trained, maintenance	1.2–1.4
Strength-trained, gain muscle mass	1.6–1.7
Endurance-trained	1.2–1.4
Intermittent, high-intensity training	1.4–1.7
Weight-restricted	1.4–1.8

The values presented represent a synthesis of those recommended by leading researchers involved in protein metabolism and exercise. Teenagers should add 10 percent to the calculated values.

To calculate body weight in kilograms, simply multiply your weight in pounds by 0.454. Then, multiply your weight in kilograms by the appropriate value in the grams per kilogram body weight column to determine the range of grams of protein intake per day. Teenagers should increase this amount by 10 percent.

▶ Timing of protein intake may be an important consideration. Consuming a protein/carbohydrate combination immediately before or after exercise training may provide a nutritional and hormonal milieu favorable to muscle anabolism and recovery. However, whether such a dietary strategy increases muscle mass or exercise performance is unknown.

▶ The National Academy of Sciences has indicated that the RDA is sufficient to meet the protein needs of athletes. However, others have suggested that physical training increases the protein requirements, but these recommended increases are well within the AMDR.

Check for Yourself

▶ Using table 6.7 as a guide, calculate how many grams of protein may be recommended for you. If you have not already done so, keep a record of your daily food intake for several days and determine if you are obtaining sufficient dietary protein.

Protein: Ergogenic Aspects

Given the potential importance of protein to optimal physical performance, a wide variety of ergogenic aids associated with protein nutrition have been used in attempts to enhance performance. Such supplements remain popular. As Lawrence and Kirby noted, protein, amino acids, and creatine were among the top five most popular sports supplements.

What types of special protein supplements are marketed to physically active individuals?

As already discussed, some investigators suggest that athletes involved in weight training to gain weight or in strenuous endurance exercise may need somewhat more than the RDA for protein to maintain or increase protein balance, particularly if energy intake (Calories) is not adequate to meet daily energy expenditure.

To provide additional protein to the diet, investigators have used high-protein diets, powdered protein sources, canned liquid meals high in protein and energy, sports drinks and bars, or special foods and concoctions high in protein content. However, the protein content is actually derived from natural protein, such as milk, egg, or soy protein. As Bucci has indicated, supplements of intact proteins, such as the proteins found in these products, offer no advantages over protein found in other food sources, since these supplements are in fact derived from natural foods. In addition, many of these protein supplements are expensive when compared to natural protein that may be obtained easily in high-protein foods such as powdered milk, skim milk, eggs, and chicken. Blending powdered milk into a glass of skim milk, with some vanilla or other flavoring, will provide substantial amounts of high-quality protein—your own personal protein supplement. Some comparative costs for different sources of protein are presented in table 6.8.

TABLE 6.8 Costs of protein found in various food sources

Source	Serving size	Grams of protein/serving	Cost per serving	Cost per 8 grams of protein
Powdered milk	23 grams	8	$0.13	$0.13
Egg	1	6	$0.10	$0.13
Turkey breast	4 ounces	28	$0.75	$0.21
Skim milk	8 fluid ounces	8	$0.20	$0.20
Protein capsules	8 capsules	8	$1.20	$1.20
MetRx Bar	3.5-ounce bar	27	$2.50	$0.74
Boost	8 fluid ounces	10	$1.10	$0.88
Avalanche Power Drink	16 fluid ounces	40	$3.00	$0.60
Whey Pro	1 scoop	23	$1.01	$0.34

Nevertheless, commercial supplements may be a convenient means for some busy athletes to secure additional protein in the diet. Many of these products contain high-quality protein, such as milk, whey, or egg protein; provide a balanced mixture of protein, carbohydrate, and fat for additional Calories; and may also contain supplemental vitamins and minerals. Although these products do not contain all of the nutrients of natural foods, they may be useful adjuncts to a balanced diet. Certain brands have been available for years, such as Nutrament, but several companies have marketed products specifically for physically active individuals, such as Mega Whey by GNC and Nutrition Shake by Gatorade. It is important to reemphasize the point that these supplements should be used as an adjunct to an otherwise balanced nutritional plan, not as a substitute.

Whey and colostrum are two forms of protein that are sold as dietary supplements and marketed as a means to enhance sport performance. Whey proteins are extracted from the liquid whey that is produced during the manufacture of cheese or casein. Whey protein isolates are more than 90 percent protein. Hayes and Cribb note that whey proteins are a rich source of essential amino acids, thus providing the foundations for preservation of muscle mass. Walzem and others note that bovine whey may contain other substances, including growth factors. Colostrum, or bovine colostrum, is the first milk secreted by cows. Standardized preparations of colostrum are available as dietary supplements. Brinkworth and others indicate that colostrum is a rich source of protein, carbohydrates, vitamins, minerals, and various biologically active components, also including growth factors. Although no mechanism has been identified, one theory involves increased levels of serum insulin-like growth factor (IGF-1), which could be anabolic. However, Kuipers and others provided 60 grams of colostrum daily for 4 weeks to endurance-trained males and found no effect on blood IGF-1 or IGF binding protein levels.

Other protein substances, such as spirulina (algae), brewer's yeast, specific enzymes, and even DNA and RNA, have been advocated as means to improve physical performance. Spirulina

and brewer's yeast are good sources of protein and a variety of vitamins and minerals but convey no magical ergogenic qualities. The enzymes DNA and RNA would be degraded in the digestive process and thus could not be utilized for the purpose for which they were ingested.

Protein/carbohydrate solutions, some marketed as sports drinks, have been theorized to enhance endurance performance above and beyond that provided by carbohydrate alone. As noted in chapter 4, carbohydrate-containing sports drinks may enhance performance in prolonged endurance exercise, but does adding protein provide any additional benefits?

Do high-protein diets or protein supplements increase muscle mass and strength in resistance-trained individuals?

Some athletes in training may need more protein, and as noted below, some may increase muscle mass and strength with resistance training and protein supplementation. Moreover, some studies suggest that protein/carbohydrate beverages consumed during resistance exercise may help reduce muscle tissue damage and soreness.

High-Protein Diets Several earlier laboratory studies have compared the effect of normal protein intake, about 0.8–1.4 grams per kilogram, to higher levels, such as 1.6–2.8 grams per kilogram, on body composition changes during a weight-training program. In general, these studies revealed that although protein balance could be maintained or even be positive with the consumption of a normal amount of protein, the body protein balance was even more positive with the larger amounts. The additional body weight also appears to be in the form of lean body mass.

Other well-designed studies have not shown any ergogenic effects on strength-type performance. Weideman and others, using nuclear magnetic resonance to measure leg volume, reported no significant increase in leg muscle hypertrophy following 13 weeks of weight training with 2.94 grams of protein per kilogram per day, nor did Lemon and others find increased muscle mass when subjects consumed 2.62 grams of protein per kilogram per day, as compared to 1.35 grams per kilogram. Additionally, neither of these two studies reported a significant effect of the high-protein intake on measures of strength. In a review, Garlick and others noted an absence of strong evidence that high-protein diets confer any advantage in terms of strength.

More recent research also indicates that protein supplementation does not appear to increase muscular strength. Andersen and others provided either protein or carbohydrate before and after resistance training over the course of 14 weeks. The protein group showed significant hypertrophy in both type I and II muscle fibers, while the carbohydrate group experienced little change from baseline. However, there were no differences between the groups regarding increases in muscle strength. Hoffman and others studied collegiate strength/power athletes stratified into three groups depending on their daily intake of protein as either below (1.0–1.4 g/kg), at (1.6–1.8 g/kg), or above (>2.0 g/kg) recommended levels. No differences in body composition or strength were noted after 12 weeks of resistance training. In a study with older men (59–76 years), Candow and others reported that although 12 weeks of resistance training increased muscle size and strength, protein supplementation (0.3 g/kg) provided either before or after each training bout had no additional effects.

As noted previously, some investigators recommend protein intake immediately following exercise. Several studies have evaluated the effect of protein supplementation on possible muscle damage during resistance training. Kraemer and others reported that amino acid supplementation may be effective as a means to attenuate muscle strength loss during a period of increased intensity of resistance training designed to produce overreaching, possibly by providing substrate for muscle anabolism and reducing muscle damage. One study reported that 15 grams of protein consumed immediately after exercise enhanced muscle repair, as measured by changes in enzyme status associated with muscle damage.

More recent research suggests that combining carbohydrate with protein may be more effective. Several studies by Bird and others have found that providing a supplement containing both carbohydrate and essential amino acids (6 grams), as compared to a placebo or carbohydrate and essential amino acids alone, reduced markers of muscle protein catabolism 48 hours after resistance training. They suggested that such a supplement may induce an anticatabolic effect and better favor conservation of muscle protein following intense resistance exercise.

Given the possibility of enhanced muscle repair, consuming some of the recommended daily amount of protein immediately following exercise may be a prudent behavior.

Whey and Colostrum Research findings reveal mixed, but generally positive, effects relative to the ergogenic potential of whey supplementation to resistance-trained individuals. However, other protein sources were often combined with the whey protein. Cribb and others found that whey isolate (1.5 g/kg/d), as compared to the same amount of casein, over the course of 10 weeks of resistance training significantly increased lean body mass and strength improvements in recreational bodybuilders. In another study, Cribb and others compared the effects of supplementation with creatine, whey protein, creatine with whey protein, or carbohydrate placebo during 11 weeks of resistance training using four groups of trained subjects; the whey protein content was approximately 100 grams. Compared to the carbohydrate group, the whey protein group and the other two groups increased muscle strength. Kerksick and others studied the effects of whey protein supplementation in resistance-trained males engaged in 10 weeks of resistance training. Three groups consumed either a carbohydrate placebo, 40 grams/day of whey protein plus casein, or 40 grams of whey protein and several other amino acids. All groups experienced similar significant increases in muscle strength, but the combination whey/casein group experienced the greatest increases in fat-free mass. Candow and others compared the effects of whey protein (1.2 g/kg) and soy protein (1.2 g/kg) versus a placebo on changes in body composition and strength over 6 weeks of resistance training in untrained individuals. They found that both the whey and soy protein supplements, compared to the placebo, induced small but significant increases in lean tissue mass and strength, but there was no difference between the two sources of protein. Finally, Coburn and others reported that supplementation with a leucine/whey combination over the course of 8 weeks of resistance training of the knee extensors significantly increased muscle strength, but had no effect on muscle hypertrophy.

Several studies have evaluated the ergogenic effect of colostrum supplementation, using whey protein as a placebo to reveal whether colostrum supplementation produced any benefits beyond those attributed to whey protein alone. Hofman and others evaluated the effect of bovine colostrum on body composition and four tests of exercise performance in elite male and female field hockey players. The tests included two shuttle sprints (50 and 300 meters total for time), a shuttle sprint test to exhaustion, and a vertical jump. The subjects consumed 60 grams of colostrum daily for 8 weeks and whey protein served as the placebo. The colostrum had no effect on body composition or three of the four exercise tests, but did appear to improve performance in the 50-meter shuttle sprint test. Antonio and others investigated the effect of 20 grams of bovine colostrum, given daily during 8 weeks of aerobic and heavy-resistance exercise training, on body composition, strength, and aerobic endurance. Whey protein was the placebo. There were no effects of the colostrum on exercise performance. The whey group significantly increased total body mass, whereas the colostrum group, although not increasing total body mass, did increase lean body mass, which was attributed to a slight decrease in body fat. Brinkworth and others, studying the effect of either bovine colostrum or whey protein supplementation (60 grams daily) during 8 weeks of resistance training, found that subjects in the colostrum group increased arm circumference and cross-sectional area, but the increase was due principally to a greater increase in skin and subcutaneous fat.

Although these studies are suggestive of some ergogenic effects associated with whey protein or colostrum supplementation, additional research is merited.

Do high-protein diets or protein supplements improve aerobic endurance performance in endurance-trained individuals?

Protein supplementation may also help reduce muscle tissue damage and soreness during aerobic endurance training, but there is little evidence to support a performance-enhancing, or ergogenic, effect on aerobic endurance following acute or prolonged protein supplementation.

High-Protein Diets or Meals The 40:30:30 "zone diet" alluded to in chapter 5 may be considered to be a high-protein diet because 30 percent of the daily Calories are derived from protein (high end of the AMDR), 40 percent are derived from carbohydrate, and 30 percent are derived from fat. The premise underlying the "zone diet" is a change in hormonal activity, resulting in vasoactive eicosanoids that permit greater oxygen delivery to the muscle, a condition referred to as the "zone." In a review, Cheuvront criticized the "zone diet" book, noting that the claims of improved sport performance are based on anecdotal reports and selectively quoted research, not on sound scientific evidence. Cheuvront states that, in actuality, reliable and abundant peer-reviewed literature is in opposition to the suggestion that such a diet can support competitive athletic endeavors, much less improve them, and even suggests that the "zone diet" may actually be ergolytic in nature. Some evidence does indicate that high-protein diets, at the expense of carbohydrate, may impair endurance performance. Jarvis and others evaluated the effects of a 7-day zone diet, compared with a normal diet, on body composition and run time to exhaustion in recreational endurance athletes. Daily energy intake was significantly reduced by about 300 Calories on the zone diet, as was body mass and run time to exhaustion at 80 percent of VO_2 max. These investigators do not recommend the zone diet for athletes unless future research validates its proposed ability to enhance athletic performance. It should be noted that subjects consumed fewer Calories while on the zone diet, a factor that may have impeded performance. However, Macdermid and Stannard conducted a study in which the caloric energy was the same in both the high-carbohydrate and high-protein diets: In a crossover design, for 7 days subjects received either a high-carbohydrate diet or a high-protein–moderate-carbohydrate diet and then completed an individually based cycling time trial that lasted more than 2 hours. Although there were no differences in various physiological measures, the high-protein diet significantly impaired cycling endurance performance by 20 percent, indicating an ergolytic effect. The subjects also indicated that it was difficult to train on the high-protein diet.

Nevertheless, for weight-restricted athletes attempting to lose body fat or maintain a low body weight for sports competition, some investigators recommend increased protein intake. With a 1,500-Calorie diet, a 30 percent protein allotment would be 450 Calories, or approximately 112 grams of protein. For a lean athlete, this amount of protein may help ensure protein adequacy and may fall in the range of recommended protein intake.

In summary, Lemon notes that although endurance athletes may need a higher protein intake (1.2–1.4 grams per kilogram body weight) than sedentary individuals, these recommendations are based on protein balance studies. Lemon further states that there are no data to indicate that such a protein intake, as compared to the RDA of 0.8 grams per kilogram, will enhance sport performance. Such studies are needed.

Moreover, protein intake might best be restricted within an hour of competition. A study by Wiles and others noted an increased oxygen consumption during various exercise intensities (an indicator of impaired efficiency), particularly the more intense levels approaching 100 percent VO_2 max, when protein was consumed 1 hour prior to the exercise task. Ratings of perceived exertion were also higher with the protein diet. The protein meal content was 0.4 gram per kilogram body weight. However, no adverse effects were noticed when the same protein intake was consumed 3 hours prior to the exercise task. These research data appear to be in accord with the dietary recommendations for precompetition meals presented in chapter 2, stressing the importance of carbohydrate.

Protein/Carbohydrate Preparations Various sports drinks containing both protein and carbohydrate have been marketed as a means to enhance performance when consumed during exercise and to facilitate recovery and improve subsequent exercise performance when consumed after exercise. In one of the first studies, Ivy and others compared the effects of adding protein to a carbohydrate solution on aerobic endurance performance. Trained cyclists, consuming 200 milliliters of solution every 20 minutes, exercised for 3 hours at intensities varying from 45 to 75 percent of VO_2 max and then exercised to exhaustion at 85 percent of VO_2 max. The carbohydrate solution (7.75 percent) significantly improved endurance performance compared to the placebo, but the carbohydrate/protein combination (7.75/1.94 percent) enhanced performance even more than the carbohydrate solution. Saunders, in a review, indicated that other studies report similar findings. However, Saunders did note limitations to these studies; the main factor was that in the studies showing improved performance, the protein supplied in the beverage was in addition to the carbohydrate, thus providing more energy.

Other studies do not support an ergogenic effect of protein/carbohydrate supplementation when compared to carbohydrate supplements containing equal energy. For example, van Essen and others reported that when trained athletes ingested a sports drink during exercise at a rate considered optimal for carbohydrate delivery, protein provided no additional performance benefit during an 80-kilometer cycling trial, an event that simulated "real life" competition. Romano-Ely and others also compared the effects of a protein/carbohydrate drink, which also included antioxidants, to an isocaloric carbohydrate drink on cycling time to exhaustion at 70 percent VO_2 max; the drinks were consumed every 15 minutes during exercise. There was no significant difference between the treatments on performance time. In his review, Gibala indicated that there is no established mechanism by which protein intake during exercise should improve acute endurance performance, and these latter studies support this viewpoint.

As noted previously, consuming protein and carbohydrate following exercise provides a milieu conducive to enhanced anabolism and muscle recovery. Some have contended that ingesting carbohydrate plus protein following prolonged exercise may restore exercise capacity more effectively than ingestion of carbohydrate alone. For example, compared to a standard commercial carbohydrate/electrolyte sports drink, Karp and others found that both low-fat chocolate milk and a commercial protein/carbohydrate sports drink, each of which contain about 34 grams of carbohydrate and 9 grams of protein per 8 fluid ounces, enhanced performance in a cycling test to exhaustion 4 hours after a hard interval workout. However, although the subjects consumed the same amount of fluid in each trial, the two protein/carbohydrate drinks contained more than twice as much carbohydrate and more than three times as much caloric energy as the carbohydrate/electrolyte sports drink.

When the energy content is similar, consuming protein/carbohydrate meals or supplements during recovery, as compared to carbohydrate alone, has no effect on subsequent exercise performance. In two separate studies, Betts and others had physically active males complete a 90-minute run at 70 percent of VO_2 max followed by a 4-hour recovery, during which they consumed either a carbohydrate or carbohydrate/protein solution with similar energy content. The recovery was followed by a run to exhaustion at either 70 or 85 percent of VO_2 max, but there was no difference between the two recovery diets. Studies by Rowlands and Millard-Stafford, along with their colleagues, have shown that consuming high-protein/carbohydrate meals or fluid supplements following intense exercise training, as compared to comparable carbohydrate feedings, does not enhance performance in intermittent, high-intensity (10 maximal 2.5-minute cycling sprints) or aerobic endurance (5-kilometer track run) the following day.

In his review, Saunders also noted that consumption of protein/carbohydrate solutions has been associated with reduced markers of muscle damage and less muscle soreness. Several studies support this viewpoint. In their study cited earlier, which involved a 21-kilometer outdoor run at a set pace followed by a treadmill run to exhaustion at 90 percent of VO_2 max, Millard-Stafford and others reported that the carbohydrate/protein mixture resulted in less muscle soreness. Romano-Ely and others also reported that subjects experienced less muscle soreness on the carbohydrate/protein drink, and blood enzyme tests indicated less muscle tissue damage. Conversely, Green and others found that a carbohydrate-protein drink consumed following an exercise task (downhill running) designed to induce muscle injury and soreness had no effect on quadriceps strength recovery or muscle soreness.

Overall these preliminary findings are promising. Nancy Rodriguez, a sports-nutrition scientist at the University of Connecticut, indicates that long-term, well-controlled diet and exercise intervention studies are essential for clarification of the relation between protein intake, endurance exercise, and skeletal-muscle protein turnover.

Colostrum   Several studies evaluated the effect of colostrum on endurance exercise performance. Brinkworth and others supplemented the daily diet of elite rowers during 9 weeks of training for the world championships with 60 grams of bovine colostrum. Whey protein was used as the placebo. Subjects completed several bouts of a rowing protocol involving both submaximal

and a 4-minute maximal test. They found that although the colostrum supplement increased the estimated buffer capacity, it had no effect on rowing performance. Coombes and others evaluated the effect of different colostrum dosages on two tests of aerobic capacity in competitive cyclists. The dosages included 60 grams of colostrum, 20 grams of colostrum plus 40 grams of whey protein, and 60 grams of whey protein, which was the placebo group. The exercise tests included two VO_2 max tests with a 20-minute interval between each, and a cycle time-trial test following 2 hours of cycling at 65 percent of VO_2 max. Although performance in the VO_2 max tests was not improved by colostrum, it did provide a small but significant improvement in the time-trial performance. Shing and others also reported some ergogenic effects of colostrum supplementation. Over the course of 10 weeks of training, including a final 5 days of high-intensity cycling, highly trained male road cyclists consumed either a placebo or a daily supplement containing 10 grams of bovine colostrum protein concentrate (CPC). A 40-kilometer time trial was done periodically to evaluate performance. The effects of the colostrum supplement on cycling time-trial performance during the first 9 weeks of regular training was unclear, but performance of the colostrum group was enhanced significantly following the 5 days of high-intensity training. They reported that the CPC helped to maintain the ventilatory threshold. As with the effects of colostrum on strength-type activities, these too should be considered preliminary data; confirmation with additional research is needed.

Are amino acid, amine, and related nitrogen-containing supplements effective ergogenic aids?

As noted previously, providing all essential amino acids during recovery from exercise may be associated with enhanced muscle protein synthesis, but whether or not this translates into enhanced exercise performance has not been determined. In recent years, however, specific amino acids have become increasingly available and popular in certain athletic circles.

Weight lifters are consuming various amino acids in attempts to stimulate the release of growth hormone from the pituitary gland, hoping that the growth hormone will then stimulate muscle development. Amino acids have also been used to stimulate the release of insulin from the pancreas; insulin is also considered to be an anabolic hormone because it facilitates the uptake of amino acids by the muscle cells. Indeed, certain amino acid mixtures have been advertised to be more potent than anabolic steroids, one of the most popular drugs used by strength and power athletes. Anabolic steroids and related substances are discussed in chapter 13. Other amino acids have been advertised in magazines for endurance athletes, suggesting that they may be utilized as a fuel during training or help prevent fatigue by altering the formation of neurotransmitters in the brain. Still other amino acid mixtures and related compounds such as creatine and inosine have been used in attempts to increase ATP or PCr levels in the muscle or to help athletes lose body weight for competition.

Scientific research has shown that individual amino acid supplements may induce specific physiological responses in the body, particularly the formation of certain chemicals in the brain needed for nerve impulse transmission as well as secretion of hormones. However, amino acid metabolism is very complex. It depends on a variety of factors, such as the concentration in the blood, competition with other amino acids, feedback control mechanisms, and the presence in the diet of other nutrients. Consumption of specific amino acid mixtures or even high-protein diets may actually lead to nutritional imbalances, as an overload of one amino acid may inhibit the absorption of others into the body.

Because purified amino acids, known as free-form amino acids, amines such as creatine, and other nitrogen-containing substances have become commercially available for athletes, they have been the focus of increased research activity by sports medicine scientists. However, although the number of studies is increasing relative to the effect of amino acid supplementation upon physical performance, with the exception of creatine the data are still somewhat limited. Moreover, some investigators combine several amino acids or use commercial supplements that may contain not only several amino acids but other nutrients as well, which may cloud the possible ergogenic effect of any one specific amino acid. The following discussion highlights some of the current key findings regarding specific amino acids, various combinations of amino acids, amines, and nitrogen-containing compounds that have been studied for their potential ergogenic effect.

Arginine and Citrulline   Arginine, a conditionally essential amino acid, has several functions in human metabolism. One of its most important is to serve as a precursor for nitric oxide (NO) synthesis. NO acts as a vasodilator to increase blood flow. Citrulline also is an amino acid, but is not one of the 20 essential or nonessential amino acids because it is not involved in protein synthesis. However, dietary citrulline is eventually taken up by the kidney and metabolized to generate large amounts of arginine. Hickner and others noted that citrulline supplementation increases plasma arginine levels to a higher level than arginine supplementation.

Arginine infusion and oral supplementation are being studied for possible health benefits, particularly in individuals with circulatory problems, because arginine may function to promote vasodilation. In their earlier review, Cheng and others reported that oral arginine supplementation has been shown to improve exercise ability in CHD patients. More recent research supports this viewpoint. For example, Doutreleau and others reported that 6 weeks of arginine supplementation to patients with chronic stable heart failure enhanced endurance exercise performance, reducing heart rate and blood lactate responses. Conversely, Wilson and others noted no beneficial effects of arginine supplementation, compared to a placebo, on treadmill walking distance to the onset of pain in patients with peripheral arterial disease. They also noted no increase in NO synthesis with arginine supplementation, which may underlie this negative finding.

There is limited research regarding the effect of arginine and citrulline supplementation on exercise performance in healthy individuals. Hickner and others used two supplementation protocols with citrulline, one using two different protocols, either 9 grams in three 3-gram doses over 24 hours or 3 grams once every 3 hours before exercise testing, which consisted of a variable speed and grade treadmill run time to exhaustion. There were no differences in treadmill run times between placebo and L-citrulline supplementation when the data were analyzed separately by dose protocol. However, the authors reported a higher rating of perceived exertion associated with citrulline supplementation and when the data from the two protocols were combined, the run time to exhaustion was actually impaired with citrulline supplementation. In a related vein, Buchman and others provided arginine or a placebo to marathon runners and speculated that arginine may be ergolytic, as the predicted times of the runners receiving arginine were slower than those receiving the placebo.

Other studies show no ergogenic or ergolytic effects of arginine supplementation. McConell and others infused arginine to endurance-trained cyclists during exercise (30 grams in one hour). Although the cyclists experienced a decrease in blood glucose, there was no effect on performance in a 15-minute maximal cycling time trial following 2 hours of cycling at 72 percent VO_2 max. Using a chronic supplementation protocol, Abel and others reported that 4 weeks of supplementation with arginine aspartate (5.7 g arginine; 8.7 g aspartate) had no effect on endocrine or metabolic responses, peak oxygen uptake, or cycling endurance to exhaustion. As noted later, aspartate salts have also been theorized to be ergogenic.

Arginine, Lysine, and Ornithine   Research has shown that infusing any of a number of amino acids into the blood potentiates the release of **human growth hormone (HGH),** a polypeptide. HGH is released from the pituitary gland into the bloodstream, affecting all tissues. One of its effects is to stimulate the production of another hormone, insulin-like growth factor-1, that spurs growth of tissue, including muscle tissue. Some amino acids may also stimulate the release of insulin, an anabolic hormone, from the pancreas. McConell reported that arginine infusion increased HGH and insulin. Such effects could be ergogenic for strength-trained individuals, and Cynober indicates that arginine and its related amino acids such as ornithine are found in dietary supplements for bodybuilders.

Although more than a half-dozen amino acids may stimulate HGH release when infused, the effect of oral supplementation is less clear. However, Jacobson has reported that the oral administration of selected amino acids may lead to HGH release similar to that promoted by infusion. Bucci, in his book on nutritional ergogenics, also notes that oral intake of amino acids, particularly arginine and ornithine, may increase HGH release, while others have suggested that lysine may elicit similar effects.

Arginine supplementation may increase HGH secretion at rest, but impair it during exercise. In one study, Collier and others found that oral arginine supplementation (7 grams) increases secretion of HGH, but not as much as a bout of resistance exercise. In a review, Kanaley concluded that arginine alone increases HGH levels by about 100 percent, while exercise can increase HGH levels by 300–500 percent. However, when arginine and exercise are combined, the increase is less than seen with exercise alone, suggesting that arginine supplementation does not augment and may actually decrease the HGH response to exercise.

Research by Bucci and his colleagues has supported the effect of ornithine to increase serum HGH levels. Using dosages of

40, 100, and 170 milligrams per kilogram body weight, only the highest dose of ornithine increased HGH levels, but it caused intestinal distress (osmotic diarrhea) in many of the subjects, and thus its use at this effective dose may be impractical. Moreover, in a related study, Bucci and others noted that ornithine did not increase the secretion of insulin.

Arginine, lysine, and ornithine, separately or in various combinations, have received the most research attention regarding an ergogenic effect for strength/power-type athletes. They have been advertised in bodybuilding magazines as being more powerful than anabolic steroids, potent drugs used by some athletes to increase muscle mass. The advertisers apparently are capitalizing on the potential of these amino acids to enhance HGH release.

Two of the earliest published studies by Elam collectively reported that arginine and ornithine supplementation in conjunction with a weight-training program reduced body fat, increased lean body mass, and increased strength over a 5-week period. The dosage was 2 grams per day (1 gram each of arginine and ornithine), 5 days per week. Unfortunately, both studies have been criticized in the literature on the grounds of the statistical procedure by which the experimental and control groups were compared. A different analysis of the same data revealed no significant difference between the experimental and control groups in the first study. The studies have also been criticized for questionable measurement techniques and for making assumptions without adequate supporting data.

Several studies with better experimental designs have not shown any significant ergogenic effect of arginine and lysine, or other similar amino acid combinations. Lambert and others, using combinations of arginine/lysine and ornithine/tyrosine, reported no significant increases in HGH, while Fogelholm and his associates noted no significant increases in HGH or insulin secretion following supplementation with arginine, ornithine, and lysine in competitive weight lifters. Hawkins and associates, using experienced male weight lifters as subjects, reported no beneficial effects of oral arginine supplementation on various measures of muscle function, including peak torque and endurance. Suminski and others reported that although a bout of weight training would increase HGH levels in noncompetitive weight lifters, supplementation with arginine and lysine provided no additional benefit. Mitchell and others, also using experienced weight lifters, reported that 8 weeks of supplementation with arginine and lysine elicited no significant effect on HGH secretion, body composition, or various strength measures. As discussed in chapter 13, increased HGH may not induce an ergogenic effect in young, resistance-trained males.

One study by Campbell and others did find some ergogenic effects of arginine supplementation when combined with alpha-ketoglutarate. Resistance-trained men consumed either a placebo or 12 grams daily (3 equal doses) of arginine alpha-ketoglutarate during 8 weeks of periodized resistance training. Compared to the placebo, the supplement group improved performance in bench press strength and anaerobic peak power in a Wingate test. However, there were no effects between groups in body composition and isokinetic quadriceps muscle endurance.

In their review, Chromiak and Antonio indicated that oral doses of arginine, lysine, and ornithine that are great enough to induce significant growth hormone release are likely to cause gastrointestinal discomfort. Moreover, they reported no studies finding that such supplementation augments HGH release, nor do any studies support an ergogenic effect to increase muscle mass and strength to a greater extent than strength training alone.

Cynober notes that, to date, there have been no studies on the safety of long-term administration of these amino acids in healthy subjects. However, Böger notes that doses of 3–8 grams per day of arginine appear to be safe and do not appear to cause acute pharmacologic effects in humans.

Tryptophan Although tryptophan is one of the amino acids that may increase the release of HGH, its theoretical ergogenic effect is based upon another function. A neurotransmitter in the brain, serotonin (5-hydroxytryptamine), is derived from tryptophan. This neurotransmitter may induce sleepiness and elicit a mellow mood, and Segura and Ventura hypothesize that it may help to decrease the perception of pain. They postulate that individuals who show the best tolerance of or resistance to pain may be able to delay the onset of fatigue, and that tryptophan supplementation therefore might improve exercise performance. In their study, 12 healthy athletes exercised to exhaustion on a treadmill at 80 percent of their VO_2 max under two conditions: A placebo was compared with a dosage of 1,200 milligrams of L-tryptophan consumed in 300-mg doses over the 24 hours prior to testing. They reported no significant improvement in peak oxygen uptake or heart rate response, but did note a significant improvement in time to exhaustion (49 percent) and a decreased rating of perceived exertion (RPE) following the L-tryptophan trial. The times to exhaustion were extremely variable among the individual subjects, ranging from 2.5–18 minutes, suggesting that some of the individuals may not have been well trained. In another study with untrained individuals, Cunliffe and others reported that tryptophan supplementation (30 mg per kilogram body weight) increased both subjective and objective measures of fatigue. Although tryptophan supplementation had no effect on grip strength, work output on a wrist ergometer increased significantly.

Stensrund and his associates challenged the results of the Segura and Ventura study, noting that a 49 percent increase in performance would be rather phenomenal in trained athletes. Thus, they decided to replicate this study using 49 well-trained male runners and better control conditions, although they had their subjects run to exhaustion at 100 percent VO_2 max, not 80 percent. In contrast to the study by Segura and Ventura, they reported no significant effect of tryptophan supplementation on performance. Other research from the University of Maastricht revealed no effect of tryptophan supplementation on endurance performance at 70–75 percent of VO_2 max, and research with horses reported a decrease in endurance performance at 50 percent of VO_2 max.

Based on these limited data, tryptophan does not appear to be an effective ergogenic in either short-term or prolonged exercise tasks in exercise-trained individuals, a finding also supported in the review by Anton Wagenmakers. Some adverse health effects have been associated with tryptophan supplementation and are discussed in the next section.

Branched-Chain Amino Acids (BCAAs) The three BCAAs are leucine, isoleucine, and valine. BCAA supplementation has been theorized to enhance exercise performance in a variety of ways. BCAAs, particularly leucine, could be used as a fuel during exercise to prevent adverse changes in neurotransmitter function, to spare the use of muscle glycogen, and to prevent or decrease the net rate of protein degradation. These effects could influence mental and physical performance, and may also favorably affect body composition, but most research has focused on the central fatigue hypothesis.

Central fatigue hypothesis Eric Newsholme, a biochemist at Oxford University, proposed the central fatigue hypothesis, postulating that high levels of serum free-tryptophan (fTRP) in conjunction with low levels of BCAA, or a high fTRP:BCAA ratio, may be a major factor in the etiology of fatigue during prolonged endurance exercise. Research with animals has shown that a high fTRP:BCAA ratio may lead to an increased production of serotonin. Newsholme suggested that serum BCAA levels eventually decrease in endurance exercise, such as marathon running, because they may be used for energy production. Such an effect would possibly increase the fTRP:BCAA ratio, facilitating the transport of tryptophan into the brain and increasing serotonin production, which could lead to fatigue because increased serotonin levels may depress central nervous system functions. Some, but not all, research with humans supports this finding. Blomstrand and others have shown in several studies that prolonged endurance exercise, such as the 26.2-mile (42.2-kilometer) marathon, increases the fTRP:BCAA ratio, but Conlay and others noted no change in this ratio in experienced runners immediately following completion of the Boston Marathon. Tanaka and others also noted no change in the fTRP:BCAA ratio in a 6-week study designed to induce overtraining.

The central fatigue hypothesis and BCAA supplementation have received considerable research attention since Newsholme proposed his hypothesis in the late 1980s, and these studies have served as the basis for several reviews. Based on these reviews, and research studies published subsequent to these reviews, the following appear to be the key points regarding the central fatigue hypothesis and the effects of nutritional interventions, particularly BCAA and carbohydrate supplementation.

Support for the hypothesis Animal studies support the concept of central fatigue during prolonged exercise tasks. Fatigue appears to be associated with increases in brain serotonin, but fatigue is also correlated with changes in other brain neurotransmitters as well, such as dopamine. Some human data also suggest that serotonin may be involved in the development of fatigue. Several drugs, approved for use with humans, may block the removal of serotonin from its active sites, thus magnifying its effects. In several studies involving running or cycling at 70 percent VO_2 max, these drugs either impaired performance or increased the psychological perception of effort, both negative findings.

However, J. Mark Davis of the University of South Carolina points out that although the central fatigue hypothesis has some

support from experimental data, the underlying mechanism has not been determined. Investigators are studying this issue, looking not only at mechanisms associated with serotonin, but other brain neurotransmitters as well, such as dopamine.

BCAA supplementation and the fTRP:BCAA ratio If serum BCAAs fall during prolonged exercise, then BCAA supplementation might be a preventive measure. It is known that BCAAs are metabolized primarily in the muscle, not the liver, and thus may provide an energy source during exercise. Some research has shown that oral supplementation with BCAAs or leucine will increase the serum levels of BCAA, the BCAAs may possibly be used as an energy source during exercise, the BCAAs may prevent or decrease the rate of endogenous protein degradation during exercise, and the BCAAs may help to maintain a normal fTRP:BCAA ratio during prolonged exercise. However, Rennie and others indicated that the total contribution of BCAAs to fuel provision during exercise is minor and insufficient to increase dietary protein requirements.

BCAA supplementation and mental performance Several sports, such as tennis and soccer, involve prolonged, high-intensity intermittent bouts of exercise in which mental alertness must be maintained. In such events, the fTRP:BCAA ratio may increase, as documented by Struder and associates in a study involving nationally ranked tennis players involved in 4 hours of continuous tournament tennis.

As evaluated by various tests of cognitive performance, reviews by Blomstrand and Meeusen and others reported that BCAA supplementation improved mental performance in national-class soccer players after a game and in runners after a 30-kilometer race. However, other investigators reported no effect of BCAA supplementation on mental acuity following a 40-kilometer cycle performance test. These are interesting field studies, and additional similar research is merited, complemented by well-controlled laboratory studies.

BCAA supplementation and perceived exertion Somewhat related to mental performance is the psychological perception of effort, or how mentally stressful the subject perceives a given exercise task to be. This psychological effort is usually evaluated by Borg's Rating of Perceived Exertion Scale, or RPE (see page 482). In their research, Blomstrand and others reported that BCAA supplementation, compared to a placebo trial, reduced the RPE and mental fatigue of endurance-trained cyclists during a 60-minute ride at 70 percent VO_2 max followed by another 20 minutes of maximal exercise. The fTRP:BCAA ratio increased in the placebo trial, but remained unchanged or even decreased in the BCAA trial. Conversely, other well-controlled studies have reported no significant effect of BCAA supplementation on RPE during intense exercise, such as during a 40-kilometer cycling performance test and 90 minutes of exercise at a 2-millimole lactate threshold.

BCAA supplementation and physical performance Investigators have studied BCAA supplementation with acute dosages administered to subjects just before and during the exercise task, and chronic dosages provided to the subject for

Several studies have reported a positive association between decreased plasma glutamine levels and overtraining. Parry-Billings and others studied 40 overtrained, international-class athletes at the British Olympic Medical Centre; most of the overtrained athletes were involved in endurance-type events. The investigators noted a decreased plasma glutamine level compared to control athletes not regarded as being overtrained. Kingsbury and others reported similar findings for overtrained elite track and field athletes, as compared to other elite athletes without symptoms of overtraining. In a review, Williams cited research indicating that plasma glutamine levels are decreased in athletes who participate in sport activities predisposing to overtraining, including marathon running and repeated bouts of intensive training. One research group indicated that plasma glutamine may be useful as an indicator of the overtrained state.

Most research with glutamine supplementation in athletes has focused on its role to affect favorably markers of immune function or to prevent signs and symptoms of overtraining, particularly upper respiratory tract infections. Williams notes that both animal and human studies provide conflicting data regarding beneficial effects of glutamine supplementation before, during, or after exercise. For example, some research revealed a lower incidence of infections during the 7 days following intense exercise bouts in various athletic groups who consumed a glutamine-supplemented drink (81 percent with no infections) compared to those taking a placebo drink (49 percent with no infections) immediately after and 2 hours after the exercise bout. The investigators suggested these effects are possibly associated with an apparent increase in specific lymphocyte cells. However, this same investigative group reported no beneficial effects of glutamine supplementation on lymphocyte distribution following the Brussels Marathon. Additionally, other investigators reported that although glutamine supplementation helped to maintain plasma glutamine levels following prolonged aerobic exercise, no beneficial effects on lymphocyte function were noted.

Although some investigators have suggested that carbohydrate intake may counter glutamine depletion, a well-controlled study by van Hall and others indicated that carbohydrate intake during prolonged exercise (cycling to exhaustion) did not prevent the normal decrease in plasma glutamine concentration during recovery. In contrast, Gleeson and others indicated that a low-carbohydrate diet over 3 days is associated with a greater fall in plasma glutamine levels during recovery from exercise. Thus, as documented previously, adequate daily carbohydrate intake appears to be a sound dietary strategy for most athletes.

Castell cited some preliminary data indicating that glutamine supplementation may reduce the self-reported incidence of illness in endurance athletes following prolonged exercise. Based on such findings, Antonio and Street speculated that glutamine has potential utility as a dietary supplement for athletes engaged in heavy exercise training. Although such a recommendation may be prudent, confirming data are needed to provide more solid scientific support. In reviews, Hargreaves and Snow, Nieman, along with Akerström and Pedersen, indicated that there is little support from controlled studies to recommend glutamine supplementation for enhanced immune function and prevention of upper respiratory tract infections.

In summary, Phillips notes that although glutamine is a popular dietary supplement consumed for purported ergogenic benefits of increased strength, quicker recovery, decreased frequency of respiratory infections, and prevention of overtraining, the available studies regarding glutamine supplementation and exercise performance show a lack of evidence for such benefits.

Aspartates Potassium and magnesium aspartate are salts of aspartic acid, a nonessential amino acid. Although the mechanism has not been clearly documented, these substances have been postulated to improve aerobic and anaerobic exercise performance, possibly by enhancing fatty acid metabolism and thereby sparing glycogen, by reducing accumulation of ammonia (metabolic by-product of protein), or simply by improving psychological motivation. The ammonia hypothesis has been tested in several studies since increases in serum ammonia have been associated with muscular fatigue, although, as noted previously, the mechanism is not clear.

Research findings relative to the ergogenic effect of acute short-term supplementation of aspartates are equivocal. A number of both early and contemporary studies have reported no beneficial effects of aspartate supplementation. For example, Maughan and Sadler had eight males ride to exhaustion on a bicycle ergometer at 75–80 percent of their VO_2 max following either a placebo or 3,000 milligrams each of potassium and magnesium aspartate consumed in the 24 hours prior to testing. No beneficial effects upon blood concentrations of energy substrates or ammonia were found, nor were any significant effects on physiological or psychological variables important to aerobic exercise performance reported. In an anaerobic exercise task, Tuttle and others reported no significant effect of aspartate supplementation (approximately 10 grams) on plasma ammonia concentrations, ratings of perceived exertion during a resistance training workout, or performance in a bench press repetition test to failure at 65 percent of maximal bench press strength. As noted earlier, chronic supplementation with aspartate (8.7 grams/day for 4 months) had no effect on peak oxygen uptake or cycling endurance to exhaustion.

However, an equal number of early and contemporary studies have found some beneficial applications of aspartates. Although several of these studies possessed flaws in experimental design, increases in aerobic endurance of 21–50 percent have been reported. Wesson and others, using a double-blind, placebo protocol, revealed that the ingestion of 10 grams of aspartates over a 24-hour period increased endurance capacity by more than 15 percent when subjects exercised at 75 percent of their VO_2 max. These researchers also reported increased blood levels of free fatty acids and decreased levels of blood ammonia.

In a review, Trudeau noted that the effect of aspartate supplementation on endurance seems generally favorable in humans, but the underlying mechanism for performance enhancement has not been confirmed. It appears that additional quality research is needed to evaluate the ability of aspartates to exert an ergogenic effect. Dosage may be a key factor, as dosages of about 10 grams have usually been associated with improved performance.

Glycine Glycine is a nonessential amino acid. Because it is involved in the formation of creatine, and hence phosphocreatine (PCr), it could theoretically be an ergogenic aid. Gelatin, an incomplete protein, is composed of approximately 25 percent glycine, and thus also has been ascribed ergogenic qualities. Several studies conducted more than a half-century ago suggested a beneficial effect of glycine or gelatin supplementation on various measures of strength, but the experiments were poorly designed. More contemporary research with proper experimental design and relatively large doses of glycine revealed no beneficial effects on physical performance. However, although glycine supplementation has not been shown to be ergogenic, direct supplementation with creatine may induce favorable effects, as noted below.

Glycine is the first-listed ingredient in glycine-arginine-alpha-ketoisocaproic acid (GAKIC), which has been theorized to enhance muscle performance by favorably modifying protein metabolism by use of amino acids (glycine, arginine) combined with ketoacids (alpha-ketoisocaproic acid). Previous research has supported its use to increase muscle strength, and a well-designed study by Buford and Koch also provides some support for its potential to enhance anaerobic performance. Subjects consumed 11.2 grams of GAKIC prior to five supramaximal 10-second cycle ergometer sprints, separated by 1-minute rest intervals. The GAKIC treatment produced a greater retention of mean power between sprints 1 and 2, but no significant differences were noted among the other trials. The investigators suggested that the data supported an ergogenic effect of GAKIC. However, these data should be considered preliminary, and additional research is merited to support these findings.

Chondroitin and Glucosamine Chondroitin and glucosamine are derived from connective tissue, and each has been marketed as a dietary supplement, either separately or in combination, to help promote healthy joints in individuals who exercise. Gelatin, also derived from connective tissue, has also been advertised to promote joint health. Although weight-bearing or resistance exercise training has not been shown to cause excessive wear-and-tear on healthy joints, and may actually improve joint health, some dietary supplement entrepreneurs may suggest otherwise. In a sense, if a dietary supplement could prevent joint pain, and thus promote optimal exercise training, it could be considered ergogenic.

Both chondroitin and glucosamine may be synthesized in the human body from amino acids and other nutrients, and both are found in human cartilage, one of the main components involved in joint health. Glucosamine is believed to help form compounds, such as proteoglycans, that form the structural basis for cartilage, while chondroitin is part of a protein that helps cartilage hold water to give it elasticity and resiliency. Cartilage serves as a kind of shock absorber, and prevents bone-to-bone contact. Excessive wear of cartilage leads to osteoarthritis, a painful joint condition. Dietary supplements of chondroitin are made from cattle cartilage, while those of glucosamine are made from shellfish. Different salt forms of supplements are available, such as sulfate and hydrochloride. Theoretically, such supplements will help maintain normal cartilage levels and prevent development of osteoarthritis. Schardt

notes that by 2030, one out of every four American adults will have doctor-diagnosed arthritis.

Numerous studies have investigated the role of chondroitin and/or glucosamine supplementation on symptoms of arthritic pain. However, the results are equivocal. For example, Hughes and Carr found that glucosamine sulfate (1,500 milligrams daily for 6 months) was no more effective than a placebo in modifying pain symptoms in patients with osteoarthritis of the knee. In contrast, in a well-controlled, 3-year study using American College of Rheumatology criteria, Pavelka and others evaluated the progression of knee osteoarthritis following either ingestion of glucosamine sulfate (1,500 mg daily) or a placebo. Given some beneficial effects on joint space narrowing and symptoms including pain, function, and stiffness, they concluded that long-term treatment with glucosamine sulfate retarded the progression of knee osteoarthritis.

The National Institutes of Health funded a large multicenter clinical study called GAIT (Glucosamine/Chondroitin Arthritis Intervention Trial) designed to provide a clearer picture of the role that these dietary supplements, both separately and in combination, may play in the treatment of osteoarthritis. Nearly 1,600 subjects, with an average age of 59 and experiencing arthritic knee pain, were assigned to receive daily either 1,500 mg of glucosamine hydrochloride, 1,200 mg of chondroitin sulfate, both glucosamine hydrochloride and chondroitin sulfate, 200 mg of an anti-inflammatory drug, or placebo for 24 weeks. Although the glucosamine/chondroitin combination did provide relief to a subset of patients with moderate-to-severe knee pain, the investigators considered these findings to be preliminary and recommended additional research. However, overall the findings indicated that glucosamine, chondroitin, or the glucosamine/chondroitin combination did not reduce knee pain in patients with osteoarthritis more than a placebo.

The NIH study was designed to provide a definitive answer regarding the efficacy of such dietary supplements to reduce arthritic pain, but it did not. In a review designed to determine why studies with glucosamine came up with such divergent findings, Vlad and others found that trials using glucosamine sulfate produced more positive results than studies using glucosamine hydrochloride. They concluded that glucosamine hydrochloride was not effective. In a meta-analysis with a similar purpose, Reginster and others noted that one of the major differences between studies with different results was the form of glucosamine, and they noted that glucosamine sulfate supplementation provided the most compelling evidence as a potential for providing symptomatic relief and inhibiting the progression of osteoarthritis. Herrero-Beaumont and others note that although the mechanism of action of glucosamine sulfate still remains to be clearly defined, it may help by reducing the effects of pro-inflammatory agents present in osteoarthritis cartilage.

In a meta-analysis of studies regarding the effects of chondroitin supplementation for osteoarthritis of the knee or hip, Reichenbach and others concluded that the benefit of chondroitin supplementation is minimal or nonexistent, and recommended that its use in clinical practice be discouraged. If these findings are valid, the supplements used in the NIH study, particularly glucosamine hydrochloride, may not have been the best choices. Current research suggests that glucosamine sulfate may possess the greatest therapeutic potential.

Most of these supplement studies have been conducted with older people; for example, the average age in the NIH study was almost 60. Few studies have been conducted with younger, athletic subjects. In a well-controlled study, Ostojic and others evaluated the effect of glucosamine sulfate administration on the functional ability and the degree of pain intensity in competitive male athletes after suffering an acute knee injury. More than 100 athletes, with an average age of 25.1 years, received either glucosamine (1,500 mg per day) or a placebo for 28 days. Testing was done weekly. The investigators found no significant differences between the glucosamine and placebo group in mean pain intensity scores for resting and walking and degree of knee swelling at any time. Knee flexibility was unaffected during the first 3 weeks, but in the final test the glucosamine group demonstrated significant improvement in knee flexion and extension as compared with the placebo group. In general, these results suggest that glucosamine supplementation is not effective as a means to treat an acute knee injury, which is not the same as arthritis. In a study of Navy Seals in training, who could certainly be considered fit athletes, a commercial supplement containing both glucosamine and chondroitin did relieve knee pain symptoms in a small group of men with arthritic pain.

Other related dietary supplements have been studied as a means to treat osteoarthritis. SAM-e, short for S-adenosylmethionine, is derived from the essential amino acid methionine, and plays some important metabolic functions in the body, including serving as a possible anti-inflammatory agent. In a recent meta-analysis of 11 studies, Soeken and others concluded that SAM-e appears to be comparable to NSAIDs for treatment of pain and functional limitations, and less likely to report adverse effects. Schardt reiterated these points, but also noted that the doses used were high and could cost as much as $20 daily. Schardt also indicated that the quality of SAM-e dietary supplements available in the United States is variable, with some brands containing less than listed on the label.

Currently, chondroitin, glucosamine, and related supplements are being marketed to those with existing arthritic pain. To our knowledge, there are no data that these supplements will prevent the development of joint pain or osteoarthritis in young, healthy athletes. However, they may be of some benefit to older athletes experiencing joint pain that limits training or competition.

For anyone, particularly those with osteoarthritis, who may want to experiment with chondroitin and glucosamine, Tufts University offers several caveats. First, although these supplements are believed to be safe, they may cause mild side effects, such as bloating or a touch of diarrhea. Second, check with your doctor because there may be some complications. For example, diabetics may react adversely to glucosamine because it may increase insulin resistance. Third, a reasonable dose would be 1,500 milligrams of glucosamine sulfate and 1,200 milligrams of chondroitin daily for about 2–4 months. If pain symptoms have not improved, they probably are not going to. Finally, remember as with most dietary supplements, purity, safety, and effectiveness are not guaranteed.

http://dietarysupplements.nlm.nih.gov/ Type in glucosamine or chondroitin in the search box. Then select the specific brand or active ingredient. Provides details on product ingredients and other information. You may use this Website to research any dietary supplement mentioned in this and other chapters.

Creatine Creatine is not an amino acid, but a nitrogen-containing compound known as an *amine*. Creatine is found in some foods, particularly meat products, and it may be formed in the kidney and liver from glycine and arginine. Creatine may be delivered to the muscle, where it may combine readily with phosphate to form phosphocreatine, a high-energy phosphagen in the ATP-PCr energy system that is stored in the muscle. As you may recall, the ATP-PCr energy system is important for rapid energy production, such as in speed and power events. Sahlin and others noted that during very high-intensity exercise, within 10 seconds maximal power output decreases considerably and coincides with depletion of PCr.

Creatine supplements have been marketed to athletes at all levels. They come in various forms (powder, pills, candy, chews, gum, gels, serum, micronized) for both strength and endurance athletes, including products specifically for men, women, and adolescent athletes age 11–19. Relative to the latter, Metzl and others, in a survey of middle and high school athletes ages 10–18 in a New York City suburb, found that creatine is being used by middle and high school athletes at all grades. Use increases with grade level and the prevalence of use by athletes in grades 11 and 12 approaches levels reported among college athletes. The most cited reasons for taking creatine were enhanced performance and appearance. Indeed, creatine continues to be one of the most popular sports supplements of all time.

Although creatine has been known for years to play an important role in energy metabolism, it is only within the past 15 years or so that considerable research has been devoted to evaluate the potential ergogenic effect of creatine supplementation. Numerous studies, several major reviews, and a book focusing on creatine supplementation have been published, and the following represent some of the key points.

Supplementation protocol, effects on total muscle creatine and phosphocreatine (PCr), and theory The average individual needs to replace about 2 grams of creatine per day to maintain normal total creatine and creatine phosphate (PCr). The normal daily intake of creatine approximates 1 gram for those who consume meat, but may be virtually zero for pure vegetarians. Endogenous formation of creatine helps complement dietary sources to achieve 2 grams, but because of inadequate dietary intake, vegetarians may have lower amounts of total creatine in the body. For example, Lukaszuk and others found that switching from a meat-eating diet to a lactoovovegetarian diet for 3 weeks significantly reduced muscle total creatine.

Several supplementation strategies have been used in attempts to increase total body creatine stores. One very effective strategy is to consume a total of 20–30 grams of creatine, usually pure creatine monohydrate, in four equal doses (5–7 grams per dose) over the course of the day (morning, noon, afternoon, evening). Significant effects have been observed even after only 2 days of creatine loading. Paul Greenhaff, one of the pioneering researchers with creatine, noted that this supplementation protocol will enhance muscle creatine storage. Excessive amounts will not be stored but, as noted by Burke and others, excesses will be excreted unchanged in the urine. Longer-term supplementation with lower doses, such as 4 weeks at a dose of 3 grams per day, has been shown to be as equally effective. However, one study providing 2 grams per day for 6 weeks showed no beneficial effects on either muscle creatine stores or PCr levels.

Subjects may be responders or nonresponders. Research by Burke and others, in a study with vegetarians, found that individuals with initially low levels of intramuscular creatine are more responsive to supplementation, while Syrotuik and Bell identified several characteristics of nonresponders, such as higher initial levels of creatine and phosphocreatine before loading and fewer type II muscle fibers. However, Green and others have shown that combining creatine with a simple carbohydrate, such as glucose, will increase creatine transport into the muscle even in subjects with near-normal levels of muscle creatine, possibly via an insulin-mediated effect. The solution used in Green's study consisted of 5 grams of creatine and about 90 grams of simple carbohydrate, consumed 4 times per day. However, Preen and others found that a smaller amount of glucose (1 gram per kilogram body weight), taken with only two of four daily 5-gram creatine doses, increased muscle creatine stores significantly more than creatine supplementation alone. This loading protocol may be useful for those who may want to cut the carbohydrate intake by 50 percent or more. Once creatine is in the muscle, it is locked there and gradually disappears over several weeks.

In general, although not all studies are in agreement, well-controlled research by Greenhaff, Harris, Casey, and their associates has shown that an appropriate creatine-loading protocol will increase total muscle creatine, including free creatine and PCr. In their book, Williams, Kreider, and Branch reviewed more than 20 studies, and reported an average 18.5 percent increase in total muscle creatine, and an average 20.7 percent increase in PCr. Preen and others found that, once loaded, total muscle creatine levels could be maintained with creatine doses of 2–5 grams per day.

Most of the creatine in the body is found in the muscles, and Casey and others suggest that any performance benefits may be related to increased creatine within type II muscle fibers. About 60 percent of the total muscle creatine is PCr, and the remainder is free creatine. Theoretically, according to Casey and Greenhaff, increasing the amount of PCr will provide more substrate for generating ATP during high-intensity exercise, and higher levels of free creatine will help resynthesize PCr. Additionally, Yquel and others, using magnetic resonance to evaluate PCr levels during repeated bouts of maximal plantar flexion exercise, found that creatine supplementation increased muscle power by about 5 percent. They noted that this effect could be attributed to a higher rate of phosphocreatine resynthesis, which would provide more PCr for ATP resynthesis.

Another theory suggests that creatine supplementation may have favorable effects on anabolic hormones, particularly human growth hormone. Schedel found that a large single dose of creatine monohydrate (20 grams) increased growth hormone secretion in the 6-hour period following ingestion, and most of the increases occurred between 2–6 hours after ingestion. However, Op 'T Eijnde and Hespel found that a standard 5-day creatine-loading protocol did not alter the responses of growth hormone, testosterone, or cortisol during the hour following a single bout of heavy resistance exercise. Because exercise itself stimulates human growth hormone release, and because creatine supplementation appears to have no additive effect, this theory appears to have little support or value for the athlete in training.

In essence, increased muscle phosphocreatine and free creatine may enhance the potential of the ATP-PCr energy system and provide the athlete with an edge in competitive events involving very high-intensity exercise performance. Moreover, the enhanced ATP-PCr energy system may permit more intensive training. Volek and others found that creatine supplementation appears to be effective for maintaining muscular performance during the initial phase of high-volume resistance training, possibly deterring overreaching and the associated small decrements in performance. Enhanced training should translate into enhanced competitive performance.

Effect on exercise performance Research regarding the effects of creatine supplementation on exercise performance continues at a solid pace. Most research has investigated the effect of creatine supplementation on short-term, maximal exercise tasks of less than 30 seconds, those highly dependent on the ATP-PCr energy system, which may be referred to as *anaerobic power*. Many studies also incorporated repetitive exercise tasks with short recovery intervals, which could evaluate the possible effect of enhanced PCr resynthesis during recovery. However, some research has also investigated the effect of creatine supplementation on exercise performance tasks of somewhat longer duration, including anaerobic endurance, that would be dependent on the lactic acid energy system (anaerobic glycolysis) and aerobic endurance that would be dependent on the oxygen energy system (aerobic glycolysis).

ATP-PCr energy system Research involving the effects of creatine supplementation on strength and power continues at a steady pace. As with most research evaluating the effectiveness of ergogenic aids, all studies are not in agreement. However, many studies with creatine, conducted at some leading universities throughout the world, have provided some strong evidence supportive of a positive ergogenic effect of creatine supplementation in certain exercise endeavors, primarily those characterized by repetitive high-intensity exercise bouts with brief recovery periods. Using appropriate research methodology, recent studies have shown significant improvement in the following exercise tasks following creatine supplementation.

- Improvement in total and maximal force in repetitive isometric muscle contractions
- Improvement in muscular strength and endurance in isotonic strength tests, including 1-RM tests

- Improvement in muscular force/torque and endurance in isokinetic strength testing
- Improvement in cycle ergometer performance in maximal tests ranging from 6 to 30 seconds

In their book, Williams, Kreider, and Branch note that approximately 75 percent of the studies reported beneficial effects of creatine supplementation on isotonic strength and endurance and cycle ergometer power and endurance, while about 50 percent of the studies revealed ergogenic effects on isometric and isokinetic tests of muscular strength, power, and endurance. All of these test protocols involved laboratory procedures, although some of the isotonic strength tests, such as the bench press, could be analogous to the sport of competitive weightlifting. Most studies involved males, but studies with females also reported improved performance. Studies continue to provide supportive evidence of the ergogenicity of creatine supplementation.

The effects of creatine supplementation on field performance tests, such as jumping, running, swimming, skating, and other miscellaneous events, are less consistent, but overall still generally favorable. For example, of 15 studies evaluating the effect of creatine supplementation on single or repetitive sprint-run, sprint-swim, or sprint-cycle performance ranging from 5 to 100 meters or up to 30 seconds duration, creatine supplementation improved performance in 8 of the trials, but had no effect in the other 7. For example, Skare and others, using a standard creatine-loading protocol with well-trained male sprinters as subjects, reported significant improvements in 100-meter sprint velocity and time to complete 6 intermittent 60-meter sprints. Additionally, Preen and others studied the effect of a 5-day creatine-loading protocol on long-term repetitive sprints, doing 10 sets of multiple 6-second bike sprints with varying periods of recovery in an 80-minute time frame. Muscle biopsies revealed increased total creatine and PCr following supplementation, and both peak power and total work production were increased significantly. Conversely, Op 'T Eijnde and others reported no significant improvement in a 70-meter shuttle run sprint power test by well-trained tennis players following a standard 5-day creatine-loading protocol.

Some of these findings have a direct application to sports competition, such as an increased 1-RM performance in weight lifting, faster 50-yard swim times, and faster 100-meter sprint run times. The laboratory findings for other types of exercise performance are also rather strong, and do support a possible application to actual field competitions. For example, Preen and others noted that the findings from their study could suggest improved performance in intermittent high-intensity sports, such as soccer.

In this regard, several investigators have designed laboratory-controlled exercise protocols designed to mimic an actual sport event. Romer and others, in a well-controlled placebo, crossover study with competitive squash players, found that creatine loading for 5 days enhanced performance in an exercise protocol involving high-intensity, intermittent exercise involving 10 sets of simulated positional play to mimic squash. Creatine supplementation improved mean set sprint time by 3.2 percent compared to the placebo condition. The authors concluded that this study provides evidence that oral creatine supplementation improves exercise performance in competitive squash players. In one of the few studies with creatine supplementation conducted with young athletes, Ostojic reported enhanced performance in various soccer-related performance tests, such as sprint-power times and dribble test times, in 16-year-old soccer players. In a related study, Cox and others studied the effects of creatine supplementation on an exercise test protocol designed to simulate match play in soccer. The test involved 5 blocks of 11-minute exercise involving sprint running, agility runs, and a precision ball-kicking drill interspersed with recovery walks, jogs, and runs. Creatine supplementation improved performance in some repeated sprint and agility tasks even though the subjects increased body mass, but the creatine had no effect on ball-kicking accuracy.

Thus, creatine supplementation might improve speed in repetitive sprints, important for many sports, but may not necessarily enhance sports skills. In support of this viewpoint, Op 'T Eijnde and others, in the study cited previously with well-trained tennis players, reported no significant effects of creatine loading on tennis stroke performance as measured by power and precision of their serves.

Kirkendall suggests the available research is not applicable to the actual style of running in soccer and indicates that because so much of the running in soccer is at less than maximal sprinting speed, creatine supplementation likely provides no benefit for match performance. It certainly is difficult to study the effect of nutritional interventions on actual game performance. However, one might rationalize that if additional phosphocreatine could provide a slight advantage in speed at a critical point during a match, it might make the difference in the outcome of the contest. In their review, Hespel and others indicated that creatine may be useful for soccer.

Available research suggests that prolonged supplementation with maintenance doses of creatine may not provide any additional performance-enhancing advantage compared to a 5-day creatine-loading protocol. Peyrebrune and others reported that 5 days of creatine loading (20 grams/day) improved performance time of elite swimmers in eight 50-yard repeat swims. Swimmers were then assigned to either a creatine-maintenance dose (3 grams/day) or placebo for 22–27 weeks of additional swim training. Following the training period, all subjects again followed the creatine-loading protocol and repeated the 50-yard swim protocol. There was no statistically significant difference in performance times between the two groups, suggesting that the maintenance protocol was not necessary if the athlete undergoes a creatine-loading protocol prior to performance.

Lactic acid energy system Theoretically, increasing muscle PCr concentration could possibly buffer acidity and mitigate the effect of lactic acid production on muscle contraction, thus improving anaerobic endurance performance in events of maximal exercise ranging from about 30 to 150 seconds. Fewer studies are available, but creatine supplementation has been reported to benefit performance in some anaerobic endurance tests, including maximal isometric and isotonic muscular work output, cycle ergometer work output, running performance in 300 meters, and treadmill run to exhaustion at intensities greater than 100 percent

e. In general, research has shown that protein supplementation above the RDA will not improve physiological performance capacity during aerobic endurance exercise.

5. In the recommendations for a healthy diet from the National Academy of Sciences, what is the Acceptable Macronutrient Distribution Range for protein as a percent of daily energy intake in Calories?

   a. 15–20
   b. 10–35
   c. 4–6
   d. 12–14
   e. 40–65

6. Which of the following statements relative to protein metabolism is false?

   a. Excess protein may be converted to glucose in the body.
   b. The liver is a critical center for the control of amino acid metabolism.
   c. Essential amino acids can be formed in the liver from carbohydrate and nitrogen from nonessential amino acids.

   d. Excess protein may be converted to fat in the body.
   e. Urea is a waste product of protein metabolism.

7. Which is most likely to be a complete, high-quality protein food?

   a. cheddar cheese
   b. peanut butter
   c. green peas
   d. corn
   e. macaroni

8. Supplementation with some amino acids has been theorized to decrease the formation of serotonin in the brain and possibly help delay the onset of central nervous system fatigue in prolonged aerobic endurance exercise. Which amino acids are theorized to do this?

   a. leucine, isoleucine, and valine
   b. arginine, ornithine, and inosine
   c. tryptophan, arginine, and creatine
   d. inosine, creatine, and alanine
   e. asparagine, aspartic acid, and glutamine

9. If an adult weighed 176 pounds, the RDA for protein would be what, in grams?

   a. 176
   b. 140.8
   c. 80
   d. 64
   e. 309.7

10. Research has suggested that creatine supplementation may enhance performance in which of the following types of physical performance tasks?

   a. an all-out power lift in 1 second
   b. high-intensity exercise lasting 6–30 seconds
   c. 10-kilometer race lasting about 30 minutes
   d. marathon running (26.2 miles)
   e. ultramarathons, such as Ironman-type triathlons

Answers to multiple-choice questions:
1. b; 2. e; 3. d; 4. d; 5. b; 6. c; 7. a; 8. a; 9. d; 10. b.

Review Questions—Essay

1. Differentiate between complete and incomplete proteins as related to essential and nonessential amino acids and indicate several specific foods that are considered to contain either complete or incomplete protein.

2. Describe the process of gluconeogenesis from protein.

3. Explain why some scientists recommend that both strength and endurance athletes may need more dietary protein than the RDA. Provide some recommended values and calculate the recommended grams of protein for a 70-kilogram athlete.

4. Explain the central fatigue hypothesis as related to BCAA supplementation for endurance athletes and summarize the research findings as to the related ergogenic efficacy of BCAA supplementation.

5. Discuss the concept of the *good* proteins in the OmniHeart diet plan and the underlying rationale as to how they may be more beneficial in helping protect against cardiovascular disease. Discuss also how the form of food protein and its preparation may influence risk for certain cancers.

References

Books

American Institute of Cancer Research. 2007. *Food, Nutrition, Physical Activity, and the Prevention of Cancer: A Global Perspective.* Washington, DC: AICR.

Bucci, L. 1993. *Nutrients as Ergogenic Aids for Sports and Exercise.* Boca Raton, FL: CRC Press.

Houston, M. 2006. *Biochemistry Primer for Exercise Science.* Champaign, IL: Human Kinetics.

National Academy of Sciences. 2005. *Dietary Reference Intakes for Energy, Carbohydrates, Fiber, Fat, Fatty Acids, Cholesterol, Protein and Amino Acids (Macronutrients).* Washington, DC: National Academies Press.

United States Anti-Doping Agency. 2005. *Optimal Dietary Intake.* Colorado Springs, CO.

Williams, M., Kreider, R., and Branch, J. 1999. *Creatine: The Power Supplement.* Champaign, IL: Human Kinetics.

Reviews

Abcouwer, S., and Souba, W. 1999. Glutamine and arginine. In *Modern Nutrition in Health and Disease,* eds. M. Shils, et al. Baltimore: Williams & Wilkins.

Akerström, T., and Pedersen, B. 2007. Strategies to enhance immune function for marathon runners: What can be done? *Sports Medicine* 37:416–19.

American College of Sports Medicine. 2000. The physiological and health effects of oral creatine supplementation. *Medicine & Science in Sports & Exercise* 32:706–17.

American College of Sports Medicine, American Dietetic Association, Dietitians of Canada. 2009. Joint position statement: Nutrition and athletic performance. *Medicine & Science in Sports & Exercise* 41:709–31.

Antonio, J., and Street, C. 1999. Glutamine: A potentially useful supplement for athletes. *Canadian Journal of Applied Physiology* 24:1–14.

Artioli, G., et al. 2010. Role of β-alanine supplementation on muscle carnosine and exercise performance. *Medicine & Science in Sports & Exercise* 42(6):1162–73.

Bailes, J., et al. 2002. The neurosurgeon in sport: Awareness of the risks of heatstroke and dietary supplements. *Neurosurgery* 51:283–86.

Barrett, S. and Herbert, V. 1999. Fads, frauds, and quackery. In *Modern Nutrition in Health and Disease,* eds. M. Shils et al. Baltimore: Williams & Wilkins.

Beelen, M., et al. 2010. Nutritional strategies to promote postexercise recovery. *International Journal of Sport Nutrition & Exercise Metabolism* 20:515–32.

Begum, G., et al. 2005. Physiological role of carnosine in contracting muscle. *International Journal of Sport Nutrition & Exercise Metabolism* 15:493–514.

Bemben, M., and Lamont, H. 2005. Creatine supplementation and exercise performance: Recent findings. *Sports Medicine* 35:107–25.

Benzi, G., and Ceci, A. 2001. Creatine as nutritional supplementation and medicinal product. *Journal of Sports Medicine & Physical Fitness* 41:1–10.

Bilsborough, S., and Mann, N. 2006. A review of issues of dietary protein intake in humans. *International Journal of Sport Nutrition & Exercise Metabolism* 16:129–52.

Blomstrand, E. 2006. A role for branched-chain amino acids in reducing central fatigue. *Journal of Nutrition* 136: 544S–47S.

Blomstrand, E. 2001. Amino acids and central fatigue. *Amino Acids* 20:25–34.

Blomstrand, E., et al. 2006. Branched-chain amino acids activate key enzymes in protein synthesis after physical exercise. *Journal of Nutrition* 136:269S–73S.

Böger, R. 2007. The pharmacodynamics of L-arginine. *Journal of Nutrition* 137:1650S–55S.

Bonjour, J. 2005. Dietary protein: An essential nutrient for bone health. *Journal of the American College of Nutrition* 24: 526S–36S.

Bonjour, J., et al. 2000. Protein intake and bone growth. *Canadian Journal of Applied Physiology* 26:S153–66.

Branch, J. 2003. Effect of creatine supplementation on body composition and performance: A meta-analysis. *International Journal of Sport Nutrition & Exercise Metabolism* 13:198–226.

Budgett, R., et al. 1998. The overtraining syndrome. In *Oxford Textbook of Sports Medicine,* eds. M. Harries, et al. Oxford: Oxford University Press.

Buford, T., et al. 2007. International Society of Sports Nutrition position stand: Creatine supplementation and exercise. *Journal of the International Society of Sports Nutrition* 4:6.

Butterfield, G. 1991. Amino acids and high protein diets. In *Perspectives in Exercise Science and Sports Medicine. Ergogenics: Enhancement of Sports Performance,* eds. D. Lamb and M. Williams. Indianapolis, IN: Benchmark Press.

Campbell, B., et al. 2007. International Society of Sports Nutrition position stand: Protein and exercise. *Journal of the International Society of Sports Nutrition* 4:8.

Candow, D., and Chilibeck, P. 2007. Effect of creatine supplementation during resistance training on muscle accretion in the elderly. *Journal of Nutrition, Health & Aging* 11(2):185–8.

Casey, A., and Greenhaff, P. 2000. Does dietary creatine supplementation play a role in skeletal muscle metabolism and performance? *American Journal of Clinical Nutrition* 72:607S–17S.

Castell, L. 2003. Glutamine supplementation in vitro and in vivo, in exercise and in immunodepression. *Sports Medicine* 33:323–45.

Cheng, J., et al. 2001. L-arginine in the management of cardiovascular disease. *Annals of Pharmacotherapy* 35:755–64.

Cheuvront, S. 1999. The zone diet and athletic performance. *Sports Medicine* 27:213–28.

Chromiak, J., and Antonio, J. 2002. Use of amino acids as growth-hormone releasing agents by athletes. *Nutrition* 18:657–61.

Clarkson, T. 2002. Soy, soy phytoestrogens and cardiovascular disease. *Journal of Nutrition* 132:566S–69S.

Clegg, D., et al. 2006. Glucosamine, chondroitin sulfate, and the two in combination for painful knee arthritis. *New England Journal of Medicine* 354:795–808.

Craig, W., and A. Mangels. 2009. Position of the American Dietetic Association: Vegetarian diets. *Journal of the American Dietetic Association* 109:1266–82.

Cynober, L. 2007. Pharmacokinetics of arginine and related amino acids. *Journal of Nutrition* 137:1646S–49S.

Dalbo, V., et al. 2008. Putting to rest the myth of creatine supplementation leading to muscle cramps and dehydration. *British Journal of Sports Medicine* 42:567–73.

Davis, J. 2000. Nutrition, neurotransmitters and central nervous system fatigue. In *Nutrition in Sport,* ed. R. J. Maughan. Oxford: Blackwell Science.

Davis, J. 1996. Carbohydrates, branched-chain amino acids and endurance: The central fatigue hypothesis. *Sports Science Exchange* 9(2):1–5.

Davis, J., et al. 2000. Serotonin and central nervous system fatigue: Nutritional considerations. *American Journal of Clinical Nutrition* 72:573S–78S.

Drummond, M., et al. 2009. Nutritional and contractile regulation of human skeletal muscle protein synthesis and mTORC1 signaling. *Journal of Applied Physiology* 106:1374–84.

Eisenstein, J., et al. 2002. High-protein weight-loss diets: Are they safe and do they work? A review of the experimental and epidemiologic data. *Nutrition Reviews* 60:189–200.

Evans, W. 2001. Protein nutrition and resistance exercise. *Canadian Journal of Applied Physiology* 26:S141–52.

Fielding, R., and Parkington, J. 2002. What are the dietary protein requirements of physically active individuals? New evidence on the effects of exercise on protein utilization during post-exercise recovery. *Nutrition in Clinical Care* 5:191–96.

Fitts, R., and Metzger, J. 1993. Mechanisms of muscular fatigue. In *Principles of Exercise Biochemistry,* ed. J. Poortmans. Basel, Switzerland: Karger.

Gaffney-Stomberg, E., et al. 2009. Increasing dietary protein requirements in elderly people for optimal muscle and bone health. *Journal of the American Geriatrics Society* 57:1073–79.

Garlick, P., et al. 1999. Adaptation of protein metabolism in relation to limits to high dietary protein intake. *European Journal of Clinical Nutrition* 53:S34–S43.

Genaro, Pde, S., and Martini, L. 2010. Effect of protein intake on bone and muscle mass in the elderly. *Nutrition Reviews* 68:616–30.

Gibala, M. 2007. Protein metabolism and endurance exercise. *Sports Medicine* 37:337–40.

Gibala, M. 2002. Dietary protein, amino acid supplements, and recovery from exercise. *Sports Science Exchange* 15(4):1–4.

Gibala, M. 2001. Regulation of skeletal muscle amino acid metabolism during exercise. *International Journal of Sport Nutrition & Exercise Metabolism* 11:87–108.

Gleeson, M. 2005. Interrelationship between physical activity and branched-chain amino acids. *Journal of Nutrition* 135:1591S–95S.

Graham, T., and MacLean, D. 1998. Ammonia and amino acid metabolism in skeletal muscle: Human, rodent and canine models. *Medicine & Science in Sports & Exercise* 30:34–46.

Graham, T., et al. 1997. Effect of endurance training on ammonia and amino acid metabolism in humans. *Medicine & Science in Sports & Exercise* 29:646–53.

Greenhaff, P. 1997. Creatine supplementation and implications for exercise performance. In *Advances in Training and Nutrition for Endurance Sports,* eds. A. Jeukendrup, M. Brouns, and F. Brouns. Maastricht, the Netherlands: Novartis Nutrition Research Unit.

Hargreaves, M., and Snow, R. 2001. Amino acids and endurance exercise. *International Journal of Sport Nutrition & Exercise Metabolism* 11:133–45.

Hayes, A., and Cribb, P. 2008. Effect of whey protein isolate on strength, body composition and muscle hypertrophy during resistance training. *Current Opinion in Clinical Nutrition & Metabolic Care* 11:40–44.

Heaney, R., and Layman, D. 2008. Amount and type of protein influences bone health. *American Journal of Clinical Nutrition* 87:1567S–70S.

Henkel, J. 2000. Soy: Health claims for soy protein, questions about other components. *FDA Consumer* 34(3):13–20.

Herrero-Beaumont, G., et al. 2007. The reverse glucosamine sulfate pathway: Application in knee osteoarthritis. *Expert Opinion on Pharmacotherapy* 8:215–25.

Hespel, P., et al. 2006. Dietary supplements for football. *Journal of Sports Sciences* 24:749–61.

Hu, F. 2005. Protein, body weight, and cardiovascular health. *American Journal of Clinical Nutrition* 82:242S–47S.

Jacobson, B. 1990. Effect of amino acids on growth hormone release. *Physician & Sportsmedicine* 18 (January):63–70.

Kanaley, J. 2008. Growth hormone, arginine and exercise. *Current Opinion in Clinical Nutrition & Metabolic Care* 11:50–54.

Kerksick, C., et al. 2008. International Society of Sports Nutrition position stand: Nutrient timing. *Journal of the International Society of Sports Nutrition* 5:17.

Kim, H., et al. 2011. Studies on the safety of creatine supplementation. *Amino Acids* 40:1409–1418.

Kirkendall, D. 2004. Creatine, carbs, and fluids: How important in soccer nutrition? *Sports Science Exchange* 17(3):1–6.

Kley, R., et al. 2007. Creatine for treating muscle disorders. *Cochrane Database of Systematic Reviews* 24 (1):CD004760.

Koopman, R. 2007. Role of amino acids and peptides in the molecular signaling in skeletal muscle after resistance exercise. *International Journal of Sport Nutrition & Exercise Metabolism* 17:S47–S57.

Krall, E., and Dawson-Hughes, B. 1999. Osteoporosis. In *Modern Nutrition in Health and Disease,* eds. M. Shils et al. Baltimore: Williams and Wilkins.

Kreider, R. 2003. Effects of creatine supplementation on performance and training adaptations. *Molecular & Cellular Biochemistry* 244:89–94.

Kreider, R., et al., 2010. ISSN exercise & sport nutrition review: Research and recommendations. *Journal of the International Society of Sports Nutrition* 7:7.

Lawrence, M., and Kirby, D. 2002. Nutrition and sports supplements: Fact or fiction? *Journal of Clinical Gastroenterology* 35:299–306.

Layman, D., et al. 2008. Protein in optimal health: Heart disease and type 2 diabetes. *American Journal of Clinical Nutrition* 87:1571S–75S.

Lemon, P. 2000. Effects of exercise on protein metabolism. In *Nutrition in Sport,* ed. R. J. Maughan. Oxford: Blackwell Science.

Lemon, P. 2000. Protein metabolism during exercise. In *Exercise and Sport Science,* eds. W. E. Garrett and D. T. Kirkendall. Philadelphia: Lippincott Williams & Wilkins.

Lemon, P. 1998. Effects of exercise on dietary protein requirements. *International Journal of Sport Nutrition,* 8:426–47.

Lesourd, B. 1995. Protein undernutrition as the major cause of decreased immune function in the elderly: Clinical and functional implications. *Nutrition Reviews* 53:S86–S94.

Lopez, R., et al. 2009. Does creatine supplementation hinder exercise heat tolerance or hydration status? A systematic review with meta-analyses. *Journal of Athletic Training* 44:215–23.

Mannion, A., et al. 1992. Carnosine and anserine concentrations in the quadriceps femoris muscle of healthy humans. *European Journal of Applied Physiology* 64:47–50.

Matthews, D. 2006. Proteins and amino acids. In *Modern Nutrition in Health and Disease,* eds. M. Shils, et al. Philadelphia: Lippincott Williams & Wilkins.

McConell, G. 2007. Effects of L-arginine supplementation on exercise metabolism. *Current Opinion in Clinical Nutrition & Metabolic Care* 10:46–51.

Meeusen, R., and Wilson, P. 2007. Amino acids and the brain: Do they play a role in "central fatigue"? *International Journal of Sport Nutrition & Exercise Metabolism* 17:S37–S46.

Meeusen, R., et al. 2006. The brain and fatigue: New opportunities for nutritional interventions? *Journal of Sports Sciences* 24:773–82.

Melis, G., et al. 2004. Glutamine: Recent developments in research on the clinical significance of glutamine. *Current Opinion in Clinical Nutrition & Metabolic Care* 7:59–79.

Miller, B. 2007. Human muscle protein synthesis after physical activity and feeding. *Exercise & Sport Sciences Reviews* 35:50–55.

Millward, D. 2004. Macronutrient intakes as determinants of dietary protein and amino acid adequacy. *Journal of Nutrition* 134:1588S–96S.

Newsholme, E., and Castell, L. 2000. Amino acids, fatigue and immunodepression in exercise. In *Nutrition in Sport,* ed. R. J. Maughan. Oxford: Blackwell Science.

Newsholme, E., et al. 1992. Physical and mental fatigue: Metabolic mechanisms and importance of plasma amino acids. *British Medical Bulletin* 48:477–95.

Nieman, D. 2001. Exercise immunology: Nutrition countermeasures. *Canadian Journal of Applied Physiology* 26:S45–55.

Paddon-Jones, D., et al. 2008. Protein, weight management, and satiety. *American Journal of Clinical Nutrition* 1558S–61S.

Palisin, T., and Stacy, J. 2005. Beta-hydroxy-beta-methylbutyrate and its use in athletics. *Current Sports Medicine Reports* 4:220–23.

Parkhouse, W. 1988. Regulation of skeletal muscle myofibrillar protein degradation: Relationships to fatigue and exercise. *International Journal of Biochemistry* 20:769–75.

Persky, A., and Brazeau, G. 2001. Clinical pharmacology of the dietary supplement creatine monohydrate. *Pharmacology Reviews* 53:161–76.

Phillips, G. 2007. Glutamine: The nonessential amino acid for performance enhancement. *Current Sports Medicine Reports* 6:265–68.

Phillips, S. 2006. Dietary protein for athletes: From requirements to metabolic advantage. *Applied Physiology, Nutrition & Metabolism* 31:647–54.

Phillips, S. 2004. Protein requirements and supplementation in strength sports. *Nutrition* 20:689–95.

Phillips, S., et al. 2007. A critical examination of dietary protein requirements, benefits, and excesses in athletes. *International Journal of Sport Nutrition & Exercise Metabolism* 17:S58–S76.

Poortmans, J. 1993. Protein metabolism. In *Principles of Exercise Biochemistry,* ed. J. Poortmans. Basel, Switzerland: Karger.

Poortmans, J., and Francaux, M. 2000. Adverse effects of creatine supplementation: Fact or fiction. *Sports Medicine* 30:155–70.

Portal, S., et al. 2010. Effect of HMB supplementation on body composition, fitness, hormonal profile and muscle damage indices. *Journal of Pediatric Endocrinology & Metabolism* 23:641–50.

Rawson, E., and Clarkson, P. 2003. Scientifically debatable: Is creatine worth its weight? *Sports Science Exchange* 16(4):1–6.

Reginster, J., et al. 2007. Current role of glucosamine in the treatment of osteoarthritis. *Rheumatology* 46:731–5.

Reichenbach, S., et al. 2007. Meta-analysis: Chondroitin for osteoarthritis of the knee or hip. *Annals of Internal Medicine* 146:580–90.

Rennie, M. 2001. Control of muscle protein synthesis as a result of contractile activity and amino acid availability: Implications for protein requirements. *International Journal of Sport Nutrition & Exercise Metabolism* 11:S170–76.

Rennie, M., and Tipton, K. 2000. Protein and amino acid metabolism during and after exercise and the effects of nutrition. *Annual Review of Nutrition* 20:457–83.

Rennie, M., et al. 2006. Branched-chain amino acids as fuels and anabolic signals in human muscle. *Journal of Nutrition* 136:264S–68S.

Reynolds, K., et al. 2006. A meta-analysis of the effect of soy protein supplementation on serum lipids. *American Journal of Cardiology* 98:633–40.

Rodriguez, N., et al. 2007. Dietary protein, endurance exercise, and human skeletal-muscle protein turnover. *Current Opinions in Clinical Nutrition & Metabolic Care* 10:40–45.

Rowlands, D., and Thomson, J. 2009. Effects of β-hydroxy-β-methylbutyrate supplementation during resistance training on strength, body composition, and muscle damage in trained and untrained young men: A meta-analysis. *Journal of Strength & Conditioning Research* 23(3):836–46.

Sacks, F., et al. 2006. Soy protein, isoflavones, and cardiovascular health: An American Heart Association Science Advisory for professionals from the Nutrition Committee. *Circulation.* 113:1034–44.

Sahlin, K., et al. 1998. Energy supply and muscle fatigue in humans. *Acta Physiologica Scandinavica* 162:261–66.

Saunders, M. 2007. Coingestion of carbohydrate-protein during endurance exercise: Influence on performance and recovery. *International Journal of Sport Nutrition & Exercise Metabolism* 17:S87–S103.

Schardt, D. 2006. Do glucosamine & chondroitin work? *Nutrition Action Health Letter* 33(7):9–11.

Schardt, D. 2002. Got soy? *Nutrition Action Health Letter* 29(9):8–11.

Schardt, D. 2001. Sam-e so-so. *Nutrition Action Health Letter* 28(2):10–11.

Shao, A., and Hathcock, J. 2006. Risk assessment for creatine monohydrate. *Regulatory Toxicology & Pharmacology* 45:242–51.

Skibola, C., and Smith, M. 2000. Potential health impacts of excessive flavonoid intake. *Free Radical Biology & Medicine* 29:375–83.

Slater, G., and Jenkins, D. 2000. Beta-hydroxy-beta-methylbutyrate (HMB) supplementation and the promotion of muscle growth and strength. *Sports Medicine* 30:105–16.

Slavin, J., et al. 1988. Amino acid supplements: Beneficial or risky? *Physician & Sportsmedicine* 16 (March):221–24.

Snow, R., and Murphy, R. 2003. Factors influencing creatine loading into human skeletal muscle. *Exercise & Sport Sciences Reviews* 31:154–58.

Soeken, K., et al. 2002. Safety and efficacy of S-adenosylmethionine (SAMe) for osteoarthritis. *Journal of Family Practice* 51:425–30.

Tarnopolsky, M. 2008. Sex differences in exercise metabolism and the role of 17-beta estradiol. *Medicine & Science in Sports & Exercise* 40:648–54.

Tarnopolsky, M. 2004. Protein requirements for endurance athletes. *Nutrition* 20:662–68.

Tarnopolsky, M., and Safdar, A. 2008. The potential benefits of creatine and conjugated linoleic acid as adjuncts to resistance training in older adults. *Applied Physiology, Nutrition & Metabolism* 33:213–27.

Tarnopolsky, M., et al. 2004. Creatine monohydrate enhances strength and body composition in Duchenne muscular dystrophy. *Neurology* 62:1771–77.

Tipton, K. 2007. Role of protein and hydrolysates before exercise. *International Journal of Sport Nutrition & Exercise Metabolism* 17:S77–S86.

Tipton, K., and Witard, O. 2007. Protein requirements and recommendations for athletes: Relevance of ivory tower arguments for practical recommendations. *Clinics in Sports Medicine* 26:17–36.

Tipton, K., and Wolfe, R. 2004. Protein and amino acids for athletes. *Journal of Sports Sciences* 22:65–79.

Tipton, K., and Wolfe, R. 1998. Exercise-induced changes in protein metabolism. *Acta Physiologica Scandinavica* 162:377–87.

Trudeau, F. 2008. Aspartate as an ergogenic supplement. *Sports Medicine* 38:9–16.

Tufts University. 2000. A look at glucosamine and chondroitin for easing arthritis pain. *Tufts University Health & Nutrition Letter* 17(11):4–5.

van Loon, L. 2007. Application of protein or protein hydrolysates to improve postexercise recovery. *International Journal of Sport Nutrition & Exercise Metabolism* 17:S104–S117.

Volek, J., et al. 2006. Nutritional aspects of women strength athletes. *British Journal of Sports Medicine* 40:742–48.

Volek, J., and Rawson, E. 2004. Scientific basis and practical aspects of creatine supplementation for athletes. *Nutrition* 20:609–14.

Wagenmakers, A. 2006. The metabolic systems: Protein and amino acid metabolism in muscle. In *ACSM's Advanced Exercise Physiology,* ed. C. M. Tipton. Philadelphia: Lippincott Williams & Wilkins.

Wagenmakers, A. 2000. Amino acid metabolism in exercise. In *Nutrition in Sport,* ed. R. J. Maughan. Oxford: Blackwell Science.

Wagenmakers, A. 1999. Amino acid supplements to improve athletic performance. *Current Opinion in Clinical Nutrition & Metabolic Care* 2:539–44.

Walberg-Rankin, J. W. 1999. Role of protein in exercise. *Clinics in Sports Medicine* 18:499–511.

Walzem, R., et al. 2002. Whey components: Millennia of evolution create functionalities for mammalian nutrition. What we know and what we may be overlooking. *Critical Reviews in Food Science & Nutrition* 42:353–75.

Williams, M. 1999. Facts and fallacies of purported ergogenic amino acid supplements. *Clinics in Sports Medicine* 18:633–49.

Wolfe, R. 2006. Skeletal muscle protein metabolism and resistance exercise. *Journal of Nutrition* 136:525S–28S.

Wolfe, R. 2001. Control of muscle protein breakdown: Effects of activity and nutritional states. *International Journal of Sport Nutrition & Exercise Metabolism* 11:S164–69.

Wolfe, R. 2001. Effects of amino acid intake on anabolic processes. *Canadian Journal of Applied Physiology* 26:S220–27.

Yoshimura, H. 1970. Anemia during physical training (sports anemia). *Nutrition Review* 28:251–53.

Specific Studies

Abel, T., et al. 2005. Influence of chronic supplementation of arginine aspartate in endurance athletes on performance and substrate metabolism: A randomized, double-blind, placebo-controlled study. *International Journal of Sports Medicine* 26:344–49.

Andersen, L., et al. 2005. The effect of resistance training combined with timed ingestion of protein on muscle fiber size and muscle strength. *Metabolism* 54:151–56.

Antonio, J., et al. 2002. The effects of high-dose glutamine ingestion on weightlifting performance. *Journal of Strength & Conditioning Research* 16:157–60.

Antonio, J., et al. 2001. The effects of bovine colostrum supplementation on body composition and exercise performance in active men and women. *Nutrition* 17:243–47.

Appel, L., et al. 2005. Effects of protein, monounsaturated fat, and carbohydrate intake on blood pressure and serum lipids: Results of the OmniHeart randomized trial. *JAMA* 294:2455–64.

Astorino, T., et al. 2005. Is running performance enhanced with creatine serum ingestion? *Journal of Strength & Conditioning Research* 19:730–34.

Bailey, S., et al. 2009. Dietary nitrate supplementation reduces the O2 cost of low-intensity exercise and enhances tolerance to high-intensity exercise in humans. *Journal of Applied Physiology* 107:1144–55.

Betts, J., et al. 2007. The influence of carbohydrate and protein ingestion during recovery from prolonged exercise on subsequent endurance performance. *Journal of Sports Sciences* 13:1–12.

Betts, J., et al. 2005. Recovery of endurance running capacity: Effect of carbohydrate-protein mixture. *International Journal of Sport Nutrition & Exercise Metabolism* 15:590–609.

Bird, S., et al. 2006. Independent and combined effects of liquid carbohydrate/essential amino acid ingestion on hormonal and muscular adaptations following resistance training in untrained men. *European Journal of Applied Physiology* 97:225–38.

Bird, S., et al. 2006. Liquid carbohydrate/protein amino acid ingestion during a short-term bout of resistance exercise suppresses myofibrillar protein degradation. *Metabolism* 55:570–77.

Blomstrand, E., et al. 1997. Influence of ingesting a solution of branched-chain amino acids on perceived exertion during exercise. *Acta Physiologica Scandinavica* 159:41–49.

Blomstrand, E., et al. 1991. Administration of branched-chain amino acids during sustained exercise—Effects on performance and on plasma concentration of some amino acids. *European Journal of Applied Physiology* 65:83–88.

Brinkworth, G., et al. 2004. Effect of bovine colostrum supplementation on the composition of resistance trained and untrained limbs in healthy young men. *European Journal of Applied Physiology* 91:53–60.

Brinkworth, G., et al. 2002. Oral bovine colostrum supplementation enhances buffer capacity, but not rowing performance in elite female rowers. *International Journal of Sport Nutrition & Exercise Metabolism* 12:349–63.

Bucci, L., et al. 1992. Ornithine supplementation and insulin release in bodybuilders. *International Journal of Sport Nutrition* 2:287–91.

Bucci, L., et al. 1990. Ornithine ingestion and growth hormone release in bodybuilders. *Nutrition Research* 10:239–45.

Buchman, A. L., et al. 1999. The effect of arginine or glycine supplementation on gastrointestinal function, muscle injury, serum amino acid concentrations and performance during a marathon run. *International Journal of Sports Medicine* 20:315–21.

Buford, B., and Koch, A. 2004. Glycine-arginine-alpha-ketoisocaproic acid improves performance of repeated cycling sprints. *Medicine & Science in Sports & Exercise* 36:583–87.

Burke, D., et al. 2003. Effect of creatine and weight training on muscle creatine and performance in vegetarians. *Medicine & Science in Sports & Exercise* 36:1946–55.

Burke, D., et al. 2001. The effect of whey protein supplementation with and without creatine monohydrate combined with resistance training on lean tissue mass and muscle strength. *International Journal of Sport Nutrition & Exercise Metabolism* 11:349–64.

Burke, D., et al. 2001. The effect of 7 days of creatine supplementation on 24-hour urinary creatine excretion. *Journal of Strength & Conditioning Research* 15:59–62.

Campbell, B., et al. 2006. Pharmacokinetics, safety, and effects on exercise performance of l-arginine alpha-ketoglutarate in trained adult men. *Nutrition* 22:872–81.

Candow, D., et al. 2006. Effect of whey and soy protein supplementation combined with resistance training in young adults. *International Journal of Sport Nutrition & Exercise Metabolism* 16:233–44.

Candow, D., et al. 2006. Protein supplementation before and after resistance training in older men. *European Journal of Applied Physiology* 97:548–56.

Candow, D., et al. 2001. Effect of glutamine supplementation combined with resistance training in young adults. *European Journal of Applied Physiology* 86:142–49.

Cao, J., et al. 2011. A diet high in meat protein and potential renal acid load increases fractional calcium absorption and urinary calcium excretion without affecting markers of bone resorption or formation in postmenopausal women. *Journal of Nutrition* 141:391–7.

Casey, A., et al. 1996. Creatine ingestion favorably affects performance and muscle metabolism during maximal exercise in humans. *American Journal of Physiology* 271:E31–E37.

Cheuvront, S., et al. 2004. Branched-chain amino acid supplementation and human performance when hypohydrated in the heat. *Journal of Applied Physiology* 97:1275–82.

Clegg, D., et al. 2006. Glucosamine, chondroitin sulfate, and the two in combination for painful knee osteoarthritis. *New England Journal of Medicine* 354:795–808.

Coburn, J., et al. 2006. Effects of leucine and whey protein supplementation during eight weeks of unilateral resistance training. *Journal of Strength & Conditioning Research* 20:284–91.

Collier, S., et al. 2006. Oral arginine attenuates the growth hormone response to resistance exercise. *Journal of Applied Physiology* 101:848–52.

Conlay, L., et al. 1989. Effects of running the Boston marathon on plasma concentrations of large neutral amino acids. *Journal of Neural Transmission* 76:65–71.

Coombes, J., et al. 2002. Dose effects of oral bovine colostrum on physical work capacity in cyclists. *Medicine & Science in Sports & Exercise* 34:1184–88.

Cox, G., et al. 2002. Acute creatine supplementation and performance during a field test simulating match play in elite soccer players. *International Journal of Sport Nutrition & Exercise Metabolism* 12:33–46.

Cribb, P., and Hayes, A. 2006. Effects of supplement timing and resistance exercise on skeletal muscle hypertrophy. *Medicine & Science in Sports & Exercise* 38:1918–25.

Cribb, P., et al. 2007. Effects of whey isolate, creatine, and resistance training on muscle hypertrophy. *Medicine & Science in Sports & Exercise* 39:298–307.

Cribb, P., et al. 2006. The effect of whey isolate and resistance training on strength, body composition, and plasma glutamine. *International Journal of Sport Nutrition & Exercise Metabolism* 16:494–509.

Crowe, M., et al. 2006. Effects of leucine supplementation on exercise performance. *European Journal of Applied Physiology* 97:664–72.

Cuisinier, C., et al. 2001. Changes in plasma and urinary taurine and amino acids in runners immediately and 24h after a marathon. *Amino Acids* 20:13–23.

Cunliffe, A., et al. 1998. A placebo controlled investigation of the effects of tryptophan or placebo on subjective and objective measures of fatigue. *European Journal of Clinical Nutrition* 52:425–30.

Davis, J., et al. 1999. Effects of branched-chain amino acids and carbohydrate on fatigue during intermittent, high-intensity running. *International Journal of Sports Medicine* 20:309–14.

Dawson-Hughes, B., and Harris, S. 2002. Calcium intake influences the association of protein intake with rates of bone loss in elderly men and women. *American Journal of Clinical Nutrition* 75:773–79.

Deldicque, L., et al. 2005. Increased IGF mRNA in human skeletal muscle after creatine supplementation. *Medicine & Science in Sports & Exercise* 37:731–36.

Doherty, M., et al. 2002. Caffeine is ergogenic after supplementation of oral creatine monohydrate. *Medicine & Science in Sports & Exercise* 34:1785–92.

Doutreleau, S., et al. 2006. Chronic L-arginine supplementation enhances endurance tolerance in heart failure patients. *International Journal of Sport Medicine* 27:567–72.

Elam, R. 1988. Morphological changes in adult males from resistance exercise and amino acid supplementation. *Journal of Sports Medicine & Physical Fitness* 28:35–39.

Elam, R., et al. 1989. Effects of arginine and ornithine on strength, lean body mass and urinary hydroxyproline in adult males. *Journal of Sports Medicine & Physical Fitness* 29:52–56.

Elliot, T., et al. 2006. Milk ingestion stimulates net muscle protein synthesis following resistance exercise. *Medicine & Science in Sports & Exercise* 38:667–74.

Esmarck, B. 2001. Timing of postexercise protein intake is important for muscle hypertrophy with resistance training in elderly humans. *Journal of Physiology* 535:301–11.

Fogelholm, G., et al. 1993. Low-dose amino acid supplementation: No effects on serum human growth hormone and insulin in male weightlifters. *International Journal of Sport Nutrition* 3:290–97.

Gill, N., et al. 2004. Creatine serum is not as effective as creatine powder for improving cycle sprint performance in competitive male team-sport athletes. *Journal of Strength & Conditioning Research* 18:272–75.

Gleeson, M., et al. 1998. Effect of low- and high-carbohydrate diets on the plasma glutamine and circulating leukocyte responses to exercise. *International Journal of Sport Nutrition* 8:45–59.

Green, A., et al. 1996. Carbohydrate ingestion augments creatine retention during creatine feeding in humans. *Acta Physiologica Scandinavica* 158:195–202.

Green, M., et al. 2008. Carbohydrate-protein drinks do not enhance recovery from exercise-induced muscle injury. *International Journal of Sport Nutrition & Exercise Metabolism* 18:1–18.

Greenhaff, P., et al. 1994. Effect of oral creatine supplementation on skeletal muscle phosphocreatine resynthesis. *American Journal of Physiology* 266:E725–E730.

Greer, B., et al. 2007. Branched-chain amino acid supplementation and indicators of muscle damage after endurance exercise. *International Journal of Sport Nutrition & Exercise Metabolism* 17:595–607.

Harris, R., et al. 1993. The effect of oral creatine supplementation on running performance during maximal short term exercise in man. *Journal of Physiology* 467:74P.

Harris, R., et al. 1992. Elevation of creatine in resting and exercised muscle on normal subjects by creatine supplementation. *Clinical Science* 83:367–74.

Hawkins, C., et al. 1991. Oral arginine does not affect body composition or muscle function in male weight lifters. *Medicine & Science in Sports & Exercise* 23:S15.

Hefler, S., et al. 1995. Branched-chain amino acid (BCAA) supplementation improves endurance performance in competitive cyclists. *Medicine & Science in Sports & Exercise* 27:S149.

Hernandez, M., et al. 1996. The protein efficiency ratios of 30:70 mixtures of animal: Vegetable protein are similar or higher than those of the animal foods alone. *Journal of Nutrition* 126:574–81.

Hespel, P., et al. 2002. Opposite actions of caffeine and creatine on muscle relaxation time in humans. *Journal of Applied Physiology* 92:513–18.

Hespel, P., et al. 2001. Oral creatine supplementation facilitates the rehabilitation of disuse atrophy and alters the expression of muscle myogenic factors in humans. *Journal of Physiology* 536:625–33.

Hickner, R., et al. 2006. L-citrulline reduces time to exhaustion and insulin response to a graded exercise test. *Medicine & Science in Sports & Exercise* 38:660–66.

Hile, A., et al. 2006. Creatine supplementation and anterior compartment pressure during exercise in the heat in dehydrated men. *Journal of Athletic Training* 41:30–5.

Hill, C., et al. 2007. Influence of beta-alanine supplementation on skeletal muscle carnosine concentrations and high intensity cycling capacity. *Amino Acids* 32:225–33.

Hoffman, J., et al. 2006. Effect of creatine and β-alanine supplementation on performance and endocrine responses in strength/power athletes. *International Journal of Sport Nutrition & Exercise Metabolism* 16:430–46.

Hoffman, J., et al. 2006. Effect of protein intake on strength, body composition and endocrine changes in strength/power athletes. *Journal of the International Society of Sport Nutrition* 3(2):12–18.

Hofman, Z., et al. 2002. The effect of bovine colostrum supplementation on exercise performance in elite field hockey players. *International Journal of Sport Nutrition & Exercise Metabolism* 12:461–69.

Houston, D., et al. 2008. Dietary protein intake is associated with lean mass change in older, community-dwelling adults: The Health, Aging, and Body Composition (Health ABC) Study. *American Journal of Clinical Nutrition* 87:150–55.

Hu, F. B., et al. 1999. Dietary protein and risk of ischemic heart disease in women.

American Journal of Clinical Nutrition 70:221–27.

Hughes, R., and Carr, A. 2002. A randomized, double-blind, placebo-controlled trial of glucosamine sulfate as an analgesic in osteoarthritis of the knee. *Rheumatology* 41:279–84.

Hultman, E., et al. 1996. Muscle creatine loading in men. *Journal of Applied Physiology* 81:232–37.

Ivy, J., et al. 2003. Effect of a carbohydrate-protein supplement on endurance performance during exercise of varying intensity. *International Journal of Sport Nutrition & Exercise Metabolism* 13:382–95.

Jacobson, B., et al. 2001. Nutrition practices and knowledge of college varsity athletes: A follow-up. *Journal of Strength & Conditioning Research* 15:63–68.

Jarvis, M., et al. 2002. The acute 1-week effects of the Zone diet on body composition, blood lipid levels, and performance in recreational endurance athletes. *Journal of Strength & Conditioning Research* 16:50–57.

Jenkins, D., et al. 2002. Effects of high- and low-isoflavone soy foods on blood lipids, oxidized LDL, homocysteine, and blood pressure in hyperlipidemic men and women. *American Journal of Clinical Nutrition* 76:365–72.

Johnson, C., et al. 2002. Postprandial thermogenesis is increased 100% on high-protein, low-fat diet versus a high-carbohydrate, low-fat diet in healthy, young women. *Journal of the American College of Nutrition* 21:55–61.

Jowko, E., et al. 2001. Creatine and beta-hydroxy-beta-methylbutyrate (HMB) additively increase lean body mass and muscle strength during a weight-training program. *Nutrition* 17: 558–66.

Karp, J., et al. 2006. Chocolate milk as a post-exercise recovery aid. *International Journal of Sport Nutrition & Exercise Metabolism* 16:78–91.

Kerksick, C., et al. 2006. The effects of protein and amino acid supplementation on performance and training adaptations during ten weeks of resistance training. *Journal of Strength & Conditioning Research* 20:643–53.

Kilduff, L., et al. 2004. The effects of creatine supplementation on cardiovascular, metabolic, and thermoregulatory responses during exercise in the heat in endurance-trained humans. *International Journal of Sport Nutrition & Exercise Metabolism* 14:443–60.

Kingsbury, K., et al. 1998. Contrasting plasma free amino acid patterns in elite athletes. *British Journal of Sports Medicine* 32:25–32.

Knitter, A., et al. 2000. Effects of beta-hydroxy-beta-methylbutyrate on muscle damage after a prolonged run. *Journal of Applied Physiology* 89:1340–44.

Koopman, E., et al. 2004. Combined ingestion of protein and carbohydrate improves protein balance during ultra-endurance exercise. *American Journal of Physiology-Endocrinology & Metabolism* 287: E712–20.

Koopman, R., et al. 2005. Combined ingestion of protein and free leucine with carbohydrate increases postexercise muscle protein synthesis in vivo in male subjects. *American Journal of Physiology. Endocrinology & Metabolism* 288:E645–53.

Kraemer, W., et al. 2006. The effects of amino acid supplementation on hormonal responses to resistance training overreaching. *Metabolism* 55:282–91.

Kreider, R., et al. 1999. Effects of calcium beta-hydroxy-beta-methylbutyrate (HMB) supplementation during resistance-training on markers of catabolism, body composition, and strength. *International Journal of Sports Medicine* 20:503–9.

Kuipers, H., et al. 2002. Effects of oral bovine colostrum supplementation on serum insulin-like growth factor-I levels. *Nutrition* 18:566–67.

Lambert, M., et al. 1993. Failure of commercial oral amino acid supplements to increase serum growth hormone concentrations in male bodybuilders. *International Journal of Sport Nutrition* 3:298–305.

Lamboley, C., et al. 2007. Effects of beta-hydroxy-beta-methylbutyrate on aerobic-performance components and body composition in college students. *International Journal of Sport Nutrition & Exercise Metabolism* 17:56–69.

Lansley, K., et al. 2011. Acute dietary nitrate supplementation improves cycling time trial performance. *Medicine & Science in Sports & Exercise* 43:1125–31.

Lemon, P., et al. 1992. Protein requirements and muscle mass/strength changes during intensive training in novice bodybuilders. *Journal of Applied Physiology* 73:767–75.

Levenhagen, D., et al. 2002. Postexercise protein intake enhances whole-body and leg protein accretion in humans. *Medicine & Science in Sports & Exercise* 34:828–37.

Levenhagen, D., et al. 2001. Postexercise nutrient intake timing in humans is critical to recovery of leg glucose and protein homeostasis. *American Journal of Physiology. Endocrinology & Metabolism* 280:E982–93.

Liappis, N., et al. 1979. Quantitative study of free amino acids in human eccrine sweat excreted from the forearms of healthy trained and untrained men during exercise. *European Journal of Applied Physiology* 42:227–34.

Lichtenstein, A., et al. 2002. Lipoprotein response to diets high in soy or animal protein with and without isoflavones in moderately hypercholesterolemic subjects. *Arteriosclerosis, Thrombosis, & Vascular Biology* 22:1852–58.

Lukaszuk, J., et al. 2002. Effect of creatine supplementation and a lactoovovegetarian diet on muscle creatine concentration. *International Journal of Sport Nutrition & Exercise Metabolism* 12:336–48.

Macdermid, P., and Stannard, S. 2006. A whey-supplemented, high-protein diet versus a high-carbohydrate diet: Effects on endurance cycling performance. *International Journal of Sport Nutrition & Exercise Metabolism* 16:65–77.

Madsen, K., et al. 1996. Effects of glucose, glucose plus branched-chain amino acids, or placebo on bike performance over 100 km. *Journal of Applied Physiology* 81:2644–50.

Maughan, R., and Sadler, D. 1983. The effects of oral administration of salts of aspartic acid on the metabolic response to prolonged exhausting exercise in man. *International Journal of Sports Medicine* 4:119–23.

Mayhew, D., et al. 2002. Effects of long-term creatine supplementation on liver and kidney functions in American college football players. *International Journal of Sport Nutrition and Exercise Metabolism* 12:453–60.

McConell, G., et al. 2006. L-arginine infusion increases glucose clearance during prolonged exercise in humans. *American Journal of Physiology. Endocrinology & Metabolism* 290:E60–E66.

McNaughton, L., et al. 1999. Inosine supplementation has no effect on aerobic or anaerobic cycling performance. *International Journal of Sport Nutrition* 9:333–44

Mendel, R., et al. 2005. Effects of creatine on thermoregulatory responses while exercising in the heat. *Nutrition* 21:301–307.

Metzl, J., et al. 2001. Creatine use among young athletes. *Pediatrics* 108:421–25.

Millard-Stafford, M., et al. 2005. Recovery from run training: Efficacy of a carbohydrate-protein beverage. *International Journal of Sport Nutrition & Exercise Metabolism* 15:610–24.

Mitchell, M., et al. 1993. Effects of supplementation with arginine and lysine on body composition, strength and growth hormone levels in weightlifters. *Medicine & Science in Sports & Exercise* 25:S25.

Mittleman, K., et al. 1998. Branched-chain amino acids prolong exercise during heat stress in men and women. *Medicine & Science in Sports & Exercise* 30:83–91.

Moore, D., et al. 2009. Ingested protein dose response of muscle and albumin protein synthesis after resistance exercise in young men. *American Journal of Clinical Nutrition* 89:161–68.

Mujika, I., et al. 2000. Creatine supplementation and sprint performance in soccer players. *Medicine & Science in Sports & Exercise* 32:518–25.

Newsholme, E., and Blomstrand, E. 1996. The plasma level of some amino acids and physical and mental fatigue. *Experientia* 52:413–15.

Nissen, S., et al. 1996. Effect of leucine metabolite β-hydroxy-β-methylbutyrate on muscle metabolism during resistance-exercise training. *Journal of Applied Physiology* 81:2095–2104.

Olsen, S., et al. 2006. Creatine supplementation augments the increase in satellite cell and myonuclei number in human skeletal muscle induced by strength training. *Journal of Physiology* 573:525–34.

Op 'T Eijnde, B., and Hespel, P. 2001. Short-term creatine supplementation does not alter the hormonal response to resistance training. *Medicine & Science in Sports & Exercise* 33:449–53.

Op 'T Eijnde, B., et al. 2001. Creatine loading does not impact on stroke performance in tennis. *International Journal of Sports Medicine* 22:76–80.

Ostojic, S. 2004. Creatine supplementation in young soccer players. *International Journal of Sport Nutrition & Exercise Metabolism* 14:95–103.

Ostojic, S., and Ahmetovic, Z. 2008. Gastrointestinal distress after creatine supplementation in athletes: Are side effects dose dependent? *Research in Sports Medicine* 16(1):15–22.

Ostojic, S., et al. 2007. Glucosamine administration in athletes: Effects on recovery of acute knee injury. *Research in Sports Medicine* 15:113–24.

Paddon-Jones, D., et al. 2001. Short-term beta-hydroxy-beta-methylbutyrate supplementation does not reduce symptoms of eccentric muscle damage. *International Journal of Sport Nutrition and Exercise Metabolism* 11:442–50.

Panton, L., et al. 2000. Nutritional supplementation of the leucine metabolite beta-hydroxy-beta-methylbutyrate (HMB) during resistance training. *Nutrition* 16:734–39.

Parry-Billings, M., et al. 1992. Plasma amino acid concentrations in the overtraining syndrome: Possible effects on the immune system. *Medicine & Science in Sports & Exercise* 24:1353–58.

Pavelka, K., et al. 2002. Glucosamine sulfate use and delay of progression of knee osteoarthritis: A 3-year, randomized, placebo-controlled, double-blind study. *Archives of Internal Medicine* 162:2113–23.

Peyrebrune, M., et al. 2005. Effect of creatine supplementation on training for competition in elite swimmers. *Medicine & Science in Sports & Exercise* 37:2140–47.

Poortmans, J., and Dellalieux, O. 2000. Do regular high protein diets have potential health risks on kidney function in athletes? *International Journal of Sport Nutrition & Exercise Metabolism* 10:28–38.

Poortmans, J., and Francaux, M. 1999. Long-term oral creatine supplementation does not impair renal function in healthy athletes. *Medicine & Science in Sports & Exercise* 31:1108–10.

Poortmans, J., et al. 2005. Effect of oral creatine supplementation on urinary methylamine, formaldehyde and formate. *Medicine & Science in Sports & Exercise* 37:1717–20.

Poortmans, J., et al. 1997. Evidence of differential renal dysfunctions during exercise in man. *European Journal of Applied Physiology* 76:88–91.

Preen, D., et al. 2003. Creatine supplementation: A comparison of loading and maintenance protocols on creatine uptake by human skeletal muscle. *International Journal of Sport Nutrition & Metabolism* 13:97–111.

Preen, D., et al. 2001. Effect of creatine loading on long-term sprint exercise performance and metabolism. *Medicine & Science in Sports & Exercise* 33:814–21.

Rockwell, J., et al. 2001. Creatine supplementation affects muscle creatine during energy restriction. *Medicine & Science in Sports & Exercise* 33:61–68.

Romano-Ely, B., et al. 2006. Effect of an isocaloric carbohydrate-protein-antioxidant drink on cycling performance. *Medicine & Science in Sports & Exercise* 38:1608–16.

Romer, L., et al. 2001. Effects of oral creatine supplementation on high intensity, intermittent exercise performance in competitive squash players. *International Journal of Sports Medicine* 22:546–52.

Rowlands, D., et al. 2007. Effect of protein-rich feeding on recovery after intense exercise. *International Journal of Sport Nutrition & Exercise Metabolism* 17:521–43.

Rutherford, J., et al. 2010. The effect of acute taurine ingestion on endurance performance and metabolism in well-trained cyclists. *International Journal of Sport Nutrition and Exercise Metabolism* 20:322–29.

Santos, R., et al. 2004. The effect of creatine supplementation upon inflammatory and muscle soreness markers after a 30 km race. *Life Sciences* 75:1917–24.

Schedel, J., et al. 2000. Acute creatine loading enhances human growth hormone secretion. *Journal of Sports Medicine & Physical Fitness* 40:336–42.

Schilling, B., et al. 2001. Creatine supplementation and health variables: A retrospective study. *Medicine & Science in Sports & Exercise* 33:183–88.

Schroeder, C., et al. 2001. The effects of creatine dietary supplementation on anterior compartment pressure in the lower leg during rest and following exercise. *Clinical Journal of Sport Medicine* 11:87–95.

Segura, R., and Ventura, J. 1988. Effect of L-tryptophan supplementation on exercise performance. *International Journal of Sports Medicine* 9:301–5.

Shing, C., et al. 2006. The influence of bovine colostrum supplementation on exercise performance in highly trained cyclists. *British Journal of Sports Medicine* 40:797–801.

Skare, O., et al. 2001. Creatine supplementation improves sprint performance in male sprinters. *Scandinavian Journal of Medicine & Science in Sports* 11:96–102.

Slater, G., et al. 2001. Beta-hydroxy-beta-methylbutyrate (HMB) supplementation does not affect changes in strength or body composition during resistive training in trained men. *International Journal of Sport Nutrition & Exercise Metabolism* 11:384–96.

Starling, R., et al. 1996. Effect of inosine supplementation on aerobic and anaerobic cycling performance. *Medicine & Science in Sports & Exercise* 28:1193–98.

Stensrund, T., et al. 1992. L-tryptophan supplementation does not improve running performance. *International Journal of Sports Medicine* 13:481–85.

Stout, J., et al. 2007. Effects of beta-alanine supplementation on the onset of neuromuscular fatigue and ventilator threshold in women. *Amino Acids* 32:381–86.

Stout, J., et al. 2006. Effects of twenty-eight days of beta-alanine and creatine monohydrate supplementation on the physical working capacity at neuromuscular fatigue threshold. *Journal of Strength & Conditioning Research* 20:928–31.

Struder, H. K., et al. 1998. Influence of paroxetine, branched-chain amino acids and tyrosine on neuroendocrine system responses and fatigue in humans. *Hormone & Metabolic Research* 30:188–94.

Suminski, R., et al. 1997. Acute effect of amino acid ingestion and resistance exercise on plasma growth hormone concentration in young men. *International Journal of Sport Nutrition* 7:48–60.

Sutton, E., et al. 2005. Ingestion of tyrosine: Effects on endurance, muscle strength, and anaerobic performance. *International Journal of Sport Nutrition & Exercise Metabolism* 15:173–85.

Syrotuik, D., and Bell, G. 2004. Acute creatine monohydrate supplementation: A descriptive physiological profile of responders vs. nonresponders. *Journal of Strength & Conditioning Research* 18:610–17.

Syrotuik, D., et al. 2001. Effects of creatine monohydrate supplementation during combined strength and high intensity rowing training on performance. *Canadian Journal of Applied Physiology* 26:527–42.

Tanaka, H., et al. 1997. Changes in plasma tryptophan/branched-chain amino acid ratio in responses to training volume variation. *International Journal of Sports Medicine* 18:270–5.

Tarnopolsky, M., et al. 2001. Creatine-dextrose and protein-dextrose induce similar strength gains during training. *Medicine & Science in Sports & Exercise* 33:2944–52.

Theodorou, A., et al. 2005. Effects of acute creatine loading with or without carbohydrate on repeated bouts of maximal swimming in high-performance swimmers. *Journal of Strength & Conditioning Research* 19:265–69.

Tipton, K., et al. 1999. Postexercise net protein synthesis in human muscle from orally administered amino acids. *American Journal of Physiology* 276:E628–E634.

Tuttle, J., et al. 1995. Effect of acute potassium-magnesium aspartate supplementation on ammonia concentrations during and after resistance training. *International Journal of Sport Nutrition* 5:102–9.

Tyler, T., et al. 2004. The effect of creatine supplementation on strength recovery after anterior cruciate ligament (ACL) reconstruction: A randomized, placebo-controlled, double-blind trial. *American Journal of Sports Medicine* 32:383–88.

Vandenberghe, K., et al. 1997. Inhibition of muscle phosphocreatine resynthesis by caffeine after creatine loading. *Medicine & Science in Sports & Exercise* 29:S249.

Vandenberghe, K., et al. 1996. Caffeine counteracts the ergogenic action of muscle creatine loading. *Journal of Applied Physiology* 80:452–57.

van Essen, M., and Gibala, M. 2006. Failure of protein to improve time trial performance when added to a sports drink. *Medicine & Science in Sports & Exercise* 38:1476–83.

van Hall, G., et al. 1998. Effect of carbohydrate supplementation on plasma glutamine during prolonged exercise and recovery. *International Journal of Sports Medicine* 19:82–86.

van Hall, G., et al. 1995. Ingestion of branched-chain amino acids and tryptophan during sustained exercise in man: Failure to affect performance. *Journal of Physiology* 486:789–94.

van Loon, L., et al. 2003. Effects of creatine loading and prolonged creatine supplementation on body composition, fuel selection, sprint and endurance performance in humans. *Clinical Science* 104:153–62.

van Someren, K., et al. 2005. Supplementation with beta-hydroxy-beta-methylbutyrate (HMB) and alpha-ketoisocaproic acid (KIC) reduces signs and symptoms of exercise-induced muscle damage in men. *International Journal of Sport Nutrition & Exercise Metabolism* 15:413–24.

Van Thienen, R., et al. 2009. β-alanine improves sprint cycling performance in endurance cycling. *Medicine & Science in Sports & Exercise* 41:898–903.

Vanhatalo, A., et al. 2010. Acute and chronic effects of dietary nitrate supplementation on blood pressure and the physiological responses to moderate-intensity and incremental exercise. *American Journal of Physiology & Regulatory, Integrative & Comparative Physiology* 299:R1121–31.

Vlad, S., et al. 2007. Glucosamine for pain in osteoarthritis: Why do trial results differ? *Arthritis & Rheumatism* 56:2267–77.

Volek, J., et al. 2004. The effects of creatine supplementation on muscular performance and body composition responses to short-term resistance training overreaching. *European Journal of Applied Physiology* 91:628–37.

Volek, J., et al. 2001. Physiological responses to short-term exercise in the heat after creatine loading. *Medicine & Science in Sports & Exercise* 33:1101–8.

Vukovich, M., et al. 2001. Body composition in 70-year-old adults responds to dietary beta-hydroxy-beta-methylbutyrate similarly to that of young adults. *Journal of Nutrition* 131:2049–52.

Watson, P., et al. 2004. The effect of acute branched-chain amino acid supplementation on prolonged exercise capacity in a warm environment. *European Journal of Applied Physiology* 93:306–14.

Weideman, C., et al. 1990. Effects of increased protein intake on muscle hypertrophy and strength following 13 weeks of resistance training. *Medicine & Science in Sports & Exercise* 22:S37.

Wesson, M., et al. 1988. Effects of oral administration of aspartic acid salts on the endurance capacity of trained athletes. *Research Quarterly for Exercise and Sport* 59:234–39.

Wiles, J., et al. 1991. Effect of pre-exercise protein ingestion upon VO_2, R, and perceived exertion during treadmill running. *British Journal of Sports Medicine* 25:26–30.

Williams, M., et al. 1990. Effect of oral inosine supplementation on 3-mile treadmill run performance and VO_2 peak. *Medicine & Science in Sports & Exercise* 22:517–22.

Willoughby, D., and Rosene, J. 2001. Effects of oral creatine and resistance training on myosin heavy chain expression. *Medicine & Science in Sports & Exercise* 33:1674–81.

Wilson, A., et al. 2007. L-arginine supplementation in peripheral arterial disease: No benefit and possible harm. *Circulation* 116:188–95.

Yaguchi, H., et al. 1998. The effect of triathlon on urinary excretion of enzymes and proteins. *International Urology & Nephrology* 30:107–12.

Yquel, R., et al. 2002. Effect of creatine supplementation on phosphocreatine resynthesis, inorganic phosphate accumulation and pH during intermittent maximal exercise. *Journal of Sports Sciences* 20:427–37.

Zhang, M., et al. 2004. Role of taurine supplementation to prevent exercise-induced oxidative stress in healthy young men. *Amino Acids* 26:203–07.

Zoeller, R., et al. 2007. Effects of 28 days of beta-alanine and creatine monohydrate supplementation on aerobic power, ventilatory and lactate thresholds, and time to exhaustion. *Amino Acids* 33:505–10.

Vitamins: The Organic Regulators

CHAPTER SEVEN

LEARNING OBJECTIVES

After studying this chapter, you should be able to:

1. Describe the various means whereby vitamins may carry out their functions in the human body.

2. Name the essential vitamins, state the RDA or AI for each, and identify several foods rich in each vitamin.

3. Describe the metabolic roles in the human body of each of the 13 essential vitamins and choline.

4. Explain the potential effects on health and sport performance associated with a deficiency of each essential vitamin and choline.

5. Identify those fat-soluble and water-soluble vitamins that are most likely to cause health risks if consumed in excess. Indicate at what doses adverse health effects may be observed, and determine how likely it is that such a dose may be obtained by consuming daily vitamin supplements and fortified foods.

6. Explain the theory as to how supplementation with each vitamin, and choline, may enhance sport performance, and highlight the research findings regarding the ergogenic efficacy of each.

7. Explain the theory as to how vitamin-like compounds may enhance sport performance, and highlight the research findings regarding the ergogenic efficacy of each.

8. Understand why health professionals recommend that we obtain our vitamins through natural foods, such as fruits and vegetables, and why some health professionals recommend that most adults also take a daily multivitamin supplement.

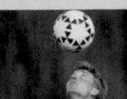

Vitamins are a diverse class of 13 known specific nutrients that are involved in almost every metabolic process in the human body. We need only minute amounts of vitamins in our daily diet, so they are classified as micronutrients. Nevertheless, they are one of our most critical nutrients. Noticeable symptoms of a deficiency may appear in 2 to 4 weeks for several of the vitamins, and major debilitating diseases may occur with prolonged deficiencies. Vitamin deficiencies appear to be widespread in many developing countries, and according to Bouis, they affect a greater number of people in the world than does protein-energy malnutrition. Hopefully, plant breeding of commonly eaten food crops, such as wheat, rice, and corn, to fortify them with vitamins and minerals may help alleviate this major health problem.

Major vitamin deficiencies are rare in industrialized societies because a wide variety of food products are available, many of them fortified with vitamins. Most health professionals recommend that we obtain the vitamins we need from the foods we eat, which is sound advice. However, some also note that certain segments of the population may not be obtaining adequate amounts of vitamins from food alone. For example, Sebastian and others note that many older adults are at risk for vitamin deficiency. Moreover, the American Institute of Cancer Research (AICR) noted that although vitamin supplements are not recommended to prevent cancer, certain groups may benefit from specific vitamin supplementation, including the elderly, women of childbearing age, and individuals not exposed to sufficient sunlight. Fairfield and Fletcher, in two studies published by the American Medical Association, go a step further and indicate that it may be *prudent* for *all adults* to take vitamin supplements.

In general, most studies reveal that athletes are obtaining adequate vitamin nutrition, probably because of the additional food energy intake associated with the increased energy expenditure of exercise. Additionally, many athletes take vitamin supplements. For example, Jacobson and others reported that vitamin/mineral pills were the most commonly used dietary supplement by female NCAA Division I collegiate athletes. However, like members of the general population, many athletes may not be obtaining optimal levels of vitamins from the diet. Moreover, certain athletic groups, particularly those who are on weight-reduction programs to qualify for competition or to enhance performance, may not receive adequate vitamin nutrition. Furthermore, individual athletes in generally well-nourished athletic groups may have a suboptimal vitamin intake.

As noted throughout this chapter, adequate vitamin nutrition is essential for both optimal health and athletic performance. But, if you do not obtain the RDA for a specific vitamin or vitamins, will your health or physical performance suffer? Will vitamin supplements above and beyond the RDA improve your health or performance? A major purpose of this chapter is to provide you with factual data, based upon the available research, to help answer these two very general questions.

A slightly different approach is used in this chapter and in chapter 8. The first section provides some basic facts about the general role of vitamins in the human body. The next two sections cover the fat-soluble and water-soluble vitamins, respectively, with each individual vitamin discussed in terms of its Dietary Reference Intake (DRI), either its Recommended Dietary Allowance (RDA) or Adequate Intake (AI); food sources that provide ample amounts; metabolic functions in the body with particular reference to health and the physically active individual; and the findings of research relative to the impact of deficiencies and supplementation. The fourth section focuses on ergogenic aspects of special vitamin or vitamin-like preparations, while the final section highlights some health implications of vitamin supplementation and provides some guidelines for selecting a multivitamin/mineral for those who choose to supplement.

Basic Facts

What are vitamins and how do they work?

Vitamins are a class of complex organic compounds that are found in small amounts in most foods. They are essential for the optimal functioning of many different physiological processes in the human body. The activity levels of many of these physiological processes are increased greatly during exercise, and an adequate bodily supply of vitamins must be present for these processes to function best.

Coenzyme Functions For the fundamental physiological processes of the body to proceed in an orderly, controlled fashion, a number of complex chemicals known as **enzymes** are necessary to regulate the diverse reactions involved. Hundreds of enzymes have been identified in the human body. Enzymes are necessary to digest our foods, to make our muscles contract, to release the energy stores in our bodies, to help us transport body gases such as carbon dioxide, to help us grow, to help clot our blood, and so on. Enzymes serve as catalysts; that is, they are capable of inducing changes in other substances without changing themselves.

Enzymes are chemicals that generally consist of two parts. One part is a protein molecule and to it is attached the second part, a **coenzyme.** For the enzyme to function properly, both parts must be present. The coenzyme often contains a vitamin or some related compound (figure 7.1). The enzyme is not used up in the chemical process that it initiates or in which it participates, but enzymes may deteriorate with time. Coenzymes also may be degraded through body metabolism. It is now known that the B complex vitamins are essential in human nutrition because of their role in the activation of enzymes, and thus a fresh supply of these water-soluble vitamins is constantly needed.

Antioxidant Functions Various oxidative reactions in the body produce substances called free radicals. **Free radicals** are chemical substances that contain a lone, unpaired electron in the outer orbit. The superoxide radical ($O_2^{\cdot-}$) and hydroxyl radical ($OH^{\cdot}$) are true free radicals. Two other related substances, referred to as non-radical oxygen species, are hydrogen peroxide (H_2O_2) and singlet oxygen ($^1O_2$). These substances are known as reactive

oxygen species (ROS), and when nitrogen is involved are known as reactive oxygen/nitrogen species (RONS). The interested reader is referred to the review by Neiss for a detailed discussion. For the purpose of our discussion, we shall refer to them collectively as free radicals.

Free radicals are unstable compounds that possess an unbalanced magnetic field that affects molecular structure and chemical reactions in the body. Free radicals may be very reactive with body tissues.

Linnane notes that formation of free radicals, such as superoxide anion and hydrogen peroxide formation during oxidative processes, are essential to normal cellular function, such as gene expression and muscle contractile force. However, although oxidative processes are essential to life, some oxidations may cause cellular damage by oxidation of unsaturated fats in cellular and subcellular membranes. Free radicals may cause such undesirable oxidations. Halliwell indicated that free radicals may damage DNA, lipids, proteins, and other molecules, and may be involved in the development of cancer, cardiovascular disease, and possibly neurodegenerative disease. Fortunately, although free radicals are formed naturally in the body, body cells produce a number of antioxidant enzymes, such as superoxide dismutase, glutathione peroxidase, and catalase, to help neutralize free radicals and prevent cellular damage. To function properly, these enzymes, often referred to as free radical-scavenging enzymes, must contain certain nutrients such as copper, zinc, and selenium. Comparable to these enzymes, as depicted in figure 7.2, vitamins E, C, and beta-carotene possess antioxidant properties. These antioxidant vitamins have received much research attention relative to effects on

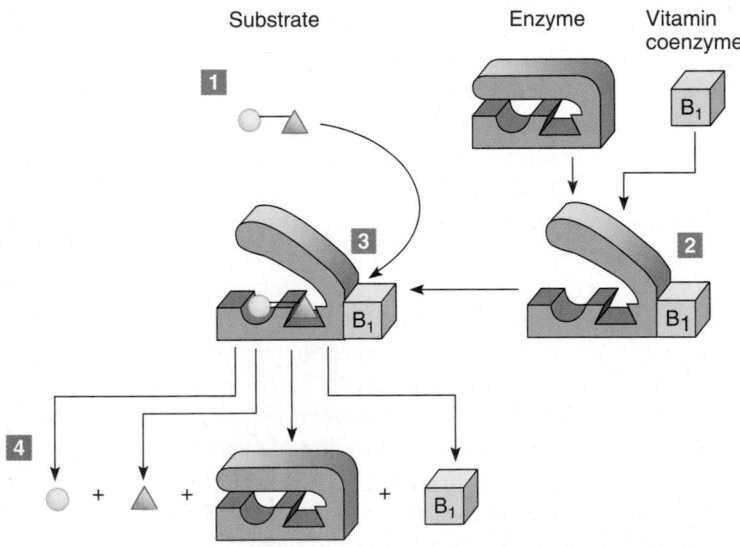

FIGURE 7.1 Role of vitamin as coenzyme. (1) Substrates, such as pyruvate, need enzymes to be converted into more usable compounds. However, many enzymes must be activated before a reaction occurs. Note that the enzyme is in a closed position. (2) An enzyme and a vitamin coenzyme (B_1) combine to form an activated complex, in essence opening up the enzyme. (3) The open, activated enzyme accepts the substrate and (4) splits it into two compounds while releasing the enzyme and coenzyme.

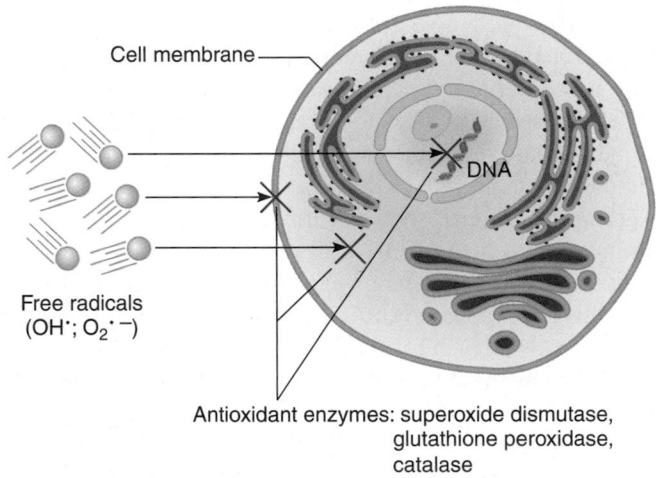

FIGURE 7.2 The antioxidant role of vitamins. To protect against the destructive nature of free radicals, such as hydroxyl radicals and superoxides, the cells contain a number of different enzymes (superoxide dismutase, glutathione peroxidase, catalase) to help neutralize them, thus helping to prevent disintegration of cell membranes or the genetic material within the cell. Additionally, several vitamins (E, C, beta-carotene) may serve as antioxidants. Such vitamins are theorized to be protective against cancer, heart disease, and adverse effects of aging.

health and physical performance and are discussed at appropriate points later in this chapter.

Hormone Functions Although vitamin D exists in vitamin form, it undergoes several conversions in the body and, in its active form, functions as a hormone. After being produced in the kidney, vitamin D circulates in the blood like other hormones and exerts its functions on various tissues to promote bone metabolism. Other vitamins, such as A and K, may be produced in the liver and intestines, respectively, and exert functions in other parts of the body. Although it is normally not referred to as a hormone, Reichrath and others indicated that vitamin A may serve a hormonal function relative to skin health. Some vitamins may be critical in the formation of various hormones—such as the role vitamin C plays in the formation of epinephrine—but are not classified as hormones. Only vitamin D is assigned hormonal status in its active form.

Energy Although vitamins are indispensable for regulating many body functions and for the maintenance of optimal health, they are not a source of energy. They do not have any caloric value. Moreover, they make no significant contribution to the structure of the body, as do protein and some minerals.

What vitamins are essential to human nutrition?

The existence of vitamins was deduced from their physiological actions before their chemical structures had been identified. In assigning names to vitamins, the alphabet was used in order of their time of discovery. In some cases, a large time gap existed between the discovery of the vitamin and determination of its chemical structure. In others, the chemical nature was discovered rapidly, and the chemical name came into early use.

An *essential vitamin* is one that cannot be synthesized in the body in sufficient quantity, causes deficiency symptoms when dietary intake is inadequate, and alleviates deficiency symptoms when added back to the diet. At present the human body is known to need an adequate supply of 13 different vitamins. Choline is a water-soluble essential nutrient, and although it is listed with the DRI alongside the B vitamins, at this time it has not been classified as a vitamin. A well-balanced diet will satisfy all the vitamin requirements of most individuals. Four of these vitamins are soluble in fat and are obtained primarily from the fat in our diet, while the other nine water-soluble vitamins are distributed rather widely in a variety of foods. Although most vitamins must be obtained from the food we eat, several of them may be formed in the body from other ingested nutrients, by the action of ultraviolet rays from sunlight on our skin, or by the activity of some intestinal bacteria.

A number of other substances have been mistakenly classified as vitamins. Included in this group are inositol, para-amino benzoic acid (PABA), vitamin B_{15} or pangamic acid, and vitamin B_{17} or laetrile. Although it has been suggested that these substances have vitamin activity, their essentiality in the diet has not been established. Other substances have been attributed vitamin-like activity and professed to enhance health or physical performance,

such as bee pollen, coenzyme Q_{10} (CoQ_{10}), and ginkgo, but these also are not essential vitamins.

Table 7.1 presents an overview of the 13 essential vitamins and choline with commonly used interchangeable synonyms, major food sources, major functions in the body, and symptoms associated with deficiencies or excessive consumption. The table also presents the RDA or AI for adults aged 19–50, as well as the Daily Value (DV). Note that the DV, which is based on older daily dietary recommendations, may vary considerably with current RDA or AI. The DV was originally set high enough to cover just about anyone but has not been updated to match current recommendations. RDA and AI values for other age groups may be found in DRI tables on the inside front cover, and the UL may be found on the inside back cover. The health and physical performance effects of the essential vitamins and selected vitamin-like substances are covered in the following sections.

Only very small amounts of vitamins are required daily. RDA or AI are usually given in milligrams (mg) or micrograms (mcg). Several vitamins come in various forms and thus the RDA may be given as activity equivalents. For example, vitamin A comes preformed as retinol, or may be derived from the conversion of beta-carotene. Thus, vitamin A requirements are technically known as retinol activity equivalents (RAE). The International Unit (IU) is an older measure of vitamin activity that may still be seen on food labels and vitamin supplements. However, it is gradually being replaced with more appropriate terminology. Because IU is still commonly used, we will include it in our discussion where relevant.

In general, how do deficiencies or excesses of vitamins influence health or physical performance?

Whether or not a vitamin deficiency affects one's health or physical performance may depend on the magnitude of the deficiency. Four stages of vitamin deficiency associated with the duration of undernourishment and inadequate vitamin intake have been described. These same four stages may apply to mineral deficiency diseases discussed in the next chapter.

1. *A preliminary stage* is associated with inadequate amount or availability of the vitamin in the diet. For example, a drastic change in the diet may influence vitamin **bioavailability** (the amount of a nutrient that the body absorbs), whereas pregnancy may increase the need for several vitamins.
2. *Biochemical deficiency.* In this stage, the body's pool of the vitamin is decreased. For a number of vitamins, biochemical deficiency can be identified by blood or tissue tests. For example, deficiencies of riboflavin may be detected by the activity of an enzyme in the red blood cells.
3. *Physiologic deficiency* is associated with the appearance of unspecific symptoms such as loss of appetite, weakness, or physical fatigue.

    These first three stages are known as latent or marginal vitamin deficiency, or **subclinical malnutrition.** Whether or not these stages impair physical performance may depend

TABLE 7.1   Essential vitamins*

Vitamin name (other terms)	RDA or AI for adults age 19–50*; Daily Value (DV)	Major sources
Fat-soluble vitamins		
Vitamin A (retinol: provitamin carotenoids)	RDA: 900 RAE ♂ 700 RAE ♀ (RAE = retinol activity equivalents) DV = 5,000 IU	Retinol in animal foods: liver, whole milk, fortified milk, cheese. Carotenoids in plant foods: carrots, green leafy vegetables, sweet potatoes, fortified margarine from vegetable oils
Vitamin D (cholecalciferol)	RDA: 600 IU or 15 mcg DV = 400 IU	Vitamin-D fortified foods like dairy products and margarine, fish oils; action of sunlight on the skin
Vitamin E (tocopherol)	RDA: 15 mg d-alpha Tocopherol DV = 30 IU	Vegetable oils, margarine, green leafy vegetables, wheat germ, vegetable oils, whole-grain products, egg yolks
Vitamin K (phylloquinone; menoquinone)	RDA: 120 mcg ♂ 90 mcg ♀ DV = 80 mcg	Pork and beef liver, eggs, spinach, cauliflower; formation in the human intestine by bacteria
Water-soluble vitamins		
Thiamin (vitamin B_1)	RDA: 1.2 mg ♂ 1.1 mg ♀ DV = 1.5 mg	Ham, pork, lean meat, liver, whole-grain products, enriched breads and cereals, legumes
Riboflavin (vitamin B_2)	RDA: 1.3 mg ♂ 1.1 mg ♀ DV = 1.7 mg	Milk and dairy products, meat, eggs, enriched grain products, green leafy vegetables, beans
Niacin (nicotinamide, nicotinic acid)	RDA: 16 mg ♂ 14 mg ♀ DV = 20 mg	Lean meats, fish, poultry, whole-grain products, beans; may be formed in the body from tryptophan, an essential amino acid
Vitamin B_6 (pyridoxal, pyridoxine, pyridoxamine)	RDA: 1.3 mg DV = 2 mg	Protein foods: liver, lean meats, fish, poultry, legumes; green leafy vegetables, baked potatoes, bananas
Vitamin B_{12} (cobalamin; cyanocobalamin)	RDA: 2.4 mcg DV = 6 mcg	Animal foods only: meat, fish, poultry, milk, eggs
Folate (folic acid)	RDA: 400 DFE (DFE = dietary folate equivalents) DV = 400 DFE	Liver, green leafy vegetables, legumes, nuts, fortified cereals
Biotin	AI: 30 mcg DV = 300 mg	Meats, legumes, milk, egg yolk, whole-grain products, most vegetables
Pantothenic acid	AI: 5 mg DV = 300 mg	Beef and pork liver, lean meats, milk, eggs, legumes, whole-grain products, most vegetables
Choline**	AI: 550 mg ♂ 425 mg ♀ DV = None	Milk, liver, eggs, peanuts; found in most foods as part of cell membranes
Vitamin C (ascorbic acid)	RDA: 90 mg ♂ 75 mg ♀ DV = 60 mg	Citrus fruits, green leafy vegetables, broccoli, peppers, strawberries, potatoes

Major functions in the body	Deficiency symptoms	Symptoms of excessive consumption*
Fat-soluble vitamins		
Maintains epithelial tissue in skin and mucous membranes; forms visual purple for night vision; promotes bone development	Night blindness, intestinal infections, impaired growth, xerophthalmia	UL is 3 milligrams/day. Nausea, headache, fatigue, liver and spleen damage, skin peeling, pain in the joints
Acts as a hormone to increase intestinal absorption of calcium and promote bone and tooth formation	Rare; rickets in children and osteomalacia in adults	UL is 4,000 IU, or 100 micrograms/day. Loss of appetite, nausea, irritability, joint pain, calcium deposits in soft tissues such as the kidney
Functions as an antioxidant to protect cell membranes from destruction by oxidation	Extremely rare; disruption of red blood cell membranes; anemia	UL is 1,000 milligrams/day. General lack of toxicity with doses up to 400 mg. Some reports of headache, fatigue, or diarrhea with megadoses
Essential for blood coagulation processes	Increased bleeding and hemorrhage	No UL set. Possible clot formation (thrombosis), vomiting
Water-soluble vitamins		
Serves as a coenzyme for energy production from carbohydrate; essential for normal functioning of the central nervous system	Poor appetite, apathy, mental depression, pain in calf muscles, beriberi	No UL set. General lack of toxicity
Functions as a coenzyme involved in energy production from carbohydrates and fats; maintenance of healthy skin	Dermatitis, cracks at the corners of the mouth, sores on the tongue, damage to the cornea	No UL set. General lack of toxicity
Functions as a coenzyme for the aerobic and anaerobic production of energy from carbohydrate; helps synthesize fat and blocks release of FFA; needed for healthy skin	Loss of appetite, weakness, skin lesions, gastrointestinal problems, pellagra	UL is 35 milligrams/day. Nicotinic acid causes headache, nausea, burning and itching skin, flushing of face, liver damage
Functions as a coenzyme in protein metabolism; necessary for formation of hemoglobin and red blood cells; needed for glycogenolysis and gluconeogenesis	Nervous irritability, convulsions, dermatitis, sores on tongue, anemia	UL is 100 milligrams/day. Loss of nerve sensation, impaired gait
Functions as a coenzyme for formation of DNA, RBC development, and maintenance of nerve tissue	Pernicious anemia, nerve damage resulting in paralysis	No UL set. General lack of toxicity
Functions as coenzyme for DNA formation and RBC development	Fatigue, gastrointestinal disorders, diarrhea, anemia, neural tube defects in newborns	UL is 1,000 micrograms/day. May prevent detection of pernicious anemia caused by B_{12} deficiency
Functions as coenzyme in the metabolism of carbohydrates, fats, and protein	Rare; may be caused by excessive intake of raw egg whites: fatigue, nausea, skin rashes	No UL set. General lack of toxicity
Functions as part of coenzyme A in energy metabolism	Rare; produced only clinically: fatigue, nausea, loss of appetite, mental depression	No UL set. General lack of toxicity
Functions as a precursor for lecithin, a phospholipid in cell membranes	Rare; liver damage	UL is 3.5 grams/day. May lead to fishy body odor, gastrointestinal distress, vomiting, low blood pressure
Forms collagen essential for connective tissue development; aids in absorption of iron; helps form epinephrine; serves as antioxidant	Weakness, rough skin, slow wound healing, bleeding gums, anemia, scurvy	UL is 2,000 milligrams/day. Diarrhea, possible kidney stones, rebound scurvy

*RDA, AI, and UL values for all age groups may be found on the inside of the front and back covers of this text.
**Not classified as a vitamin.

upon the nature of the sport, but weakness or physical fatigue would certainly be counterproductive to optimal performance.

4. *Clinically manifest vitamin deficiency.* In this final stage, specific clinical symptoms are observed. For example, anemia is a clinical symptom associated with a deficiency of several vitamins, such as folic acid, vitamin B$_6$, and B$_{12}$. Both health and performance would be adversely affected with a clinically manifest vitamin deficiency.

In the past, RDA for vitamins have been established to prevent vitamin-deficiency diseases. However, recommendations are beginning to incorporate the role of vitamins in health promotion. For example, as noted later, the new Adequate Intake (AI) for vitamin D has been modified to help prevent osteoporosis, while the folic acid RDA is designed to prevent damage to the nervous system of the unborn child during pregnancy. When scientific evidence is deemed sufficient, vitamin recommendations may be modified to help prevent chronic diseases. If the RDA for some vitamins are increased as a possible means of achieving health promotion objectives, the most likely recommendation will be to obtain the increased amounts from natural foods. However, food fortification or supplementation may be recommended for a few vitamins, such as folic acid.

In general, it is very difficult to obtain excessive amounts of vitamins through the diet to the point that health or physical performance is impaired. Even when supplements are taken, the body may excrete several vitamins, keeping body functions normal. However, overconsumption of some vitamins may induce **hypervitaminosis,** a condition in which a vitamin may function comparable to a drug, not a nutrient, and induce toxic reactions. An excessive intake of vitamin supplements may be a common cause of hypervitaminosis, but some dietary practices may also lead to excessive vitamin intake. As shall be noted later in this chapter, consuming a vitamin supplement and vitamin-fortified foods, such as cereals, on a regular basis could induce vitamin functions that are hypothesized to increase health risks. A Tolerable Upper Intake Level (UL) has been established for seven of the thirteen essential vitamins.

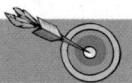

Key Concepts

▶ Vitamins are complex organic compounds that function in the body in a variety of ways. Some act as coenzymes to help regulate metabolic processes; others are antioxidants that protect cell membranes; and one is even classified as a hormone. Vitamins do not contain energy *per se,* such as Calories, but they do help regulate energy processes in the body.

▶ The RDA for vitamins have been established to prevent vitamin-deficiency diseases like scurvy, but the new DRI may be modified to help prevent chronic diseases, such as osteoporosis, or excessive intake and associated adverse health effects.

▶ There may be four stages in a vitamin deficiency: the preliminary stage, the biochemical deficiency stage, the physiologic deficiency stage, and the clinically manifest deficiency stage.

Fat-Soluble Vitamins

The four fat-soluble vitamins are A, D, E, and K. Because they are soluble in fat but not in water, dietary sources include foods that have some fat content. The body may contain appreciable stores of each fat-soluble vitamin, and several of them may be manufactured by the body, so deficiencies are relatively rare in industrialized societies. On the other hand, excessive intake may be toxic. With the exception of vitamin E, very little research has been conducted relative to deficiency or supplementation effects upon physical performance.

Vitamin A (retinol)

Vitamin A is a fat-soluble, unsaturated alcohol. The physiologically active form of vitamin A is known as **retinol.** The human body is capable of forming retinol from provitamins known as carotenoids, primarily **beta-carotene.** Both preformed vitamin A, or retinol, and carotenoids are found in the foods we eat.

DRI The RDA for vitamin A may be obtained by consuming preformed retinol, beta-carotene and other carotenoids, or a combination of the two. The RDA may be expressed in several ways, usually as **retinol equivalents (RE), retinol activity equivalents (RAE)** as a combination of retinol and carotenoids, or as international units. In brief, 1 RAE equals 1 microgram of retinol, or 12 micrograms of beta-carotene, or about 3.3 IU. The RDA is 900 RAE, or 3,000 IU for adult males and 700 RAE, or 2,300 IU for adult females. See the DRI table on the inside cover for more details on vitamin A requirements derived from either retinol or the carotenoids. The Daily Value (DV) for use on food labels is 5,000 IU, but should be set at 3,000. The UL for adults is 3 milligrams RAE/day from retinol, or 10,000 IU; no UL has been established for carotenoids. See the UL table on the inside of the back cover for more details.

Food Sources Preformed vitamin A is found in substantial amounts in some animal foods such as liver, butter, cheese, egg yolks, fish liver oils, and fortified milk. Provitamin A, as beta-carotene, is found in dark-green leafy and yellow-orange vegetables, as well as in some fruits such as oranges, limes, pineapples, prunes, and cantaloupes. Fortified margarine also contains beta-carotene. One glass of milk provides about 15 percent of the RDA, while one medium carrot will supply nearly 200 percent and a serving of liver a whopping 1,000 percent or more of the RDA.

Major Functions Vitamin A is essential for maintenance of the epithelial cells, those cells covering the outside of the body and lining the body cavities. It is also essential for proper visual function, such as night vision and peripheral vision. Vitamin A also has a variety of other physiological roles in the body that are not well understood, although it is considered essential in proper bone development and for maintaining optimal function of the immune system. Vitamin A and beta-carotene may function as antioxidants and have been theorized by some scientists to confer some health benefits.

Deficiency: Health and Physical Performance Vitamin A is stored in the body in relatively large amounts. However, an inadequate intake of vitamin A could have serious health implications if prolonged. The gradual loss of night vision is one of the first symptoms of vitamin A deficiency. Other symptoms of mild deficiencies include increased susceptibility to infection and skin lesions. Epidemiological research also has suggested that a deficient intake of beta-carotene could predispose the individual to the development of cancer in the epithelial tissues such as the skin, lungs, breasts, and intestinal lining. Although severe deficiencies are not common in industrialized nations, they do occur in some parts of the world and lead to blindness through destruction of the cornea of the eye, a condition known as **xerophthalmia.** Vitamin A deficiency has been associated with higher mortality rates in children of developing countries, with several million childhood deaths annually. Some, but not all, studies have shown that vitamin A supplementation to such children may decrease the death rate, possibly by strengthening the immune system.

Theoretically, vitamin A deficiency could affect physical performance. Some investigators have suggested that a deficiency may impair the process of gluconeogenesis in the liver, which may be an important consideration for the endurance athlete in the latter stages of competition. Others have implied a reduction in the synthesis of muscle protein and impaired vision, which could negatively affect strength athletes or those involved in sports requiring eye alertness. Very little research is available to support these theoretical views.

Supplementation: Health and Physical Performance Vitamin A in supplements can come from retinol (vitamin A palmitate or acetate) or beta-carotene, or both. Check the label; it may or may not list the separate components. The UL for adults is set at 3,000 RAE, or 10,000 IU. The UL applies only to preformed vitamin A, or retinol, not to carotenoids. In general, supplements of vitamin A as retinol are not recommended unless under the guidance of a health professional. Excessive amounts of vitamin A, generally caused by self-medication with megadoses, can cause a condition known as hypervitaminosis A. Symptoms may include weakness, headache, loss of appetite, nausea, pain in the joints, and peeling of skin. Similar symptoms were reported in a young soccer player who took about 100,000 IU daily for 2 months in an attempt to improve performance. The symptoms were relieved when he stopped taking the supplements.

Excess vitamin A may also weaken the bones. Binkley and Krueger reported that excess vitamin A stimulates bone resorption and inhibits bone formation, leading to bone loss and contributing to osteoporosis. Feskanich and others found that women with the highest intake of vitamin A as retinol, greater than 3,000 micrograms daily, had double the risk of hip fractures compared to women with the lowest intake, less than 1,250 micrograms per day.

As noted by Ross, excessive vitamin A during pregnancy may be teratogenic, causing deformities in the developing embryo or fetus. Research by Rothman and others has indicated that vitamin A doses as low as four times the RDA can markedly increase a pregnant woman's chances of having a baby with birth defects, such as a cleft palate, heart defects, or other problems. Although this amount would not be consumed with a normal diet, it could be obtained by someone who takes a daily supplement, drinks substantial amounts of milk, eats liver, and has several servings of fortified cereals. Additionally, Zachman and Grummer indicated that consuming alcohol during pregnancy may worsen these teratogenic effects of vitamin A. Finally, extremely large doses of vitamin A may lead to severe liver damage, especially with concomitant alcohol intake, and may be fatal.

Beta-carotene supplements are not believed to be toxic but may cause harmless yellowing of the skin when taken in excess because the beta-carotene may accumulate in the fat tissues. The supplements may also cause adverse health effects in some individuals, particularly smokers, discussed later in this chapter.

There appears to be little theoretical value in using vitamin A supplementation for ergogenic purposes, and no scientific evidence supports its use as a means to enhance physical performance. However, beta-carotene has been combined with other antioxidants in an attempt to prevent muscle damage during exercise, and this research is discussed later.

Prudent Recommendations In summary, vitamin A supplementation to the diet of the active individual does not have a sound theoretical basis. Moreover, the research conducted with vitamin A and physical performance has shown no beneficial effect. Hence, there appears to be no advantage for the active individual to supplement the diet with vitamin A, particularly not with megadoses that may have undesirable effects. The advisability of beta-carotene supplementation for its antioxidant properties is discussed in the later sections of this chapter dealing with ergogenic and health issues. As shall be noted, individuals should not consume high doses of beta-carotene.

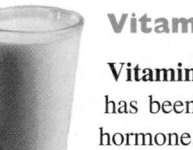

Vitamin D (cholecalciferol)

Vitamin D, a term representing a number of compounds, has been classified as both a fat-soluble vitamin and as a hormone. The physiologically active form is calcitriol, which is the hormone of this vitamin. In brief, the ultraviolet rays from sunshine initiate a process that eventually converts a provitamin found in the skin (7-dehydrocholesterol) into **cholecalciferol (vitamin D$_3$),** a prohormone, which is released into the blood and is eventually converted by the liver and kidneys into the active hormone, calcitriol (1,25-dihydroxycholecalciferol). Figure 7.3 illustrates the formation of vitamin D from sunlight.

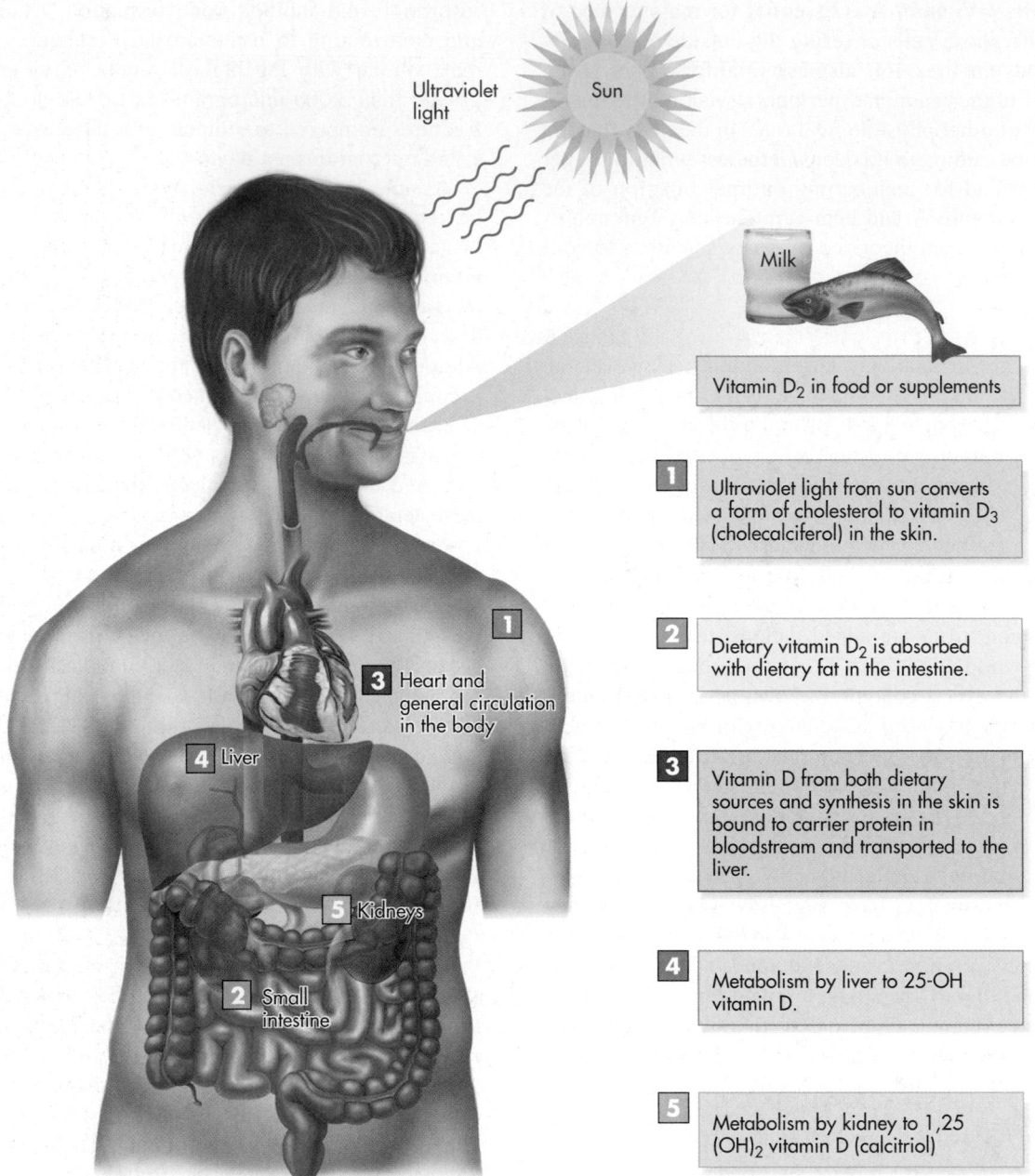

Ultraviolet light

Sun

Milk

Vitamin D₂ in food or supplements

1 Ultraviolet light from sun converts a form of cholesterol to vitamin D₃ (cholecalciferol) in the skin.

2 Dietary vitamin D₂ is absorbed with dietary fat in the intestine.

3 Vitamin D from both dietary sources and synthesis in the skin is bound to carrier protein in bloodstream and transported to the liver.

4 Metabolism by liver to 25-OH vitamin D.

5 Metabolism by kidney to 1,25 (OH)₂ vitamin D (calcitriol)

3 Heart and general circulation in the body

4 Liver

5 Kidneys

2 Small intestine

1

FIGURE 7.3 The many facets of vitamin D metabolism. Whether synthesized in the skin or obtained from dietary sources, vitamin D ultimately functions as a hormone: calcitriol.

Dietary supplements contain vitamin D_2 (ergocalciferol) and vitamin D_3. For those who take vitamin D supplements, health professionals recommend vitamin D_3 because it is more effective in raising the serum marker (25-hydroxyvitamin D) of vitamin D status. Check supplement labels for "Vitamin D as cholecalciferol" or the ingredients list for vitamin D_3 or cholecalciferol.

DRI The RDA for vitamin D is given in micrograms of cholecalciferol or as IU; one microgram of cholecalciferol is the equivalent of 40 IU. Even though sunlight is a major source of vitamin D

for some people, the RDA is based on minimal exposure to sunlight. For infants zero to twelve months old, the AI is 10 mcg (400 IU); for ages 1 to 70 years, the RDA is 15 mcg (600 IU); and for 70 years and older, the RDA is 20 mcg (800 IU). The DV is 400 IU. The UL for those over age 9 is 100 mcg (4000 IU). See the DRI tables on the inside front and back covers for more details. Despite the fact that the RDA and UL for vitamin D were recently increased, there is considerable debate as to whether the standards were increased enough to support health. For instance, Hollis and colleagues recommend vitamin D supplementation of 4,000 IU per day for pregnant women, and noted that a supplement of 400 IU per day was comparatively ineffective at raising serum 25-hydroxyvitamin D levels.

Part of the vitamin D controversy is due to the fact that cut points of serum 25-hydroxyvitamin D levels associated with deficiency or insufficiency in terms of bone health, optimal concentration for health or athletic performance, and levels associated with toxicity have not been developed. Larson-Meyer and Willis describe the different thresholds of vitamin D status as follows:

- Deficiency is 25-hydroxyvitamin D <20 ng/mL (ng is nanogram or one-billionth of a gram)
- Insufficiency is <32 ng/mL
- Toxicity is >50 ng/mL when coupled with increased elevated serum calcium

The Office of Dietary Supplements describes vitamin D status as follows:

- <12 ng/mL is deficient and leads to rickets in infants and children and osteomalacia in adults
- 12 to 20 ng/mL is inadequate for bone and overall health in healthy individuals
- ≥20 ng/mL is adequate for bone and overall health in healthy individuals
- 50 ng/mL is linked to potential adverse effects (especially if >60 ng/mL)

Larson-Meyer reports that optimal concentrations may lie between 40 and 70 ng/mL, which is the concentration at which the human genome evolved.

Food Sources

Most foods do not contain any vitamin D. Fatty fish, such as wild salmon, mackerel, sardines, and catfish, are good sources and may contain about 200–500 IU in 3 ounces. Shitake mushrooms are also a good source, containing about 250 IU in four mushrooms. Small amounts are found in egg yolks, about 25 IU. Several foods are fortified with vitamin D, such as milk, margarine, and some breakfast cereals. One glass of fortified milk will provide 100 IU, which is 25 percent of the AI for infants and 17 percent of the RDA for children and adults to age 70.

The Consumers Union notes that we normally get about 90 percent of our vitamin D from sunlight and the remaining 10 percent from food. Liebman notes that a light-skinned person out in the sun in a bathing suit, with no sunscreen, can make 20,000 to 30,000 IU in 30 minutes. However, African-Americans may need up to ten times as much sunlight as Caucasians to make similar amounts of vitamin D. Clothes block the action of the sun, but the RDA for vitamin D may be obtained by exposing the hands, arms, and face to 10–20 minutes of summer sunshine about 2–3 times per week. The ultraviolet-B (UV-B) radiation waves promote vitamin D formation in the skin, but Gilchrest notes that UV-B waves also cause wrinkles and skin cancer. Total sunblocking agents prevent vitamin D formation, but their use by individuals concerned with skin cancer due to sun exposure is still recommended because even very small amounts of sunshine will promote vitamin D formation. Longer periods of exposure may be necessary in the winter, and it may be difficult to obtain adequate vitamin D by sunlight in northern latitudes. Vieth and Fraser indicated this was especially true for the northern latitudes of Canada during winter, and it may also apply to the northern parts of the United States. Formation of vitamin D from sunlight is also decreased in the elderly and in individuals with dark skin. Fortunately, as Gilchrest points out, we can buy vitamin D at the corner store.

Major Functions

Most tissues and cells in the body have receptors for the hormonal form of vitamin D, and between 200 and 2,000 genes are controlled by vitamin D. In particular, vitamin D plays a central role in bone metabolism through its effect on calcium and phosphorus, whose roles in bone metabolism are discussed in the next chapter. It works in conjunction with several other hormones, particularly parathormone secreted by the parathyroid gland. Vitamin D helps to absorb calcium from the intestinal tract and the kidneys, helping to maintain normal serum calcium levels and proper bone metabolism. Vitamin D also helps regulate phosphorus metabolism, another mineral essential in bone formation. Verhaar and others note that besides the classical actions of vitamin D in bone metabolism, it also appears to be important for muscle function. Vitamin D status has been associated with chronic, nonskeletal diseases, including cardiovascular disease, hypertension, multiple sclerosis, arthritis, infection, autism, and certain cancers. A meta-analysis by Autier and Gandini demonstrated that taking vitamin D supplements is associated with decreased mortality. For a detailed review of vitamin D metabolism, the interested reader is referred to the review by Holick.

Deficiency: Health and Physical Performance

Deficiencies of vitamin D are unusual in most temperate climates because the body possesses adequate stores in the liver and can manufacture it through exposure to the sun. Children normally get adequate sun exposure if they play outdoors during daylight. However, deficiencies may occur in individuals who have little exposure to sunshine, such as elderly people who are homebound. Many elderly are more concerned with health, and are more likely to wear more clothing and use sunscreen lotions, possibly blocking vitamin D formation. Vegans who avoid sunlight may also be at risk for vitamin D deficiency, but may obtain some vitamin D from shiitake mushrooms and fortified products.

Vitamin D deficiency may be related to a variety of health problems. In particular, a deficiency leads to increased serum levels of parathyroid hormone, which removes calcium from bones. Thus, deficiencies may lead to inadequate calcium metabolism and bone deformities known as rickets, especially in children. This was a major concern years ago, but it has nearly been eradicated through the use of vitamin D-fortified foods, primarily milk. However, Calvo and others noted that hypovitaminosis D may occur in various groups, such as those living in northern latitudes. Infants who breast-feed may also be deficient if their mothers have inadequate vitamin D. Thus, Raiten and Picciano noted that there is a reemergence of vitamin-D-deficient rickets in young children.

Moreover, in a recent interview, Holick indicated that adults do not drink much milk and many are not getting enough vitamin D to satisfy their body requirements, predisposing them to bone loss. Loss of bone tissue may occur in adults, leading to **osteomalacia,** or a softening of the bones, accompanied by muscular weakness. The muscle weakness has been theoretically linked with an impairment of calcium metabolism in the muscle, possibly due to inadequate activation of vitamin D receptors in muscle. Some research notes a decrease in muscle strength in institutionalized elderly patients who are deficient in vitamin D.

Larson-Meyer and Willis, experts in vitamin D and athletes, report that numerous studies have documented vitamin D deficiency and insufficiency in the general population, but that much less is known about athletes. In a review of seven studies, they noted vitamin D deficiency or insufficiency in athletes from all over the world. In a year-long study of 41 athletes (12 indoor and 29 outdoor), Halliday and others showed that 64 percent of athletes were vitamin D deficient or insufficient in the winter, 12 percent in the fall, and 20 percent in the spring. Low vitamin D status was correlated with upper respiratory infections, colds, influenza, and gastroenteritis. In this study, indoor sport athletes (e.g, wrestling, basketball) had lower serum levels of 25-hydroxyvitamin D than did outdoor sport athletes (football, cross-country). Cannell and others reviewed the effects of vitamin D on performance and made the following observations. Studies from the 1950s showed improved performance following exposure to ultraviolet light; peak performance is seasonal and is related to serum 25-hydroxyvitamin D levels; and vitamin D increases type II fiber size and number and muscle function in older adults. Cannell and colleagues concluded that vitamin D may improve performance in vitamin D deficient athletes, and that peak performance may occur when 25-hydroxyvitamin D levels approach 50 ng/mL. More recently, preliminary data were presented at the annual meeting of the American Orthopaedic Society for Sports Medicine by Shindle and others. Of 89 professional football players, 30 percent were vitamin D deficient (<20 ng/mL) and 50 percent had vitamin D insufficiency (20 to 31.9 ng/mL). African-American players and players who suffered muscle injuries had significantly lower vitamin D levels. Thus, there is increasing evidence that athletes should be concerned with their vitamin D status.

http://ods.od.nih.gov/factsheets/vitamind/ Find the "Vitamin D Dietary Supplement Fact Sheet" from the NIH Office of Dietary Supplements at this site.

Vitamin D may help inhibit cell proliferation, so a deficiency could lead to increased cell proliferation, a key characteristic in cancer growth. Grant and others reported that solar UVB irradiance and/or vitamin D have been found inversely correlated with incidence, mortality, and/or survival rates for breast, colorectal, ovarian, and prostate cancer and Hodgkin's and non-Hodgkin's lymphoma, and also noted that evidence is emerging that more than 17 different types of cancer are likely to be vitamin D-sensitive. Schwartz and Skinner reported that epidemiologic studies over the past year lend additional support for important roles for vitamin D in the natural history of several cancers.

Holick and Chen state that vitamin D deficiency is a worldwide problem with serious health consequences. Low levels of serum vitamin D_3 appear to increase health risks. In a large prospective study, Giovannucci and others reported that low levels of vitamin D are associated with higher risk of myocardial infarction in a graded manner, even after controlling for factors known to be associated with coronary artery disease. Dobnig and others recently reported that low vitamin D levels are independently associated with all-cause and cardiovascular mortality. However, a causal relationship has yet to be proved by intervention trials using vitamin D.

Chiu and others reported that a low level of vitamin D in the blood is associated with insulin resistance and increased risk of diabetes. Additionally, vitamin D deficiency may lead to an increased production of renin by the kidney, which could lead to an increased blood pressure.

Scientists have hypothesized that vitamin D, obtained either via sunlight or dietary intake, may reduce the risk of various chronic diseases.

Supplementation: Health and Physical Performance Vitamin D supplementation research has focused primarily on bone health and related issues, but the effect on other chronic diseases has also received increased research attention.

Bone health Although some studies have shown that vitamin D and calcium supplementation did not prevent bone fractures, Bischoff-Ferrari and Dawson-Hughes noted such studies had several limitations. In particular, they used the relatively less potent vitamin D_2 or a too low dose of D_3 (400 IU) that may have limited the increase in vitamin D status necessary to prevent bone fractures. More recent extensive reviews indicate that considerable evidence supports the role of both calcium and vitamin D in protecting the skeleton. For example, in the NIH report on multivitamin/mineral supplements and chronic disease prevention, Hyang noted that vitamin D *alone* does not increase bone mineral density or decrease fracture risk, but it does work in combination with calcium to decrease the risk of fractures in postmenopausal women. Each nutrient is necessary to maximize the benefits of the other in bone health. Heaney supports this viewpoint in his review on bone health.

Additionally, research suggests vitamin D supplementation may lower the risk of bone fractures in older people by increasing muscular strength, which helps maintain balance and prevent falls. In a meta-analysis, Jackson and others reported a trend toward a reduction in the risk of falls among patients treated with vitamin D_3 compared with placebo.

Cancer Lips, in a review of vitamin D physiology, indicated it has an antiproliferative effect that can regulate cell differentiation and function, which may explain how a vitamin D deficiency can play a role in the pathogenesis of certain diseases, such as cancer. Epidemiologic studies have shown a reduced risk of colorectal cancer with increased intake of calcium and vitamin D. Some randomized controlled studies, such as the report by Wactawshi-Wende and others, revealed no effect of supplementation with 1,000 mg of calcium and 400 IU of vitamin D_3, for 7 years, on the development of colorectal cancer in postmenopausal women.

However, Lappe and others, using a supplemental dose of 1,400–1,500 milligrams of calcium plus 1,100 IU of vitamin D_3, did find a substantial reduction in all-cancer risk in postmenopausal women. Moreover, in a meta-analysis, Gorham and others reported that a 50 percent lower risk of colorectal cancer was associated with elevated serum vitamin D levels that could be obtained with a daily intake of 1,000–2,000 IU/day of vitamin D$_3$. Research is ongoing to help understand the role of vitamin D$_3$ supplementation as a possible means to help prevent cancer. Dosage may be important.

Diabetes   Vitamin D may enhance immune cell functions to help prevent autoimmune diseases, like type I diabetes. Harris indicated that doses of 2,000 IU and higher daily may have a strong protective effect in children at risk for type I diabetes.

Kidney stones and other adverse health effects   In the NIH report, Hyang reported that supplementation with calcium and vitamin D may increase the risk for kidney stones. The elevated serum calcium levels may combine with other substances, such as oxalates or phosphates, to form the kidney stones which may pass through the urinary tract and cause considerable pain. The calcium may also become incorporated into plaque in the arteries, leading to calcified or hardened plaque. Additionally, hypervitaminosis D may lead to vomiting, diarrhea, weight loss, and loss of muscle tone.

To help promote health, primarily bone health, scientists suggest that a healthy serum D (25-hydroxyvitamin D) concentration should be about 30–60 nanograms per liter (ng/L), which may require 1,000–2,000 IU of vitamin D$_3$ daily. However, many vitamin D scientists are recommending that the UL be increased. In support of this viewpoint, Hathcock and others recently assessed the risk of vitamin D supplementation and noted the absence of toxicity in trials conducted in healthy adults who used vitamin D$_3$ doses up to 10,000 IU daily, which supports the selection of this value as the UL.

Heaney indicated that the nutrient status for both vitamin D and calcium tends to be deficient in the adult population of the industrialized nations. Given the health implications of adequate vitamin D and calcium intake, he believes that fortification with both nutrients is appropriate and, given contemporary diets and sun exposure, probably necessary because people normally do not adhere to a regimen of taking supplements daily.

Physical performance   Although there may be some rationale for using vitamin D supplementation as a means to enhance health status, and although Ardestani and colleagues reported that serum 25-hydroxyvitamin D levels are correlated with VO$_2$ max, there is little support for athletes to take vitamin D supplements. Only a few studies have been conducted with vitamin D supplementation and physical performance, and they revealed no beneficial effect, either through single megadoses or supplementation over a 2-year period. Some research has revealed that weight training increases the serum concentration of vitamin D, and the investigators theorized that this could be related to the increased bone mass which is developed through exercise. Others indicate that the exercising elderly need to obtain adequate vitamin D. However, these studies do not suggest that vitamin D supplementation

would be ergogenic in those with normal vitamin D status. Nevertheless, Willis and others reported that little is known about the vitamin D status of athletes, but suggested sports nutritionists should advise athletes on the wisdom of obtaining adequate amounts, either through safe sun exposure or dietary supplementation with 1,000–2,000 IU vitamin D$_3$ daily. Also, given data demonstrating vitamin D deficiency and insufficiency in athletes, perhaps athletes should consider having their vitamin D levels checked.

There are sound medical reasons for individuals to obtain adequate amounts of both vitamin D and calcium. As noted earlier, they function together. Dietary calcium recommendations are presented in the next chapter.

Prudent Recommendations   Based on the current data, Liebman notes that many health professionals are recommending an intake of 1,000 to 2,000 IU of vitamin D daily for most individuals. Such an amount may be obtained in the diet, but you must select foods rich in vitamin D, such as fatty fish and vitamin-D-fortified products like milk, cereals, and orange juice. Check food labels for vitamin D content, preferably D$_3$. Remember, the DV is 400 IU, but a food with 100 IU only contains 17 percent of the RDA. Supplements may be recommended for those who do not obtain sufficient vitamin D through sunshine or the diet. In 2007, Canada included the recommendation that people over age 50 should take a daily vitamin D$_3$ supplement. Liebman also indicates that you take in no more than 2,000 IU daily. Individuals at risk for kidney stones should discuss vitamin D intake with their physician.

Vitamin E (alpha-tocopherol)

Vitamin E is a fat-soluble vitamin. In its natural form, it is a complex family of eight compounds including tocopherols and tocotrienols, both with alpha, beta, gamma, and delta forms. The two major forms are **RRR-alpha-tocopherol** and **RRR-gamma-tocopherol.** Alpha-tocopherol alone is the basis for the RDA and it is the most common form in the bloodstream and dietary supplements. You may see it listed as d-alpha-tocopherol (natural form) or dl-alpha-tocopherol (synthetic form).

DRI   The RDA for vitamin E is 15 mg of natural and other forms of alpha-tocopherol, although you might see the RDA expressed as IU. One mg RRR-alpha-tocopherol is equivalent to about 1.5 IU. The RDA is slightly less for children. See the DRI table on the inside of the front cover for more details. The DV is 30 IU. The UL for adults is 1,000 mg/day, which is equal to 1,500 IU.

Food Sources   Vitamin E is found primarily in the small fat content in various vegetables. The most common dietary sources are polyunsaturated vegetable oils such as corn, soybean, and safflower oils, and margarines made from these oils; one tablespoon contains about 3–5 IU. The amount of the different tocopherols and tocotrienols varies among different oils. Other good sources of vitamin E include fortified ready-to-eat cereals,

of the average individual or to improve performance in athletes. Some research suggests that vitamin K supplementation may help promote bone health by increasing bone mineral content. Typical multivitamin tablets may contain about 0–120 micrograms of vitamin K. Individuals desiring to take vitamin K supplements are recommended to do so under the guidance of a physician.

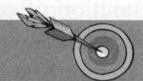

Key Concepts

▶ The fat-soluble vitamins are A, D, E, and K. Although most vitamins must be obtained from the food we eat, several fat-soluble vitamins may be manufactured in the body. Vitamin A may be produced from dietary beta-carotene, vitamin D from exposure to the sun, and vitamin K from intestinal bacterial activity.

▶ Current research suggests that some individuals, particularly the elderly, need to obtain more vitamin D and calcium from their diet. Although obtaining these nutrients through consumption of health foods is the ideal, supplements may be recommended for some. Some health professionals recommend daily intake from food and supplements of 1,000–2,000 IU of vitamin D and 1,000–1,300 milligrams of calcium. D_3 is preferable.

▶ Although research is somewhat limited, in general, supplementation with fat-soluble vitamins has not been shown to enhance sports performance.

Water-Soluble Vitamins

There are nine water-soluble vitamins, including eight in the vitamin B complex and vitamin C (ascorbic acid). The B complex vitamins include thiamin, riboflavin, niacin, B_6, B_{12}, folate, biotin, and pantothenic acid. Choline, although included in the DRI for the B vitamins, has not been classified as a vitamin at this time. Being water soluble, they are not, with a few exceptions, stored to any significant extent in the body. The effects of a deficiency may be noted in 2–4 weeks for some of these vitamins, often reducing physical performance capacity. Excess supplements of these vitamins are usually excreted in the urine and are generally considered to be relatively harmless. However, there are some exceptions.

Because several of the B vitamins work closely together in energy metabolism, many studies have investigated the effect of a deficiency or supplementation of multiple vitamins from the *B complex*. A summary of this research follows a discussion of each individual vitamin.

Figure 7.4 provides a broad perspective on the major sites of activity of the water-soluble vitamins, highlighting sites for vitamin E and other antioxidants as well.

Thiamin (vitamin B₁)

Thiamin, also known as **vitamin B₁,** is a water-soluble vitamin and is also known as the antiberiberi or antineuritic vitamin. It was one of the first vitamins discovered.

DRI   The RDA for thiamin varies according to the intake of Calories, being approximately 0.5 mg per 1,000 Calories. The average adult male needs approximately 1.2 mg/day, while the adult female needs about 1.1 mg/day. See the DRI table on the inside front cover for more details. The DV is 1.5 mg. No UL has been established.

Food Sources   Thiamin is widely distributed in both plant and animal tissues. Excellent sources include whole-grain cereals, beans, and pork. One lean pork chop contains more than 50 percent of the RDA. Several fortified ready-to-eat cereals contain 100 percent of the RDA for thiamin, as well as most of the other B vitamins.

Major Functions   Thiamin has a central role in the metabolism of glucose. It is part of a coenzyme known as thiamin pyrophosphate, which is needed to convert pyruvate to acetyl CoA for entrance into the Krebs cycle. Thiamin is essential for the normal functioning of the nervous system and energy derivation from glycogen in the muscles.

Deficiency: Health and Physical Performance   Deficiency symptoms may occur in several weeks, and may include loss of appetite, mental confusion, muscular weakness, and pain in the calf muscles. Prolonged deficiencies lead to beriberi, a serious disease involving damage to the nervous system and the heart. Fortunately, thiamin deficiency is not very common, although it may be rather prevalent among the homeless, alcoholics, and other special groups.

Of importance to the athlete, two factors that increase the need for thiamin are exercise and high-carbohydrate intake. A deficiency of thiamin could prove to be detrimental to the active individual who might rely on high levels of carbohydrate metabolism for aerobic energy production during exercise, such as endurance athletes. Indeed, some well-controlled research conducted during World War II to evaluate military nutrition needs in combat noted decreased endurance capacity after several weeks of a thiamin-deficient diet. More contemporary research has also investigated the role of thiamin deficiency upon exercise performance, but in conjunction with riboflavin and niacin deficiencies. These reports are discussed under vitamin B complex.

Supplementation: Health and Physical Performance   Thiamin supplementation apparently has no health benefits for a well-nourished individual. Tanphaichitr found no evidence of thiamin toxicity with oral administration, as the excess will be excreted in the urine. No UL has been set for thiamin.

No contemporary research appears to exist relative to the effect of thiamin supplementation upon physical performance, although results from a number of studies conducted more than 50 years ago are available. Following a careful review of these studies, many of which had problems in establishing a proper experimental design, there appears to be no conclusive evidence to support the contention that vitamin B₁ intake above and beyond the normal RDA will enhance performance.

Although not using thiamine, Doyle and others reported that 5 days of supplementation with allithiamine, a thiamin derivative, did not improve muscular strength and endurance. In several

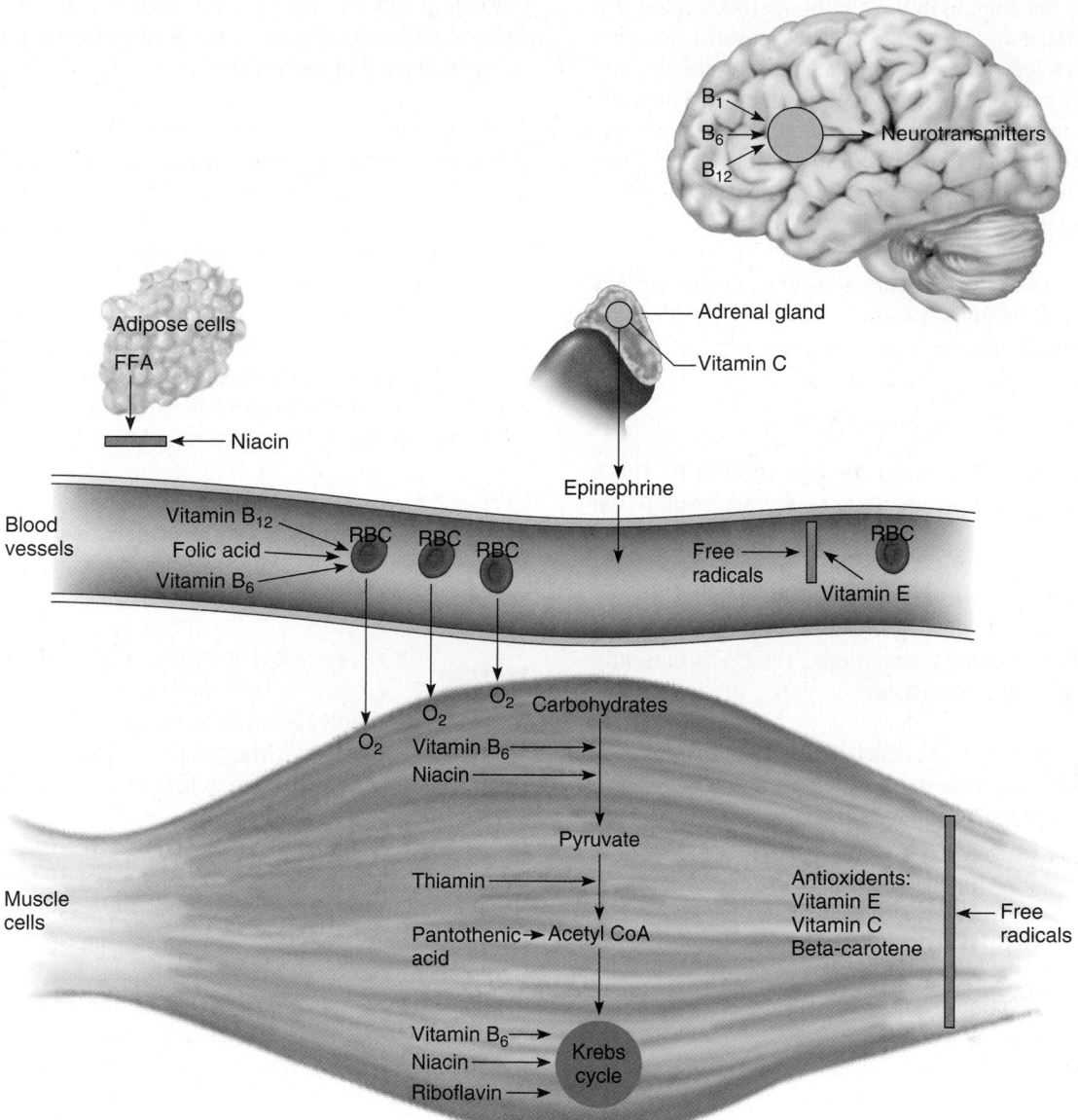

FIGURE 7.4 Roles of vitamins important to sports performance. A number of B vitamins, including thiamin, riboflavin, niacin, B$_6$, and pantothenic acid, are essential for the conversion of carbohydrate into energy for muscular contraction. Vitamin B$_{12}$ and folic acid are essential for the development of the red blood cells (RBCs), which deliver oxygen to the muscle cell. Vitamin E helps protect the RBC membrane from destruction by free radicals. Vitamin E and other antioxidant vitamins are theorized to prevent free radical damage in muscle cells during exercise. Vitamin C is needed for the formation of epinephrine (adrenaline), a key hormone during strenuous exercise. Niacin may actually block the release of free fatty acids from the adipose tissue, which could be a disadvantage for ultraendurance athletes. Finally, several of the B vitamins are also involved in the formation of neurotransmitters in the brain, which may induce a relaxation effect.

well-controlled studies, Michael Webster reported no significant effects of thiamin derivatives on metabolic, physiologic, or psychologic responses to various cycling exercise tasks in well-trained cyclists. In both studies, performance time in a 2,000-meter time trial (in one study after a 50-kilometer ride) was not affected by the thiamine derivatives.

Thiamin, as indicated, is important for normal neurological functions. In a study from Japan, Suzuki and Itokawa reported that 100 milligrams of thiamine for 3 days increased serum thiamin

levels and reduced subjective complaints of fatigue from subjects following a strenuous exercise task. As noted later under the B-complex section, thiamin was one of the vitamins proposed to improve neurological function in pistol shooting. These are interesting observations and merit additional research.

As noted previously, physical activity, particularly high-intensity, endurance-type activity, increases the need for thiamin in the diet; this exercise training also increases the need for caloric intake. With proper selection of foods, the increased thiamin need may be met by the content in the additional foods eaten. An adequate thiamin intake is one of the reasons physically active individuals need to select foods that are dense in nutrients, and in general to avoid foods that provide Calories but few nutrients. Woolf and Manore, in their review of B vitamins and exercise performance, concluded that thiamin intake of most athletes, even those in weight-control sports, appears to be adequate and consistent with recommendations.

Prudent Recommendations Thiamin supplements are not needed by the individual who is consuming an adequate diet, and they do not appear to enhance exercise performance.

Riboflavin (vitamin B$_2$)

Riboflavin is also known as **vitamin B$_2$.** It is a water-soluble vitamin and is a component of the B complex.

DRI The RDA for riboflavin is 1.3 mg for the adult male and 1.1 mg for the adult female. The DRI table on the inside front cover contains the RDA for other age groups. The DV is currently 1.7 mg and no UL has been established.

Food Sources Riboflavin is distributed widely in foods. A major source is milk and other dairy products; one glass of milk contains 20 percent of the RDA. Other good sources include liver, eggs, dark-green leafy vegetables, wheat germ, yeast, whole-grain products, and enriched breads and cereals.

Major Functions Riboflavin is important for the formation of several oxidative enzymes known as *flavoproteins*, which are involved in energy production from carbohydrate and fats in the body cells. It is also involved in protein metabolism and maintenance of healthy skin tissue.

Deficiency: Health and Physical Performance Deficiencies are very rare but have been seen in alcoholics and those adhering to various fad diets. Early signs of deficiency may include glossitis (an inflammation of the tongue), cracks at the corners of the mouth, and dry, scaly skin at the corners of the nose, symptoms common in individuals who experience multiple nutrient deficits.

Although the effect of a riboflavin deficiency upon physical performance has not been studied directly, research from Cornell University suggests that physically untrained women who initiate an aerobic training program may need a higher intake of riboflavin to synthesize more flavoproteins in the muscles. Using a blood test, the investigators determined that the RDA did not maintain proper riboflavin status in the early stages of training, but they suggested that a value of about 1.1 mg per 1,000 Calories would be sufficient. It should be noted that no data were reported relative to the effect of this deficiency upon performance. Haralambie also reported a possible deficiency in trained athletes but did not relate it to performance. Most recently, Woolf and Manore reported that although athletes may need more riboflavin than the general population and the current RDA, they can satisfy these increased needs if adequate energy is consumed and they currently appear to be meeting recommendations.

Supplementation: Health and Physical Performance Riboflavin supplementation apparently has no health benefits for a well-nourished individual. McCormick indicates that toxicity for excess riboflavin intake is doubtful. Excesses will not be stored but will be excreted in the urine. No UL has been set for riboflavin.

Reviews by Keith and van der Beek reveal only one reputable study of the effects of riboflavin supplementation on physical performance. Tremblay and others, studying elite swimmers, reported that 60 mg of riboflavin daily for 16 to 20 days did not improve VO$_2$ max, anaerobic (lactate) threshold, or swim performance.

Prudent Recommendations Considering the available research data and the absence of riboflavin deficiency in most individuals, one must conclude that riboflavin supplementation will not enhance health or physical performance.

Niacin

Niacin is also known as nicotinic acid, nicotinamide, or the antipellagra vitamin. It is a water-soluble vitamin in the B complex and is sometimes erroneously referred to as vitamin B$_3$.

DRI Niacin is found naturally in many foods, but it also may be formed in the body from excess amounts of dietary tryptophan, an essential amino acid. Therefore, the RDA is expressed in **niacin equivalents,** or **NE.** One NE equals 1 mg of niacin or 60 mg of tryptophan, because 1 mg of niacin can be produced from that amount of tryptophan. The RDA for niacin is 16 NE for adult males and 14 NE for adult females. The requirement is different for other age groups, and specific values may be obtained from the DRI table on the inside front cover. The DV is 20 mg. Because excess niacin intake may cause some health problems, as we will note, an UL of 35 mg/day has been set for adults, and even lesser amounts for younger individuals.

Food Sources Niacin is found in foods that have a high protein content. It is most abundant in lean meats, organ meats, fish, poultry, whole-grain cereal products, legumes such as beans and peanuts, and enriched foods. Milk and eggs contain small amounts of niacin, but they contain sufficient tryptophan. One-half of a chicken breast contains more than 60 percent of the RDA of niacin.

Major Functions Niacin serves as a component of two coenzymes concerned with energy processes within the cell. One of these coenzymes (nicotinamide adenine dinucleotide; NAD$^+$) is important in the process of glycolysis, which is the means by which muscle glycogen produces energy both aerobically and anaerobically. The other coenzyme is involved in fat metabolism by promoting fat synthesis in the body, which may block release of free fatty acids from adipose cells.

Deficiency: Health and Physical Performance Although niacin deficiency was prevalent in the past, the enrichment of foods with niacin has nearly eliminated this problem. Deficiency symptoms include loss of appetite, skin rashes, mental confusion, lack of energy, and muscular weakness. Serious deficiencies lead to pellagra, a disease characterized by severe dermatitis, diarrhea, and symptoms of mental illness.

In theory, physical performance would be impaired by a niacin deficiency because the production of energy from carbohydrate could be impaired. Both aerobic- and anaerobic-type performances could be affected. However, no research has been uncovered that has directly studied the effects of niacin deficiency alone on exercise performance.

Supplementation: Health and Physical Performance Megadoses of niacin may function like drugs and have been used in attempts to treat several health problems, being relatively ineffective in the treatment of mental disease and somewhat successful in reducing high serum lipid levels. McKenney noted that niacin favorably affects all components of the lipid profile to a significant degree, as it has consistently been shown to significantly reduce levels of total cholesterol, LDL-cholesterol, triglycerides, and lipoprotein (a). In particular, niacin has a very potent effect to increase HDL-cholesterol by blocking the uptake of apolipoprotein A1 by the liver; some indicate that it is the best drug for this purpose. Niacin may be useful as a therapeutic treatment of dyslipidemia. In several reviews of clinical studies, Hunninghake and Bourgeois revealed that niacin, either alone or combined with other agents, can result in regression of atherosclerosis and reduce patient mortality. However, results from the AIM-HIGH trial showed that niacin did not provide any additional protection against heart attacks when taken with the cholesterol-lowering drug Zocor®, but did increase risk of stroke. Surprisingly, patients ingesting niacin and Zocor® had increased HDL levels and decreased triglycerides, but there was no benefit in terms of disease outcomes. Although medications that reduce LDL are clearly beneficial, there is less evidence that nutrients and medications that increase HDL and decrease triglycerides are as effective at reducing heart disease risk. Given these rather contradictory research findings, individuals with cardiovascular disease should adhere to their physician's recommendations.

Although niacin is generally considered to be nontoxic, large doses in the form of nicotinic acid may cause flushing, with burning and tingling sensations around the face, neck, and hands occurring within 15 to 20 minutes after ingestion (i.e., the histamine-like effect). Taken over long periods, niacin may contribute to liver problems such as hepatitis and peptic ulcers. Pieper noted that niacin comes in three formulations: immediate-release, sustained-release, and extended-release. Niaspan, an extended-release niacin preparation, appears to minimize the flushing effects seen with the immediate-release form and the hepatotoxic effects seen with the sustained-release form. In their review, Guyton and Bays concluded that, overall, the perception of niacin side effects is often greater than the reality and thus, as a result, a valuable medication for cardiovascular risk is underused. Nevertheless, the American Heart Association and the National Institutes of Health recommend that no one take niacin to lower blood cholesterol without guidance from a physician.

Because of the role of niacin in energy metabolism, a number of experiments have been conducted relative to niacin supplementation and physical performance capacity. However, several reviews concluded that niacin supplementation has not been shown to be an effective ergogenic aid for well-nourished athletes, having no effect on various exercise endeavors, including performance in a 10-mile run and in a 3.5-mile cycle time trial following 2 hours of cycling.

As a matter of fact, niacin supplementation is not recommended for most athletes, particularly those involved in endurance-type exercise such as marathon running, because excessive niacin intake (3–9 grams/day) influences fat metabolism, blocking the release of FFA from the adipose tissue. This will decrease the supply of FFA to the muscle, which may lead to an increased dependence on carbohydrate as an energy source during exercise, as shown by Heath and others. This could lead to a more rapid depletion of muscle glycogen, an important energy source during exercise. As noted by Bulow, niacin supplements may reduce endurance capacity.

Niacin supplements may also increase blood flow to the skin due to a histamine-like effect. In one experiment, Kolka and Stephenson found that such an effect could lower the sweat rate and decrease body heat storage during exercise. These effects could possibly be ergogenic to athletes exercising in the heat, but further investigation is needed.

Prudent Recommendations Unless recommended under the treatment of a physician, niacin supplements are not recommended for a physically active individual on a balanced diet. Excessive intake may actually impair certain types of athletic performance and elicit adverse health effects.

Vitamin B$_6$ (pyridoxine)

Vitamin B$_6$ is a collective term for three naturally occurring substances that are all metabolically and functionally related: pyridoxine, pyridoxal, and pyridoxamine. Pyridoxine is most often used as a synonym. Vitamin B$_6$ is water soluble.

DRI The adult RDA for vitamin B$_6$ is 1.3 mg/day for ages 19 to 50, and then increases to 1.7 mg for males and 1.5 for females above age 51. Slightly different amounts are needed at different age levels. Consult the DRI table on the inside front cover for specific RDA. Actually, the RDA for vitamin B$_6$ is based on protein intake, so requirements may increase with high-protein diets. The DV is 2 mg. As excess B$_6$ intake may cause some health problems, as noted in this section, a UL of 100 mg/day has been set for adults, and even lesser amounts for younger individuals.

Food Sources Vitamin B$_6$ is widely distributed in foods. The most reliable sources are protein foods such as meats, poultry, fish, wheat germ, whole-grain products, brown rice, and eggs. One-half of a chicken breast contains more than 25 percent of the RDA.

Major Functions In its coenzyme form (primarily pyridoxal phosphate; PLP), vitamin B_6 is critically involved in the metabolism of protein, but it is also involved in carbohydrate and fat metabolism. It functions with more than 60 enzymes in such processes as the synthesis of dispensable amino acids, the conversion of tryptophan to niacin, the formation of neurotransmitters in the nervous system, and the incorporation of amino acids into body proteins such as hemoglobin, myoglobin, and oxidative enzymes. It is also involved in the breakdown of muscle glycogen, as well as gluconeogenesis in the liver. Interested readers are directed to the review by Woolf and Manore for more details on the metabolic functions of vitamin B_6.

Deficiency: Health and Physical Performance Vitamin B_6 deficiency is not considered to be a major health problem. The average American diet appears to provide an adequate amount of the vitamin, but poor diets do not. The use of diuretics and oral contraceptives has been associated with deficiencies. Woolf and Manore reported that studies have found poor vitamin B_6 status in some athletes, particularly in endurance athletes. Female athletes on low-energy diets may also have low vitamin B_6 intakes. Deficiency symptoms include nausea, impaired immune function, skin disorders, mouth sores, weakness, mental depression, anemia, and epileptic-like convulsions.

Theoretically, a B_6 deficiency could adversely affect endurance activities dependent upon oxygen, for it is involved in the formation of protein compounds, such as hemoglobin, that are essential to oxidative processes. Its role in carbohydrate metabolism, particularly muscle glycogen utilization, is also important to the endurance athlete. Its role in the formation of neurotransmitters could be important to athletes engaged in fine motor control sports, such as archery and riflery. In addition, the requirement for B_6 increases with protein intake, which may have some implications for athletes who may be on high-protein diets. However, because B_6 is found in protein products, it should be easily obtainable in such a diet.

No research has been uncovered that has directly studied the effect of a B_6 deficiency upon physical performance. One report did suggest that runners who covered 5 to 10 miles per day appear to use more B_6 than their sedentary counterparts, but these investigators also noted that exercise may actually promote storage of the vitamin in the athlete, thus helping to prevent a deficiency state. Serum levels of B_6 actually increase during exercise. Woolf and Manore indicate that exercise increases plasma levels of PLP, which can be converted into an acid and lost in the urine during exercise; thus, exercise may increase the turnover and loss of vitamin B_6 from the body.

In general, exercise does not appear to cause excessive losses of vitamin B_6 from the body. However, prolonged aerobic endurance exercise tasks may lead to increased B_6 losses. Rokitzki reported loss of 1 milligram from running a marathon, which approximates the daily RDA. In contrast, Leonard and Leklem found that plasma pyridoxal phosphate levels fell following a 50-kilometer ultramarathon, results that are not consistent with those reported in previous studies involving shorter length endurance tasks. However, whether or not ultraendurance athletes are at risk for vitamin B_6 deficiency has not been determined. These vitamin B_6 losses could easily be replaced during recovery from endurance exercise with consumption of meals rich in protein and carbohydrate.

Supplementation: Health and Physical Performance Vitamin B_6 supplementation has been used to treat the nausea of pregnancy, mental depression associated with the use of oral contraceptives, and premenstrual syndrome (PMS), but its effectiveness for these purposes has received mixed reviews. For example, in a systematic review, Wyatt and others found that conclusions are limited due to the poor quality of most studies, but doses of 100 mg per day of B_6 (which coincides with the UL) are likely to yield benefits in the treatment of PMS symptoms.

As discussed later, folate supplementation may decrease plasma homocysteine levels, which has been studied as a risk factor for CHD. McKinley and others noted that although not as effective as folate, low doses of B_6 (1.6 milligrams/day) may provide additional homocysteine-lowering benefits to elderly individuals who have adequate intake of the other B vitamins. Vitamin B_6 has also been studied as part of B-complex supplementation for prevention of CHD, and the results are presented later in this chapter.

Woolf and Manore suggest that some active individuals, depending on training level, may require 1.5 to 2.5 times the current RDA for B_6 to maintain good B_6 status. Several reports relative to the effect of B_6 supplementation upon physical performance are available. Although the muscle may store B_6, Coburn and others noted that B_6 supplementation did not markedly increase muscle stores. Moreover, in general, the studies reveal no significant effect upon metabolic functions during exercise or the capacity to do more work. One investigator suggested that B_6 may actually be detrimental to endurance athletes because it may facilitate the use of muscle glycogen and lead to earlier depletion in prolonged events. However, in a study from the laboratory at Oregon State University, Virk and others reported that B_6 supplementation (20 g/day for 9 days) did not influence, either positively or negatively, performance of trained males in an exhaustive aerobic endurance exercise task just under 2 hours in duration.

There appears to be little or no toxicity associated with moderate doses, but Bender noted that at high levels, B_6 supplementation can cause peripheral nerve damage, evidenced by such problems as loss of natural sensation from the limbs and an impaired gait. The National Research Council noted neurological symptoms with smaller dosages, averaging 117 mg per day for 6 months to 5 years.

Prudent Recommendations Vitamin B_6 supplementation does not appear to be warranted for the physically active individual, and may be associated with some health risks if consumed in large doses for prolonged periods.

Vitamin B_{12} (cobalamin)

Vitamin B_{12} (cobalamin) is a water-soluble vitamin. It is part of the B complex and is the latest vitamin to be discovered.

DRI The adult RDA for B_{12} is 2.4 micrograms per day. The average diet contains about 5–15 micrograms. Slightly different allowances are made for other age groups; see the DRI table on the inside front cover. Note that recommendations for individuals over age 50 are to obtain the RDA from fortified foods or supplements. The DV is 6 micrograms. No UL is available.

Food Sources Vitamin B_{12} is found in good supply only in animal foods such as meat, fish, poultry, cheese, eggs, and milk. One glass of milk contains nearly 30 percent of the RDA. It is not found in natural plant foods such as fruits, vegetables, beans, and grains, but vitamin-fortified cereals may be an excellent source. It is present in microorganisms such as bacteria and yeast, which may be found in some plant foods, but the bioavailability of B_{12} from these sources is uncertain. Although B_{12} may be produced by microorganisms in the human bowel, the site of production is below the point of absorption.

Major Functions Vitamin B_{12} is a part of coenzymes present in all body cells and is essential in the synthesis of DNA. It works closely with folic acid, and both have important roles in the development of red blood cells. Vitamin B_{12} is also essential for the formation of the protective sheath around nerve fibers (the myelin sheath) and for the metabolism of homocysteine.

Deficiency: Health and Physical Performance Deficiency of vitamin B_{12} in humans due to inadequate dietary intake is rare. Even strict vegetarians appear to receive enough in their diet, either through the consumption of microorganisms or the use of fortified products. The body also stores a considerable amount in the liver, which may last for years; the body contains about 2,500 micrograms, but loses only about one microgram daily. A deficiency normally is caused by the inability to release cobalamin from food or a deficiency of intestinal absorption due to decreased transport proteins. The major symptoms are a severe form of anemia, known as megaloblastic (pernicious) anemia, and nerve damage that may cause paralysis. Pregnant women, particularly vegans, need to obtain adequate B_{12} because a deficit may impair myelination and cause birth defects in the newborn. Aging affects the absorption of B_{12} when it is present in food and bound to protein.

Because of its role in the formation of RBC, a deficiency of B_{12} resulting in pernicious anemia would be theorized to decrease aerobic endurance capacity. No research is available relative to the effect of a vitamin B_{12} deficiency upon performance, but other types of anemia have been shown to impair exercise performance.

Supplementation: Health and Physical Performance B_{12} megadoses may be an effective medical treatment for pernicious anemia, but do not appear to benefit the active individual who eats a balanced diet. However, as noted below, lower-dose supplements may be recommended for some individuals.

Relative to sports, vitamin B_{12} has been one of the most abused vitamins in the athletic world, with some reports of athletes receiving large amounts by injection just prior to competition. The belief probably exists that if a little vitamin B_{12} can prevent anemia,

then a lot of it will do something magical to increase performance capacity. However, several well-controlled studies conducted with B_{12} supplementation reached the general conclusion that it will not help to increase metabolic functions, such as VO_2 max or endurance performance. B_{12} supplements appear to be safe, but do not appear to benefit the active individual on a balanced diet.

Prudent Recommendations Individuals who consume animal products normally do not need vitamin B_{12} supplements, and there are no sound data that supplementation will enhance sport performance. However, vegans should consume food products fortified with vitamin B_{12}. Additionally, individuals over age 50, including senior athletes, may have decreased intrinsic factor and limited B_{12} absorption from natural B_{12} food sources, so they are advised to get about 2.4 mcg of B_{12} from fortified food products, such as cereals, or supplements. One serving of B_{12}-fortified cereal contains about 1.5 mcg, whereas a senior multivitamin usually contains 25 mcg.

Folate (folic acid)

Folate, or **folic acid,** is a water-soluble vitamin. It is part of the B complex. Folate is found naturally in some foods, but folic acid is a synthetic form found in fortified foods and dietary supplements; collectively they are called *folacin.*

DRI The RDA for folate is given as micrograms of **dietary folate equivalents (DFE).** One DFE equals 1 microgram of food folate, 0.6 microgram of folic acid in fortified foods, or 0.5 microgram of folic acid supplements taken on an empty stomach. One microgram of folic acid in fortified foods equals 1.7 DFE, while one microgram folic acid in a supplement equals 2 DFE, because these forms are better absorbed. The RDA for folate is 400 micrograms of DFE/day. During pregnancy the RDA is increased to 600 micrograms of DFE per day, and it is 500 micrograms DFE during the early stages of lactation. The DV is 400 micrograms of DFE. An UL of 1,000 micrograms DFE/day has been set for adults, and even lesser amounts for younger individuals.

Food Sources Folate derives its name from foliage because it is found in green leafy vegetables like spinach. Other good sources include organ meats such as liver and kidney, dry beans, whole-grain products, and some fruits like oranges and bananas. One cup of cooked black or navy beans contains about 60–75 percent of the folate RDA. One banana provides almost 10 percent of the RDA. Currently, all cereal and grain products in the United States are fortified with folic acid to reduce the occurrence of neural tube defects. The average fortification is 140 micrograms per 100 grams of food product. Studies indicate that such fortification has increased daily dietary folic acid intake by 100 micrograms or more.

Major Functions Folate serves as part of a coenzyme that plays a critical role in the metabolism of methionine, an essential amino acid. In this regard, folic acid is critical to the formation of DNA, the genetic material that regulates cell division. It is essential for maintaining normal production of RBC, one of the most rapidly dividing cells in the body. Folate is also critical during the very early stages of pregnancy when cells in the fetus divide rapidly. Researchers indicate during periods of rapid cell division large amounts of folate are needed to make DNA.

Folate is also involved in the metabolism of **homocysteine,** an amino acid derived in a conversion from methionine. Folate is necessary for the reformation of methionine from homocysteine.

Deficiency: Health and Physical Performance One national survey has reported folate intakes below the RDA for some Americans. Individuals who consume large quantities of alcohol and women who take oral contraceptives may experience deficiencies in folic acid, as these drugs may impair absorption of the vitamin. A folic acid deficiency may impair DNA formation, or lead to an increase in homocysteine.

Due to its effect on DNA synthesis, one of the major effects of folate deficiency is pernicious anemia, attributed to inadequate RBC regeneration. Anemia could impair delivery of oxygen and significantly impair performance in aerobic endurance events.

DNA and chromosomal damage caused by folic acid deficiency has been suggested to increase the risk of cancer. For example, in a Tufts University review, a low level of folate in large intestine cells was associated with an increased risk of colon cancer, a finding one of the authors reported to be consistent with the results of 20 other epidemiologic studies which have found that people who eat the most folic acid are the least likely to get colon cancer. Zhang and others also reported that for women who consume alcohol, those with the lowest dietary folic acid intake were at the highest risk for developing breast cancer.

Either due to DNA damage or the adverse neural effects of homocysteine, women who are folate-deficient and become pregnant may give birth to children with neural tube defects (NTD) such as spina bifida, an incomplete closure of the tissue surrounding the spinal cord. Such defects may cause paralysis and severe disabling conditions in the child. Approximately 2,500 infants in the United States are affected each year.

Elevated plasma levels of homocysteine are thought to damage the lining of the blood vessels or initiate growth of cells that form the framework of plaque, increasing the risk for several vascular diseases, including coronary heart disease (CHD), stroke, peripheral vascular disease (PVD), and Alzheimer's disease. However, Wierzbicki contended that it is simply a marker for CHD, not a cause. As an aside, Joubert and Manore, in a review of exercise, nutrition, and homocysteine, noted that no consistent relationship exists between physical activity and plasma homocysteine concentrations. The American Heart Association has not yet classified a high blood level of homocysteine as a major risk factor for CHD.

Supplementation: Health and Physical Performance In a review, Eichholzer and others reported irrefutable evidence that adequate folic acid helps prevent neural tube defects. In countries mandating fortification of flour with folic acid, the incidence of neural tube defects decreased by 31 to 78 percent. The NIH report on vitamin supplementation also noted that multiple studies have supported the effectiveness of folic acid use by women of child-bearing age to prevent neural tube defects in offspring. All women who have the potential to become pregnant should consume 400 micrograms of synthetic folic acid daily. The 400 micrograms should be consumed as folic acid in fortified foods or dietary supplements, in addition to normal food folate intake. When pregnancy is confirmed, the RDA is increased to 600 micrograms DFE. Currently, only 1 in 3 women consume 400 micrograms DFE daily, so many women need to increase their intake of folic acid-fortified foods or dietary supplements, a recommendation of many health professionals. Some researchers suggest that women at high risk for neural tube defects should take 4,000 micrograms daily, but only in consultation with their physicians.

Although folic acid supplementation is effective in preventing neural tube defects, there is ongoing debate relative to beneficial vascular effects associated with homocysteine lowering by folic acid supplementation. For example, Wang and others conducted a meta-analysis of eight studies and found that folic acid supplementation significantly reduced the risk of a first stroke by 18 percent, particularly when supplemented over the course of 3 years and reducing homocysteine levels by more than 20 percent. Conversely, Bazzano and others did a meta-analysis of 12 randomized controlled studies and reported that folic acid supplementation has not been shown to reduce risk of cardiovascular diseases or all-cause mortality among participants with prior history of vascular disease. Most recently, Clarke and others, based on a meta-analysis of 37,485 individuals, reported that although folic acid supplementation reduces homocysteine, it has no effects on cardiovascular disease, cancer, or mortality in those with increased cardiovascular disease risk.

Research suggests caution with excessive folic acid supplementation. Cole and others conducted a double-blind, placebo-controlled study over 10 years to study the effects of supplementation with folic acid (1 mg/day) or placebo on the development of colorectal adenoma. Folic acid supplementation did not reduce colorectal adenoma risk, but was associated with higher risks of having more adenomas and noncolorectal cancers. The investigators indicated that further research is needed to investigate the possibility that folic acid supplementation might increase the risk of colorectal neoplasia. The dosage used in this study was the UL of 1 milligram.

A UL of 1,000 micrograms/day has been established for folic acid from fortified foods or supplements because megadoses could mask a vitamin B_{12} deficiency by preventing the development of anemia that would otherwise be discovered by a blood test. Unfortunately, folic acid does not prevent nerve damage, so the B_{12} deficiency may lead to paralysis if not detected. Rothenberg indicated that this may be a problem associated with the mandatory folic acid fortification of grain products. Thus, individuals who may be prone to a vitamin B_{12} deficiency are advised to take a B_{12} supplement or consume B_{12}-fortified foods.

One advocate of vitamin supplementation to athletes has reported that runners need additional folic acid to replace RBC that may be destroyed in heavy training programs. Unfortunately, no evidence is available to support this theory, nor are there any data showing that folic acid supplements will benefit physical performance. Only one study has been uncovered related to folate supplementation to athletes. Matter and her colleagues provided folate therapy (5 mg/day for 11 weeks) to female marathon runners who were diagnosed as being folate deficient. Although the folate therapy restored serum folate levels to normal, no improvements were noted in VO_2 max, maximum treadmill running time, peak lactate levels, or running speed at the lactate anaerobic threshold.

To be sure, anemia resulting from a folate deficiency could have serious consequences for endurance performance, but a balanced diet including fortified grain products should prevent this condition from developing.

Prudent Recommendations All individuals should increase their intake of folate-rich foods, particularly vegetable sources, not only to obtain adequate folate but other healthful nutrients as well. Women in their childbearing years should obtain 400 micrograms DFE daily from a supplement to complement natural dietary sources, a recommendation approved by the American Academy of Pediatrics. Given the importance of adequate DFE, the National Academy of Sciences, in establishing the new RDA, indicated that women should get folic acid from fortified foods or supplements. Relative to the theoretical risk of vascular diseases, 400 micrograms DFE again appears to be a reasonable amount that may be obtained through the diet, particularly with folic acid-fortified cereals, or with the use of a daily supplement. However, because several studies have linked daily intake of 1,000 micrograms of folic acid with increased risk for cancer, Liebman and Schardt suggested that although women of childbearing age are recommended to obtain 400 micrograms of folic acid daily, males and postmenopausal women who take multivitamins might be advised to take one every other day and also to try to avoid cereals, such as Total, that are fortified with 100 percent of the Daily Value for folic acid.

Folic acid has been combined with other B vitamins to evaluate health benefits of supplementation, which is covered in the section on the Vitamin B Complex.

Pantothenic acid

Pantothenic acid is a water-soluble vitamin. It is a factor in the B complex. Pantothenate is a salt of pantothenic acid.

DRI The adult AI for pantothenic acid is 5 mg, with lesser amounts for younger age groups and greater amounts during pregnancy and lactation. The DV is 10 mg and no UL has been established.

Food Sources Pantothenic acid is distributed widely in foods. It is found in all natural animal and plant products, but best sources include organ meats, eggs, legumes, yeasts, and whole grains. It should also be noted that highly refined, processed foods have lost most of the pantothenate content.

Major Functions Pantothenic acid is an essential component of coenzyme A (CoA), which plays a central role in energy metabolism. You may recall that acetyl CoA, which may be derived from carbohydrate, fat, and protein metabolism, is the principal substrate for the Krebs cycle. Pantothenic acid is also involved in gluconeogenesis, in the synthesis and breakdown of fatty acids, modification of proteins, and in the synthesis of acetylcholine, a chemical released by the motor neuron to initiate muscle contraction.

Deficiency: Health and Physical Performance Except under experimentally induced conditions, deficiencies are not seen in humans. In such cases deficiencies have been reported to cause a variety of symptoms, including fatigue, muscle cramping, and impairment of motor coordination.

On a theoretical basis, pantothenic acid appears crucial to the active individual because it has an important function at the center of energy pathways. Several investigators have suggested that a deficiency would decrease the availability of acetyl CoA for the Krebs cycle and thus shift energy production to anaerobic glycolysis, which is less efficient. Because deficiencies of pantothenic acid have not been observed, such effects upon physical performance have not been studied.

Supplementation: Health and Physical Performance Pantothenic acid supplementation apparently has no health benefits for a well-nourished individual. Liebman, in her review on how to select a multivitamin, indicated that you can ignore it on the label.

Research findings regarding the effect of pantothenic acid supplementation on physical performance are equivocal. Data from one well-designed study with supplements of pantothenic acid—2 grams per day for 14 days—suggested a beneficial effect by reducing oxygen consumption and lactate production during a submaximal exercise task at 75 percent VO_2 max for 40 minutes. This would suggest that pantothenic acid increased the efficiency of the exercise task. No data on maximal performance were provided. Unfortunately this report was available only as a brief abstract, and very few details were presented. Conversely, another well-designed study revealed that 1 gram of pantothenic acid given daily for 2 weeks had no effect upon various blood measures or maximal performance in highly trained distance runners. Most recently, Webster, using six highly trained cyclists, reported no significant effects of pantothenic acid supplementation (1.8 grams per day for 7 days, combined with allithiamin) on a 2,000-meter time trial following a 50-kilometer steady-state ride. There also were no significant metabolic, physiologic, or psychologic effects.

Supplements of pantothenic acid appear to be relatively nontoxic. However, large doses of 10 to 20 grams have been known to cause diarrhea.

Prudent Recommendations Given the fact that pantothenic acid deficiency is rather nonexistent and there is little research to support a beneficial effect on health or physical performance at this time, supplementation is not recommended. A balanced diet should provide adequate pantothenic acid for the healthy, physically active individual.

Biotin

Biotin is a water-soluble vitamin in the B complex.

DRI The adult AI for biotin is 30 micrograms, with somewhat lesser amounts for younger age groups, and greater amounts during lactation. The DV is 300 micrograms, and no UL is available.

Food Sources Good dietary sources of biotin include organ meats such as liver, egg yolk, legumes such as peas and beans, and dark-green leafy vegetables. It is also synthesized in significant amounts in the intestines by bacteria.

Major Functions McMahon noted recent research suggests that biotin may be involved in the regulation of gene expression, which may be related to its role as a coenzyme for a variety of enzymes involved in amino acid metabolism. Biotin is also involved in the synthesis of glucose and fatty acids. Because biotin is an important coenzyme for gluconeogenesis, it may have some implications relative to endurance performance.

Deficiency: Health and Physical Performance Deficiency states are rare but may occur when the diet contains large amounts of raw egg whites; a protein in the raw egg white binds biotin and prevents its absorption into the body. In such cases symptoms include loss of appetite, mental depression, dermatitis, and muscle pain. For athletes who consume eggs for their protein content, it may be important to know that cooking the egg white eliminates this problem while providing the same amount of high-quality protein. It should also be mentioned in passing that raw eggs pose a risk of salmonella, a type of bacteria associated with food poisoning.

Although a biotin deficiency could impair physical performance, no data are available to support this hypothesis.

Supplementation: Health and Physical Performance No research into the effects of biotin supplementation on health or physical performance has been uncovered. Thus, there is no evidence that biotin supplementation improves health or increases physical performance capacity. Supplements of biotin appear to be harmless, as Mock reports no adverse effects in doses ranging up to 200 mg daily.

Prudent Recommendations It would appear that biotin supplements are unnecessary for the physically active individual.

Choline

Choline, an amine, is a water-soluble essential nutrient listed in the DRI report with the B vitamins, but has not been classified as a vitamin. Commercial choline products are available as lecithin or choline salts, but the actual choline content may vary. Check the labels for actual choline content. Choline is also marketed as a powder with carbohydrate and electrolytes to make a sports drink for athletes.

DRI An AI has recently been set at 550 and 425 milligrams/day for male and female adults, respectively. Lesser amounts have been established for adolescents and children. No DV has been established. The UL is 3.5 grams/day.

Food Sources Choline is found in most foods, particularly as lecithin (phosphotidylcholine) in animal foods and free choline in plants. Milk, liver, and eggs are good animal sources, while good plant sources include vegetables, legumes, nuts, seeds, and wheat germ. Zeisel and Niculescu note that normal diets deliver sufficient choline.

Major Functions Choline functions as a precursor for lecithin, a phospholipid in cell membranes. Choline is also involved in the formation of acetylcholine, an important neurotransmitter in the central nervous system.

Deficiency: Health and Physical Performance As choline is found in most foods as part of cell membranes, choline deficiency is very rare. The only research available, involving individuals fed a choline-deficient solution, revealed the development of fatty livers and liver damage. Plasma choline levels have been reported to be significantly reduced following exhaustive exercise such as marathon running, and thus a possible reduction in acetylcholine levels in the nervous system may be theorized to be a contributing factor to the development of fatigue. However, exercise performance was not evaluated in these reports. Penry and Manore suggested that choline supplementation might only increase endurance performance in activities that reduce circulating choline levels below normal.

Supplementation: Health and Physical Performance As choline deficiency is very rare, the effect of choline supplementation on health status has received little research attention. However, its effect on exercise performance has been the focus of several studies in recent years. According to Zeisel and Niculescu, several reports indicate that choline administration accelerated synthesis and release of acetylcholine by neurons.

Research has shown that choline supplementation, either as choline salts or lecithin preparations, will increase blood choline levels at rest and during prolonged exercise. Some preliminary field and laboratory research has suggested increased plasma choline levels are associated with a significantly decreased time to run 20 miles and improved mood states of cyclists 40 minutes after completion of a cycle ergometer ride to exhaustion. In contrast, well-controlled laboratory research has revealed that choline supplementation, although increasing plasma choline levels, exerted no effect on either brief, high-intensity anaerobic cycling tests lasting about 2 minutes, or on more prolonged aerobic exercise tasks lasting about 70 minutes.

Based on these equivocal findings, several reviewers recommended more research with choline supplementation, particularly controlled laboratory research involving prolonged aerobic endurance exercise tasks greater than 2 hours duration. In this regard, Warber and others, in a double-blind, placebo-controlled, crossover study, evaluated the effect of choline supplementation

(6 g total free choline) on performance of trained Army Rangers during and after 4 hours of strenuous exercise. Although choline supplementation increased plasma choline levels by 128 percent, there were no significant effects on any exercise performance measure, including a treadmill run to exhaustion following the 4-hour treadmill exercise protocol. In a short-term supplementation field study, Buchman and others had 12 marathoners consume either a lecithin supplement or placebo one day prior to the Houston marathon. The lecithin supplement provided approximately 1.1 grams of choline on a daily basis, or 2.2 grams total. Although the lecithin supplementation increased plasma choline concentration while the placebo group experienced a significant decrease, there were no significant differences between marathon running times.

Excessive choline intake may lead to a fishy body odor, gastrointestinal distress, vomiting, and low blood pressure. A UL of 3.5 grams/day has been set for adults, and smaller amounts have been set for adolescents and children.

Prudent Recommendations   Given the evidence that choline deficiency states are very rare, and that supplementation does not appear to enhance health or exercise performance, choline supplementation is not recommended. A balanced diet will provide adequate choline.

Vitamin B complex

There are eight vitamins in the B complex, and because several of the vitamins in the B complex work together in energy metabolism, a number of studies have investigated the effect of either a deficiency or supplement of more than one vitamin upon health or physical performance.

Deficiency: Health and Physical Performance   As noted previously, a deficiency of folate has been associated with elevated homocysteine levels. Deficiencies in several other B vitamins, vitamin B_6 and B_{12}, have also been associated with increased plasma homocysteine. The Consumers Union cited an analysis of 72 studies concluding that very high levels of homocysteine can predict heart attack and stroke. As noted previously, elevated levels of homocysteine may be a marker, or result, of disease, but not a cause.

As might be expected from evidence presented on deficiencies of individual vitamins, a deficiency of several B vitamins together would negatively affect physical performance. This theory has been supported by studies in which daily intake was reduced to less than 50 percent of the RDA, such as well-controlled starvation experiments conducted during World War II. Several more contemporary studies detailed by van der Beek, in his review from the Netherlands, have shown that a daily intake of less than one-third of the Dutch RDA for several of the B vitamins (B_1, B_2, B_6) and vitamin C leads to a dramatic decrease of VO_2 max and the anaerobic threshold in less than 4 weeks. The reduction in performance occurred even when other vitamins in the diet were supplemented at twice the RDA. In the most recent study, VO_2 max decreased by 10 percent and

the onset of blood lactate accumulation (anaerobic threshold) decreased approximately 20 percent after 8 weeks of a deficient diet. The findings support earlier research showing a significant decrease in endurance capacity with a B complex deficiency.

Supplementation: Health and Physical Performance   In 2004, the Consumers Union noted a growing body of research involving the role of various B vitamins as a means to help prevent heart disease and other serious cardiovascular problems. At that time, some research had reported cardiovascular health benefits, such as a reduction in blood pressure, associated with folic acid and vitamin B_6 supplementation. However, subsequent research findings were not as promising. In the largest clinical trial, the Vitamin Intervention for Stroke Prevention (VISP) study, B vitamin supplementation (folic acid, 2 mg; vitamin B_6, 400 mcg; vitamin B_{12}, 400 mcg) modestly lowered serum homocysteine levels, but had no effect on recurrent stroke, coronary events, or death. Furthermore, in a study with heart attack survivors, those taking a combination of folic acid (800 mcg) and vitamin B_6 (40 mg) actually had an increased risk of heart attack and stroke. However, Schwammenthal and Tanne noted that the VISP study had some limitations, and both studies involved individuals with cardiovascular disease.

Similar studies with healthy individuals are limited, but indicate no cardiovascular health benefits of vitamin B supplementation. McMahon and others studied the effects of folate (1 mg), vitamin B_{12} (500 mcg), and vitamin B_6 (10 mg), or a placebo on the blood pressure responses over the course of 2 years in healthy older individuals with elevated homocysteine levels. Although the vitamin B supplementation lowered plasma homocysteine levels, there was no effect on blood pressure. Bleys and others, in a meta-analysis, reported no effect of B vitamin supplements on the progression of atherosclerosis, which is one of the theoretical means whereby vitamin B supplementation may help prevent cardiovascular diseases. Based on the available evidence, the American Heart Association does not recommend widespread use of folic acid and B vitamin supplements to reduce the risk of heart disease and stroke.

In their review of B vitamins and exercise, Woolf and Manore cite several reasons why athletes may need more vitamin B. First, the metabolic pathways that produce energy are stressed during physical activity, and thus requirements for several vitamins may increase; second, biochemical adaptations that occur with training in the tissues may increase requirements; third, strenuous exercise may also increase the turnover or loss of a particular micronutrient in sweat, urine, or feces; and finally, additional micronutrients may be required to repair and maintain the higher lean tissue mass of some athletes and active individuals. A diet rich in healthy carbohydrates and protein will provide an adequate amount of the B vitamins.

In general, research supports the idea that individuals who obtain adequate vitamins through a balanced diet will not improve performance through the use of B complex supplements. However, a number of earlier studies, several with children, have shown that when a deficiency state is corrected by vitamin supplements, physical performance is restored to normal. Moreover, some research with large dosages of B_1, B_6, and B_{12} (about 60–200 times the RDA) has shown increases in fine motor control and performance in pistol shooting. Bonke suggested that the beneficial effect was related to the role of these vitamins in promoting the development of neurotransmitters that induce relaxation. Additional research is needed to confirm this finding.

Several of the principal Dutch investigators in this area, such as van Erp-Baart and Saris, suggest that B complex supplementation may be useful in sports with a high energy expenditure if these athletes consume large amounts of foods with empty Calories—high-sugar and high-fat foods. This again stresses the importance of eating foods that are high in nutrient value.

Prudent Recommendations Vitamin B complex supplementation does not appear to be needed for the individual consuming a balanced diet of wholesome, natural foods. However, consuming fortified foods or supplements to provide adequate amounts of all B vitamins for potential health benefits may be prudent. In particular, women of childbearing age should obtain adequate amounts of folic acid. Moreover, athletes involved in intensive training for endurance-type sports and consuming highly processed foods may benefit from a B complex supplement.

Vitamin C (ascorbic acid)

Vitamin C, or **ascorbic acid,** is a water-soluble vitamin. Its alleged effects upon health and physical performance have been the subject of much controversy.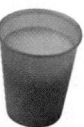

DRI The vitamin C RDA for adult males is 90 mg/day and 75 mg/day for adult females. Slightly lower amounts are recommended for children, whereas somewhat larger amounts are recommended during pregnancy and lactation. The DV is only 60 mg, but the UL has been set at 2,000 mg/day for adults and lower amounts for children and adolescents. For current DRI, see the tables on the inside front and back covers.

Food Sources The best food sources of vitamin C are fruits and vegetables, primarily the citrus fruits and the leafy parts of green vegetables. Excellent sources include oranges, grapefruit, broccoli, and salad greens. Other good sources are green peppers, potatoes, strawberries, and tomatoes. One orange contains the RDA. Milk, meats, and grain products are low in vitamin C. Some products are fortified with vitamin C. Keep in mind when reading food labels that the DV is only 60 milligrams, while the RDA is 75 and 90 for adult females and males, respectively. A food label indicating that one serving is 100 percent of the vitamin C RDA would contain only about 67 percent of the current RDA for males.

Major Functions Although vitamin C does not directly participate in enzyme-catalyzed conversions of substrate to product, Jacob suggests that it modifies mineral ions in the enzymes to make them active. Vitamin C has a number of different functions in the body, some of which have important implications for the physically active individual. Its principal role is in the synthesis of collagen, which is necessary for the formation and maintenance of the connective tissues of the body, such as cartilage, tendon, and bone. Vitamin C is also involved in the formation of certain hormones and neurotransmitters, such as epinephrine (adrenaline), which are secreted during stressful situations like exercise. It helps absorb some forms of iron from the intestinal tract—about a two to fourfold increased absorption—and is involved in the synthesis of RBC. Vitamin C helps regulate the metabolism of folic acid, cholesterol, and amino acids. It is also important in the healing of wounds through the development of scar tissue. Finally, vitamin C is a powerful antioxidant, which helps it contribute to normal function of the immune system.

Deficiency: Health and Physical Performance Serious deficiencies of vitamin C are rare in industrialized societies because fresh or frozen fruits and vegetables are abundant. Also, the human body has a pool of vitamin C ranging from 1.5–3.0 grams. However, smoking, aspirin, oral contraceptives, and stress may increase the need for this vitamin, and a study by Johnston and others reported marginal vitamin C status in 12–16 percent of college students. The major deficiency disease is scurvy, a disintegration of the connective tissue in the gums, skin, tendons, and cartilage that may develop in a month on a vitamin C-free diet. Typical symptoms include bleeding gums, rupture of blood vessels in the skin, impaired wound healing, muscle cramps, and weakness. Anemia also may develop.

Observations by Ness and others indicate that adequate vitamin C intake is associated with increased serum HDL-cholesterol levels, reduced serum triglycerides, and lower blood pressure. Adequate vitamin C is also needed to maintain optimal antioxidant functions. Thus, inadequate vitamin C may increase the risk for various chronic diseases. Some epidemiological research has indicated that individuals with low plasma levels of vitamin C, most often associated with a vitamin deficiency, had a higher incidence of CHD and stroke. For example, Kurl and others evaluated the effect of serum levels of vitamin C on the incidence of stroke over a 12-year period, and found that those with the lowest levels had a 2.4-fold greater risk of stroke than those with the highest levels, especially among hypertensive and overweight men. Additionally, the Consumers Union noted that men with the lowest levels of plasma vitamin C had a 57 percent higher risk of dying from any cause, and a 62 percent higher risk of cancer death, than men with the highest levels. The effects were not seen in women, possibly because they had far more hormone-sensitive cancers, which seem to be unaffected by the vitamin. However, other research from Japan has shown similar benefits, and the vitamin C was consumed mainly from foods, not supplements. Thus, the Consumers Union indicated that the health benefits may be from other substances in foods that accompany vitamin C.

It is obvious that many of the symptoms of a vitamin C deficiency we have cited would impair physical performance. Sensations of weakness could adversely affect all types of performance, whereas anemia would hamper aerobic endurance. Data available from several studies with vitamin C-deficient subjects do suggest such an effect, particularly the widely known Minnesota starvation experiments during World War II, directed by Ancel Keys.

Supplementation: Health and Physical Performance Vitamin C supplementation has been claimed to have significant health benefits, most notably the prevention of CHD and cancer. Because vitamin C is an antioxidant, and because many related supplementation studies have included other antioxidant vitamins (beta-carotene and vitamin E), we will discuss its effects on chronic disease and prevention of muscle tissue damage in physically active individuals later in this chapter.

There is some debate regarding the safety of megadoses of vitamin C. Several investigators have found that excessive amounts of vitamin C, such as 5–10 grams daily, may produce some undesirable side effects such as diarrhea; destruction of vitamin B_{12} in the diet; excessive excretion of vitamin B_6; decreased copper bioavailability; predisposition to gout, creating pain in the joints; and formation of kidney stones from oxalate salts, one of the breakdown products of vitamin C. Although for some individuals, increased iron absorption is a beneficial effect of vitamin C, it may be a major health problem for individuals prone to iron-storage disease, discussed in the next chapter. Moreover, one study reported increased markers of oxidative DNA damage in some subjects when vitamin C and iron supplements were taken together. Excess vitamin C may potentiate the oxidative effects of iron. Excessive amounts of vitamin C also may interfere with the correct interpretation of certain blood and urine tests. Finally, several case studies revealed the development of a condition known as rebound scurvy when the individual stopped taking the supplements. The researchers suggested a mechanism whereby the increased activity of an enzyme in the body that destroys excess vitamin C during the supplement stages continued after the supplements were stopped, leading to a deficiency and symptoms of scurvy.

Conversely, others have reported megadoses to be relatively harmless because excessive amounts are excreted by the kidneys. They criticize the research upon which claims of adverse effects are based, noting that some of the conclusions rest on isolated case studies. Others support a middle viewpoint, noting that larger doses may be harmless to many, but certain individuals may be prone to problems, such as those who have a family history of kidney stones. For example, a highly controlled supplementation study by Massey and others reported that large daily intakes of vitamin C (2,000 mg) increased the excretion of urinary oxalate and increased the risk for calcium oxalate kidney stones in 40 percent of study participants, both stoneformers and non-stoneformers. Levine and others reported evidence of oxalates appearing in the urine when subjects were supplemented with only 1,000 milligrams of vitamin C per day. These were short-term studies and no observations of kidney stones were detected, but increased oxalates could lead to stone formation over time in those at risk. However, in a longer prospective study involving men between the ages of 40 and 75 with no history of kidney stones, Curhan and others found that after 6 years of follow-up there was no association between vitamin C intake—up to levels of 250–1,500 milligrams per day— and kidney stone formation. Nevertheless, Gerster notes that those at risk for kidney stones should restrict daily vitamin C intake to about 100 mg. The National Academy of Sciences recommends against the routine use of large supplements. Megadose supplementation with vitamin C remains controversial, and the interested reader is referred to the opposing viewpoints presented by Herbert and Enstrom.

The effect of vitamin C supplementation upon physical performance has received considerable attention, mainly because it is one of the vitamins that athletes consume in rather substantial quantities. Both early and contemporary research have shown that vitamin C supplementation improves physical performance in subjects who were vitamin C-deficient, but a thorough analysis of these studies supports the general conclusion that vitamin C supplementation does not increase physical performance capacity in subjects who are not vitamin deficient. Bell and others found that vitamin C, 500 milligrams daily for 30 days, did not increase VO_2 max or cardiac output in either young or older men. No solid experimental evidence supports the use of megadoses of 5–10 grams that some athletes take. The interested reader may consult the reviews by Gerster, Keith, and Peake.

Because exercise is a stressor, some investigators have recommended that the active individual may need slightly more vitamin C than the RDA, for example, 200–300 milligrams per day. Some research with runners doing 5–10 miles a day does not support this viewpoint; in any case, this amount could easily be obtained by wise selection of foods high in vitamin C content. Keith also suggests that vitamin C supplementation may be beneficial to heat acclimation, a topic that merits additional research with trained athletes.

Although exercise normally promotes health benefits, Nieman notes that in contrast to moderate levels of physical activity, prolonged and intensive exertion, such as running an ultramarathon, causes numerous changes in the human immune system that may predispose to certain illnesses, such as upper respiratory tract infection (URTI). Large doses of vitamin C have been claimed to strengthen the immune system and prevent URTI. Some early research suggests that the antihistamine effects of vitamin C may decrease the severity of some symptoms of a cold. For example, Peters and others reported that 600 milligrams of vitamin C supplementation for 21 days prior to an ultramarathon reduced symptoms of respiratory tract infections, while Douglas and others reported that doses greater than 200 milligrams may also help prevent URTI in heavy physical exercise in cold environments, such as soldiers in subartic weather conditions. However, more recent research revealed that 200 milligrams of vitamin C daily will lead to full saturation of plasma and white blood cells, which should optimize immune functions associated with vitamin C. It may be possible that smaller amounts of vitamin C, such as 200 milligrams, may provide effects comparable to those seen with larger doses.

In general, although the duration of the symptoms may be reduced slightly, a review and meta-analysis by Douglas and others indicated that vitamin C (>200 milligrams per day) supplementation had no effect on developing a cold or its severity. Moreover, vitamin C supplementation does not appear to benefit immune function, even in ultraendurance athletes. David Nieman, an international expert in exercise and immune function, along with his colleagues, reported no effect of 7 days of vitamin C supplementation (1,500 mg/day) on oxidative and immune responses in runners both during and after a competitive ultramarathon race.

Two studies by Davison and Gleeson also reported no beneficial effects of vitamin C supplementation, either alone or with carbohydrate, on immune functions following 2.5 hours of cycling at 60 percent VO_2 max. In a review of his own and other research, Nieman indicated that vitamin C supplementation, as well as combined antioxidant vitamin supplementation, is not an effective countermeasure to exercise-induced immunosuppression.

Prudent Recommendations A review by Weber and others suggests that adequate vitamin C intake may be associated with various health benefits for certain individuals. The amounts recommended approximate 200 milligrams per day, an amount easily obtained in the diet. Currently, the Consumers Union indicates it is premature to recommend vitamin C supplements, but it does recommend a diet rich in fruits and vegetables, which (as previously noted) contain not only substantial amounts of vitamin C but other healthful substances as well. Eating the recommended 5–9 fruits and vegetables daily should supply about 200–350 milligrams of vitamin C. This is a solid recommendation for both the sedentary and physically active individual.

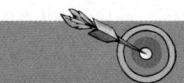

Key Concepts

▶ The water-soluble vitamins consist of those in the B complex and vitamin C. Choline is also a water-soluble nutrient for which DRI have been established.

▶ In general, water-soluble vitamins are not toxic in excess. However, excess niacin may interfere with proper liver function and excess vitamin B_6 has been associated with neurological problems.

▶ Water-soluble vitamin deficiencies are rare in developed countries. However, supplements may be advised for some individuals. Women of childbearing age should consume 400 micrograms of folic acid daily to prevent the possibility of birth defects in the newborn. Elderly individuals should obtain adequate vitamin B_{12} through fortified foods or vitamin supplements.

▶ A water-soluble vitamin deficiency may impair physical performance, usually by interfering with some phase of the energy-producing process. In some cases, impairment may be seen in 2–4 weeks on a deficient diet.

▶ Supplementation with water-soluble vitamins has not been shown to enhance sports performance.

Vitamin Supplements: Ergogenic Aspects

Like the general population, the vast majority of athletes receive the RDA for most vitamins in their daily diet. It is true that some studies report that certain groups of athletes receive less than the RDA for some vitamins or even have indicators of a biochemical deficiency, but other studies, such as that by Ziegler and others involving athletes in weight-control sports with low energy intake, find that biochemical indexes of nutritional status are usually within normal limits. Sarah Short of Syracuse University, in her exhaustive review of dietary surveys with athletes, and Larry Armstrong and Carl Maresh in their review, found that vitamin deficiency symptoms rarely are reported. Moreover, in his review, Michael Fogelholm reported that, at least in developed countries, dietary vitamin intake by athletes is more than required for maximal exercise performance. Nevertheless, elite endurance athletes, such as Tour de France cyclists, and the majority of both high school and college athletes believe that vitamins are essential for success, and it is a matter of fact that many consume vitamin supplements either as nutritional insurance or in the hope of improving performance. For example, in a review of more than 51 studies involving data on more than 10,000 male and female athletes in 15 sports, Sobol and Marquart reported that the overall mean prevalence of athletes' supplement use was 46 percent, a finding supported in a survey by Krumbach and others. Elite athletes use supplements more than college or high school athletes, and women more often than men. Athletes appear to use supplements more than the general population, and some take high doses that may lead to nutritional problems.

In recent years some vitamin manufacturers have turned their attention to the physically active individual, including older athletes, suggesting through advertisements that their special product enhances athletic performance. In her review, Priscilla Clarkson of the University of Massachusetts suggested such advertisements were a major reason for the use of vitamin supplements by athletes.

Should physically active individuals take vitamin supplements?

In her review, Stella Volpe, an expert in sport nutrition at Drexel University, commented that the vitamin and mineral needs of athletes have always been a topic of discussion. Although Volpe notes that researchers disagree as to whether athletes need more micronutrients, she indicates that the intensity, duration, and frequency of the sport or exercise training and the overall energy and nutrient intakes of the individual all have an impact on whether micronutrients are required in greater amounts.

There may be some good reasons for physically active individuals to take vitamin supplements. For example, in certain types of athletic activity, such as wrestling, gymnastics, and ballet, participants may undertake prolonged semi-starvation or starvation diets. As discussed in chapter 10, this is not a recommended procedure, but some athletes may do it to obtain or maintain an optimal body weight for competition. In such cases, when the energy intake may be well below 1,200–1,600 Calories per day, many surveys have shown that the athlete may not be receiving enough vitamins. Research suggests that vitamin depletion, mainly the water-soluble vitamins, can occur rapidly in humans on low-Calorie diets and that these vitamins should be replaced daily. Athletes may also need vitamin supplementation if they are subsisting on poor diets, as discussed in the next section. Moreover, some vitamin requirements are increased in pregnant women and the elderly, so those who exercise need to consume vitamin-rich diets. Sacheck and Roubenoff recommended vitamin supplements for elderly athletes when adequate dietary intakes cannot be obtained. In general, however, individuals should consult appropriate health professionals before self-prescribing vitamin supplements, particularly megadoses of individual vitamins.

As is obvious from the evidence presented in this chapter, the athlete who is on a balanced diet has no need for vitamin supplementation to improve performance. Nevertheless, some interesting hypotheses suggest that antioxidant vitamin supplements may help prevent muscle tissue damage during training, and a variety of special vitamin-like compounds have been marketed specifically for athletes.

Can the antioxidant vitamins prevent fatigue or muscle damage during training?

Aerobic exercise induces oxidative stress in the body, increasing the production of free radicals. Finaud and others indicate that the effects of the free radicals may be positive or negative. On the positive side, Neiss indicates growing evidence that regular aerobic exercise training enhances the functional capacity of the antioxidant network, upgrading the capacity of the natural antioxidant enzymes in the muscles. Reviews by Ji and Powers noted that *chronic* exercise training increased the activity of superoxide dismutase and glutathione peroxidase in response to free radical generation. These enzymes are important to muscle cell survival during increased oxidative stress. In particular, Knez and others reported that the volumes and intensities of exercise associated with ultraendurance training, such as for Ironman-type triathlon competition, induce favorable changes in innate antioxidant defenses against free radical damage, resulting in improved oxidative balance. One possible benefit is improved immune functions. On the negative side, excessive exercise-induced oxidative stress may occur if the generation of free radicals overwhelms tissue antioxidative defenses, which may disturb cellular homeostasis and cause fatigue or lipid peroxidation and muscle tissue damage.

Antioxidant supplements have been studied as a means to enhance physical performance. However, as noted previously, individual supplementation with either vitamin C or E has not been shown to enhance exercise performance, with the possible exception of vitamin E at altitude. Moreover, reviews by Powers and Sen and their colleagues concluded that antioxidants, including antioxidant cocktails containing several vitamins, have not been shown to reliably improve physical performance. For example, Zoppi and others found that supplementation with vitamins C (1000 mg/day) and E (800 mg/day) to professional soccer players over the course of 3 months of training had no effect on strength, speed, and aerobic capacity.

Atalay and others suggested that performance should not be the only criterion to evaluate the success of antioxidant supplementation. Faster recovery and minimization of injury time could also be affected by antioxidant therapy. Although Zoppi and others found no performance enhancement with antioxidant supplementation to the soccer players, supplementation was associated with reduced levels of blood markers for muscle tissue damage.

It has been known for years that certain forms of physical training for sports, particularly intense training, can induce muscle

damage and soreness. Eccentric muscle contractions, such as those incurred in the quadriceps muscle when running downhill, may cause mechanical trauma to the muscle and connective tissue resulting in soreness during the following days. Neiss indicates that although an *acute* bout of exercise increases the activity of antioxidant enzymes in the body, strenuous exercise may generate reactive oxygen species to a level to overwhelm tissue antioxidant defense systems. The result is oxidative stress. The magnitude of the stress depends on the ability of the tissues to detoxify ROS. Excessive production of free radicals may induce lipid peroxidation, possibly damaging the integrity of cellular and subcellular membranes in the muscles, leading to muscle injury and muscle soreness.

Most of the research with antioxidant supplements to athletes has focused on prevention of muscle tissue damage and soreness. Theoretically, prevention of muscle tissue damage may enable the athlete to train more effectively, the desired result being improvement in competition. Some endurance athletes will train at altitude in attempts to enhance their oxygen-delivery ability, and as noted earlier in this chapter, vitamin E supplements may convey some benefits when exercising at altitude. Additionally, older individuals may be more susceptible to oxidative stress during exercise, for optimal functioning of the free radical-scavenging enzymes appears to decline with the aging process. Millions of older individuals perform aerobic exercise for the related health benefits and often become involved in various forms of athletic competition, including local, national, and international competition for athletes over age 40. Companies are now marketing *Super Antioxidants* to speed recovery in athletes during sport training. Do they help?

Numerous studies have been conducted to evaluate the effect of antioxidant supplements on exercise-induced muscle damage and, in some studies, on performance. The designs of these studies have varied, including differences in subjects (animals versus humans, young and old), methods to induce muscle soreness (e.g., downhill running versus level running; resistance exercise), the type and amount of supplement given, and the biochemical markers used to assess muscle damage. The most common supplements used were vitamins E and C, and beta-carotene, but coenzyme Q_{10}, selenium, and other substances have also been used. Some studies used "antioxidant cocktails" consisting of approximately 800 IU of vitamin E, 1,000 milligrams of vitamin C, and 10–30 milligrams of beta-carotene. The markers of muscle tissue damage include serum enzymes that may leak from the muscle, such as creatine kinase (CK) and lactic acid dehydrogenase (LDH); end products of lipid peroxidation, such as malondialdehyde (MDA); myoglobin leakage from the muscle tissue; and others.

Overall, the results of these studies may be regarded as promising. A number of studies, such as the report by Itoh and others, have shown some beneficial effects of antioxidant supplementation, that is, reduced markers of muscle tissue damage when compared to the placebo treatment. Benefits have been reported for both young and old physically active individuals. Most studies used multiple markers of muscle tissue damage, and in some cases one marker of muscle damage would be improved by the antioxidant supplements but another would be unaffected. Some studies compared different antioxidants, for example, C versus E, reporting a beneficial effect of one but not the other.

In contrast, more recent studies have reported no significant benefits of antioxidant supplementation to prevent muscle tissue damage during exercise. For example, Mastaloudis and others reported that supplementation with vitamin C (1,000 mg) and vitamin E (300 mg alpha-tocopheryl acetate) before a 50-kilometer ultramarathon had no effect on leg muscle damage or recovery following the race and up to 6 days afterwards. Machefer and others investigated the effect of moderate supplementation with vitamin C, vitamin E, and beta-carotene on muscle tissue damage during and following the Marathon des Sables, a 6-day, 156-mile (254 kilometers) ultramarathon race across the Sahara desert. The supplement elevated serum vitamin levels, but had no effect on markers of muscle tissue damage. Bryer and Goldfarb found that prolonged vitamin C supplementation (3 grams) both before and after eccentric exercise designed to induce muscle soreness produced divergent results on markers of muscle damage and measures of muscle soreness. In general, there were lower levels of creatine kinase 48 hours after testing, but no effect on muscle soreness.

Some studies actually reported adverse effects of supplementation. Nieman and others found that vitamin E supplementation actually promoted lipid peroxidation and inflammation during an Ironman-distance triathlon. In a similar fashion, Close and others also reported that consuming 1 gram of ascorbic acid 2 hours before and 14 days after completing a downhill run did not prevent the delayed onset of muscle soreness (DOMS). Muscle function was impaired in both the vitamin C and placebo groups, but more so in the supplement group, suggesting that vitamin C supplementation may actually inhibit the recovery of muscle function. Moreover, in a small study, Gomez-Cabrera and others reported that vitamin C supplementation during training may actually impair training adaptations, possibly by decreasing production of mitochondria.

The role of antioxidants to prevent exercise-induced muscle tissue damage was the subject of several recent reviews, and the opinions are mixed regarding their efficacy. Adams and Best indicated that although animal studies have shown some promising effects of antioxidant supplementation to lessen exercise-induced oxidative stress damage, studies with humans are less convincing. Relative to vitamin E, Jackson and others concluded that supplements are unlikely to reliably reduce the severity of muscle damage. Viitala and Newhouse also concluded that vitamin E supplementation does not appear to decrease exercise-induced lipid peroxidation in humans. Clarkson and Thompson noted that whether the body's own natural antioxidant defense system is sufficient to combat oxidative stress during prolonged exercise or whether antioxidant supplements are needed is unknown, but trained athletes who received antioxidant supplements have shown evidence of reduced oxidative stress. Ji notes that the aging process lessens the exercise training-induced improvement in natural antioxidant enzymes and suggests that exercise training in older athletes might be assisted with antioxidant supplementation in attempts to optimize antioxidant defense. Sacheck and Blumberg concluded that the use of dietary antioxidants like vitamin E to reduce exercise-induced muscle injury have met with mixed success, which seems to be the prevailing viewpoint. All reviewers agree that more research is needed to address this issue and to provide guidelines for recommendations to athletes.

Prudent Recommendations In a review, McGinley and colleagues report that there is little evidence to suggest that high doses of antioxidants, and in particular vitamin E, can reduce muscle damage. For this reason, and because of the potential dangers of long-term antioxidant supplement use, the authors do not suggest the use of high-dose antioxidant supplements for athletes. The meta-analysis of antioxidant supplements by Bjelakovic and others showed that supplementation with beta carotene, vitamin A, and vitamin E may increase mortality, while the effects of vitamin C and selenium on longevity required more research. However, others note that the prudent use of antioxidant supplementation can provide insurance against a suboptimal diet and/or the elevated demands of intense physical activity, and thus may be recommended to limit the effects of oxidative stress in individuals performing regular, heavy exercise. For example, Takanami and others are convinced that vitamin E contributes to preventing exercise-induced lipid peroxidation and possible muscle tissue damage, and recommend that athletes supplement with 100–200 milligrams of vitamin E daily to help prevent exercise-induced oxidative damage.

Most experts in this area recommend that physically active individuals obtain antioxidant vitamins naturally from food. Increasing the consumption of fruits, fruit juices, and vegetables will enable athletes to obtain the proposed beneficial amounts of beta-carotene (10–30 milligrams) and vitamin C (250–1,000 milligrams) but it would be difficult to obtain 100–200 IU of vitamin E through natural dietary sources. Watson and others indicate that there seems no valid reason to recommend antioxidant supplements to most athletes, except in those known to be consuming a low-antioxidant diet for prolonged periods. For the athlete who wants to supplement vitamin E, inexpensive over-the-counter preparations are available in 100 and 200 IU capsules. For health benefits, remember that most research documents beneficial effects when these vitamins, along with other phytochemicals, are obtained through natural foods, primarily fruits and vegetables.

How effective are the special vitamin supplements marketed for athletes?

Special athletic vitamin packs have been appearing on the market—even in single packets at your local convenience store—that have been advertised as a means for the athlete to increase energy and reach peak performance. Many of these have simply been multivitamin-mineral supplements, while others have been special concoctions that contain ingredients like bee pollen and ginseng. Three such products will be highlighted.

Multivitamin-Mineral Supplements Because in human metabolism vitamins often work together, and often in conjunction with minerals, the ergogenic potential of multivitamin-mineral compounds has been studied for half a century. In a review of the older research, Williams reported that although results of a number of studies suggested ergogenic effects, the experimental designs were usually poorly controlled. In contrast, contemporary research indicates that such supplements, consumed for substantial periods, are not ergogenic for the athlete on a balanced diet. From Timothy Noakes's laboratory in South Africa, Weight conducted a thorough 9-month double-blind, placebo, crossover study. Although multivitamin-mineral supplements did raise blood levels of some vitamins, the authors reported that 3 months of supplementation did not improve maximal oxygen uptake, the anaerobic (lactate) threshold, treadmill run time to exhaustion, or running performance in a 15-kilometer time trial. Anita Singh and her colleagues provided either a high-potency multivitamin-mineral supplement or a placebo to 22 healthy, physically active males for 90 days. The vitamin dosages ranged from 300 to 6,000 percent of the RDA. Although serum levels of many of the vitamins increased, there were no significant effects on physiological variables during a 90-minute run, nor were there any effects on maximal heart rate, VO_2 max, or time to exhaustion. Finally, Richard Telford and his colleagues matched 82 nationally ranked Australian athletes in training at the Australian Institute of Sport and assigned them to either a supplement or placebo treatment. The supplement contained an assortment of vitamins and minerals, ranging from about 100 to 5,000 percent of the RDA. The supplement was taken for approximately 7–8 months, and the subjects were tested on a variety of sport specific tests (e.g., swim bench) as well as common tests of strength (torque), anaerobic power (400-meter run), and aerobic endurance (12-minute run and VO_2 max). These investigators reported no significant effect of the supplement on any measure of physical performance when compared with athletes whose vitamin and mineral RDA were met by dietary intake.

Vitamins and minerals recently have also been marketed to physically active individuals in liquid forms, such as sports drinks. Although research is limited, Fry and others reported no significant improvement in two tests of anaerobic exercise performance (30-second cycle sprint and one set of squats) following 8 weeks of supplementation with a multivitamin/mineral liquid. Thus, all of the current reputable research refutes an ergogenic effect of multivitamin-mineral supplements in adequately nourished athletes.

Prudent recommendations   Although multivitamin-mineral supplements may not enhance athletic performance in well-nourished athletes, those involved in weight-control sports with limited caloric intake might consider taking a simple one-a-day supplement with no more than 100 percent of the RDA for the essential vitamins and minerals. Moreover, the U.S. Anti-Doping Agency, in its booklet on optimal dietary intake, indicated that an athlete who takes a simple one-a-day type of vitamin or mineral that does not exceed the nutrient levels of the RDA/DRI is probably not doing any harm.

Bee Pollen   **Bee pollen** has been marketed almost specifically for athletes, primarily runners, as a means to improve performance.

Chemical analysis of bee pollen reveals that it is a mixture of vitamins, minerals, amino acids, and other nutrients. Although no specific physiological effects of bee pollen have been documented, theoretical ergogenic effects are based on some of the roles that vitamins have in the body. Advertising claims for bee pollen cite questionable research: a field study showing faster recovery rates in athletes who took pollen supplements. However, six well-designed studies using double-blind placebo protocols revealed that supplementation with bee pollen had no significant effect upon VO_2 max, other physiological responses to exercise, endurance capacity, or rate of recovery from exhausting exercise.

Prudent recommendations   Bee pollen supplements are not recommended for physically active individuals. Moreover, caution is necessary, as some individuals may experience an allergic reaction.

CoQ₁₀   The compound **CoQ₁₀**, also known as coenzyme Q_{10} and ubiquinone, is actually a lipid but has characteristics common to vitamins; its chemical structure is similar to vitamin K. CoQ_{10} is found in the mitochondria of all mammalian tissues, but concentrations are relatively high in the heart and other organs in humans. It plays an important role in oxidative metabolism within the mitochondria, facilitating the aerobic generation of ATP as part of the electron transfer system. CoQ_{10} also functions as an antioxidant. It has been used therapeutically for treatment of cardiovascular disease since 1965 because it may protect heart tissue from damage associated with inadequate oxygen, although Webb noted that not all scientists agree it has shown beneficial applications. Tran and others noted that if used therapeutically, coenzyme Q_{10} should be used only in conjunction with other drugs and not relied on by itself for the treatment of any cardiovascular health problem.

Because some studies have shown that CoQ_{10} may improve heart function, maximal oxygen uptake, and exercise performance in cardiac patients, it has been theorized to be ergogenic for athletes. Moreover, Bucci has cited a number of studies indicating that CoQ_{10} levels are lower in trained athletes compared to sedentary controls and that oral supplementation with CoQ_{10} will increase tissue levels, two factors providing theoretical support for its role as an ergogenic. Theoretically, CoQ_{10} should benefit endurance performance because of its role in aerobic metabolism.

Are CoQ_{10} supplements ergogenic? In his book on nutritional ergogenics, Bucci cites results from six studies with sedentary young men, sedentary middle-aged women, aerobically trained volleyball players, male professional basketball players, and endurance runners supporting an ergogenic effect of CoQ_{10}, noting improvements in one or more of the following: VO_2 max, exercise performance, indicators of enhanced aerobic capacity, and improved antioxidant function. Most of these studies were presented in a book entitled *Biomedical and Clinical Aspects of Coenzyme Q* and do not appear to have been published in refereed scientific journals. Moreover, a careful review of these studies revealed that each suffered one or more flaws in proper experimental design, including no control group, no placebo, no randomization of order in which CoQ_{10} or placebo was given, and use of a submaximal heart rate exercise task to predict maximal oxygen uptake.

To be effective, the CoQ_{10} must get into the muscle and mitochondria. However, studies by Svensson and Zhou and their associates reported that although CoQ_{10} supplementation significantly increased CoQ_{10} plasma concentrations, there was no corresponding increase in the skeletal muscle or mitochondria.

There are several published studies regarding the effect of CoQ_{10} on exercise performance, but most that are available do not support its effectiveness as an ergogenic. For example, Weston and others, using 1 milligram of CoQ_{10} per kilogram body weight daily for 28 days, reported no beneficial effects on oxygen uptake, substrate use, or cycle ergometer exercise time to exhaustion in trained male cyclists and triathletes. Although serum CoQ_{10} levels were increased, Braun and others reported no effect of 100 milligrams daily for 8 weeks on submaximal physiological indicators of enhanced aerobic capacity, VO_2 max, time to exhaustion on a bicycle ergometer, or lipid peroxidation, indicating no effect on either aerobic metabolism or antioxidant function. Bonetti and others also found no effect of CoQ_{10} supplementation for 8 weeks on the aerobic power, including VO_2 peak and anaerobic threshold, of trained middle-aged cyclists. In a well-designed, double-blind, placebo, crossover study, Laaksonen and others supplemented both young and old physically trained males with 120 milligrams of CoQ_{10} per day for 6 weeks, and reported no significant effect on maximal oxygen uptake or on time to exhaustion in a progressive cycling task following 60 minutes of submaximal cycling. Actually, performance time in the placebo trial was significantly greater than the CoQ_{10} trial. Additionally, there were no effects of the CoQ_{10} supplement on MDA, a marker of lipid peroxidation. In yet another study from the Karolinska Institute in Sweden, Malm and others reported that CoQ_{10} supplementation (120 milligrams per day for 20 days) exerted no effect on fifteen high-intensity, anaerobic 10-second sprint tests on a cycle ergometer with 50 seconds recovery between each sprint. These investigators noted that, compared to the placebo groups, subjects taking the CoQ_{10} supplement showed evidence of muscle tissue damage. In actuality, the placebo group improved their performance in the cycle sprints, but the supplement group did not, suggesting that CoQ_{10} might be ergolytic. In contrast, Ylikoski and others reported that CoQ_{10} supplementation (90 mg/day) improved several measures of performance, such as VO_2 max, in Finnish cross-country skiers, but they did not evaluate its effect on actual exercise performance. Gül and Gökbel and colleagues showed that eight weeks of CoQ_{10} supplementation (100 mg/d) resulted in small reductions in malondialdehyde (a marker of oxidative stress) and increases in mean cycling power.

CoQ_{10} is also one of the ingredients in a supplement (also containing vitamin E, inosine, and cytochrome C) that has been widely advertised for endurance athletes, particularly triathletes. In a double-blind, placebo, crossover study, Snider and others reported that 4 weeks of supplementation with this commercial product had no ergogenic effect on an endurance task that consisted of a 90-minute treadmill run at 70 percent VO_2 max followed by a cycling test to exhaustion at 70 percent VO_2 max. Zhou and others reported no effect of 4 weeks of CoQ_{10} supplementation (150 mg/day), either separately or combined with vitamin E (1,000 IU/day), on VO_2 max. Using the same supplements, Kaikkonen and others found that supplementation with both CoQ_{10} and vitamin E to marathon runners for 3 weeks had no beneficial effects on lipid peroxidation or muscle damage induced by running the marathon.

At present, the most contemporary published well-designed studies do not support an ergogenic effect of CoQ_{10} supplementation.

Prudent recommendations   Although promising, the majority of research studies still suggest that CoQ_{10} is not an effective ergogenic aid, and thus it is not recommended as a supplement for physically active individuals.

Quercetin   Quercetin is a dietary flavonol, part of polyphenolic compounds, that functions as an antioxidant and may also be an anti-inflammatory agent. Some energy drinks marketed to physically active individuals contain quercetin. Some research has evaluated the effects of quercetin supplementation relative to various aspects of exercise.

David Nieman and his associates conducted four studies on quercetin supplementation (1 gram/day) regarding immune responses and inflammation. Several studies revealed that quercetin supplementation for about 3 weeks could favorably affect immune responses after exercise or reduce the incidence of upper respiratory tract infections during a 2-week recovery from 3 days of intense cycling. However, in a subsequent study with ultraendurance runners, quercetin supplementation for 3 weeks before and 2 weeks after a 160-km mountain run did not favorably affect immune responses or illness rates, while another study reported no protection from exercise-induced oxidative stress and inflammation.

In a comprehensive review, Williams identified six studies of the effects of quercetin supplementation on various endurance tasks, metabolic outcomes, and perceived exertion in trained individuals. It was concluded that quercetin does not perform as claimed, especially in trained individuals. Williams also identified four studies of quercetin supplementation on exercise performance in untrained individuals, and noted that the findings were equivocal. While future studies may be needed to determine if quercetin is effective in untrained persons or those just starting a training program, it could be concluded that quercetin does not perform as claimed, especially in trained individuals.

Prudent Recommendations   At this point, quercetin is not recommended as a supplement to improve exercise performance, although data on the prevention of URTI are promising. More data are needed on the effects of quercetin in untrained individuals and those beginning an endurance training program. Williams suggests that, in the future, researchers focus on flavonoid "cocktails," as flavonoids such as kaempferol, hesperidin, and others may have synergistic effects. Quercetin may interact with medications, such as aspirin, so a health care practitioner should be consulted before taking this supplement.

What's the bottom line regarding vitamin supplements for athletes?

Given the available scientific data, there does not appear to be a very strong case supporting an ergogenic effect of any single vitamin, vitamin-mineral combinations, or the various vitamin-like compounds. As noted, additional research is warranted for those that have some limited support as an ergogenic, for example, the effect of vitamin E on performance at altitude.

At present, the recommended advice is to obtain adequate vitamin nutrition through a well-planned diet. For example, Melinda Manore noted that athletes involved in heavy training may need more of several vitamins, such as thiamin, riboflavin, and B$_6$, because they are involved in energy production, but the amount needed is only about twice the RDA and that may be easily obtained through the increased food intake associated with heavy training.

Dan Benardot and other sports nutrition experts indicate that some athletes, such as those in weight control sports, those who do not have adequate exposure to sunlight, and those who do not eat a well-balanced diet, may be at risk for vitamin deficiency. Thus, some health professionals recommend vitamin supplementation, not only to prevent a deficiency that may impair sport performance, but also for beneficial health reasons, as noted in the next section.

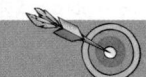

Key Concepts

▶ Although research findings regarding the ability of antioxidant vitamin supplements to prevent muscle tissue damage following intense exercise are somewhat equivocal, in general the benefits are minor. Antioxidant vitamin supplementation has not been shown to enhance sport or exercise performance.

▶ Results from well-controlled research generally indicated that multivitamin/mineral supplements and vitamin-like compounds, such as coenzyme Q$_{10}$, are not effective ergogenic aids.

Check for Yourself

▶ Use a search engine on the Internet, such as www.google.com, and search for "sports vitamins." Check out the advertisements and claims, and compare to the text discussion.

Vitamin Supplements: Health Aspects

Vitamins are big business, being the most popular of all the dietary supplements. They are marketed to all segments of the population, from infant formulas to geriatric preparations, and for a wide variety of health reasons, ranging from combating the stress of everyday life to helping prevent heart disease and cancer. Surveys indicate that vitamin-supplement users have strong beliefs about their effectiveness, and this is evident in the multibillion-dollar sales annually by the vitamin industry.

In the preceding sections, we have already covered each individual vitamin and the possible effects of deficiencies and supplementation upon health (review table 7.1 for a broad overview). This section summarizes prudent dietary recommendations for overall optimal vitamin nutrition, including the possible use of supplements, relative to health.

Can I obtain the vitamins I need through my diet?

Some advertisements for vitamin supplements may leave you with the impression that it is difficult, if not impossible, to obtain adequate vitamin nutrition through the typical American diet. In contrast, most health professional organizations focusing on nutrition, such as the American Dietetic Association (ADA), support the view that a balanced diet will satisfy all nutrient needs of the healthy individual. There is some truth to both positions, for the typical diet of some individuals may not be a balanced diet. Our selection, storage, and preparation of food may lead to poor vitamin intake.

Vitamin intake may be inadequate for several reasons. First, the refining process of many foods removes vitamins. For example, the preparation of flour for white bread removes many of the vitamins found in the outer parts of the grain. Although some of these vitamins are returned by an enrichment process, not all are restored. Thus, many processed foods may be lower in total vitamin content than their natural counterparts. In some cases, however, processing actually increases the vitamin content of foods. Examples include the fortification of milk with vitamins A and D, grain products with folic acid, and the use of vitamin C as an antioxidant preservative in some foods. Second, improper storage of foods may lead to vitamin losses. Once fruits and vegetables are harvested, the vitamin content begins to diminish. In general, such foods should be refrigerated or frozen in airtight containers as applicable, and stored in dark places to minimize vitamin losses caused by exposure to air, heat, and light. Third, improper preparation may also lead to significant vitamin losses from foods. Prolonged cooking, excessive heat, and cooking vegetables in water should be avoided. Steaming, microwave cooking, and the use of boiling bags and waterless cookware will help retain the natural vitamin content of foods. Thus, the individual who consumes a diet high in processed foods with empty Calories and does not store or prepare foods properly may receive less than the RDA for several vitamins.

The key to adequate vitamin nutrition is to consume a balanced diet of natural foods that have a high nutrient density. Buy foods in their natural state and store them properly as soon as possible. Prepare them to eat so as to minimize vitamin losses.

The position of the ADA is that the best nutritional strategy for promoting optimal health and reducing the risk of chronic disease is to obtain essential nutrients through a wide variety of foods. In this way, other nutrients, particularly minerals and other phytonutrients, will be obtained at the same time, as they also are natural constituents of the food we eat. Vitamins often work in conjunction with minerals, such as vitamin D and calcium, vitamin B$_6$ and magnesium, and vitamin E and selenium. By obtaining vitamins through the selection of a balanced diet containing wholesome, natural foods, we may be assured of receiving sufficient amounts of other nutrients necessary for optimal physiological functioning, in addition to various phytochemicals that may also confer some health benefits. The Consumers Union estimates there are about 5,000 phytochemicals in plant foods.

Moreover, it is recommended that the active individual be selective in choosing foods. The stress of exercise can increase

For example, comparing the vegan diet to the typical American diet provides some dietary guidance for the prevention of CHD. In recent years, the vitamin content of the diet, particularly antioxidant vitamins, has been studied as a means to prevent chronic diseases by reducing oxidative damage in the body.

As discussed earlier in this chapter, free radicals may be very reactive with body tissues, causing cellular damage by oxidation of unsaturated fats in cellular and subcellular membranes. Free radicals are theorized to contribute to the aging process and to the development of more than 60 diseases, including cardiovascular disease and cancer. Discussing the free radical theory of aging, Koltover estimated that our life span could be 250 years but for the damage caused by free radicals. Various antioxidant enzymes in the cells counteract undesirable effects of free radicals, but there is increasing evidence that what we eat may also help to prevent certain adverse health effects associated with free radicals.

Fruits and vegetables, along with whole grains, nuts, and seeds, are rich in antioxidants, including vitamins C and E and carotenoids (beta-carotene, lycopene, lutein, zeaxanthin), as well as other micronutrients and phytochemicals. Mehta indicated that there is no doubt that antioxidants and other micronutrients, taken in their proper form in vegetables and fruits, confer a number of overall health benefits. Prevention of cancer and cardiovascular disease appear to be the two major health benefits. Several reviews, including those by Lee, Gaziano and Hennekens, and by Steinmetz and Potter indicated that the evidence for a protective effect of increased consumption of vegetables and fruits, foods rich in antioxidant vitamins, is consistent for cancers of the stomach, esophagus, lung, endometrium, pancreas, and colon, and that the most effective are raw vegetables. The precise mechanism underlying this possible protective effect is not known, although phytochemicals found in some vegetables may block tumor formation. Other investigators believe the antioxidant vitamins (vitamin C, vitamin E, beta-carotene) found naturally in vegetables and fruits may confer the protective effect, for various epidemiologic studies have shown that high serum levels of some antioxidant vitamins are associated with a decreased risk of cancer. In a review, Gladys Block presented biochemical data suggesting that optimal antioxidant intake may protect against environmental factors, such as cigarette smoke and polluted air, that may generate free radicals and subsequent cancer. Antioxidant vitamins may also strengthen the immune system, a major defense against cancer, particularly as we grow older. Meydani indicated that cells of the immune system have a very high content of polyunsaturated fatty acids, which makes them susceptible to oxidative damage. When oxidized, polyunsaturated fats may produce PGE_2, an eicosanoid that may suppress immune function by interfering with several major functions, such as the activity of T cells. Dietary antioxidant vitamins may help prevent this undesirable oxidation.

Universally, all reviewers recommend diets rich in fruits, vegetables, whole grains, and other vitamin-rich foods as the best means of obtaining the antioxidant vitamins, and along with other potential health-promoting phytochemicals, as the most effective dietary strategy to promote health and prevent disease. In this regard, the National Cancer Institute has sponsored a campaign called "Five a Day for Better Health," meaning to eat at least five servings of fruits and vegetables daily. The point is stressed that five is the minimum number of servings and more should be consumed, hopefully five servings *each* of fruits and vegetables.

www.fruitsandveggiesmatter.org   Check to obtain tips on how to incorporate more fruits and vegetables into your daily diet.

However, the health benefits of a diet rich in antioxidant-containing nutrients presented here are based on epidemiological studies. Such diets appear to protect against CHD and other chronic diseases, but the underlying mechanism is not known. Fruits and vegetables are rich in various vitamins that may exert beneficial health effects, such as the antioxidant vitamins, folate, and vitamins B_6, and these vitamins may individually or collectively account for such positive health effects. As noted, these foods also contain other micronutrients and phytochemicals, and vitamins may interact with them, either individually or collectively, to provide the apparent health benefits. Thus, controlled randomized studies have been conducted in attempts to determine whether vitamins are the health-promoting nutrient.

www.ars.usda.gov/nutrientdata/ORAC   Check foods for antioxidant content. The database presents amount of antioxidants, as measured by Oxygen Radical Absorbance Capacity (ORAC), per 100 grams of food, about 3 ounces.

Do vitamin supplements help deter disease?

If the epidemiological evidence suggests that diets rich in vitamins, particularly antioxidant vitamins, may provide some protection against the development of chronic diseases, such as cancer and heart disease, will supplements provide any additional benefit? Scientists have used a variety of research techniques to evaluate the effect of antioxidant supplementation to prevent disease.

Basic research studies, using *in vitro* techniques or animal models, have evaluated the effects of antioxidants on underlying mechanisms of disease. These studies provide evidence in relation to the theory underlying the beneficial effects of supplementation.

Both retrospective and prospective epidemiological studies of various populations have compared differences in the incidence of disease between supplement users and nonusers. These studies provide evidence of a relationship between supplement use and disease, but do not establish a cause-and-effect relationship. Moreover, as Patterson and others have noted, vitamin supplement users are more likely to engage in other healthy behaviors, such as exercising regularly, that may confound the relationship.

Randomized, clinical intervention studies with humans, providing antioxidant supplements to some and placebos to others for years, have evaluated the effect of supplementation on disease. These trials provide cause-and-effect evidence and are considered to be the gold standard in diet-health research.

Nevertheless, as mentioned previously, results from a single study are insufficient to support or refute a theory. The totality of evidence must be considered. In 2006 the National Institutes of Health (NIH) convened a state-of-the-science conference on vitamin and mineral supplements and chronic disease prevention.

The conference planning committee chose to focus the evidence report on nutrients for which the potential for impact had been most strongly suggested and on conditions for which supplements were thought to have the most potential influence. The planning committee also limited the scope of the evidence report to consideration of randomized controlled trials (RCTs). The following sections contain some data from basic and epidemiological studies with vitamin supplements, some of the key conclusions of the 2006 NIH conference, and some other relevant and subsequent research findings.

www.ahrq.gov/clinic/tp/multivittp.htm   Check the full report of the National Institutes of Health state-of-the-science conference on vitamin and mineral supplements and chronic disease prevention.

Cardiovascular Disease and Stroke   Basic research using *in vitro* techniques and biomarkers of oxidation appears to support the theoretical mechanisms underlying the beneficial effects of antioxidant supplementation on cardiovascular disease. In a review, Diplock indicated that there is substantial basic research evidence that vitamin E may prevent undesirable free radical oxidation associated with the development of disease processes. In support of this point, Devaraj and Jialal cite several studies showing that vitamin E decreases the susceptibility of LDL to oxidation, and by becoming part of cell membranes, vitamin E may also inhibit other factors, such as platelet adhesion and resultant clotting, that contribute to atherosclerosis. Singh and Devaraj also note that inflammation may play a role in atherogenesis, and vitamin E is anti-inflammatory. However, Meagher and others questioned whether vitamin E does prevent lipid oxidation in healthy individuals, as they reported no significant effect of 8 weeks supplementation (200, 400, 600, 800, or 1,000 IU/day) on three indices of lipid peroxidation. Moreover, in a meta-analysis, Bleys and others found no evidence of a protective effect of antioxidant, or B vitamin, supplements on the progression of atherosclerosis, suggesting such supplements may not prevent CHD via this mechanism.

Diplock also notes a large body of epidemiological evidence suggesting that the incidence of cardiovascular disease is lower in populations having a high level of antioxidants, even those taking supplements. However, these effects may be specific to vitamin E. Mayne concluded that beta-carotene supplements do not prevent cardiovascular disease. In addition, Rimm and Stampfer noted that epidemiological data do not support a cardiovascular benefit from vitamin C. However, they did note that in several large prospective studies, the greatest reduction in cardiovascular risk was associated with those groups of subjects who took vitamin E supplements, usually in doses greater than 100 IU daily. Epidemiological research has also found that vitamin E supplementation may also help to prevent stroke. In a longitudinal study, Paganini-Hill and Perez Barreto found that individuals who took antioxidant vitamin supplements decreased the risk of cerebral occlusion. It should be noted that not all epidemiological studies reveal positive findings. For example, Ascherio and others, in a study covering 8 years, found that neither vitamin C, nor vitamin E, nor beta-carotene prevented stroke.

Tufts University notes that about a decade ago, the scientific community was flush with findings from large population studies that diets high in antioxidants, vitamin E in particular, could help stave off heart disease. But those studies, though they included tens of thousands of people, were simply observations of the way people ate and lived.

The NIH report, which analyzed only RCTs, concluded that the effects of multivitamin/mineral supplementation on cardiovascular disease are inconsistent. Although some positive findings were reported with vitamin E supplementation, the NIH indicated there is insufficient evidence to make any recommendations. In reviews related to physically active individuals, Hamilton also concluded that studies with humans relative to the cardioprotective effects of antioxidant supplements are conflicting, and more research is needed to determine if various antioxidant supplements may help prevent oxidative damage to the heart following exercise when oxygen radical formation is accelerated. Williams also reported that at this time there is currently insufficient evidence to recommend antioxidant supplements for endurance athletes because the types of long-term studies needed to more adequately assess the health benefits of antioxidant supplements in athletes have not been done.

However, some research suggests that antioxidant supplementation to heart disease patients may be harmful. Miller and others, in a meta-analysis of 19 clinical trials involving vitamin E alone or combined with other antioxidants, reported an increased risk of all-cause mortality with dosages greater than 150 IU/day, and concluded that high-dosage vitamin E supplements (equal to or greater than 400 IU daily) may increase all-cause mortality and should be avoided. The increased mortality may be due to heart failure, as reported in a recent study by Lonn and others. Bjelakovic and others, in a meta-analysis of 68 randomized trials, reported no effect of antioxidant supplementation on overall mortality. However, when the data from only the best-designed studies were analyzed, the investigators concluded that supplementation with antioxidants might actually increase mortality by 4–16 percent, dependent on the specific antioxidant.

Although most recent RCTs and meta-analyses do not support a protective effect of vitamin supplementation against the development of CHD, Rodrigo and others questioned the methodology of the studies. One criticism was the selection of subjects. Tufts University noted that most of the studies analyzed in the meta-analysis by Bjelakovic and others dealt with people who already have a disease, so the conclusions do not apply to a healthy population. Miller and others noted this limitation in their meta-analysis of vitamin E suggesting an increased all-cause mortality, and indicated that the generalizability of their findings to healthy adults is uncertain. Another criticism by Rodrigo and others was the nature of the antioxidant sources of vitamins. For example, supplementation studies with vitamin E have mostly involved alpha-tocopherol. Most recently, however, Sen and Das, along with their associates, have indicated that other forms of vitamin E, particularly the tocotrienols, may have specific health benefits independent of alpha-tocopherol, such as powerful cholesterol-lowering properties.

Given the overall evidence currently available, the American Heart Association does not recommend widespread use of B vitamin supplements to reduce the risk of heart disease and stroke. The Consumers Union also notes that the AHA now recommends *against* taking antioxidant supplements.

In a their review, Futterman and Lemberg make an excellent point. They note that even if antioxidants prove to be effective, their place on the therapeutic ladder of cardiovascular disease prevention should be low. Modifying other risk factors, such as treating hypertension and achieving a normal body weight, should have a higher priority.

Cancer   Antioxidants are theorized to prevent cancer in several ways, primarily by preventing DNA damage and strengthening the immune system, as noted previously.

In a review, Prasad and others noted that extensive *in vitro* studies and some *in vivo* studies have revealed that individual antioxidants may affect animal and human cancer cells by complex mechanisms, and that multiple antioxidant-vitamin supplementation, together with other lifestyle modifications, may improve the efficacy of cancer therapies.

Epidemiological data suggest that antioxidant supplementation, particularly vitamin E, may help in the fight against cancer. Gridley and others indicated that individuals who took supplements of individual vitamins, such as C and E, had a significantly lower risk of oral and pharyngeal cancer, whereas Losonczy and others reported that vitamin E supplementation was associated with about a 50 percent reduction in overall cancer mortality. However, in a review of the relationship between vitamin E and breast cancer, Kimmick and others noted that the epidemiologic study results have been inconsistent.

Experimental studies do not appear to support a cancer-protective effect of antioxidant supplementation. The NIH concluded that the effects of multivitamin/mineral supplementation on cancer are inconsistent and claimed there were not enough data to recommend for or against multivitamins based on cancer data. In another major report dealing with nutrition and prevention of cancer, the American Institute of Cancer Research indicated that although high-dose dietary supplements can modify the risk of some cancers, usually in high-risk groups, these findings may not apply to the general population. Greenwald and others noted that several large randomized clinical trials are underway, including the Physicians' Health Study II, to help clarify the health effects of multivitamin supplements. The Selenium and Vitamin E Cancer Prevention Trial (SELECT) to detect possible prevention of prostate cancer was scheduled to end in 2012, but the National Cancer Institute stopped the study prematurely in 2008. Data analysis indicated that the supplements did not prevent prostate cancer; moreover, there was a small increase, but not statistically significant, in the number of prostate cancer cases in the men taking vitamin E. The antioxidant effects of selenium are discussed in chapter 8.

The AICR noted that there may be some adverse effects, possibly an increased risk of some cancers, associated with vitamin supplementation. In the NIH report, Hyang and others noted that two large trials designed to test lung cancer prevention with beta-carotene found a surprising increase in lung cancer incidence and deaths in smokers and recommend that smokers avoid beta-carotene supplementation. Cole and others, in a 10-year study with the effects of folic acid supplementation on the development of colorectal adenoma, reported a higher risk of having three or more adenomas and of noncolorectal cancers, and indicated research that is needed to investigate the possibility that folic acid supplementation might increase cancer risk. Lawson and others reported that although taking more than one multivitamin daily was not associated with an increased risk of developing localized prostate cancer, excessive multivitamin intake did increase the risk of developing advanced prostate cancer, suggesting that such supplementation may promote tumor growth in men who already have the disease.

Fairfield and Stampfer, in a review of issues and evidence relative to vitamin and mineral supplements for cancer prevention, highlighted the numerous difficulties in studying the effects of vitamin and mineral supplementation on cancer development. For example, given the length of time that it takes cancer to develop, existing studies may not have been long enough. They recommended long-term prospective cohort studies, especially with repeated measures and high follow-up, to help provide useful data as the basis for rational recommendations.

Given the overall evidence currently available, the NIH does not provide a recommendation for or against vitamin supplementation to prevent cancer. Based on its worldwide report on nutrition and prevention of cancer, the AICR indicated that individuals should aim to meet nutritional needs through diet alone, and concluded that dietary supplements are not recommended for cancer prevention.

Eye Health   According to Christen, basic research studies suggest that oxidative mechanisms may play an important role in the pathogenesis of cataract and age-related macular degeneration (ARMD), the two most important causes of visual impairment in older adults. In the United States, more than 1.3 million cataract extractions are performed annually. Jacques theorized that these eye problems may be prevented by optimal antioxidant nutrition, particularly vitamin E. Johnson also noted that the carotenoids, including lycopene and lutein, particularly from natural foods, may play a role in prevention of macular degeneration. Christen notes that findings from several epidemiological studies are generally compatible with a possible protective effect of antioxidant vitamins, but the data are inconsistent. Evans and Henshaw, in a review of three randomized controlled trials, concluded there was no evidence that supplementation with vitamin E and beta-carotene prevented or delayed the onset of ARMD.

Although the NIH indicated that results from trials investigating the effects of multivitamin/mineral supplementation on ARMD are inconsistent, evidence was cited from one well-designed trial (Age-Related Eye Disease Study; AREDS) that might support use of antioxidants and zinc in adults with intermediate-stage ARMD. Evans indicates that data from this single study provides the main support for such use and that more research is needed. Nevertheless, Coleman and Chew indicated that a multivitamin/mineral supplement with a combination of vitamin C, vitamin E, beta-carotene, and zinc (with cupric oxide) may be recommended for ARMD, but not cataract. The Consumers Union recommends that those who are in the intermediate stages of the disease take 400 IU vitamin E daily, along with 500 milligrams of vitamin C, 15 milligrams of beta-carotene, 80 milligrams of zinc, and 2 milligrams of copper. Note that this recommendation is for those who already have ARMD, not for the general public. The Consumers Union recommends that individuals taking such supplements do so under a doctor's supervision. As shall be noted in the next chapter, the recommended zinc intake exceeds the UL.

Seddon indicates that other antioxidants, particularly lutein and zeaxanthin, may be beneficial for ARMD and possibly cataract. However, Trumbo and Ellwood noted that the FDA, in an evidence-based review, concluded that no credible evidence exists for a health claim about the intake of lutein or zeaxanthin and the risk of ARMD or cataracts. The Age-Related Eye Disease Study II is currently evaluating the role of these supplements in ARMD.

Mental Health   Brain cells are also susceptible to oxidative damage, which may contribute to neurologic disease such as Alzheimer's, a devastating disease developing primarily in the elderly. In an epidemiological study, Morris and others found that of individuals 65 years of age and older who used vitamin C or vitamin E supplements, none developed Alzheimer's disease during a 4.3 year follow-up, whereas several cases developed in nonusers. The authors suggested that the use of these antioxidant supplements may lower the risk of Alzheimer's disease. In a more recent study, Englehart and others also found that high dietary intake of vitamin C and vitamin E may lower the risk of Alzheimer's disease. However, in a subsequent study, Morris and others reported that vitamin E from food, but not other antioxidants, may be associated with a reduced risk of Alzheimer's disease. Both of these latter studies followed healthy older adults, aged 55 or 65 and above for a period of 4–7 years.

Results from RCTs are mixed. In one intervention study, using 2,000 IU vitamin E daily for 2 years, the onset of the major debilitating effects associated with Alzheimer's disease was delayed by 7 months. However, in another study, Petersen and others reported that 2,000 IU daily for 3 years did not affect the rate of development of Alzheimer's disease in older people with mild cognitive impairment.

Although research findings are still considered preliminary, several reviews suggest that vitamin E supplementation may be useful in the prevention and treatment of Alzheimer's disease. Munoz and others indicate that vitamin E may decrease the vascular damage caused by peptides involved in development of Alzheimer's, while Berman and Brodaty suggest current clinical practice favors its use during treatment.

General Health   The theory of a health-protective effect of vitamin supplementation is enticing, but the available scientific data are somewhat indecisive. The NIH, in its summarization, concluded that the present evidence is insufficient to recommend either for or against the use of multivitamins/minerals by the American public to prevent chronic disease. The resolution of this important issue will require, among other things, advances in research and improved communication and collaboration among scientists. As noted earlier, several large-scale clinical trials are currently underway and, hopefully, will provide us with some findings to provide more specific recommendations. Keep in mind, given possible gene-nutrient interactions, recommendations may become specific to the individual as human genome research advances with the possible individualization of nutrient requirements.

In the meantime, as noted previously, most health professionals recommend that we obtain our antioxidants from healthful foods. Traber makes the point that, in hindsight, clinical trials of a single nutrient, such as vitamin E, have been overly optimistic in their expectation that a vitamin could reverse poor dietary habits and a sedentary lifestyle in treating heart disease. Again, it may be the whole food and its array of nutrients, rather than a single isolated nutrient, that provides health benefits. In an American Heart Association scientific advisory based on its analysis of clinical trials, Kris-Etherton and others concluded that vitamin supplements do not have the same heart-protective effects as a healthy diet rich in fruits, vegetables, whole grains, and legumes.

How much of a vitamin supplement is too much?

As noted throughout this chapter, vitamins play some very important roles in helping us maintain our health. They are the most popular of all the dietary supplements. However, can we get too much of a good thing? Based on possible adverse health effects of excess vitamin intake, the National Academy of Sciences has established the UL, which is the highest level of a vitamin that can be safely taken without any risk of adverse effects. In general, the higher above the UL, the greater the risk. Exceeding the UL on an occasional basis may not pose any significant health risks, but doing so on a daily basis eventually will. An UL has been set for choline and for seven of the thirteen vitamins for which DRI have been developed. These data can be found on the inside of the back cover of this book. For some vitamins, such as niacin and folate, the UL is only about twice the RDA, whereas for others, such as vitamins C and E, the UL is about 20–60 times greater than the RDA.

In general, it is difficult to exceed the UL for any given vitamin by eating natural, wholesome foods. However, in its report, the NIH noted that this can occur not only in individuals consuming high-potency single-nutrient supplements but also in individuals who consume a healthy diet rich in fortified foods in combination with multivitamin/mineral supplements. For example, the adult UL for niacin is 35 milligrams, but only synthetic niacin derived from fortified foods or supplements and not from niacin in nonfortified foods. Some breakfast cereals may be fortified with 100 percent of the DV for various vitamins, which for niacin would be 20 milligrams, or nearly half the UL. Consumption of a vitamin supplement or other fortified foods could easily lead to excess niacin intake.

If the vitamin content of the body is adequate, excessive vitamin intake serves no useful purpose and may even be harmful in certain situations. As noted previously, vitamins function primarily as coenzymes. When a vitamin enters the body, it travels through the bloodstream to a particular body cell and then forms part of the enzyme complex within that cell. The cell has a limited capacity to produce these enzymes, and when that capacity is reached, the vitamin cannot be used for its basic purpose. It may now have other fates. It may be excreted from the body if in excess, particularly if it is a water-soluble vitamin; it may be stored in some body tissue, particularly if it is a fat-soluble vitamin; or it may begin to function in uncharacteristic ways, as a drug instead of a nutrient.

Mulholland and Benford indicated that the risk of harm occurring from taking vitamin and mineral supplements will depend on the safe intake range of the nutrient concerned, the susceptibility of the individual, and the likely intake of the same nutrient from other supplements or the rest of the diet, such as fortified foods. The NIH panel expressed concern that with the strong trends of increasing multivitamin/mineral and other dietary supplement consumption, and the increasing fortification of the U.S. diet, a growing proportion of the population may be consuming levels considerably above the UL, thus increasing the possibility of adverse effects. Adverse events from multivitamin/minerals appear with some frequency in both the reports of the American Association of Poison Control Centers and the FDA's Med-Watch system.

As noted throughout this chapter, megadoses of several vitamins may be pathological, particularly A, D, niacin, and B_6, when not taken under medical supervision. There are more than 4,000 cases of vitamin/mineral overdose in the United States each year, resulting in about 30 fatalities. Although most of these cases occur in children, the literature contains some case reports of serious health problems with adults, including athletes taking vitamin megadoses in attempts to improve athletic performance. A good review of possible adverse effects of excessive vitamin supplementation is presented by Hathcock.

http://www.fda.gov/medwatch/ Check the safety of specific vitamin or other supplements. Type in the name of the supplement in the search box.

If I want to take a vitamin-mineral supplement, what are some prudent guidelines?

Unfortunately, scientific data are not available to provide specific guidelines relative to the amounts of each particular vitamin or mineral needed to promote optimal health. Although individual vitamin and mineral supplements are available, health professionals do not generally recommend their use. To reiterate, excess amounts of some vitamins (A, D, niacin, and B_6) can be toxic, as can excess amounts of some minerals (calcium, phosphorus, iron, chromium, selenium, and zinc) as discussed in the next chapter. Although antioxidant supplements are hot sellers, the Consumers Union states that there is currently no reason for the average person to take supplements of nutrients such as vitamins A, C, E, or beta-carotene because of their antioxidant potential. Nor is there any reason to eat concentrated antioxidant-rich foods. As noted

previously, the American Heart Association now recommends *against* taking antioxidant supplements.

In general, health professionals who do recommend vitamin and mineral supplements suggest multivitamin/mineral combinations. Minerals are covered in detail in the next chapter, but because they are found in most multivitamin/mineral preparations, it was deemed appropriate to include them in this discussion. For those who desire to take vitamin supplements, the American Dietetic Association recommends low levels that do not exceed the RDA or AI. The Center for Science in the Public Interest (CSPI), an organization promoting healthful nutrition, used an educated-guess approach to offer some prudent guidelines. The following are the highlights of the CSPI recommendations, as reported in an article written by Bonnie Liebman, with some modifications based on advice from the Consumers Union, publishers of *Consumer Reports on Health,* and other nutrition health professionals.

General Points

1. Check the Daily Value (DV). The amounts of vitamins and minerals listed on food and dietary supplement labels are based on the Daily Value (DV) for each nutrient, a value based on the RDA that has not been changed since the 1970s. For example, the DV for vitamin C is 60 milligrams, and yet the new RDA for adult males is 90 milligrams. For zinc, the DV is set at 15 milligrams, yet the new RDA for adult males is 11 milligrams. Thus, supplements that contain 100 percent of the DV may contain less than the current RDA, in the case of vitamin C, or more than the current RDA, as in the case of zinc. In general, these differences are not substantial, but may be for certain vitamins. For example, the DV for vitamin A is 5,000 IU, while the UL is only twice this amount, or 10,000 IU. A Supplement Facts label is presented in figure 7.5.

2. Buy the inexpensive house brand of vitamins that contains about 100 percent of the DV for most vitamins and minerals. There usually is no need to buy special brands, such as those labeled with catchy terms, such as *High Potency.* However, as Yetley notes, multivitamin/mineral products may have widely varied compositions and characteristics. Actual vitamin and mineral amounts often deviate from label values. The Consumers Union warned that you should be leery of bargain-basement brands, such as those found in dollar stores, as tests revealed that more than half did not contain the labeled amount of at least one nutrient. The best buys may be at major drug stores and warehouse stores, which are more likely to carry higher quality products. Most companies that market vitamins buy their vitamins from the same manufacturers, so the contents in national brands and house brands are similar. Look for labels with USP (United States Pharmacopeia), or better yet, USP-Verified, which means that the product meets standards for quality and purity.

   In an evaluation of vitamin supplements, the Consumers Union and CSPI recommended that if you decide to take vitamins, including antioxidants, avoid high-priced products.

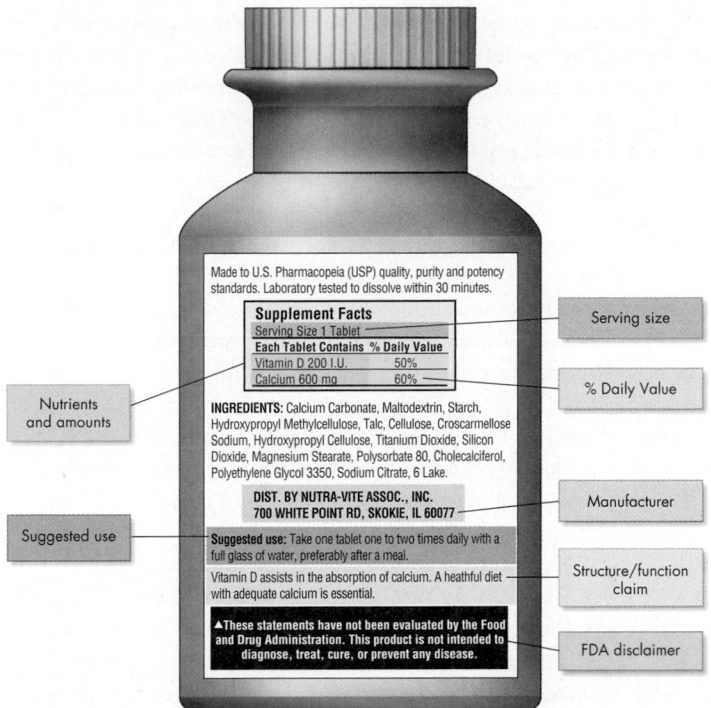

Nutrients and amounts

Suggested use

Made to U.S. Pharmacopeia (USP) quality, purity and potency standards. Laboratory tested to dissolve within 30 minutes.

Supplement Facts
Serving Size 1 Tablet
Each Tablet Contains % Daily Value
Vitamin D 200 I.U.   50%
Calcium 600 mg   60%

INGREDIENTS: Calcium Carbonate, Maltodextrin, Starch, Hydroxypropyl Methylcellulose, Talc, Cellulose, Croscarmellose Sodium, Hydroxypropyl Cellulose, Titanium Dioxide, Silicon Dioxide, Magnesium Stearate, Polysorbate 80, Cholecalciferol, Polyethylene Glycol 3350, Sodium Citrate, 6 Lake.

DIST. BY NUTRA-VITE ASSOC., INC.
700 WHITE POINT RD, SKOKIE, IL 60077

Suggested use: Take one tablet one to two times daily with a full glass of water, preferably after a meal.

Vitamin D assists in the absorption of calcium. A healthful diet with adequate calcium is essential.

▲These statements have not been evaluated by the Food and Drug Administration. This product is not intended to diagnose, treat, cure, or prevent any disease.

Serving size

% Daily Value

Manufacturer

Structure/function claim

FDA disclaimer

FIGURE 7.5 Nutrient supplements display a nutrition label that is different from that of foods. This Supplement Facts label must list the ingredient(s), amount(s) per serving, serving size, suggested use, and % Daily Value if one has been established. Note that this label also includes structure/function claims. Thus, it also must include the FDA warning that these claims have not been evaluated by the agency.

In particular, Schardt recommends against purchasing vitamin supplements endorsed by celebrities on television infomercials and on the Internet. The Center for Science in the Public Interest went to one celebrity's website and clicked on "Vitamin Advisor" to get advice on vitamin supplements. They answered the questionnaire in a variety of ways, representing individuals whose diets ranged from very poor to individuals in top health consuming a stellar diet rich in fruits and vegetables, dairy, and fish. Even the healthiest individuals received recommendations to buy vitamins sold at the website, to the tune of about $45–$50 a month.

3. Stick with the basics. The Consumers Union indicates that all most people need is a pill containing 18 nutrients, about 11 vitamins and 7 minerals, in amounts approximating the RDA.

Fat-Soluble Vitamins

1. Buy a supplement low in vitamin A, particularly one with preformed retinol. CSPI recommends limiting vitamin A to no more than 3,000 IU of retinol, preferably less. Select supplements containing vitamin A from beta-carotene. If the supplement is beta-carotene, 15,000 IU is a recommended limit. Obtain most of your vitamin A as beta-carotene in

fruits and vegetables, a recommendation especially important to smokers. Smokers should not take beta-carotene supplements.

2. Buy a supplement with 400–600 IU of vitamin D if you are elderly, a vegan, or a postmenopausal woman, particularly if you do not drink adequate amounts of vitamin D-fortified milk or do not get enough sunshine. Look for supplements with vitamin D_3, which is more effective than D_2.

3. Buy a supplement containing at least the DV for vitamin E, which is 30 IU. The Consumers Union states you should not take vitamin E to prevent chronic disease; doses of 400 IU or more per day may cause harm. Daily intake of 100–200 IU would appear to pose little risk to most healthy adults. Given the current research data, it may be prudent to limit intake of high-dose vitamin E supplements.

4. Buy a supplement that contains vitamin K. Not all supplements include vitamin K, so check the label. The AI for an adult male is 120 micrograms, but the DV is only 80 micrograms. Multivitamins contain about 25 micrograms.

Water-Soluble Vitamins

1. Buy a supplement that contains 100–200 percent of thiamin, riboflavin, niacin, folic acid, B_6 and B_{12}. You can ignore biotin and pantothenic acid. Check the label to ensure that the supplement contains at least 200–400 micrograms of folic acid, which should complement the diet to provide about 400–600 micrograms per day.

2. Buy a B_{12} supplement that contains 6 micrograms of vitamin B_{12} if you are a vegan, and 25 micrograms if you are elderly. The DV for B_{12} is 6 micrograms, so many supplements contain this amount. Some preparations for seniors may contain the 25 micrograms.

3. Buy a supplement that contains 100–200 percent of vitamin C. The RDA for an adult male is 90 milligrams, yet the DV is only 60 milligrams. The supplement should complement vitamin C intake from a variety of fruits and vegetables.

Minerals

1. Buy a supplement with calcium if you are female or elderly and do not consume adequate dietary calcium. Most multivitamin/mineral tablets contain about 200–300 milligrams of calcium, which can substitute for a serving of low-fat milk. If you consume no dairy products and few calcium-rich foods, you may consider buying a separate calcium supplement.

2. Buy a supplement limited in iron, copper, and zinc, with no more than 100 percent of the RDA for each. The DV for iron is 18 milligrams, while the RDA for young women is 15–18 milligrams. The RDA for adult males and women over age 50 is only 8 milligrams, so men and postmenopausal women may want to select supplements without iron since the diet should provide ample amounts.

3. Buy a supplement that provides no more than 100 milligrams of magnesium and is limited in phosphorus. Magnesium should be obtained primarily from foods, and we normally consume too much phosphorus from foods already.

4. Buy a supplement containing 100 percent of the RDA for chromium and selenium. Selenium is one of the supplements in the SELECT study, mentioned previously, and selenium supplement intake should be limited as suggested in the next chapter.

Food Vitamins and Minerals   Think food first! Although the CSPI published some of these recommendations, they, along with most investigators researching the health implications of vitamin supplementation, note that there is no guarantee of improved health. Almost all health professionals agree we should obtain our vitamin nutrition through consumption of a wide variety of healthful, natural foods, particularly fruits and vegetables. Remember, vitamin supplements do not supply all of the nutrients and other substances, such as phytochemicals, present in foods that are believed to be important to health.

through their natural sources—fruits, vegetables, and other wholesome, natural foods. Such foods also provide other non-essential nutrients that may possess health benefits. Epidemiologic data strongly suggest that diets rich in fruits and vegetables are associated with lower risks of certain chronic diseases, such as heart disease and cancer.

▶ Megadoses of some vitamins are potentially harmful.

▶ In general, health professionals indicate that vitamin supplements are not necessary for the individual on a well-balanced diet, but they may be recommended for certain individuals, such as the elderly, vegans, and women of childbearing age. Moreover, some health professionals note that most people do not consume an optimal amount of vitamins by diet alone and indicate that it appears prudent for all adults to take a vitamin supplement. For most individuals who desire to take vitamin or mineral supplements, a basic multivitamin/mineral tablet should suffice.

Key Concepts

▶ Although several national surveys have reported that some Americans and Canadians are receiving less than the RDA for several vitamins, actual vitamin deficiencies resulting in disease are rare.

▶ Vitamins certainly are essential for good health, but most health professionals recommend that vitamins should be obtained

Check for Yourself

▶ Use a search engine on the Internet, such as www.google.com, and search for "antioxidant vitamins health." Check out the advertisements and claims, and compare to the text discussion.

APPLICATION EXERCISES

Construct a brief, one-page survey regarding vitamin supplements, and other supplements as well, if you like. For example, you might use some of the following questions:

1. Do you take a vitamin supplement?
   _____ Yes _____ No
2. What type of supplement do you take?
   _____ Multivitamin
   _____ Multivitamin/mineral
   _____ Vitamin B Complex
   _____ Vitamin E
   _____ Other

3. How often do you take the supplement?
   _____ Two or more times a day
   _____ Daily
   _____ Several times a week
   _____ Once a week
   _____ Several times a month
   _____ Once a month
   _____ Never
4. Why do you take the vitamin supplement?
   _____ To help guarantee good health
   _____ To enhance my sport or exercise performance
   _____ Other

Once your survey is developed, get permission to administer it to some physically active individuals or athletes, such as participants in recreational sports activities or sports at your school, members of a local cycling or running club, or members of a commercial fitness facility. Share the findings with your class.

Review Questions—Multiple Choice

1. Vitamin A toxicity is most likely to occur from:
   a. consuming too many dark green and deep orange vegetables
   b. eating liver more than once per week
   c. consuming high-dosage vitamin A supplements

   d. drinking too much vitamin A fortified milk
   e. eating rabbit meat two days per week

2. The task of acquiring enough vitamin B_{12} may pose a problem to vegans who do not eat fortified foods because:

   a. fibers in vegetables inhibit its absorption
   b. vegans lack the intrinsic factor
   c. B_{12} is found only in animal products
   d. a deficiency may occur from excess intake of soy products
   e. folacin retards its absorption

3. Which of the following statements is not true about vitamin B_6?

   a. The term vitamin B_6 refers to a family of compounds: pyridoxine, pyridoxal, and pyridoxamine.
   b. As a coenzyme, it acts in the conversion of the amino acid tryptophan to one of the essential vitamins.
   c. It is fat soluble and therefore can be stored in the body.
   d. Foods containing it should be included in the diet daily.
   e. The richest food sources are meats, liver, vegetables, and whole grains.

4. A deficiency of either of these two vitamins produces a similar anemia:

   a. thiamin and riboflavin
   b. riboflavin and niacin
   c. thiamin and vitamin B_2
   d. pantothenic acid and biotin
   e. vitamin B_{12} and folate

5. If an individual is on a well-balanced diet, which of the following vitamin supplements will increase physical performance at sea level competition?

   a. thiamin
   b. niacin

   c. vitamin C
   d. vitamin E
   e. none will

6. Most of the B vitamins function in human metabolism as:

   a. coenzymes
   b. hormones
   c. antioxidants
   d. a source of Calories
   e. activators of mineral metabolism

7. Although athletes on weight reduction diets normally may not need vitamin supplementation, which athletes, based on the nature of their sport, may be best advised to take a supplement?

   a. swimmers
   b. wrestlers
   c. baseball players
   d. field hockey players
   e. sprinters

8. Which of the following are fat-soluble vitamins?

   a. vitamins B, C, D, niacin
   b. vitamin E, niacin, thiamin, riboflavin
   c. vitamins A, D, E, K
   d. vitamins A, B, C, D
   e. vitamins B_1, B_2, B_6, C

9. Which of the following are true B vitamins? (1) inositol (2) choline (3) biotin (4) lipoic acid (5) PABA (6) niacin (7) bioflavinoids (8) ubiquinone (9) vitamin B_6 (10) thiamin (11) laetrile (12) pantothenic acid (13) vitamin B_{15} (14) vitamin P (15) vitamin B_{17}

   a. 1, 2, 3, 5, 7
   b. 2, 4, 7, 8, 9
   c. 3, 6, 9, 10, 12
   d. 5, 9, 11, 13, 15
   e. 7, 11, 12, 14, 15

10. The main function of vitamin E in the body is to act as a(n):

   a. antioxidant
   b. superoxide
   c. free radical
   d. hormone
   e. source of energy

Answers to multiple-choice questions:
1. c; 2. c; 3. c; 4. e; 5. e; 6. a; 7. b; 8. c; 9. c; 10. a.

Review Questions—Essay

1. Explain at least three ways whereby vitamins function in metabolic processes in the human body.
2. Name the four fat-soluble vitamins and describe the metabolic function of each in the human body.

3. Name the nine water-soluble vitamins, and, along with choline, describe their major metabolic functions in the human body.
4. What is coenzyme Q_{10}, why is it purported to be an ergogenic aid, and does

research support its efficacy as an ergogenic?
5. Would you consider taking antioxidant vitamin supplements, such as beta-carotene, E, and C? If so, why so? If not, why not?

References

Books

American Institute of Cancer Research. 2007. *Food, Nutrition, Physical Activity, and the Prevention of Cancer: A Global Perspective.* Washington, DC: AICR.

Bucci, L. 1993. *Nutrients as Ergogenic Aids for Sports and Exercise.* Boca Raton, FL: CRC Press.

Driskell, J., and Wolinsky, I. 2006. *Vitamins and Trace Elements.* Boca Raton, FL: CRC Press.

Keys, A. 1950. *Human Starvation.* Minneapolis, MN: West.

National Academy of Sciences. 2002. *Dietary Reference Intakes for Vitamin A, Vitamin K, Arsenic, Boron, Chromium,*

Copper, Iodine, Iron, Manganese, Molybdenum, Nickel, Silicon, Vanadium, and Zinc. Washington, DC: National Academy Press.

National Academy of Sciences. 2000. *Dietary Reference Intakes for Vitamin C, Vitamin E, Selenium, and Carotenoids.* Washington, DC: National Academy Press.

National Academy of Sciences. 2000. *Dietary Reference Intakes for Thiamin, Riboflavin, Niacin, Vitamin B6, Folate, Vitamin B12, Pantothenic Acid, Biotin, and Choline*. Washington, DC: National Academy Press.

National Academy of Sciences. 1999. *Dietary Reference Intakes for Calcium, Phosphorus, Magnesium, Vitamin D, and Fluoride*. Washington, DC: National Academy Press.

National Academy of Sciences. Institute of Medicine, Food, and Nutrition Board. 2010. *Dietary Reference Intakes for Calcium and Vitamin D*. Washington, DC: National Academy Press.

Shils, M., et al. 2006. *Modern Nutrition in Health and Disease*. Philadelphia: Lippincott Williams & Wilkins.

United States Anti-Doping Agency. 2005. *Optimal Dietary Intake*. U.S. Anti-Doping Agency. Colorado Springs, CO.

Walter, P., et al. eds. 1989. Elevated dosages of vitamins: Benefits and hazards. *International Journal for Vitamin and Nutrition Research,* Supplement 30.

Reviews

Adams, A., and Best, T. 2002. The role of antioxidants in exercise and disease prevention. *Physician and Sportsmedicine* 30 (5):37–44.

American Academy of Pediatrics. 1999. Folic acid for the prevention of neural tube defects. *Pediatrics* 104:325–27.

American Dietetic Association. 2001. Position of the American Dietetic Association: Food fortification and dietary supplements. *Journal of the American Dietetic Association* 101:115–25.

American Dietetic Association. 1996. Position of the American Dietetic Association: Vitamin and mineral supplementation. *Journal of the American Dietetic Association* 96:73–77.

Armstrong, L., and Maresh, C. 1996. Vitamin and mineral supplements as nutritional aids to exercise performance and health. *Nutrition Reviews* 54:S148–S158.

Atalay, M., et al. 2006. Dietary antioxidants for the athlete. *Current Sports Medicine Reports* 5:182–86.

Autier, P., and Gandini, S. 2007. Vitamin D supplementation and total mortality: A meta-analysis of randomized controlled trials. *Archives of Internal Medicine* 167:1730–7.

Bazzano, L., et al. 2006. Effect of folic acid supplementation on risk of cardiovascular diseases: A meta-analysis of randomized controlled trials. *Journal of the American Medical Association* 296:2720–26.

Benardot, D., et al. 2001. Can vitamin supplements improve sport performance? *Sports Science Exchange Roundtable* 12 (3):1–4.

Bender, D. 1999. Non-nutritional uses of vitamin B6. *British Journal of Nutrition* 81:7–20.

Berman, K., and Brodaty, H. 2004. Tocopherol (vitamin E) in Alzheimer's disease and other neurodegenerative disorders. *CNS Drugs* 18:807–25.

Binkley, N., and Krueger, D. 2000. Hypervitaminosis A and bone. *Nutrition Reviews* 58:138–44.

Bischoff-Ferrari, H., and Dawson-Hughes, B. 2007. Where do we stand on vitamin D? *Bone* 41:S13–S19.

Bischoff-Ferrari, H., et al. 2005. Fracture prevention with vitamin D supplementation: A meta-analysis of randomized controlled trials. *JAMA* 293:2257–64.

Bjelakovic, G., et al. 2007. Mortality in randomized trials of antioxidant supplements for primary and secondary prevention: Systematic review and meta-analysis. *Journal of the American Medical Association* 297:842–57.

Bleys, J., et al. 2006. Vitamin-mineral supplementation and the progression of atherosclerosis: A meta-analysis of randomized controlled trials. *American Journal of Clinical Nutrition* 84:880–87.

Block, G. 1992. The data support: A role for antioxidants in reducing cancer risk. *Nutrition Reviews* 50:207–13.

Bouis, H. 1996. Enrichment of food staples through plant breeding: A new strategy for fighting micronutrient malnutrition. *Nutrition Reviews* 54:131–37.

Bourgeois, C., et al. 2006. Niacin. In *Modern Nutrition in Health and Disease,* eds. M. Shils, et al. Philadelphia: Lippincott Williams & Wilkins.

Bügel, S. 2008. Vitamin K and bone health in adult humans. *Vitamins and Hormones* 78:393–416.

Bulow, J. 1993. Lipid metabolism and utilization. In *Principles of Exercise Biochemistry,* ed. J. Poortmans. Basel, Switzerland: Karger.

Calvo, M., et al. 2004. Vitamin D fortification in the United States and Canada: Current status and data needs. *American Journal of Clinical Nutrition* 80:1710S–16S.

Cannell, J., et al. 2009. Athletic performance and vitamin D. *Medicine and Science in Sports and Exercise* 41:1102–10.

Carmel, R. 2006. Folic acid. In *Modern Nutrition in Health and Disease,* eds. M. Shils, et al. Philadelphia: Lippincott Williams & Wilkins.

Chen, J. 2000. Vitamins: Effects of exercise on requirements. In *Nutrition in Sport,* ed. R. Maughan. Oxford: Blackwell Science.

Christen, W. 1999. Antioxidant vitamins and age-related eye disease. *Proceedings of the Association of American Physicians* 111:16–21.

Clarke, R., et al. 2010. Effects of lowering homocysteine levels with B vitamins on cardiovascular disease, cancer, and cause-specific mortality: Meta-analysis of 8 randomized trials involving 37,485 individuals. *Archives of Internal Medicine* 170:1622–31.

Clarkson, P. 1991. Vitamins, iron and trace minerals. In *Perspectives in Exercise Science and Sports Medicine. Ergogenics: The Enhancement of Sports Performance,* eds. D. Lamb and M. Williams. Indianapolis, IN: Benchmark.

Clarkson, P., and Thompson, H. 2000. Antioxidants: What role do they play in physical activity and health? *American Journal of Clinical Nutrition* 72:637S–46S.

Cockayne, S., et al. 2006. Vitamin K and the prevention of fractures: Systematic review and meta-analysis of randomized controlled trials. *Archives of Internal Medicine* 166:1256–61.

Coleman, H., and Chew, E. 2007. Nutritional supplementation in age-related macular degeneration. *Current Opinion in Ophthalmology* 18:220–23.

Consumers Union. 2007. Antioxidant reality check. *Consumer Reports on Health* 19 (9):1, 4–5.

Consumers Union. 2006. Multivitamins: What to avoid, how to choose. *Consumer Reports* 71 (2):19–20.

Consumers Union. 2005. Vitamin E pills: What to do now? *Consumer Reports on Health* 17 (7):3.

Consumers Union. 2004. Disease-fighting B vitamins. *Consumer Reports on Health* 16 (1):10.

Consumers Union. 2002. Do you need more vitamin D? *Consumer Reports on Health* 14 (11):1, 4–5.

Consumers Union. 2001. Surprising health risk from low vitamin C? *Consumer Reports on Health* 13 (5):7.

Consumers Union. 2001. Vitamin A: How much is too much? *Consumer Reports on Health* 13 (10):1, 4–5.

Das, S., et al. 2007. Tocotrienols in cardioprotection. *Vitamins and Hormones* 76:419–33.

Devaraj, S., and Jialal, I. 1998. The effects of alpha-tocopherol on critical cells in atherogenesis. *Current Opinion in Lipidology* 9:11–15.

Diplock, A. 1997. Will the 'good fairies' please prove to us that vitamin E lessens human degenerative disease? *Free Radical Research* 26:565–83.

Douglas, R., et al. 2007. Vitamin C for preventing and treating the common cold. *Cochrane Database of Systematic Reviews* 18(3):CD000980.

Eichholzer, M., et al. 2006. Folic acid: A public-health challenge. *Lancet* 367:1352–61.

Enstrom, J. 1993. Counterpoint: Vitamin C and mortality. *Nutrition Today* 28 (May/June):39–42.

Evans, J. 2006. Antioxidant vitamin and mineral supplements for slowing the progression of age-related macular degeneration. *Cochrane Database of Systematic Reviews* (2):CD000254.

Evans, J., and Henshaw, K. 2008. Antioxidant vitamin and mineral supplements for age-related macular degeneration. *Cochrane Database of Systematic Reviews* (1):CD000253.

Fairfield, K., and Fletcher, R. 2002. Vitamins for chronic disease prevention in adults: Scientific review. *JAMA* 287:3116–26.

Fairfield, K., and Stampfer, M. 2007. Vitamin and mineral supplements for cancer prevention: Issues and evidence. *American Journal of Clinical Nutrition* 85:289S–292S.

Fletcher, R., and Fairfield, K. 2002. Vitamins for chronic disease prevention in adults: Clinical applications. *JAMA* 287:3127–29.

Fogelholm, M. 2000. Vitamins: Metabolic functions. In *Nutrition in Sport*, ed. R. J. Maughan. Oxford: Blackwell Science.

Futterman, L., and Lemberg, L. 1999. The use of antioxidants in retarding atherosclerosis: Fact or fiction? *American Journal of Critical Care* 8:130–33.

Gaziano, J., and Hennekens, C. 1996. Update on dietary antioxidants and cancer. *Pathological Biology* 44:42–45.

Gerster, H. 1997. No contribution of ascorbic acid to renal calcium oxalate stones. *Annals of Nutrition and Metabolism* 41:269–82.

Gerster, H. 1989. Review: The role of vitamin C in athletic performance. *Journal of the American College of Nutrition* 8:636–43.

Gilchrest, B. 2007. Sun protection and Vitamin D: Three dimensions of obfuscation. *Journal of Steroid Biochemistry and Molecular Biology* 103:655–63.

Gorham, E., et al. 2007. Optimal vitamin D status for colorectal cancer prevention: A quantitative meta-analysis. *American Journal of Preventive Medicine* 32:210–6.

Grant, W., et al. 2007. An estimate of cancer mortality rate reductions in Europe and the US with 1,000 IU of oral vitamin D per day. *Recent Results in Cancer Research* 174:225–34.

Greenwald, P., et al. 2007. Clinical trials of vitamin and mineral supplements for cancer prevention. *American Journal of Clinical Nutrition* 85:314S–317S.

Guyton, J., and Bays, H. 2007. Safety considerations with niacin therapy. *American Journal of Cardiology* 99:22C–31C.

Halliwell, B. 1996. Oxidative stress, nutrition and health: Experimental strategies for optimization of nutritional antioxidant intake in humans. *Free Radical Research* 25:57–74.

Hamilton, K. 2007. Antioxidants and cardioprotection. *Medicine and Science in Sports and Exercise* 39:1544–53.

Harris, S. 2005. Vitamin D in type 1 diabetes prevention. *Journal of Nutrition* 135:323–25.

Hathcock, J. 1997. Vitamins and minerals: Efficacy and safety. *American Journal of Clinical Nutrition* 66:427–37.

Hathcock, J., and Shao, A. 2006. Risk assessment of coenzyme Q_{10} (Ubiquinone). *Regulations in Toxicology and Pharmacology* 45:282–88.

Hathcock, J., et al. 2007. Risk assessment for vitamin D. *American Journal of Clinical Nutrition* 85:6–18.

Hathcock, J., et al. 2005. Vitamins E and C are safe across a broad range of intakes. *American Journal of Clinical Nutrition* 81:736–45.

Heaney, R., 2007. Bone health. *American Journal of Clinical Nutrition* 85:300S–303S.

Heaney, R. 2005. The vitamin D requirement in health and disease. *Journal of Steroid Biochemistry and Molecular Biology* 97:13–19.

Hemila, H. 2004. Vitamin C supplementation and respiratory infections: A systematic review. *Military Medicine* 169:920–25.

Herbert, V. 1993. Viewpoint: Does mega-C do more good than harm, or more harm than good? *Nutrition Today* 28 (January/February):28–32.

Holick, M. 2006. Vitamin D. In *Modern Nutrition in Health and Disease*, eds. M. Shils, et al. Philadelphia: Lippincott Williams & Wilkins.

Holick, M., and Chen, T. 2008. Vitamin D deficiency: A worldwide problem with health consequences. *American Journal of Clinical Nutrition* 87:1080S–86S.

Hunninghake, D. 1999. Pharmacologic management of triglycerides. *Clinical Cardiology* II44–II48.

Hyang, H., et al. 2006. The efficacy and safety of multivitamin and mineral supplement use to prevent cancer and chronic disease in adults: A systematic review for a National Institutes of Health state-of-the-science conferences. *Annals of Internal Medicine* 145:372–85.

Jackson, C., et al. 2007. The effect of cholecalciferol (vitamin D3) on the risk of fall and fracture: A meta-analysis. *QJM* 100:185–92.

Jackson, H., and Sheehan, A. 2005. Effect of vitamin A on fracture risk. *Annals of Pharmacotherapy* 39:2086–90.

Jackson, M., et al. 2004. Vitamin E and the oxidative stress of exercise. *Annals of the New York Academy of Sciences* 1031:158–68.

Jacob, R. 1999. Vitamin C. In *Modern Nutrition in Health and Disease*, eds. M. Shils et al. Baltimore: Williams & Wilkins.

Jacques, P. 1999. The potential preventive effects of vitamins for cataract and age-related macular degeneration. *International Journal of Vitamin and Nutrition Research* 69:198–205.

Ji, L. 2008. Modulation of skeletal muscle antioxidant defense by exercise: Role of redox signaling. *Free Radicals in Biology and Medicine* 44:142–52.

Ji, L. 2002. Exercise-induced modulation of antioxidant defense. *New York Academy of Sciences* 959:82–92.

Ji, L. 2000. Free radicals and antioxidants in exercise and sports. In *Exercise and Sport Science*, eds. W. Garrett and D. Kirkendall. Philadelphia: Lippincott Williams & Wilkins.

Johnson, E. 2002. The role of carotenoids in human health. *Nutrition in Clinical Care* 5:56–65.

Joubert, L., and Manore, M. 2006. Exercise, nutrition, and homocysteine. *International Journal of Sport Nutrition and Exercise Metabolism* 16:341–61.

Keith, R. 1994. Vitamins and physical activity. In *Nutrition in Exercise and Sport*, eds. I. Wolinsky and J. Hickson. Boca Raton, FL: CRC Press.

Kimmick, G., et al. 1997. Vitamin E and breast cancer: A review. *Nutrition and Cancer* 27:109–17.

Koltover, V. 1992. Free radical theory of aging: View against the reliability theory. *EXS* 62:11–19.

Kontush, K., and Schekatolina, S. 2004. Vitamin E in neurodegenerative disorders: Alzheimer's disease. *Annals of the New York Academy of Sciences* 1031:249–62.

Kris-Etherton, P., et al. 2004. Antioxidant vitamin supplements and cardiovascular disease. *Circulation* 110:637–41.

Lachance, P. 1998. Overview of key nutrients: Micronutrient aspects. *Nutrition Reviews* 56:S34–S39.

Larson-Meyer, D., and Willis, K. 2010. Vitamin D and athletes. *Current Sports Medicine Reports* 9:220–6.

Lawson, K., et al. 2007. Multivitamin use and risk of prostate cancer in the National Institutes of Health-AARP Diet and Health Study. *Journal of the National Cancer Institute* 99:754–64.

Lee, I. 1999. Antioxidant vitamins in the prevention of cancer. *Proceedings of the American Association of Physicians* 111:10–15.

Levine, M., et al. 2006. Vitamin C. In *Modern Nutrition in Health and Disease,* eds. M. Shils et al. Philadelphia: Lippincott Williams & Wilkins.

Liebman, B. 2006. Are you deficient? *Nutrition Action Health Letter* 33 (9):1–7.

Liebman, B. 2006. Folic acid. *Nutrition Action Health Letter* 33 (1):8–11.

Liebman, B. 2004. Eye wise: Seeing into the future. *Nutrition Action Health Letter* 31 (9):1–7.

Liebman, B. 2003. Spin the bottle: How to pick a multivitamin. *Nutrition Action Health Letter* 30 (1):1–9.

Liebman, B. 2002. Antioxidants: No magic bullets. *Nutrition Action Health Letter* 29 (3):1–8.

Liebman, B., and Hurley, J. 2002. Vegetables: Vitamin K weighs in. *Nutrition Action Health Letter* 29 (6):13–15.

Liebman, B., and Schardt, D. 2008. Multi-Complex: Picking a multivitamin gets tricky. *Nutrition Action Health Letter* 35(5):1–9.

Linnane, A., et al. 2007. The essential requirement for superoxide radical and nitric oxide formation for normal physiological function and healthy aging. *Mitochondrion* 7:1–5.

Lukaski, H. 2004. Vitamin and mineral status: Effects on physical performance. *Nutrition* 20:632–44.

Manore, M. 2001. Vitamins and minerals: Part I. How much do I need? *ACSM's Health and Fitness Journal* 5 (3):33–35.

Manore, M. 2001. Vitamins and minerals: Part II. Who needs to supplement? *ACSM's Health and Fitness Journal* 5 (4):30–34.

Manore, M. 2001. Vitamins and minerals: Part III. Can you get too much? *ACSM's Health and Fitness Journal* 5 (5):26–28.

Manore, M. 1994. Vitamin B$_6$ and exercise. *International Journal of Sport Nutrition* 4:89–103.

Mansfield, L., and Goldstein, G. 1981. Anaphylactic reaction after ingestion of local bee pollen. *Annals of Allergy* 47:154–56.

Mayne, S. 1996. Beta-carotene, carotenoids, and disease prevention in humans. *FASEB Journal* 10:690–701.

McCormick, D. 2006. Riboflavin. In *Modern Nutrition in Health and Disease,* eds. M. Shils et al. Philadelphia: Lippincott Williams & Wilkins.

McGinley, C., et al. 2009. Does antioxidant vitamin supplementation protect against muscle damage? *Sports Medicine* 39:1011–32.

McKenney, J. 2004. New perspectives on the use of niacin in the treatment of lipid disorders. *Archives of Internal Medicine* 164:697–705.

McMahon, R. 2002. Biotin in metabolism and molecular biology. *Annual Review of Nutrition* 22:221–39.

Mehta, J. 1999. Antioxidants are useful in preventing cardiovascular disease: A debate. Con antioxidants. *Canadian Journal of Cardiology* 15:26B–28B.

Meydani, S. 1995. Vitamin E enhancement of T cell-mediated function in healthy elderly: Mechanisms of action. *Nutrition Reviews* 53:S52–S58.

Miller, E., et al. 2005. Meta-analysis: High-dosage vitamin E supplementation may increase all-cause mortality. *Annals of Internal Medicine* 142:37–46.

Mock, D. 2006. Biotin. In *Modern Nutrition in Health and Disease,* eds. M. Shils, et al. Philadelphia: Lippincott Williams & Wilkins.

Moon, J., et al. 1992. Hypothesis: Etiology of atherosclerosis and osteoporosis: Are imbalances in the calciferol endocrine system implicated? *Journal of the American College of Nutrition* 11:567–83.

Mulholland, C., and Benford, D. 2007. What is known about the safety of multivitamin-multimineral supplements for the generally healthy population? Theoretical basis for harm. *American Journal of Clinical Nutrition* 85:318S–322S.

Munoz, F., et al. 2005. The protective effect of vitamin E in vascular amyloid beta-mediated damage. *Subcellular Biochemestry* 38:147–65.

National Institutes of Health. 2006. National Institutes of Health State-of-the-Science conference statement: Multivitamin/mineral supplements and chronic disease prevention. *Annals of Internal Medicine* 145:364–71.

Neiss, A. 2005. Generation and disposal of reactive oxygen and nitrogen species. In *Molecular and Cellular Exercise Physiology,* eds. F. Mooren and K. Völker. Champaign, IL: Human Kinetics.

Ness, A., et al. 1997. Vitamin C and blood pressure: An overview. *Journal of Human Hypertension* 11:342–50.

Nieman, D. 2001. Exercise immunology: Nutritional countermeasures. *Canadian Journal of Applied Physiology* 26:S45–55.

Office of Dietary Supplements. National Institutes of Health. 2011. Dietary Supplement Fact Sheet: Vitamin D. http://ods.od.nih.gov/factsheets/vitamind/

Peake, J. 2003. Vitamin C: Effects of exercise and requirements with training. *International Journal of Sport Nutrition and Exercise Metabolism* 13:125–51.

Penry, J., and Manore, M. 2008. Choline: An important micronutrient for maximal endurance-exercise performance. *International Journal of Sport Nutrition and Exercise Metabolism* 18:191–203.

Pieper, J. 2002. Understanding niacin formulations. *American Journal of Management Care* 8:S308–14.

Powers, S., et al. 2004. Dietary antioxidants and exercise. *Journal of Sports Sciences* 22:81–94.

Prasad, K., et al. 1999. High doses of multiple antioxidant vitamins: Essential ingredients in improving the efficacy of standard cancer therapy. *Journal of the American College of Nutrition* 18:13–25.

Prentice, R. 2007. Clinical trials and observational studies to assess the chronic disease benefits and risks of multivitamin-multimineral supplements. *American Journal of Clinical Nutrition* 85:308S–13S.

Pryor, W., et al. 2000. Beta carotene: From biochemistry to clinical trials. *Nutrition Reviews* 58:39–53.

Raiten, D., and Picciano, M. 2004. Vitamin D and health in the 21st century: Bone and beyond. *American Journal of Clinical Nutrition* 80:1673S–77S.

Reichrath, J., et al. 2007. Vitamins as hormones. *Hormone and Metabolic Research* 39:71–84.

Rimm, E., and Stampfer, M. 1997. The role of antioxidants in preventive cardiology. *Current Opinion in Cardiology* 12:188–94.

Rock, C. 2007. Multivitamin-multimineral supplements: Who uses them? *American Journal of Clinical Nutrition* 85:277S–79S.

Rodrigo, R., et al. 2007. Clinical pharmacology and therapeutic use of antioxidant vitamins. *Fundamental and Clinical Pharmacology* 21:111–27.

Rosenberg, I. 2007. Challenges and opportunities in the translation of the science of vitamins. *American Journal of Clinical Nutrition* 85:325S–27S.

Ross, A. 2006. Vitamin A and retinoids. In *Modern Nutrition in Health and Disease,* eds. M. Shils, et al. Philadelphia: Lippincott Williams & Wilkins.

Rothenberg, S. 1999. Increasing the dietary intake of folate: Pros and cons. *Seminars in Hematology* 36:65–74.

Sacheck, J., and Blumberg, J. 2001. Role of vitamin E and oxidative stress in exercise. *Nutrition* 17:809–14.

Sacheck, J., and Roubenoff, R. 1999. Nutrition in the exercising elderly. *Clinics in Sports Medicine* 18:565–84.

Schardt, D. 2006. Supplementing their income: How celebrities turn trust into cash. *Nutrition Action Health Letter* 33 (1):1–6.

Schürks, M., et al. 2010. Effects of vitamin E on stroke subtypes: Meta-analysis of randomised controlled trials. *British Medical Journal* 341:c5702.

Schwammenthal, Y., and Tanne, D. 2004. Homocysteine B-vitamin supplementation, and stroke prevention: From observational to interventional trials. *Lancet Neurology* 3:493–95.

Schwartz, B., and Skinner, H. 2007. Vitamin D status and cancer: New insights. *Current Opinion in Clinical Nutrition and Metabolic Care* 10:6–11.

Seddon, J. 2007. Multivitamin-multimineral supplements and eye disease: Age-related macular degeneration and cataract. *American Journal of Clinical Nutrition* 85:304S–307S.

Sen, C., et al. 2007. Tocotrienols: The emerging face of natural vitamin E. *Vitamins and Hormones* 76:203–61.

Sen, C., et al. 2006. Tocotrienols: Vitamin E beyond tocopherols. *Life Sciences* 78:2088–98.

Sen, C., et al. 2000. Exercise-induced oxidative stress and antioxidant nutrients. In *Nutrition in Sport,* ed. R. Maughan. Oxford: Blackwell Science.

Short, S. 1994. Surveys of dietary intake and nutrition knowledge of athletes and their coaches. In *Nutrition in Exercise and Sport,* eds. I. Wolinsky and J. Hickson. Boca Raton, FL: CRC Press.

Simon-Schnass, I. 1993. Vitamin requirements for increased physical activity: Vitamin E. In *Nutrition and Fitness for Athletes* 71:144–53, eds. A. Simopoulos and K. Pavlou. Basel, Switzerland: Karger.

Singh, U., and Devaraj, S. 2007. Vitamin E: Inflammation and atherosclerosis. *Vitamins and Hormones* 76:519–49.

Sobol, J., and Marquart, L. 1994. Vitamin/mineral supplement use among athletes:
A review of the literature. *International Journal of Sport Nutrition* 4:320–34.

Steinmetz, K., and Potter, J. 1996. Vegetables, fruit, and cancer prevention: A review. *Journal of the American Dietetic Association* 96:1027–39.

Stipanuk, M. 2006. Homocysteine, cysteine and taurine. In *Modern Nutrition in Health and Disease,* eds. M. Shils et al. Philadelphia: Lippincott Williams & Wilkins.

Suttie, J. 2006. Vitamin K. In *Modern Nutrition in Health and Disease,* eds. M. Shils et al. Philadelphia: Lippincott Williams & Wilkins.

Takanami, Y., et al. 2000. Vitamin E supplementation and endurance exercise: Are there benefits? *Sports Medicine* 29:73–83.

Tanphaichitr, V. 1999. Thiamin. In *Modern Nutrition in Health and Disease,* eds. M. Shils et al. Philadelphia: Lippincott Williams & Wilkins.

Tiidus, P., and Houston, M. 1995. Vitamin E status and response to exercise training. *Sports Medicine* 20:12–23.

Traber, M. 2007. Heart disease and single-vitamin supplementation. *American Journal of Clinical Nutrition* 85:293S–99S.

Traber, M. 2006. Vitamin E. In *Modern Nutrition in Health and Disease,* eds. M. Shils et al. Philadelphia: Lippincott Williams & Wilkins.

Tran, M., et al. 2001. Role of coenzyme Q_{10} in chronic heart failure, angina, and hypertension. *Pharmacotherapy* 21:797–806.

Trumbo, P., and Ellwood, K. 2006. Lutein and zeaxanthin intakes and risk of age-related macular degeneration and cataracts: An evaluation using the Food and Drug Administration's evidence-based review system for health claims. *American Journal of Clinical Nutrition* 84:971–74.

Tufts University. 2007. Antioxidant supplements—Now what? *Tufts University Health and Nutrition Letter* 25 (4):4–5.

Tufts University. 2007. Are you getting enough vitamin D? *Tufts University Health and Nutrition Letter* 25 (10):1–2.

Tufts University. 2002. Antioxidant supplements lose promise as disease preventers. *Tufts University Health and Nutrition Letter* 20 (1):4–5.

Tufts University. 2002. Eating for eye health. *Tufts University Health and Nutrition Letter* 19 (11):4–5.

van der Beek, E. 1991. Vitamin supplementation and physical exercise performance. *Journal of Sports Sciences* 92:77–79.

Vieth, R. 1999. Vitamin D supplementation, 25-hydroxyvitamin D concentrations,
and safety. *American Journal of Clinical Nutrition* 69:842–56.

Vieth, R., and Fraser, D. 2002. Vitamin D insufficiency: No recommended dietary allowance exists for this nutrient. *Canadian Medical Association Journal* 166:1541–42.

Viitala, P., and Newhouse, I. 2004. Vitamin E supplementation, exercise and lipid peroxidation in human participants. *European Journal of Applied Physiology* 93:108–15.

Volpe, S. 2007. Micronutrient requirements for athletes. *Clinics in Sports Medicine* 26:119–30.

Wang, X., et al. 2007. Efficacy of folic acid supplementation in stroke prevention: A meta-analysis. *Lancet* 369:1876–82.

Webb, D. 1997. Coenzyme Q_{10}: Miracle nutrient or merely promising? *Environmental Nutrition* 20 (11): 1, 4.

Weber, P. 2001. Vitamin K and bone health. *Nutrition* 17:880–87.

Weber, P. 1996. Vitamin C and human health: A review of recent data relevant to human requirements. *International Journal of Vitamin and Nutrition Research* 66:19–30.

Wierzbicki, A. 2007. Homocysteine and cardiovascular disease: A review of the evidence. *Diabetes and Vascular Disease Research* 4:143–50.

Williams, M. 2011. Sports supplements: Quercetin. *ACSM Health & Fitness Journal* 15(5):17–20.

Williams, M. 1989. Vitamin supplementation and athletic performance. *International Journal for Vitamin and Nutrition Research,* Supplement 30:161–91.

Williams, S., et al. 2006. Antioxidant requirements of endurance athletes: Implications for health. *Nutrition Reviews* 64:93–108.

Willis, K., et al. 2008. Should we be concerned about the vitamin D status of athletes? *International Journal of Sport Nutrition and Exercise Metabolism* 18:204–24.

Woolf, K., and Manore, M. 2006. B-vitamins and exercise: Does exercise alter requirements? *International Journal of Sport Nutrition and Exercise Metabolism* 16:453–84.

Yetley, E. 2007. Multivitamin and multimineral dietary supplements: Definitions, characterization, bioavailability, and drug interactions. *American Journal of Clinical Nutrition* 85:269S–76S.

Zachman, R., and Grummer, M. 1998. The interaction of ethanol and vitamin A as a potential mechanism for the pathogenesis of Fetal Alcohol Syndrome. *Alcoholism, Clinical and Experimental Research* 22:1544–56.

Zeisel, S., and Niculescu, M. 2006. Choline and phosphatidylcholine. In *Modern Nutrition in Health and Disease,* eds. M. Shils, et al. Philadelphia: Lippincott Williams & Wilkins.

Zittermann, A. 2001. Effects of vitamin K on calcium and bone metabolism. *Current Opinion in Clinical Nutrition and Metabolic Care* 4:483–87.

Specific Studies

AIM-HIGH Investigators. 2011. The role of niacin in raising high-density lipoprotein cholesterol to reduce cardiovascular events in patients with atherosclerotic cardiovascular disease and optimally treated low-density lipoprotein cholesterol: Rationale and study design. The Atherothrombosis Intervention in Metabolic syndrome with low HDL/high triglycerides: Impact on global health outcomes (AIM-HIGH). *American Heart Journal* 161:471–77.

Ardestani, A., et al. 2011. Relation of vitamin D level to maximal oxygen uptake in adults. *American Journal of Cardiology* 107:1246–9.

Ascherio, A., et al. 1999. Relation of consumption of vitamin E, vitamin C, and carotenoids to risk for stroke among men in the United States. *Annals of Internal Medicine* 130:963–70.

Bell, C., et al. 2005. Ascorbic acid does not affect the age-associated reduction in maximal cardiac output and oxygen consumption in healthy adults. *Journal of Applied Physiology* 98:845–49.

Bloomer, R., et al. 2006. Oxidative stress response to aerobic exercise. *Medicine and Science in Sports and Exercise* 38:1098–1105.

Bonetti, A., et al. 2000. Effect of ubidecarenone oral treatment on aerobic power in middle-aged trained subjects. *Journal of Sports Medicine and Physical Fitness* 40:51–57.

Bonke, D. 1986. Influence of vitamin B_1, B_6 and B_{12} on the control of fine motoric movements. *Bibliotheca Nutritio et Dieta* 38:104–9.

Braam, L., et al. 2003. Factors affecting bone loss in female endurance athletes: A two-year follow-up study. *American Journal of Sports Medicine* 31:889–95.

Braun, B., et al. 1991. The effect of coenzyme Q_{10} supplementation on exercise performance, VO_2 max, and lipid peroxidation in trained cyclists. *International Journal of Sport Nutrition* 1:353–65.

Broe, K., et al. 2007. A higher dose of vitamin D reduces the risk of falls in nursing home residents: A randomized, multiple-dose study. *Journal of the American Geriatric Society* 55:234–39.

Bryer, S., and Goldfarb, A. 2006. Effect of high dose vitamin C supplementation on muscle soreness, damage, function, and oxidative stress to eccentric exercise. *International Journal of Sport Nutrition and Exercise Metabolism* 16:270–80.

Buchman, A., et al. 2000. The effect of lecithin supplementation on plasma choline concentrations during a marathon. *Journal of the American College of Nutrition* 19:768–70.

Chandler, J., and Hawkins, J. 1984. The effect of bee pollen on physiological performance. *International Journal of Biosocial Research* 6:107–14.

Chiu, K., et al. 2004. Hypovitaminosis D is associated with insulin resistance and β cell dysfunction. *American Journal of Clinical Nutrition* 79:820–25.

Close, G., et al. 2006. Ascorbic acid supplementation does not attenuate post-exercise muscle soreness following muscle-damaging exercise but may delay the recovery process. *British Journal of Nutrition* 95:976–81.

Coburn, S., et al. 1990. Effect of vitamin B_6 intake on the vitamin content of human muscle. *FASEB Journal* 4:A365.

Cole, B., et al. 2007. Folic acid for the prevention of colorectal adenomas: A randomized clinical trial. *Journal of the American Medical Association* 297:2351–59.

Craciun, A., et al. 1998. Improved bone metabolism in female elite athletes after vitamin K supplementation. *International Journal of Sports Medicine* 19:479–84.

Curhan, G., et al. 1996. A prospective study of the intake of vitamin C and B_6, and the risk of kidney stones in men. *Journal of Urology* 155:1847–51.

Davison, G., and Gleeson, M. 2006. The effect of 2 weeks vitamin C supplementation on immunoendocrine responses to 2.5 h cycling exercise in man. *European Journal of Applied Physiology* 97:454–61.

Davison, G., and Gleeson, M. 2005. Influence of acute vitamin C and/or carbohydrate ingestion on hormonal, cytokine, and immune responses to prolonged exercise. *International Journal of Sport Nutrition and Exercise Metabolism* 15:465–79.

Davison, G., et al. 2007. Antioxidant supplementation and immunoendocrine responses to prolonged exercise. *Medicine and Science in Sports and Exercise* 39:645–52.

Dawson, B., et al. 2002. Effect of vitamin C and E supplementation on biochemical and ultrastructural indices of muscle damage after a 21-km run. *International Journal of Sports Medicine* 23:10–15.

Dhesi, J., et al. 2004. Vitamin D supplementation improves neuromuscular function in older people who fall. *Age and Ageing* 33:589–95.

Dobnig, H., et al. 2008. Independent association of low serum 25-hydroxyvitamin D and 1,25-dihydroxyvitamin D levels with all-cause and cardiovascular mortality. *Archives of International Medicine* 168:1340–9.

Doyle, M., et al. 1997. Allithiamine ingestion does not enhance isokinetic parameters of muscle performance. *International Journal of Sport Nutrition* 7:39–47.

Englehart, M., et al. 2002. Dietary intake of antioxidants and risk of Alzheimer disease. *JAMA* 287:3223–29.

Feskanich, D., et al. 2002. Vitamin A intake and hip fractures among postmenopausal women. *JAMA* 287:47–54.

Finaud, J., et al. 2006. Oxidative stress: Relationship with exercise and training. *Sports Medicine* 36:327–48.

Fry, A., et al. 2006. Effect of a liquid multivitamin/mineral supplement on anaerobic exercise performance. *Research in Sports Medicine* 14:53–64.

Gauche, E., et al. 2006. Vitamin and mineral supplementation and neuromuscular recovery after a running race. *Medicine and Science in Sports and Exercise* 38:2110–17.

Giovannucci, E., et al. 2008. 25-hydroxyvitamin D and risk of myocardial infarction in men: A prospective study. *Archives of Internal Medicine* 168:1174–80.

Gökbel, H., et al. 2010. The effects of coenzyme Q_{10} supplementation on performance during repeated bouts of supramaximal exercise in sedentary men. *Journal of Strength and Conditioning Research* 24:97–102.

Gomez-Cabrera, M., et al. 2008. Oral administration of vitamin C decreases muscle mitochondrial biogenesis and hampers training-induced adaptions in endurance performance. *American Journal of Clinical Nutrition* 87:142–49.

Gomez-Cabrera, M., et al. 2006. Oxidative stress in marathon runners: Interest in antioxidant supplementation. *British Journal of Nutrition* 96:S31–S33.

Gridley, G., et al. 1992. Vitamin supplement use and reduced risk of oral and pharyngeal cancer. *American Journal of Epidemiology* 135:1083–92.

Gül, I., et al. 2011. Oxidative stress and antioxidant defense in plasma after repeated bouts of supramaximal exercise: The effect of coenzyme Q$_{10}$. *Journal of Sports Medicine and Physical Fitness* 51:305–12.

Halliday, T., et al. 2011. Vitamin D status relative to diet, lifestyle, injury, and illness in college athletes. *Medicine and Science in Sports and Exercise* 43:335–43.

Haralambie, G. 1976. Vitamin B$_2$ status in athletes and the influence of riboflavin administration on neuromuscular irritability. *Nutrition and Metabolism* 20:1–8.

Heath, E., et al. 1993. Effect of nicotinic acid on respiratory exchange ratio and substrate levels during exercise. *Medicine and Science in Sport and Exercise* 25:1018–23.

Henson, D., et al. 2008. Post-160-km race illness rates and decreases in granulocyte respiratory burst and salivary IGA output are not countered by quercetin ingestion. *International Journal of Sports Medicine* 29:856–63.

Hollis, B., et al. 2011. Vitamin D supplementation during pregnancy: Double-blind, randomized clinical trial of safety and effectiveness. *Journal of Bone Mineral Research* Epub June 27.

Itoh, H., et al. 2000. Vitamin E supplementation attenuates leakage of enzymes following 6 successive days of running training. *International Journal of Sport Medicine* 21:369–74.

Jackson, R., et al. 2006. Calcium plus vitamin D supplementation and the risk of fractures. *New England Journal of Medicine* 354:669–83.

Jacobson, B., et al. 2001. Nutrition practices and knowledge of college varsity athletes: A follow-up. *Journal of Strength and Conditioning Research* 15:63–68.

Johnston, C., et al. 1998. Vitamin C status of a campus population: College students get a C minus. *Journal of the American College of Health* 46:209–13.

Kaikkonen, J., et al. 1998. Effect of combined coenzyme Q$_{10}$ and d-alpha-tocopheryl acetate supplementation on exercise-induced lipid peroxidation and muscular damage: A placebo-controlled double-blind study in marathon runners. *Free Radical Research* 29:85–92.

Kim, I., et al. 1993. Vitamin and mineral supplement use and mortality in a U.S. cohort. *American Journal of Public Health* 83:546–50.

Knez, W., et al. 2007. Oxidative stress in half and full ironman triathletes. *Medicine and Science in Sports and Exercise* 39:283–88.

Kobayashi, Y. 1974. Effect of vitamin E on aerobic work performance in man during acute exposure to hypoxic hypoxia. Unpublished doctoral dissertation. University of New Mexico.

Kolka, M., and Stephenson, L. 1990. Skin blood flow during exercise after niacin ingestion. *FASEB Journal* 4:A279.

Krumbach, C., et al. 1999. A report of vitamin and mineral supplement use among university athletes in a Division I institution. *International Journal of Sport Nutrition* 9:416–25.

Kurl, S., et al. 2002. Plasma vitamin C modifies the association between hypertension and risk of stroke. *Stroke* 33:1568–73.

Laaksonen, R., et al. 1995. Ubiquinone supplementation and exercise capacity in trained young and older men. *European Journal of Applied Physiology* 72:95–100.

Lappe, J., et al. 2007. Vitamin D and calcium supplementation reduces cancer risk: Results of a randomized trial. *American Journal of Clinical Nutrition* 85:1586–91.

Lee, I., et al. 2005. Vitamin E in the primary prevention of cardiovascular disease and cancer: The Women's Health Study: a randomized controlled trial. *Journal of the American Medical Association* 294:56–65.

Leonard, S., and Leklem, J. 2000. Plasma B-6 vitamer changes following a 50-km ultra-marathon. *International Journal of Sport Nutrition and Exercise Metabolism* 10:302–14.

Lonn, E., et al. 2005. Effects of long-term vitamin E supplementation on cardiovascular events and cancer: A randomized controlled trial. *JAMA* 293:1338–47.

Losonczy, K., et al. 1996. Vitamin E and vitamin C supplement use and risk of all cause and coronary heart disease mortality in older persons: The Established Populations for Epidemiologic Studies of the Elderly. *American Journal of Clinical Nutrition* 64:190–96.

Machefer, G., et al. 2007. Multivitamin-mineral supplementation prevents lipid peroxidation during "the Marathon des Sables." *Journal of the American College of Nutrition* 26:111–20.

MacRae, H., and Mefferd, K. 2006. Dietary antioxidant supplementation combined with quercetin improves cycling time trial performance. *International Journal of Sport Nutrition and Exercise Metabolism* 16:405–19.

Malm, C., et al. 1996. Supplementation with ubiquinone-10 causes cellular damage during intense exercise. *Acta Physiologica Scandinavica* 157:511–12.

Massey, L., et al. 2005. Ascorbate increases human oxaluria and kidney stone risk. *Journal of Nutrition* 135:1673–77.

Mastaloudis, A., et al, 2006. Antioxidants did not prevent muscle damage in response to an ultramarathon run. *Medicine and Science in Sports and Exercise* 38:72–80.

Matter, M., et al. 1987. The effect of iron and folate therapy on maximal exercise performance in female marathon runners with iron and folate deficiency. *Clinical Science* 72:415–22.

McAnulty, S., et al. 2008. Chronic quercetin ingestion and exercise-induced oxidative damage and inflammation. *Applied Physiology, Nutrition and Metabolism* 33:254–62.

McKinley, M., et al. 2001. Low-dose vitamin B-6 effectively lowers fasting plasma homocysteine in healthy elderly persons who are folate and riboflavin replete. *American Journal of Clinical Nutrition* 73:759–64.

McMahon, J., et al. 2007. Lowering homocysteine with B vitamins has no effect on blood pressure in older adults. *Journal of Nutrition* 137:1183–87.

Meagher, E., et al. 2001. Effects of vitamin E on lipid peroxidation in healthy persons. *JAMA* 285:1178–82.

Morris, M., et al. 2002. Dietary intake of antioxidant nutrients and the risk of incident Alzheimer disease in a biracial community study. *JAMA* 287:3230–37.

Morris, M., et al. 1998. Vitamin E and vitamin C supplement use and risk of incident Alzheimer disease. *Alzheimer Disease and Associated Disorders* 12:121–26.

Murray, R., et al. 1995. Physiological and performance responses to nicotinic-acid ingestion during exercise. *Medicine and Science in Sport and Exercise* 27:1057–62.

Nielsen, A., et al. 1999. No effect of antioxidant supplementation in triathletes on maximal oxygen uptake, 31P-NMRS detected muscle energy metabolism and muscle fatigue. *International Journal of Sports Medicine* 20:154–58.

Nieman, D., et al. 2007. Quercetin ingestion does not alter cytokine changes in athletes competing in the Western States Endurance Run. *Journal of Interferon and Cyokine Research* 27:1003–11.

Nieman, D., et al. 2007. Quercetin reduces illness, but not immune perturbations after intensive exercise. *Medicine and Science in Sports and Exercise* 39:1561–69.

Nieman, D., et al. 2007. Quercetin's influence on exercise-induced changes in plasma cytokines and muscle and leukocyte cytokine mRNA. *Journal of Applied Physiology* 103:1728–35.

Nieman, D., et al. 2004. Vitamin E and immunity after the Kona Triathlon World Championship. *Medicine and Science in Sports and Exercise* 36:1328–35.

Nieman, D., et al. 2002. Influence of vitamin C supplementation on oxidative and immune changes after an ultramarathon. *Journal of Applied Physiology* 92:1970–77.

Paganini-Hill, A., and Perez Barreto, M. 2001. Stroke risk in older men and women: Aspirin, estrogen, exercise, vitamins, and other factors. *Journal of Gender-Specific Medicine* 4:18–28.

Patterson, R., et al. 1998. Cancer-related behavior of vitamin supplement users. *Cancer Epidemiology, Biomarkers and Prevention* 7:79–81.

Peters, E., et al. 1993. Vitamin C supplementation reduces the incidence of postrace symptoms of upper-respiratory-tract infection in ultramarathon runners. *American Journal of Clinical Nutrition* 57:170–74.

Petersen, R., et al. 2005. Vitamin E and donepezil for the treatment of mild cognitive impairment. *New England Journal of Medicine* 352:2379–88.

Pincemail, J., et al. 1988. Tocopherol mobilization during intensive exercise. *European Journal of Applied Physiology* 57:188–91.

Rokitzki, L., et al. 1994. Acute changes in vitamin B_6 status in endurance athletes before and after a marathon. *International Journal of Sport Nutrition* 4:154–65.

Rokitzki, L., et al. 1994. α-tocopherol supplementation in racing cyclists during extreme endurance training. *International Journal of Sport Nutrition* 4:253–64.

Rothman, K., et al. 1995. Teratogenicity of high vitamin A intake. *New England Journal of Medicine* 333:1369–73.

Sebastian, R., et al. 2007. Older adults who use vitamin/mineral supplements differ from nonusers in nutrient intake adequacy and dietary attitudes. *Journal of the American Dietetic Association* 107:1322–32.

Shindle, M., et al., 2011. Vitamin D status in a professional American football team. *Proceedings from the AOSSM Annual Meeting* ID 46-9849.

Simon-Schnass, I., and Pabst, H. 1988. Influence of vitamin E on physical performance. *International Journal for Vitamin and Nutrition Research* 58:49–54.

Singh, A., et al. 1992. Chronic multivitamin-mineral supplementation does not enhance physical performance. *Medicine and Science in Sport and Exercise* 24:726–32.

Snider, I., et al. 1992. Effects of coenzyme athletic performance system as an ergogenic aid on endurance performance to exhaustion. *International Journal of Sport Nutrition* 2:272–86.

Suzuki, M., and Itokawa, Y. 1996. Effects of thiamine supplementation on exercise-induced fatigue. *Metabolism in Brain Diseases* 11:95–106.

Svensson, M., et al. 1999. Effect of Q_{10} supplementation on tissue Q_{10} levels and adenine nucleotide catabolism during high-intensity exercise. *International Journal of Sport Nutrition* 9:166–80.

Telford, R., et al. 1992. The effect of 7 to 8 months of vitamin/mineral supplementation on athletic performance. *International Journal of Sport Nutrition* 2:135–53.

Telford, R., et al. 1992. The effect of 7 to 8 months of vitamin/mineral supplementation on the vitamin and mineral status of athletes. *International Journal of Sport Nutrition* 2:123–34.

Tremblay, A., et al. 1984. The effects of a riboflavin supplementation on the nutritional status and performance of elite swimmers. *Nutrition Research* 4:201.

Troppman, L., et al. 2002. Supplement use: Is there any nutritional benefit? *Journal of the American Dietetic Association* 102:818–25.

van Erp-Baart, A., et al. 1989. Nationwide survey on nutritional habits in elite athletes. *International Journal of Sports Medicine* 10 (Suppl 1):S11–S16.

Verhaar, H., et al. 2000. Muscle strength, functional mobility and vitamin D in older women. *Aging* 12:455–60.

Virk, R., et al. 1999. Effect of vitamin B-6 supplementation on fuels, catecholamines, and amino acids during exercise in men. *Medicine and Science in Sports and Exercise* 31:400–8.

Wactawshi-Wende, J., et al. 2006. Calcium plus vitamin D supplementation and the risk of colorectal cancer. *New England Journal of Medicine* 354:684–96.

Warber, J., et al. 2000. The effects of choline supplementation on physical performance. *International Journal of Sport Nutrition and Exercise Metabolism* 10:170–81.

Watson, T., et al. 2005. Antioxidant restriction and oxidative stress in short-duration exhaustive exercise. *Medicine and Science in Sports and Exercise* 37:63–71.

Webster, M. 1998. Physiological and performance responses to supplementation with thiamin and pantothenic acid derivatives. *European Journal of Applied Physiology* 77:486–91.

Webster, M., et al. 1997. The effect of a thiamin derivative on exercise performance. *European Journal of Applied Physiology* 75:520–24.

Weight, L., et al. 1988. Vitamin and mineral supplementation: Effect on the running performance of trained athletes. *American Journal of Clinical Nutrition* 47:192–95.

Weston, S., et al. 1997. Does exogenous coenzyme Q_{10} affect aerobic capacity in endurance athletes? *International Journal of Sport Nutrition* 7:197–206.

Wyatt, K., et al. 1999. Efficacy of vitamin B-6 in the treatment of premenstrual syndrome: Systematic review. *British Medical Journal* 318:1375–81.

Ylikoski, T., et al. 1997. The effect of coenzyme Q_{10} on the exercise performance of cross-country skiers. *Molecular Aspects of Medicine* 18:S283–S290.

Zhang, S., et al. 1999. A prospective study of folate intake and the risk of breast cancer. *Journal of the American Medical Association* 281:1632–37.

Zhou, S., et al. 2005. Muscle and plasma coenzyme Q_{10} concentration, aerobic power and exercise economy of healthy men in response to four weeks of supplementation. *Journal of Sports Medicine and Physical Fitness* 45:337–46.

Ziegler, P., et al. 2002. Nutritional status of teenage female competitive figure skaters. *Journal of the American Dietetic Association* 102:374–79.

Zoppi, C., et al. 2006. Vitamin C and E supplementation effects in professional soccer players under regular training. *Journal of the International Society of Sports Nutrition* 3:37–44.

Minerals: The Inorganic Regulators

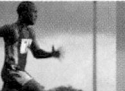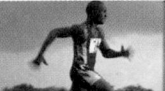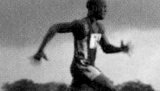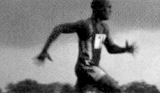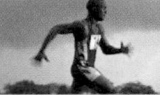

CHAPTER EIGHT

LEARNING OBJECTIVES

After studying this chapter, you should be able to:

1. Describe the various means whereby minerals may carry out their functions in the human body.

2. Name the essential minerals, state the RDA or AI for each, and identify several foods rich in each mineral.

3. Describe the metabolic roles in the human body of calcium, phosphorus, magnesium, iron, copper, zinc, chromium, selenium, fluoride, and iodine.

4. Explain the role of calcium in bone metabolism and identify the factors that may contribute to bone health and those that may contribute to osteoporosis.

5. Explain the theory as to how phosphate salt supplementation may enhance sport performance, and highlight the research findings regarding its ergogenic efficacy.

6. Explain the potential effects on health and sport performance associated with a deficiency of each trace mineral.

7. Explain the theory as to how iron, zinc, chromium, selenium, boron, and vanadium may enhance sport performance, and highlight the research findings regarding the ergogenic efficacy of each.

8. Understand why health professionals may recommend mineral supplements under certain circumstances to improve the health of some individuals.

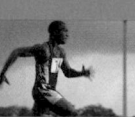

Introduction

You may recall the periodic table of the elements hanging on the wall in your high school or college chemistry class. At latest count there were 118 known elements, 78 of them occurring naturally and the remainder being synthetic. Many of the natural elements, including a wide variety of minerals, are essential to human bodily structure and function.

Much research attention is currently being devoted to the role of mineral nutrition in health and disease, including both epidemiological and laboratory research. For example, using the RDA as a basis for comparison, national surveys among the general population have revealed that either an inadequate dietary intake of some minerals or an excessive dietary intake of others in certain small segments of the population may be contributing to several health problems. Laboratory studies using either animals or humans as subjects have explored the roles of both deficiencies and supplementation of minerals on human health and disease processes.

An increasing number of research studies have been conducted with athletes to evaluate the effect of mineral nutrition on physical performance and the converse—the effect of exercise on mineral metabolism. Because some minerals function similarly to vitamins,

a deficiency state could adversely affect performance. Moreover, exercise in itself may be a contributing factor to mineral deficiencies or impaired mineral metabolism in some types of athletes. Additionally, several mineral supplements are being marketed specifically for physically active individuals.

This chapter is especially important to all females and young athletes because it addresses two of their major dietary concerns: obtaining sufficient calcium and obtaining sufficient iron. These key minerals are of particular interest to females who participate in sports or are otherwise physically active. The female athlete triad—disordered eating, amenorrhea, and osteoporosis—is introduced in this chapter with the major focus on osteoporosis because of its relationship to calcium metabolism. An expanded discussion of eating disorders is presented in chapter 10. Female endurance athletes also need to obtain adequate dietary iron

intake because of its important role in the oxygen energy system.

The major purpose of this chapter is to analyze the available data relative to the effect of mineral nutrition on physical performance and health. The first section discusses some basic facts about the general role of those minerals that are essential to human nutrition. The second and third sections cover, respectively, the major minerals and the trace minerals. In these two sections, each of the minerals is discussed in terms of its Dietary Reference Intake (DRI), good dietary sources, metabolic functions in the body with particular reference to the physically active individual, an evaluation of the research pertaining to the effects of deficiencies or supplementation on health or exercise performance, and prudent recommendations. The last section summarizes dietary mineral nutrition guidelines for those who exercise for health or sport.

Basic Facts

What are minerals, and what is their importance to humans?

A **mineral** is an inorganic element found in nature, and the term is usually reserved for those elements that are solid. Hence, a mineral is an element, but an element is not necessarily a mineral. For example, oxygen is an element, but it is not classified as a mineral. In nutrition, the term *mineral* is usually used to classify those dietary elements essential to life processes.

Minerals are found in the soil and are eventually incorporated in growing plants. Most animals get their mineral nutrition from the plants they eat, whereas humans obtain their supply from both plant and animal food. Drinking water may also be a good source of several minerals. As minerals are excreted daily from the body in sweat, urine, or feces, they must be replaced.

Minerals serve two of the three basic functions of nutrients in foods.

Growth and Development Many minerals are used as the building blocks for body tissues, such as bones, teeth, muscles, and other organic structures. In particular, calcium and phosphorus are important to bone health. Iron is an important component of hemoglobin, which is needed for optimal oxygen transport during aerobic endurance exercise.

Metabolic Regulation A number of minerals are involved in regulation of metabolic processes. Many are components of enzymes known as **metalloenzymes,** such as the cytochrome enzymes in the mitochondria that facilitate ATP production. Others, such as zinc and copper, are part of the natural antioxidant enzymes discussed in chapter 7. Still others exist as **ions,** or

electrolytes, which are small particles carrying electrical charges. They are important components or activators of several enzymes and hormones. Speich and others reviewed the physiological roles of minerals important to athletes, noting that minerals are involved in muscle contraction, normal heart rhythm, nerve impulse conduction, oxygen transport, oxidative phosphorylation, enzyme activation, immune functions, antioxidant activity, bone health, acid-base balance of the blood, and maintenance of body water supplies. Figure 8.1 provides a broad overview of mineral function in the body.

Energy Minerals are comparable to vitamins. Although minerals may play a significant role in the generation of energy via their metabolic functions, they do not provide a source of calorie energy.

Inadequate mineral nutrition has been associated with impairment of normal physiological functions, as well as with a variety of human diseases, including anemia, high blood pressure, obesity diabetes, cancer, tooth decay, and osteoporosis. However, excessive intake of minerals may also contribute to significant health risks. Thus, proper dietary intake of essential minerals is necessary for optimal health and physical performance.

What minerals are essential to human nutrition?

Of all the elements in the periodic table, only 25 are currently known to be, or presumed to be, essential in humans. Five of these elements, which make up the carbohydrate, fat, and protein that we eat and the water we drink, constitute more than 96 percent of the body weight. In varying combinations, hydrogen, oxygen, carbon, sulfur, and nitrogen are the components of the body water, protein, fat, and carbohydrate stores. The remaining 20 minerals compose less than 4 percent of the body weight but are equally important.

Table 8.1 lists those minerals for which the National Academy of Sciences (NAS) has established a DRI or other recommendation. The DRIs include the Recommended Dietary Allowance (RDA), the Adequate Intake (AI), and the Tolerable Upper Intake Level (UL). The NAS has established the RDA or AI for most minerals discussed in this chapter, and for sodium, chloride, and potassium, elements that are discussed in the next chapter. Sulfur is found in the diet mainly as a component of the sulfur-containing amino acids (methionine and cysteine), and body needs are satisfied by the RDA for these amino acids.

Other minerals, such as boron, nickel, silicon, and vanadium, among others, are found in animal tissues and also may be important to human nutrition, but their roles have not yet been completely elucidated, and thus no RDA or AI have yet been established. However, UL have been set for boron, nickel, and vanadium.

In general, how do deficiencies or excesses of minerals influence health or physical performance?

Similar to vitamin deficiencies, mineral deficiencies may occur in several stages. The first three stages (preliminary, biochemical deficiency, and physiological deficiency) may be termed subclinical malnutrition and may or may not have significant effects on health or physical performance. In the clinically manifest deficiency state, however, health and performance most likely will suffer.

The interaction of exercise and mineral nutrition may pose some special health problems, as we shall see in later sections of this chapter. In regard to the preliminary stage, some athletes may reduce their mineral intake as they shift toward a low-Calorie diet.

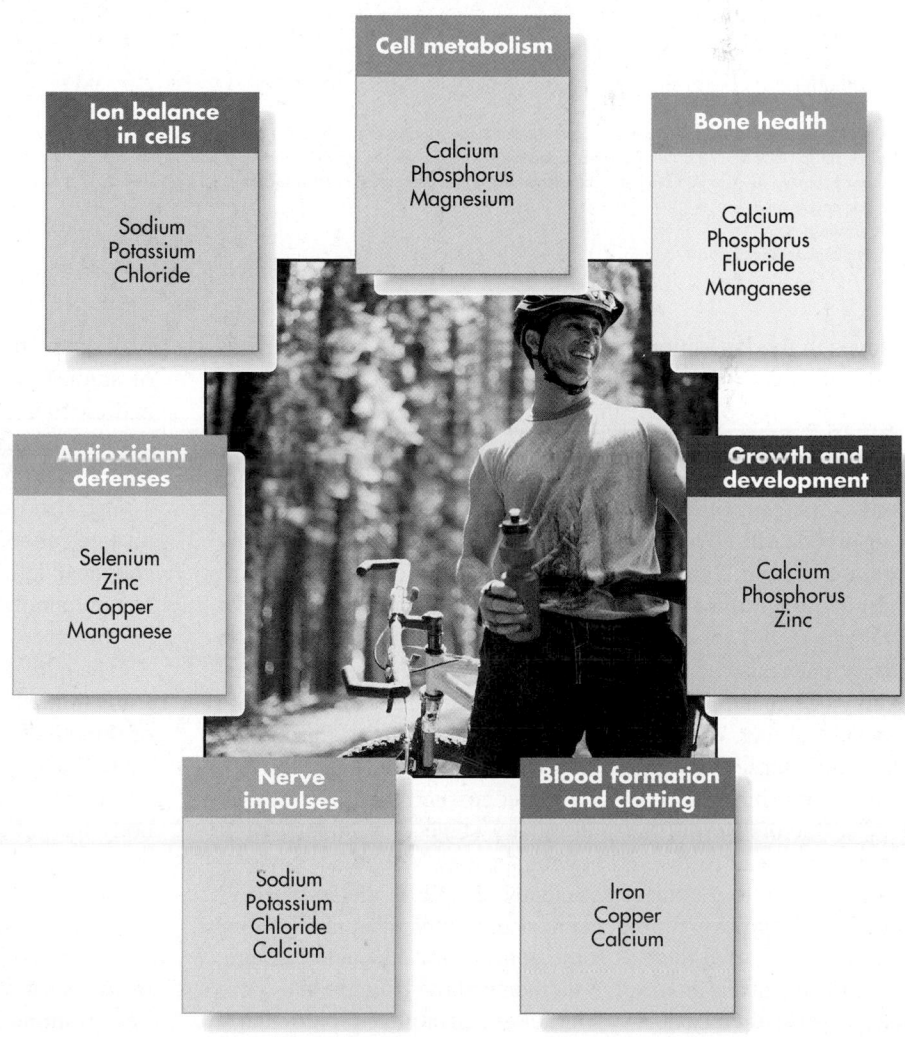

FIGURE 8.1 Minerals contribute to many functions in the body. Mineral deficiencies therefore lead to a variety of health problems and may impair physical performance.

TABLE 8.1   Mineral Dietary Reference Intakes for adults aged 19–50*

Mineral	Symbol	RDA or AI (mg)		Daily value (mg)	UL (mg)	Amount in adult body (g)
Calcium (2)	Ca	1,000♂	1,000♀	1,000	2,500	1,500
Phosphorus (1)	P	700♂	700♀	1,000	4,000	850
Potassium (2)	K	4,700♂	4,700♀	3,500	ND	180
Chloride (2)	Cl	2,300♂	2,300♀	3,400	3,500	75
Sodium (2)	Na	1,500♂	1,500♀	< 2,400	2,300	65
Magnesium (1)	Mg	420♂	320♀	400	350***	25
Iron (1)	Fe	8♂	18♀	18	45	5
Fluoride (2)	F	4♂	3.0♀	**	10	2.5
Zinc (1)	Zn	11♂	8♀	15	40	2
Copper (1)	Cu	0.9♂	0.9♀	2	10	0.1
Selenium (1)	Se	0.055♂	0.055♀	0.70	0.4	0.013
Manganese (2)	Mn	2.3♂	1.8♀	2	11	0.012
Iodine (1)	I	0.15♂	0.15♀	0.15	1.1	0.011
Molybdenum (1)	Mo	0.045♂	0.045♀	0.075	2	0.009
Chromium (2)	Cr	0.035♂	0.025♀	0.12	ND	0.006

*Different terms are used to quantify the recommended dietary intake of minerals: (1) Recommended Dietary Allowance (RDA); (2) Adequate Intake (AI). The UL listed is for adult males; lower values are set for females and other age groups. See the DRI tables on the inside of the front and back covers for more details. Arsenic, boron, nickel, silicon, and vanadium are also covered in the DRI reports, but no RDA or AI have been established. A UL has been set for nickel and vanadium.

ND = not determined

**Not established

***Only pharmacological form

Changes in food selection may also be important, for the bioavailability of many minerals is markedly influenced by the form in which they are consumed. In general, most minerals are poorly absorbed from the intestine. For example, the RDA for iron is ten times the amount actually needed by the body, because only about 10 percent of dietary iron from the average American diet is absorbed. Moreover, mineral absorption may be inhibited by certain compounds in foods, and supplementation with one mineral may impair the absorption of another. In athletes, factors that lower intake and absorption may be compounded because athletic activity may raise some mineral requirements. Additional minerals may be needed for the synthesis of new tissues associated with physical training, or to replace losses often observed during and following intense exercise training via sweat, urine, and feces.

Sports nutritionists are becoming concerned that the presence of these factors during the preliminary stage of a mineral deficiency could lead to the subsequent stages of subclinical malnutrition, or even to a clinical deficiency. Based on dietary surveys and clinical studies with biochemical measures of mineral status, Pennington reported there is some concern for adequate calcium, iron, and zinc nutrition in some segments of the United States population. Most dietary surveys indicate that athletes, particularly

males, are obtaining the RDA for all minerals. However, a number of studies have reported athletes with inadequate dietary intake and biochemical deficiencies of several minerals, predominately athletes involved in weight control sports such as gymnastics, figure skating, and wrestling. Switching to a vegetarian diet for 1 year also decreased plasma levels of several minerals. Experts disagree about the potential adverse effects of such dietary or biochemical deficiencies, but certain physiologic and clinically manifest mineral deficiencies are known to have impaired physical performance.

The human body possesses a very effective control system for some minerals. When a deficiency occurs, the body absorbs more of the mineral from the food in the intestine and excretes less via routes such as the urine. When an excess is consumed, the opposite is true; less is absorbed and more is excreted. However, the body has a limited ability to excrete certain minerals, so excessive consumption may override these natural control systems and cause a number of health problems, even in relatively small dosages. Additionally, a few minerals not important to human nutrition, such as lead, mercury, cadmium, arsenic, and some industrial forms of chromium, may be extremely toxic to the human body. For example, as discussed in chapter 5, mercury in polluted waterways may accumulate in fish, which if eaten may damage the nervous system of unborn or young children.

Let us now detail the role of various macrominerals and trace minerals in health and exercise performance.

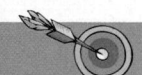

Key Concepts

▶ Minerals perform two of the three major functions of nutrients in food, including the formation of several body tissues and the regulation of numerous physiological processes. Minerals do not contain energy *per se*, such as Calories, but they do help regulate energy processes in the body.

▶ RDA or AI have been established for 15 different minerals. UL have also been established for most minerals, including several for which no RDA or AI have been established. Like vitamins, the mineral DRI have been modified to help prevent chronic diseases such as osteoporosis.

▶ Mineral deficiencies or excess may have adverse effects on both health and physical performance.

Check for Yourself

▶ Check the food labels for various foods you have in the cupboard to see what minerals are listed. If the DV is provided, compare the amount of the mineral provided and its DV with the current RDA or AI. Relate your findings to the text discussion.

Macrominerals

The seven **macrominerals** (major minerals) are calcium, phosphorus, magnesium, potassium, sodium, chloride, and sulfur. Minerals are classified as macrominerals if the RDA or AI is greater than 100 mg per day or the body contains more than 5 grams. In general, the human body maintains a proper balance of these minerals through precise hormonal control mechanisms, but deficiencies or excesses may occur and disturb normal physiological functions, thus impairing health or physical performance. Sulfur, an integral component of several amino acids and vitamins, is not discussed here because its functions are associated with those nutrients. Because potassium, sodium, and chloride are the major electrolytes in sweat, and in some sports drinks, they are covered in the following chapter dealing with water and temperature regulation.

Calcium (Ca)

Calcium, a silver-white metallic element, is the most abundant mineral in the body, representing almost 2 percent of the body weight.

DRI   The AI for calcium is intended to provide optimal amounts for health, particularly for bone health and the prevention of osteoporosis. The daily recommendations, in parentheses, are given for several selected age groups: children 1 to 3 years (700 mg); youths 4 to 8 years (1000 mg); youths and adolescents 9 to 18 years (1,300 mg); adults 19 to 50 (1,000 mg); adults 51 to 70 (1,000 mg for men and 1,200 mg for women); adults over 71 (1,200 mg). Pregnant and breastfeeding women should get the amount recommended for their age group. The DV is 1,000 mg. The UL, for adults 19 to 50 is 2,500 mg.

Food Sources   Calcium content is highest in dairy products. One 8-ounce glass of skim milk, which contains about 300 mg of calcium, supplies about one-third of the RDA for adults and men over 50 and about one-quarter of the RDA for adolescents and women over 50. It is used as the basis of comparison for other foods. Other equivalent dairy foods are 1½ ounces of cheese, 1 cup of yogurt, and 1¾ cups of ice cream. Dairy products supply almost 80 percent of daily calcium intake for adults. Other good sources are fish with small bones, such as sardines and canned salmon, dark-green leafy vegetables (particularly broccoli, kale, and turnip greens), calcium-set tofu, legumes, and nuts. Incorporation of milk or cheese into foods such as soups, pasta dishes, and pizza is an excellent way to obtain dietary calcium. For individuals with lactose intolerance, the use of yogurt, lactase enzymes, or smaller portions of milk may be helpful. Calcium is also used as a preservative in some foods, such as breads, which may provide small amounts. Additionally, some food products such as fruit juice and cereals are now being fortified with calcium; one serving of orange juice may contain 300–350 milligrams while one brand of cereal contains 100 percent of the calcium DV. Foods high in calcium are listed in table 8.2.

Calcium is one of the key nutrients listed on food labels, and although the food label does not indicate the milligrams of calcium per serving, you can calculate the amount fairly easily. The Daily Value (DV) for calcium is 1,000 milligrams, and the label will provide you with the percentage of the calcium DV contained in one serving. All you need to do is multiply the percentage, as a decimal, times 1,000 milligrams. For example, if a glass of calcium-fortified orange juice provides you with 30 percent of the DV, then it contains 300 milligrams of calcium ($0.30 \times 1,000$ milligrams = 300 milligrams). Both the United States and Canada have approved food label health claims for calcium if one serving contains 20 percent of the Daily Value, or 200 milligrams.

Titchenal and Dobbs developed a system to assess the quality of food sources for calcium. The system is based on two criteria: the amount of calcium per serving including nutrient density, and its absorbability.

Some nutrients in food may influence calcium absorption or excretion. The calcium in milk appears to be absorbed more readily because vitamin D and lactose in milk facilitate absorption. Straub indicates that absorption from calcium-fortified beverages varies and in general is not equal to that of milk. Calcium absorption from broccoli, cabbage, and kale is good, but the calcium content per serving is much less than that for milk. Phytates (phytic acid compounds) found in legumes and oxalates in spinach may diminish somewhat the absorption of calcium from those foods. Thus, Titchenal and Dobbs indicated that foods like beans are poor sources of calcium because of poor absorption. Dietary fiber may reduce calcium absorption, although the effect is rather variable and presumably small. Dietary phosphorus may also decrease calcium absorption, but decreases its excretion by the kidney as

TABLE 8.2 Major minerals: calcium, phosphorus, and magnesium

Major mineral	Major food sources	Major body functions	Deficiency symptoms	Symptoms of excessive consumption
Calcium (Ca)	All dairy products: milk, cheese, ice cream, yogurt; egg yolk; dried beans and peas; dark-green leafy vegetables; soy milk; calcium-fortified food products	Bone formation; enzyme activation; nerve impulse transmission; muscle contraction; cell membrane potential	Osteoporosis; rickets; impaired muscle contraction; muscle cramps	Constipation; inhibition of trace mineral absorption. In susceptible individuals: heart arrhythmias; kidney stones; calcification of soft tissues
Phosphorus (P)	All protein products: meat, poultry, fish, eggs, milk, cheese, dried beans and peas; whole-grain products; soft drinks	Bone formation; acid-base balance; cell membrane structure; B vitamin activation; organic compound component, e.g., ATP-PCr, 2, 3-DPG	Rare. Deficiency symptoms parallel calcium deficiency. Muscular weakness	Rare. Impaired calcium metabolism; gastrointestinal distress from phosphate salts
Magnesium (Mg)	Milk and yogurt; dried beans; nuts; whole-grain products; fruits and vegetables, especially green leafy vegetables	Protein synthesis; metalloenzyme; 2, 3-DPG formation; glucose metabolism; smooth muscle contraction; bone component	Rare. Muscle weakness; apathy; muscle twitching; muscle cramps; cardiac arrhythmias	Nausea; vomiting; diarrhea

well, so its effect on calcium balance is somewhat neutral. Excess sodium intake increases calcium excretion. Dawson-Hughes indicates that for every 500-mg increase in urinary sodium excretion, there is about a 10-mg increase in urinary calcium loss. As mentioned in chapter 6, excessive protein intake may lead to calcium excretion, an estimate cited by the National Dairy Council being 1 milligram of calcium lost for every gram of protein consumed. However, as also noted, adequate protein intake is needed to optimize calcium bone metabolism.

Overall, however, calcium balance in the body is attributed mostly to adequate calcium intake. Although certain food constituents may impair the absorption of calcium, the effect is not as great as once believed. In general, the amounts of protein, phosphorus, fiber, phytates, and oxalates found in the average North American diet do not appear to pose a problem for calcium absorption. For example, research has revealed that vegetarian diets provide adequate calcium nutrition as measured by body stores. Nevertheless, non-lactovegetarian females should be sure to include calcium-rich foods in their diet. High intakes of coffee and alcohol may increase calcium loss from the body, although studies have shown that up to five cups of coffee and moderate alcohol consumption appear to have little effect on calcium balance.

As we shall see, the major factor underlying calcium deficiency is inadequate calcium intake, and although some of these other dietary factors may adversely influence calcium balance if taken to excess, their effect is lessened if calcium intake is adequate.

Major Functions The vast majority of body calcium, 98 percent, is found in the skeleton, where it gives strength by the formation of salts such as calcium phosphate. One percent is used for tooth formation. The remainder, which exists in an ionic state or in combination with certain proteins, exerts considerable influence over human metabolism. Intracellular calcium ions (Ca^{2+}) are involved in all types of muscle contraction, including that of the heart, skeletal muscle, and smooth muscle found in blood vessels such as the arteries. Calcium activates a number of enzymes; in this capacity it plays a central role in both the synthesis and breakdown of muscle glycogen and liver glycogen. Calcium also helps regulate nerve impulse transmission, blood clotting, and secretion of hormones. It should be noted that the skeletal content of calcium is not inert. The physiological functions of calcium, such as nerve cell transmission, take precedence over formation of bone tissue. If the diet is low in calcium for a short time, the body can mobilize some from the skeleton through the action of hormones, such as parathormone and calcitriol (hormonal form of vitamin D), to maintain an adequate amount in ionic form.

Deficiency: Health and Physical Performance Calcium balance in the human body is rather complex. Figure 8.2 depicts the fate of an intake of 1,000 mg. Only 300 mg (about 30 percent) is absorbed, while the remaining 700 mg is excreted in the feces. The calcium that is absorbed into the blood interacts with the current body stores, the net result being the excretion of 300 mg through the intestines, kidneys, and sweat to balance the amount originally absorbed. Calcium deficiency may develop from inadequate dietary intake or increased excretion.

Nationwide surveys have revealed that many Americans, particularly females, are not obtaining adequate dietary calcium. Recent data indicate that 75 percent of women do not consume the AI for calcium and more than 50 percent do not even consume half of the new AI. However, surveys with athletic groups reveal that some athletes are getting well above the recommended amount, particularly males. Nevertheless, Clarkson and Haymes indicated that many female athletes are also consuming less than the AI, and in a Canadian study, Webster and Barr noted that although the mean value of calcium intake for a group of gymnasts met the Canadian recommendations, many individual gymnasts within the group consumed considerably less. Many

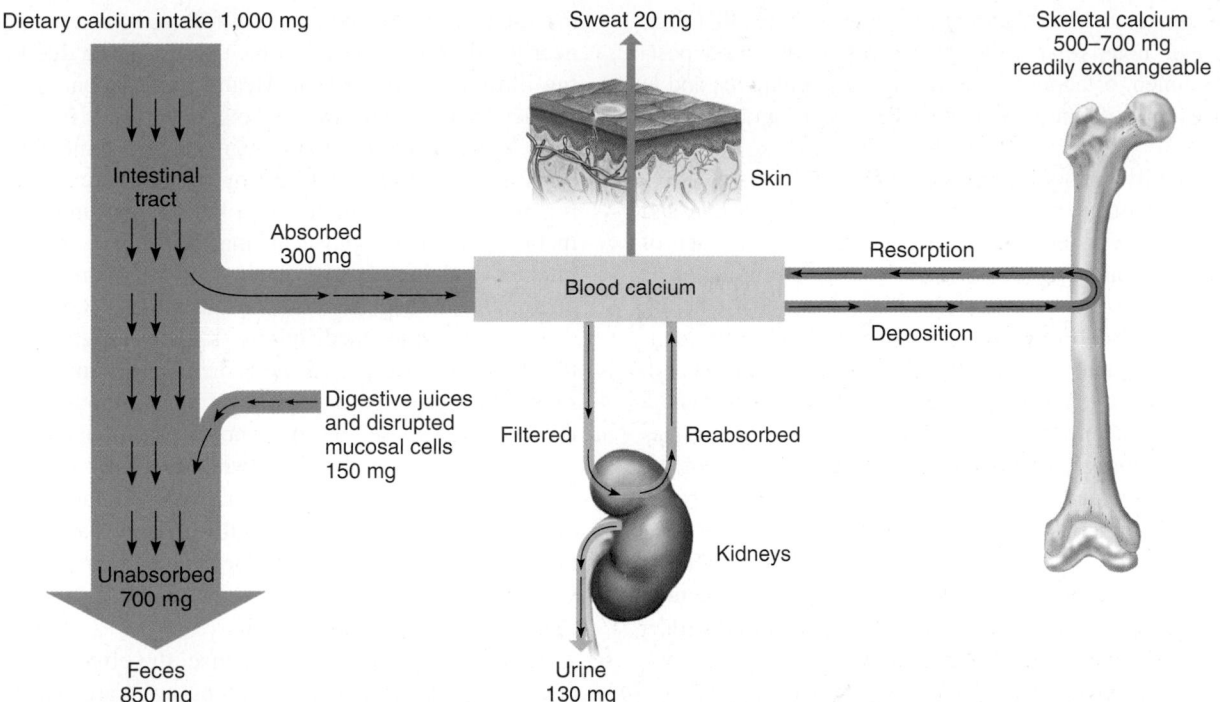

Dietary calcium intake 1,000 mg

Intestinal tract

Absorbed 300 mg

Blood calcium

Digestive juices and disrupted mucosal cells 150 mg

Unabsorbed 700 mg

Feces 850 mg

Sweat 20 mg

Skin

Filtered

Reabsorbed

Kidneys

Urine 130 mg

Skeletal calcium 500–700 mg readily exchangeable

Resorption

Deposition

FIGURE 8.2 Calcium balance in an adult who requires 1,000 mg daily. On an intake of 1,000 mg, only about 30 percent, or 300 mg, are absorbed into the body, the remaining 700 mg being excreted in the feces. To maintain calcium balance, 300 mg are excreted including an additional 150 mg in the feces, 130 mg through the kidneys to the urine, and 20 mg in sweat. See text for further discussion.

athletes trying to obtain a low body weight for competition, such as female gymnasts, long-distance runners, and figure skaters, have substandard intakes.

Exercise may increase sweat or urinary loss of calcium. Bullen and others noted that moderate exercise (80 percent HR_{max} for 45 minutes in a warm environment) induced a loss of 45 mg calcium via sweating. Montain and others also reported small sweat calcium losses, about 16 milligrams per liter of sweat, in an intermittent 7-hour walking exercise task. Martin and others also reported that exercise increases sweat calcium losses only slightly in women who exercised at about 65–70 percent of maximum heart rate reserve for one hour. More strenuous exercise may also increase sweat losses of calcium. In another study, Klesges and others, studying primarily African-American basketball players, reported losses of greater than 400 milligrams of calcium per daily training session. Such a loss would match or exceed the amount normally absorbed from the daily diet. However, Chinevere and others reported that following 10 days of acclimation, total sweat losses of calcium were significantly reduced, as were those of several other minerals. Dressendorfer and others examined the effect of 10-week intense endurance training, including volume, interval, and tapering phases, on serum and urinary mineral levels. The training did not affect magnesium, iron, zinc, or copper metabolism, but urinary calcium increased and serum calcium decreased below the clinical norm following the high-intensity interval phase. However, these changes were reversed following the tapering phase. Thus, it appears that calcium excretion may be increased with high-intensity training.

Relative to health, an inadequate dietary intake or increased excretion of calcium has been associated with several health problems, most notably colon cancer, high blood pressure, and osteoporosis.

Some epidemiologic evidence indicates that low levels of dietary calcium may contribute to the development of cancer of the colon. Calcium is believed to combine with bile salts or fatty acids, forming an insoluble complex and helping to excrete them in the feces, thereby reducing their potential carcinogenic effect on the walls of the colon, something akin to the role of dietary fiber. As noted later, although the evidence is somewhat equivocal, a major review suggests that calcium intake may influence risk of cancer.

One theory also suggests that calcium deficiency is involved in the development of high blood pressure through the mechanism of contraction of the smooth muscles in the arterioles. However, the National Academy of Sciences reports that the relationship of dietary calcium to high blood pressure is weak and the data are inconclusive.

The major health problems associated with impaired calcium metabolism involve diseases of the bones. A number of factors are involved in the formation, or mineralization, of bone tissue, including mechanical stresses such as exercise; hormones such as parathormone, calcitonin, vitamin D (calcitriol), and estrogen; and dietary calcium. An imbalance in any one of these factors could lead to bone demineralization, resulting in the development of rickets in children and osteoporosis in adults.

Osteoporosis (thinning and weakening of the bones related to loss of calcium stores) is a debilitating disease that is primarily age- and gender-related. A National Institutes of Health (NIH) consensus panel noted that although prevalent in white post-menopausal women, osteoporosis occurs in all populations and at all ages and has significant physical, psychosocial, and financial consequences.

A positive family history, or heredity, and low levels of estrogen are the two primary risk factors in women. Caucasian and Asian women are at higher risk for osteoporosis than women of African ancestry. Following menopause, estrogen production is diminished. Estrogen is a hormone essential for optimal calcium balance in women. Bone receptors for estrogen have been identified, indicating an active role in bone metabolism. In general, reduced levels of estrogen lead to negative calcium balance and a rapid onset of bone demineralization. This softening of the bones predisposes to fractures, particularly in the spine, the end of the radius in the forearm, and the neck of the femur at the hip joint, as illustrated in figure 8.3. These latter two fractures may be completely debilitating to the older individual. The spinal fracture is more common because the vertebrae are composed of **trabecular bone,** a spongy type of bone more susceptible to calcium loss than the more dense compact bone. However, both types of bone may be lost during osteoporosis, as depicted in figure 8.4.

The FDA indicated that during their lifetimes half of American women older than 50 will be at risk of fractures from thinning bones. Each year, osteoporosis causes 1.5 million fractures, including 300,000 hip and 700,000 vertebral fractures. Although more common in women, more than 2 million American men suffer from osteoporosis, and millions more are at risk. Each year 80,000 men suffer a hip fracture. Osteoporosis is known as the silent killer. The disease itself causes no pain, but following a serious bone fracture nearly a third or more of women and men die due to accompanying illnesses within a year. Health professionals recommend that women aged 65 and over, and others with risk factors for osteoporosis, routinely have measurements of bone mineral density.

Although heredity and estrogen status are strong risk factors for osteoporosis, some lifestyle factors may impair optimal bone metabolism. Both physical inactivity and inadequate dietary intake of calcium are risk factors for osteoporosis, and so too are cigarette smoking, excess consumption of coffee and alcohol, stress, and various medications. Table 8.3 highlights the risk factors for osteoporosis. All these factors may influence **peak bone mass** (the highest bone mass in young adulthood). Modifying your lifestyle to increase your peak bone mass is like putting money in the bank for later in life. However, Modlesky and Lewis note that although the idea that the growing years are an opportune time to optimize bone mass and strength certainly has merit, the importance of these gains depends largely on their permanence. Thus, you need to continue to practice good dietary and exercise habits to maintain optimal bone health.

Relative to physical performance, the effect of a calcium deficiency depends on whether calcium levels are low in the blood or in the bones. Serum calcium levels are usually regulated by several hormones in the average individual. The body can adapt to low dietary intake by increasing the rate of absorption from the intestines and decreasing the rate of excretion by the kidneys. Because the skeleton is a large reservoir of body calcium, low serum levels are rare. When they do occur, it usually is because of hormonal imbalances rather than dietary deficiencies.

Nevertheless, owing to the diverse physiological roles of calcium, a low serum level reflecting low calcium concentration in the tissues could be expected to cause a number of problems. For the athlete, impaired muscular contraction would certainly affect sport performance. One symptom may be muscle cramping due to an imbalance of calcium in the muscle and in the surrounding body fluids. Fortunately, serious deficiencies of serum calcium are rare in athletes because hormones may extract calcium from the bone as needed.

Supplementation: Health and Physical Performance

Although most research with calcium supplementation has focused on bone health, the effect on several other chronic diseases has also been studied. Many more recent studies have also combined calcium with vitamin D supplements, particularly in studies evaluating the effects on bone health. Heaney notes that each nutrient is necessary for the full expression of the effect of the other, and while their actions are independent, their effects on skeletal health are complementary.

Cancer Research findings relative to the intake of dietary calcium, either as food or as supplements, are equivocal relative to the effects on various forms of cancer. Most research has focused on prevention of colorectal cancer. Dairy products are rich sources of calcium, but Parodi reported that evidence from more than 40 case-control and 12 cohort studies does not support an association between dairy product consumption and the risk of

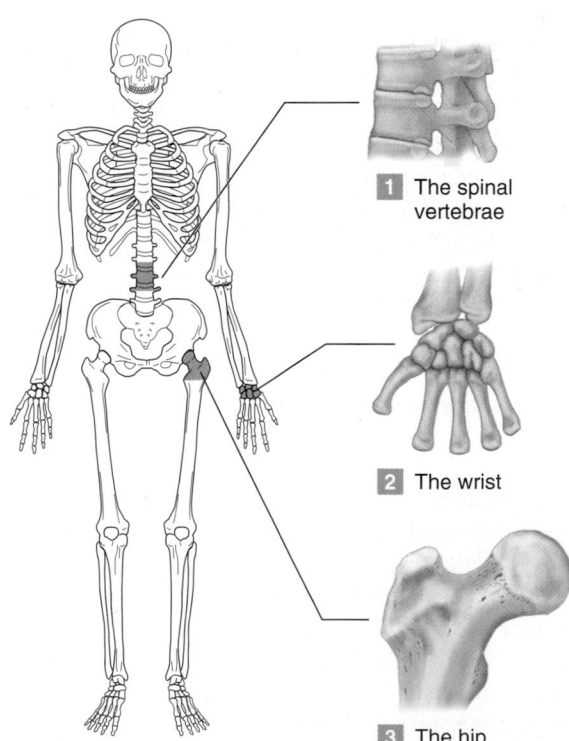

1 The spinal vertebrae

2 The wrist

3 The hip

FIGURE 8.3 Three principal sites of osteoporosis fractures.

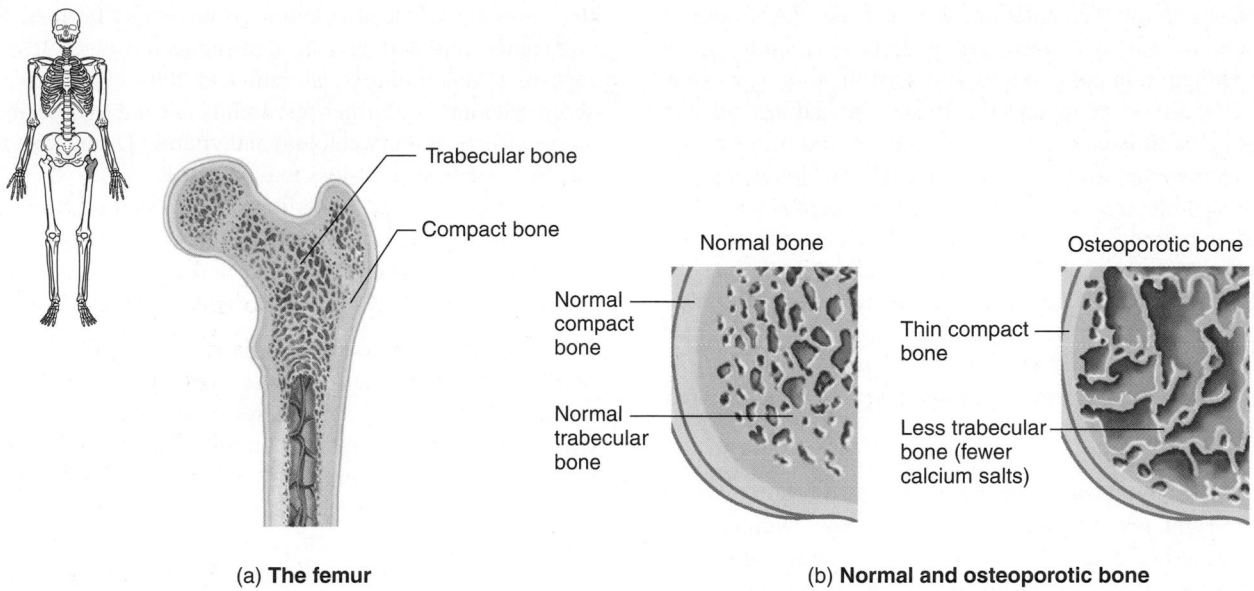

(a) **The femur** (b) **Normal and osteoporotic bone**

FIGURE 8.4 In osteoporosis, impaired calcium metabolism may decrease the external compact bone thickness and the strength of the internal trabecular bone lattice network.

TABLE 8.3	**Risk factors for osteoporosis**
Heredity	Positive family history
Race	White or Asian
Gender	Female
Menstrual status	Postmenopausal; amenorrheic
Age	Advanced age
Exercise	Physical inactivity; bed rest
Diet	Inadequate calcium; inadequate vitamin D; excessive coffee; excessive alcohol
Tobacco	Cigarette smoking
Alcohol	Excessive use
Stress	Excessive stress; anxiety
Medications	Certain medications increase calcium losses
Hormonal status	Low estrogen; low testosterone

breast cancer. Weingarten and others, although noting that two studies produced evidence that calcium supplementation may contribute to a moderate degree to the prevention of colorectal polyps, commented that this does not constitute sufficient evidence to recommend the general use of calcium supplements to prevent colorectal cancer. Wactawski-Wende and others also reported that although epidemiologic studies have shown a reduced risk of colorectal cancer with increased intake of calcium and vitamin D, their experimental study did not. In a large study with more than 36,000 healthy postmenopausal women, they reported that daily supplementation of calcium (1,000 mg) with vitamin D_3 (400 IU) had no effect on the development of colorectal cancer, but noted that the 7-year time frame may have been too short due to the long latency for the development of colorectal cancer. The study is ongoing. In a meta-analysis of six studies, Carroll and others noted that supplemental calcium was effective in preventing adenoma reoccurrence in patients with a history of adenomas, but had no effect on risk of colon cancer. Bonjour and others actually hypothesized that high calcium consumption could promote prostate cancer by reducing the production of calcitriol, the hormone form of vitamin D. However, they also noted that the plausibility of the hypothesis is not supported by the analysis of available clinical data.

Some research has shown some beneficial effects. Lappe and others supplemented the diets of healthy postmenopausal women with either 1,400–1,500 milligrams of supplemental calcium per day, supplemental calcium plus 1,100 IU vitamin D_3 per day, or placebo for a period of 4 years. They found that improving calcium and vitamin D nutritional status substantially reduces all-cancer risk in postmenopausal women. However, it was a short-term study. In its worldwide review on nutrition and cancer, the American Institute of Cancer Research analyzed 10 cohort studies and reported a 22 percent reduction in colorectal cancer risk for those groups with the highest calcium intake (dietary and supplemental sources). They also noted that dietary calcium may possess growth-restraining effects on normal and cancer cells. The AICR concluded that the evidence from cohort studies is generally consistent, the mechanism is plausible, and calcium probably protects against colorectal cancers. However, their overall recommendation for nutrition to prevent cancer is to obtain the nutrients from foods.

High blood pressure Several extensive reviews have concluded that calcium may have small, but weak, beneficial effects on blood pressure. van Mierlo and others, in a meta-analysis of 40 studies, found that calcium supplementation, with a mean daily dose of 1,200 milligrams, was associated with a slight (1–2 mmHg), but significant, reduction in both systolic and diastolic blood pressure, and the effect was more pronounced in those who had low calcium intakes prior to supplementation. Dickinson and others also conducted a meta-analysis of 13 randomized controlled trials and concluded that subjects receiving calcium supplements, compared to controls, experienced a small but significant reduction in systolic, but not diastolic, blood pressure. However, they noted that these results may be related to the poor quality of some studies and thus concluded that the evidence supporting a beneficial effect of calcium supplementation in hypertensive individuals is weak. Investigators recommend additional research to help clarify these findings.

Weight loss   Calcium supplementation has also been theorized to promote weight loss. Zemel indicated that low-calcium diets cause an increase in calcitriol, the vitamin D hormone, which can stimulate adipose cell calcium influx, promoting fat accumulation; he also notes the converse, that higher calcium diets inhibit the formation of body fat. Zemel and others, in several studies, have shown that supplementing a reduced-Calorie diet with calcium, in particular calcium-rich dairy products, led to greater weight loss compared to placebo groups. A long-term study by Caan and others provides some supportive data, not for weight loss but for prevention of weight gain. Over the course of 7 years, they found that supplementation with calcium (1,000 mg) and vitamin D (400 IU) had a small effect on the prevention of weight gain, which was observed primarily in women who reported inadequate calcium intakes.

However, most other studies comparable to those of Zemel report no beneficial effects of high-calcium diets or supplements on weight loss. For example, Harvey-Berino and others reported that a high-dairy calcium diet does not substantially improve weight loss beyond what can be achieved in a behavioral intervention. The low-dairy diet contained 500 mg calcium versus the high-dairy diet with 1,200–1,400 mg. Thompson and others found no evidence that diets higher than 800 mg of calcium in dairy products enhance weight reduction beyond what is seen with caloric restriction alone. Lorenzen and others found that a supplement containing 500 milligrams of calcium, provided for 1 year to young girls, had no effect on body weight or percentage body fat. Moreover, Trowman and others conducted a meta-analysis of 13 studies and concluded that calcium supplementation has no statistically significant association with a reduction in body weight. Given this evidence, Severson reported that the Federal Trade Commission indicated that a national advertising campaign associating dairy products with weight loss will be curtailed because research does not support the claim. However, in a narrative review, van Loan highlights observational studies that demonstrate an inverse relationship between dairy or calcium intake and body mass, body fat, and body mass index; when increased dairy or calcium intakes are combined with energy restriction in overweight and obese persons, randomized clinical trials demonstrate greater weight and fat loss; also, initially high calcium or dairy intake may explain the findings of randomized clinical trials

that show no effect of calcium on weight or fat loss. Shahar and colleagues reported greater diet-induced weight loss in people ingesting higher dairy calcium and those who have increased serum vitamin D. Further research is needed to describe the interactive effects of dairy calcium and vitamin D status on weight loss and ultimately, weight-loss maintenance.

Although dairy products may not be helpful, in and of themselves, for weight loss, there certainly are other healthy benefits that may accrue from a calcium-rich diet, such as one derived from low-fat dairy products and other dietary sources of calcium.

Bone health   Although genetic factors are involved in optimal bone health, so too are lifestyle factors, such as diet, including dietary supplements, and exercise. In two separate consensus conferences, one on multivitamin/mineral supplementation and one on osteoporosis, the National Institutes of Health indicated that supplementation with calcium, along with vitamin D, may be necessary in persons not achieving the recommended dietary intake. Specifically, the NIH panel concluded that calcium and vitamin D supplements could protect and even improve bone mineral density as well as reduce fracture risk in postmenopausal women. The NIH panel on osteoporosis also indicated that regular exercise—especially resistance and high-impact activities—contributes to development of maximal peak bone mass. Additionally, the panel noted that gonadal hormones are important determinants of peak and lifetime bone mass in men, women, and children. The role of vitamin D in bone health was discussed in chapter 7. This discussion will focus on calcium supplements, exercise, and hormone replacement or nonhormonal drug therapy. However, it is important to reemphasize the current opinion that calcium and vitamin D supplementation for bone health work more effectively when combined.

Calcium supplements   Calcium supplements come in a variety of forms, such as calcium carbonate, calcium citrate, calcium lactate, and calcium gluconate, and are found in certain antacids, such as Tums. The Consumers Union indicates that calcium citrate may offer a few advantages over calcium carbonate because the body appears to absorb it better and it is less likely to cause gastrointestinal side effects, but also notes that the absorption difference is small, so most people should look for calcium supplements that deliver calcium at the lowest price. Straub notes that calcium carbonate is the most effective form, but should be taken with a meal to ensure optimal absorption. The Consumers Union also suggests that people over age 50 may do better with a chewable calcium-carbonate supplement, such as *Caltrate Plus Chewables,* or calcium-antacid tablets like *Rolaids Calcium Rich* and *Tums.* Be sure to check the label for the calcium content per tablet, which may range from 50–600 mg depending on the brand. Be aware that some forms of calcium supplements are contaminated with lead, particularly calcium from oyster shells, bone meal, and dolomite.

For those who desire to take a calcium supplement, it may be wise to take a tablet with about 200 mg with snacks and small meals three times a day, rather than one tablet with 600 mg, as it appears that more calcium is absorbed when the intake is spread throughout the day. Moreover, when the supplement is combined with meals, gastric acidity and slower transit time in the gut promote calcium absorption. A daily total supplement of 600 mg calcium, combined with a dietary intake of 500–600 mg, should provide adequate calcium nutrition for most individuals. Multivitamin/mineral tablets normally contain about 200 milligrams of calcium, or 20 percent of the AI. However, three tablets are needed to provide 600 milligrams of calcium and may not be the best means to obtain calcium, because the three tablets may provide excess amounts of other nutrients, such as vitamin A. However, the point should be stressed that careful selection of foods will provide all of the calcium you need from the daily diet, thus eliminating the need for supplements. Nevertheless, as Straub points out, most Americans do not meet the AI for calcium, and supplements can help meet requirements.

Weaver and Heaney note that hypercalcemia essentially never occurs from ingestion of natural food sources, but only with supplements. Although supplements up to 600 mg per day do not appear to pose much danger, excessive amounts may contribute to abnormal heart contractions, constipation, and the development of kidney stones in susceptible individuals, particularly those with a family history of kidney problems. For those susceptible to kidney stones, data from the Nurses' Health Study revealed that dietary calcium does not contribute to kidney stone formation because it reduces the absorption of oxalate in foods, preventing the formation of calcium oxalates, or kidney stones. However, calcium supplements taken without food do not retard oxalate absorption, and thus may contribute to kidney stone formation. Moreover, excessive dietary calcium or calcium supplements may interfere with the absorption of other key minerals, notably iron and zinc. The calcium AI for some age groups (1,000–1,300 milligrams) may require supplementation for some individuals, but the National Academy of Sciences recommends against supplementation to a total much above the AI. The UL is 2,500 mg, which may be exceeded if one takes supplements and consumes too many calcium-fortified foods. Meal replacement powders and food bars, popular dietary supplements in strength-power athletes, often have 1,000 mg of calcium per serving. A large athlete who consumes three of these products per day for extra calories and protein can very easily exceed the UL for calcium. As noted previously, some health professionals recommend that you not exceed 1,500 milligrams of calcium per day, as excess calcium may promote prostate cancer by interfering with the ability of vitamin D to prevent cell proliferation in the prostate.

Although calcium is the major structural mineral for bone, Heaney notes that adequate amounts of both calcium and vitamin D are needed to optimize bone health. The NIH, in its state-of-the-science consensus report on vitamin and mineral supplementation, indicated that for most vitamins and minerals the evidence was insufficient to make a recommendation for or against supplementation. However, in one of the few exceptions, the NIH panel did indicate that calcium and vitamin D supplements could protect and even improve bone mineral density as well as reduce fracture risk in postmenopausal women.

One of the key purposes of calcium supplementation is to prevent fractures in older people. Boonen and others, in a review, noted that the data are consistent that calcium and vitamin D supplementation may enhance bone mineral density in individuals with insufficient calcium and/or vitamin D intake, particularly those with osteoporosis. Additionally, calcium and vitamin D supplementation significantly improves body sway and lower extremity strength, reducing the risk of falls. Although not all studies have reported reduced incidence of bone fracture in the elderly following supplementation with calcium alone or combined with vitamin D, a review suggests beneficial effects. Tang and others, in a meta-analysis of 29 randomized studies with individuals aged 50 years or older, found that those taking calcium, either alone or combined with vitamin D, reported a 12 percent risk reduction in fractures of all types. Moreover, the fracture risk reduction was significantly greater (24 percent) in trials in which compliance with taking the supplement was high. For best therapeutic effect, they recommend minimum doses of 1,200 mg of calcium and 800 IU of vitamin D.

As a potential side benefit to females, well-controlled research by Thys-Jacobs and others has indicated that a daily 1,200-mg calcium supplement significantly decreased some adverse side effects of the premenstrual syndrome (PMS), including psychological symptoms, food craving, and water retention.

Exercise Exercise places a mechanical stress on the bone, stimulating mechanical receptors that facilitate the deposition of calcium salts and an increase in bone mass and density. In a review of exercise regimens to increase bone strength, Turner and Robling indicated that mechanical loading through exercise will add bone, and a small amount of added new bone results in dramatic increases in bone strength because the location of the new bone through exercise is where mechanical stresses in the bone will cause fracture. However, they note that not all exercises are equally effective. Dynamic exercise, as compared to static exercise, creates a unique stress on the bone to stimulate bone strength gains. Dynamic, high-impact exercise, such as running and jumping, may stimulate bone growth more than low-impact exercise. Kato and others found that young college women who did 10 maximal vertical jumps for 3 days a week over the course of 6 months increased bone mineral density in the hip and spinal bones. Studies find that female athletes in high-impact sports have greater bone mineral density than athletes in low-impact sports. Maimoun and others note that nonimpact aerobic exercise, such as cycling, may increase markers of bone cell activity and bone turnover, but it has to be intense, such as beyond the anaerobic threshold. However, this is controversial. As Beatty and colleagues describe in their review, road cyclists are at risk of osteopenia and osteoporosis.

Age is an important consideration in optimizing bone mass with exercise, and youth is the age of opportunity. Turner and Robling also indicate that although exercise has clear benefits for the skeleton, engaging in exercise during skeletal growth is clearly more osteogenic than exercise during skeletal maturity. Periosteal expansion occurs predominantly during growth, and consequently, the childhood and adolescent years provide a window of opportunity to enhance periosteal growth with exercise.

As Bloomfield notes, you should get bone in your bone bank by age 30. Exercise is an important means of doing so, and Bloomfield also notes that you should engage in multiple brief bouts of activity during the day, focusing on weight-bearing activities and a variety of movements.

Although adult bone health is dependent on maximal attainment of peak bone mass in youth and the prevention of bone loss during young adulthood, whether or not exercise prevents bone loss after menopause appears to be debatable. Numerous studies have indicated that resistance strength training can increase bone density in postmenopausal women. Such findings were reported in a study by Cussler and others, and they also noted that the increase in bone mineral density in the femur at the hip was linearly related to the amount of weight lifted in the leg squat exercise. Miller and others, in a review of 13 studies, concluded that the findings provide support for regular aerobic activity in postmenopausal women as a means to offset age-related declines in bone mineral density. Additionally, in a meta-analysis of 18 randomized controlled trials, Bonaiuti and others concluded that aerobics, weight-bearing, and resistance exercises are all effective in increasing the bone mineral density of the spine in postmenopausal women, and walking is also effective on the hip. Moreover, Michaelsson and others noted that men who maintained the highest levels of physical activity had the fewest fractures, and those with the lowest levels had the most. This was true for all fractures, especially for hip fractures.

However, others suggest that exercise provides minimal, if any, benefits. Turner and Robling note that in elderly adults with low bone mass, exercise constitutes only a moderately effective bone-building therapy and may elicit only minor reductions in bone mineral density loss per year. The American College of Sports Medicine (ACSM), in a position statement on physical activity and bone health, indicated that although physical activity for optimal bone health is important across the age spectrum, currently there is no strong evidence that even vigorous physical activity attenuates the menopause-related loss of bone mineral in women.

Adequate calcium intake may be the answer to these varying viewpoints, as it may be needed to complement the effects of exercise. Zernicke and others indicate that exercise produces increases in bone mineral density only when calcium intake exceeds 1,000 mg daily, and it is generally accepted that chronic exercise and dietary calcium can improve bone mass to a greater extent than calcium intake alone. Candow and Chilibeck, experts on the dietary supplement creatine, report that although long term data are lacking, short-term studies show that creatine supplementation alone or in combination with resistance training can improve bone health.

The current position statement by the ACSM, complemented by recent reviews, offers the following points relative to exercise and prevention of osteoporosis.

1. Dynamic exercises, such as resistance training through a range of motion and high-impact weight-bearing aerobic exercise, are effective means to stimulate development of bone.

2. Development of peak bone mass through exercise is best achieved during the developmental years of youth; high-impact exercises are more effective.

3. Exercise may increase bone mass slightly in adulthood, but the primary benefit of exercise at this time of life may be the avoidance of further loss of bone that occurs with inactivity.

4. The optimal program for older women would include moderate- to high-impact activities that improve strength, flexibility, and coordination that may increase postural stability and decrease the incidence of osteoporotic fractures by lessening the likelihood of falling.

5. Exercise will stimulate bone development, but optimal calcium intake approximating 1,000 milligrams or more daily appears to be equally important.

Although the ACSM does recommend exercise throughout the life span for bone health, it also indicates that pharmacologic therapy for the prevention of osteoporosis may be indicated even for those postmenopausal women who are habitually physically active.

Hormone replacement or nonhormonal drug therapy In the past, hormone replacement therapy (HRT) involving estrogen, possibly combined with progesterone, was commonly used for prevention and treatment of osteoporosis and, as noted by the Consumers Union, a host of other health benefits. However, in a report from the NIH Women's Health Initiative, the biggest hormone study ever done, women on estrogen-progestin therapy were at increased risk for breast cancer, heart attacks, and strokes as compared to women not taking these hormones. Following this report, Bern highlighted the updated FDA recommendations for postmenopausal women and the use of estrogen-containing drugs. The recommendations vary depending on the health condition, and if a woman and her healthcare provider decide that estrogen-containing products are appropriate, they should be used at the lowest doses for the shortest duration to reach treatment goals. Some health benefits already seem to have been realized following this recommendation. Ravdin and others suggested that the decrease in breast-cancer incidence seems to be related to the Women's Health Initiative report and the ensuing drop in the use of HRT among postmenopausal women in the United States.

The FDA recommended that when estrogen was being taken primarily for the prevention of postmenopausal osteoporosis, estrogen and combined estrogen-progestin products should be considered only for women with significant risk of osteoporosis, a risk that outweighs other risks of the drug. The FDA recommended that women should carefully consider using approved non-estrogen treatments.

Various non-estrogen drugs are available to help treat or prevent osteoporosis. In 2006, the Consumers Union indicated that bisphosphonates remain the optimal treatment for osteoporosis. Bisphosphonates represent a class of drugs that inhibit the osteoclasts, thereby decreasing resorption of bone, but they do not inhibit bone mineralization. Thus, they prevent bone loss and possibly increase bone mineral density. Brand names for bisphosphonates include Fosamax, Boniva, and Reclast. Some forms, such as Boniva, may need to be taken orally only once a month. The FDA approved Reclast (zoledronic acid), that requires only a yearly 15-minute infusion, which may help women who do not adhere to other regimens where pills must be taken on a regular basis. However, in 2008 the FDA reported that bisphosphonates can trigger severe bone, joint, and muscle pain, and may also increase the risk of a serious heartbeat abnormality. The FDA alert includes Fosamax, Reclast, and others. Given this risk, the Consumers Union recommends non-drug therapy, including exercise and a diet adequate in calcium and vitamin D, and also recommends that if you do take bisphosphonates and experience problems, consult with your physician about switching to another type of bone-building drug. Bisphosphonates also may cause deterioration of bone in the jaw, so individuals need to check periodically with their physician or dentist.

Other nonhormonal drugs are available. Evista (raloxifene), a selective estrogen receptor modulator, appears to act like estrogen on the skeleton but blocks estrogen's effect on the breast, and may actually decrease the risk of breast cancer. Calcitonin, a hormone secreted by the thyroid gland, helps deposit calcium in the bone and may be useful as a means of deterring bone loss. Nasal calcitonin is available. Forteo (teriparatide) stimulates the activity of osteoblasts, the cells that build bone, but is recommended for use only in cases of severe osteoporosis. Hansen and Tho indicate that androgens (male sex hormones) may also be useful as an adjunct to hormone replacement therapy. Moreover, phytoestrogens in soy foods may also reduce bone loss through their estrogen-like activity.

Osteoporosis in sports Although osteoporosis occurs primarily in older individuals, investigators are expressing serious concern regarding disturbed calcium metabolism in young female athletes, particularly endurance athletes and those involved in weight-control sports. The **female athlete triad**—*disordered eating, amenorrhea, osteoporosis*—has been reported in numerous studies. As noted previously, a properly planned exercise program may actually help to prevent osteoporosis and is one of the three major components of a treatment program. However, when research first began to show that amenorrhea and osteoporosis were associated with excessive exercise, such as in female distance runners, exercise was thought to be one of the causative factors.

However, other theories prevail today. Although the exact cause has not been identified, the underlying behavior appears to be disordered eating, as will be discussed in chapter 10. Females who attempt to lose body weight in order to improve their appearance or competitive ability in sports may modify their diets, decreasing energy and protein intake. They may also exercise excessively to burn Calories. Restrictive diets and excessive exercise regimens may affect hormone status in various ways, including disturbed functioning of the hypothalamus and pituitary gland, two glands that significantly influence overall hormone status in the body including female reproductive hormones, and decreased levels of body fat, which may lead to a reduced production of estrone, a form of estrogen. **Secondary amenorrhea** (cessation of menses for prolonged periods) is a classic sign of disturbed hormonal status associated with disordered eating in postpubertal females, as seen in patients with anorexia nervosa. When observed in athletic females, secondary amenorrhea is often referred to as **athletic amenorrhea** and it may involve oligomenorrhea, or intermittent periods of amenorrhea. In young female athletes, athletic amenorrhea is often associated with osteoporosis. In her review, Anne Loucks reported that competitive endurance, aesthetic, and weight class female athletes had the bone density of 60-year-old women.

Sophisticated techniques have been used to assess bone density, or bone mineral content. In a number of these studies, amenorrheic and oligomenorrheic athletes were found to have significantly less bone mineral content in the spine and other bones, including the femur, than sedentary women and athletes who were menstruating normally. For example, Gremion and others reported that long-distance runners with oligomenorrhea had greater decreases in bone mineral density in the spine than in the femur, even though they had similar energy, calcium, and protein intakes compared to eumenorrheic runners. Moreover, these young, amenorrheic athletes had a higher incidence of stress fractures. As with postmenopausal women, the decreased estrogen is believed to be the causative factor in loss of bone density. However, Zanker and Swaine evaluated the effect of energy restriction during running, and reported significant decreases in IGF-1 when compared to normal energy intake. They suggested that lower levels of IGF-1 could be associated with the decreased bone density that has been observed in some male and female distance runners. Some evidence suggests that when amenorrheic athletes resume normal menstruation, bone mineral content increases. In contrast, Warren and Stiehl indicated that some bone loss in amenorrheic athletes is irreversible.

Although these premenopausal athletes do not need any more exercise, one investigator recommended a daily intake of 1,200–1,500 milligrams of calcium as a possible means of helping to prevent osteoporosis. For premenopausal athletes who become amenorrheic and estrogen depleted, oral contraceptive pills have been suggested as a practical means of getting additional estrogen. However, Cobb and others reported that the effect of oral contraceptives taken over the course of 2 years on bone mass and stress fractures in 150 female distance runners was inconclusive. The medical treatment suggested for this condition depends on the point of view of the individual endocrinologist, and may include individualized hormone/drug therapy. An appropriate physician, such as a sports-oriented gynecologist, should be consulted.

Males are at less risk for developing osteoporosis than females; however, reviews by Seeman and by Bennell and others noted that low calcium intake, weight loss, low body fat, and excess alcohol intake, along with other risk factors, may adversely affect bone density in males. Low levels of testosterone, the male sex hormone, are also associated with decreased bone density in males. Interestingly, Bilanin and Ormerod, along with their colleagues, reported decreased spinal bone mass in male long-distance runners, suggesting that the decreased levels of testosterone or increased levels of cortisol often seen in endurance runners could be the cause. Smathers and colleagues, however, reported decreased spine bone mineral density in elite cyclists relative to control subjects, but no differences in testosterone. Klesges and others also reported a decrease in total-body bone mineral content in male basketball players involved in intense training from pre-season to midseason. However, these investigators also reported that calcium supplementation was associated with significant increases in bone mineral content. Androgen therapy may also be recommended.

Sports Performance Research   Research regarding the effect of calcium supplementation on physical performance is almost nonexistent. In one of the only studies, White and others studied the acute effect of calcium on fat metabolism and exercise performance in trained female runners. The subjects consumed either a high-calcium (500 mg) or low-calcium (80 mg) drink 60 minutes prior to a 90-minute run at 70 percent VO_2 max, which was followed by a 10-kilometer treadmill time trial. The high-calcium drink did not affect carbohydrate or fat metabolism during the 90-minute run or 10-kilometer run time.

Low serum levels may impair neuromuscular functions, but such conditions are rare because the body will draw from calcium reserves in the skeleton to restore serum levels. In a review, Kunstel concluded that increased physical activity alone does not necessarily demand an increased intake of dietary calcium. Thus, acute or chronic calcium supplementation is not recommended as a means to enhance sports performance. However, calcium supplementation may be useful to help maintain bone mass in some female and male athletes, particularly those who do not consume adequate calcium from foods.

Prudent Recommendations   Adequate daily calcium intake and weight-bearing exercise are very important during the developmental years of childhood and adolescence to maximize peak bone mass, and such practices should be continued throughout adult life.

To help prevent osteoporosis, postmenopausal women and elderly men should obtain about 1,200 milligrams of calcium per day, along with adequate vitamin D (200–600 IU). Both weight-bearing aerobic and resistance strength-training exercises are recommended. Postmenopausal women should consult with their physicians relative to hormone replacement or drug therapy. Older men should also obtain adequate calcium, exercise, and consult their physicians for appropriate drug therapy if warranted.

For younger, premenopausal women, the nonpharmacological approach is recommended. The key with younger women, and men as well, is prevention. They need to develop peak bone mass, the optimal amount within genetic limitations, prior to age 25–30, and attempt to keep the bone mass high in the advancing years. Health professionals note that because evidence suggests that osteoporosis is easier to prevent than to treat, initiating sound health behaviors early in life and continuing them throughout life is the best approach. As the venerable Fred Astaire once noted, "Old age is like everything else. To make a success of it, you've got to start young." Thus, it would appear prudent for young women to develop a lifetime exercise program and obtain the AI of 1,000–1,300 milligrams for calcium in the diet. The earlier the better, for research has suggested a greater increase in bone mass when calcium supplements are given to prepubertal children, but adequate calcium intake is critical for adolescents as well.

Weight-bearing exercises, such as walking or jogging, promote bone mineralization by stressing the hips and spine, while resistance strength training and modified push-ups are also excellent for the spine and for the radial bone at the wrist joint.

Dairy products often are not consumed because they are believed to be high in fat and Calories. However, research with young girls has shown that a low-Calorie, calcium-rich diet mainly from dairy products can promote bone health and is not necessarily associated with excess weight gain. Although some dairy products may contain significant amounts of fat, four glasses of skim milk provide 1,200 mg of calcium. In addition, the milk (or its equivalent) would provide 32 grams of protein, which is about 80 percent of the protein RDA for the average woman, and a variety of other vitamins and minerals in less than 400 Calories.

It should also be noted that a balanced intake of multiple nutrients is needed for optimal bone health. Ilich and Kerstetter note that although approximately 80–90 percent of bone is comprised of calcium and phosphorus, other nutrients such as protein, magnesium, zinc, copper, iron, fluoride, and vitamins A, C, D, and K are also required for bone metabolism. Bonjour stresses the importance of adequate dietary protein, indicating that it is as essential as calcium and vitamin D for bone health and osteoporosis prevention.

Because coffee, alcohol, and tobacco use are secondary risk factors associated with the development of osteoporosis, moderation or abstinence is advocated.

The Consumers Union recommends a bone density test for women at risk, indicating that women over age 65 should be tested every two years. For younger women, whether or not to be tested depends on individual risks, such as a family history, being underweight, low calcium intake, little weight-bearing physical activity, and cigarette smoking. Amenorrheic athletes may also be at risk. Men over age 65 should also be tested. A dual energy x-ray absorptiometry (DEXA) test is recommended, not the ultrasound of the heel at your local drugstore.

Phosphorus (P)

Phosphorus is a nonmetallic element and is the second most abundant mineral in the body after calcium.

DRI   The adult RDA is 700 mg for both men and women. Higher amounts are needed between ages 9 and 18. Specific values for different age groups may be found in the DRI table on the inside of the front cover. The DV is 1,000 mg. The UL for adults is 4 grams, but only 3 grams between ages 1–8 and over 70.

Food Sources   As noted earlier in table 8.2, phosphorus is distributed widely in foods, mainly as phosphate salts in conjunction with animal protein. Excellent sources include seafood, meat, eggs, milk, cheese, nuts, dried beans and peas, grain products, and a wide variety of vegetables. Phosphate is a common food additive, and soft drinks have a relatively high phosphate content. In some foods, phosphorus is also a part of phytate, which may diminish the absorption of minerals like calcium, iron, zinc, and copper by forming insoluble phosphate salts in the intestine.

However, as noted previously, this is not a major problem with the typical North American diet.

Most Americans consume more than the RDA for phosphorus, and as noted previously, too little calcium. The recommended calcium:phosphorus ratio is about 1:1, that is equal amounts of each. In a review, Anderson and Barrett indicated that too much dietary phosphorus, which may occur because of phosphate additives in food, may impair calcium metabolism and predispose to osteoporosis. Too much phosphorus may also stimulate the release of parathyroid hormone. Anderson and Barrett noted that a ratio of up to 1:1.6 may be compatible with bone health, but ratios of 1:4 may be associated with osteoporosis. Conversely, Heaney and Nordin found that high intakes of dietary calcium may impair phosphorus absorption and eventually lead to phosphorus insufficiency and osteoporosis. A high dietary calcium:phosphorus ratio can occur with the use of calcium supplements and calcium-fortified foods.

Major Functions Knochel notes that phosphorus is a critically important element in every cell in the body. In the human body, phosphorus occurs only as the salt phosphate, which exists as inorganic phosphate or is coupled with other minerals or organic compounds. Phosphates are extremely important in human metabolism. About 80–90 percent of the phosphorus in the body combines to form calcium phosphate, which is used for the development of bones and teeth. As with calcium, the bones represent a sizable store of phosphate salts. Other phosphate salts, such as sodium phosphate, are involved in acid-base balance.

The remainder of the body phosphates are found in a variety of organic forms, including the phospholipids, which help form cell membranes, and DNA. Several other organic phosphates are of prime importance to the active individual. For example, organic phosphates are essential to the normal function of most of the B vitamins involved in the energy processes within the cell. They are also part of the high-energy compounds found in the muscle cell, such as ATP and PCr, which are needed for muscle contraction. Glucose also must be phosphorylated in order to proceed through glycolysis. Organic phosphates also are a part of a compound in the RBC known as 2,3-DPG (2,3-diphosphoglycerate), which facilitates the release of oxygen to the muscle tissues.

Deficiency: Health and Physical Performance Because phosphorus is distributed so widely in foods and because hormonal control is very effective, deficiency states are rare. They have been known to occur in hospital patients with serious illnesses, recovering alcoholics, and in those who use antacid compounds for long periods, as the antacid decreases the absorption of phosphorus. Symptoms parallel those of calcium deficiency, such as loss of bone material resulting in rickets or osteomalacia. Other symptoms include muscular weakness. Extreme muscular exercise may increase phosphorus excretion in the urine but has not been reported to cause a deficiency state. Phosphorus deficiency could theoretically impair physical performance, but it has not been the subject of study because such deficiencies are rare.

Supplementation: Health and Physical Performance Although various health problems, most notably osteoporosis, could occur with a phosphate deficiency, supplementation for health-related benefits has not received research attention because deficiency states are rare. However, phosphate salt supplementation has been studied as a means of enhancing exercise performance.

Phosphate salt supplements, such as sodium phosphate and potassium phosphate, were reported to relieve fatigue in German soldiers during World War I. Other research in Germany during the 1930s suggested that phosphate salts could improve physical performance. More than 50 years ago, one reviewer discredited much of this early research, but he did note that phosphates probably could increase human work output when consumed in quantities exceeding the amounts found in the normal diet. Indeed, they still are advertised today in some European sports-medicine journals and continue to be a favorite among European athletes. They have also been marketed as an ergogenic aid in the United States, most recently as the main ingredient in PhosFuel. Although phosphate salt supplementation may influence various physiological processes associated with physical performance, its effects to increase 2,3-DPG and related oxygen dynamics during aerobic endurance exercise have received most research attention. Bremner and others found that a 7-day phosphate loading protocol would increase erythrocyte phosphate pools and 2,3-DPG.

The results of contemporary research relative to the ergogenic effect of phosphate supplementation are somewhat equivocal. A number of studies, using appropriate experimental methods and the recommended phosphate dosages, have shown no effects of phosphate supplementation on a variety of performance variables. For example, Mannix and others reported that although phosphate supplementation did increase 2,3-DPG levels, it did not improve cardiovascular function or oxygen efficiency in subjects exercising at 60 percent of VO_2 max. These investigators generally concluded that phosphate salts were not ergogenic in nature, at least in relation to the type of performance tested in their studies.

In contrast, the results of other contemporary, well-designed studies suggest that phosphate salts may enhance exercise performance. One of the first studies reported was conducted by Robert Cade and his associates at the University of Florida. In a double-blind, placebo, crossover study, highly trained runners took 1 gram of sodium phosphate four times a day during the experimental phase. The phosphate salts increased the 2,3-DPG in the RBC, which related very closely to an increase in VO_2 max. The amount of lactate produced at a standard exercise workload decreased, suggesting more efficient oxygen delivery to the muscles. Although no performance data were presented, the authors did report that the subjects ran longer on the treadmill during the phosphate trials. This University of Florida research group also noted a reduced sensation of psychological stress while exercising at a standard workload.

Other investigators, using a protocol similar to that of Cade and his associates, have also revealed ergogenic effects. Richard Kreider and his colleagues, using highly trained cross-country runners as subjects, found that 4 grams of trisodium phosphate for 6 days produced a significant increase in VO_2 max, approximately

10 percent—very similar to the improvement noted in Cade's study. Changes in 2,3-DPG were not the mechanism for this increase, as these values did not increase. However, performance in a 5-mile competitive run on a treadmill did not improve. Ian Stewart and his associates from Australia, using trained cyclists, reported that 3.6 grams of sodium phosphate for 3 days did significantly increase 2,3-DPG levels and also increased VO_2 max by 11 percent and time to exhaustion on a progressive workload test on a bicycle ergometer by nearly 16 percent. In a follow-up to his previous study, Kreider looked at the effect of 4 grams of trisodium phosphate, 1 gram four times daily for 3–4 days, on physiological and performance factors during a maximal cycling test and a 40-kilometer bike race on a Velodyne. The study followed a double-blind, placebo, crossover protocol. Kreider and his colleagues noted a significant 9 percent increase in VO_2 max, a significantly faster 40-km time (improving from 45.75 to 42.25 minutes), and enhanced myocardial efficiency as monitored by echocardiographic techniques. These investigators suggested that phosphate salt supplementation could possess ergogenic qualities. However, Tremblay and others addressed methodological differences between studies (e.g., calcium versus sodium phosphate supplements) that could contribute to the equivocal results and also recommended additional research employing rigorous methodological control. These viewpoints have been reiterated in subsequent reviews by Horswill and Clarkson, although Clarkson did indicate that several studies have documented ergogenic effects, and the degree to which performance improved was similar among the studies.

Studies with phosphate supplementation conducted following these reviews revealed equivocal effects. Goss and others examined the effect of potassium phosphate supplementation (4 grams per day for 2 days) on ratings of perceived exertion (RPE) and physiological responses during a maximal graded exercise test in highly trained endurance runners. They found that although the phosphate supplementation did not affect physiological responses during exercise, the RPE was lower, suggesting that phosphate supplementation may have a beneficial effect on perceived exertion during moderately intense exercise at about 70–80 percent VO_2 max. Galloway and others provided an acute dose (22.2 grams) of calcium phosphate to trained cyclists and untrained subjects 90 minutes prior to a submaximal cycle test followed by a maximal exercise test, and reported no significant effects on heart rate, ventilation, oxygen uptake, or time to exhaustion. In another study, Kraemer and others had recreationally trained cyclists and untrained subjects consume a commercial product (PhosFuel) for 3.5 days and evaluated its effect on anaerobic performance in four 30-second cycle Wingate tests with 2 minutes rest between. The supplement provided no advantage over the placebo relative to peak power or mean power. However, these studies employed procedures (acute dose and calcium or potassium phosphate; commercial supplement and anaerobic performance) unlike those studies reporting beneficial effects, which used sodium phosphate, a more prolonged supplementation protocol, and more aerobic exercise performance tests.

The effect of 5–6 days of sodium phosphate supplementation on aerobic performance merits additional research.

Adenosine triphosphate (ATP), as you may recall, is the immediate source of energy for muscle contraction. Although some entrepreneurs have marketed ATP supplements for athletes, there is no available evidence that they enhance physical performance. Jordan and others studied the effect of 14 days of low-dose (150 milligrams) or high-dose (225 milligrams) oral ATP supplementation on indices of anaerobic capacity as measured by a 30-second Wingate power test and muscular strength. Although the investigators noted within-group differences in the high ATP group suggesting some small ergogenic effects on muscular strength, the finding of no differences between groups supports the conclusion that the ATP supplementation did not enhance performance.

Creatine phosphate is used to replenish ATP rapidly as a component of the ATP-PCr energy system. As noted in chapter 6, research with oral creatine supplementation has suggested some ergogenic effects on muscular strength and running speed. In a study with patients over 60 years of age who experienced muscular atrophy following fracture of the femur, creatine phosphate supplements, as compared to a placebo, significantly increased muscle mass during a rehabilitation program. As noted in chapter 6, similar benefits have been associated with creatine supplementation alone.

Excesses of phosphorus in the body are excreted by the kidneys. Phosphorus excess per se does not appear to pose any problems, with the exception of individuals who have limited kidney function. Subjects consuming phosphate supplements may experience gastrointestinal distress, which may be alleviated by mixing the salts in a liquid and consuming with a meal. Excessive amounts of phosphate over time may impair calcium metabolism and balance.

Prudent Recommendations Consuming a concentrated amount of phosphate salts, such as 4–5 grams, could cause gastrointestinal distress. Moreover, phosphate supplements are not recommended on a long-term basis as they may create calcium imbalances, possibly leading to osteoporosis. Some evidence suggests that sodium phosphate salt supplementation may enhance aerobic endurance performance. An accepted protocol appears to be a total of 4 grams of trisodium phosphate per day, consumed in 1-gram portions with food and drink, for 5–6 days. If you decide to experiment with phosphate supplementation, do so in training before using it in conjunction with competition. Given the association with possible calcium imbalances, this procedure should be used sparingly. Currently, the International Olympic Committee does not prohibit the use of phosphate salts.

Magnesium (Mg)

Magnesium is the sixth most abundant mineral found in the body; it is a positive ion and is related to calcium and phosphorus.

DRI The adult RDA for magnesium is 400–420 mg for men and 310–320 mg for women. Slightly different amounts, found in the DRI table on the inside front cover, are required by children and adolescents. The DV is 400 mg. The UL of 350 mg for magnesium, which is greater than the RDA for females, applies only to pharmacological forms of magnesium, as in supplements and fortified foods. There are no restrictions in obtaining magnesium via natural food sources.

Food Sources Magnesium is widely distributed in foods, particularly nuts, seafood, green leafy vegetables, other fruits and vegetables, black beans, and whole-grain products. One-half cup of shrimp or cooked spinach contains about 20 percent of the RDA, and a glass of skim milk has 10 percent. Many other foods contain about 2–10 percent of the RDA per serving. Areas with hard water may contain up to 20 mg of magnesium per liter, and some bottled waters may contain more than 100 mg per liter. About 25–60 percent of dietary magnesium is absorbed, depending on the amount consumed. See table 8.2.

Major Functions The body stores about 50–60 percent of its magnesium in the skeletal system, which may serve as a reserve during short periods of dietary deficiency. Sojka and Weaver indicate that magnesium influences bone metabolism and helps prevent bone fragility. Only about 1 percent is in the serum, but the remainder is found in soft tissues such as muscle, where it is a component of more than 300 enzymes. As such, magnesium plays a key role in a variety of physiological processes, many of which are important to the physically active individual, including neuromuscular, cardiovascular, and hormonal functions. For example, as a part of ATPase it is involved in muscle contraction and all body functions involving ATP as an energy source. Magnesium helps regulate the synthesis of protein and other compounds, such as 2,3-DPG, which may be essential for optimal oxygen metabolism, and glutathione, an antioxidant. It is a part of an enzyme that facilitates the metabolism of glucose in the muscle and is involved in gluconeogenesis. It is required in lipid metabolism. Magnesium also helps block some of the actions of calcium in the body, such as contraction in both the skeletal and smooth muscles.

Deficiency: Health and Physical Performance In a review, Rude and Shils noted that almost three of every four Americans fail to get the RDA of magnesium. The mean magnesium intake for males and females is 323 and 228 milligrams daily, respectively, which is about 100 milligrams less than the RDA. However, the National Academy of Sciences has reported that magnesium deficiency is rare. No purely dietary magnesium deficiency has been reported in people consuming normal diets, probably because of its wide availability in a variety of foods, an effective system of conservation by the kidneys and intestines, and a substantial storage in the bone tissue. However, certain health conditions such as kidney malfunction and prolonged diarrhea, as well as the use of diuretics and excessive alcohol, may contribute to a deficiency state. Durlach and others note that primary magnesium deficiency is due to inadequate magnesium intake, and certain athletic groups may have diets deficient in magnesium. Henry Lukaski reported that dietary survey findings were somewhat mixed; some studies indicated that although most male athletes equaled or exceeded the RDA for magnesium, many female athletes were obtaining only about 60–65 percent of the RDA, while athletes in weight-control

sports were getting only 30–35 percent. In one study, Nuviala and others reported that no group of female athletes in their survey consumed the RDA for magnesium. Over time, such low dietary intakes may lead to a magnesium deficiency.

Deficiency symptoms include apathy, muscle weakness, muscle twitching and tremor, muscle cramps (particularly in the feet), and cardiac arrhythmias. The muscular symptoms may occur because the low levels of magnesium are not able to block the stimulating effect of calcium on muscle contraction. In this sense, magnesium deficiency may be related to high blood pressure because excessive calcium may cause the muscles in the arterioles to constrict. Indeed, in a review, Mizushima and others suggested that a low dietary intake of magnesium is associated with increased blood pressure. Additionally, Lima and others note that low serum magnesium is associated with type 2 diabetes. Given the possible relationship of magnesium deficiency to cardiac arrhythmias, high blood pressure, and type 2 diabetes, Durlach and others suggested that magnesium deficiency may be a cardiovascular disease risk factor.

Exercise appears to influence magnesium metabolism, but in an unknown way. Deuster has noted that one of the most common research observations is a decrease in plasma levels of magnesium following exercise, a finding confirmed by Buchman and others who measured magnesium levels following a marathon run. It is thought that magnesium enters the tissues in response to exercise-related requirements, for example, of the muscle tissue for energy metabolism and the adipose tissue for lipolysis. Some investigators also suggested that prolonged exercise increases magnesium losses from the body via urine and sweat. Although the reported sweat losses of 4–15 mg per liter are relatively small in comparison to body stores and daily intake, Nielsen and Lukaski stated that strenuous exercise apparently increases urinary and sweat losses that may increase magnesium requirements by 10–20 percent. Keep in mind that to replace 15 milligrams of magnesium lost from the body, one would need to consume about 40 milligrams at a 40 percent rate of absorption. That is almost 10 percent of the male RDA. Casoni and others reported significantly lower serum magnesium levels in Italian endurance athletes as compared with sedentary individuals, but the serum values were well within the normal range. One study reported a correlation between plasma levels of magnesium and VO_2 max in trained individuals, but this finding has not been replicated. Other research suggests that magnesium deficiency may be associated with an impaired immune function and chronic fatigue syndrome, characterized by unexplained fatigue or easy fatigability lasting longer than 6 months. On the basis of some of these findings, several reports have recommended that individuals undergoing prolonged, intensive physical training should increase their daily intake of magnesium, but these recommendations are within range of the new RDA. The extra Calories consumed when energy expenditure increases during exercise should provide the additional magnesium.

Lukaski indicates that a magnesium deficiency increases oxygen requirements to complete submaximal exercise and reduces endurance performance. Although there is little evidence showing a magnesium deficiency in athletes severe enough to impair physical performance, Nielsen and Lukaski indicate that magnesium intakes of less than 260 mg/day for males and 220 mg/day for female athletes may result in a magnesium-deficient status over time, and such could be the case with athletes on strict diets in weight control sports.

Supplementation: Health and Physical Performance Relative to health, some epidemiological research from Europe and the United States has indicated that males who consume hard drinking water, which is high in magnesium, experience fewer deaths from myocardial infarction. Rubenowitz and others reported a 35 percent reduction in death for those who consumed the most magnesium from municipal water supplies. High blood pressure is one of the major risk factors for heart disease. Antinoro noted that magnesium may help reduce blood pressure, but usually as part of a healthful diet, such as the DASH (Dietary Approaches to Stop Hypertension) diet discussed in chapter 9. However, magnesium supplementation appears to have little effect on blood pressure. Dickinson and others analyzed data from 12 randomly controlled trials and found no effect of magnesium supplementation over the course of 8 to 26 weeks on systolic blood pressure, although there was a small but significant reduction in diastolic blood pressure. However, the investigators indicated that the evidence in favor of a causal association between magnesium supplementation and blood pressure reduction is weak and probably due to bias. Although magnesium supplementation may benefit individuals with deficiencies, there appears to be little research to support health benefits of magnesium supplementation in well-nourished individuals.

In an earlier review, McDonald and Keen indicated that they are not aware of any data showing a positive effect of magnesium supplementation on exercise performance in individuals who are in adequate magnesium status. However, several studies published subsequent to their review have provided some preliminary data, although the results are equivocal. For example, relative to aerobic endurance, Brilla and Gunter reported that magnesium enhanced running economy at 90 percent VO_2 max because the oxygen cost of running was lower compared to a placebo condition. However, magnesium did not significantly increase run time to exhaustion in this study. Additionally, Terblanche and others, matching 20 marathon runners into two groups based on performance time, provided either a placebo or 365 milligrams of magnesium per day to the subjects 4 weeks prior to and 6 weeks after running a marathon. Their dependent variables were marathon performance and several tests of quadriceps muscular strength and fatigue during the recovery phase after the marathon. They reported no significant effects of magnesium supplementation on muscle or serum levels of magnesium, marathon performance, muscle function, or muscle recovery. They suggested that excess magnesium in the diet may not be absorbed by those with normal levels in the body. More recently, Weller and others confirmed these findings. In a double-blind, placebo-controlled study, athletes who received 500 mg magnesium oxide for 3 weeks experienced no significant increase in serum or muscle magnesium levels, nor did the athletes improve performance on three exercise protocols (cycle ergometer; arm ergometer; treadmill run) to exhaustion.

These three studies appear to be well designed, and, in general, indicate that magnesium supplements were not helpful. Indeed, in their meta-analysis of human supplementation studies, Newhouse and Finstad noted that the strength of the evidence favors those studies finding no effect of magnesium supplementation on any form of exercise performance, including aerobic, anaerobic-lactic acid, and strength activities. In the most recent review, Nielsen and Lukaski also concluded that magnesium supplementation of physically active individuals with adequate magnesium status has not been shown to enhance physical performance. However, it may be possible that if a magnesium deficiency is corrected, exercise performance may be improved. For example, Lukaski noted that some earlier studies have shown that magnesium supplementation improved strength and cardiorespiratory function in healthy persons and athletes, but also noted that it is unclear as to whether these observations related to improvement of an impaired nutritional status or a pharmacologic effect. In a case study, magnesium supplementation also helped resolve muscle cramps in a tennis player, which may be part of the reason some sport drinks contain magnesium. However, at present the data are too limited to support an ergogenic effect of magnesium supplementation, and additional well-controlled research is justified.

As noted, an UL of 350 mg has been established for magnesium supplements or fortified foods. Mildly excessive intakes of magnesium may cause nausea, vomiting, and diarrhea. In individuals with kidney disorders who cannot excrete the excess, increased serum levels of magnesium may lead to coma and death.

Prudent Recommendations Physically active individuals should obtain adequate magnesium from a balanced diet containing foods rich in magnesium. For those trying to lose body weight for competition, dietary magnesium may be compromised. In particular, Newhouse and Finstad indicate that female athletes are at risk for magnesium deficiency. In such cases, magnesium from supplements and/or fortified foods is recommended, but not to exceed 350 milligrams daily. There is no need for larger doses, as they may be associated with some adverse effects.

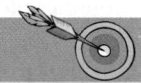

Key Concepts

- ▶ Calcium is most prevalent in the milk food group. One glass of low-fat milk provides about 30 percent of the daily AI.
- ▶ Calcium intake is important for everyone, but in particular, children, adolescents, and all women should obtain adequate dietary calcium. Children and adolescents should obtain adequate calcium to increase their peak bone mass; women need calcium to help prevent losses during aging.
- ▶ Two keys to the prevention of osteoporosis are weight-bearing or resistance exercise and adequate calcium and vitamin D in the diet. Appropriate drug therapy may be recommended for some women.
- ▶ Phosphate salts have been used for more than 80 years in attempts to improve athletic performance, but research findings are equivocal. The most recent studies supporting ergogenic effects need confirmation by additional research.
- ▶ A deficiency of magnesium may be associated with muscle cramps. At the present time, the data are too limited to support an ergogenic effect from magnesium supplementation.

Trace Minerals

The **trace minerals** (trace elements) are those needed in quantities less than 100 mg per day. These minerals are often known as *microminerals*. For several, the body needs only extremely minute amounts, such as a few micrograms (millionth of a gram) per day. The term *ultratrace* is applied to these minerals.

Iron (Fe)

Iron is a metallic element that exists in two general forms, ferrous (Fe^{2+}) and ferric (Fe^{3+}).

DRI Depending upon age and sex, the average individual needs to replace about 1.0–1.5 mg of iron that is lost from the body daily. However, because the bioavailability of iron is very low, with only about 10 percent of food iron being absorbed, the RDA is ten times the need. Currently the RDA is 8 mg for men, 11 mg for males age 14–18, and 15 mg for female teenagers and 18 mg for female adults. Slightly different amounts are needed by other age groups and may be found in the DRI table on the inside front cover. Pregnant women need 27 mg, whereas postmenopausal women need only 8 mg. The current DV is 18 mg. The UL range is 40–45 mg/day.

Food Sources Dietary iron comes in two forms. **Heme iron** is associated with hemoglobin and myoglobin and thus is found only in animal foods, such as meat, chicken, and fish. About 35–55 percent of the iron found in meat is heme iron, the percentage being somewhat higher in beef as compared to chicken and fish. **Nonheme iron** is found in both animal and plant foods. About 20–70 percent of the iron in animal foods and 100 percent in plant foods is in the nonheme form. Heme iron has greater bioavailability: about 10–35 percent of it is absorbed from the intestines compared to only 2–10 percent for nonheme iron. The percent absorbed depends on the iron needs of the individual. Those with higher needs will absorb more and those with lower needs will absorb less.

Excellent animal sources of dietary iron include liver, heart, lean meats, oysters, clams, and dark poultry meat. One ounce of lean meat provides about 1 mg of heme iron. Good sources of nonheme iron include dried fruits such as apricots, prunes, and raisins; vegetables such as broccoli and peas; legumes; and whole-grain products. Six dried apricot halves or one-half cup of beans provides about 3 mg of nonheme iron, and some breakfast cereals are fortified to provide 100 percent of the RDA. Cooking in iron pots or skillets also contributes some iron to the diet. On a balanced diet, about 6 mg of iron is provided in every 1,000 Calories ingested. See table 8.4 for foods high in iron.

Certain factors in food may affect the amount of iron absorbed into the body. A muscle protein factor (MPF) found in meat, fish, poultry is an unknown agent that facilitates the absorption of both heme and nonheme iron. The existence of such a factor is suggested by the fact that small amounts of meat added to vegetable or grain products enhance nonheme absorption. Certain peptides in meat may cause this increased absorption. For example, iron absorption from beans is almost doubled when mixed with small amounts of meat, as in dishes such as chili. Baech and others even found that small amounts of meat significantly increase nonheme iron absorption in a meal low in vitamin C and rich in phytates, two factors that would limit iron absorption. Vitamin C prevents the oxidation of ferrous iron to the ferric form (ferrous iron is more readily absorbed) and thus facilitates nonheme iron absorption, but it has no effect on absorption of heme iron. Thus, for breakfast, drinking orange juice improves the bioavailability of iron in toast.

However, substances found naturally in some foods, such as tannins in tea, phytic acid in grains, oxalic acid in vegetables, and excessive fiber, may decrease the bioavailability of nonheme iron by forming insoluble salts (phytates, oxalates) or by promoting rapid transport and excretion through the intestines. Tea, for example, which is high in tannins, decreases iron absorption by 60 percent. However, if the diet is balanced these factors should not pose a major problem for adequate iron nutrition. Certain mineral supplements, particularly calcium, and even the calcium in milk, when taken with a meal, may impair absorption of nonheme iron. This effect may be lessened by ingestion of vitamin C with the meal. As mentioned previously, calcium supplements may be recommended for some individuals, including youth, who also need more dietary iron. Molgaard and others noted increasing evidence suggesting that high calcium intake does not impair iron status. In a study they found that consuming a 500-mg calcium supplement at the evening meal over the course of a year had no effect on the iron status of adolescent girls.

Major Functions The major function of iron in the body is the formation of compounds essential to the transportation and utilization of oxygen. The vast majority is used to form hemoglobin, a protein-iron compound in the RBC that transports oxygen from the lungs to the body tissues. Other iron compounds include myoglobin, the cytochromes, and several Krebs-cycle metalloenzymes, which help use oxygen at the cellular level. The remainder of the body iron is stored in the tissues, principally as protein compounds called **ferritins.** The iron in the blood, serum ferritin, is used as an index of the body iron stores, as are a number of other markers such as transferrin, protoporphyrin, and hemoglobin. Other major storage sites include the liver, spleen, and bone marrow. When ferritin levels become excessive in the liver, the iron is stored as hemosiderin, an insoluble form. Approximately 30 percent of the body iron is in storage form, while the remaining 70 percent is involved in oxygen metabolism. Because iron is so critical to oxygen use in humans, it is essential that those individuals engaged in aerobic endurance-type exercises have an adequate dietary intake. Figure 8.5 represents a brief outline of iron metabolism in humans. For a comprehensive review of iron metabolism and regulation, the interested reader is referred to the review by Wood and Ronnenberg.

Deficiency: Health and Physical Performance According to Zimmermann and Hurrell, iron deficiency is one of the leading risk factors for disability and death worldwide, affecting an estimated 2 billion people, particularly in the developing world. Denic and Agarwal suggest that iron deficiency is so prevalent because, in the evolutionary process, it conferred some protection against many infectious diseases, such as malaria and the plague. Thus, there may be a genetic predisposition to iron deficiency, and it may be

TABLE 8.4 Trace minerals: iron, copper, zinc, chromium, selenium

Trace mineral*	Major food sources	Major body functions	Deficiency symptoms	Symptoms of excessive consumption
Iron (Fe) RDA: 8 mg♂ 18 mg♀ DV: 18 mg	Organ meats such as liver; meat, fish, and poultry; shellfish, especially oysters; dried beans and peas; whole-grain products; green leafy vegetables; spinach; broccoli; dried apricots, dates, figs, raisins; iron cookware	Hemoglobin and myoglobin formation; electron transfer; essential in oxidative processes	Fatigue; anemia; impaired temperature regulation; decreased resistance to infection	Hemochromatosis; liver damage
Copper (Cu) RDA: 900 mcg DV: 2 mg	Organ meats such as liver; meat, fish, and poultry; shellfish; nuts; eggs; whole-grain breads; bran cereals; avocado; broccoli; banana	Proper use of iron and hemoglobin in the body; metalloenzyme involved in connective tissue formation and oxidations	Rare; anemia	Rare; nausea; vomiting
Zinc (Zn) RDA: 11 mg♂ 8 mg♀ DV: 15 mg	Organ meats; meat, fish, poultry; shellfish, especially oysters; dairy products; nuts; whole-grain products; vegetables, asparagus, spinach	Cofactor of many enzymes involved in energy metabolism, protein synthesis, immune function, sexual maturation, and sensations of taste and smell	Depressed immune function; impaired wound healing; depressed appetite; failure to grow; skin inflammation	Increased LDL- and decreased HDL-cholesterol; impaired immune system; nausea; vomiting; impaired copper absorption
Chromium (Cr) AI: 35 mcg♂ 25 mcg♀ DV: 120 mcg	Organ meats such as liver; meats; oysters; cheese; whole-grain products; asparagus; beer	Enhances insulin function as glucose tolerance factor	Glucose intolerance; impaired lipid metabolism	Rare from dietary sources
Selenium (Se) RDA: 55 mcg DV: 70 mcg	Meat, fish, poultry; organ meats such as kidney, liver; seafood; whole grains and nuts from selenium-rich soil	Cofactor of glutathione peroxidase, an antioxidant enzyme	Rare; cardiac muscle damage	Nausea; vomiting; abdominal pain; hair loss

*RDA or AI: adults age19–50 DV: Daily Value

prevalent even in countries where adequate amounts of dietary iron are available. Iron is one of the few nutrients commonly found to be slightly deficient in the diet of many Americans and Canadians. Cooper and others noted that poor dietary intake and iron deficiency exist in Canada, and may approximate 10 percent of women 50 and younger.

The body normally loses very little iron through such routes as the skin, gastrointestinal tract, hair, and sweat. About 8 mg of dietary iron daily will replace these losses. Females also lose some additional iron in the blood flow during menstruation. They need about 15–18 mg of dietary iron per day to replace their total losses. Adolescent boys need about 11 mg, as they are increasing muscle tissue and blood volume during this rapid period of growth. With 6 mg of iron per 1,000 Calories, the adult male has no problem meeting his requirement of 8 mg per day. With a normal intake of 2,900 Calories, he will receive 17.4 mg. With 2,200 Calories, the average intake for females, only 13.2 mg iron would be provided. This is somewhat short of the 15–18 mg needed.

The main factor underlying iron deficiency in Western diets is inadequate dietary intake. Fairbanks indicates that the diet has

evolved so that many individuals consume iron-poor diets, such as snack foods, white bread, and soft drinks. However, most females have normal hemoglobin and serum ferritin status. Because the normal loss of iron from the body is relatively low, and because excessive amounts in the body may be harmful, the intestine limits the amount absorbed from the diet. In contrast, when an individual becomes iron deficient, the intestines may increase the amount of dietary iron absorbed to above 30 percent. Nevertheless, Looker and others reported that iron deficiency and iron deficiency anemia are still relatively common in adolescent girls and women of childbearing age. The National Academy of Sciences has reported that the frequency of iron deficiency without anemia is much greater than that of iron-deficiency anemia. Nevertheless, about 3–5 percent of the female population has iron-deficiency anemia, a common nutrient-deficiency disorder in the United States and Canada.

Deficiency stages Iron deficiency occurs in stages. The first stage involves depletion of the bone marrow stores and a decrease in serum ferritin. It is referred to as the stage of iron depletion. The second stage involves a further decrease in serum ferritin and

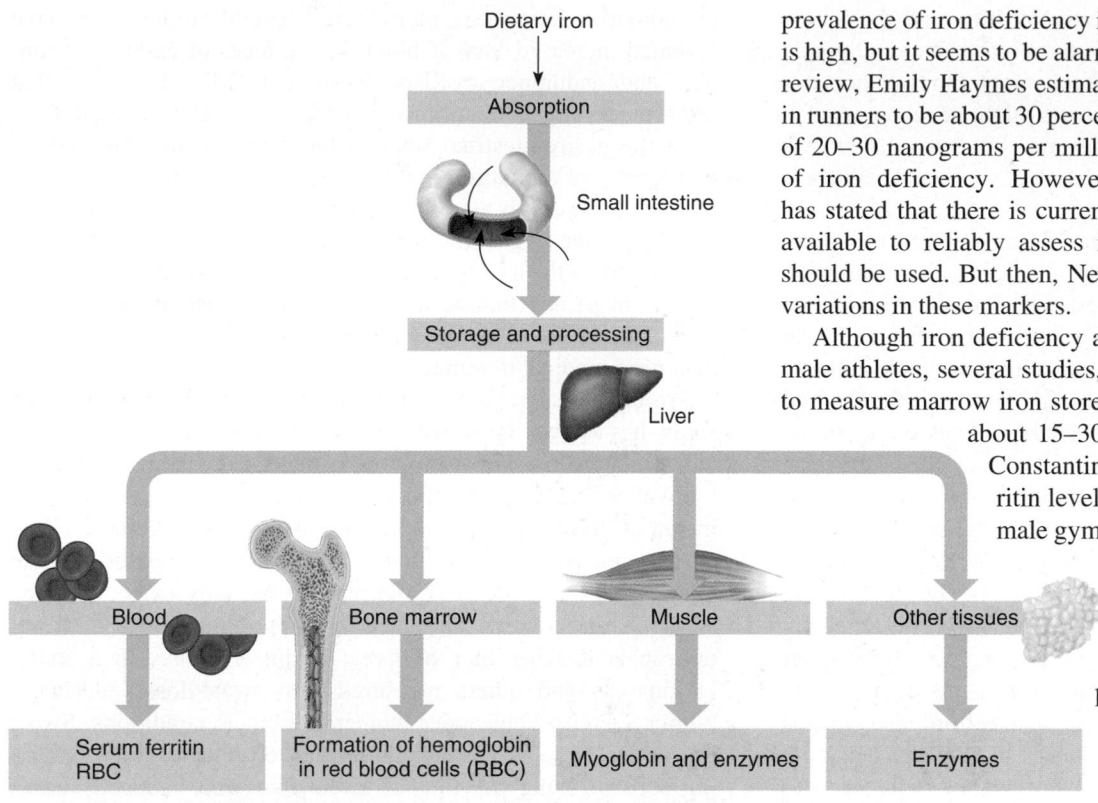

Dietary iron

Absorption

Small intestine

Storage and processing

Liver

Blood

Bone marrow

Muscle

Other tissues

Serum ferritin RBC

Formation of hemoglobin in red blood cells (RBC)

Myoglobin and enzymes

Enzymes

FIGURE 8.5 Simplified diagram of iron metabolism in humans. After digestion, iron is used in the formation of hemoglobin, myoglobin, and certain cellular enzymes, all of which are essential for transportation of oxygen in the body.

less iron in the hemoglobin, or less circulating iron. Other markers are used to evaluate iron stores in this stage, including free erythrocyte protoporphyrin (FEP), which is used to form hemoglobin. FEP in the blood increases when adequate iron is not available. Serum transferrin, a protein that carries iron in the blood, also increases. This is the stage referred to as iron-deficiency erythropoiesis. In these first two stages the hemoglobin concentration in the blood is still normal. Collectively, these stages are often alluded to as **iron deficiency without anemia.** The third stage consists of a very low level of serum ferritin and decreased hemoglobin concentration, or **iron-deficiency anemia.** Symptoms of iron-deficiency anemia include paleness, tiredness, and low vitality, and impaired ability to regulate body temperature in a cold environment. Most notably, iron-deficiency anemia impairs muscular performance. In their review of 29 research reports, Haas and Brownlie noted a strong causal effect of iron-deficiency anemia to impaired work capacity in both humans and animals.

Deficiency in athletes Because iron is so critical to the oxygen energy system, it is essential for endurance athletes to have adequate iron in the diet to maintain optimal body supplies. There are some differences of opinion about the magnitude of iron deficiency in athletes. A substantial number of studies, using serum ferritin levels as a basis of iron status, revealed that 50–80 percent of female athletes, particularly gymnasts and endurance runners, were at risk of iron deficiency. In other sports, such as soccer (football), Maughan and Shirreffs reported that the

prevalence of iron deficiency in male and female players generally is high, but it seems to be alarmingly high in female players. In her review, Emily Haymes estimated the prevalence of iron depletion in runners to be about 30 percent. Serum ferritin levels in the range of 20–30 nanograms per milliliter have been considered markers of iron deficiency. However, the National Research Council has stated that there is currently no single biochemical indicator available to reliably assess iron adequacy, so several markers should be used. But then, Newhouse and Clement reported wide variations in these markers.

Although iron deficiency appears not to be a problem in most male athletes, several studies, including one using a bone biopsy to measure marrow iron stores, have reported poor iron status in about 15–30 percent of male distance runners. Constantini and others reported low serum ferritin levels in a high percentage of adolescent male gymnasts.

After reviewing the literature, Priscilla Clarkson reported that iron deficiency to the point of decreased RBC and hemoglobin production does not appear to be prevalent in the athletic population. Some studies have reported iron-deficiency anemia occuring in female athletes at the same rate as in the general U.S. female population (about 3–5 percent) or at a higher rate. However, in a review, Beard and Tobin indicated that the prevalence of iron-deficiency anemia is likely to be higher in athletic groups, especially younger female athletes, than in healthy sedentary individuals. One recent study reported iron-deficiency anemia in 14 percent of female national basketball team players, and 3 percent of male players. In a study of elite women soccer players six months before the FIFA Women's World Cup, Landahl and others reported that 57 percent had iron deficiency and 29 percent had iron deficiency anemia.

The normal hemoglobin level is 14–16 grams per deciliter (100 ml) of blood for males and 12–14 grams for females. Males have been classified as anemic with less than 13 grams, whereas values less than 11 grams, and in some cases 12 grams, have been used as the criterion for anemia in females. Randy Eichner, a hematologist involved in sports medicine, poses the interesting question of whether an athlete whose usual hemoglobin is 16 grams per deciliter is anemic if his level decreases to 14 grams.

Although there may be some debate about the magnitude of the problem of iron deficiency in athletes, most investigators concede that it may be important to monitor the diet and iron status of certain athletes, particularly if performance begins to suffer without any obvious explanation. One report noted that Greg Lemond was struggling in the first stages of the Tour of Italy until his trainer suggested iron therapy. Following several injections, Lemond finished strong in the Tour, winning the last trial race. A month later he won the Tour de France in a remarkable finish.

The International Center for Sports Nutrition and the Sports Medicine and Science Division of the United States Olympic Committee recommend screening for hemoglobin and hematocrit twice yearly. Other tests of iron stores might be recommended for menstruating female athletes. Some, but not all, NCAA Division I-A schools screen for iron deficiency in female athletes.

Causes of deficiency in athletes There may be a number of causes for the low iron or hemoglobin levels found in some athletes. Although adult male athletes appear to obtain sufficient dietary iron, numerous studies have revealed that dietary intake of iron may be inadequate in female and adolescent male athletes. The type of dietary iron may also be important. Ann Snyder and her colleagues noted that although female athletes on a normal mixed diet or a modified vegetarian diet had the same iron intake (14 mg/day), the modified vegetarian diet was associated with significantly lower iron stores in the body, suggestive of a beneficial effect of heme iron. In a study by Wilson and Ball of male Australian athletes, although vegetarians consumed more iron than omnivores, their serum ferritin levels were significantly lower. Other studies, such as by Weight and Lyle, and their colleagues, have confirmed the value of meat to help prevent decreases in iron stores during training, and Telford also stresses the value of dietary protein. Three ounces of beef per day were effective. Vegetarian athletes should be aware of the need to incorporate plant foods with high iron content in their diets, a viewpoint supported by the American Dietetic Association in its position stand on vegetarian diets. Athletes who begin to train at altitude will need to ensure adequate dietary iron intake, because the increased production of red blood cells at altitude will draw upon the body reserves.

Exercise, particularly running, may contribute to iron loss in both sexes for a variety of reasons. In their review, Jones and Newhouse report a common condition often seen in distance runners, **hematuria,** the presence of hemoglobin or myoglobin in the urine. This may be caused by repeated foot contact with the ground, rupturing some RBC and releasing hemoglobin (a process called **hemolysis**), some of which may be excreted by the kidneys. For example, in a well–controlled study Jones and others examined the effect of intense training in middle-distance track athletes on urine markers of hematuria over a 4-week period. Hematuria was reported after 45 percent of the workouts observed, and 90 percent of the athletes experienced post-workout hematuria at least once. The highest incidence of hematuria was observed after interval workouts run at high intensity over distances ranging from 400–3,000 meters. Moreover, Schumacher and others compared blood markers of iron status among various male athletic groups and found a marker in endurance runners, as compared to endurance cyclists, that suggested runners may experience more hemolysis due to foot impact.

Prolonged running may also lead to ruptured muscle cells, releasing myoglobin, which may have the same fate. An irritation of the inner lining of the urinary bladder may also be a source of RBC loss. Even nonimpact athletes like rowers and weight lifters have experienced hemolysis, possibly due to the mechanical stress developed in the muscles or hand-grip hemolysis, similar to foot-strike hemolysis in runners. Several studies also have revealed increased loss of blood in the feces of endurance runners and endurance cyclists. Horn and Feller indicated that intense prolonged endurance exercise may shunt blood flow from the gastrointestinal tract to the skin and muscles, which may cause inflammation and bleeding in the GI tract. They cite several studies with marathon runners that found hemoglobin in the feces after races. Another contributing factor may be bleeding caused by the use of aspirin or other anti-inflammatory drugs to control pain. Athletes who detect blood loss in the urine or feces should see a physician, as there may be other causes that may need medical treatment.

An additional source of iron loss is the sweat. Although one study has shown that sweat losses of iron are relatively low when induced by sauna (0.02 mg per liter), according to a study by Waller and Haymes, the total amount of iron lost in sweat increases during exercise, more so in males than in females. This may be related to the fact that serum iron may actually increase during an exercise session and may be partially excreted in the sweat. Earlier studies suggested that approximately 0.3–0.4 mg of iron is lost per liter of sweat during exercise. In a study, DeRuisseau and others measured iron sweat losses during a 2-hour exercise bout under temperate climate conditions. Sweat iron losses were higher during the first 60 minutes, approximating 0.18–0.20 mg per liter of sweat, but were reduced almost by half during the second 60 minutes. These do not appear to be substantial iron losses, but if an athlete loses 2 liters of sweat in a heavy workout, and if we use a value of 0.20 milligrams of iron per liter, then 0.4 milligrams of iron would be lost. At a 10 percent rate of absorption, it would take 4 milligrams of iron to replace these sweat iron losses, which is 50 percent of the adult male RDA.

In summary, athletes in training may lose more iron than nonathletes. In another review, Weaver and Rajaram noted that when compared to the reference value of sedentary individuals, iron losses in the feces, urine, and sweat may be 75 percent greater in male athletes (1.75 versus 1.0 milligrams) and about 65 percent greater in female athletes (2.3 versus 1.4 milligrams). In less-athletic women engaging in a moderate exercise training program for 6 months, Rajaram and others found that training at 60–75 percent of the heart rate reserve had little effect on serum ferritin levels, although they remained below normal from the beginning to the end of the study.

Sports anemia As would be expected, the problem of concern to the endurance athlete is the development of iron-deficiency anemia. A number of studies have shown that anemia causes a significant reduction in the ability to perform prolonged high-level exercise. The donation of blood causes a drop in hemoglobin, which may also decrease performance capacity. This is, of course, related to the decreased ability to transport and use oxygen in the body.

One form of anemia associated with endurance training is sports anemia, mentioned previously in chapter 6. Sports anemia is not a true anemia. Although the hemoglobin concentration is toward the lower end of the normal range, the other indices of iron status are normal. Whether sports anemia is a beneficial physiological response to endurance exercise or a condition that will hinder performance is not known. Short-term sports anemia appears to develop in some individuals during the early phases of training or when the magnitude of training increases drastically. One of the effects of endurance training is to increase both the plasma volume and the number of RBC. However, the plasma expansion appears to be greater, so there is a dilution of the RBC and a lowering of the hemoglobin concentration. This effect is believed to be beneficial to the athlete, however, because it reduces the viscosity, or thickness, of the blood and allows it to flow more easily. In many athletes the hemoglobin concentration returns to normal after the first month or so of training. Long-term sports anemia is often seen in highly trained endurance athletes. One theory proposes that the production of RBC by the bone marrow is decreased in endurance athletes because the RBC become so efficient in releasing oxygen to the tissues. The authors of this theory suggest that sports anemia is not due to poor iron status. Moreover, in a review relating hematological factors to aerobic power, Norman Gledhill and his associates indicated that an increase in blood volume can compensate for a moderate reduction in hemoglobin concentration.

Eichner noted that the term *sports anemia* is a pseudoanemia, or a false anemia in athletes who are aerobically fit. Weight also indicated that the term is misleading and its use should be discouraged because athletes who develop anemia do so not because of exercise, but for the same reasons that nonathletes do, primarily inadequate dietary iron.

Iron deficiency without anemia   As reinforced in a study at the Australian Institute of Sport, rigorous physical training may lead to a decreased iron status, but not to the point of anemia. The effect of iron deficiency without anemia on physical performance is controversial and still under study. Lukaski and others had 11 females live in a metabolic ward for 80–100 days to induce iron deficiency without anemia. They observed a decreased rate of oxygen uptake and reduced energy production during exercise. Other research with iron-deficient, nonanemic human subjects revealed an increased lactate production during maximal exercise, indicative of reduced oxygen utilization in the muscle cells. Other research by Khaled and others indicates that a mild iron deficiency in elite athletes could be associated with an increased subjective feeling of exercise overload. Based on their reviews, Lukaski indicated that iron deficiency without anemia impairs muscle function and limits exercise capacity, while Suedekum and Dimeff concluded that iron deficiency without anemia may adversely affect athletic performance.

Nevertheless, research has shown that it is possible to maintain VO_2 max, endurance capacity, and maximal functioning of the muscle oxidative enzymes even when the body iron stores are severely diminished or depleted. Swedish investigators, as cited by Celsing, withdrew blood over a 4-week period to create an iron deficiency. They then infused the blood back into the subjects so that they were in a condition of iron deficiency without anemia. Even though the iron status was poor, physiological

functioning and endurance performance were not impaired. These investigators noted that low serum ferritin levels may not reflect low iron levels in the muscles.

One might speculate that differences between these studies, that is, poor iron status due to diet versus blood withdrawal, could influence the results. As many athletes may be iron deficient, yet nonanemic, this continues to be an important research topic.

Supplementation: Health and Physical Performance
The importance of iron to oxygen transport and endurance capacity and the possibility that many athletes, particularly females, may be iron deficient have led a number of investigators in the area of sport nutrition to recommend that more athletes take dietary iron or supplements. Others discourage the indiscriminate use of iron supplements by athletes.

Does iron supplementation improve physical performance? Many studies have been conducted in attempts to answer this question, and the answer appears to be dependent upon the iron status of the individual.

Iron-deficiency anemia   If the individual suffers from iron-deficiency anemia, iron therapy could help correct this condition and concomitantly increase performance capacity. In their review, Rodenberg and Gustafson concluded that athletes who are found to be anemic secondary to iron deficiency do benefit and show improved performance with appropriate iron supplementation.

Iron deficiency without anemia   The effect on exercise performance of iron supplementation to iron-deficient, nonanemic individuals is somewhat more controversial.

Several studies have shown beneficial effects. In some cases small increases in hemoglobin levels have been associated with an increased VO_2 max. For example, Magazanik and others reported that 160 mg of a daily oral iron supplement to young women in training had a more favorable effect on hemoglobin status and VO_2 max during the first 21 days of training, but there were no differences between the supplemented and placebo group after 42 days of training. Beneficial effects on exercise performance have also been observed in several well-designed studies with iron deficient, nonanemic subjects. One double-blind, placebo study did note an improvement in running performance when iron-deficient, yet nonanemic, female high school distance runners were treated with iron supplements for 1 month. Hudgins and others found that 65 milligrams of iron per day improved the 5-kilometer performance of 12 female cross-country runners. Rowland and associates reported significant improvements in treadmill endurance time in competitive runners following 4 weeks of ferrous sulfate supplementation. Compared to a placebo group, Hinton and others from Cornell University reported a significantly improved 15-kilometer cycle ergometer performance in iron-deficient females who received 100 milligrams ferrous sulfate daily during six weeks of strenuous exercise training. In a similarly designed follow-up study from the Cornell University research group, Brownlie and others reported that untrained, iron-depleted, nonanemic women who received an iron supplement had significantly greater increases in VO_2 max as compared to the placebo group. Based on these two studies, the investigators suggested that iron deficiency without anemia impairs favorable adaptation to aerobic exercise.

Conversely, most research with iron-deficient, nonanemic subjects has shown that iron supplementation may improve iron status, for example by increasing serum ferritin, but appears to have little effect upon maximal physiological functioning as measured by VO_2 max. Additionally, other researchers have observed no beneficial effect of iron supplementation on physical performance in subjects who had iron deficiency without anemia. Lamanca and Haymes revealed a 38 percent improvement in an endurance task following iron supplementation as compared with a 1 percent decrease in the control group; although this difference is impressive, it was not statistically significant. Matter and her associates found no improvement in the treadmill endurance performance of female marathon runners following either 1 week or 10 weeks of iron supplementation, which was combined with a folate supplement. Also, Newhouse and others reported no improvement in performance on a variety of exercise tests, both aerobic and anaerobic, in physically active females following 8 weeks of oral iron supplementation. In a single-blind, placebo, crossover study, Powell and Tucker provided a placebo or 130 mg of elemental iron per day for 2 weeks to ten highly trained female cross-country runners. The supplementation had no significant effect on metabolic variables related to running performance, but the authors noted that serum iron indices were also unaffected by the supplements. Fogelholm and others studied the effect of 100 mg iron daily for 8 weeks, versus a placebo, on a bicycle ergometer ride to exhaustion in two groups of female athletes. The supplement did increase serum ferritin levels but had no effect on performance. Klingshirn and others matched 18 distance runners on endurance time, giving half of them 100 mg elemental iron per day and the other half a placebo for 8 weeks. The supplement improved serum iron status but did not enhance endurance capacity in a treadmill run to exhaustion, nor did it improve VO_2 max. Similar findings were reported in a study by Karamizrak and others, who supplemented both male and female athletes with iron for 3 weeks. Peeling and others reported that although five intramuscular injections of elemental iron (100 mg) increased serum ferritin levels in female athletes, there were no significant effects on submaximal or maximal aerobic-exercise performance.

Thus, the research relative to the beneficial effects of iron supplementation to those athletes who are iron deficient, yet nonanemic, is contradictory, but the majority of the studies indicate that although iron supplementation will improve iron status, performance does not appear to be enhanced. Indeed, in a critical review of the scientific evidence relating low iron stores to endurance performance, Garza and others concluded that although iron supplementation can raise serum ferritin levels, increases in ferritin concentration unaccompanied by increases in hemoglobin concentration have not been shown to improve endurance performance. Rodenberg and Gustafson reached a similar conclusion in their review, indicating that supplementation for the iron-depleted nonanemic athlete does not appear to be justified solely to improve performance. Nevertheless, although Nielsen and Nachtigall agree with this finding, they note that many of the studies reporting no benefit of iron supplementation did not meet the general recommendations for the optimal clinical management of iron deficiency, and recommend more research with appropriate supplementation protocols to resolve this issue.

Iron saturated Iron supplementation offers no benefits to individuals with normal hemoglobin and iron status. Some well-controlled research on highly active, nonanemic, females with normal iron status has shown no effect of iron supplementation on hemoglobin concentration or exercise performance.

However, endurance athletes with normal hemoglobin status who attempt to increase their red blood cells (RBC) and hemoglobin levels may benefit from iron supplementation. Increased hemoglobin levels increase the ability to transport oxygen to the muscles, with the goal of enhancing performance. Previously, athletes used blood doping techniques (reinfusion of one's own blood previously drawn or from a blood-matched donor) or injection of recombinant erythropoietin (rEPO), a hormone that stimulates RBC and hemoglobin production. However, both blood doping and rEPO have been prohibited by the International Olympic Committee, not only because they may provide an unfair advantage, but also because their use may be lethal.

The technique of "Live high, train low" may be an effective alternative. When one ascends to altitude, such as 2,500 meters (8,225 feet) or so, the atmospheric oxygen pressure decreases, leading to lower oxygen pressure in the blood. The body immediately begins to adapt. The kidneys produce natural EPO, which stimulates the bone marrow to produce more RBC. Over time, the RBC and hemoglobin concentration are elevated. This is the benefit of "Live high." However, given the decreased oxygen pressure, athletes may not train as intensely at altitude, and thus may not train optimally as they could at sea level, the "Train low" component. Some athletes may reside in geographical locations where it is possible to live high and train low by driving an hour or so to a lower altitude. Such is not the case for most athletes, so scientists have constructed houses at sea level whose inside atmosphere has been manipulated to resemble one of high altitude. Thus, the athlete can "Live high" in the house and produce EPO naturally, but can also step outside and "Train low" at sea-level atmosphere.

Research supports the efficacy of a "Live high, train low" protocol to enhance aerobic endurance performance. Wilber and others suggest that the optimal dose is to live at a natural elevation of 2,000–2,500 meters for at least 4 weeks with more than 22 hours a day at that altitude. Mazzeo and Fulco recommend living at about 2,100 meters for at least 20 days and about 16 hours per day while maintaining high-intensity training. Wehrlin and others recently studied Swiss national team orienteers who for 24 days, 18 hours a day, trained at 1,000 to 1,800 meters. Compared to a sea-level control group, these athletes experienced significant increases in hemoglobin, maximal oxygen uptake, and 5-kilometer run times.

Although living at natural altitude is effective, Mazzeo and Fulco contended that the results from using alternative means, such as altitude houses or sleeping tents, are equivocal. For example, Robach and others found that Nordic skiers who lived in an altitude house (2,500 to 3,500 meters simulated altitude) for

11 hours a day for 18 days, although responding with elevated EPO levels, did not increase hemoglobin levels, VO_2 max, or maximal aerobic performance.

Runner's World magazine reported that many elite athletes have been reported to use such methods, including the women's world record holder in the marathon, Paula Radcliffe, and multiple Tour de France champion Lance Armstrong. Malloy and others note that although the World Anti-Doping Agency (WADA) has considered placing "artificially induced hypoxic conditions" on its doping list, their use is not currently banned. However, their use is prohibited in the Olympic villages for athletes. Systems are available commercially to adapt rooms or sleeping chambers to high atmospheric conditions.

For athletes who use this strategy, iron supplementation may be necessary to provide substrate for hemoglobin synthesis. Mazzeo and Fulco note that this is true particularly for women who come to altitude with inadequate or borderline iron stores. Iron supplementation prior to and during their stay at altitude will increase hematocrit similarly to men. Thus, they recommend that prior to coming to altitude, women (and men) should ensure that they have adequate iron stores, especially for athletes who plan on training or competing at high elevations.

Interestingly, two studies reported that elite and professional cyclists were found to have abnormally high serum ferritin levels, suggestive of an excessive intake of iron. Such excess supplementation with iron may be dangerous over time.

Excess Iron   Iron is both an essential nutrient and a potentially harmful toxicant to cells. If you plan to take iron supplements, you should have your serum ferritin checked, because some danger is associated with iron supplements if they lead to excessive iron in the body. Prolonged consumption of large amounts can cause a disturbance in iron metabolism in susceptible individuals. Iron then tends to accumulate in the liver as hemosiderin, which in excess can cause **hemochromatosis** in those genetically predisposed. This condition causes cirrhosis and may lead to the ultimate destruction of the liver. Of every 1,000 Americans, approximately two to three have a genetic predisposition to hemochromatosis.

Other health problems associated with excessive iron intake have been detailed by Emery, and some preliminary epidemiological data reported by Wurzelmann and others suggest that high levels of iron intake may confer an increased risk for colon cancer. However, the American Institute of Cancer Research (AICR), in its worldwide report on nutrition and cancer, reported that the evidence linking foods containing iron with colorectal cancer is sparse, of poor quality, and inconsistent. However, the AICR also noted convincing evidence that red meat and processed meat may cause colorectal cancer. As noted previously, the cause may be linked to methods of food preparation, such as excessive charring by grilling.

Additionally, high iron intakes may interfere with the absorption of other essential minerals, such as copper and zinc. Excessive iron may be fatal to young children; more than 30 deaths occur each year from overdoses of iron obtained by eating large amounts of candy-flavored vitamin tablets with iron.

Dietary iron has also been associated with heart disease. In their review, deValk and Marx indicate there is growing epidemiologic evidence for a relationship between iron levels and cardiovascular disease. One hypothesis suggests that inflammatory processes in the coronary arteries provoke increased numbers of white blood cells, which may release iron. Iron is a pro-oxidant, and may possibly oxidize LDL-cholesterol, a reaction believed to be one of the causes of atherosclerosis. Other observations have suggested a link between serum iron and coronary heart disease; for example, females have lower serum iron levels due to menstruation and also have lower incidence rates of heart attack compared to men, and aspirin reduces the risk of heart attack, possibly because it causes gastrointestinal bleeding and increased loss of iron.

However, Derstine and others, using a controlled diet for 4 to 8 weeks to vary iron status in the blood, reported no relationship between iron status and LDL-oxidative susceptibility, a possible risk factor for CHD. Moreover, a meta-analysis by Danesh and Appleby, based on 12 prospective studies, indicated that there is no good evidence supporting an association between iron status and cardiovascular disease. Individuals who may be concerned about high serum levels of iron should consult a physician for advice.

Prudent Recommendations   In summary, it would be wise for developing adolescent males and females of all ages to be aware of the iron content in their diets. This concern is especially important to endurance athletes, although it would appear that the extra Calories they eat to meet the additional energy requirements of training would provide the necessary iron. All active males and females should be aware of heme iron-rich foods, such as lean red meat, and be sure to include them in the daily diet, or at least two to three times a week. Mixing small amounts of meat with iron-rich plant foods, such as lean beef and chili beans, will enhance iron nutrition. Eating foods rich in vitamin C with nonheme iron-containing foods and using iron cookware also will increase iron bioavailability. Heath and others found that an intensive 16-week dietary program, one that includes an increased intake of meat, heme iron, vitamin C, and foods cooked using cast-iron cookware, along with decreased phytate and calcium intakes, could significantly increase serum ferritin in women with iron deficiency, but the increase was less than that in women who took a 50-milligram iron supplement daily.

Iron supplementation by commercial preparations may be recommended for certain individuals who have or who are at high risk of having low serum ferritin levels, including female distance runners, some vegetarian athletes, those who experience heavy menstrual blood flow, athletes who initiate altitude training, and athletes who are on restricted caloric intake. Over-the-counter multivitamin/mineral preparations vary in iron content. Some contain none, such as those marketed to men and postmenopausal women, while others contain the Daily Value of 18 mg iron, which is 100 percent of the RDA for adult females and 120 percent for adolescent girls. One tablet a day may be advisable for these individuals, and it should be consumed on an empty stomach to minimize adverse effects of some foods on absorption. According to Schmid and others, ingestion of iron together with physical exercise increased serum iron concentrations more than supplementation and rest. For women who have iron deficiency without anemia who want a rapid restoration of serum iron, injections may be preferable. Dawson and others had women consume either an iron tablet (105 mg iron) for 30 days or receive five intramuscular injections (100 mg elemental iron) over a 10-day period. The iron injections were significantly more effective (both in time and degree of increase) in improving serum ferritin levels over the course of 30 days. The individual with iron-deficiency anemia should consult a physician for iron therapy, which may consist of 100–200 mg of elemental iron per day until the condition is corrected.

It is important to reemphasize that iron supplementation should not be done indiscriminately, but preferably only after determination of one's iron status. In an investigation of iron status in marathoners, Mettler and Zimmermann showed signs of iron overload in 17 percent of male runners. Health professionals indicate that iron supplements should be given to athletes only by prescription, primarily only in cases of iron-deficiency anemia.

Copper (Cu)

Copper is an essential mineral whose function is closely associated with the function of iron.

DRI The RDA for copper is 900 micrograms, or 0.90 mg, for adults age 19–50, but amounts vary for other age groups and may be found in the DRI table on the inside of the front cover. The DV is 2 mg, or about twice the amount of the RDA. The UL for adults is 10 milligrams/day.

Food Sources Copper is widely distributed in foods and is high in seafoods, meats, nuts, beans, and whole-grain products. One cup of whole-grain cereal contains about 8 percent of the DV, or nearly 18 percent of the adult RDA. Copper also may be found in drinking water, particularly soft water, which leaches it from copper pipes. Some good food sources are listed in table 8.4. About 30–40 percent of dietary copper is absorbed, but this percentage may increase or decrease depending on body copper stores.

Major Functions Copper functions in the body as a metalloenzyme and works closely with iron in oxygen metabolism. It is needed for the absorption of iron from the intestinal tract, helps in the formation of hemoglobin, and is involved in the activity of a specific cytochrome, an oxidative enzyme in the mitochondria. Copper is also a component of ceruloplasmin, a glycoprotein in the plasma, and is in superoxide dismutase (SOD), an enzyme that functions as an antioxidant to quench free radicals. Lowe and others indicate that copper is also involved in bone formation, being an essential cofactor in enzymes involved in the synthesis of various bone matrix constituents.

Deficiency: Health and Physical Performance Copper deficiency due to inadequate dietary intake is not known to exist in humans, although a deficiency has occurred in some patients receiving prolonged intravenous feeding of a copper-free solution and in malnourished infants. The major deficiency symptom is anemia, but osteoporosis, neurological defects, and heart disease may also develop.

Available surveys indicate that most athletes consume ample amounts of copper. The effects of exercise or exercise training on serum copper levels are variable, with studies showing increases, decreases, or no changes. Several studies have reported decreases in serum copper in athletes involved in prolonged training or after an endurance exercise task. The authors theorized that the decreased levels were due to sweat or fecal losses. However, no deficiency symptoms were noted. In his review, Lukaski indicated that physical training does increase the copper-containing SOD, and normal body stores of copper are apparently adequate to support the increase of this antioxidant enzyme.

Supplementation: Health and Physical Performance No research is available relative to copper supplementation and health or physical performance. Although copper (2 mg) is used in a supplement being studied to help prevent age-related macular degeneration, it is not because it plays a role in eye health, but rather to help counter the effect of the high zinc content that could reduce copper absorption. Supplements are not recommended because excessive copper intake, even 5–10 milligrams, may cause nausea and vomiting. The National Academy of Sciences reports that toxicity from dietary sources is rare. However, Turnlund indicates that copper poisoning can result from excess intake via supplements.

Prudent Recommendations Copper supplements are not recommended for the physically active individual.

Zinc (Zn)

Zinc is a blue-white metal that is an essential nutrient for humans.

DRI The RDA for zinc is 11 mg per day for adult males and 8 mg per day for adult females. The DV is 15 mg per day. The UL for adults is 40 mg per day.

Food Sources Good sources of zinc are found in animal protein, such as meat, milk, and seafood, particularly oysters. Three ounces of meat contain approximately 30–50 percent of the RDA, whereas only one oyster will provide more that 70 percent. Whole-grain products also contain significant amounts of zinc, but the phytate and fiber content will slightly decrease its bioavailability. Zinc is lost in the milling process of wheat, but some breakfast cereals are fortified to 25–100 percent of the RDA. In general, if you receive enough protein in the diet you will obtain the RDA for zinc. The MPF enhances zinc absorption. About 20–50 percent of dietary zinc is absorbed. Table 8.4 presents foods high in zinc.

Major Functions Zinc is found in virtually all tissues in the body and, according to Micheletti and others, is required for the activity of more than 300 enzymes. Several of these enzymes are involved in the major pathways of energy metabolism, including lactic acid dehydrogenase (LDH), which is important for the lactic acid energy system. Zinc also is involved in a wide variety of other body functions such as protein synthesis, insulin synthesis, the growth process, bone formation, and wound healing. Zinc is also associated with immune functions, including optimal functioning of white blood cells and the lymphatic system.

Deficiency: Health and Physical Performance

Maret and Sandstead noted that about 25 percent of the world's population is at risk of zinc deficiency, mostly the poor who could benefit from supplementation. However, Helen Lane has noted that zinc nutritional status appears to be well maintained in the average U.S. population, even with marginal intakes. For example, Hunt and others reported that although some vegetarians have both decreased dietary zinc and zinc absorption, the inclusion of whole grains and legumes in the diet helps them maintain normal zinc balance. However, several zinc researchers have indicated that a mild dietary zinc deficiency is not uncommon in the United States, particularly in areas where animal protein intake is relatively low and consumption of grain products is high. King and Cousins note that zinc deficiency states have been observed in young children with symptoms of impaired wound healing, depressed appetite, and failure to grow properly.

Most research indicates that athletes who obtain sufficient dietary Calories generally meet the RDA for zinc, but Micheletti and others indicated that endurance athletes who adopt a diet rich in carbohydrate, but low in protein and fat, may decrease zinc intake, which over time may lead to a zinc deficiency with loss of body weight, latent fatigue, decreased endurance, and increased risk of osteoporosis. Female athletes are more likely to have inadequate zinc intake as compared to males. Zinc deficiency could be a problem for certain athletes, particularly young athletes in sports that stress weight loss for optimal performance or competition. Very low-Calorie or starvation-type diets may induce significant zinc losses. In addition, sweat also may contain substantial amounts of zinc. DeRuisseau and others measured sweat losses of zinc during a 2-hour exercise bout under temperate climate conditions. Sweat zinc losses were higher during the first 60 minutes, approximating 0.8–1.0 mg per liter of sweat, but were reduced by about 40 percent the second 60 minutes. The authors indicated that the zinc sweat losses approximated 9 percent and 8 percent of the RDA for men and women, respectively.

Although few experimental data are available, young wrestlers and gymnasts who use both dieting and sweating techniques to induce weight loss may be at risk for zinc deficiency and possible impairment of optimal growth, as suggested by Brun and others. Several studies also have reported a low serum zinc level in endurance runners, triathletes, and other athletes, and the cause was attributed to high sweat losses, increased urinary excretion, or low-Calorie diets. Low dietary zinc intake has been shown to depress testosterone levels, which may be related to the decreased serum testosterone often observed in endurance athletes and wrestlers. Zinc deficiency may also depress immune functions. However, no zinc deficiency symptoms were noted in these athletes or wrestlers; the authors suggested that low serum levels do not necessarily reflect low levels of zinc in the muscles. In this regard,

Hambidge noted that there is a lack of ideal biomarkers for mild zinc deficiency states. Following her review of the available literature, which is limited, Lane noted that, in general, there is no evidence that exercise causes a poor zinc status or that a marginal deficiency impairs performance. A more recent review by Lukaski supports this viewpoint.

Supplementation: Health and Physical Performance

In a meta-analysis of 33 randomized, intervention controlled trials, Brown and others concluded that zinc supplementation produced highly significant, positive responses in height and weight increments in prepubertal children. They note that interventions to improve children's zinc nutriture should be considered in populations at risk for zinc deficiency.

Zinc supplementation has been advocated as a means of enhancing immune functions, particularly treatment of the common cold, a health problem that could impair exercise training. Nearly a dozen clinical studies have evaluated the effect of zinc lozenges as a means to reduce the duration of symptoms of the common cold, but a review by Nieman and a meta-analysis by Jackson and others concluded that evidence supporting its effectiveness in this regard is still lacking. Diets rich in zinc may be associated with a decreased risk of macular degeneration, and clinical trials are underway to evaluate the effect of zinc supplementation (80 mg) combined with several other micronutrients.

Beletate and others indicated that zinc plays a key role in the synthesis and action of insulin, both physiologically and in diabetes mellitus. Hypothetically, zinc supplementation may help prevent type 2 diabetes. However, in their review, research was very limited and they concluded that there is currently no evidence to suggest the use of zinc supplementation in the prevention of type 2 diabetes mellitus.

Given the potential ergogenic importance of zinc, it is unusual that only limited research has been uncovered that has investigated the effect of zinc supplementation upon physical performance. In one study, Van Loan and others used a zinc-deficient diet (0.3 mg zinc for 33–41 days) to induce a zinc deficiency in apparently untrained males, and reported a significant decrease in muscular endurance in some, but not all, muscle groups. However, the zinc deficiency had no effect on peak muscle force. Following three weeks of zinc repletion, muscular endurance did not return to normal even though serum zinc levels did. In the most cited study by Krotkiewski and others, subjects were untrained women with an average age of 35 years. In a series of tests for both isometric and isokinetic strength and endurance, zinc supplements improved performance in isometric endurance and in isokinetic strength at one speed. However, performance was not affected in isokinetic endurance or in isokinetic strength at two other speeds of muscle contraction. Although the authors reported a beneficial effect of zinc supplementation and theorized that it helped optimize the function of LDH in the muscle during fast contractions, it would appear additional research is needed to confirm this finding. Both of these studies provide some important data, but the findings are somewhat equivocal. In his review, Lukaski noted that study designs limit our ability to provide recommendations regarding zinc supplementation to athletes. Zinc supplementation studies are needed, particularly using physically trained subjects.

Maret and Sandstead indicated that individuals in affluent countries may experience the problem of chronic zinc toxicity caused by excessive consumption of zinc supplements. Small amounts of zinc supplements do not appear to pose any major problems to the healthy individual, but larger doses may. Research has shown that zinc supplements, even 25–50 mg per day, may impair the absorption of other essential minerals, such as copper and iron. Supplements of more than 100 mg/day may increase the amount of LDL-cholesterol and decrease the HDL-cholesterol level, increasing the risk of coronary artery disease. Anemia may also result from such doses. Higher doses may impair the immune system and cause nausea and vomiting; they may even be fatal.

Prudent Recommendations On the basis of available evidence, zinc supplementation is not warranted for most athletes. Foods rich in zinc, similar to the animal protein rich in iron, should be selected to replace the increased Calories expended through exercise. However, athletes such as wrestlers and others incurring weight losses, as well as older endurance athletes whose immune system normally declines, should be exceptionally aware of high-zinc foods. Zinc-fortified foods may provide the RDA for zinc. Check the food label. If a supplement for these athletes is recommended, it should not exceed the RDA. Keep in mind that the current DV used on food labels is 15 milligrams, or nearly twice the RDA for females and almost 40 percent higher than the RDA for males. Eating several servings of fortified foods daily could provide enough zinc to exceed the UL.

Chromium (Cr)

Chromium is a very hard metal essential in human nutrition.

DRI The AI for chromium is 35 and 25 micrograms per day, respectively, for adult males and females. The DV is 120 micrograms. Thus, a vitamin pill containing 100 percent of the DV for chromium will provide about 3 to 5 times the RDA for adult males and females. No UL is currently available.

Food Sources Good sources of chromium include brewer's yeast, whole grains, baked beans, nuts, molasses, cheese, mushrooms, and asparagus. Beer also contains some chromium. One slice of whole wheat bread provides approximately 15 percent of the daily requirement of chromium. Cooking acidic foods in stainless steel cookware provides negligible additional chromium. Chromium is poorly absorbed from the intestinal tract, less than 1 percent being absorbed with intakes in the AI range. At lower dietary intakes, absorption is somewhat increased.

Major Functions Chromium is considered to be an essential component of the glucose-tolerance factor associated with insulin in the proper metabolism of blood glucose. In her review, Stoecker notes that chromium potentiates the activity of insulin and thus may also influence lipid and protein metabolism. In addition to maintenance of blood glucose levels, it may be involved in the formation of glycogen in muscle tissue and may facilitate the transport of amino acids into the muscles. Chromium may also affect cholesterol metabolism.

Deficiency: Health and Physical Performance Clinically manifest deficiencies of chromium are rare, but abnormally high blood glucose levels have been reported in hospital patients receiving prolonged intravenous nutrition containing no chromium. Richard Anderson, one of the principal investigators in chromium metabolism, observed that the average American intake of chromium may not be optimal and also noted that the role of chromium in the development of diabetes is currently being studied.

Chromium deficiency could be a problem with both endurance- and strength-type athletes. Impairment in carbohydrate metabolism would not be conducive to optimal performance in endurance events, whereas decreased amino acid transport into the muscle could limit the benefits from a weight-training program. On the basis of animal experiments, Anderson has linked chromium to carbohydrate and protein metabolism during exercise, noting, for example, that chromium-deficient rats use muscle glycogen at a faster rate. Anderson believes that strenuous exercise may increase the need for chromium in humans. He noted that chromium losses are associated with stress, such as exercise, and reported increased excretion of chromium in the urine following a strenuous run. Lefavi speculated that athletes may incur a negative chromium balance under various conditions. One, increased intensity and duration of exercise may increase chromium excretion. Two, athletes who consume substantial amounts of carbohydrates may need more chromium to process glucose. And three, athletes who lose weight for competition may decrease dietary intake of chromium.

Supplementation: Health and Physical Performance Given the potential role of chromium in glucose metabolism, supplementation has been studied for possible benefits on blood sugar and glucose tolerance, particularly in individuals with type 2 diabetes. In a meta-analysis of 41 studies, Balk and others noted that although chromium supplementation significantly improved blood glucose control among patients *with* diabetes, they noted that future studies that address the limitations in the current evidence are needed before definitive claims can be made about the effect of chromium supplementation. Althius and others, in their meta-analysis, reached a similar conclusion, and Trumbo and Ellwood reported that the FDA conducted an evidence-based review and concluded that the relationship between chromium picolinate intake and insulin resistance is highly uncertain. In their meta-analysis, Balk and others reported no significant effect of chromium on lipid or glucose metabolism in people *without* diabetes.

Other research has suggested that chromium may help lower total cholesterol and LDL-cholesterol while raising HDL-cholesterol in individuals with unhealthy serum cholesterol levels. Grant and others did find that chromium nicotinate supplementation, when combined with exercise training, significantly reduced body weight in young, obese women and improved their glucose tolerance, but that chromium picolinate supplementation actually increased body weight in similar subjects. However, Anderson has noted that chromium supplements can correct only that part of a health problem which is associated with a deficiency. In other words, individuals who have a health problem in which chromium deficiency plays a part will benefit if the deficiency is corrected, just like any nutrient-deficiency-related health problem. Anderson noted that chromium acts as a nutrient, not a therapeutic agent. Unfortunately, there is currently no reliable measure of chromium status in the body. Thus, individuals who are chromium deficient and who might benefit from chromium supplementation cannot be identified.

Theoretically, chromium supplementation might benefit the endurance athlete by improving insulin sensitivity and carbohydrate metabolism during exercise. Also, because chromium may enhance the anabolic effect of insulin, it may increase amino acid uptake into the muscle and modify the body composition, hopefully increasing muscle mass and decreasing body fat. Given the potential commercial application of this latter theoretical possibility to both athletes and the general population, most of the research to date has focused on the effect of chromium supplementation on body composition, but several recent studies have evaluated its effect on strength. Most studies have used chromium picolinate.

In the first published report of the effects of chromium supplementation on body composition, Gary Evans, a chemistry professor at Bemidji State University in Minnesota, used chromium picolinate as an adjunct to a weight-training program to investigate its effect upon body composition. Picolinate is a natural derivative of tryptophan, an amino acid, and apparently facilitates the absorption of chromium into the body. In a review article, Evans described two of his studies. In the first study, ten male volunteers from a weight-training class were assigned to either a placebo or a chromium supplement group. The chromium dosage was 200 micrograms. Body fat and lean body mass were determined by skinfold and girth measurements. The subjects trained with weights for 40 days, and at the conclusion Evans found that the chromium group had increased their body weight by 2.2 kilograms, mostly as lean body mass. The placebo group had also increased their body weight slightly, but Evans noted this increase was due almost totally to body fat. The second study was similar to the first, but 32 football players at Bemidji State University served as subjects. After a 42-day training period, the chromium group actually lost body weight, but most of it was fat so their proportion of lean body mass increased. The placebo group also lost body weight, but their lean body mass increased only slightly. In both studies, Evans noted that the results were statistically significant, suggesting that chromium picolinate supplementation enhanced body composition by decreasing body fat and increasing lean body mass. The findings of this report are certainly interesting, but it should be noted that the studies were reported in a review article on the health benefits of chromium and do not appear to have been published previously in a refereed scientific journal.

Following the publicity associated with this report, chromium picolinate was billed in certain muscle magazines as the alternative to anabolic steroids. The advertisers suggested that chromium's insulin-like effects may elicit significant anabolic hormone effects in the body. Advertisements also appeared in magazines targeted for the general population, suggesting that chromium picolinate would facilitate the loss of body fat.

However, well-controlled research does not support these advertisement claims. For example, Hallmark and others conducted a study with 16 untrained males, matching the subjects based on initial levels of strength and giving half of them a placebo and the other half 200 micrograms chromium picolinate daily for 12 weeks of progressive resistance training. Dependent variables included measures of body composition as determined by underwater weighing, and strength. The authors reported no significant effects of chromium picolinate supplementation on lean body mass, body fat, or strength. Clancy and others randomly placed 21 football players into either a placebo group or an experimental group receiving 200 micrograms chromium picolinate daily while involved in intensive resistance training over a 9-week period. A number of dependent variables were studied, including body composition determined by underwater weighing, anthropometrical measurements such as muscle girth, and strength. Chromium picolinate supplementation had no effect on lean body mass, body fat percentage, or strength. The studies by Hallmark and Clancy and their associates paralleled those conducted by Evans, yet the results were diametrically opposite.

Other studies have not found any significant effect of chromium supplementation on body composition, either with or without exercise training. In a well-controlled energy balance study, Lukaski and others evaluated the effect of chromium picolinate (200 mcg/d) on body weight and composition in nonexercising women over the course of 12 weeks. Compared to both a placebo and picolinate-supplemented group, they reported no changes. In another study, Lukaski and others compared the effects of two different types of chromium supplements, chromium chloride and chromium picolinate (about 200 micrograms each), with a placebo on body composition changes during 8 weeks of supplementation and controlled resistance strength training. Using several measures of body composition, they found no significant effects of the chromium supplements on body fat or lean muscle mass. Trent and Thieding-Cancel also reported no significant effects of chromium picolinate (400 micrograms for 16 weeks) on body weight, body fat, or lean muscle mass in either men or women engaging in aerobic exercise for 30 minutes three times a week. Compared to a placebo group, Volpe and others reported that chromium picolinate supplementation (400 micrograms/day) during a 12-week walking and resistance exercise program had no effect on body composition, resting metabolic rate, blood glucose and insulin concentrations, and other related factors in moderately obese women aged 27 to 51. In a similar fashion, Campbell and others found no significant effect of high-dose chromium picolinate supplementation (924 micrograms/ day) on strength or body composition of older women (54 to 71 years) following 12 weeks of resistance training. In a review, Vincent noted that more than a decade of human studies with chromium picolinate indicate that the supplement has not demonstrated effects on the body composition of healthy individuals, even when taken in combination with an exercise training program. In general, these studies did not use athletes as subjects.

Several other studies evaluated the effect of chromium picolinate on performance of highly trained athletes and physically active individuals. In a very well-designed study, Walker and others reported no beneficial effects of chromium supplementation (200 mg chromium picolinate for 14 weeks) on body composition, or on neuromuscular or metabolic performance, in highly trained NCAA Division-I wrestlers. In a placebo, randomized study, Livolsi and others reported no significant ergogenic effect of chromium picolinate supplementation (500 micrograms/day) on muscular strength and body composition in 15 female softball players during 6 weeks of resistance training. In a well-designed, crossover study with physically active males, Davis and others evaluated the effects of adding chromium to a carbohydrate-electrolyte sports drink on prolonged intermittent high-intensity exercise to fatigue, and found that the chromium picolinate provided no additional advantage above that provided by the carbohydrate.

Contemporary well-designed studies have not shown any beneficial effects of chromium picolinate supplementation on lean body mass, body fat, strength, or intermittent, high-intensity, prolonged endurance performance in athletes or untrained individuals involved in exercise training programs. These findings argue against an ergogenic effect of chromium supplementation.

The safety of chromium picolinate has been questioned. In its recent review, the Institute of Medicine reported that no consistent, frequent adverse events were evident from human studies, but also noted that most of these studies were not long-term. Vincent noted that recent *in vitro* cell culture and *in vivo* animal studies have indicated that chromium picolinate probably generates oxidative damage of DNA and is mutagenic, but the significance of these results on humans taking the supplement for prolonged periods of time is unknown. The Institute of Medicine does note that there is a lack of information on the long-term effects of chronic chromium picolinate supplementation at the recommended doses, and does recommend additional research to resolve any uncertainties. Current data suggest that using up to 200 micrograms of chromium picolinate daily for 3 to 6 months appears to be safe. Several case studies have shown that using larger doses (1,200–2,400 mg) of chromium picolinate for several months could lead to liver damage and other health problems.

Prudent Recommendations In a review of chromium supplementation by Schardt and Schmidt, the Center for Science in the Public Interest provided a bottom-line recommendation, which appears to be in accord with this presentation of the scientific data. If you are glucose intolerant or a type 2 diabetic, consult your physician about chromium supplementation. In general, chromium supplementation will not help you lose weight or gain muscle. If you insist on taking a chromium supplement, it should not exceed 200 micrograms and might best be taken as part of an inexpensive multivitamin-mineral tablet containing the other essential vitamins and minerals. Keep in mind, however, that the best sources of chromium are whole grains, fruits, and vegetables.

Selenium (Se)

Selenium is a chemical element resembling sulfur.

DRI The RDA for selenium is 55 micrograms per day for males and females, with lower amounts for children. The DV currently is 70 micrograms. The UL has been set at 400 micrograms/day for adults, but somewhat lower levels for children and adolescents.

Food Sources Most selenium found in nature is a part of protein. Foods rich in selenium include Brazil nuts, seafoods, organ meats like kidney and liver, other meats, and grains grown in soil abundant in selenium. About 3 ounces of meat contain more than 30 micrograms of selenium, as does 3 ounces of wheat bread.

Major Functions Selenium, as a part of selenoproteins in the body, is essential for the functioning of numerous enzymes, particularly glutathione peroxidase, an antioxidant enzyme that helps catabolize free radicals and prevent damage to cellular structures, such as the membranes of RBC. As mentioned chapter 7, selenium works with vitamin E as an antioxidant. Selenium is also involved in thyroid hormone metabolism and immune functions and has been theorized to be important in the prevention of cancer.

Deficiency: Health and Physical Performance The selenium content of plants depends on the selenium content of the soil. Selenium deficiency is rare in industrialized countries because foods in the diet are obtained from diverse geographical areas. For example, Burk notes that in the United States more than 99 percent of subjects are selenium replete. Estimates of daily intake approximate 80 micrograms. However, deficiency diseases may be noted in geographical areas where the selenium content in the soil is low. Keshan disease, a cardiomyopathy, is evident in parts of China because the primary sources of food are plants grown locally in selenium-depleted soil. Other possible health effects of selenium deficiency include heart disease, possibly because of a diminished ability to prevent oxidation of LDL-cholesterol. Selenium deficiency has also been linked to an impaired immune system and to cancer. Rayman and Rayman cite studies showing that those with the lowest consumption of selenium, as compared to those with the highest dietary intake, were almost five times more likely to develop prostate cancer. The interested reader is referred to the review by Burk and Levander.

For the athlete, selenium deficiency may impair antioxidant functions during intense exercise, possibly leading to muscle tissue or mitochondrial damage, thus impairing physical performance. However, there are no data to support this notion.

Supplementation: Health and Physical Performance Intervention trials in China have shown that selenium supplementation may help prevent Keshan disease by preventing a deficiency. But can selenium supplementation help prevent cardiovascular disease or cancer in Western populations with better nutritional status? In theory, selenium supplementation may help protect cell membranes from peroxidation. Preventing LDL oxidation may help prevent cardiovascular disease. However, in a meta-analysis of 25 studies, Flores-Mateo and others noted that while, in general, selenium concentrations were inversely associated with coronary heart disease risk in observational studies, the validity of this association is uncertain given recent experimental research with other antioxidants, such as vitamin E, showing no protection against heart disease. They conclude that, currently, selenium supplements should not be recommended for cardiovascular disease prevention.

Selenium, as an antioxidant, may also be theorized to prevent cancer. Reviews by Combs and Bjelakovic suggested that selenium can play a role in cancer prevention, particularly cancers of the gastrointestinal tract. Ward notes that a large number of epidemiological studies have shown that the higher the body selenium levels, the lower the risk of prostate cancer. In a long-term (4.5 years) study, Clark and others found that selenium supplementation (200 micrograms/day) reduced prostate cancer by 63 percent. However, subsequent reviews of the data from this study, as reported by Burk and Levander, suggested some uncertainty in the findings. Two major reviews also expressed some degree of uncertainty. The National Institutes of Health concluded there is a suggestion that selenium may reduce risk for prostate cancer, while the American Institute of Cancer Research noted that there is limited evidence to suggest that selenium protects against colorectal cancer. Thus, current investigators indicate that the role of selenium supplementation in cancer prevention is unclear, and recommend additional research.

In this regard, the National Cancer Institute (NCI) is conducting a long-term study (SELECT; Selenium and Vitamin E Cancer Prevention Trial) to evaluate the effect of selenium supplementation (200 micrograms/day), separately and in combination with vitamin E, on the development of prostate cancer. However, the NCI stopped the study prematurely in 2008 after the data indicated that neither supplement, either alone or in combination, prevented prostate cancer. Moreover, there was a small increase in the number of cases of type 2 diabetes in the men taking selenium, but the NCI indicated that this could be a chance finding because the data were analyzed early.

As noted chapter 7, selenium was often combined with vitamin antioxidants as a combined antioxidant supplement to evaluate the effect on muscle tissue damage. The effects of selenium supplementation by itself on physical performance has received only limited research attention. Although antioxidant supplements have not universally been shown to prevent peroxidation of lipids in cell membranes and other cell structures, some studies by Tessier and his associates have shown that selenium supplementation will enhance glutathione peroxidase status and reduce lipid peroxidation during prolonged aerobic exercise. Although these findings are intriguing, selenium supplementation did not improve actual physical performance, as evaluated by VO_2 max or running performance of an aerobic/anaerobic nature. In a subsequent study, Margaritis and others reported that selenium supplementation (180 micrograms/day) had no effect on muscle antioxidant capacity or exercise performance during 10 weeks of endurance training.

Selenium supplements within RDA levels under 100 micrograms appear to be safe, and investigators in the United States using supplements up to 200 micrograms saw no problems. However,

Vinceti and others noted that dietary intake of around 300 micrograms of selenium daily could lead to adverse health effects, such as impaired synthesis of thyroid hormones. Accidental intakes of large amounts (more than 25 milligrams per day) have been associated with nausea, vomiting, abdominal pain, hair loss, and unusual fatigue.

Prudent Recommendations Adequate selenium may be obtained on a healthful, balanced diet containing substantial amounts of grain products. In the United States and Canada, most grains are produced in the upper Great Plains, where the soil is rich in selenium. Selenium in foods is present in an organic form, which may be more effectively used by the body than inorganic selenium salt supplements. Selenium supplements do not appear to enhance exercise training or performance, but if you decide to take a selenium supplement, note that most experts agree such a supplement, or a multivitamin-mineral supplement, should not exceed 200 micrograms. Larger doses are not recommended at the present time. Moreover, Liebman and Schardt from the Center for Science in the Public Interest recommend caution, possibly limiting selenium to 100 micrograms a day.

Boron (B)

Boron is a nonmetallic element.

DRI Although boron is an essential nutrient for plants, no RDA or AI has been established. However, some scientists suggest that it is of nutritional and clinical importance and most likely is an essential nutrient for humans. In a review, Nielsen indicated that establishment of a DRI for boron is justified, and suggested that an acceptable safe range for adults could well be 1–13 mg/day. A UL of 20 mg/day has been set for adults.

Food Sources Boron is found naturally in many plant foods, particularly dried fruits, nuts, peanut butter, legumes, fresh vegetables, apple sauce, milk and dairy products, grape juice, and wine. One ounce of almonds contains about 0.75 milligram of boron. Five servings of fruits and vegetables, along with legumes and some nuts, could easily provide 3 milligrams.

Major Functions Boron is believed to influence cell membrane structure and function in some unknown way to influence mineral metabolism, and to be involved in the metabolism of steroid hormones, such as estrogen. Nielsen indicated that the effects of boron on calcium and estrogen metabolism could favorably affect bone development. Some investigators indicate that boron may also influence testosterone metabolism.

Deficiency: Health and Physical Performance Barr and others noted that evidence on boron deficiency is scanty. Rainey and others reported that the mean boron intake by Americans approximates 1.0–1.5 mg per day. Because the mean represents 50 percent of the population, Nielsen indicates that a significant number of Americans do not consistently consume this amount. However, Rainey and others concluded that we need more data to determine whether our daily intake of boron is adequate. Although boron deficiency has been studied in relation to bone metabolism—possibly because of its potential role in estrogen metabolism—its role is poorly understood. Other than its potential role in bone health, Nielsen noted that low intakes of boron may be associated with impaired brain function and immune response.

If a boron deficiency would impair testosterone production, muscle development could be compromised.

Supplementation: Health and Physical Performance

Boron supplementation may not increase body stores. Hunt and others reported that a boron supplement of 3 milligrams did not accumulate in the body. Recent research indicates that increases in dietary boron intake are rapidly excreted by the kidney, suggesting that the human body maintains a stable boron level.

In his review, Nielsen presents an excellent example of how the results of a single study may be distorted by nutritional supplement entrepreneurs to market new products. In their study, Nielsen and his colleagues designed a diet for 12 postmenopausal women to deprive them of adequate dietary boron for nearly 4 months, and then fed them the same diet for 48 days but supplemented with 3 milligrams of boron daily, an amount found in a diet high in fruits and vegetables. The authors reported that the boron supplements reduced the plasma concentration of calcium and the urinary excretion of calcium and magnesium, at the same time elevating the serum concentration of one form of estrogen and testosterone. The authors concluded that correcting a boron deficiency with boron supplements elicits physiological effects associated with the prevention of calcium loss and bone demineralization, suggesting that dietary boron may play an important nutritional role in the prevention of osteoporosis. The major focus of this study was on the effects of boron deprivation and deficiency, not boron supplementation. The authors simply created a boron deficiency to see its physiological effects, and then restored normal dietary boron to evaluate its effects.

Nielsen notes that these findings were completely misinterpreted, the media reporting erroneously that boron could end bone disease. Commercial enterprises immediately began marketing boron supplements for prevention of osteoporosis. In his review, Nielsen negates the sensational claims the media propagated, but did indicate that boron may be one of a number of nutrients that may play a role in the prevention of osteoporosis.

One of the other findings of this study, the elevated serum testosterone levels in these postmenopausal women, was also sensationalized. Advertisements began to appear in muscle magazines indicating that boron supplements could act pharmacologically like anabolic steroids. However, Nielsen indicated that this was an erroneous extrapolation of the research data, noting that boron supplementation increased serum testosterone only after these postmenopausal women had been deprived of boron for nearly 4 months; continuation of boron supplementation did not further elevate serum testosterone levels. Moreover, Nielsen conducted other studies with males and reported no significant changes in serum testosterone levels when dietary boron intake was modified. Nevertheless, although noting more research is needed, Naghii indicated that boron supplementation could increase serum testosterone, suggesting that it could be used safely as an ergogenic aid by athletes.

Limited research data are available relative to the ergogenic efficacy of boron supplementation. Ferrando and Green randomly assigned 19 nonsteroid-using, male bodybuilders to receive either a placebo or 2.5 milligrams of a commercial boron supplement daily for 7 weeks. The bodybuilders maintained their normal diets and consumed no other supplements. The authors found that although boron supplements increased serum boron levels, there were no significant effects on total and free testosterone, lean body mass, or strength. In his review, Kreider concluded that currently there is no evidence that boron supplementation promotes muscle growth during resistance training. These limited findings indicate that boron supplements are not ergogenic, but additional research is desirable.

Nielsen notes that 10 milligrams per day may possibly be obtained in the diet, and that this amount is probably not too high. However, he cautions that an intake of 50 milligrams per day may be toxic.

Prudent Recommendations
Based on the available scientific evidence, boron supplementation does not enhance athletic performance and is not recommended. However, a leading expert on boron indicated that boron deprivation for 3 weeks or more may have a negative impact on the ability to exercise. A balanced diet containing adequate amounts of plant foods will provide sufficient dietary boron, so physically active individuals who consume a typical diet should have no problem with boron deprivation.

Vanadium (V)

Vanadium is a light gray metallic element.

DRI
No RDA or AI has been established for vanadium because it has not been deemed essential for human metabolism. Nevertheless, based on some animal research, Nielsen estimated that about 10 micrograms per day would meet any postulated requirement. An UL of 1.8 mg/day has been set for adults.

Food Sources
Good sources of vanadium include shellfish, grain products, parsley, mushrooms, and black pepper. The average North American diet supplies 15–30 micrograms of vanadium daily, and approximately 5 percent of that is absorbed into the body.

Major Functions
Research with animals suggests that vanadium may be involved in several enzymatic reactions in the body, including the metabolism of carbohydrate and lipids. Nielsen noted that the action of vanadium receiving the most attention is its insulin-like effect on glucose and protein metabolism, which Mehdi indicated was attributed to its activation of several key components of insulin-signaling pathways.

Deficiency: Health and Physical Performance
Nielsen indicated that a vanadium deficiency has not been detected in

humans. However, if vanadium does induce an insulin-like effect, a deficiency could impair glucose metabolism.

Supplementation: Health and Physical Performance

Vanadium supplements are available as vanadyl salts, primarily vanadyl sulfate, and in various organic vanadium complexes that are regarded as being more readily absorbed, more effective, and safer. Verma and others noted a growing body of experimental and clinical research indicating that vanadium, when supplemented in pharmacological doses, may exert a potent insulin-like effect and improve glucose status in humans with noninsulin-dependent diabetes mellitus. However, similar effects may not occur in healthy individuals. Jentjens and Jeukendrup evaluated the effect of vanadyl sulfate supplementation (100 milligrams for 6 days) on insulin sensitivity in healthy adults, and reported no significant effects of vanadyl sulfate supplementation on plasma glucose and insulin concentrations, indicating no significant effects on insulin sensitivity.

Vanadyl salts have been marketed to athletes as a means to favorably modify body composition, comparable to the proposed effects of chromium supplementation. However, there are very limited research data with vanadium supplementation. In a well-controlled study, Fawcett and others found that supplementation with 0.5 milligrams per kilogram body weight (about 40 milligrams daily) of vanadyl sulfate to subjects undertaking strength training for 12 weeks had no effect on body fat or lean muscle mass. The investigators also studied strength gains in four tasks, a 1-repetition and 10-repetition maximal test for both the bench press and leg extension. There were no significant effects of vanadyl sulfate on three of the tests. Although subjects taking vanadyl sulfate did gain more strength on the 1-repetition maximal leg extension test during the first 4 weeks of the study, the investigators suggested that this may be attributed to low scores on the pretest. The investigators concluded that vanadyl sulfate supplementation was ineffective in changing body composition, and any modest performance-enhancing effect requires further investigation.

Although Jentjens and Jeukendrup noted that short-term supplementation with vanadyl sulfate resulted in no adverse side effects, they indicated that long-term safety studies are needed. The National Academy of Sciences set the UL for vanadium at 1.8 milligrams/day for adults. Vanadium constitutes about one-third of the atomic weight of vanadyl sulfate, so it could constitute 33 milligrams in a 100 milligram tablet, and thus greatly exceed the UL.

Adverse side effects of vanadyl salt supplementation when taken in milligram doses may include gastrointestinal distress, primarily diarrhea. Excess supplementation may also cause damage to both the liver and kidney.

Prudent Recommendations

Type 2 diabetics should consult with their physicians regarding the use of vanadyl salt as a therapeutic agent to control blood glucose. Vanadyl salt supplementation is not recommended for the physically active individual, as it has not been found to enhance either body composition or physical performance. Moreover, excess amounts may be toxic.

Other trace minerals

A number of other trace minerals have physiological roles that may have important implications for health or physical performance. Food sources, RDA or AI, major physiological functions, and the effects of deficiencies or excesses are summarized in table 8.5. Only trace minerals for which an RDA or AI have been developed are included. Other elements, such as nickel, tin, silicon, and arsenic, may prove to be essential. It should be noted that deficiencies and excesses due to dietary sources for most of these nutrients are extremely rare. However, to help prevent a deficiency it is important to consume unprocessed foods, because many of the trace elements that are removed during processing are not returned. For example, as already noted, one slice of whole wheat bread provides about 15 percent of the daily requirement of chromium, whereas a slice of white bread contains only 1 percent. Excesses may occur with use of supplements or through industrial exposure, and an UL has been set for nickel.

Two of these trace elements deserve mention because they have been shown to prevent health problems in humans.

Fluoride

A fluoride AI has been established, ranging from about 1 to 4 mg/day from childhood through adulthood. Featherstone indicates that fluoride may prevent dental caries, possibly by inhibiting bacterial enzymes and demineralization of the tooth. In a meta-analysis of 20 studies, Griffin and others indicated the findings suggest that fluoride, either through water fluoridation or application by oneself or a health professional, prevents dental caries among adults of all ages. In its position stand regarding the impact of fluoride on health, the American Dietetic Association (ADA) noted that the use of systemic and topical fluoride for oral health has resulted in major reductions in dental caries. Thus, fluoridation of public water supplies has been endorsed by more than 90 professional health organizations as the most effective dental public health measure in existence. Brushing teeth with fluoride toothpaste may also be beneficial, as may sucking on fluoride-containing tablets or lozenges. In these cases the fluoride is applied topically, mixing in the saliva and around the teeth. Excess fluoride use may contribute to fluorosis, or varying shades of whiteness (known as mottling) in the outer tooth enamel. Although the underlying mechanism is not known, DenBesten indicates that fluorosis may occur when excess fluoride interferes in some way with the maturation of dental enamel. Ismail and Bandekar, using a meta-analysis, concluded that children in non-fluoridated communities who use fluoride supplements during childhood are at an increased risk of developing dental fluorosis. In such communities, dental health professionals should be consulted for appropriate advice on use of fluoride supplements.

Fluoride may possess other health benefits, as it is believed to work with calcium and other minerals in bone mineralization. The ADA notes that although fluoride plays a role in bone health, the role of high doses of fluoride for prevention of osteoporosis is undergoing active study and thus should be considered experimental at this point. Osteoporotic patients should consult with their physicians regarding use of fluoride supplements.

TABLE 8.5 Trace minerals: cobalt, fluoride, iodine, manganese, molybdenum

Trace mineral	RDA or AI*	Major food sources	Major body functions	Deficiency symptoms	Symptons of excessive consumption	Recommended as dietary supplement
Cobalt (Co)	**	Meat, liver, milk	Component of vitamin B_{12}; promotes development of red blood cells	Not found in humans	Nausea, vomiting, death	No
Fluoride (F)	3.0–4.0 mg	Milk, egg yolks, drinking water, seafood	Helps form bones and teeth	Higher incidence of dental cavities	Discolored teeth	No
Iodine (I)	150 micrograms	Iodized salt, seafood, vegetables	Helps in formation of thyroid hormones	Goiter, an enlarged thyroid gland	Depressed thyroid gland activity	No
Manganese (Mn)	1.8–2.3 mg	Whole-grain products, dried peas and beans, leafy vegetables, bananas	Many enzymes involved in energy metabolism; bone formation; fat synthesis	Poor growth	Weakness; nervous system problems; mental confusion	No
Molybdenum (Mo)	45 micrograms	Liver, organ meats, whole-grain products, dried beans and peas	Works with riboflavin in enzymes involved in carbohydrate and fat metabolism	Not found in humans	Rare	No

*For adults. RDA or AI for other age groups may be found in the DRI table on the inside front cover.
**Essential as part of vitamin B_{12}.

Iodine Iodine is used in the formation of thyroxine and triiodo-thyronine, two hormones produced in the thyroid gland. Decreased production of these hormones would lower the body's metabolism, a possible contributing factor to the development of obesity. The use of iodized salt has nearly eliminated iodine deficiency in the United States and has thereby greatly reduced the incidence of goiter, a serious iodine-deficiency disease. However, some health professionals are concerned that individuals who restrict salt intake in attempts to prevent the development of high blood pressure may be at risk for iodine deficiency, and thus recommend that such individuals use dietary supplements containing iodine. In developing countries, iodine deficiency is a major problem worldwide, with nearly 750 million people suffering from goiter. In such cases, iodized salts could help.

Research literature relative to the effect of exercise on the metabolic fates of these trace nutrients is almost nonexistent, nor are any studies available regarding the effects of supplements on performance. This may be understandable, as deficiencies are rare.

Key Concepts

▶ Iron deficiency, particularly among women and young children, is a major nutritional health concern, so iron-rich foods such as lean meats and beans should be stressed in the diet.

▶ Iron status is important to aerobic endurance athletes because insufficient hemoglobin or other factors associated with iron deficiency may impair performance. Athletes may have poor iron status due to inadequate dietary iron and increased losses of iron in the urine, sweat, and feces.

▶ Iron supplementation may improve performance in individuals with iron-deficiency anemia, but not in individuals with normal iron status. Although individuals who have iron deficiency without anemia may experience less favorable responses to aerobic training, findings from studies are equivocal as to the efficacy of iron supplementation to improve performance, and investigators recommend additional research. Athletes who train at altitude may consider iron supplementation.

▶ Zinc deficiency has been shown to impair the growth process in children, so it may be a problem for young athletes who incur heavy sweat losses and are on low-Calorie diets, such as wrestlers, dancers, or gymnasts.

▶ Chromium supplements have been marketed to increase muscle mass and decrease body fat, but research does not support those claims.

▶ There does not appear to be much valid scientific evidence to support an ergogenic effect of trace mineral supplementation including zinc, copper, boron, selenium, and vanadium.

Mineral Supplements: Exercise and Health

Following her extensive review of dietary surveys, Sarah Short noted that both athletes and health professionals are becoming more concerned with mineral deficiencies. Perusal of athletic and health magazines marketed for the general public reveals a variety of articles and advertisements suggesting that supplementation of certain minerals will enhance athletic performance or health. As the foregoing discussion indicates, individuals who have a mineral deficiency may experience improved health or physical performance if that deficiency is corrected. In general, however, supplementation has little effect on the individual whose mineral status is adequate. This last section summarizes some key points relative to mineral nutrition, focusing on the need for supplementation.

Does exercise increase my need for minerals?

Exercise may induce mineral losses from the body by several mechanisms. Many minerals appear to be mobilized into the circulation during exercise, probably being released from body stores in the muscles or elsewhere. As they circulate, some may be removed by the kidneys and excreted in the urine, whereas others may appear in the sweat, particularly in a warm environment. Losses from the gastrointestinal tract may also occur during exercise, although the mechanism is not totally understood.

Other body changes mediated by exercise may influence mineral requirements. The female athlete who develops secondary amenorrhea may need additional calcium, as might the male endurance athlete in whom trabecular bone mass is decreased. The need for iron in the female athlete may decrease somewhat with the cessation of menses in secondary amenorrhea.

Because of potential mineral losses, at least one investigator in sport nutrition has suggested that mineral supplementation should be considered for athletes. Although supplementation may be helpful for some, the first concern should be to educate the athlete about obtaining adequate mineral nutrition through dietary means.

Can I obtain the minerals I need through my diet?

As many dietary surveys have shown, many Americans are not obtaining the RDA or AI for a variety of minerals, including iron, zinc, calcium, and chromium. Similar dietary deficiencies have been noted in surveys with athletes, but mainly with athletes who participate in activities such as wrestling, distance running, ballet, and gymnastics, where weight control is a concern. Let us briefly highlight the dietary recommendations that will help ensure adequate amounts of nutrients in the diet.

In general, as with all other nutrients, a balanced diet is essential. Select a wide variety of foods from all the food groups and within each group. Table 8.6 presents the percentage of the DV provided by servings of different foods from several food groups. Keep in mind that the DV, the value used on food labels, may vary with the RDA and AI, being higher for some minerals and lower for others. But the purpose of this table is simply to support the value of eating a wide variety of foods to obtain adequate mineral nutrition.

Note that the percentage values for the minerals differ not only between food groups but also for some minerals in foods within the same group. For example, note that calcium is high in dairy foods but low in meats. Conversely, iron is high in meats but low in dairy products. Also, in the meat group, an oyster is high in copper, but lean beef is relatively low, even more so if you consider the caloric value of each. It is also important to eat foods in their natural state as much as possible. The milling of flour removes many minerals, but only iron is replaced in the enrichment process. Note the differences between whole wheat and enriched white bread in table 8.6. Some food products rich in other healthful nutrients, such as orange juice and whole-grain cereal, are fortified with minerals and may be an effective means to ensure adequate mineral nutrition.

TABLE 8.6 Approximate percentages of the DV in various foods for selected minerals

Food	Serving	Calories	Ca (1,000 mg)	P (1,000 mg)	Mg (400 mg)	Fe (18 mg)	Cu (2 mg)	Zn (15 mg)
Milk, skim	1 glass	90	30	25	7	1	2	7
Cheese, cheddar	1 ounce	114	21	15	2	1	0	6
Oyster	1 ounce	20	1	4	4	11	40	166
Liver, beef	3 ounces	150	1	34	4	32	150	35
Beef, lean sirloin	3 ounces	230	1	18	6	13	7	33
Potato, baked	medium	220	2	11	14	15	15	4
Beans, kidney, cooked	1/2 cup	110	1	12	9	14	12	5
Broccoli	1/2 cup	25	4	5	5	4	2	2
Bread, whole wheat	1 slice	70	2	5	5	4	14	3
Bread, enriched white	1 slice	70	2	2	2	4	6	1

A basic principle of mineral nutrition is to eat natural foods that are rich in calcium and iron. If you select a diet to provide your RDA for these two minerals, you should receive adequate amounts of the other major and trace minerals at the same time. Dairy products and meats are excellent sources of these minerals, but other foods such as legumes and dark-green leafy vegetables also may provide significant amounts if selected wisely. Note the foods rich in calcium and iron in tables 8.2 and 8.4, and compare the similarity to the foods listed for the other minerals in these two tables and table 8.5.

Are mineral megadoses or some nonessential minerals harmful?

One of the generally accepted facts relative to mineral nutrition in the healthy individual is that the levels associated with toxicity can normally be obtained only through the use of supplements or fortified foods, not through natural dietary sources. Because they hope to improve health or physical performance, many individuals purchase supplements containing minerals. However, surveys indicate that the most common preparations purchased contain the RDA or less, which should pose no health problems to the healthy individual. Unfortunately, as indicated in the last chapter, many individuals self-prescribe and may consume more than the recommended daily dosage. Although the toxicity and possible health problems associated with excessive intake of several minerals, such as calcium, iron, zinc, and copper, are fairly well documented, the level of safety for intake of a variety of other minerals, particularly some of the trace minerals suggested to be therapeutic in nature, has been more difficult to document. Nevertheless, the National Academy of Sciences has noted that all trace minerals are toxic if consumed at high doses for a long enough time.

Several nonessential minerals may be consumed inadvertently and cause significant health problems, even in small amounts. Lead can displace other minerals, such as calcium and zinc, in various enzymes and thus interfere with intracellular processes involving protein and gene expression. Industrial chromium is regarded as a carcinogen. Of recent concern is mercury, which may be found in foods that we normally think of as healthy: Fish!

Methylmercury, an industrial waste product, has been dumped into the seas where it may be consumed by fish. As noted in chapter 5, high levels of mercury may accumulate more in larger, older, predatory fish, such as shark, swordfish, king mackerel, and tilefish. Tuna may contain somewhat less mercury. However, the Consumers Union cites new FDA data indicating that some light tuna, which normally has lower levels of mercury than white (Albacore) tuna, may have as much as or more.

Houston indicates that mercury may displace other minerals, such as zinc and copper, thus reducing the effectiveness of various metalloenzymes, including antioxidant enzymes, inducing numerous pathological effects. In particular, too much mercury may damage the nervous system, especially the brain during its formative years prior to birth and the first 7 years of life. Thus, the FDA advises women who are or who can become pregnant and small children should not eat any shark, swordfish, king mackerel, or tilefish. Additional information is presented on page xxx.

Should physically active individuals take mineral supplements?

In general, the answer to this question for most athletes is *no*—for several reasons. First, contrary to advertising claims of mineral-supplement manufacturers, you can obtain adequate mineral nutrition from the diet if you adhere to some of the guidelines presented throughout this chapter. Second, although some athletes may not be obtaining the recommended amounts of several minerals, such as zinc and calcium, mineral deficiencies to the point of impairing physical performance are rare. Very few data are available on this topic, but the evidence that is available with most minerals suggests that though serum levels may be low, physical performance is not affected. An exception may be low levels of serum iron for, as noted previously, supplementation, although controversial, has been helpful to some athletes. Third, many minerals may be harmful when taken in excess. As noted throughout this chapter, the absorption rate for most minerals is relatively low. Only 40 percent of calcium is absorbed from the intestinal tract, while the percentages for iron and chromium are, respectively, 10 and 1–2 percent. Also, a high dietary intake of several minerals that are easily absorbed increases their excretion rate by the kidney. Thus, a low absorption or high excretion rate prevents the accumulation of excess amounts of minerals in the body, which may interfere with normal metabolism. However, large supplemental doses may overload the body and cause numerous health problems and, as noted for several minerals, may be fatal.

Nevertheless, it is recognized that certain athletes may not be obtaining adequate mineral nutrition from their diets and may possibly benefit from supplementation. As noted previously, athletes who are attempting to lose weight for performance are at most risk for developing a mineral deficiency. Because many of the dietary surveys of these athletes have reported intakes lower than the RDA for iron and calcium, it may be assumed that their diets are also low in other trace minerals.

If there is concern for the nutritional status of the athlete, the ideal situation would be to consult a sport nutritionist or nutritionally oriented physician. Unfortunately, this approach does not appear to be common among athletes who may be in need of nutritional counseling, although the situation is improving. Some elite athletes take medically prescribed iron supplements, and dietitians with specialties in exercise physiology and sport nutrition are becoming increasingly available.

For athletes who cannot or will not seek professional advice, it may be prudent to recommend a one-a-day vitamin-mineral supplement to those who are known to have poor nutritional habits. The tablet should contain no more than 50–100 percent of the RDA for any mineral. Additionally, the point should be made to the athlete that the supplement is being recommended to help prevent a deficiency, not for any ergogenic purposes. As noted in chapter 7, large doses of multivitamin-mineral supplements taken over prolonged periods of time have not been shown to enhance physical performance. In the meantime, efforts should be undertaken to educate the athlete concerning sound nutritional practices.

For those considering mineral supplementation for health reasons, the new DRI being developed by the National Academy of Sciences reflect a new paradigm in which the determination of nutrient requirements include consideration of the total health effects of nutrients, not just their roles in preventing deficiency pathology. For example, the updated AI for calcium and vitamin D as a possible means to prevent osteoporosis reflect this new paradigm. Although much research is needed before concrete recommendations may be made relative to mineral supplementation and purported health benefits, the recommendations presented on page 299 may be useful guidelines for healthy sedentary and physically active individuals to use in the meantime.

▶ groups, will provide adequate amounts of both the major and trace minerals.
▶ Mineral supplements may be recommended for some individuals as a means to improve health or sports performance, but excessive intake is not recommended because of potential health problems.

Key Concepts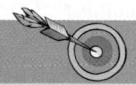

▶ Health professionals recommend that individuals obtain their mineral needs from healthful foods. A diet that provides the RDA for iron and the AI for calcium, as well as Calories from a balanced selection of foods throughout the different food

Check for Yourself

▶ Calcium and iron are two of our key nutrients for health and sport performance. If you obtain adequate amounts of each through natural dietary sources, you should obtain adequate amounts of most other essential minerals. Using food labels or computerized dietary analyses, calculate the calcium and iron intake of your typical daily diet to determine if you are obtaining the RDA for your gender and age.

APPLICATION EXERCISE

Your municipal water supply may contain a variety of minerals, such as calcium, magnesium, fluoride, and sodium. Contact the appropriate governmental authorities in your community to see if you may obtain a detailed water quality report highlighting the mineral content of city drinking water. Calculate the amount of various minerals you consume with each quart of water.

Mineral Content of Municipal Drinking Water

Minerals	Calcium	Magnesium	Fluoride	Sodium	Other	Other
Mineral content in 1 quart of water						

Review Questions—Multiple Choice

1. Which statement does *not* describe the role of major minerals in the body?
   a. They give teeth and bone their rigidity and strength.
   b. They regulate body processes.
   c. They are constituents of soft tissues.
   d. They provide a source of caloric energy.
   e. They help to maintain the acid-base balance.

2. Who has the lesser need for iron as specified by the RDA?
   a. adolescent boys
   b. adolescent girls
   c. young adult females

   d. adult males
   e. female distance runners

3. To help prevent the development of osteoporosis in later life, females should consume adequate quantities of which nutrient during the years in which they are developing peak bone mass?
   a. calcium
   b. iron
   c. retinol
   d. vitamin E
   e. ascorbic acid

4. Which mineral is theorized to be an effective ergogenic aid for runners, because it may possibly increase the delivery of

oxygen to the muscle cell by facilitating its release from hemoglobin?
   a. calcium
   b. phosphorus
   c. zinc
   d. magnesium
   e. chromium

5. Excessive intake of iron can lead to a condition called hemachromatosis, which damages which organ in the body?
   a. arterial walls
   b. kidney
   c. heart
   d. liver
   e. lungs

6. Approximately how much calcium is found in one glass (8 ounces) of skim milk?

    a. 50 milligrams
    b. 100 milligrams
    c. 300 milligrams
    d. 800 milligrams
    e. 1200 milligrams

7. Which of the following would not contain heme iron?

    a. liver
    b. dried beans
    c. fish
    d. chicken
    e. beef

8. Which of the following contains the least amount of calcium?

    a. milk
    b. meat
    c. dried beans
    d. dark-green leafy vegetables
    e. cheese

9. Which food exchange is the best source of zinc, iron, and copper in regards to the concept of bioavailability?

    a. milk
    b. meat
    c. starch/bread
    d. fruit
    e. vegetable

10. Which of the following statements concerning trace minerals is false?

    a. Copper and iron are needed for optimal functioning of the red blood cell.
    b. Selenium works as an antioxidant with one of the vitamins.
    c. Chromium appears to be essential in the use of blood glucose.
    d. Zinc is a part of numerous metalloenzymes.
    e. Mercury is essential for carbohydrate metabolism.

Answers to multiple-choice questions:
1. d; 2. d; 3. a; 4. b; 5. d; 6. c; 7. b; 8. b; 9. b; 10. e.

Review Questions—Essay

1. Explain several ways whereby minerals function in metabolic processes in the human body.
2. Name three macrominerals and at least five trace minerals and describe the metabolic function of each in the human body.
3. Osteoporosis is a significant health problem in the United States and Canada. Discuss the risk factors for osteoporosis and provide specifics as to how life-style behaviors may help prevent its development.
4. Discuss the role that iron supplementation may play if provided to an athlete under three conditions: (a) normal iron and hemoglobin status; (b) iron deficiency without anemia; (c) iron-deficiency anemia.
5. Several minerals have been alleged to possess ergogenic potential. Select two of the following, explain the theoretical rationale underlying their purported ergogenic effects, and highlight the current research findings regarding their efficacy:

    chromium   phosphate salts
    boron   vanadium

References

Books

American Institute of Cancer Research. 2007. *Food, Nutrition, Physical Activity, and the Prevention of Cancer: A Global Perspective.* Washington, DC: AICR.

Celsing, F. 1987. *Influence of Iron Deficiency and Changes in Hemoglobin Concentration on Exercise Capacity in Man.* Stockholm: Repro Print.

Emery, T. 1991. *Iron and Your Health.* Boca Raton, FL: CRC Press.

Institute of Medicine. 2005. *Dietary Supplements: A Framework for Evaluating Safety.* Washington, DC: National Academies Press.

National Academy of Sciences. 2002. *Dietary Reference Intakes for Vitamin A, Vitamin K, Arsenic, Boron, Chromium, Copper, Iodine, Iron, Manganese, Molybdenum, Nickel, Silicon, Vanadium, and Zinc.* Washington, DC: National Academy Press.

National Academy of Sciences. 2000. *Dietary Reference Intakes for Vitamin C, Vitamin E, Selenium and Carotenoids.* Washington, DC: National Academy Press.

National Academy of Sciences. 1999. *Dietary Reference Intakes for Calcium, Phosphorus, Magnesium, Vitamin D, and Fluoride.* Washington, DC: National Academy Press.

National Academy of Sciences. Institute of Medicine, Food, and Nutrition Board. 2010. *Dietary Reference Intakes for Calcium and Vitamin D.* Washington, DC: National Academy Press.

Nelson, M. 2005. *Strong Women, Strong Bones.* New York: Penguin Putnam.

Reviews

Althuis, M., et al. 2002. Glucose and insulin responses to dietary chromium supplements: A meta-analysis. *American Journal of Clinical Nutrition* 76:148–55.

American College of Sports Medicine. 2004. Physical activity and bone health. *Medicine & Science in Sports & Exercise* 36:1985–96.

American Dietetic Association. 2000. Position of the American Dietetic Association: The impact of fluoride on health. *Journal of the American Dietetic Association* 100:1208–13.

American Dietetic Association. 1997. Position of the American Dietetic Association: Vegetarian diets. *Journal of the American Dietetic Association* 97:1317–21.

Anderson, J., and Barrett, C. 1994. Dietary phosphorus: The benefits and the problems. *Nutrition Today* 29 (2):29–34.

Anderson, R. 1988. Selenium, chromium, and manganese. (B) Chromium. In *Modern Nutrition in Health and Disease,* eds. M. Shils and V. Young. Philadelphia: Lea and Febiger.

Anderson, R. 1998. Chromium, glucose intolerance and diabetes. *Journal of the American College of Nutrition* 17: 548–55.

Anderson, R. 1998. Effects of chromium on body composition and weight loss. *Nutrition Reviews* 56:266–70.

Antinoro, L. 2002. Marvelous magnesium offers health benefits: From heart to bones. *Environmental Nutrition* 25 (9):1, 6.

Balk, E., et al. 2007. Effect of chromium supplementation on glucose metabolism and lipids: A systematic review of randomized controlled trials. *Diabetes Care* 30:2154–63.

Beard, J., and Tobin, B. 2000. Iron status and exercise. *American Journal of Clinical Nutrition.* 72:594S–97S.

Beatty, T., et al. 2010. Bone density in competitive cyclists. *Current Sports Medicine Reports* 9:352–55.

Beletate, V., et al. 2007. Zinc supplementation for the prevention of type 2 diabetes mellitus. *Cochrane Database of Systematic Reviews* 24:CD005525.

Bennell, K., et al. 1996. Effect of altered reproductive function and lowered testosterone levels on bone density in male endurance athletes. *British Journal of Sports Medicine* 30:205–8.

Bern, L. 2003. The estrogen and progestin dilemma: New advice, labeling guidelines. *FDA Consumer* 37 (2):10–11.

Bjelakovic, G., et al. 2004. Antioxidant supplements for prevention of gastrointestinal cancers: A systematic review and meta-analysis. *Lancet* 364:1219–28.

Bloomfield, S. 2001. Optimizing bone health: Impact of nutrition, exercise, and hormones. *Sports Science Exchange* 14 (3):1–4.

Bonaiuti, D., et al. 2002. Exercise for preventing and treating osteoporosis in postmenopausal women. *Cochrane Database of System Reviews* 3:CD000333.

Bonjour, J. 2005. Dietary protein: An essential nutrient for bone health. *Journal of the American College of Nutrition* 24: 526S–36S.

Bonjour, J., et al. 2007. Calcium intake and vitamin D metabolism and action, in healthy conditions and in prostate cancer. *British Journal of Nutrition* 97:611–6.

Boonen, S., et al. 2006. Addressing the musculoskeletal components of fracture risk with calcium and vitamin D: A review of the evidence. *Calcified Tissue International* 78:257–70.

Brilla, L., and Lombardi, V. 1999. Magnesium in exercise and sport. In *Macroelements, Water, and Electrolytes in Sports Nutrition,* eds. J. Driskell and I. Wolinsky. Boca Raton, FL: CRC Press.

Brown, K., et al. 2002. Effect of supplemental zinc on the growth and serum zinc concentrations of prepubertal children: A meta-analysis of randomized controlled trials. *American Journal of Clinical Nutrition* 75:1062–71.

Burk, R. 2002. Selenium, an antioxidant nutrient. *Nutrition in Clinical Care* 5:75–79.

Burk, R., and Levander, O. 2006. Selenium. In *Modern Nutrition in Health and Disease,* eds. M. Shils et al. Philadelphia: Lippincott Williams & Wilkins.

Candow, D., and Chilibeck, P. 2010. Potential of creatine supplementation for improving aging bone health. *Journal of Nutrition Health and Aging* 14:149–53.

Carroll, C., et al. 2010. Supplemental calcium in the chemoprevention of colorectal cancer: A systematic review and meta-analysis. *Clinical Therapeutics* 32:789–803.

Clarkson, P. 1997. Effects of exercise on chromium levels: Is supplementation required? *Sports Medicine* 23:341–49.

Clarkson, P. 1996. Nutrition for improved sports performance. *Sports Medicine* 21:393–401.

Clarkson, P., and Haymes, E. 1995. Exercise and mineral status of athletes: Calcium, magnesium, phosphorus, and iron. *Medicine & Science in Sports & Exercise* 27:831–45.

Combs, G. 2005. Current evidence and research needs to support a health claim for selenium and cancer prevention. *Journal of Nutrition* 135:343–47.

Consumers Union. 2008. New concerns for bone-building drugs. *Consumer Reports on Health* 20 (4):3.

Consumers Union. 2006. Mercury in tuna. *Consumer Reports on Health* 71 (7):20–21.

Consumers Union. 2006. Bone-building drugs. *Consumer Reports on Health* 18 (5):3.

Consumers Union. 2004. Stronger bones without the hype. *Consumer Reports on Health* 16 (5):1, 4–5.

Cooper, M., et al. 2006. The iron status of Canadian adolescents and adults: Current knowledge and practical implications. *Canadian Journal of Dietary Practice and Research* 67:130–38.

Danesh, J., and Appleby, P. 1999. Coronary heart disease and iron status: Meta-analysis of prospective studies. *Circulation* 99:852–54.

Dawson-Hughes, B. 2006. Osteoporosis. In *Modern Nutrition in Health and Disease,* eds. M. Shils et al. Philadelphia: Lippincott Williams & Wilkins.

DenBesten, P. 1999. Biological mechanisms of dental fluorosis relevant to the use of fluoride supplements. *Community Dentistry and Oral Epidemiology* 27:41–47.

Denic, S., and Agarwal, M. 2007. Nutritional iron deficiency: An evolutionary perspective. *Nutrition* 23:603–14.

Deuster, P. 1989. Magnesium in sports medicine. *Journal of the American College of Nutrition* 8:462.

DeValk, B., and Marx, J. 1999. Iron, atherosclerosis, and ischemic heart disease. *Archives of Internal Medicine* 159: 1542–48.

Dickinson, H., et al. 2006. Calcium supplementation for the management of primary hypertension in adults. *Cochrane Database of Systematic Reviews* (2):CD004639.

Dickinson, H., et al. 2006. Magnesium supplementation for the management of essential hypertension in adults. *Cochrane Database of Systematic Reviews* (19):CD004640.

Durlach, J., et al. 1999. Cardiovasoprotective foods and nutrients: Possible importance of magnesium intake. *Magnesium Research* 12:57–61.

Eichner, E. 2001. Anemia and blood boosting. *Sports Science Exchange* 14 (2):1–4.

Eichner, E. 1992. Sports anemia, iron supplements, and blood doping. *Medicine & Science in Sports & Exercise* 24:S315–S318.

Evans, G. 1989. The effect of chromium picolinate on insulin controlled parameters in humans. *International Journal of Biosocial and Medical Research* 11:163–80.

Fairbanks, V. 1999. Iron in medicine and nutrition. In *Modern Nutrition in Health and Disease,* eds. M. Shils et al. Baltimore: Williams and Wilkins.

Featherstone, J. 1999. Prevention and reversal of dental caries: Role of low-level fluoride. *Community Dentistry and Oral Epidemiology* 27:31–40.

Flores-Mateo, G., et al. 2006. Selenium and coronary heart disease: A meta-analysis. *American Journal of Clinical Nutrition* 84:762–73.

Food and Drug Administration. 2005. Americans over 50 at risk of bone fractures. *FDA Consumer* 39 (1):10–11.

Garza, D., et al. 1997. The clinical value of serum ferritin tests in endurance athletes. *Clinics in Sport Medicine* 7:46–53.

Gledhill, N., et al. 1999. Haemoglobin, blood volume, cardiac function, and aerobic power. *Canadian Journal of Applied Physiology* 24:54–65.

Griffin, S., et al. 2007. Effectiveness of fluoride in preventing caries in adults. *Journal of Dental Research* 86:410–5.

Haas, J., and Brownlie, T. 2001. Iron deficiency and reduced work capacity: A critical review of the research to determine a causal relationship. *Journal of Nutrition* 131:676S–88S.

Hambidge, M. 2000. Human zinc deficiency. *Journal of Nutrition* 130:1344S–49S.

Hansen, K., and Tho, S. 1998. Androgens and bone health. *Seminars in Reproductive Endocrinology* 16:129–34.

Haymes, E. 1993. Dietary iron needs in exercising women: A rational plan to follow in evaluating iron status. *Medicine, Exercise, Nutrition, and Health* 2:203–12.

Heaney, R. 2007. Bone health. *American Journal of Clinical Nutrition* 85:300S–303S.

Horn, S., and Feller, E. 2003. Gastrointestinal (GI) bleeding in endurance runners. *AMAA Journal* 16 (1):5–6, 11.

Horswill, C. 1995. Effects of bicarbonate, citrate, and phosphate loading on performance. *International Journal of Sport Nutrition* 5:S111–S119.

Houston, M. 2007. The role of mercury and cadmium heavy metals in vascular disease, hypertension, coronary heart disease, and myocardial infarction. *Alternative Therapies in Health and Medicine* 13:S128–S133.

Hunt, C., et al. 1997. Metabolic responses of postmenopausal women to supplemental dietary boron and aluminum during usual and low magnesium intake: Boron, calcium, and magnesium absorption and retention and blood mineral concentrations. *American Journal of Clinical Nutrition* 65:808–13.

Ilich, J., and Kerstetter, J. 2000. Nutrition in bone health revisited: A story beyond calcium. *Journal of the American College of Nutrition* 19:715–37.

Ismail, A., and Bandekar, R. 1999. Fluoride supplements and fluorosis: A meta-analysis. *Community Dentistry and Oral Epidemiology* 27:48–56.

Jackson, J., et al. 2000. Zinc and the common cold: A meta-analysis revisited. *Journal of Nutrition* 130:1512S–1515S.

Jones, G., and Newhouse, I. 1997. Sport-related hematuria: A review. *Clinical Journal of Sports Medicine* 7:119–25.

King, J., and Cousins, R. 2006. Zinc. In *Modern Nutrition in Health and Disease,* eds. M. Shils et al. Philadelphia: Lippincott Williams & Wilkins.

Knochel, J. 2006. Phosphorus. In *Modern Nutrition in Health and Disease,* eds. M. Shils et al. Philadelphia: Lippincott Williams & Wilkins.

Kreider, R. 1999. Dietary supplements and the promotion of muscle growth with resistance exercise. *Sports Medicine* 27:97–110.

Kunstel, K. 2005. Calcium requirements for the athletes. *Current Sports Medicine Reports* 4:203–206.

Lane, H. 1989. Some trace elements related to physical activity: Zinc, copper, selenium, chromium, and iodine. In *Nutrition in Exercise and Sport,* eds. J. Hickson and I. Wolinsky. Boca Raton, FL: CRC Press.

Lefavi, R. 1992. Efficacy of chromium supplementation in athletes: Emphasis on anabolism. *International Journal of Sport Nutrition* 2:111–22.

Levine, J. 2006. Pharmacologic and nonpharmacologic management of osteoporosis. *Clinical Cornerstone* 8(1):40–53.

Liebman, B. 2007. Confusion at the vitamin counter. *Nutrition Action Health Letter* 34 (9):1–8.

Liebman, B., and Schardt, D. 2008. MultiComplex: Picking a multivitamin gets tricky. *Nutrition Action Health Letter* 35 (5):1–9.

Loucks, A. 2006. The endocrine system: Integrated influences on metabolism, growth, and reproduction. In *ACSM's Advanced Exercise Physiology,* ed. C. Tipton. Philadelphia: Lippincott Williams & Wilkins.

Lowe, N., et al. 2002. Is there a potential therapeutic value of copper and zinc for osteoporosis? *Proceedings of the Nutrition Society* 61:181–85.

Lukaski, H. 2004. Vitamin and mineral status: Effects on physical performance. *Nutrition* 20:632–44.

Lukaski, H. 2001. Magnesium, zinc, and chromium nutrition and athletic performance. *Canadian Journal of Applied Physiology* 26:S13–22.

Lukaski, H. 1995. Micronutrients (magnesium, zinc, and copper): Are mineral supplements needed for athletes? *International Journal of Sport Nutrition* 5:S74–S83.

Lukaski, H. 1999. Chromium as a supplement. *Annual Reviews in Nutrition* 19:279–302.

Malloy, D., et al. 2007. The spirit of sport, morality, and hypoxic tents: Logic and authenticity. *Applied Physiology, Nutrition and Metabolism* 32:289–96.

Manore, M. 2001. Vitamins and minerals: How much do you need? *ACSM's Health & Fitness Journal* 5 (1):33–35.

Maret, W., and Sandstead, H. 2006. Zinc requirements and the risks and benefits of zinc supplementation. *Journal of Trace Elements in Medicine and Biology* 20:3–18.

Maughan, R., and Shirreffs, S. 2007. Nutrition and hydration concerns of the female football player. *British Journal of Sports Medicine* 41 (Supplement 1):60–63.

Mazzeo, R., and Fulco, C. 2006. Physiological systems and their responses to conditions of hypoxia. In *ACSM's Advanced Exercise Physiology,* ed. C. Tipton. Philadelphia: Lippincott Williams & Wilkins.

McDonald, R., and Keen, C. 1988. Iron, zinc and magnesium nutrition and athletic performance. *Sports Medicine* 5:171–84.

Mehdi, M., et al. 2006. Insulin signal mimicry as a mechanism for the insulin-like effects of vanadium. *Cell Biochemistry and Biophysics* 44:73–81.

Micheletti, A., et al. 2001. Zinc status in athletes: Relation to diet and exercise. *Sports Medicine* 31:577–82.

Miller, L., et al. 2004. Bone mineral density in postmenopausal women. *Physician and Sportsmedicine* 32 (2):18–24.

Mizushima, S., et al. 1998. Dietary magnesium intake and blood pressure: A qualitative overview of the observational studies. *Journal of Human Hypertension* 12:447–53.

Modlesky, C., and Lewis, R. 2002. Does exercise during growth have a long-term effect on bone health? *Exercise and Sport Sciences Reviews* 30:171–76.

Naghii, M. 1999. The significance of dietary boron, with particular reference to athletes. *Nutrition and Health* 13:31–37.

National Institutes of Health. 2006. National Institutes of Health State-of-the-Science conference statement: Multivitamin/mineral supplements and chronic disease prevention. *Annals of Internal Medicine* 145:364–71.

Newhouse, I., and Finstad, E. 2000. The effects of magnesium supplementation on exercise performance. *Clinical Journal of Sport Medicine* 10:195–200.

Newhouse, I., and Clement, D. 1988. Iron status in athletes: An update. *Sports Medicine* 5:337–52.

Nielsen, F. 2008. Is boron nutritionally relevant? *Nutrition Reviews* 66:183–91.

Nielsen, F. 1999. Ultratrace minerals. In *Modern Nutrition in Health and Disease,* eds. M. Shils et al. Philadelphia: Lippincott Williams & Wilkins.

Nielsen, F. 1998. The justification for providing dietary guidance for the nutritional intake of boron. *Biological Trace Element Research* 66:319–30.

Nielsen, F. 1992. Facts and fallacies about boron. *Nutrition Today* 27:6–12.

Nielsen, F., and Lukaski, H. 2006. Update on the relationship between magnesium and exercise. *Magnesium Research* 19:180–89.

Nielsen, P., and Nachtigall, D. 1998. Iron supplementation to athletes: Current recommendations. *Sports Medicine* 26:207–16.

Nieman, D. 2001. Exercise immunology: Nutritional countermeasures. *Canadian Journal of Applied Physiology* 26:S45–S55.

NIH Consensus Development Panel on Osteoporosis Prevention, Diagnosis, and Therapy. 2001. Osteoporosis prevention, diagnosis, and therapy. *JAMA* 285:785–95.

Parodi, P. 2005. Dairy product consumption and the risk of breast cancer. *Journal of the American College of Nutrition* 24: 556S–68S.

Pennington, J. 1996. Intakes of minerals from diets and foods: Is there a need for concern? *Journal of Nutrition* 126:2304S–2308S.

Pittler, M., et al. 2003. Chromium picolinate for reducing body weight: Meta-analysis of randomized trials. *International Journal of Obesity and Related Metabolic Disorders* 27:522–29.

Rayman, M., and Rayman, M. 2002. The argument for increasing selenium intake. *Proceedings of the Nutrition Society* 61:203–15.

Rodenberg, R., and Gustafson, S. 2007. Iron as an ergogenic aid: Ironclad evidence? *Current Sports Medicine Reports* 6:258–64.

Rude, R., and Shils, M. 2006. Magnesium. In *Modern Nutrition in Health and Disease,* eds. M. Shils et al. Philadelphia: Lippincott Williams & Wilkins.

Runner's World. 2003. Live high, train low. *Runner's World* 38 (1):64.

Schardt, D., and Schmidt, S. 1996. Chromium. *Nutrition Action Healthletter* 23 (4):10–11.

Seeman, E. 1999. The structural basis of bone fragility in men. *Bone* 25:143–47.

Severson, K. 2007. Dairy Council to end ad campaign that linked drinking milk to weight loss. *New York Times* May 11.

Sharman, I. 1984. Need for micro-nutrient supplementation with regard to physical performance. *International Journal of Sports Medicine* 5 (Suppl):22–24.

Shaskey, D., and Green, G. 2000. Sports haematology. *Sports Medicine* 29:27–38.

Short, S. 1994. Dietary surveys and nutrition knowledge. In *Nutrition in Exercise and Sport,* eds. I. Wolinsky and J. Hickson. Boca Raton, FL: CRC Press.

Sojka, J., and Weaver, C. 1995. Magnesium supplementation and osteoporosis. *Nutrition Reviews* 53:71–80.

Specker, B., and Vukovich, M. 2007. Evidence for an interaction between exercise and nutrition for improved bone health during growth. *Medicine and Sport Science* 51:50–63.

Speich, M., et al. 2001. Minerals, trace elements and related biological variables in athletes and during physical activity. *Clinical Chimica Acta* 312:1–11.

Stearns, D., et al. 1995. A prediction of chromium (III) accumulation in humans from chromium dietary supplements. *FASEB Journal* 9:1650–57.

Stoecker, B. 2006. Chromium. In *Modern Nutrition in Health and Disease,* eds. M. Shils et al. Philadelphia: Lippincott Williams & Wilkins.

Straub, D. 2007. Calcium supplementation in clinical practice: A review of forms, doses, and indications. *Nutrition in Clinical Practice* 22:286–96.

Suedekum, N., and Dimeff, R. 2005. Iron and the athlete. *Current Sports Medicine Reports* 4:199–202.

Tang, B., et al. 2007. Use of calcium or calcium in combination with vitamin D supplementation to prevent fractures and bone loss in people aged 50 years and older: A meta-analysis. *Lancet* 370:657–66.

Titchenal, C., and Dobbs, J. 2007. A system to assess the quality of food sources of calcium. *Journal of Food Composition and Analysis* 20:717–24.

Tremblay, M., et al. 1994. Ergogenic effects of phosphate loading: Physiological fact or methodological fiction? *Canadian Journal of Applied Physiology* 19:1–11.

Trowman, R., et al. 2006. A systematic review of the effects of calcium supplementation on body weight. *British Journal of Nutrition* 95:1033–38.

Trumbo, P., and Ellwood, K. 2006. Chromium picolinate intake and risk of type 2 diabetes: An evidence-based review by the United States Food and Drug Administration. *Nutrition Reviews* 64:357–63.

Tufts University. 2007. Selenium may help protect aging brain. *Tufts University Health & Nutrition Letter* 25 (3):1–2.

Turner, C., and Robling, A. 2003. Designing exercise regimens to increase bone strength. *Exercise and Sport Sciences Reviews* 31:45–50.

Turnlund, J. 2006. Copper. In *Modern Nutrition in Health and Disease,* eds. M. Shils et al. Philadelphia: Lippincott Williams & Wilkins.

Van Loan, M. 2009. The role of dairy foods and dietary calcium in weight management. *Journal of the American College of Nutrition* 28:120S–9S.

van Mierlo, L., et al. 2006. Blood pressure response to calcium supplementation: A meta-analysis of randomized controlled trials. *Journal of Human Hypertension* 20:571–80.

Verma, S., et al. 1998. Nutritional factors that can favorably influence the glucose/insulin system: Vanadium. *Journal of the American College of Nutrition* 17:11–18.

Vincent, J. 2003. The potential value and toxicity of chromium picolinate as a nutritional supplement, weight loss agent and muscle development agent. *Sports Medicine* 33:213–30.

Vinceti, M., et al. 2001. Adverse effects of selenium in humans. *Reviews on Environmental Health* 16:233–51.

Ward, E. 2007. Selenium protects joints, prostate: Could it do more? *Environmental Nutrition* 30 (3):1, 6.

Warren, M., and Stiehl, A. 1999. Exercise and female adolescents: Effects on the reproductive and skeletal systems. *Journal of the American Medical Women's Association* 54:115–20.

Weaver, C. 2000. Calcium requirements of physically active people. *American Journal of Clinical Nutrition* 72:579S–84S.

Weaver, C., and Heaney, R. 2006. Calcium. In *Modern Nutrition in Health and Disease,* eds. M. Shils et al. Philadelphia: Lippincott Williams & Wilkins.

Weaver, C., and Rajaram, S. 1992. Exercise and iron status. *Journal of Nutrition* 122:782–87.

Weight, L. 1993. "Sports anemia": Does it exist? *Sports Medicine* 16:1–4.

Weingarten, M., et al. 2005. Dietary calcium supplementation for preventing colorectal cancer and adenomatous polyps. *Cochrane Database of Systematic Reviews* (3) CD003548.

Wilber, R., et al. 2007. Effect of hypoxic "dose" on physiological responses and sea-level performance. *Medicine & Science in Sports & Exercise* 39:1590–99.

Wood, R., and Ronnenberg, A. 2006. Iron. In *Modern Nutrition in Health and Disease,* eds. M. Shils et al. Philadelphia: Lippincott Williams & Wilkens.

Wurzelmann, J., et al. 1996. Iron intake and the risk of colorectal cancer. *Cancer Epidemiology and Biomarkers of Prevention* 5:503–7.

Zemel, M. 2005. The role of dairy in weight management. *Journal of the American College of Nutrition* 24:537S–46S.

Zernicke, R., et al. 2006. The skeletal-articular system. In *ACSM's Advanced Exercise Physiology,* ed. C. Tipton. Philadelphia: Lippincott Williams & Wilkins.

Zimmermann, M., and Hurrell, R. 2007. Nutritional iron deficiency. *Lancet* 370:511–20.

Specific Studies

Anderson, R., et al. 1995. Acute exercise effects on urinary losses and serum concentrations of copper and zinc of moderately trained and untrained men consuming a controlled diet. *Analyst* 120:867–70.

Baech, S., et al. 2003. Nonheme-iron absorption from a phytate-rich meal is increased by the addition of small amounts of pork meat. *American Journal of Clinical Nutrition* 77:173–79.

Barr, S., et al. 1998. Spinal bone mineral density in premenopausal vegetarian and nonvegetarian women: Cross-sectional and prospective comparisons. *Journal of the American Dietetic Association* 98:760–5.

Bilanin, J., et al. 1989. Lower vertebral bone density in male long distance runners. *Medicine & Science in Sports & Exercise* 21:66–70.

Bremner, K., et al. 2002. The effect of phosphate loading on erythrocyte 2,3-bisphophoglycerate levels. *Clinical Chimica Acta* 323:111–14.

Brilla, L., and Gunter, K., 1994. Magnesium ameliorates aerobic contribution at high intensity. *Medicine & Science in Sports & Exercise* 26:S53.

Brownlie, T., et al. 2002. Marginal iron deficiency without anemia impairs aerobic adaptation among previously untrained women. *American Journal of Clinical Nutrition* 75:734–42.

Brun, J., et al. 1995. Serum zinc in highly trained adolescent gymnasts. *Biological Trace Element Research* 47:273–78.

Buchman, A., et al. 1998. The effect of a marathon run on plasma and urine mineral and metal concentrations. *Journal of the American College of Nutrition* 17:124–27.

Bullen, D., et al. 1999. Calcium losses resulting from an acute bout of moderate-intensity exercise. *International Journal of Sport Nutrition* 9:275–84.

Caan, B., et al. 2007. Calcium plus vitamin D supplementation and the risk of postmenopausal weight gain. *Archives of Internal Medicine* 167:893–902.

Cade, R., et al. 1984. Effects of phosphate loading on 2,3-diphosphoglycerate and maximal oxygen uptake. *Medicine & Science in Sports & Exercise* 16:263–68.

Campbell, W., et al. 2002. Effects of resistive training and chromium picolinate on body composition and skeletal muscle size in older women. *International Journal of Sport Nutrition and Exercise Metabolism* 12:125–35.

Casoni, I., et al. 1990. Changes in magnesium concentrations in endurance athletes. *International Journal of Sports Medicine* 11:234–37.

Chinevere, T., et al. 2008. Effect of heat acclimation on sweat minerals. *Medicine & Science in Sports & Exercise* 40:886–91.

Clancy, S., et al. 1994. Effects of chromium picolinate supplementation on body composition, strength, and urinary chromium loss in football players. *International Journal of Sport Nutrition* 4:142–53.

Clark, L., et al. 1998. Decreased incidence of prostate cancer with selenium supplementation: Results of a double-blind cancer prevention trial. *British Journal of Urology* 81:730–34.

Cobb, K., et al. 2007. The effect of oral contraceptives on bone mass and stress fractures in female runners. *Medicine & Science in Sports & Exercise* 39:1464–73.

Constantini, N., et al. 2000. Iron status of highly active adolescents: Evidence of depleted stores in gymnasts. *International Journal of Sport Nutrition and Exercise Metabolism* 10:62–70.

Cussler, E., et al. 2003. Weight lifted in strength training predicts bone change in postmenopausal women. *Medicine & Science in Sports & Exercise* 35:10–17.

Davis, J., et al. 2000. Effects of carbohydrate and chromium ingestion during intermittent high-intensity exercise to fatigue. *International Journal of Sport Nutrition and Exercise Metabolism* 10:476–85.

Dawson, B., et al. 2006. Iron supplementation: Oral tablets versus intramuscular injection. *International Journal of Sport Nutrition and Exercise Metabolism* 16:180–86.

Derstine, J., et al. 2003. Iron status in association with cardiovascular disease risk in 3 controlled feeding studies. *American Journal of Clinical Nutrition* 77:55–62.

DeRuisseau, K., et al. 2002. Sweat iron and zinc losses during prolonged exercise. *International Journal of Sport Nutrition and Exercise Metabolism* 12:428–37.

Deugnier, Y., et al. 2002. Increased body iron stores in elite road cyclists. *Medicine & Science in Sports & Exercise* 34:876–80.

Dressendorfer, R., et al. 2002. Mineral metabolism in male cyclists during high-intensity endurance training. *International Journal of Sport Nutrition and Exercise Metabolism* 12:63–72.

Dubnov, G., and Constantini, N. 2004. Prevalence of iron depletion and anemia in top-level basketball players. *International Journal of Sport Nutrition and Exercise Metabolism* 14:30–37.

Dunn, B., et al. 2010. A nutrient approach to prostate cancer prevention: The Selenium and Vitamin E Cancer Prevention Trial (SELECT). *Nutrition and Cancer* 62:896–918.

Fawcett, J., et al. 1996. The effect of oral vanadyl sulfate on body composition and performance in weight-training athletes. *International Journal of Sport Nutrition* 6:382–90.

Ferrando, A., and Green, N. 1993. The effect of boron supplementation on lean body mass, plasma testosterone levels, and strength in male bodybuilders. *International Journal of Sport Nutrition* 3:140–49.

Fogelholm, M., et al. 1992. Effect of iron supplementation in female athletes with low serum ferritin concentration. *International Journal of Sports Medicine* 13:158–62.

Galloway, S., et al. 1996. The effects of acute phosphate supplementation in subjects of different aerobic fitness levels. *European Journal of Applied Physiology* 72:224–30.

Goss, F., et al. 2001. Effect of potassium phosphate supplementation on perceptual and physiological responses to maximal graded exercise. *International Journal of Sport Nutrition and Exercise Metabolism* 11:53–62.

Grant, K., et al. 1997. Chromium and exercise training: Effect on obese women. *Medicine & Science in Sport & Exercise* 29:992–98.

Gremion, G., et al. 2001. Oligo-amenorrheic long-distance runners may lose more bone in spine than in femur. *Medicine & Science in Sports & Exercise* 33:15–21.

Hallmark, M., et al. 1996. Effects of chromium and resistive training on muscle strength and body composition. *Medicine & Science in Sports & Exercise* 28:139–44.

Harvey-Berino, J., et al. 2005. The impact of calcium and dairy product consumption on weight loss. *Obesity Research* 13:1720–26.

Heaney, R., and Nordin, B. 2002. Calcium effects on phosphorus absorption: Implications for the prevention and co-therapy of osteoporosis. *Journal of the American College of Nutrition* 21:239–44.

Heath, A., et al. 2001. Can dietary treatment of non-anemic iron deficiency improve iron status? *Journal of the American College of Nutrition* 20:477–84.

Hinton, P., et al. 2000. Iron supplementation improves endurance after training in iron-depleted, nonanemic women. *Journal of Applied Physiology* 88:1103–11.

Hudgins, P., et al. 1990. Effects of iron supplementation on hematologic profile and performance in female endurance athletes. *FASEB Journal* 4:A1197.

Hunt, J., et al. 1998. Zinc absorption, mineral balance, and blood lipids in women consuming controlled lactoovovegetarian and omnivorous diets for 8 weeks. *American Journal of Clinical Nutrition* 67:421–30.

Jackson, R., et al. 2006. Calcium plus vitamin D supplementation and the risk of fractures. *New England Journal of Medicine* 354:669–83.

Jentjens, R., and Jeukendrup, A. 2002. Effect of acute and short-term administration of vanadyl sulphate on insulin sensitivity in healthy active humans. *International Journal of Sport Nutrition and Exercise Metabolism* 12:470–79.

Jones, G., et al. 2001. The incidence of hematuria in middle distance track running. *Canadian Journal of Applied Physiology* 26:336–49.

Jordan, A., et al. 2004. Effects of oral ATP supplementation on anaerobic power and muscular strength. *Medicine & Science in Sports & Exercise* 36:983–90.

Karamizrak, S., et al. 1996. Evaluation of iron metabolism indices and their relation with physical work capacity in athletes. *British Journal of Sports Medicine* 30:15–19.

Kato, T., et al. 2006. Effect of low-repetition jump training on bone mineral density in young women. *Journal of Applied Physiology* 100:839–43.

Khaled, S., et al. 1998. Increased blood viscosity in iron-depleted elite athletes. *Clinical Hemorheology and Microcirculation* 18:309–18.

Klesges, R., et al. 1996. Changes in bone mineral content in male athletes. *Journal of the American Medical Association* 276:226–30.

Klingshirn, L., et al. 1992. Effect of iron supplementation on endurance capacity in iron-depleted female runners. *Medicine & Science in Sports & Exercise* 24:819–24.

Kraemer, W., et al. 1995. Effects of multibuffer supplementation on acid-base balance and 2,3-diphosphoglycerate following repetitive anaerobic exercise. *International Journal of Sport Nutrition* 5:300–314.

Kreider, R., et al. 1992. Effects of phosphate loading on metabolic and myocardial responses to maximal and endurance exercise. *International Journal of Sport Nutrition* 2:20–47.

Kreider, R., et al. 1990. Effects of phosphate loading on oxygen uptake, ventilatory anaerobic threshold, and run performance. *Medicine & Science in Sports & Exercise* 22:250–56.

Krotkiewski, M., et al. 1982. Zinc and muscle strength and endurance. *Acta Physiologica Scandinavica* 116:309–11.

Lamanca, J., and Haymes, E. 1993. Effects of iron repletion on VO$_2$ max, endurance, and blood lactate in women. *Medicine & Science in Sports & Exercise* 25:1386–92.

Landahl, G., et al. 2005. Iron deficiency and anemia: A common problem in female elite soccer players. *International Journal of Sport Nutrition and Exercise Metabolism* 15:689–94.

Lappe, J., et al. 2007. Vitamin D and calcium supplementation reduces cancer risk: Results of a randomized trial. *American Journal of Clinical Nutrition* 85:1586–91.

Lappe, J., et al. 2004. Girls on a high-calcium diet gain weight at the same rate as girls on a normal diet: A pilot study. *Journal of the American Dietetic Association* 104:1361–67.

Lima, M., et al. 1998. The effect of magnesium supplementation in increasing doses on the control of type 2 diabetes. *Diabetes Care* 21:682–86.

Liu, I., et al. 1983. Hypomagnesemia in a tennis player. *Physician and Sportsmedicine* 11 (May):79–80.

Livolsi, J., et al. 2001. The effect of chromium picolinate on muscular strength and body composition in women athletes. *Journal of Strength and Conditioning Research* 15:161–66.

Looker, A., et al. 1997. Prevalence of iron deficiency in the United States. *Journal of the American Medical Association* 277:973–76.

Lorenzen, J., et al. 2006. Calcium supplementation for 1 y does not reduce body weight or fat mass in young girls. *American Journal of Clinical Nutrition* 83:18–23.

Lukaski, H., et al. 2007. Chromium picolinate supplementation in women: Effects on body weight, composition, and iron status. *Nutrition* 23:187–95.

Lukaski, H., et al. 1996. Chromium supplementation and resistance training: Effects on body composition, strength, and trace element status of men. *American Journal of Clinical Nutrition* 63:954–65.

Lukaski, H., et al. 1991. Altered metabolic response of iron deficient women during graded, maximal exercises. *European Journal of Applied Physiology* 63:140–45.

Lyle, R., et al. 1992. Iron status in exercising women: The effect of oral iron therapy vs increased consumption of muscle foods. *American Journal of Clinical Nutrition* 56:1049–55.

Magazanik, A., et al. 1991. Effect of an iron supplement on body iron status and aerobic capacity of young training women. *European Journal of Applied Physiology* 62:317–23.

Maimoun, L., et al. 2006. The intensity level of physical exercise and the bone metabolism response. *International Journal of Sports Medicine* 27:105–11.

Mannix, E., et al. 1990. Oxygen delivery and cardiac output during exercise following oral phosphate-glucose. *Medicine & Science in Sports & Exercise* 22:341–47.

Margaritis, I., et al. 1997. Effects of endurance training on skeletal muscle oxidative capacities with and without selenium supplementation. *Journal of Trace Elements in Medicine and Biology* 11:37–43.

Martin, B., et al. 2007. Exercise and calcium supplementation: Effects on calcium homeostasis in sportswomen. *Medicine & Science in Sports & Exercise* 39:1481–86.

Matter, M., et al. 1987. The effect of iron and folate therapy on maximal exercise performance in female marathon runners with iron and folate deficiency. *Clinical Science* 72:415–22.

Mettler, S., and Zimmermann, M. 2010. Iron excess in recreational marathon runners. *European Journal of Clinical Nutrition* 64:490–4.

Michaelsson, K., et al. 2007. Leisure physical activity and the risk of fracture in men. *PLoS Medicine* 4(6): e199.

Molgaard, C., et al. 2005. Long-term calcium supplementation does not affect the iron status of 12–14-y-old girls. *American Journal of Clinical Nutrition* 82:98–102.

Montain, S., et al. 2007. Sweat mineral-element responses during 7 h of exercise-heat stress. *International Journal of Sport Nutrition and Exercise Metabolism* 17:574–82.

Newhouse, I., et al. 1993. Effects of iron supplementation and discontinuation on serum copper, zinc, calcium, and magnesium levels in women. *Medicine & Science in Sports & Exercise* 25:562–71.

Nuviala, R., et al. 1999. Magnesium, zinc, and copper status in women involved in different sports. *International Journal of Sport Nutrition* 9:295–309.

Ormerod, S., et al. 1990. The relationship between weekly mileage and bone density in male runners. *Medicine & Science in Sports & Exercise* 22:562.

Peeling, P., et al. 2007. Effect of iron injections on aerobic-exercise performance of iron-depleted female athletes. *International Journal of Sport Nutrition and Exercise Metabolism* 17:221–31.

Powell, P., and Tucker, A. 1991. Iron supplementation and running performance in female cross-country runners. *International Journal of Sports Medicine* 12:462–67.

Rainey, C., et al. 1999. Daily boron intake from the American Diet. *Journal of the American Dietetic Association* 99: 335–40.

Rajaram, S., et al. 1995. Effects of long-term moderate exercise on iron status in young women. *Medicine & Science in Sports & Exercise* 27:1105–10.

Ravdin, P., et al. 2007. The decrease in breast-cancer incidence in 2003 in the United States. *New England Journal of Medicine* 356:1670–74.

Robach, P., et al. 2006. Living high-training low: Effect on erythropoiesis and maximal aerobic performance in elite Nordic skiers. *European Journal of Applied Physiology* 97:695–705.

Rowland, T., et al. 1988. The effect of iron therapy on the exercise capacity of non-anemic iron-deficient adolescent runners. *American Journal of Diseases in Children* 142:165–69.

Rubenowitz, E., et al. 1996. Magnesium in drinking water and death from acute myocardial infarction. *American Journal of Epidemiology* 143:456–62.

Schmid, A., et al. 1996. Effect of physical exercise and vitamin C on absorption of ferric sodium citrate. *Medicine & Science in Sports & Exercise* 28:1470–73.

Schumacher, Y., et al. 2002. Hematological indices and iron status in athletes of various sports and performances. *Medicine & Science in Sports & Exercise* 34: 869–75.

Shahar, D., et al. 2010. Dairy calcium intake, serum vitamin D, and successful weight loss. *American Journal of Clinical Nutrition* 92:1017–22.

Smathers, A., et al. 2009. Bone density comparisons in male competitive road cyclists and untrained controls. *Medicine and Science in Sports and Exercise* 41:290–6.

Snyder, A., et al. 1989. Influence of dietary iron source on measures of iron status among female runners. *Medicine & Science in Sports & Exercise* 21:7–10.

Stewart, I., et al. 1990. Phosphate loading and the effects on VO_2 max in trained cyclists. *Research Quarterly for Exercise and Sport* 61:80–84.

Telford, R., et al. 1993. Iron status and diet in athletes. *Medicine & Science in Sports & Exercise* 25:796–800.

Terblanche, S., et al. 1992. Failure of magnesium supplementation to influence marathon running performance or recovery in magnesium-replete subjects. *International Journal of Sport Nutrition* 2:154–64.

Tessier, F., et al. 1995. Selenium and training effects on the glutathione system and aerobic performance. *Medicine & Science in Sports & Exercise* 27:390–96.

Thompson, W., et al. 2005. Effect of energy-restricted diets high in dairy products and fiber on weight loss in obese adults. *Obesity Research* 13:1344–53.

Thys-Jacobs, S., et al. 1998. Calcium carbonate and the premenstrual syndrome. *American Journal of Obstetrics and Gynecology* 179:444–52.

Trent, L., and Thieding-Cancel, D. 1995. Effects of chromium picolinate on body composition. *Journal of Sports Medicine and Physical Fitness* 35:273–80.

Van Loan, M., et al. 1999. The effects of zinc depletion on peak force and total work of knee and shoulder extensor and flexor muscles. *International Journal of Sport Nutrition* 9:125–35.

Volpe, S., et al. 2001. Effect of chromium supplementation and exercise on body composition, resting metabolic rate and selected biochemical parameters in moderately obese women following an exercise program. *Journal of the American College of Nutrition* 20:293–306.

Wactawski-Wende, J., et al. 2006. Calcium plus vitamin D supplementation and the risk of colorectal cancer. *New England Journal of Medicine* 354:684–96.

Walker, L., et al. 1998. Chromium picolinate effects on body composition and muscular performance in wrestlers. *Medicine & Science in Sports & Exercise* 30:1730–37.

Waller, M., and Haymes, E. 1996. The effects of heat and exercise on sweat iron loss. *Medicine & Science in Sports & Exercise* 28:197–203.

Ward, K., et al. 2007. Calcium supplementation and weight bearing physical activity: Do they have a combined effect on the bone density of pre-pubertal children? *Bone* 41:496–504.

Webster, B., and Barr, S. 1995. Calcium intake of adolescent female gymnasts and speed skaters: Lack of association with dieting behavior. *International Journal of Sport Nutrition* 5:2–12.

Wehrlin, J., et al. 2006. Live high-train low for 24 days increases hemoglobin and red cell volume in elite endurance athletes. *Journal of Applied Physiology* 100:1938–45.

Weight, L., et al. 1992. Dietary iron deficiency and sports anaemia. *British Journal of Nutrition* 68:253–60.

Weller, E., et al. 1998. Lack of effect of oral Mg-supplementation on Mg in serum, blood cells, and calf muscle. *Medicine & Science in Sports & Exercise* 30: 1584–91.

White, K., et al. 2006. The acute effects of dietary calcium intake on fat metabolism during exercise and endurance exercise performance. *International Journal of Sport Nutrition and Exercise Metabolism* 16:565–79.

Wilson, A., and Ball, M. 1999. Nutrient intake and iron status of Australian male vegetarians. *European Journal of Clinical Nutrition* 53:189–94.

Zanker, C., and Swaine, I. 2000. Responses of bone turnover markers to repeated endurance running in humans under conditions of energy balance or energy restriction. *European Journal of Applied Physiology* 83:434–40.

Zemel, M. 2005. Dairy augmentation of total and central fat loss in obese subjects. *International Journal of Obesity and Related Metabolic Disorders* 29:391–97.

Zemel, M., et al. 2005. Effects of calcium and dairy on body composition and weight loss in African-American adults. *Obesity Research* 13:1218–25.

Ziegler, P., et al. 2002. Nutritional status of teenage female competitive figure skaters. *Journal of the American Dietetic Association* 102:374–79.

Zotter, H., et al. 2004. Abnormally high serum ferritin levels among professional road cyclists. *British Journal of Sports Medicine* 38:704–8.

Water, Electrolytes, and Temperature Regulation

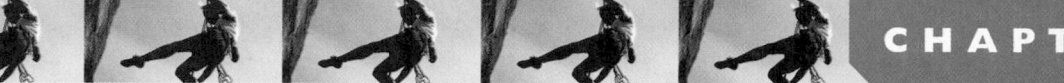

CHAPTER NINE

LEARNING OBJECTIVES

After studying this chapter, you should be able to:

1. Identify the principal water compartments in the body, describe the general function of each, and explain how your body maintains overall water balance.

2. Identify foods that are high or low in sodium and potassium, and explain the physiological responses of your body to restore normal serum sodium levels following a high salt intake.

3. List the four components of environmental heat stress recorded by the wet-bulb globe temperature (WBGT), and explain how each may affect the heat balance equation during exercise under hot, humid environmental conditions.

4. Describe how exercise in the heat may impair endurance performance as compared to exercise in a cooler environment, and explain the physiological responses your body would make to promote heat loss.

5. Outline the key guidelines for consuming water, electrolytes, and carbohydrate before, during, and after exercise under warm or hot environmental conditions, and offer general recommendations to athletes participating in such events.

6. Describe the theory underlying the use of glycerol as an ergogenic aid, and understand the current research findings regarding its efficacy in enhancing exercise performance.

7. Learn various strategies to reduce the risk of heat illness while exercising in a hot environment, but also be able to identify the various heat illnesses along with their causes, clinical findings, and appropriate treatment.

8. Understand the meaning of high blood pressure and associated health risks, and describe the role that diet and exercise may play in its prevention and treatment.

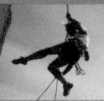

Water is a clear, tasteless, odorless fluid. It is a rather simple compound composed of two parts hydrogen and one part oxygen (H_2O). Of all the nutrients essential in the chemistry and functioning of living forms, it is the most important. Although humans may survive about seven days without water under optimal conditions, rapid losses of body water through dehydration may prove fatal in a relatively short time, even within hours when young children with diarrhea lose large amounts of water and electrolytes.

Water provides no food energy, but most of the other nutrients essential to life can be used by the human body only because of their reaction with water. Water constitutes most of the body weight and provides the medium within which the other nutrients may function. Water has a number of diverse functions in human metabolism; one of the most important, particularly for the athletic individual, is the regulation of body temperature. In a review of food and drink in sport, Macdonald noted that fluid is still the priority constituent that one needs to monitor.

When the body loses fluids by any route, it loses not only water but electrolytes as well. Electrolytes, particularly those discussed in this chapter (sodium, chloride, and potassium), are involved in numerous physiological functions, such as muscle contraction. Sodium is particularly involved in fluid balance, a major determinant of blood pressure. An abnormal electrolyte status may adversely affect both health and physical performance.

Proper fluid replacement is important for both health and sport. To help decrease mortality from diarrhea, a major health problem associated with cholera in undeveloped countries, medical scientists developed oral rehydration therapy (ORT) solutions to help replace lost fluids rapidly. Today, the standard ORT solution contains sodium chloride, potassium chloride, trisodium citrate, glucose, and water, and its application has effectively decreased mortality during epidemics of cholera. In the 1950s and 1960s, heat illnesses were widespread among military personnel and athletes, primarily because of regulations that restricted fluid intake. Research by sports medicine scientists during this time helped to identify risk factors associated with exercise under warm or hot environmental conditions, and with application of appropriate guidelines, the incidence of heat injuries declined. During these studies, scientists also noted that endurance-exercise performance declined with excessive exercise-induced sweating and fluid loss, and research into sport ORT as a means of helping delay fatigue due to fluid losses increased dramatically, leading to our sports drinks of today.

Of the factors that may influence physical performance on any given day, one of the major concerns is the environmental temperature. Anyone who is physically active for prolonged periods is probably aware of the effect that temperature changes have on performance ability. In particular, as the temperature increases, the combination of the environmental heat and the increased body heat from exercise metabolism may disturb body-water supplies, electrolyte status, and temperature regulation, which at the least may prove detrimental to endurance capacity and at the extreme may have fatal consequences.

Given the seriousness of this topic, the primary focus of this chapter will be upon those problems that may confront you when exercising in the heat and how you may prevent or correct them. Topics covered include the role of water and selected electrolytes in human metabolism, the regulation of body temperature, the effect of fluid and electrolyte losses upon performance, methods of fluid and electrolyte replacement, ergogenic aids, and health-related problems such as heat illnesses and high blood pressure (hypertension).

Water

How much water do you need per day?

Manz and others note that water is recognized as the most essential nutrient, and an AI for total water from beverages and food has been established. The requirement for body water depends on the body weight of the individual. The requirement varies in different stages of the life cycle. Under normal environmental temperatures and activity levels, the AI for adult males and females age 19 and over is, respectively, 3.7 and 2.7 liters (3.9 and 2.9 quarts). Somewhat lesser AI have been established for teenagers and children. Water requirements may be increased substantially during exercise, particularly under warm environmental conditions, and will be discussed later in this chapter. All in all, how much water one needs daily involves a number of factors and thus is highly individualized. Heinz Valtin, an expert on body water balance, in general noted that thirst is a good guide to help maintain normal body water balance.

Body water balance is maintained when the output of body fluids is matched by the input of water. A small amount of water is lost in the feces and through the exhaled air in breathing. **Insensible perspiration** on the skin, which is not visible, is almost pure water and accounts for about 30 percent of body-water losses. Perspiration, or sweat, losses may be increased considerably during exercise and/or hot environmental conditions. Urinary output is the main avenue for water loss. It may increase somewhat through the use of diuretics, including alcohol and caffeine. Stookey indicates that we lose about 1 milliliter of water for every milligram of caffeine, and 10 milliliters for every gram of alcohol. Also, use of a high-protein diet produces urea, which has to be excreted by the kidneys and may increase urine output.

Fluid intake of beverages, such as water, soda, milk, juice, coffee, and tea, provides about 80 percent of total water needed to replenish losses. Valtin notes that we obtain significant amounts of fluid from caffeinated and alcoholic beverages, such as coffee and beer. Although both beverages contain diuretics, the Consumers Union noted that if you are used to drinking caffeinated or alcoholic beverages, the diuretic effect of each may be offset by the amount of fluid in the beverage and you probably gain more fluid from beverages, such as colas, coffee and beer, than you lose. About 20 percent of our daily total water intake comes from the foods we eat. Solid foods also contribute as a water source, and in two different ways. First, food contains water in varying amounts; certain foods such as lettuce, celery, melons, and most fruits contain about 80–90 percent water; meats and seafood contain about 60–70 percent water; even bread, an apparently dry food, contains 36 percent water. Second, the metabolism of foods for energy also produces water. Fat, carbohydrate, and protein all produce water when broken down for energy. You may recall the reaction when glucose is metabolized to produce energy, with one of the by-products being **metabolic water:**

$$C_6H_{12}O_6 + 6O_2 \rightarrow Energy + 6CO_2 + 6H_2O$$

Figure 9.1 summarizes the daily water loss and intake for the maintenance of water balance for an adult female. Amounts would be greater for an adult male. As shall be seen later, however, these amounts may change drastically under certain conditions.

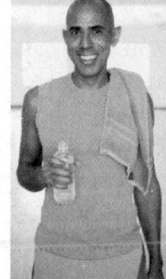

What else is in the water we drink?

In general, the tap water we drink daily is safe. However, it should be noted that most of the water we drink contains more than just water, including substances added from natural geological formations, discharge or runoff from industry or farming, water processing, and pipes in our homes. In some areas, water may contain substantial amounts of various minerals, including calcium, sodium, magnesium, iron, zinc, arsenic, and lead. Some minerals, like excess sodium, arsenic, and lead, may lead to various health problems, whereas others, such as calcium and magnesium, may be beneficial. Other substances find their way into our water supply as well. Lefferts reported that more than 700 contaminants have been found in public drinking water, including organic chemicals like pesticides. Under the Safe Drinking Water Act, the Environmental Protection Agency (EPA) has set maximum contaminant levels for the most harmful substances, and most, but not all, municipal water treatment facilities conform to these standards. The Consumers Union notes that, in general, most community water systems meet federal health-based standards, but also notes that some contaminants found in water systems may not be appropriate for vulnerable populations, such as pregnant women, infants, and the elderly.

If you are concerned about your tap water, know that some health professionals suggest a water filter as the best alternative. Water filters added to your tap may help remove unwanted substances, such as chlorine or chlorinated by-products; some water filters are designed to eliminate lead and mercury, and others can even trap parasites. Many types of water filters are on the market, so, if interested, have your water analyzed and then seek an appropriate filter to help purify your tap water. To get information on the quality of your water supply, you may contact your local water utility and ask for the latest water quality or Consumer Confidence Report, or contact the EPA Website.

water.epa.gov/drink/index.cfm **The Environmental Protection** Agency provides information on the quality of your water supply. Click on *Local Drinking Water Information.*

Bottled water is the current rage. Not only do we have artesian, spring, or purified water, we also have vitamin water, herbal water, nutraceutical water, oxygen water, and fitness water, to name a few of the specialty beverages available. The Food and Drug Administration (FDA) has set guidelines for defining bottled waters. Artesian water is drawn from a well that taps a confined aquifer; mineral water comes from a protected underground source and must contain minerals distinguishing it from other waters; spring water flows naturally from an underground source; purified water is produced by distillation or some comparable process. Bottled waters must conform to the same safety standards as municipal water supplies. About 85 percent of bottled-water manufacturers belong to the International Bottled Water Association (IBWA), which sets even tougher standards for its members than the FDA. Individuals who drink bottled water should be aware that approximately 25 percent is simply tap water that has undergone a purification process. The nation's two best-selling bottled waters, Aquafina and Dasani, are purified municipal water. Also, surveys have shown that most bottled waters do not contain fluoride. For example, Lalumandier and Ayers reported that only 5 percent of 57 samples of bottled water contained fluoride within the recommended range. Check bottled water labels for mineral content. The FDA is also seeking legislation requiring that bottled water manufacturers list contaminant levels on bottle labels.

Bottled water isn't cheap. One *gourmet* bottled water, Bling, is marketed at $40 or more per bottle. Other specialty waters are less expensive, but a bottle of vitamin water may cost well over a dollar, whereas a glass of water with an inexpensive

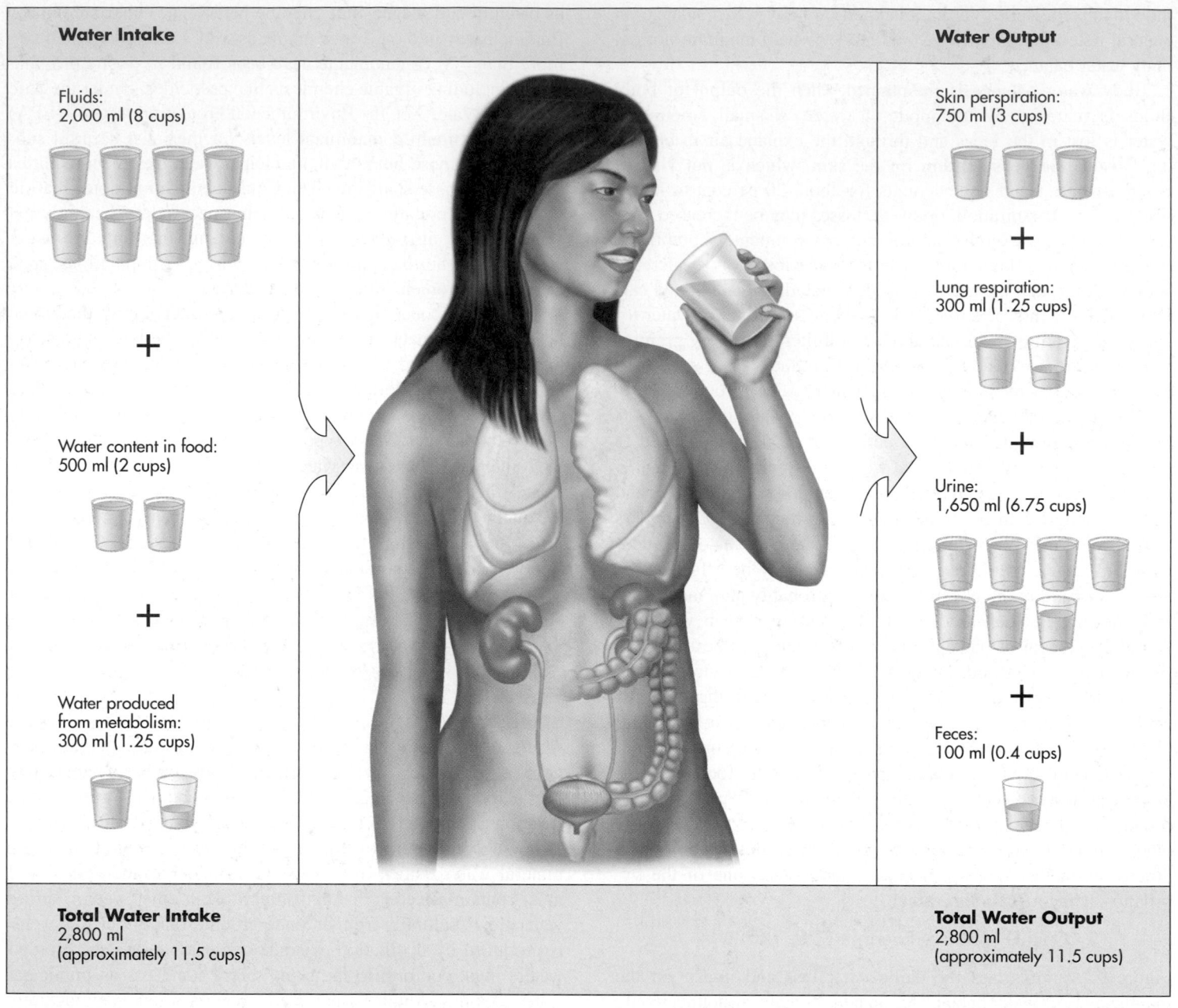

Water Intake

Fluids:
2,000 ml (8 cups)

+

Water content in food:
500 ml (2 cups)

+

Water produced
from metabolism:
300 ml (1.25 cups)

Water Output

Skin perspiration:
750 ml (3 cups)

+

Lung respiration:
300 ml (1.25 cups)

+

Urine:
1,650 ml (6.75 cups)

+

Feces:
100 ml (0.4 cups)

Total Water Intake
2,800 ml
(approximately 11.5 cups)

Total Water Output
2,800 ml
(approximately 11.5 cups)

FIGURE 9.1 Estimate of water balance—intake versus output—in a woman. We primarily maintain our volume of body fluids by adjusting water output to intake. As you can see, most water comes from the liquids we consume. Some comes from the moisture in more solid foods, and the remainder is manufactured during metabolism. Water output includes losses from the lungs, urine, skin, and feces.

multivitamin/mineral tablet will provide the same benefits but cost ten times less. The Consumers Union indicates that you do not need any of the specialty waters to replenish fluids, but if their taste encourages you to drink more, they may be worthwhile, especially if you normally do not drink adequate fluids.

Where is water stored in the body?

Water is stored in several body compartments but moves constantly between compartments. About 60–65 percent of body water is stored inside body cells as **intracellular water.**

The remaining 35–40 percent is outside the cells and is termed **extracellular water.** The extracellular water is further subdivided into the **intercellular** (interstitial) **water** between or surrounding the cells, the **intravascular water** within the blood vessels, and miscellaneous water compartments such as the cerebrospinal fluid. Figure 9.2 represents the distribution of water in the body.

Water is held in the body in conjunction with protein, carbohydrate, and electrolytes. The protein content in the muscles, blood, and other tissues helps bind water to those tissues. As discussed in chapter 4, muscle glycogen has considerable amounts of water bound to it (about 3 grams of water per gram of

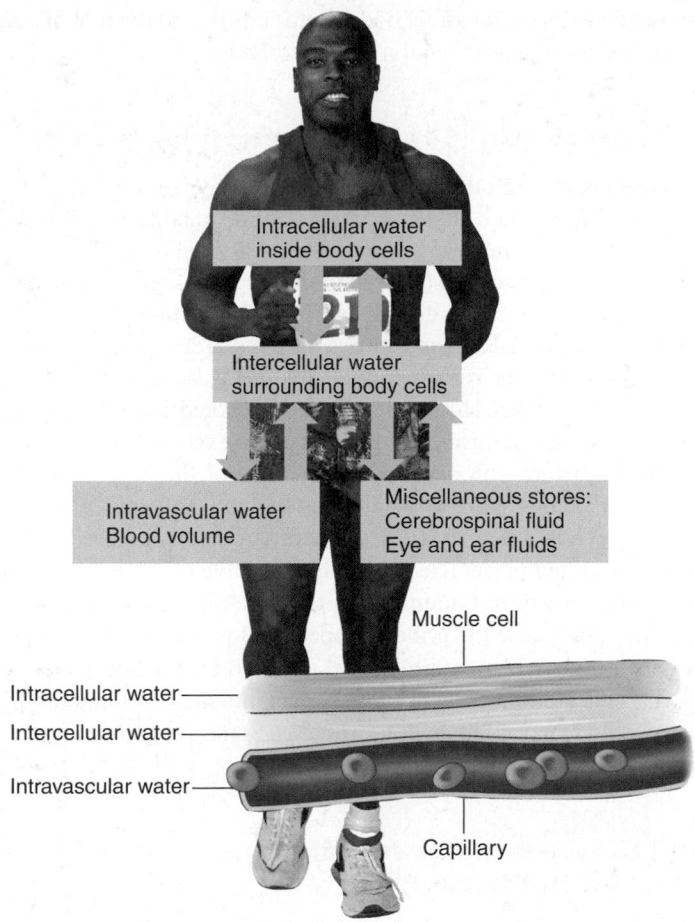

FIGURE 9.2 Body-water compartments. There is a constant interchange among the different body-water compartments. The water inside the body cells, the intracellular water, is important for cell functions. The other three compartments (intercellular, intravascular, and miscellaneous) are known collectively as the extracellular water. The intracellular water constitutes about 60–65 percent of the total body water, while the extracellular water constitutes the remaining 35–40 percent. In the blood, some of the water is intracellular in the blood cells, while the remainder is extracellular in the plasma. Decreases in blood volume (intravascular water) may adversely affect endurance capacity.

glycogen), which may prove to be an advantage when exercising in the heat. In essence, the metabolism of 350 grams of carbohydrate during exercise will provide nearly 1 liter of water for body functions, as documented by Rogers and others. The sodium in the extracellular fluid, including sodium in the circulatory system, attracts water.

Proper water and electrolyte balance within these compartments is of extreme importance to the athletic individual. Fluid shifts such as decreases in blood volume and cellular dehydration, both of which may develop during exercise in the heat, could contribute to the onset of fatigue or heat illness.

Water constitutes about 60 percent of the body weight in the average adult male and 50 percent in the adult female, but this percentage may be as low as 40 percent in obese individuals and as high as 70 percent or more in muscular individuals. The reason is that fat tissue is low in water content and muscle tissue is high in water content.

How is body water regulated?

Johnson notes that maintaining body water and sodium balance is so critical to health that the central nervous system has developed specific neural patterns fostering an appetite for both water and salt. Body water is maintained at a normal level through kidney function. Normal body-water level is called **normohydration,** or **euhydration. Dehydration,** the loss of body water, results in a state of **hypohydration,** or low body-water level. **Hyperhydration** represents a condition in which the body retains excess body fluids. Normal kidneys function very effectively to eliminate excess water during hyperhydration and conserve water during hypohydration.

Because water is so essential to life, it is indeed fortunate that the body possesses an efficient mechanism to maintain proper water balance. **Homeostasis** is the term used to describe the maintenance of a normal internal environment so that the body has the proper distribution and use of water, electrolytes, hormones, and other substances essential for life processes. Homeostatic mechanisms are extremely complex, and a full discussion is beyond the scope of this book. However, in essence, all homeostatic mechanisms work by a series of feedback devices. If these feedback devices are functioning properly, the body usually has no problem in maintaining the normal physical and chemical composition of its fluid compartments.

The main feedback device for the control of body water is the osmolality of the various body fluids. **Osmolality** refers to the amount, or concentration, of dissolved substances, known as *solute,* in a solution. In the body, a number of different substances affect osmolality, including glucose, protein, and several electrolytes, most notably sodium. These substances are dissolved in the body water. One mole of a nonionic substance, such as glucose, dissolved in a liter of water is one osmole. One millimole (1/1,000 mole) is one milliosmole. However, a mole of a substance that can dissociate into two ions, such as sodium chloride, is equivalent to two osmoles. One millimole of sodium chloride would be two milliosmoles (mOsm).

A term often used in conjunction with osmolality is **tonicity,** which means tension or pressure. When two solutions have the same osmotic pressure they are said to be *isosmotic* or, more commonly, *isotonic.* Iso means "same." When two solutions with different solute concentrations are compared, the one with the higher osmotic pressure is called hypertonic and the other is hypotonic.

When two solutions with different solute concentrations are separated by a permeable membrane, as in the human body between the fluid compartments, a potential pressure difference may develop between the solutions that will allow for water movement. This pressure is known as *osmotic pressure.* Water moves through cell membrane proteins, known as aquaporin water channels, from the hypotonic solution (low solute concentration and high water content) to the hypertonic solution (high solute concentration and low water content). In essence, high solute concentrations create high osmotic pressures and tend to draw water into their compartments. Figure 9.3 depicts this mechanism between the blood and the body cells.

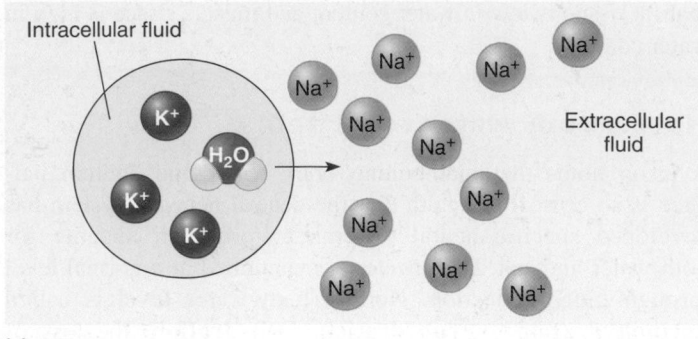

(a)

(b)

FIGURE 9.3 Osmosis and tonicity. *(a)* When the extracellular fluid contains more electrolytes or other osmotic substances, it is hypertonic to the intracellular fluid. In this case, water will flow from the interior of the cell to the outside, or to an area of greater osmotic pressure. *(b)* When the intracellular fluid contains more electrolytes or greater osmotic pressure, water will flow into the cell from the extracellular fluid.

To briefly illustrate the feedback mechanism for control of body water, let us look at what happens when you become dehydrated owing to excessive body-water losses or lowered water intake. The blood then becomes more concentrated, or hypertonic. Because maintenance of a normal blood volume is of prime importance, the blood tends to draw water from the body cells. Certain cells in the hypothalamus, called *osmoreceptors,* are sensitive to changes in osmotic pressure. These cells react to the more concentrated body fluids by stimulating the release of a hormone from the pituitary gland, the so-called master gland of the body. This hormone is called the **antidiuretic hormone (ADH),** also known as vasopressin. The ADH travels by the blood to the kidneys and directs them to reabsorb more water. Hence, urinary output of water is diminished considerably. Figure 9.4 illustrates this feedback process that helps conserve body water and blood volume. During hyperhydration, which would produce a hypotonic condition in the body fluids, a reverse process would occur leading to increased water excretion.

Because maintenance of euhydration is critical for health and physical performance, it is important to note that ADH is only one of several hormones that help to regulate body-water balance. Other hormones are involved in the maintenance of sodium and potassium, which also affect body-water levels, and the role of one is discussed in the next section on electrolytes.

How do I know if I am adequately hydrated?

Osmoreceptors and other mechanisms also may stimulate the sensation of thirst, which is usually a good guide to body-water needs and is effective in restoring body water to normal on a day-to-day basis. Some sport scientists contend that thirst may also be a good guide to hydration status during exercise. For example, Fudge and others studied elite Kenyan runners during a 5-day training period and found that they remained well hydrated day-to-day with *ad libitum* fluid intake. However, as shall be noted later, it may be advisable to start consuming fluids during exercise under warm conditions before you become thirsty. One of the best guides to indicate a state of normohydration is the color of your urine. In general, it should be a clear, pale yellow. A deeply colored urine, usually excreted in small amounts, is indicative of a state of hypohydration. However, vitamin supplements containing riboflavin (B$_2$) may also cause the urine to appear yellow and suggest a state of dehydration when the individual is euhydrated. Cheuvront and Sawka indicate that change in body weight is also a reliable and easy method to evaluate hydration status. Some guidelines are presented later in this chapter.

What are the major functions of water in the body?

Water is essential if the other nutrients are to function properly within the human body; it is the solvent for life. It has a number of diverse functions that may be summarized as follows:

1. Water provides the essential building material for cell protoplasm, the fundamental component of all living matter.
2. Because water cannot be compressed, it serves to protect key body tissues such as the spinal cord and brain.
3. Water is essential in the control of the osmotic pressure in the body, or the maintenance of a proper balance between water and the electrolytes. Any major changes in the electrolyte concentration may adversely affect cellular function. A serious departure from normal osmotic pressure cannot be tolerated by the body for long.
4. Water is the main constituent of blood, the major transportation mechanism in the body for conveying oxygen, nutrients, hormones, and other compounds to the cells for their use, and for carrying waste products of metabolism away from the cells to organs such as the lungs and kidneys for excretion from the body.
5. Water is essential for the proper functioning of our senses. Hearing waves are transmitted by fluid in the inner ear. Fluid in the eye is involved in the reflection of light for proper vision. For the taste and smelling senses to function, the foods and odors must be dissolved in water.
6. Of primary importance to the active individual is the role that water plays in the regulation of body temperature. Water is the major constituent of sweat, and through its evaporation

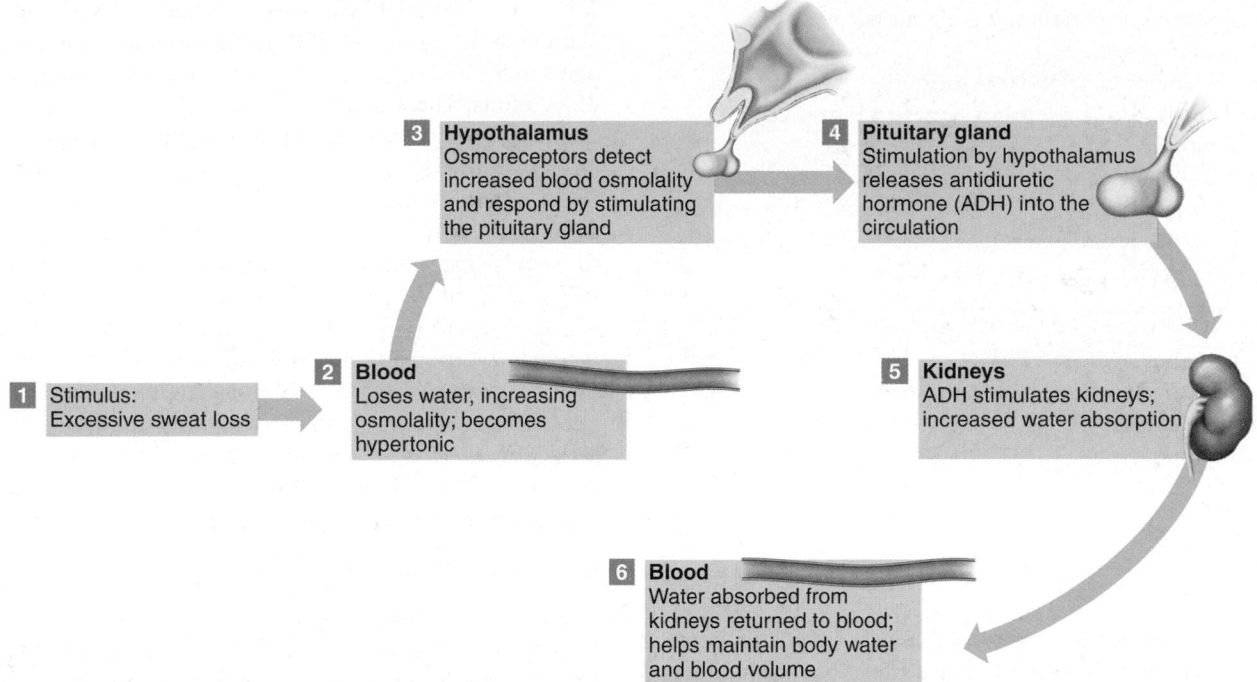

FIGURE 9.4 One feedback mechanism for homeostatic control of body water and blood volume. Other feedback mechanisms operate concurrently. For example, the hypothalamus also stimulates the thirst response to increase fluid intake.

from the surface of the skin, it can help dissipate excess body heat. Of all the nutrients, water is the most important to the physically active person and is one of several that may have beneficial effects on performance when used in supplemental amounts before or during exercise. Hence, the athletic individual should know what is necessary to help maintain proper fluid balance, a topic covered in detail later in this chapter.

Can drinking more water or fluids confer any health benefits?

Although the major functions of water have been long known, nutrition scientists now theorize that drinking enough water may have specific health benefits. For example, Michaud and others found that men who consumed the most water had a decreased risk of bladder cancer, while the Consumers Union indicated a similar relationship between water intake and colon cancer. Theoretically, increased water intake could flush carcinogens from the bladder and colon. Some dietitians indicated that increased water intake may help one reduce excess fat in a body-weight control program by increasing the sensation of fullness and suppressing hunger. Research suggests that this may be the case: de Castro reported that subjects consumed fewer Calories, at least on a short-term basis, when eating foods with high water content; as discussed in chapter 11, high-volume, low-energy foods may be an integral part of a weight control diet. Other benefits might include less chance of kidney stones, fewer asthma attacks, and better oral health, all of which are attributed to better hydration. Although you can consume water in a variety of beverages, such as juices, soda, or coffee, scientists recommend water itself. It is cheap and Calorie free.

However, most of us do obtain our daily water needs from beverages other than water. Some beverages, such as pure fruit juices, may provide some health benefits associated with their vitamin, mineral, and phytonutrients content. Other beverages have been suggested to pose health threats, such as alcoholic beverages, which are discussed in chapter 13. Popkin and other health professionals formed a Beverage Guidance Panel to provide guidance to consumers on the relative health and nutritional benefits and risks of various beverage categories. In essence, the major concern was the increased incidence of overweight and obesity in the United States, which some studies suggested could be associated with excess consumption of high-Calorie beverages. In general, the panel recommends that the consumption of beverages with no or few Calories should take precedence over the consumption of beverages with more calories, and concluded that drinking water was ranked as the preferred beverage to fulfill daily water needs. As this issue deals with weight control, additional information will be presented in the next two chapters.

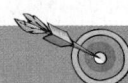

Key Concepts

▶ The average adult, who needs 2 to 3 quarts of water per day, maintains fluid balance primarily by drinking liquids, but substantial amounts of water are also obtained from solid foods in the diet. Caffeine is not as potent a diuretic as once thought, and beverages containing caffeine, such as coffee and cola sodas, may augment daily fluid intake.

▶ Normal water levels in the various body fluid compartments are maintained by a feedback mechanism involving specific receptors for osmotic pressure, the antidiuretic hormone (ADH), and the kidneys.

▶ Water has a number of functions in the body. One of its most important benefits for people who exercise is the control of body temperature.

▶ Plain water is an effective and inexpensive means to help maintain fluid balance in the body. Some beverages, such as pure fruit juices, may provide healthful nutrients, whereas others, such as alcoholic beverages, may pose a health risk.

Check for Yourself

▶ Use a measuring cup and accurately measure the amount of fluids you drink for a day.

Electrolytes

What is an electrolyte?

An **electrolyte** is defined as a substance which, in solution, conducts an electric current. The solution itself may be referred to as an electrolyte solution. Acids, bases, and salts are common electrolytes, and they usually dissociate into ions, particles carrying either a positive (cation) or a negative (anion) electric charge. The major electrolytes in the body fluids are sodium, potassium, chloride, bicarbonate, sulfate, magnesium, and calcium. Electrolytes can act at the cell membrane and generate electrical current, such as in a nerve impulse. Electrolytes can also function in other ways, activating enzymes to control a variety of metabolic activities in the cell. In chapter 8 we covered some of the important metabolic functions of calcium, phosphorus, and magnesium; in this chapter the focus is on sodium, chloride, and potassium because of their presence in sports drinks, popular beverages used to replace fluid losses in physically active people.

The concentration of all elements in the body may be expressed in a variety of ways, such as milligrams per unit volume, millimoles, and milliequivalents. The equivalencies for sodium, chloride, and potassium will be provided, as you may often see these various terms in the literature.

In later sections we shall look at the interaction of these electrolytes with exercise in warm environmental conditions and their role in the etiology of high blood pressure. But first, let us briefly cover the function of each of these electrolytes in the human body.

Sodium (Na)

Sodium is a mineral element also known as natrium, from which the symbol *Na* is derived. It is one of the principal positive ions, or electrolytes, in the body fluids. The gram atomic weight of sodium is 23 grams, so the milligram atomic weight for sodium is 23 milligrams. One millimole of sodium is 23 milligrams, as is one milliequivalent. One millimole of sodium chloride (salt) is 58.5 milligrams, as is one milliequivalent, containing 23 milligrams of sodium and 35.5 milligrams of chloride.

DRI The National Academy of Sciences (NAS) set an AI for sodium at 1.5 grams (1,500 milligrams) for males and females age 9 to 50, and somewhat lower amounts for young children and older adults. There is no evidence that higher intakes confer any additional health benefits. However, this AI contains no allowance for large sodium losses through exercise-induced sweating. Common table salt (sodium chloride) is about 40 percent sodium, so only about 3.8 grams (3,800 milligrams) is needed to supply the minimum requirement. The NAS also established a UL at 2.3 grams, or the equivalent of about 5.8 grams of salt. Currently, the amount used as the Daily Value for food labels is 2.4 grams (2,400 milligrams), which is higher than the UL. Keep this in mind when purchasing foods if you are attempting to limit sodium intake. According to the *Dietary Guidelines for Americans 2010*, the average intake of sodium for all Americans age 2 years and older is 3,400 milligrams daily, or more than twice the recommended amount.

Food Sources Sodium is distributed widely in nature but is found in rather small amounts in most natural foods. However, significant amounts of salt, and hence sodium, are usually added from the salt shaker for flavor. One teaspoon of salt contains about 2,000 milligrams of sodium. Moreover, processing techniques add significant amounts of salt to the foods we buy. For example, a serving of fresh or frozen green peas contains only 2 milligrams of sodium, but increases to 240 milligrams in the canning process. In general, natural foods are low in sodium, whereas processed foods are relatively high.

The Center for Science in the Public Interest has indicated that the FDA is investigating means to lower sodium content in food, and some companies are being proactive and decreasing sodium content. For example, canned soups may contain more than 1,300 milligrams of sodium per serving, but some brands are available that contain much less, only 40–60 milligrams of sodium per serving. Nevertheless, most Americans obtain about 75–80 percent of their sodium intake from processed and restaurant foods. Table 9.1 highlights the sodium content in several foods within the major food groups and some restaurant fast foods. Note the difference in sodium content between fresh and processed foods. Checking food labels is the best means to control sodium intake. Food labels must list the sodium content, both in milligrams and in percent of the Daily Value, and may carry claims such as "sodium free" if the product meets certain restrictions (see table 9.2).

Cooking your own food can help reduce salt intake. With some canned vegetables, draining and rinsing the product with fresh water removes some of the sodium. Herbs and other spices can add flavor and be used to replace salt added to home-prepared meals. Salt substitutes are available, such as Morton Salt Substitute which is 100 percent sodium-free, containing only potassium. Light salts are also available, such as Morton's Lite Salt, that contain less than 50 percent sodium.

Major Functions Sodium is an important element in a number of body functions. As the principal electrolyte in the extracellular fluids, it serves primarily to help maintain normal body-fluid balance and osmotic pressure. In this regard it is essential in the control of normal blood pressure through its effect on

TABLE 9.1   Sodium content of common foods

Food exchange item	Amount	Sodium (mg)
Milk		
Low-fat milk	1 c	120
Cottage cheese		
Creamed	1/2 c	320
Unsalted	1/2 c	30
Cheese, American	1 oz	445
Vegetables		
Beans, cooked fresh	1 oz	5
Beans, canned	1 oz	150
Pickles, dill	1 medium	900
Potato, baked	1 medium	6
Fruits		
Banana	1 medium	1
Orange	1 medium	1
Starch		
Bread, whole wheat	1 slice	130
Bran flakes	3/4 c	340
Oatmeal, cooked	1 c	175
Pretzels	1 oz	890
Meat		
Luncheon meats	1 oz	450
Chicken	3 oz	40
Beef, steak	3 oz	70
Tuna, low sodium	3 oz	35
Tuna, in oil	3 oz	800
Fats		
Butter, salted	1 tsp	50
Margarine, salted	1 tsp	50
Canned foods and prepared entrees		
Spaghetti, canned	1 c	1,220
Turkey dinner, frozen	1	1,735
Chicken noodle soup	5 oz	655
Chicken noodle soup, low sodium	5 oz	120
Restaurant fast foods		
Arby's chicken breast fillet sandwich	1	1,220
McDonald's Big Mac	1	1,010
Subway club (6 inches)	1	1,310
Taco Bell bean burrito	1	1,220
Condiments		
Mustard	1 tbsp	195
Tomato catsup	1 tbsp	155
Soy sauce	1 tbsp	1,320

As you can see in this table, the sodium content of foods can vary greatly. In general, canned and processed foods have a much higher sodium content than do fresh foods. Eat fresh meats, fruits, vegetables, and bread products whenever possible and prepare them with little or no salt. Avoid highly salted foods like pickles, pretzels, soy sauce, and others. Look for "sodium free" or "low sodium" labels when shopping for canned foods.

Source: U.S. Department of Agriculture.

TABLE 9.2   Nutrition facts label terms for sodium*

Sodium-Free or Salt-Free
  Less than 5 milligrams per serving

Very Low Sodium
  35 milligrams or less per serving

Low Sodium
  140 milligrams or less per serving

Reduced-Sodium or Less Sodium
  At least 25 percent less than the regular product

No Salt Added
  Amount of sodium per serving must be listed

*Food labels must list the milligrams of sodium and the percent of the Daily Value, which is 2,400 mg.

the blood volume. The role of sodium in the etiology of high blood pressure is discussed in a later section.

In conjunction with several other electrolytes, sodium is critical for nerve impulse transmission and muscle contraction. It is also a component of several compounds, such as sodium bicarbonate, that help maintain normal acid-base balance and, as noted in chapter 13, may be an effective ergogenic aid. An overview of sodium is presented in table 9.3.

Deficiency and Excess   Because the maintenance of normal blood pressure is critical to life, and because sodium is critical to maintenance of blood volume and pressure, Geerling and Loewy indicate that humans have developed a sodium appetite, a behavioral drive to ingest salt. The human body has also developed an effective regulatory feedback mechanism allowing for a wide range of dietary sodium intake. The hypothalamus helps regulate sodium as well as water balance in the body. If the sodium concentration decreases in the blood, a series of complex reactions leads to the secretion of **aldosterone,** a hormone produced in the adrenal gland, which stimulates the kidneys to retain more sodium. In contrast, excesses of serum sodium will lead to decreased aldosterone secretion and increased excretion of sodium by the kidneys in the urine. Other hormones, notably ADH via its effect on water absorption in the kidneys, help maintain normal sodium equilibrium in the body fluids. During exercise, particularly intense exercise, sodium concentration increases in the blood, which helps to maintain blood volume. Exercise also leads to increased secretion of ADH and aldosterone, which helps conserve body water and sodium supplies.

Because this regulatory mechanism is so effective, deficiency states due to inadequate dietary intake of sodium are not common. Indeed, humans even have a natural appetite for salt, assuring adequate sodium intake and sodium balance over time. Nevertheless, excessive losses of sodium from the body, usually induced by prolonged sweating while exercising in the heat, may lead to short-term deficiencies that may be debilitating to the athletic individual. These problems are discussed later in this chapter in the sections on fluid and electrolyte replacement and health aspects.

TABLE 9.3 Major electrolytes: sodium, chloride, and potassium*

Major electrolyte	Adequate intake	Major functions in the body	Deficiency symptoms	Symptoms of excess consumption
Sodium	1,500 milligrams	Primary positive ion in extracellular fluid; nerve impulse conduction; muscle contraction; acid-base balance; blood volume homeostasis	Hyponatremia; muscle cramps; nausea; vomiting; loss of appetite; dizziness; seizures; shock; coma	Hypertension (high blood pressure) in susceptible individuals
Chloride	2,300 milligrams	Primary negative ion in extracellular fluid; nerve impulse conduction; hydrochloric acid formation in stomach	Rare; may be caused by excess vomiting and loss of hydrochloric acid; convulsions	Hypertension, in conjunction with excess sodium
Potassium	4,700 milligrams	Primary positive ion in intracellular fluid; same functions as sodium, but intra-cellular; glucose transport into cell	Hypokalemia; loss of appetite; muscle cramps; apathy; irregular heartbeat	Hyperkalemia; inhibited heart function

*Food sources for sodium and potassium may be found in tables 9.2 and 9.4, respectively; food sources for chloride are similar to those for sodium.

Chloride (Cl)

Chloride is the major negative ion in the extracellular fluids. The gram atomic weight of chloride is 35.5 grams, so the milligram atomic weight for chloride is 35.5 milligrams. One millimole of chloride is 35.5 milligrams, as is one milliequivalent.

DRI The chloride AI for individuals age 9–50 is 2.3 grams, or the equivalent of about 3.8 grams of salt. The UL is 3.5 grams, or 5.8 grams of salt. The DV for food label use is 3,500 milligrams, which is the UL.

Food Sources Chloride is distributed in a variety of foods. Its dietary intake is closely associated with that of sodium, notably in the form of common table salt, which is 60 percent chloride.

Major Functions Chloride ions have a variety of functions in the human body. They work with sodium in the regulation of body-water balance and electrical potentials across cell membranes. They also are involved in the formation of hydrochloric acid in the stomach, which is necessary for certain digestive processes.

Deficiency Under normal circumstances chloride deficiency is rather rare. However, because the losses of sodium and chloride in sweat are directly proportional, the symptoms of chloride loss during excessive dehydration through sweating parallel those of sodium loss. The effects of sweat electrolyte losses and replacement on physical performance and health are covered in later sections of this chapter. An overview of chloride is presented in table 9.3.

Potassium (K)

Potassium is a mineral element also known as kalium, from which the symbol K is derived. It is a positive ion. The gram atomic weight of potassium is 39 grams, so the milligram atomic weight for potassium is 39 milligrams. One millimole of potassium is 39 milligrams, as is one milliequivalent.

DRI The potassium AI for individuals age 14 and above is 4.7 grams (4,700 milligrams), and somewhat less for children. No UL has been established for potassium from foods. Supplements are not recommended. The DV used for food labels is 3.5 grams, which is less than the AI. American adults take in much less, only about 2,500 milligrams a day.

Food Sources Potassium is found in most foods and is especially abundant in bananas, citrus fruits, fresh vegetables, milk, meat, and fish. Table 9.4 provides some data on the potassium content of several common foods in the major food groups.

Major Functions As the major electrolyte inside the body cells, potassium works in close association with sodium and chloride in the maintenance of body fluids and in the generation of electrical impulses in the nerves and the muscles, including the heart muscle. Potassium also plays an important role in the energy processes in the muscle; it helps in the transport of glucose into the muscle cells, the storage of glycogen, and the production of high-energy compounds.

Deficiency and Excess Potassium balance, like sodium balance, is regulated by aldosterone but in a reverse way. A high serum potassium level stimulates the release of aldosterone from the adrenal cortex, leading to an increased excretion of potassium by the kidneys into the urine. A decrease in serum potassium levels elicits a drop in aldosterone secretion and hence a greater conservation of potassium by the kidneys. Because a potassium imbalance in the body may have serious health consequences, potassium regulation is quite precise. Deficiencies or excessive accumulation are extremely rare under normal circumstances.

Although potassium deficiencies are rare, they may occur under certain conditions such as during fasting, diarrhea, and the use of diuretics. In such cases **hypokalemia,** or low serum potassium levels, could lead to muscular weakness and even cardiac arrest due to a decreased ability to generate nerve impulses and

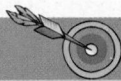

TABLE 9.4 Potassium content in some common foods in the major food exchanges

Food	Amount	Milligrams of potassium
Milk		
Skim milk	8 oz glass	410
Yogurt, low-fat	1 c	530
Cheese, cheddar	1 oz	28
Meat		
Chicken breast	1 oz	70
Beef, lean	1 oz	100
Fish, flounder	1 oz	160
Starch		
Bread, whole wheat	1 slice	65
Cereal, Cheerios	1 oz	110
Fruit		
Banana	1 medium	460
Orange	1 avg	260
Apple	1 avg	35
Vegetables		
Potato, baked	1 avg	780
Broccoli	1 stalk	270
Carrot	1 medium	275

an irregular heartbeat. Several deaths of individuals on unbalanced liquid-protein fasting diets several years ago were associated with potassium deficiencies.

Excessive body potassium stores also are not very common, occurring mainly in conjunction with several disease states or in individuals who overdose on potassium supplements. **Hyperkalemia,** or excessive potassium in the blood, may disturb electrical impulses, causing cardiac arrhythmias and possible death. Parisi and others reported a case study of a young soccer player who suffered from premature ventricular arrhythmia while consuming a supplement giving him about 5 grams (5,000 milligrams) of potassium daily. The hyperkalemia and arrhythmia resolved when he stopped using the supplements. More than 18,000 milligrams may cause a heart attack. For this reason, individuals should never take potassium supplements in large doses without the consent of a physician. An overview of potassium is presented in table 9.3.

In theory, a potassium deficiency could adversely affect physical performance capacity. However, given the potential risks associated with excess potassium supplementation, there is very little research evaluating its ergogenic effects. The role of potassium in the etiology of high blood pressure has also been studied. The results of this research are presented in later sections of this chapter.

Regulation of Body Temperature

What is the normal body temperature?

The temperature of different body parts may vary considerably. The skin may be very cold but the body internally is much warmer. When we speak of body temperature, we mean the internal, or **core temperature,** and not the external shell temperature. **Shell temperature,** which represents the temperature of the skin and the tissues directly under it, varies considerably depending upon the surrounding environmental temperature.

In humans, normal body temperature is approximately 98.6°F (37°C). This core temperature may be measured in a variety of ways. The two most common methods are orally and rectally. For research purposes, a thermocouple is inserted through the nose down into the esophagus to provide a more precise measure of core temperature. Capsules, containing miniature electronic thermometers, may be swallowed and use wireless telemetry to transmit core temperatures during rest or exercise, an excellent means to study temperature responses in athletes during actual sport competition. Normal body temperature at rest varies and may range from 97–99°F (36.1–37.2°C). At rest, the rectal temperature is normally about 0.5–1.0°F higher than the oral temperature; however, assessing temperature following a road race, one study reported that the rectal temperature was 5.5°F higher than the oral temperature, suggesting that an oral reading may not be an accurate reflection of the true body temperature in an assessment of heat injury. Shell temperatures may be measured by adhesive thermometer pads attached to the skin.

Humans can survive a range of core temperatures for a short time, but optimal physiological functioning usually occurs within a range of 97–104°F (36.1–40.0°C). A variety of factors may affect body temperature. Here we are concerned with the effect exercise has on the core temperature and how the body adjusts to help maintain heat balance.

What are the major factors that influence body temperature?

Humans are warm-blooded animals and are able to maintain a constant body temperature under varying environmental temperatures. To do this, the body must constantly make adjustments to either gain or lose heat.

Humans are heat-producing machines. The basal metabolic heat production is provided through normal burning (oxidation) of the three basic foodstuffs in the body—carbohydrate, fat, and protein. A higher basal metabolic rate, infectious diseases, shivering, and exercise are several factors that might increase heat production.

The human body also has a variety of means to lose heat. Heat loss is governed by four physical means—conduction, convection, radiation, and evaporation.

Conduction—Heat is transferred from the body by direct physical contact, as when you sit on a cold seat.
Convection—Heat is transferred by movement of air or water over the body.
Radiation—Heat energy radiates from the body into the surrounding air.
Evaporation—Heat is lost from the body when it is used to convert sweat to a vapor, known as the heat of vaporization. The lungs also help to dissipate heat through evaporation.

During rest and under normal environmental temperatures, body heat is transported from the core to the shell by way of conduction and convection, the blood being the main carrier of the heat. The vast majority of the heat escapes from the body by radiation and convection, with a smaller amount being carried away by the evaporation of insensible perspiration. A cooler environment, increased air movement such as a cool wind, increased blood circulation to the skin, or an increased radiation surface would facilitate heat loss.

In contrast, under certain environmental conditions, such as exercising in the sunlight on a hot day, some of these processes may be reversed with the body gaining heat instead of losing it. For example, radiant energy from the sun could add heat to the body.

The well-known **heat-balance equation** may be used to illustrate these interrelationships:

$$H = M \pm W \pm C \pm R - E$$

where H = heat balance, M = resting metabolic rate, W = work done (exercise), C = conduction and convection, R = radiation, E = evaporation.

If any of these factors governing heat production or heat loss is not balanced by an opposite reaction, heat balance will be lost and the body will deviate from its normal value. During exercise, W increases heat production. Hence, compensating adjustments in C, R, and E must be made to dissipate the extra heat. Figure 9.5 illustrates heat stress factors and mechanisms of heat loss during exercise.

How does the body regulate its own temperature?

Body temperature is controlled by the autonomic division of the central nervous system. The hypothalamus is an important structure in the brain that is involved in the control of a wide variety of physiological functions, including body temperature. The hypothalamus is thought to function pretty much like the thermostat in your house. If your house gets too cold, the heat comes on; if it gets too warm, the air conditioning system starts. The human body makes similar adjustments.

The temperature-regulating center in the hypothalamus receives input from several sources. First, receptors in the skin can detect temperature changes and send impulses to the hypothalamus. Second, the temperature of the blood can directly affect the hypothalamus as it flows through that structure.

In general, if the skin receptors detect a warmer temperature or the blood temperature rises, the body will make adjustments in an

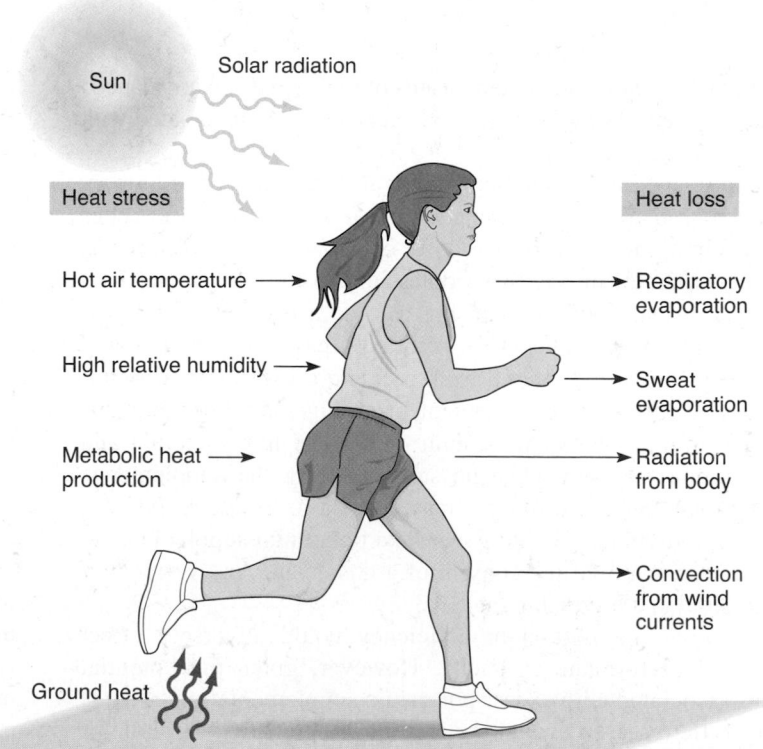

FIGURE 9.5 Sources of heat gain and heat loss to the body during exercise. See text for details.

attempt to lose heat. Two major adjustments may occur. First, the blood will be channeled closer to the skin so that the heat from within may get closer to the outside and radiate away more easily. Second, sweating will begin and evaporation of the sweat will carry heat away from the body.

If the skin receptors detect a colder temperature or the blood temperature is lowered, then the body will react to conserve heat or increase heat production. First, the blood will be shunted away from the skin to the central core of the body. This decreases heat loss by radiation and helps keep the vital organs at the proper temperature. Second, shivering may begin. Shivering is nothing more than the contraction of muscles, which produces extra heat by increasing the metabolic rate. Figure 9.6 is a simplified schematic of body temperature control.

The hypothalamus is usually very effective in controlling body temperature. However, certain conditions may threaten temperature control. For example, an individual who falls into cold water will lose body heat rapidly, for water is an excellent conductor of heat. Such a situation may lead to **hypothermia** (low body temperature) and a rapid loss of temperature control. Hypothermia may also develop in slower runners during the latter part of a road race under cold, wet, and windy environmental conditions when heat is lost more rapidly than it is produced through exercise. Muscular incoordination and mental confusion are early signs of hypothermia.

On the other hand, the most prevalent threat to the athletic individual is **hyperthermia,** or the increased body temperature that occurs with exercise in a warm or hot environment. Hyperthermia is one of the major factors limiting physical performance and one of the most dangerous.

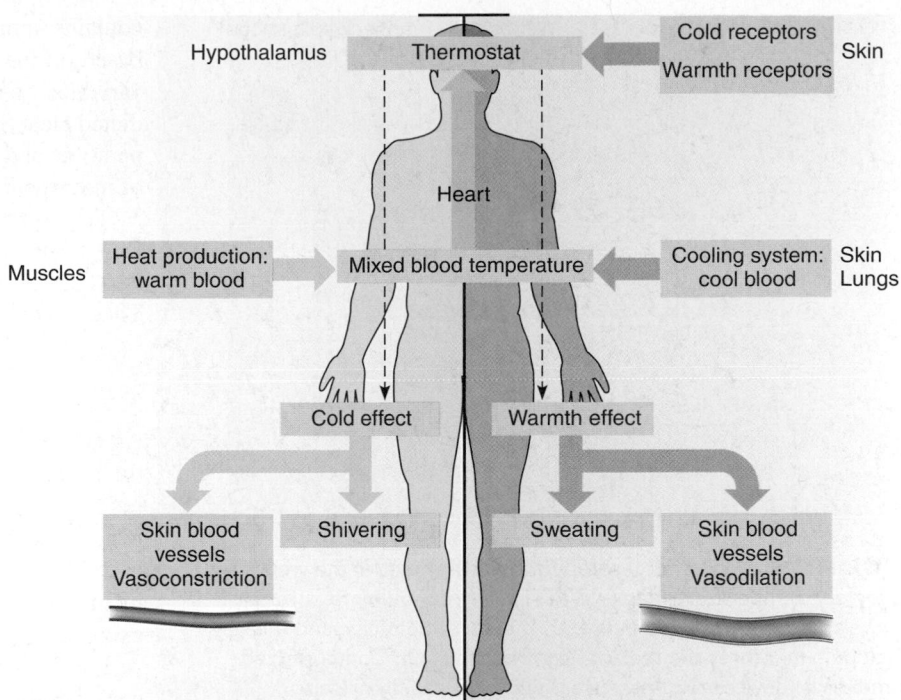

FIGURE 9.6 Simplified schematic of body temperature control. The temperature of the blood returning from the muscles and the skin stimulates the temperature regulation center (thermostat) in the hypothalamus, as do nerve impulses from the warmth and cold receptors in the skin. An overall cold effect will elicit a constriction of the blood vessels near the body surface and muscular shivering, thus helping to conserve body heat. An overall warmth effect will elicit a dilation of blood vessels near the skin and sweating, thus increasing the loss of body heat.

What environmental conditions may predispose an athletic individual to hyperthermia?

The interaction of four environmental factors are important determinants of the heat stress imposed on an active individual:

1. Air temperature. Caution should be advised when the air temperature is 80°F (27°C) or above. However, if the relative humidity and solar radiation are high, lower air temperatures, even 70°F, may pose a risk of heat stress during exercise.
2. Relative humidity. As the water content in the air increases, the relative humidity rises, which impairs the ability of sweat on the skin to vaporize and cool the body. Evaporation of sweat is the body's main cooling system during exercise. Baker and Kenney note that with a high relative humidity, 70 percent and above, sweat evaporation is decreased. With humidity levels from 90–100 percent, heat loss via evaporation nears zero. Some note that caution should be used when the relative humidity exceeds 50–60 percent, especially when accompanied by warmer temperatures.
3. Air movement. Still air limits heat carried away by convection. Even a small breeze may help keep body temperature near normal by moving heat away from the skin surface.
4. Radiation. Radiant heat from the sun may create an additional heat load.

Some useful guidelines have been developed taking these four factors into consideration. The wet-bulb globe temperature (WBGT) thermometer, illustrated in figure 9.7, measures all four. Small hand-held WBGT thermometers are available. The dry-bulb thermometer (DB) measures air temperature, the globe thermometer (G) measures radiant heat, and the wet-bulb thermometer (WB) evaluates relative humidity and air movement as they influence air temperature. The **WBGT Index** is computed as follows:

$$\text{WBGT Index} = 0.7\,\text{WB} + 0.2\,\text{G} + 0.1\,\text{DB}$$

For example, if the WB reads 70, the G is 100, and the DB is 80, then the WBGT = (0.7 × 70) + (0.2 × 100) + (0.1 × 80) = 77°F. It is important to note that 70 percent of the heat stress is associated with the effects of humidity to decrease heat loss from the body.

Another indicator of heat stress is the **heat index** (figure 9.8), which combines the air temperature and relative humidity to determine the apparent temperature, or how hot it feels. Figure 9.8 also

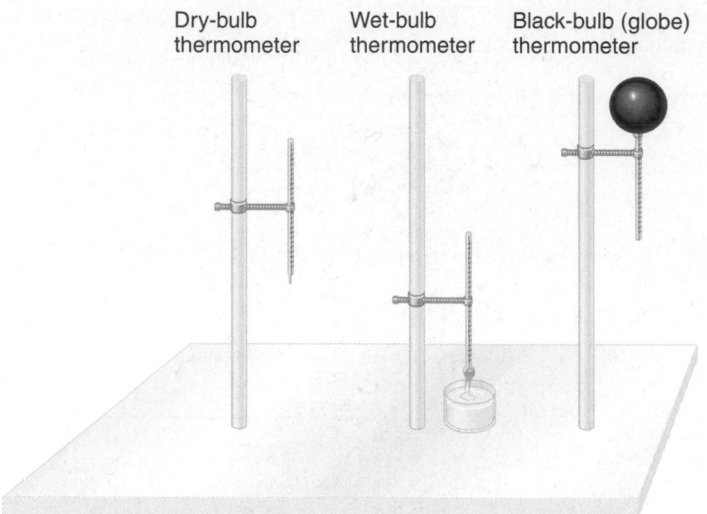

Dry-bulb thermometer Wet-bulb thermometer Black-bulb (globe) thermometer

FIGURE 9.7 A typical setup for measurement of the wet-bulb globe temperature index (WBGT). The dry bulb measures air temperature, the wet bulb indirectly measures humidity, and the black bulb measures the radiant heat from the sun. Computerized commercial devices that measure the WBGT rapidly are also available.

contains some temperature levels predisposing to heat disorders based on the heat index. Other models incorporate physiological variables of interest to assess heat stress. For example, the Predicted Heat Strain model incorporates core temperature, skin temperature, and sweat rate, and may take into consideration the effect of movement and clothing.

The American College of Sports Medicine (ACSM) has published a position statement with guidelines for the prevention of heat illness during distance exercise training and competition. These guidelines are incorporated in the last section of this chapter.

How does exercise affect body temperature?

As noted in chapter 3, exercise increases the metabolic rate and the production of energy. Under a normal mechanical efficiency ratio of 20–25 percent, the remaining 75–80 percent of energy is released as heat. The total amount of heat produced in the body depends on the intensity and duration of the exercise. A more intense exercise will produce heat faster, while the longer the exercise lasts, the more total heat is produced.

For illustrative purposes only, let us look at a hypothetical example of the body temperature changes that might occur in an exercising individual who was unable to dissipate heat. A physically conditioned person may be able to perform in

Heat Index

Relative Humidity (%)	70°	75°	80°	85°	90°	95°	100°	105°	110°
100	72°	80°	91°	108°					
90	71°	79°	88°	102°	122°				
80	71°	78°	86°	97°	113°	136°			
70	70°	77°	85°	93°	106°	124°	144°		
60	69°	76°	82°	90°	100°	114°	132°	149°	
50	70°	75°	81°	88°	96°	107°	120°	135°	150°
40	68°	74°	79°	86°	93°	101°	110°	123°	137°
30	67°	73°	78°	84°	90°	96°	104°	113°	123°
20	66°	72°	77°	82°	87°	93°	99°	105°	112°
10	65°	70°	75°	80°	85°	90°	95°	100°	105°
0	64°	69°	73°	78°	83°	87°	91°	95°	99°

Air Temperature (°F)

Heat index	Heat disorders possible with prolonged exposure and/or physical activity
80° – 89°	Fatigue
90° – 104°	Sunstroke, heat cramps, and heat exhaustion
105° – 129°	Sunstroke, heat cramps, or heat exhaustion likely and heatstroke possible
130° or higher	Heatstroke/sunstroke highly likely

NOTE: Direct sunshine increases the heat index by up to 15°F

FIGURE 9.8 Possible heat disorders in runners and other high-risk groups based on the heat index (air temperature and relative humidity versus apparent temperature).

a steady state for prolonged periods. If a normal-sized male, 154 lbs or 70 kg, were to jog for about an hour, he could expend approximately 900 Calories. Assuming a mechanical efficiency rate of 20 percent, 80 percent, or 720 Calories (0.80 × 900), would be released in the body as heat.

Specific heat is defined as the heat in Calories required to raise the temperature of 1 kilogram of a substance by 1 degree Celsius. Because the specific heat of the body is 0.83, that is, 0.83 Calorie will raise 1 kg of the body 1°C, then 58 Calories (70 kg × 0.83) would raise the body temperature 1°C in this person. Thus, if this excess heat were not dissipated, his body temperature would increase by more than 12.4°C (720/58), or 22°F, resulting in a body temperature of 120°F, a fatal condition. Although the core temperature does rise during exercise, it rarely hits these extreme levels. The average core temperature during exercise, even during moderately warm temperatures, may reach about 102.2–104.0°F (39–40°C). This is because of the body's cooling system.

How is body heat dissipated during exercise?

During exercise in a cold or cool environment, body heat is lost mainly through radiation and convection via the air movement around the body. Some evaporation of sweat and evaporative heat loss from the lungs may also contribute to maintenance of heat balance.

However, when the environmental temperature rises, the evaporation of sweat becomes the main means of controlling an excessive rise in the core temperature. For example, evaporation of sweat may account for about 20 percent of total heat loss when exercising in an ambient temperature of 50°F (10°C), but increases to about 45 percent at 68°F (20°C) and 70 percent at 86°F (30°C). Although variable, the maximal evaporation rate is about 30 milliliters of sweat per minute, or 1.8 liters per hour. However, greater sweat rates may occur when sweat drops off the skin without vaporizing. Only sweat that evaporates has a cooling effect. One liter of sweat, if perfectly evaporated, will dissipate about 580 C. In our previous example, the evaporation of 1.24 liters of sweat (720/580) would prevent a rise in the core temperature. However, the evaporation of sweat from the body is not perfect, as sweat can drip off the body and not carry away body heat, so more than 1.24 liters may be lost. If we assume that 2.0 liters were lost, then this individual would have lost 4.4 lbs of body fluids during the 1-hour run; 1 liter of sweat weighs 1 kg or 2.2 lbs. It should be noted that sweat rates may vary considerably between individuals. Ron Maughan, an environmental physiologist from England, studied two marathoners who completed a race in the same time and had the same fluid intake; one lost only 1 percent of his body weight while the other lost 6 percent.

Under most warm environmental circumstances, the evaporative mechanisms and the body's natural warning signals are able to keep the core temperature during exercise below 104°F (40°C) and prevent heat injuries. However, an excessive rise in the core temperature, above 104°F, or excessive fluid and electrolyte losses may lead to diminished performance or serious thermal injury in some individuals.

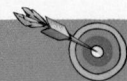

Exercise Performance in the Heat: Effect of Environmental Temperature and Fluid and Electrolyte Losses

Athletes train and compete in all types of weather conditions, as do many individuals who exercise for fitness and health. Not all types of physical performance are impaired when performed under warm or hot environmental conditions, but some are. In general, performance in strength, power, or speed events that last less than a minute or so does not appear to be affected adversely by warm environmental conditions. However, as noted later, some research suggests otherwise. The major concern is performance in prolonged exercise and whether or not the core body temperature is maintained. Sawka and Young noted that with **compensated heat stress,** a condition in which heat loss balances heat production, a set body temperature is maintained and the individuals can continue to exercise. In contrast, if heat loss is insufficient to offset heat production, a condition known as **uncompensated heat stress,** the body temperature continues to rise and exhaustion eventually occurs. Environmental heat stress itself may contribute to impaired performance, but so too can fluid and electrolyte losses over time.

How does environmental heat affect physical performance?

Performance in more prolonged aerobic endurance activities is normally worse when compared to performance in cooler temperatures. In their reviews, Febbraio, Hargreaves and Febbraio, and Maughan noted that the cause of fatigue during prolonged exercise in the heat has not been clearly established, but changes in brain function, blood circulation, skeletal muscle function, hyperthermia, and dehydration, either separately or collectively, could impair performance. Much of the research evaluating the effect of heat on endurance performance has been conducted with runners. In this regard, McCann and Adams reported a significant linear relationship between the WBGT and decreased performance in endurance events such as the 10,000-meter run. Montain and others analyzed data of elite runners from 140 race-years of major marathons and found that as environmental temperature increased, so too did finishing times. Slower runners suffered even greater performance decrements in warmer weather. In general, Sawka and Young note that marathon running performance declines by about 1 minute for each 1°C increase in air temperature beyond 8–15°C (each 1.8°F increase in air temperature beyond 46–59°F).

Environmental heat may affect exercise performance in various ways:

- Central neural fatigue caused by increased brain temperature
- Cardiovascular strain caused by changes in blood circulation
- Muscle metabolism changes caused by increased muscle temperature
- Dehydration caused by excessive sweat losses

Central Neural Fatigue   The brain appears to play an important role in the development of fatigue during exercise in the heat. Cheung and Sleivert suggest that fatigue occurs when the brain reaches a critical core temperature. In his latest review on heat stress and central nervous system (CNS) fatigue, Nybo indicated that the main factor adversely affecting muscle tissue activation appears to be elevated brain temperature. Subjects exercising in the heat seem to reach the point of voluntary fatigue at similar and consistent core body temperatures despite various experimental manipulations. In essence, the elevated brain temperature impairs central arousal of voluntary activation of muscle. Although environmental heat normally does not affect muscle power production, Tucker and others reported reductions in both neuromuscular stimulation and power output during exercise in the heat before there was any abnormal increase in rectal temperature, heart rate, or perception of effort; in other words, the brain apparently anticipates heat stress and reduces heat production (by decreasing muscle contraction) accordingly. Theoretically, this may be the reason Drust and others reported a decrease in mean power output during five 15-second maximal cycle ergometer sprints when exercising in the heat as compared to exercising in normal temperature. These investigators note that an elevated muscle temperature normally is expected to improve sprint performance. Central fatigue is discussed in more detail in chapter 3.

Cardiovascular Strain   Cheung and Sleivert noted that other factors may also inhibit performance in the heat, such as high levels of cardiovascular strain. For example, in a 5-kilometer race the runner will be performing at a rather high metabolic rate and thus will be producing heat rapidly. To prevent hyperthermia, blood flow to the skin will increase so as to dissipate heat to the environment. This shifting of blood to the skin will result in a lesser proportion of blood, and hence oxygen, being delivered to the active musculature. Young found that under these conditions cellular metabolism changes somewhat, with greater accumulation of lactic acid if the athlete attempts to maintain the pace normally done in a cooler environment. Yaspelkis and others reported similar lactate findings but found no increase in muscle glycogen utilization. They speculated that the increased lactic acid could be associated with decreased clearance by the liver. Nevertheless, increased lactic acid could be associated with a greater sensation of stress. In some individuals, the circulatory adjustments may not be adequate and the body temperature will rise rapidly, leading to hyperthermia and symptoms of weakness. Because of these changes, and possibly others not yet identified, the runner normally must slow the pace.

Muscle Metabolism   In two reviews, Mark Febbraio indicated that exercise in the heat may adversely affect muscle metabolism with possible reduction in physical performance. He indicated that exercising in the heat appears to shift energy metabolism toward increased carbohydrate use and decreased fat use. In particular, muscle glycogen use is accelerated, possibly due to an augmented sympatho-adrenal response and intramuscular temperature increases. A more rapid depletion of muscle glycogen could impair prolonged endurance performance. Depletion of muscle glycogen as a cause of fatigue is discussed in chapter 4. Febbraio also indicated that increased intramuscular temperature may in some way lead to dysfunction of skeletal muscle contraction, which could decrease performance capacity. Supportive of this viewpoint is the review by Marino, who notes that precooling the body prior to exercise, such as by taking a cold shower or bath to lower the body temperature, may be beneficial for endurance exercise tasks up to 30–40 minutes. Body cooling techniques as an ergogenic aid are discussed later in this chapter.

Dehydration   Dehydration may also impair exercise performance. Although the 5-kilometer runner will sweat heavily, the duration of the event is usually short, so an excessive loss of body fluids does not occur. However, in more prolonged events, athletes may suffer the problems noted previously plus the adverse effects of dehydration. Marathoners may lose 5 percent or more of their body weight (mostly water) during a race, which may not only deteriorate performance but have serious health consequences as well.

How do dehydration and hypohydration affect physical performance?

The effect of dehydration on physical performance has been studied from two different viewpoints. Voluntary dehydration is often used by athletes such as wrestlers and boxers to qualify for lower weight classes prior to competition. In other athletes, dehydration occurs involuntarily during training or competition as the body attempts to maintain temperature homeostasis. Dehydration leads to hypohydration.

Hypohydration may affect numerous physiological processes that may impair physical performance. Michael Sawka and others noted that hypohydration may lead to decreases in both intracellular and extracellular fluid volumes (particularly blood volume) with associated decreases in stroke volume and cardiac output. Body heat storage may increase by reducing sweating rate and skin blood flow responses. Kenefick and others found that hypohydration induced an earlier onset of the lactate threshold during exercise, an adverse effect relative to aerobic endurance performance. Hypohydration could also lead to electrolyte imbalances in the muscle, with subsequent adverse effects.

Voluntary Dehydration Voluntary dehydration techniques used by wrestlers have included exercise-induced sweating, thermal-induced sweating such as the use of saunas, diuretics to increase urine losses, and decreased intake of fluids and food.

Much of the research with voluntary dehydration has been conducted with wrestlers. Evaluation criteria have emphasized factors such as strength, power, local muscular endurance, and performance of anaerobic exercise tasks designed to mimic wrestling. In one review, Barr noted that the effects of hypohydration on muscle strength and endurance are not consistent and require further study. Many studies conducted in this area suggest that hypohydration, even up to levels of 8 percent of the body weight, will not affect these physical performance factors in events involving brief, intense muscular effort. For example, Greiwe and others reported that 4 percent reduction in body weight had no effect on isometric muscle strength or endurance. In its position stand on fluid replacement, the ACSM indicated that dehydration of 3–5 percent of body weight does not degrade either anaerobic performance or muscular strength.

In contrast, Schoffstall and others reported that passive dehydration resulting in approximately 1.5 percent loss of body mass adversely affected bench press 1-repetition maximal performance, but these adverse effects seem to be overcome by a 2-hour rest period and water consumption. Judelson and others reported that dehydration by 5 percent significantly decreased total work during four of six sets of a back-squat protocol, but dehydration by 2.5 percent diminished total work in only one set. Neither level of dehydration affected performance in vertical jump height or peak lower-body power. Other studies have reported significant impairments in such tasks with body weight losses of 4 percent or higher. The adverse effects on strength are not consistent, but anaerobic muscular endurance tasks lasting longer than 20–30 seconds have been impaired when subjects were hypohydrated. For example, Montain and others recently reported that a 4 percent decrease in body weight decreased knee-extension endurance by 15 percent. Suggested mechanisms of impairment include loss of potassium from the muscle, higher muscle temperatures during exercise, and decreased central drive, or the ability of the central nervous system to stimulate the musculature. It should also be noted that there is no evidence that hypohydration improves performance in these exercise tasks. Investigators recommend more research.

Involuntary Dehydration Involuntary dehydration is most common during prolonged physical activity. Dehydration may occur during exercise in cold or temperate environments, but the ACSM, in its position stand on fluid replacement, indicated that dehydration (3 percent body weight) has marginal influence on degrading aerobic exercise performance when exercising in colder environments. However, the adverse effects of involuntary dehydration are most severe on aerobic endurance performance when exercising in warm, humid environmental conditions. The following represent the major highlights of the ACSM position stand on fluid replacement relative to dehydration and prolonged endurance exercise performance.

- Dehydration increases physiologic strain and perceived effort to perform the same exercise task, and is accentuated in warm-hot weather.
- Dehydration can degrade aerobic exercise performance, especially in warm-hot weather.
- The greater the dehydration level, the greater the physiologic strain and aerobic exercise performance impairment.
- The critical water deficit and magnitude of exercise performance degradation are related to the heat stress, exercise task, and the individual's unique biological characteristics.

In several major reviews, Michael Sawka, Kent Pandolf, and John Greenleaf have suggested that the deterioration in aerobic endurance performance appears to be related to adverse effects on cardiovascular functions and temperature regulation. Reduction in the plasma volume may reduce cardiac output and blood flow to the skin and the muscles. Reductions in skin blood flow have been shown to lower the sweat rate and raise the core temperature. In his review, Coyle reported some of the effects of dehydration in endurance-trained cyclists. In general, he reported that skin blood flow decreased with dehydration and that the greater the level of dehydration, the greater the rise in the core temperature and heart rate and the greater the decrease in the stroke volume (amount of blood pumped by the heart per beat). Montain and others noted that hypohydration decreased cardiac output, and the greater the intensity of the exercise, the greater the decrease. The effects of dehydration on cardiovascular dynamics are depicted in figure 9.9.

One of the key points of the ACSM position stand is the effect an individual's unique biological characteristics and the exercise task may play regarding hydration status and exercise performance, and some research suggests that highly trained endurance runners may be able to better tolerate some, but not all, of the adverse effects of dehydration. In an article on marathon runners, Tim Noakes, an international authority in hydration for endurance athletes, contends that there is no evidence that athletes who drink according to thirst are at any significant disadvantage from the 3–5 percent level of dehydration that they may develop. In support of this viewpoint, Armstrong and others found that dehydration up to 5.7 percent had no adverse effect on running economy in highly trained collegiate distance runners during 10 minutes of running at 70 or 85 percent VO_2 max. Further, Byrne and others suggested that the effects of body weight loss (used as the measure for dehydration via sweat loss) on temperature regulation may

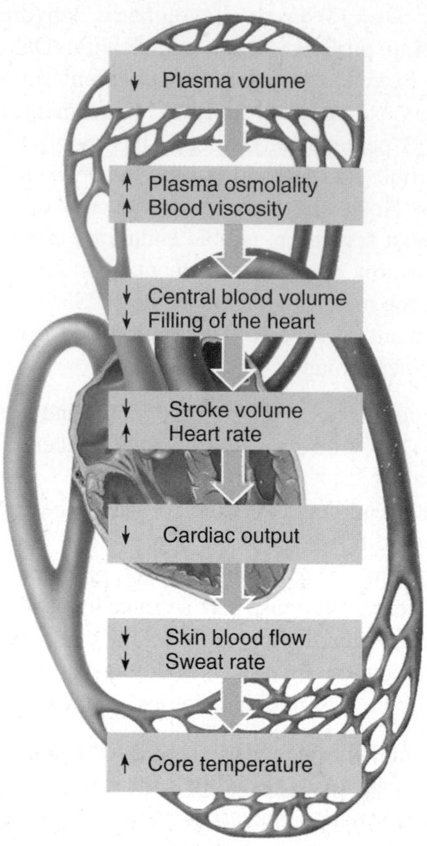
↓ Plasma volume
↑ Plasma osmolality
↑ Blood viscosity
↓ Central blood volume
↓ Filling of the heart
↓ Stroke volume
↑ Heart rate
↓ Cardiac output
↓ Skin blood flow
↓ Sweat rate
↑ Core temperature

FIGURE 9.9 Some physiological effects of dehydration. The decreased blood volume and increased core temperature may contribute to premature fatigue and heat illness.

vary in actual outdoor race competition under warm conditions, as compared to controlled laboratory conditions. They reported that core temperature after running a half-marathon was not affected by level of dehydration, which ranged from 1.62 to 4.0 liters in 18 nonelite runners. However, the authors did not appear to evaluate the effect of weight loss on performance time, as they had no measures of running speed during the race. Although, as noted previously, Armstrong and others reported that dehydration did not affect running economy, dehydration did result in increased heart rate and rectal temperature, concurrent with reduced stroke volume and cardiac output; over time, these physiological responses would lead to impaired performance. As noted previously, there is a strong relationship between higher environmental temperatures and slower running times in elite and slower runners. As one champion commented years ago at the start of the Olympic marathon on a hot day, "Men, today we die a little."

The ACSM also noted that dehydration might degrade mental/cognitive performance, which may be caused by adverse effects of hyperthermia on mental processes. In several reports, Baker and others reported that dehydration may impair vigilance in dynamic sports environments, such as basketball, leading to increased errors of omission and commission and impaired reaction time. In one study, skilled basketball players were dehydrated by 1, 2, 3, and 4 percent prior to taking a test mimicking basketball skills in a fast-paced game. The players experienced a progressive deterioration in performance as dehydration progressed from 1 to 4 percent, but performance was not significantly impaired until dehydration reached 2 percent. Dougherty and others also reported impaired basketball skill performance, including sprint times and shooting percentage, in young (12–15 years) skilled basketball players who were dehydrated by 2 percent prior to a simulated 48-minute basketball game. Edwards and colleagues studied the impact of dehydration on sport specific activities in male soccer players. The athletes performed the protocol in a random order with no fluid intake, fluid intake, and a mouth rinse. The protocol included 45 minutes of pre-match cycling, a 45-minute soccer match, followed by a sport-specific test (Yo-Yo Intermittent Recovery Test) and a mental concentration test. After the soccer match, body mass was reduced by 2.14 percent in the mouth-rinse trial, 2.4 percent in the no-fluid trial, and only 0.7% in the fluid trial. Although dehydration had no impact on the mental concentration tests, sport-specific performance was decreased by 13–15 percent when fluid was not ingested. Additional research would appear to be warranted to explore the effects of dehydration on other mental aspects of sports performance.

Dehydration may also be a major factor in the onset of gastrointestinal (GI) distress, according to Nancy Rehrer and her associates. GI symptoms include nausea, vomiting, bloating, GI cramps, flatulence, diarrhea, and GI bleeding, many of which could impair performance if severe enough. However, Peters and others contend that the causes of GI distress during exercise are currently unknown and may vary depending on the individual.

The ACSM indicated that dehydration is also a risk factor for various heat illnesses, which are covered in a later section of this chapter.

How fast may an individual dehydrate while exercising?

Mack, in his review, indicated that sweat rates as high as 3–4 liters per hour, or a loss of about 6.5 to 9.0 pounds, have been reported. Most athletes may lose somewhat less, maybe 2–3 liters, when exercising strenuously in the heat, but even then it will not take long to incur a 2–3 percent decrease in body weight. Two liters of sweat is the equivalent of 4.4 pounds (1 liter = 1 kg = 2.2 pounds), so a 150-pound runner could experience a loss of 3 percent body weight in 1 hour ($4.4/150 = 0.03$; $0.03 \times 100 = 3$ percent), which could cause premature fatigue. Research has shown that some athletes, like football players, may lose up to 10 kg (22 pounds) over a day with multiple daily workouts.

There may be some gender and age differences in sweating. White and others report significantly greater sweat losses, almost twofold greater, per unit body mass in male compared to female athletes. Meyer and Bar-Or indicate that while children may sweat somewhat less than adults, they still may reach hypohydration levels comparable to adults. Young tennis players may lose 1–2 liters of sweat per hour in tournament play, and some older adolescents as much as 3 liters per hour. Excessive dehydration may not only impair one's physical performance, but possibly also one's health, as discussed later in this chapter.

How can I determine my sweat rate?

The rate of sweating varies among different individuals, so some may be more prone to dehydration than others. Cheuvront and Sawka indicated that there are a number of methods to evaluate your sweat loss and hydration status, but body weight change is reliable and easy to do. However, Maughan and others note that although sweat rate and hydration status are often estimated from body weight loss, several sources of error may give rise to misleading results. For example, respiratory water losses can be substantial during hard work in dry environments and body mass loss also results from substrate oxidation, such as fat. Additionally, water produced as a by-product of oxidation, and possible water released from muscle glycogen, may add to the body-water pool. Mack notes that burning 100 grams of glycogen per hour could liberate about 0.3 to 0.4 liter of water into the total body-water pool. Other factors may also be involved so that an individual may lose body weight but maintain total body water. Nevertheless, although body weight loss may not always be a reliable marker of changes in hydration status, when adjusted for fluid intake and urine losses, Cheuvront and Sawka indicate that it is primarily a function of sweat losses.

The Gatorade Sports Science Institute has presented a method to calculate the sweat rate during exercise. To do so, one must accurately measure body weight before and after exercise, measure the amount of fluid consumed during exercise, and the amount of urine excreted, if any, during exercise. You may use the following examples as a guide to calculate your own sweat rate during exercise (See the Application Exercise at the end of this chapter). The sweat rate for athlete A is calculated in the metric measurement system and for athlete B in the English system. Remember, 1 gram equals about 1 milliliter, and 1 pound equals 16 ounces.

	Athlete A	Athlete B
A. Body weight before exercise	70.5 kg	180 lbs
B. Body weight after exercise	68.9 kg	174 lbs
C. Change in body weight	−1.6 kg 1,600 g	−6 lbs 96 oz
D. Drink volume	+300 ml	16 oz
E. Urine volume	−100 ml	0 oz
F. Sweat loss (C + D − E)	1,800 ml	112 oz
G. Exercise time	60 min	90 min
H. Sweat rate (F ÷ G)	30 ml/min	1.25 oz/min

What is the composition of sweat?

The human body contains two different types of sweat glands. The apocrine sweat glands are located in hairy areas of the body, such as the armpits, and secrete an oily mixture to decrease friction. We are all aware of the odor that may be generated from these sweat glands under certain conditions. Our concern here is with the eccrine sweat glands, about 2–3 million over the surface of the body, which are primarily involved in temperature regulation.

Sweat is mostly water (about 99 percent), but a number of major electrolytes and other nutrients may be found in varying amounts. Sweat is hypotonic in comparison to the fluids in the body. This means that the concentration of electrolytes is lower in sweat than in the body fluids.

The composition of sweat may vary somewhat from individual to individual and will even be different in the same individual when acclimatized to the heat, as contrasted to the unacclimatized state. The major differences are the concentrations of the solid matter in the sweat, the electrolytes or salts.

The major electrolytes found in sweat are sodium and chloride, as sweat is derived from the extracellular fluids, such as the plasma and intercellular fluids, which are high in these electrolytes. You may actually note the formation of dried salt on your skin or clothing after prolonged sweating. Mack has reported that the concentration of salt in sweat is variable but averages about 55 mEq (3.2 grams) per liter of sweat during exercise with sweat losses of about 1–1.5 liters per hour.

Other minerals lost in small amounts include potassium, magnesium, calcium, iron, copper, and zinc. As noted in chapter 8, certain athletes, especially those who lose large amounts of sweat, may need to increase their dietary intake of certain trace minerals, such as iron and zinc, to replace losses during exercise.

Small quantities of nitrogen (N), amino acids, and some of the water-soluble vitamins also are present in sweat, but these amounts are easily restored by consuming a balanced diet.

Is excessive sweating likely to create an electrolyte deficiency?

There are two ways to look at this question. What happens to electrolyte balance during exercise? And what happens during the recovery period on a day-to-day basis?

The concentration of electrolytes in the blood during exercise with excessive sweating has been studied under laboratory conditions, as well as immediately after endurance events such as the Ironman triathlon and a marathon run. In general, exercise raises the concentration of several electrolytes in the blood. Sodium and potassium concentrations are elevated; the sodium increase may be due to greater body-water loss than sodium loss, so a concentration effect occurs. The potassium may leak from the muscle tissue to the blood, thereby increasing the blood concentration of this ion. Calcium ion concentration remains relatively unchanged during exercise. Magnesium levels usually fall, possibly because the active muscle cells and other tissues need this ion during exercise and it passes from the blood into the tissues. Thus, during acute, prolonged bouts of exercise, even in marathon running, it appears that an electrolyte deficiency will not occur.

This is not to say that electrolyte replacement is not important. As we shall see in the next section, an electrolyte imbalance may occur in the body during extremely prolonged endurance events, such as ultramarathoning and Ironman-type triathlons, if proper fluid replacement techniques are not used. Moreover, what happens during the recovery period after excessive sweating may contribute to an electrolyte deficiency. Prolonged sweating has been shown to decrease the body content of sodium and chloride by

5–7 percent and potassium by about 1 percent. If these electrolytes are not replaced daily, an electrolyte deficiency may occur over time. The next section deals with the need for water and electrolyte replacement.

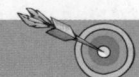

Key Concepts

▶ Both hyperthermia and dehydration may impair endurance capacity.

▶ Sweat consists mainly of water and some minerals, primarily sodium and chloride. It is hypotonic compared to the body fluids.

Exercise in the Heat: Fluid, Carbohydrate, and Electrolyte Replacement

Maintenance of an optimal body-water balance is believed to be an important means to delay the onset of fatigue during prolonged exercise and thus has been one of the most studied areas of sport nutrition over the years. Various guidelines for fluid replenishment for athletes during and after exercise have been provided in the past, but have been criticized because they were not based on scientifically proven evidence. For example, Noakes criticized the 1996 ACSM guidelines because they recommended that athletes drink "as much as tolerable" during exercise, which may have contributed to excess fluid intake and serious consequences, as noted later. Noakes also has criticized the International Olympic Committee guidelines, indicating that they too are not based on appropriately controlled, randomized, prospective studies. Most research underlying fluid replacement guidelines has been conducted under laboratory conditions, not in actual sports competition.

In 2007, the ACSM replaced its 1996 guidelines, in part, with its position stand on fluid replacement. These current guidelines represent a synthesis of the best research available, and provide recommendations that are considered to be prudent. They are more likely to help delay the onset of premature fatigue during prolonged exercise in the heat, may help in the prevention of exercise-associated heat illness, and are less likely to cause other exercise-associated health problems.

Which is most important to replace during exercise in the heat—water, carbohydrate, or electrolytes?

In the 1960s Robert Cade, a scientist-physician working at the University of Florida, developed an oral fluid replacement for athletes that was designed to restore some of the nutrients lost in sweat. This product was eventually marketed as Gatorade (Gator is the nickname for University of Florida athletes) and was the first glucose-electrolyte solution (GES) to appear as a sports drink in the athletic marketplace. The three main ingredients in sports drinks are water, carbohydrates, and electrolytes, and because the

source of carbohydrate in a sports drink may vary, it is known as a **carbohydrate-electrolyte solution (CES).** Maughan classifies the CES as a functional food for athletes.

CES were the first commercial fluid-replacement preparations designed to replace both fluid and carbohydrate. Common brands today include Accelerade, All-Sport, Gatorade, and PowerAde. Other than water, the major ingredients in these solutions are carbohydrates, usually in various combinations of glucose, glucose polymers, sucrose, or fructose, and some of the major electrolytes. As noted in chapter 4, sports drinks containing multiple carbohydrates, such as glucose, fructose, sucrose, and maltodextrins (glucose polymer), may be a good choice. The sugar content ranges from about 5–10 percent depending on the brand. The caloric values range from about 6–12 Calories per ounce. The major electrolytes include sodium, chloride, potassium, and phosphorus. These ions are found in varying amounts in different brands. Some brands may also include a variety of other substances, including vitamins (B vitamins and C), minerals (calcium and magnesium), amino acids (BCAA), drugs (caffeine), herbals (ginseng), and artificial coloring and flavoring. Do not confuse the standard sports drinks with the newer "Energy" or "Sports Energy" drinks in the marketplace, which contain considerably more carbohydrate and numerous other ingredients. However, other beverages that appear to be sports drinks may contain minimal carbohydrate content. Nutrition Facts labels on sports drinks will provide you with the actual content, including source of carbohydrates. The contents of selected ingredients for several CES and GES are presented in table 9.5.

Each of the components of CES and GES may be important to the athlete, depending on the circumstances. When dehydration or hyperthermia is the major threat to performance, water replacement is the primary consideration. In prolonged endurance events, where muscle glycogen and blood glucose are the primary energy sources, carbohydrate replacement, as noted in chapter 4, may help improve performance. In very prolonged exercise in the heat with heavy sweat losses, such as ultramarathons, electrolyte replacement may be essential to prevent heat injury. Although the beneficial effects of carbohydrate intake during exercise were covered in chapter 4, the role of carbohydrate as a component of the CES is stressed in this chapter.

The following questions focus on the importance and mechanisms of water, carbohydrate, and electrolyte replacement for the individual incurring sweat losses while exercising under heat stress conditions.

What are some sound guidelines for maintaining water (fluid) balance during exercise?

Proper hydration is probably the most important nutritional strategy an athlete can use in training and competition. As compared to hypohydration, adequate hydration will help decrease fluid loss, reduce cardiovascular strain, enhance performance, and prevent some heat illnesses. Athletes have used several strategies to help prevent hypohydration and excessive

TABLE 9.5 Fluid-replacement and high-carbohydrate* beverage comparison chart per 8 oz. serving

Beverage	Carbohydrate ingredient	Carbohydrate (% concentration)	Carbohydrate (grams)	Sodium (mg)	Potassium (mg)
Gatorade Thirst Quencher (Gatorade Company)	Sucrose, glucose, fructose	6	14	110	30
Gatorade Endurance Formula	Sucrose, glucose, fructose	6	14	200	90
Accelerade (Pacific Health Laboratories)	Sucrose, trehalose (disaccharide), fructose	6	14	127	43
PowerAde (The Coca-Cola Company)	High-fructose corn syrup	6	14	100	25
Lucozade Sport (GlaxoSmithKline)	Glucose; maltodextrin	6	15	Trace	Trace
Ultima (Ultima Replenisher)	Maltodextrin	1.5	3	37	75
Cytomax Performance Plus (Cytosport)	alpha-l-polylactate	9	13	55	30
Coca-Cola	High-fructose corn syrup, sucrose	11	27	30	0
Diet soft drinks	None	0	0	0–25	Low
Orange juice (100% juice)	Fructose, sucrose	11	26	0	450
Water	None	0	0	Low	Low
Gatorade Carb Energy Drink (Gatorade Company)	Maltodextrin, glucose, fructose	24	55	147	0

*Compiled from product labels and sources provided by the Gatorade Company; some products are in powdered form to be mixed with water.

increases in body temperature associated with certain types of sport competition. Depending on the sport, three commonly used practices are skin wetting, hyperhydration, and rehydration. Another procedure, body cooling, is discussed in the section on ergogenic aids.

Skin Wetting   Skin wetting techniques, such as sponging the head and torso with cold water or using a water spray, have been shown to decrease sweat loss. This could be an important consideration in a long run, as body-water supplies may be depleted less rapidly. These techniques also cool the skin and offer an immediate sense of psychological relief from the heat stress, which may help to improve performance. However, skin wetting techniques as they may be used in athletic competition have not been shown to cause any major reductions in core temperature or cardiovascular responses. Moreover, some researchers have theorized that skin wetting techniques may be potentially harmful: the psychological sense of relief may encourage athletes to accelerate their pace, increasing heat production without providing for control of the body temperature. If the core temperature increases, heat illness may occur. Although some scientists suggest that skin wetting is not beneficial, many endurance athletes claim that it helps. Additional research appears to be warranted.

Hyperhydration   Hyperhydration, also known as superhydration, is simply an increase in body fluids by the voluntary ingestion of water or other beverages. It is an attempt to ensure that the body-water level is high before exercising in a hot environment. In a review of hyperhydration strategies, Lamb and Shehata noted that increasing body water above normal by drinking fluids before exercise is likely to improve cardiovascular functions and temperature regulation when it is impossible to ingest sufficient fluids during exercise. Although these effects would appear to help prevent fatigue, Lamb and Shehata also indicated that there was insufficient evidence to support the claim that pre-exercise hyperhydration improves exercise performance. Sawka and others support this viewpoint, noting that hyperhydration provides no advantages over euhydration regarding thermoregulation and exercise performance in the heat.

However, given its potential benefits, the American College of Sports Medicine recommends that hyperhydration be used prior to exercise in heat stress environments. If you plan to compete or do any prolonged exercise in the heat, it may be wise for you to hyperhydrate. Either cold water or a CES may be used to hyperhydrate, although the CES will provide some carbohydrate and sodium that may be helpful. The ACSM guidelines relative to hyperhydration are presented later in this section.

Glycerol supplementation may help retain more water with hyperhydration, an effect which has been theorized to improve endurance performance. The proposed ergogenic effects of glycerol-induced hyperhydration are discussed later in this chapter.

Rehydration Of the various techniques used, research has shown that rehydration is the most effective to enhance performance. Rehydration techniques have been used to replenish fluid loss associated with both voluntary and involuntary dehydration in sports such as wrestling and distance running, respectively.

One laboratory research approach to evaluate the effects of rehydration is related to the sport of wrestling, in which athletes dehydrate to qualify for a weight class and then attempt to rehydrate rapidly prior to competition. In this approach, subjects performed some exercise or mental task, such as a measure of strength, power, anaerobic endurance, or cognitive function, were then dehydrated and tested again, and finally were rehydrated and tested one more time to see if rehydration could improve performance back to the predehydration level. The results of such research are mixed. In some studies, no effect of rehydration was found, probably because as some studies have shown, dehydration may not impair strength, power, or local muscular endurance. Thus, rehydration would not improve performance as measured by these criteria beyond that usually seen in normohydration. However, some studies reported a partial improvement in endurance performance after rehydration, but usually not all the way back to normal. In one study rehydration returned cognitive functions to normal. Because rehydration may possibly bring about performance improvements beyond the dehydrated level, it is therefore recommended for wrestlers when feasible.

A second approach in studying rehydration is to have subjects ingest fluids during prolonged endurance exercise, particularly in warm environments. Rehydration has been shown to minimize the rise in core temperature, to reduce stress on the cardiovascular system by minimizing the decrease in blood volume, and to help maintain an optimal race pace for a longer period. This beneficial effect is usually attributed to decreased dehydration and the maintenance of a better water balance in the blood and other fluid compartments. Rehydration techniques, both with water alone or with CES solutions, have been shown to improve performance in exercise tasks of 1 hour or more in the heat. Although not all studies have shown improved performance with rehydration, Jeukendrup and Martin, in their review of techniques to improve cycling performance, indicate that carbohydrate-electrolyte drinks may decrease 40-kilometer (25-mile) cycling time by 32–42 seconds. Hargreaves and others also reported that water intake may help reduce muscle glycogen use in prolonged exercise, another benefit.

If fluid replacement is to be effective, water has to be absorbed into the circulating blood so that the reduction in blood volume and sweat production that occurs during prolonged endurance exercise will be minimized. Research in which water was labeled with radionuclides showed that water ingested during exercise may appear in plasma and sweat within 10–20 minutes. However, the amount of the ingested fluid that enters the circulation to benefit the athlete depends on two factors: gastric emptying and intestinal absorption.

The ACSM position stand on fluid replacement during exercise focuses mainly on replacing fluid losses during exercise in the heat, and the related recommendations are presented later in this section.

What factors influence gastric emptying and intestinal absorption?

In a later section we will discuss factors, such as palatability, that may influence how much fluid you drink during exercise. For any fluid to be of benefit during exercise, it must first empty from the stomach and then be absorbed into the bloodstream from the intestines.

Gastric Emptying A number of factors may influence the gastric emptying rate, including volume, solute or caloric density, osmolality, drink temperature, exercise intensity, mode of exercise, and dehydration.

Volume is one of the most important factors affecting gastric emptying. In a review, Gisolfi noted that the larger the volume of fluid ingested, up to approximately 700 milliliters, the greater the rate of gastric emptying. However, large volumes consumed during exercise may cause discomfort to the athlete because of abdominal distention.

Although some preliminary data by Murray and others indicated that an 8 percent GES, as compared to 0, 4, and 6 percent GES, decreased gastric emptying, the decrease was only 6 ounces over 90 minutes. Gant and others compared a CES (6.2 percent) with flavored water during repetitive sprint performance of male soccer players over 60 minutes and reported no differences in gastric emptying. Other studies have shown that GES up to 8 percent carbohydrate had no adverse effect on gastric emptying of fluids, a finding in accord with the ACSM position stand on fluid replacement during exercise. Thus, 6 to 8 percent carbohydrate solutions may provide the athlete with the best of both worlds, water and carbohydrate. However, solutions with higher concentrations, particularly above 10 percent, may impair gastric emptying. The mechanism is not known, but may be related to the effects of carbohydrate on osmolality.

Fluids with a higher osmolality generally inhibit gastric emptying. Adding electrolytes and carbohydrates to fluids increases their osmolality, and Gisolfi indicated that this effect may be attributed mostly to the carbohydrate content. Although glucose polymers have a lesser effect on osmolality than glucose, some investigators have observed little difference in gastric emptying of fluids that had marked differences in osmotic pressure created by adding electrolytes, glucose, or glucose polymers. Nevertheless, more recent research has found that some hypotonic glucose polymers emptied from the stomach more rapidly than hypertonic solutions, about 80 percent faster in the first 10 minutes. In general, cold fluids empty rapidly and may also help cool the body core.

Moderate exercise intensity facilitates emptying, whereas intense exercise greater than 70–75 percent VO_2 max has been reported to exert an inhibitory effect. Little difference is noted in gastric emptying between cycling and running during the first hour even at an exercise intensity of 75 percent VO_2 max, but some research suggests that more fluids appear to be emptied during the later stages of prolonged cycling.

Ryan and others noted that hypohydration to approximately 3 percent of body weight does not impair gastric emptying. However, excessive dehydration may inhibit gastric emptying, and may be associated with gastric discomfort experienced by some athletes who consume large amounts of fluids during prolonged exercise in warm environmental conditions.

Intestinal Absorption Factors affecting intestinal absorption of ingested fluids during exercise have not been studied as extensively as gastric emptying, but several important findings have been presented by key investigators in this area, particularly Carl Gisolfi. The review by Murray and Shi presents a detailed review of gastrointestinal system functions during exercise and fluid intake.

Gisolfi indicated that the absorptive capacity of the intestines is not likely to limit the effectiveness of an oral rehydration solution. Water is absorbed fairly readily by passive diffusion, and theoretically water absorption may actually be helped by concurrent absorption of glucose and sodium. As highlighted in figure 9.10(a), glucose and sodium interact in the intestinal wall; glucose stimulates sodium absorption, and sodium is necessary for glucose absorption. When glucose and sodium are absorbed, these solutes tend to pull fluid with them via an osmotic effect, thus facilitating the absorption of water from the intestine into the circulation. However, research by Hargreaves and others noted

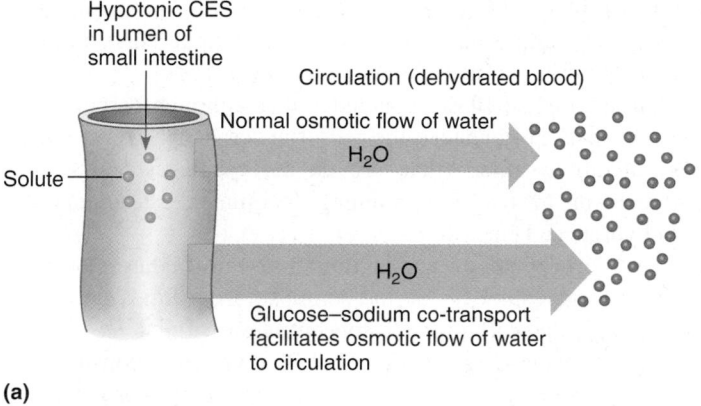

(a)

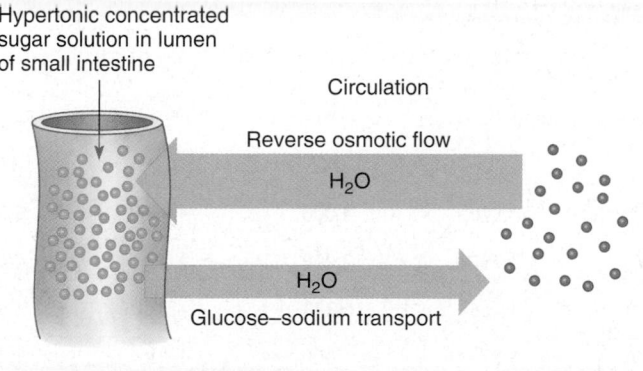

(b)

FIGURE 9.10 (*a*) Water normally diffuses from the intestine to the circulation via osmosis. Glucose and sodium in a CES enhance osmosis, as shown by the larger arrow. (*b*) A hypertonic solution may actually reverse osmosis, moving fluid from the circulatory system to the intestines, possibly leading to gastrointestinal distress symptoms such as diarrhea.

that beverage sodium content of either 0, 25, or 50 mmol per liter had no effect on plasma glucose levels during exercise. Gisolfi indicated that the intestines themselves contain enough sodium from body fluids, so that adding sodium to the rehydration solution provides no additional benefits. Gisolfi and others also noted no difference in intestinal fluid absorption or plasma volume changes during exercise when consuming either a hypotonic or isotonic 6 percent carbohydrate beverage with or without sodium. Murray and Shi noted that when compared to a single form of carbohydrate, using multiple, different forms, such as glucose, fructose, and polymers, enhanced intestinal absorption of water. Each form of carbohydrate may have its own receptor for absorption and pull water with it.

However, as discussed in chapter 4, excess carbohydrate in the intestine may cause a reverse osmotic effect, as depicted in figure 9.10(b). Highly concentrated sugars in the intestine draw water from the blood, leading to gastrointestinal distress with symptoms such as abdominal cramping and diarrhea. In her review, Leslie Bonci notes that this may be one of the problems associated with some of the "energy" drinks available, as they may be too highly concentrated with simple sugars. Distance runners have coined the term *Runner's Trots* to characterize one of the adverse effects.

Whether exercise impairs intestinal absorption is controversial. High-intensity exercise may compromise blood flow to the intestine, which might impair absorption. Gisolfi, in his review, noted some of the methodological difficulties in studying this problem, citing studies showing that exercise either reduced or had no effect on intestinal absorption.

It should be noted that individual differences in both gastric emptying and intestinal absorption may be significant. In reviewing studies of gastric emptying, Costill noted some subjects could empty 80–90 percent of the ingested solution in 15–20 minutes, whereas others emptied only 10 percent. As noted previously, some subjects may also develop diarrhea caused by ineffective intestinal absorption of fluids. Training to drink during exercise is recommended as a possible means of enhancing tolerance to consuming larger amounts of fluids. For endurance athletes, training your stomach to handle fluids during exercise is an important consideration.

How should carbohydrate be replaced during exercise in the heat?

The value of carbohydrate intake during exercise as a means to improve performance was detailed in chapter 4, primarily in relationship to performance in a cool environment. Keep in mind that carbohydrate intake may be useful primarily in prolonged exercise, under conditions where one is exercising at a high level of intensity for an hour or more. Carbohydrate is the primary fuel during such exercise tasks, and research suggests that warm environmental conditions may accelerate the use of muscle glycogen. Thus, carbohydrate intake may also improve performance during exercise in the heat, but if temperature regulation is of prime importance, water replacement should receive top priority. Hence, one of the goals of researchers has been to develop a fluid that will help replace carbohydrate during exercise in the heat without affecting water absorption. As discussed previously, carbohydrate-electrolyte solutions have been developed for this purpose.

Research indicates that an appropriate amount of carbohydrate in solution may maintain body temperature as effectively as water and may enhance performance during prolonged exercise. Water and carbohydrate complement each other to improve physical performance. In a unique study, Fritzsche and others, from Coyle's laboratory at the University of Texas, investigated the individual and combined effects of water and carbohydrate intake on power, thermoregulation, cardiovascular function, and metabolism in endurance-trained cyclists exercising for 2 hours in a hot environment. They found that although water alone attenuated the decline in power, ingestion of water with carbohydrate was even more effective. Similar findings have been reported for exercise tests of about an hour duration. Below and others found that water alone and carbohydrate alone improved 1-hour cycling performance in the heat, but the beneficial effects were additive when both were consumed. Mindy Millard-Stafford also reported that a carbohydrate solution, in comparison to water alone, improved performance in highly trained runners in a 15-kilometer run.

Scores of studies have compared the effectiveness of different carbohydrate combinations and concentrations in enhancing physical performance during prolonged endurance tasks. Most of this research is discussed in chapter 4. The following are the pertinent general findings relative to CES intake during prolonged exercise under warm environmental conditions.

In general, CESs between 5 to 10 percent seem to empty from the stomach as effectively as water during prolonged exercise in a hot environment, a finding supported by Rogers and others. They may possibly also be absorbed more readily from the intestinal tract. No significant adverse effects of these solutions upon plasma volume, sweat rate, or temperature regulation, when compared to water ingestion, have been observed. Actually, they may help maintain plasma volume, liver glycogen, and blood glucose levels during prolonged exercise, and, as noted, most investigators report that carbohydrate intake during exercise enhances endurance capacity in a variety of prolonged tasks in the heat.

Numerous studies from Asker Jeukendrup's laboratory at the University of Birmingham have shown that using a mixture of carbohydrates may be the best choice. Jentjens and others reported that ingestion of a glucose/fructose drink (1.0 g/0.5 g per minute), as compared to a glucose drink (1.5 g per minute) increased exogenous carbohydrate oxidation rates approximately 36 percent. Other studies from Jeukendrup's laboratory suggest that about 1.5–1.7 grams of carbohydrate per minute may be oxidized if a mixture of carbohydrates, such as glucose, fructose and sucrose, is used.

Although higher concentrations of carbohydrates deliver more glucose to the intestine, solutions higher than 10–12 percent may significantly delay gastric emptying, decrease intestinal absorption, and possibly cause gastrointestinal distress, as noted previously. High concentrations of fructose in some fruit juices or juice blends may be particularly debilitating. However, ultraendurance athletes may experiment with higher concentrations of carbohydrate in training and may adapt to such concentrated solutions for use during competition. In a case study, Alice Lindeman noted that one cyclist involved in the Race Across America (RAAM) consumed a 23 percent carbohydrate solution with no gastrointestinal problems. In such competitions, where cyclists may ride 20 hours or more a day, such high carbohydrate concentrations may be necessary to meet the high energy demands.

In brief, Louise Burke concludes that although carbohydrate ingestion may not enhance the performance of all events undertaken in hot weather, there are no disadvantages to the consumption of beverages containing recommended amounts of carbohydrate and electrolytes.

The ACSM position stand on fluid replacement during exercise includes some guidelines on the composition of fluids to be consumed, including carbohydrate concentration.

Table 9.6 calculates the amount of fluid you must consume, for a given concentration, to obtain 30–100 grams of carbohydrate.

TABLE 9.6 Fluid consumption (milliliters) at a given percent carbohydrate concentration to obtain desired grams of carbohydrate

Percent concentration	Grams of carbohydrate delivered							
	30	40	50	60	70	80	90	100
2%	1,500	2,000	2,500	3,000	3,500	4,000	4,500	5,000
4%	750	1,000	1,250	1,500	1,750	2,000	2,250	2,500
6%	500	666	833	1,000	1,166	1,333	1,500	1,666
8%	375	500	625	750	875	1,000	1,125	1,250
10%	300	400	500	600	700	800	900	1,000
12%	250	333	417	500	583	667	750	833
15%	225	300	375	450	525	600	675	750
20%	150	200	250	300	350	400	450	500

For example, if you wanted to get 60 grams of carbohydrate per hour, you would need to drink 1 liter (1,000 ml) of a 6 percent solution, but only one-half liter (500 ml) of a 12 percent solution. Additional strategies for carbohydrate intake before and after exercise are presented in chapter 4.

How should electrolytes be replaced during or following exercise?

Because the major solid component of sweat consists of electrolytes, considerable research has been conducted relative to the need for replacement of these lost nutrients, primarily sodium and potassium. We shall look at this question from two points of view, one dealing with the need for replacement during exercise and the other involving daily replacement.

During Exercise   Because sweat is hypotonic to the body fluids, the concentration of electrolytes in the blood and other body fluids actually increases during exercise and makes the body fluids hypertonic. Thus, electrolyte replacement during moderately prolonged exercise is not necessary. In a study of cyclists who exercised 90 minutes at 60 percent VO_2 max, Sanders and others concluded that a 40 millimole sodium solution (Gatorade is about 20 millimole), compared to plain water, may not be of much advantage to athletes who practice normal fluid replacement during such exercise tasks. Several studies have reported that even during strenuous prolonged exercise with high levels of sweat losses, like marathon running for several hours, water alone is the recommended fluid replacement to help maintain electrolyte balance, although added carbohydrate may provide some needed energy.

However, electrolyte replacement, particularly sodium, may be necessary for some athletes participating in very prolonged bouts of physical activity, such as marathons, ultramarathons, Ironman-type triathlons, or tennis tournaments where one might play off and on all day. A number of medical case studies following such events have reported complications resulting from an electrolyte imbalance in the blood, which is the topic of a subsequent question.

Daily Replacement   In general, heavy daily sweat losses do not lead to an electrolyte deficiency. If body levels of sodium and potassium begin to decrease, the kidneys begin to reabsorb more of these minerals and less are excreted in the urine. Research has shown that water alone, in combination with a balanced diet, will adequately maintain proper body electrolyte levels from day to day, even when an individual is exercising and is losing large amounts of sweat.

However, if electrolytes are not adequately replaced because of poor dietary intake, a deficit may occur over 4–7 days of very hard training, especially in hot environmental conditions where fluid losses will tend to be high. Thus, in a review, Maughan noted that exercising individuals who experience heavy daily sweat losses need both adequate fluids and sodium to ensure adequate rehydration. For such individuals, adding salt to meals and drinks may help. Ray and others reported that consuming high-sodium foods, such as chicken broth or chicken noodle soup, improved fluid retention following dehydration. The sodium is needed in the body to help retain water and maintain normal osmotic pressures.

A good method of checking on the adequacy of fluid replenishment on a day-to-day basis is to check your body weight in the morning; it should be nearly the same every day. If you weigh several pounds less from one day to the next, it is likely that you are hypohydrated. Conversely, if you weigh several pounds more, you may be overhydrated.

What is hyponatremia and what causes it during exercise?

Hyponatremia is a condition of subnormal levels of sodium in the blood. It can occur at rest simply by consuming too much water, and may also be known as *water intoxication*. Hyponatremia can also occur following prolonged exercise, in which case it may be known as *exercise-associated hyponatremia (EAH)*. An international consensus conference on EAH defined it as a serum sodium concentration below the normal reference range, or less than 135 mmol/liter. Milder forms are 130–134 mmol/liter and may be asymptomatic, but not always. Signs and symptoms of mild hyponatremia usually occur when serum sodium goes below 130 mmol/liter and may include the following:

- Bloating
- Puffiness of hands and feet
- Nausea
- Vomiting
- Headache

Severe cases, below 120 mmol/liter, may cause massive brain swelling, which may be associated with the following:

- Seizures
- Coma
- Respiratory arrest
- Permanent brain damage
- Death

In a study from a Boston marathon, Almond and others tested 488 runners following the race; 13 percent, or one in eight, had a serious fluid and salt imbalance from drinking too much water or sports drinks, and one 28-year-old woman died from hyponatremia. In addition to affecting endurance athletes exercising in the heat, according to Rogers and Hew-Butler, EAH has been documented in hikers, climbers, trekkers, and cold-climate endurance athletes. Treatment of individuals with symptomatic hyponatremia is a medical emergency, and transportation to a hospital is essential. Infusion of hypertonic solutions may be necessary.

Various risk factors have been identified that predispose individuals to development of EAH in marathons and other endurance events, including the following:

- Excessive drinking of fluids before, during, and after the event
- Considerable weight gain over the course of the event
- Slower finishers
- Females
- Low body weight

- Heat-unacclimatized, poorly trained competitors
- High sweat sodium losses
- Race inexperience
- NSAID use; altered kidney functions to excrete fluids

Hyponatremia may be caused by water dilution, excess sodium losses, or both. The EAH consensus conference committee indicated that dilutional hyponatremia, caused by an increase in total body water relative to the amount of total body sodium, is the current etiology of EAH. The ACSM, in its position stand on fluid replacement, indicates that fluid consumption that exceeds sweating rate is the primary factor leading to exercise-associated hyponatraemia. Additionally, factors that normally control body water balance, mainly hormones and the kidney, may malfunction. Nonsteroidal anti-inflammatory drugs (NSAIDs) interfere with normal kidney function. Wharam and others reported that Ironman triathletes using NSAIDs experienced significantly lower serum sodium levels upon completion of an Ironman triathlon.

Many of these factors may interact to contribute to the development of EAH. For example, females may be of lower body weight, generally run slower marathon times than males, may be more conscientious about consuming fluids given the old adage *to drink as much as you can,* and thus have more time to consume more fluids and gain proportionately more weight. The weight gain is water, which dilutes the serum sodium concentration. The ACSM advises athletes to not excessively overhydrate during and after exercise, the main contributing factor to hyponatremia.

Although sports drinks do contain some sodium, the EAH consensus committee notes that ingesting sports drinks does not prevent the development of EAH in athletes who drink to excess, because all such drinks are hypotonic. Indeed, sports drinks are constituted to be palatable so athletes will drink more. In a recent study, Passe and others reported that exercising individuals consumed more fluid as sport drinks as compared to water and orange juice. However, the EAH consensus committee did note some studies showing that consuming sports drinks can decrease the severity of EAH.

Twenty milliequivalents (20 mEq; 20 mmol/liter) of sodium may be found in some commercial sports drinks, but research by Barr and others suggests that this amount may be inadequate to prevent a decrease in plasma sodium during prolonged exercise in the heat. Higher amounts approaching the salt content of sweat (about 30–50 mEq per liter) have been suggested by Nancy Rehrer. In their study, Twerenbold and others reported that consuming sodium, in a solution approximating 30 mEq (680 milligrams/liter), minimized hyponatremia in female endurance athletes running for 4 hours; two athletes in the water control trial developed hyponatremia (<130 mmol serum sodium). Anatasiou and colleagues investigated the effectiveness of sports drinks with different sodium content to prevent hyponatremia. They found that if sports drinks were consumed at a rate equal to body mass change, a relatively small amount of sodium (19.9 mmol/l) was effective in preventing the decrease in plasma sodium frequently seen when sodium-free beverages are consumed during exercise in the heat. Some commercial sports drinks may contain higher amounts of sodium. For example, the Gatorade Endurance Hydration Formula contains more than 800 milligrams of sodium per liter, or about 35 mEq. The point should be stressed, however, that although sports drinks may help replace some lost sodium, drinking to excess may still lead to hyponatremia.

Treatment for hyponatremia varies. Chorley recommends that for mild symptomatic hyponatremia, drinking of hypotonic fluids should be restricted until the athlete is urinating. Hypertonic solutions may be provided if the athlete can drink fluids. For severe hyponatremia, intravenous sodium chloride solutions will speed recovery and improve outcomes. Athletes who do not recover rapidly should be sent to the nearest medical emergency facility.

Individual differences may dictate who may be prone to developing hyponatremia during prolonged exercise, but given the current evidence, it appears that athletes involved in ultraendurance events should consume adequate salt in their diet the days before competition to help assure normal serum sodium levels and consume fluids with added sodium during the event. More research is needed to help refine current recommendations. In the meantime, experiment with salty solutions during practice. You can carry some fluids with you in competition, and in others you may have personal beverages located at specific aid stations on the course.

www.overhydration.info **The International Exercise-Associated Hyponatremia Registry contains educational materials on EAH and preventative strategies for those engaged in endurance exercise.**

Are salt tablets or potassium supplements necessary?

In general, the use of salt tablets to replace lost electrolytes, primarily sodium, is not necessary. As noted, an adequate diet will replace, on a daily basis, electrolytes lost in sweat.

The concentrations of salt in sweat may vary. Some individuals who have a high amount of salt in their sweat are sometimes referred to as "salty sweaters." According to Maughan and Shirreffs, a rough self-assessment may be done by wearing a black t-shirt during exercise and looking for salt stains when the sweat has evaporated. We have noted previously that the average salt concentration may be about 3.2 grams of salt per liter, although there are reports as high as 4.5 grams per liter in unacclimatized individuals, and as low as 1.75 grams per liter in the heat-acclimatized individual. Because salt is 40 percent sodium and 60 percent chloride, the sodium content in 3.2 grams of salt is 1.3 grams, in 4.5 grams of salt is 1.8 grams, and in 1.75 grams of salt is 0.7 gram. If an athlete lost about 8–9 pounds of body fluids during an exercise period, a total of 4 liters of fluid (about 4 quarts) would be lost because a liter weighs 2.2 pounds. Four liters of sweat would contain, at the most, 7.2 grams of sodium in the unacclimatized individual, but less than 3 grams in one who was acclimatized. Because the average meal contains about 2–3 grams of sodium if well salted, three meals a day would offer 6–9 grams, about enough to just cover the losses in the sweat. However, sodium is lost through other means, primarily in the urine; thus, a slight increase in sodium intake may be reasonable for the unacclimatized athlete. Doug Hiller, a physician who has worked extensively with endurance athletes, suggests that during the week or two of acclimatization to exercising in the heat, athletes should consume about 10–25 grams of salt daily, or 4–10 grams of sodium. Consuming more high-sodium foods or a more liberal salting of the food should provide an adequate amount; 1 teaspoon of salt contains about 5 grams of salt, or 2 grams of sodium. Although this recommendation is much greater than the UL of 2.3 grams recommended by the National Academy of Sciences, that recommendation is based on the sedentary individual, not an athlete losing copious amounts of sodium during a period of acclimatization. However, once an athlete is acclimatized to the heat, sodium intake may be reduced to normal.

Common salt tablets contain only sodium and chloride. They are not necessary to replace lost sodium but may be recommended for unacclimatized athletes who do not replace sodium through normal dietary means in the early stages of an acclimatization program. Salt tablets should be taken only if the athlete loses substantial amounts of weight via sweat losses during a workout. Checking the body weight before and after a workout provides a good estimate of sweat loss. If we switch to the English system, 1 quart of sweat equals 2 pounds; one-half quart, or a pint, is 1 pound. One recommendation is that salt tablets should be taken only if the athlete needs to drink more than 4 quarts of fluid per day to replace that lost during sweating; that is, an 8-pound weight loss. The general rule is to take two salt tablets with each additional quart of fluid beyond the 4 quarts; this would be equal to 1 gram of sodium (the average tablet has one-half gram of sodium) per quart. Another way to look at it is to take one pint of water with every salt tablet. The use of salt tablets should be discontinued after the athlete is acclimatized, usually about 6–9 days.

Potassium supplements are not recommended—for several reasons. First, research by David Costill and his associates has revealed that a deficiency of potassium is rare, even with large sweat losses and a diet low in potassium. Second, as noted previously, excessive potassium may be lethal as it can disturb the electrical rhythm of the heart. The moderate use of substitutes, such as potassium chloride for common table salt, may be helpful in assuring potassium replacement, but investigators recommended particular attention to the diet, citing citrus fruits and bananas as two of the many foods high in potassium. For example, a large glass of orange juice will replace the potassium lost in 2 liters of sweat.

What are some prudent guidelines relative to fluid replacement while exercising under warm or hot environmental conditions?

In sport nutrition, no other area has received as much research attention as the objective of determining the optimal formulation of an oral rehydration solution (sports drink) for individuals doing prolonged exercise under warm or hot environmental conditions. This may be because water and carbohydrates are two nutrients that may enhance performance in such events, and water and electrolytes may also help to prevent heat-related illnesses. As discussed previously in relation to the need for fluid, carbohydrate, or electrolytes, a number of factors—in particular, the intensity and duration of the exercise task, the prevailing environmental conditions,

and individual differences in sweat rate, gastric emptying, and intestinal absorption—may influence the desired composition of the sports drink. Given these considerations, many of the leading investigators in exercise-hydration research indicate that there is no agreement on the optimal formulation of an oral rehydration solution that would suit the needs of all individuals who engage in a variety of prolonged exercise tasks. Indeed, as noted previously, the ACSM identified the individual's unique biological characteristics as a factor affecting hydration status and exercise performance.

Through their concerted research efforts over the years, sports scientists such as Louise Burke, Edward Coyle, Ronald Maughan, Timothy Noakes, Michael Sawka, and Scott Montain have provided us with a sound basis to promote prudent recommendations regarding fluid replacement before, during, and after exercise. The latest guidelines on fluid replacement for exercise have been published by the ACSM, which serve as the basis for these prudent recommendations.

journals.lww.com/acsm-msse **Access the American College of Sports Medicine 2007 position stand on fluid replacement by clicking on the link for ACSM Position Stands and Joint Position Statements.**

Before Competition and Practice The goal of the ACSM guidelines is to start in a state of euhydration with normal plasma electrolyte levels. Unfortunately, not all athletes come to practice adequately hydrated. Osterberg and colleagues examined pregame hydration in players from five teams in the National Basketball Association and found that 52 percent began the game dehydrated. National Collegiate Athletic Association Division I athletes were assessed for their prepractice hydration status by Volpe and others. They found that 66 percent of the college athletes hypohydrated prior to practice, with a greater percentage of men in a hypohydrated state compared to women. Here are some key points:

1. Be sure you are adequately hydrated the day before competition. Minimize consumption of alcoholic beverages the night before competition, for they may lead to hypohydration in the morning.
2. Drink slowly about 5–7 milliliters/kilogram (0.08–0.11 ounce/pound) body weight at least 4 hours prior to exercise.
   - Fluid palatability (temperature, sodium, flavoring) will enhance fluid intake.
   - If the exercise task is to be prolonged, carbohydrate may be added. A concentration of 6–8 percent is advisable, but concentrations of 20 percent and higher have been used by some individuals without adverse effects.
   - Beverages with sodium (20–50 mEq/L) and/or salty foods or snacks will help stimulate thirst and retain fluids.
3. If no urine is produced, or urine is dark or highly concentrated, drink another 3–5 ml/kg body weight about 2 hours prior to exercise. Your urine should be a clear pale yellow before competition or practice.
4. Do not excessively overhydrate, which may increase the risk of dilutional hyponatremia if fluids are aggressively replaced during and after exercise.

www.urinecolors.com/dehydration.php Provides a Dehydration Urine Color Chart to help estimate your level of dehydration.

During Competition and Practice The goal of the ACSM guidelines is to prevent excessive dehydration (> 2 percent body weight loss from water deficit). The amount and rate of fluid replacement depends on individual sweating rate, exercise duration, and opportunities to rehydrate. Here are some key considerations:

1. Individuals should monitor body weight changes during training/competition sessions to estimate fluid losses during a particular exercise task.

2. It is important to start rehydrating early in endurance events because thirst does not develop until about 1–2 percent of body weight has been lost. The ACSM guidelines recommend a possible starting point for marathon runners is to drink *ad libitum* about 0.4–0.8 liter of fluids per hour, smaller runners might consume 0.4 liter while bigger runners consume 0.8 liter. Consuming 0.4 liter (about 14 ounces) per hour could be accomplished by drinking 3–4 ounces every 15 minutes, while drinking about 7 ounces every 15 minutes would provide 0.8 liter per hour. These amounts may be adjusted to individual preferences and to increase carbohydrate content, as discussed later.

   It is important to realize that during periods of heavy sweating, it is very difficult to consume enough fluids to replace those lost. Costill has noted that, per minute, 50 milliliters or more of fluid may be lost though sweating (3 liters per hour), but only 20–30 milliliters per minute may be absorbed from the intestines. The sweating rate in this case simply outweighs the absorption of ingested fluids. Although some dehydration will occur, rehydration will help maintain circulatory stability and heat balance, thereby delaying deterioration of endurance capacity. Cheuvront and Haymes reported that replacing 60–70 percent of sweat losses helps to maintain thermoregulatory responses during hot and warm weather conditions. By calculating your typical sweat losses, as discussed on page 369 and determined in the Application Exercise at the end of this chapter, you may be able to estimate how much fluid you should consume per hour.

3. Cold water is effective when carbohydrate intake is of little or no concern, for example, in endurance events lasting less than 50–60 minutes. Sports drinks with 6–8 percent carbohydrates and normal electrolyte content may also be consumed but, in general, provide no advantages over water alone.

4. The composition of the fluid is considered important for prolonged endurance events. Carbohydrates and electrolytes may provide some advantages, and these components may be in the drink or nonfluid sources such as gels or energy bars. Palatability and the presence of other ingredients may also be important considerations.

   • Carbohydrate provides energy for longer duration events. If carbohydrate is desired in the drink, the concentration should not be excessive. A 6–10 percent concentration is recommended. Concentrations greater than 10–12 percent may retard gastric emptying and contribute to gastrointestinal distress. Use a sports drink containing multiple sources of carbohydrate, including glucose, sucrose, fructose, and maltodextrins. Such a mixture may enhance absorption and utilization of the exogenous carbohydrate, possibly up to 1.2–1.7 grams per minute. Check the food label for ingredients.

   The ACSM recommends that athletes consume enough fluid to provide about 30–80 grams of carbohydrate per hour. Similarly, Bob Murray indicates that the consumption of about 1 gram of carbohydrate per kilogram body weight per hour appears sufficient to improve performance in prolonged exercise. On average, sports drinks containing 6–8 percent carbohydrate provide about 2 grams of carbohydrate for every ounce of fluid consumed. Thus, you need to drink about 15–16 ounces of a sports drink per hour to obtain about 30 grams of carbohydrate, or about one liter per hour to obtain 60 grams. See table 9.6 for guidelines.

   It may be difficult for some athletes, such as marathon runners, to consume the amount of fluid during exercise to obtain the recommended grams of carbohydrate. Many runners do not consume a liter per hour, which is needed to provide 60 grams from a 6 percent sports drink. However, consuming other sources of carbohydrate with the sports drink, such as sports gels or sports beans, can provide the additional grams of carbohydrate.

   Athletes in prolonged, intermittent high-intensity sports, such as soccer, may use various rehydration procedures. Clarke and others provided the same total amount of a CES to soccer players during a 90-minute soccer specific protocol. In one trial, the CES was given at 0 and 45 minutes, while in a second trial it was provided in smaller volumes at 0, 15, 30, 45, 60, and 75 minutes. There were no differences in metabolic responses during the soccer protocol, and sprint power was not different, suggesting that the two methods of providing fluids were equally effective.

   • The fluid should contain small amounts of electrolytes, particularly sodium and potassium, to help replace lost electrolytes. The ACSM recommends about 20–30 mEq of sodium and 2–5 mEq of potassium, which are amounts present in many commercial sports drinks. However, for athletes involved in very prolonged endurance events under warm environmental conditions, some recommend a range of about 700–1,150 milligrams of sodium per liter (approximately 30–50 mmol per liter) and 120–225 milligrams of potassium per liter (approximately 3–6 mmol per liter). Some commercial sports drinks contain electrolytes comparable to this range. For example, for each 8-ounce serving, Gatorade Endurance Formula contains 200 milligrams of sodium and 90 milligrams of potassium, which is more than 800 milligrams of sodium (about 36 mmol) and 360 milligrams of potassium (about 10 mmol) per liter.

   • The fluid should be palatable and not interfere with normal gastrointestinal functions. Research has shown that the voluntary intake of fluids increases when they are tasty.

Being cold and sweet enhances palatability. In contrast, Lambert and others noted that subjects exercising in the heat consumed less fluid when it was carbonated, suggesting a lower palatability compared to noncarbonated beverages. Carbonated beverages do not appear to inhibit gastric emptying, nor does the use of the artificial sweetener aspartame, but Zachwieja and others noted that certain flavorings, such as citric acid, may impair gastric emptying by as much as 25 percent.

- Caffeine is found in some sports drinks and may help sustain performance. Detailed information on caffeine and exercise performance is presented in chapter 13. In brief, however, caffeine supplementation appears to be an effective ergogenic aid for aerobic endurance performance, and its use is currently not prohibited by the World Anti-Doping Agency (WADA). Moreover, caffeinated sports drinks maintain hydration and metabolic and thermoregulatory functions as well as standard sports drinks.

- Some sports drinks include protein, but they do not appear to enhance performance more than typical CESs. Van Essen and Gibala, in a well-designed study, compared the effects of a carbohydrate/protein drink (6 percent with 2 percent protein added) to a carbohydrate drink (6 percent) on performance of well-trained cyclists in a laboratory 80-kilometer time trial. Although performance time was significantly faster with the two sports drinks, as compared to the placebo, there was no difference between them. As noted in chapter 6, other studies have not reported performance enhancement associated with protein-containing CESs when compared to typical CESs. However, several studies, such as that by Bird and others, did provide evidence suggestive of reduced muscle tissue damage. Review pages 231–232 for details.

After Competition and Practice The goal of the ACSM guidelines is to fully replace any fluid and electrolyte deficit. Replacement may have to be rapid, such as in preparation for a subsequent exercise endeavor on the same day. For example, tennis players may compete in two or more events daily with a short recovery period, while some athletes may also train twice daily. In other situations, fluid replacement may be more leisurely if time permits.

1. If time is short to the next exercise session, aggressive rehydration is important.
   - Drink 1.5 liter of fluid for every kilogram of body weight loss, or about 1.5 pints for each pound loss. The additional fluid is needed to compensate for increased urine output.
   - Consume adequate carbohydrates and electrolytes as well. Fruit juices and sports drinks are helpful when you need to replenish both fluids and carbohydrates. Pretzels and other salty snacks may provide sodium, as well as carbohydrate. This may be especially important for competition. Osterberg and others found that the inclusion of carbohydrate (3 percent, 6 percent, and 12 percent) to an electrolyte beverage enhanced the retention of fluid following exercise-induced dehydration. Bilzon and others found that

provided adequate hydration status is maintained, inclusion of carbohydrate within an oral rehydration solution will delay the onset of fatigue in subsequent prolonged exercise.
   - Some preliminary research suggests that consuming a sports drink with protein may help. Seifert and others reported that a CES with protein, as compared to a CES and water, restored more fluids in a 3-hour recovery period following a 2.5 percent dehydration; the protein solution helped retain 88 percent, the carbohydrate 75 percent, and water only 53 percent.

2. If recovery time permits (24 hours), normal meal and water intake will restore euhydration, provided sodium intake is adequate. Nancy Rehrer also notes that sodium is necessary in the recovery period to restore fluid balance.
   - A diet rich in wholesome, natural foods adhering to healthy eating practices will help replenish needed electrolytes.
   - Sodium replacement is important, particularly if your sweat contains significant amounts. Check your skin and clothing for traces of dried salt after exercise; if white streaks occur, you may be losing substantial amounts of sodium during exercise.
   - Extra salt may be added to meals when sodium losses are high.
   - Drink fluids with added sodium or consume salty foods or snacks.

3. Minimize alcohol intake. Shirreffs and Maughan noted that drinks containing 4 percent alcohol or more, such as beer, tend to delay the recovery process, as measured by restoration of blood and plasma volume.

In Training

1. Practice consuming fluids while you train. Use a trial-and-error approach. Some research indicates that consuming CESs during training, particularly high-intensity training, may result in a more effective workout, which could lead to better performance in competition. By consuming various formulations while you train, particularly during training comparable to the intensity and duration experienced in competition, you will be able to determine what fluids work specifically for you. Consuming fluids during training may help you overcome some of the factors that inhibit fluid intake during exercise, such as the uncomfortable sensation of fluid in the stomach, and lead to increased fluid intake during competition. This is especially important for older athletes, who tend to drink less than their younger counterparts.

2. If you sip sports drinks throughout the day to stay hydrated, be sure to practice sound dental hygiene. As noted in chapter 4, some research has shown that sports drinks may exert significant eroding effects on dental enamel.

A summary of guidelines for fluid, carbohydrate, and electrolyte replacement during exercise under warm environmental conditions is presented in table 9.7. In brief, the ACSM guidelines present three key points to prevent hypohydration during exercise. Hydrate well before the exercise task; drink according to your personal

TABLE 9.7 Fluid intake guidelines before, during, and after exercise in warm or hot environmental conditions

Before competition and practice

The goal of the ACSM guidelines is to start in a state of euhydration with normal plasma electrolyte levels.

- Drink slowly about 5–7 milliliters/kilogram (0.08–0.11 ounce/pound) body weight at least 4 hours prior to exercise. For an athlete weighing 70 kg (154 pounds), this would approximate 350–490 milliliters, or 12–17 ounces of fluids. Athletes weighing more or less will drink accordingly.
- Drink another 3–5 ml/kg body weight about 2 hours prior to exercise if no urine is produced or the urine is dark or highly concentrated. Your urine should be a clear pale yellow before competition or practice.
- Drink water. However, carbohydrate-electrolyte solutions (CESs) also may be used if preferred.
- Drink beverages with carbohydrate (6–8 percent) to help increase body stores of glucose and glycogen for use in prolonged exercise bouts.
- Drink beverages with sodium (20–50 mEq/L) and/or consume salty foods or snacks to help increase body stores of sodium and water for prolonged exercise.
- Do not drink excessively, which may increase the risk of dilutional hyponatremia if fluids are aggressively replaced during and after exercise.

During competition and practice

The goal of the ACSM guidelines is to prevent excessive dehydration (> 2% body weight loss from water deficit).

- Determine your sweat loss for a given intensity and duration of exercise in the heat. This will provide you with an estimate for fluid intake during exercise. A procedure is presented on page 369.
- Drink about 0.4 to 0.8 liters of fluids per hour, which is about 14 to 28 ounces. Smaller athletes may consume 14 ounces or about 3–4 ounces every 15 minutes. Larger athletes my consume 28 ounces, or about 7 ounces every 15 minutes. However, the fluids may be consumed at your pleasure, or adlibitum, on other time schedules as conditions permit. Athletes can adjust the amounts according to personal needs.
- Drink cold water when carbohydrate intake is of little or no concern, such as in endurance events of less than 50–60 minutes. CESs may be consumed during such events if preferred, but provide no advantages over water alone.
- Drink fluids with carbohydrates for longer-duration events.
  - Select a CES with a 6–8 percent concentration.
  - Use a CES containing multiple sources of carbohydrate, including glucose, sucrose, fructose, and maltodextrins.
  - Consume enough fluid to provide about 30–80 grams of carbohydrate per hour. One ounce of a CES provides about 2 grams of carbohydrate.
  - Use sports gels or sports beans to provide additional carbohydrate if the necessary fluid intake would be unreasonable. Sports gels and beans may provide about 25–30 grams of carbohydrate per serving.
- Drink fluids with small amounts of electrolytes, particularly sodium and potassium. Many CESs contain about 20–30 mEq of sodium and 2–5 mEq of potassium, which amounts to about 110–160 grams of sodium and 19–45 grams of potassium in an 8-ounce serving.

After competition and practice

The goal of the ACSM guidelines is to fully replace any fluid and electrolyte deficit.

- Rapid replacement
  - Drink 1.5 liter of fluid for every kilogram of body weight loss, or about 1.5 pints for each pound loss.
  - Consume about 1.0 to 1.5 grams of carbohydrate per kilogram body weight (about 0.5 to 0.7 grams per pound body weight) each hour for 3–4 hours. For a 60-kg athlete, this would represent about 60–90 grams of carbohydrate per hour.
  - Consume adequate sodium. Salty carbohydrate snacks, such as pretzels, may provide both sodium and carbohydrate.
- Leisurely replacement (24-hour recovery)
  - Eat a diet rich in wholesome, natural foods adhering to healthy eating practices to help replenish needed electrolytes.
  - Extra salt may be added to meals when sodium losses are high.
  - Drink fluids with added sodium or consume salty foods or snacks.

These guidelines have been adapted from the position stand on fluid replacement developed by the American College of Sports Medicine. The guidelines are appropriate for athletes competing or training for endurance or high-intensity intermittent sports, such as 10-kilometer races, marathons and ultramarathons, endurance cycling races, Olympic- to Ironman-distance triathlons, soccer and field hockey games, and tennis matches. These guidelines are approximations and may be modified based on individual preferences derived through personal experience in both training and competition. See text for additional information.

needs; and rehydrate rapidly in preparation for subsequent exercise bouts on the same day, or more leisurely if recovery time permits. Use of sports drinks may be helpful. In their review, Coombes and Hamilton concluded that in studies where a practical protocol has been used along with a currently available sports beverage (less than 10 percent carbohydrate solutions), there is evidence to suggest that consuming a sports drink will improve performance compared with consuming a placebo beverage.

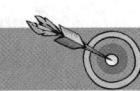

Key Concepts

▶ Hyperhydration before exercise is important, but rehydration is the most important nutritional consideration when exercising in the heat.
▶ Rehydration with cold water is effective in moderating body temperature during exercise in the heat, but carbohydrate

solutions may be equally effective and also provide a source of energy for more prolonged endurance exercise.

▶ An effective rehydration solution is one that optimizes gastric emptying and intestinal absorption of fluid.

▶ Electrolyte replacement generally is not needed during exercise, but may be helpful during very prolonged exercise tasks. Water alone, in combination with a balanced diet including adequate sodium and potassium, will adequately restore normal electrolyte levels in the body on a day-to-day basis.

▶ Current research suggests that 6–10 percent solutions of glucose, fructose, sucrose, glucose polymers, or combinations of these different carbohydrates, may be effective for athletes who need carbohydrate replacement during exercise.

▶ Excessive fluid consumption during very prolonged exercise, coupled with inadequate salt intake, may contribute to hyponatremia, a potentially dangerous condition.

▶ One ounce of a typical 6–8 percent carbohydrate-electrolyte solution (CES) contains about 2 grams of carbohydrate. Drinking 20 ounces of a CES per hour during exercise will provide about 40 grams of carbohydrate.

▶ Individuals who desire to rehydrate rapidly following exercise should consume about 120–150 percent of the fluid lost. Added salt will help the body retain the ingested fluids.

Ergogenic Aspects

If preventing or correcting a nutrient deficiency is seen as an ergogenic technique, then certainly water could be construed to be an ergogenic aid. Compared to taking in no fluid during exercise, rehydration has been shown to enhance temperature regulation or exercise performance by optimizing hydration status. However, some athletes have attempted to lose body water for ergogenic purposes. Although we have seen that hypohydration generally does not improve performance, and indeed may actually impair performance in endurance-type events, certain athletes such as high jumpers may use drugs like diuretics to lose weight rapidly without losses in power. Research has shown that diuretic-induced weight losses may improve vertical jumping ability because the athlete can develop the same power to move a lower body weight. Detailed coverage of these drugs is beyond the scope of this text. Moreover, the use of diuretics is banned by most athletic governing bodies, such as the United States Olympic Committee and the National Collegiate Athletic Association.

Over the years, athletes have attempted to modify body water stores or body temperature using various ergogenic techniques, including supplementation with various nutrients, in attempts to enhance sport performance.

Does oxygen water enhance exercise performance?

Oxygen water, or water oxygenated before bottling, has been marketed to physically active individuals. One brand claims to be a *performance water,* suggesting that tests show that it positively affects cardiovascular and muscular performance and endurance. However, there is the question as to whether oxygen bound in water would actually be absorbed into the bloodstream for delivery to the muscles. Peer-reviewed research does not support marketing claims that oxygen water enhances energy and boosts athletic performance. For example, Hampson and others reported no effect of oxygenated water on oxygen consumption during exercise, and noted that the amount of oxygen contained in the bottle would last only about two seconds in an individual doing moderate exercise. Wing-Gaia and others theorized that oxygenated water might be more beneficial in an hypoxic environment, so they studied its effects on recreational cyclists who completed two cycling time trials in hypoxic conditions with either regular or oxygenated water. There was no significant effect on blood oxygenation, physiological responses, or cycling time-trial performance.

The available scientific evidence does not support an ergogenic effect of oxygen water.

Do pre-cooling techniques help reduce body temperature and enhance performance during exercise in the heat?

Pre-cooling may be an effective ergogenic strategy for some athletes competing in the heat, and there may be several possible reasons. For example, Sawka and Young indicated that cooling the skin will decrease skin blood flow, so theoretically more blood could be shuttled to the muscles during exercise. In their review, Quod and others reported that a number of pre-cooling methods have been used; the main theory is that an increased heat storage capacity will allow an athlete to complete a greater amount of work before a critical body temperature is reached. Research supports this viewpoint. Hunter and others tested the effects of wearing an ice-vest on body core temperatures of collegiate female distance runners participating in two major distance running events. The runners ingested radiotelemetry temperature sensors 4 hours before the race, and core temperature was monitored before and after the race. The investigators found that runners using the vest during the warm-up period, in comparison to runners not wearing the vest, experienced a significantly lower core temperature prior to the start and a lesser increase in core temperature at the finish.

Although not all studies have shown beneficial effects of body-cooling techniques on exercise performance, several have. For example, Yeargin and others reported that cold water immersion following 90 minutes of cross-country running improved performance in a 2-mile run. The authors noted that the research supports its potential role as an ergogenic aid in athletic performance. Uckert and Joch, in a crossover design, had subjects complete three treadmill runs to exhaustion (5 days apart) either after a 20-minute warm-up, after wearing a cooling vest for 20 minutes, or without any particular preparation (control). During the first 30 minutes of exercise, the heart rate, core temperature, and skin temperature were significantly lower after the pre-cooling than after the warm-up. The use of an ice-cooling vest also improved running performance. Webster and others evaluated the effect of a lightweight cooling vest on endurance running performance. The subjects wore the cooling vest during stretching and warm-up, but not during the running tests. The vest cooled the body core temperature by 0.5° Celsius and decreased sweat rate by approximately 10–23 percent during a 30-minute run at 70 percent of VO_2 max, and also improved endurance time by 49 seconds when running at 95 percent of VO_2 max.

Hunter and others reported that American and Australian athletes were provided with ice vests in the 2004 Olympic Games in Athens, where the environment was hot and humid. The vest appeared to be effective in keeping body temperatures down and improving the performance of the marathoners. Additional research is recommended for specific applications to athletes. For example, Castle and others found that leg cooling (ice bags to legs) improved peak power output in cycling more than total body or upper body cooling.

Does sodium loading enhance endurance performance?

An electrolyte deficiency could impair physical performance, but supplements above and beyond normal electrolyte nutrition have not been recommended for ergogenic purposes. However, sodium concentration is one of the main determinants of blood volume, acting like a sponge to attract water into the circulatory system. As Gledhill and others note, an increased blood volume may increase VO_2 max. Luetkemeier and others noted that ingestion, or infusion, of a saline solution before exercise (**sodium loading**) may expand the plasma volume, leading to cardiovascular responses that could benefit exercise performance, but at the time they also noted that such advantages have yet to be reported.

Subsequently, Sims and others studied the effect of sodium loading on the plasma volume and the physiological strain of moderately trained males running in the heat. In a crossover design, subjects consumed either a high-sodium (164 mmol/L) or low-sodium (10 mmol/L) beverage before running to exhaustion at 70 percent VO_2 max in warm conditions (32°C). About 0.75 liter was consumed over the course of 60 minutes, with an additional 45 minutes of rest before testing. The high sodium increased plasma volume before exercise, reduced ratings of perceived exertion during exercise, and involved greater time to exhaustion when stopped because of an ethical end point (core temperature at 39.5°C). The authors concluded that consuming the high-sodium beverage involved less thermoregulatory and perceived strain during exercise and increased exercise capacity in warm conditions. However, because subjects were stopped at a preestablished core body temperature, technically the subjects did not run to exhaustion. Nevertheless, the data are supportive of an ergogenic effect. Moreover, using a similar research protocol with trained female cyclists who cycled to exhaustion at 70 percent VO_2 max in warm conditions (32°C), Sims and others reported again that consumption of the high sodium beverage increased plasma volume, reduced thermoregulatory strain, and increased exercise performance.

These data are supportive of an ergogenic effect of sodium loading *before* exercising in a hot environment. In chapter 13,

sodium bicarbonate supplementation has been shown to enhance endurance performance in some studies when provided before exercise, which could be related to the sodium content in the bicarbonate preparation. However, consuming sodium tablets *during* exercise does not appear to enhance performance. Hew-Butler and others, in a study of more than 400 triathletes, reported no ergogenic effect from consuming additional sodium in tablet form (a total of 3.6 grams more than the placebo and control groups) on finishing time in Ironman competition.

Does glycerol supplementation enhance endurance performance during exercise under warm environmental conditions?

Glycerol, as noted in chapter 5, is an alcohol that combines with fatty acids to form a triglyceride. Years ago, glycerol had been studied as an ergogenic aid because it may be a source of energy during exercise or used as a substrate for gluconeogenesis. However, Massicotte and others reported that only a small portion, about 4 percent, of glycerol consumed during exercise is converted to glucose for oxidation or directly oxidized for energy. Results of studies have not supported an ergogenic effect of glycerol when used for its energy content.

More recently, however, glycerol supplementation has been studied in attempts to enhance endurance performance in warm environments. Glycerol has been combined with water during hyperhydration prior to exercise to study its potential ergogenic effects on performance in prolonged endurance events, often under warm environmental conditions. Theoretically, glycerol-induced hyperhydration will increase osmotic pressure in the body fluids, helping to retain more total body water and also possibly increase the plasma volume, factors that could enhance temperature regulation and exercise performance.

Various techniques have been used to hyperhydrate subjects with glycerol. The amount used was based on either the subject's body weight, lean body mass, or body-water content. On average, for each kilogram body weight, subjects consumed 1 gram of glycerol combined with about 20–25 milliliters of water. Thus, a 70-kilogram male would consume 70 grams of glycerol in about 1.4–1.75 liters of water or similar fluid. In some studies, glycerol was also provided with carbohydrate solutions. Glycerol-induced hyperhydration protocols were normally compared to water-induced hyperhydration techniques.

Research data are equivocal regarding the effects of glycerol-induced hyperhydration, compared to water-induced hyperhydration, on body-water levels. For example, Freund and his associates from the U.S. Army Research Institute of Environmental Medicine found that glycerol-induced hyperhydration as compared to water hyperhydration resulted in a greater retention of fluids in the body. The investigators noted that the glycerol helped to maintain the osmolality of the blood, leading to better preservation of serum ADH levels, which they suggested may have contributed to the lower urinary output of water. Conversely, using similar hyperhydration protocols, two reports by Latzka and others have not shown any advantage of glycerol-induced hyperhydration over water-induced hyperhydration on total body water. Overall, however, glycerol hyperhydration does appear to increase body water. Goulet and others conducted a meta-analysis of 14 studies and concluded that glycerol hyperhydration significantly increased body fluid retention compared to water rehydration.

Research data regarding the effects of glycerol-induced hyperhydration on temperature regulation and on performance are also equivocal. Lyons and others found that glycerol-induced hyperhydration was more effective than water-induced hyperhydration in reducing the thermal stress of moderate exercise in the heat. Montner and others reported that glycerol-induced hyperhydration significantly improved performance in a cycling endurance test to exhaustion at 65 percent VO_2 max in a neutral laboratory environment. The authors also noted a lower heart rate and rectal temperature response during the glycerol trial and speculated that the benefits were due to an increased plasma volume. Scheett and others found that, compared to water alone, glycerol hyperhydration significantly increased plasma volume restoration following dehydration and increased cycle exercise time to exhaustion in the heat. Anderson and others, using a standard glycerol hyperhydration protocol, studied its effects on a 15-minute cycling test following 1 hour of steady-state cycling in the heat at 98 percent of the lactate threshold. Compared to the placebo hyperhydration, the glycerol hyperhydration resulted in greater fluid retention, a lower heart rate, and a lower rectal temperature during the steady-state ride, and a significantly improved cycle test performance. The authors suggested that the improved performance resulted from reducing cardiovascular strain and enhancing thermoregulation. Kavouras and others evaluated the effects of a glycerol-induced hyperhydration on performance of eight highly trained male cyclists. Subjects were dehydrated about 4 percent of body weight by exercise and water restriction, and then rehydrated with water alone or a glycerol-water combination prior to cycling to exhaustion (74 percent VO_2 peak) in a hot and humid environment. Although the glycerol protocol did not provide any thermoregulatory benefits, it did increase plasma volume, which was associated with an increased cycling exercise time to exhaustion compared to the water trial. In a field study involving a crossover protocol, Coutts and others studied the effects of glycerol hyperhydration on competitive Olympic distance triathlon performance. The triathlon was conducted outdoors. The weather on the day of the first competitive triathlon was classified as hot (WBGT, 30.5°), while on the day of the second triathlon it was classified as warm (WBGT, 25.4°). The glycerol hyperhydration induced a significantly greater plasma expansion compared to the placebo, and the increase in the triathlon completion time between the hot and warm conditions was significantly less than the placebo trial. Based on this finding, the authors suggested that glycerol hyperhydration prior to triathlon competition in high ambient temperatures may provide some protection against the negative performance effect of competing in the heat. Although competitive field studies such as this one are important, the rather substantial temperature difference on the two days of competition may have confounded the results.

In contrast, Latzka and others reported that glycerol-induced hyperhydration did not affect sweating dynamics, body temperature, or physiological responses during exercise in two studies. In one of these studies, they reported that although glycerol-induced hyperhydration did improve exercise performance in the heat at 55 percent VO_2 max compared to control conditions, the improvement was not significantly greater than that noted in the water-induced hyperhydration trial. Goulet and others, in a crossover study with a placebo control, found that a standard glycerol-loading protocol did not affect sweat rate, heart rate, or thermal regulation during cycling for 2 hours at 66 percent VO_2 max, nor did it enhance performance in a subsequent cycling test to exhaustion. In a well-designed crossover study, Magal and others evaluated the effect of glycerol hyperhydration, as compared to water hyperhydration, on tennis-related performance in highly skilled male tennis players. Each trial consisted of three phases: hyperhydration with or without glycerol over 150 minutes; 120 minutes of exercise-induced dehydration; and rehydration with or without glycerol over 90 minutes. After each phase subjects performed various tests, including short sprints, repeated agility drills, and tennis skills. Compared to the placebo trial, the glycerol hyperhydration protocol provided a better hydration status and greater plasma volume after both the initial hydration phase and the rehydration phase, but no performance benefits were observed. Wingo and others reported that although glycerol hyperhydration resulted in less dehydration and post-race thirst during a 30-mile mountain-bike race in the heat, there was no significant difference in final race time even though the cyclists completed the final 10-mile loop five minutes faster during the glycerol trial. Compared to water hyperhydration, Marino and others also reported no significant effect of a standard glycerol-hyperhydration protocol on a 60-minute cycling time trial under hot, humid conditions.

The ergogenic effect of glycerol-induced hyperhydration has been the subject of several reviews, and even the conclusions of these reviewers are somewhat equivocal. Some reviewers concluded that glycerol hyperhydration is an effective ergogenic for endurance athletes exercising in the heat, whereas others concluded that it is ineffective and should be avoided. Still others concluded that the research findings are equivocal. For example, in its position stand on fluid replacement, the ACSM indicated that although hyperhydration, including use of glycerol, does not provide any thermoregulatory advantages, it can delay the onset of dehydration, which may be responsible for any small performance benefits that are occasionally reported. A meta-analysis supports this qualified appraisal. Goulet and others analyzed 14 studies comparing glycerol hyperhydration with water hyperhydration. However, only four studies met the criteria for comparing the two treatments on endurance performance. The meta-analysis indicated that glycerol hyperhydration significantly improved performance by 2.6 percent, but due to the limited research available, more research is needed before more definitive conclusions can be drawn as to the ergogenic effects of glycerol hyperhydration. Several magazines targeted to cyclists and runners have suggested that glycerol may be an effective ergogenic. Additionally, articles in bodybuilding magazines suggest that glycerol-induced hyperhydration may enhance vascularity during judged competition, providing a "cut" appearance for aesthetic purposes. Glycerol-containing products have been marketed to both endurance and strength athletes. Glycerate and ProHydrator were aimed at endurance athletes; however, these products no longer appear to be available. GlycerGrow and Liquid Muscle and other such products have been or are advertised on Websites for strength athletes.

There may be several caveats for individuals who use glycerol supplements, including health and performance issues. Although the dosages used in these studies appear to be safe, researchers indicate that if larger doses are used there may be some concern with the possibility of excess fluid being retained in the intracellular spaces, leading to abnormal pressures and possible tissue damage. Some investigators suggest that glycerol-induced hyperhydration may predispose individuals to hyponatremia. Additionally, reviewers indicate that glycerol supplementation may cause nausea, vomiting, and headaches in some subjects, all of which are symptoms of hyponatremia. From a health perspective, van Rosendal and others advise against glycerol supplementation for certain populations, including pregnant females, and those with diabetes, renal disease, migraine and headache disorders, cardiovascular disease, and liver disorders. This recommendation is due to the actions of glycerol on liver gluconeogenesis, kidney filtration, cardiovascular homeostasis, and hydration homeostasis.

For some athletes, glycerol supplementation may be ergolytic, not ergogenic. Studies showing ergogenic effects of glycerol-induced hyperhydration have used cycling protocols. Although hyperhydration may be ergogenic for cyclists, who need not be too concerned with the additional body weight associated with water retention, runners may be at a slight disadvantage because they need to expend energy to move the extra water weight. If the potential benefits of hyperhydration do not counteract the potential adverse effects of the extra weight, exercise performance may not be improved and may be impaired. However, a report in *Runner's World* magazine indicated that several elite U.S. marathon runners used glycerol in some of their best marathons run in the heat.

For those who want to experiment, glycerol is sold in drug stores as glycerine (glycerin). Glycerine is not to be taken internally as sold, but should be diluted. One recommendation presented in *FitNews,* a publication of the American Running and Fitness Association, is to mix 36 milliliters of glycerol with 955 milliliters of water for each 100 pounds of body weight. This recommendation is in accord with amounts used in research. Roughly, this would be about 1.25 ounces of glycerol per quart of water. Thus, a 150-pound runner would need to consume 1.5 quarts of this concoction to hyperhydrate prior to performance.

Key Concept
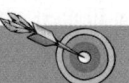

▶ Glycerol supplementation appears to enhance hyperhydration, increase blood volume, and produce favorable physiological responses during exercise. However, research findings are equivocal regarding its effects as a means of improving endurance performance. Glycerol hypohydration, if abused, may also be associated with several adverse health effects.

Health Aspects: Heat Illness

Heat illness, as the name implies, involves various health problems associated with environmental heat stress. As noted previously, excessive dehydration may impair physical performance, and individuals who overhydrate in attempts to prevent dehydration during exercise may experience exercise-associated hyponatremia, which could have serious health consequences. Dehydration and loss of electrolytes may also cause health problems during exercise, some more serious than others.

However, high environmental heat stress poses one of the most serious health threats to athletes and others who exercise, and such individuals should use caution when exercising in the heat.

Should I exercise in the heat?

Given the potential health threats of exercising in the heat, the American College of Sports Medicine published a position stand on exertional heat illness during training and competition, which is available on the ACSM Website. In general, this position stand presents guidelines targeted to sports medicine personnel, such as athletic trainers, and other sport administrators who should be aware of environmental heat conditions that suggest modification or cancellation of competition or practice. However, individuals may also use these guidelines to determine when to modify exercise protocols in the heat. The guidelines are based on the WBGT, which may not be readily available to most individuals. However, local television stations or various Websites usually can provide a heat index, which is a good approximation of the WBGT when exercising in the shade; exercising in the sun adds to the heat index. Table 9.8 presents a modification of the ACSM guidelines.

www.weather.com

www.wunderground.com   Various Websites may provide you with the temperature, humidity, wind, and possibility of sunshine. They also generally provide a heat index, indicating that although the air temperature is only 85°F, it may feel like 95°F due to humidity.

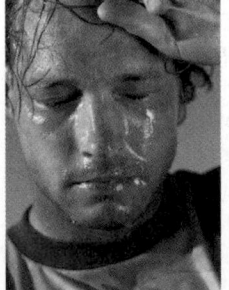

What are the potential health hazards of excessive heat stress imposed on the body?

One of the most serious threats to the performance and health of the physically active individual is heat illness, which is often referred to as exertional heat illness or exercise-associated heat illness when it occurs with exercise. Barrow and Clark indicated that heat-related illnesses cause 240 deaths annually, often in athletes. Any athlete who exercises in a warm environment is susceptible to heat injury, but the increasing popularity of road racing has generated concern for runners who are not prepared for strenuous exercise in the heat, or who participate in races that are poorly organized in regard to preventing and treating heat injuries. Marathon running is becoming increasingly popular,

TABLE 9.8 American College of Sports Medicine guidelines for modifying or canceling competition or training to help prevent heat illness

WBGT (°F)	WBGT (°C)	Continuous activity and competition	Training and noncontinuous activity
<50–65	(10–18.3)	Generally safe	Normal activity
65.1–72.0	(18.4–22.2)	Risk of heat illness begins to rise; *High-risk:* Should be monitored or not compete	*Low-risk:* Normal activity *High-risk:* Increase rest: exercise ratio and monitor fluid intake
72.1–78.0	(22.3–25.6)	Risk for all competitors is increased	*Low-risk:* Normal activity and monitor fluid intake *High-risk:* Increase the rest: exercise ratio and decrease total duration of activity
78.1–82.0	(25.7–27.8)	*High-risk:* Risk is high	*Low-risk:* Normal activity and monitor fluid intake *High-risk:* Increase the rest: exercise ratio and decrease intensity and total duration of activity
82.1–86.0	(27.9–30.0)	Cancel for those at risk of exertional heat stroke	*Low-risk:* Plan intense or prolonged exercise with discretion* *High-risk:* Increase the rest:exercise ratio to 1:1 and decrease intensity and total duration of activity*
86.1–90.0	(30.1–32.2)		*Low-risk:* Limit intense exercise and total daily exposure to heat and humidity *High-risk:* Cancel or stop practice and competition
>90	(>32.3)		Cancel exercise when uncompensable heat stress exists for all athletes*

Low-risk: Individuals acclimatized to the heat for 3 weeks; high fitness level.
High-risk: Individuals nonacclimatized to the heat; unfit; using certain medications; dehydrated; recent illness; previous heat illness, particularly exertional heat stroke.
*Differences of local climate and individual heat acclimatization status may allow activity at higher levels than outlined in the table. Athletes and coaches should consult with sports medicine staff and be cautious when exercising in extreme heat conditions.
The WBGT is the wet-bulb globe thermometer temperature. Commercial devices are available to quickly and accurately measure the WBGT and should be used to help assess environmental heat stress and modify training or competition as recommended. For those who wish to construct an inexpensive WBGT device, consult the reference cited by Spickard at the end of this chapter.

with some major races having tens of thousands of runners. Even well-organized events may experience problems in providing for the needs of runners when the environmental heat stress becomes excessive, as occurred recently during an unexpected heat wave in races that normally have cooler weather.

The individual who exercises unwisely under conditions of environmental heat stress may experience one or several of a variety of heat injuries. Three factors may contribute to these injuries: increased core temperature, loss of body fluids, and loss of electrolytes. However, other factors may also be involved, as Noakes noted that several of the heat illnesses, such as muscle cramps, also occur during exercise in cold environments.

Figure 9.11 represents a simple flow chart of heat disorders. When a combination of exercise and environmental heat stress is imposed on the body, vasodilation and sweating increase as the body tries to cool itself. When these two adjustments begin to falter, problems develop. In essence, the circulation is attempting to regulate both body temperature and blood pressure at the same time, and when stressed excessively, control of blood pressure wins and body temperature regulation is impaired. In addition, if the exercise metabolic load is very great, heat injuries may develop independent of circulatory and sweating inadequacies.

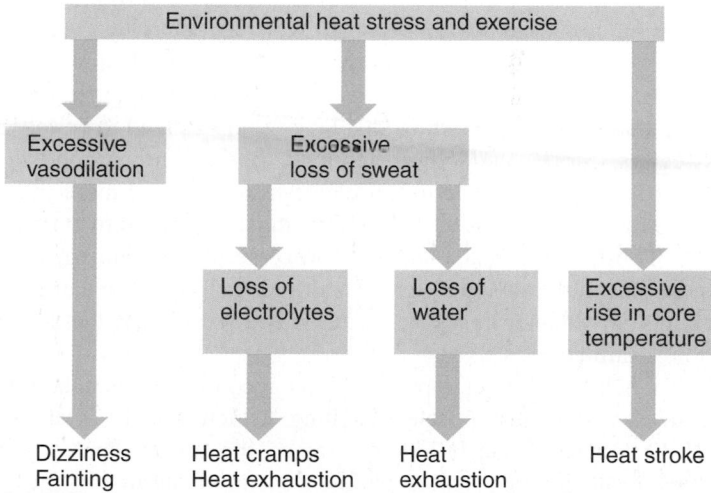

FIGURE 9.11 Basic flow chart for heat illnesses. The combination of environmental heat and exercise may cause an excessive vasodilation or pooling of blood. These conditions may decrease blood return to the heart and brain, causing dizziness and fainting. Excessive loss of sweat may cause significant losses of body water and electrolytes, leading to various heat illnesses. See text for details.

Heat Syncope   Excessive vasodilation may contribute to circulatory instability. The blood vessels expand and have a much greater capacity. Owing to a decreased relative blood volume, cardiac output may decrease and the blood pressure will fall, reducing blood flow to the brain. Dizziness and fainting may occur. This condition is called **heat syncope,** and is usually associated with heat exhaustion as discussed later; a newer term, *exercise-associated collapse,* has been introduced, of which simple fainting may be a mild form, whereas more severe forms may include heat stroke or hyponatremia.

Kenefick and Sawka also note that fainting after a race may be due to the reduced muscle pump activity. When the runner stops, blood may pool in the legs and reduce blood return to the heart and, subsequently, to the brain. Runners are advised to keep the legs moving at the completion of the race. If dizzy, lie down with feet elevated.

Heat Cramps   The ACSM indicates that exercise-associated muscle cramping can occur with exhaustive work in any temperature range, but appears to be more prevalent in hot and humid conditions (**heat cramps**). Although no conclusive evidence is available, one theory postulates that heat cramps may be caused by excessive loss of sodium, potassium, calcium, or magnesium through profuse sweating. However, Schwellnus indicates that there is little scientific evidence to support the hypothesis that exercise-associated muscle cramping is related to serum electrolyte changes. He indicates that the development of premature muscle fatigue appears to be a more plausible explanation for such cramping. Schwellnus also indicated that the cause of muscle cramps may be due to abnormal spinal nerve control of the muscles. Possibly normal neural activity may be disturbed by an electrolyte imbalance.

Conversely, Eichner notes that although not all cramps are alike, he indicates three lines of evidence suggesting that heat cramping is caused by "salty sweating," specifically by the triad of salt loss, fluid loss, and muscle fatigue. First, historically, heat cramping in industrial workers is alleviated by salt. Second, field studies of athletes show that heat-crampers tend to be salty sweaters. Stofan and others reported that American football players who were prone to muscle cramps averaged more than twice the amount of sodium loss than those not prone to cramping. Third, intravenous saline can reverse heat cramping, and more salt in the diet and in sports drinks can help prevent heat cramping. Eichner concludes that for heat cramping, the solution is saline.

To help prevent cramps, Bergeron recommends that at the first sign of subtle muscle twitching, which usually is about 20–30 minutes before full-blown cramps, the athlete should consume a salt solution, such as half a teaspoon of salt in 16 ounces of a sport drink. The athlete should then continue to drink small amounts of a similar solution (the same amount of salt in 32 ounces of a sports drink) at regular intervals for the remainder of the exercise session. Several case studies with tennis players who consistently experienced heat cramps have shown that increased intake of either sodium or magnesium, along with adequate fluids, was effective in preventing muscle cramping during exercise.

Several electrolyte products have been developed for athletes who are prone to muscle cramps. Products such as EnduroLyte and GatorLYTES contain sodium, potassium, calcium, and magnesium, all of which may be helpful in the prevention of muscle cramping. However, Sulzer and others, studying triathletes who were either prone to muscle cramping or not, reported that serum electrolytes (sodium, chloride, potassium, and magnesium) did not appear to be associated with muscle cramps. The cause of muscle cramping still remains a mystery. Nevertheless, the ACSM notes that muscle cramping usually responds to rest and replacement of fluid and salt (sodium).

Heat Exhaustion   **Heat exhaustion** is a common heat illness during exercise. Dehydration is the main risk factor for exercise-associated heat exhaustion. Inadequate salt replacement over the course of several days may also be a contributing factor, as blood volume may decrease. A high body mass index (BMI) also increases the risk. Heat exhaustion is a cause of heat syncope. Fatigue and weakness are key signs of heat exhaustion, which may be associated with dizziness and fainting; other signs and symptoms include rapid pulse, headache, nausea, vomiting, unsteady walk, muscle cramps, chills or goose bumps. The rectal temperature is usually less than 104°F(40°C), which the ACSM notes may be the only discernable difference between severe heat exhaustion and exertional heat stroke in on-site evaluations. Heat exhaustion may incapacitate the individual for a few hours, but will generally resolve with body cooling and fluid intake.

Heat Stroke   **Heat stroke** may occur under heat stress conditions even when resting, particularly in older individuals. When heat stroke occurs during exercise, it is known as **exertional heat stroke,** as illustrated in figure 9.12. The ACSM indicates that exertional heat stroke can affect seemingly healthy athletes even when the environment is relatively cool. However, it occurs more during exercise in heat stress environments, and dehydration is a major risk factor. Along with dehydration, Randy Eichner, a prominent sports medicine physician, indicated that heat stroke in sport is caused by a combination of the following:

- Hot environment
- Strenuous exercise
- Clothing that limits evaporation of sweat
- Inadequate adaptation to the heat
- Too much body fat
- Lack of fitness

Although inconvenient, Ronneberg and others reported that rectal temperature was very effective in diagnosing hyperthermic runners. Other techniques, such as oral temperature or temporal artery temperature, are not effective. The ACSM defines exertional heat stroke as a rectal temperature greater than 40°C (104°F) accompanied by symptoms or signs of organ system failure, most frequently central nervous system changes such as confusion, disorientation, agitation, aggressiveness, blank stare, apathy, irrational behavior, staggering gait, delirium, convulsions, unresponsiveness, or coma. Other signs of possible heat stroke include weak and rapid pulse, vomiting, involuntary bowel movement, and hyperventilation.

What are the symptoms and treatment of heat injuries?

As noted, the symptoms of impending heat injury are variable. Among those reported are weakness, feeling of chills, pilo-erection (goose pimples) on the chest and upper arms, tingling arms, nausea, headache, faintness, disorientation, muscle cramping, and cessation of sweating. Continuing to exercise in a warm environment when experiencing any of these symptoms may lead to heat injury. Table 9.9 presents the major heat injuries along with principal causes, clinical findings, and treatment. In general, treatment of heat syncope, heat cramps, and heat exhaustion involves resting (preferably lying down), cooling the body if overheated, and drinking fluids, preferably with sodium. Most individuals recover fairly rapidly, but should be monitored until in a safe environment.

The ACSM indicates that early recognition and rapid cooling can reduce both the morbidity and mortality associated with exertional heat stroke. Doug Casa and his associates at the University of Connecticut, experts in exercise and thermoregulation research, indicate that cold-water immersion is the *gold standard* for exertional heat stroke. In the field, such as at marathon races, Roberts indicates that the optimal treatment of heat stroke is immediate, total-body cooling with ice-water tub immersion. If not available, rapidly rotating ice-water towels to the trunk, extremities, and head, combined with ice packing of the neck, axillae, and groin, may be very effective.

For collapsed athletes, Sallis indicates that it is essential to check vital signs (especially rectal temperature if heat stroke is suspected), assess fluids status (dehydrated versus fluid overload), and perform laboratory tests when needed. He notes that the most common cause of collapse is low blood pressure due to blood pooling in the legs after cessation of exercise, which is benign and resolves upon rest. However, both hyponatremia, mentioned previously, and heat stroke are serious medical problems and require prompt medical attention. It is critical to differentiate between heat exhaustion or heat stroke and hyponatremia. Providing hypotonic fluids to individuals with hyponatremia will exacerbate the condition because they are already overhydrated.

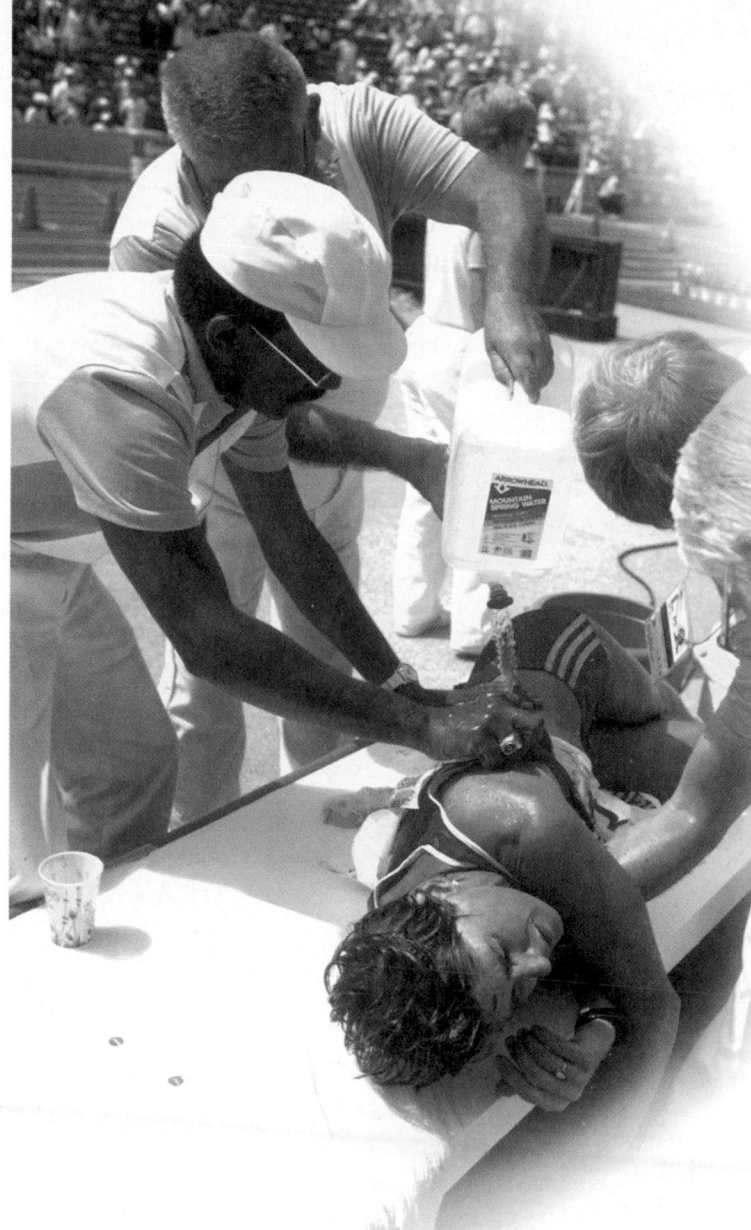

FIGURE 9.12 Heat stroke may be caused by exercising in the heat without taking proper precautions. Rapid cooling of the body is high priority.

William Roberts, former ACSM president and medical director of the Twin Cities Marathon, stated that the skin appearance is usually ashen and sweaty, can be either warm or cool to touch, and is rarely pink, hot, and dry as described in text books.

Heat stroke is the most dangerous heat injury, as it may be fatal. Several deaths of professional and collegiate athletes have been associated with such circumstances, and one involved the use of ephedrine, which as noted in chapter 13 can stimulate metabolism and heat production and predispose to heat stress. Exertional heat stroke may lead to rhabdomyolysis, damaged muscle tissue that leaks its contents into the blood, eventually leading to kidney damage and possible death.

www.acsm-msse.org For the American College of Sports Medicine Position Stand on heat illness during exercise and training, click on *Position Stands* on the right side of the page, then click on *Exertional Heat Illness during Training and Competition*.

Do some individuals have problems tolerating exercise in the heat?

A number of predisposing factors have been associated with heat injury, including gender, level of physical fitness, age, body composition, previous history of heat injury, and degree of acclimatization.

Poor Physical Fitness One of the major factors contributing to exertional heat illness is poor physical fitness. For example, in a study of Marine Corps recruits in training, Gardner and others

TABLE 9.9 Heat injuries: causes, clinical findings, and treatment

Heat injury	Causes	Clinical findings	Treatment*
Heat syncope (Exercise-associated collapse)	Excessive vasodilation: pooling of blood in the skin	Fainting Weakness Fatigue	Place on back in cool environment; give cool fluids
Heat cramps	Excessive loss of electrolytes in sweat; inadequate salt intake	Muscle cramps	Rest in cool environment; oral ingestion of salt drinks; salt foods daily; medical treatment in severe cases
Heat exhaustion	Excessive loss of water and salt; inadequate fluid and salt intake	Fatigue Nausea Cool, pale, moist skin Weakness Dizziness Chills Rectal temperature lower than 104°F (40°C)	Rest in cool environment; replace fluids and salt by mouth; medical treatment if serious
Heat stroke (Exercise-associated heat stroke)	Excessive body temperature	Headache Confusion Blank stare Disorientation Unconsciousness Rectal temperature greater than 104°F (40°C)	Cool body immediately to 102°F (38.9°C), preferably with cold-water immersion; if not, cool body areas with ice packs, ice, or cold water; give cool drinks with glucose if conscious; administer intravenous fluids if available; get medical help immediately
Hyponatremia (Exercise-associated hyponatremia)	Excessive fluid intake	Confusion Lethargy Agitation Coma **Need to determine by serum sodium level lower than 135 mmol/L	Mild cases may be treated with hypertonic fluids; more severe cases may need intravenous fluids, and possible hospitalization

*Begin treatment as soon as possible. In cases of heat stroke, begin immediately.

**Symptoms of hyponatremia may be similar to other heat illnesses; determination must be made by measurement of serum sodium levels less than 135 mmol/L. Providing hypotonic fluids to individuals with hyponatremia could exacerbate the condition.

found that one of the major predictors of exertional heat illness was poor aerobic fitness as measured by 1.5-mile run performance. In general, the better the physical fitness, the better tolerance to a given heat stress. However, even highly trained athletes may experience heat illnesses when using unsafe training practices. NCAA Division I wrestlers have died from heat stroke or related causes in attempts to reduce body weight for competition through exercise-induced sweating in a hot environment. For example, one of the wrestlers was wearing a rubber suit while riding a stationary bicycle in a steam-filled shower.

Gender   In earlier studies, investigators found that female subjects tolerated exercise in the heat less well than males. These findings may have been related to the higher percentage of body fat and the generally lower level of physical fitness of women in those studies. However, in their review, Baker and Kenney reported that when women and men are matched for fitness, acclimation state, adiposity, and body size, there do not appear to be gender-related differences in thermoregulatory function other than

a lower sweating rate in women as compared to men. They note that the latter may be a disadvantage in hot-dry environments, but an advantage in hot-humid conditions because they are less likely to dehydrate. Previous studies have also suggested that increased progesterone levels during the luteal phase of the menstrual cycle could alter the core temperature at which sweating begins, but Baker and Kenney indicated that the menstrual cycle has minimal effects on tolerance to exercise-heat stress. They also noted that while hyponatremia occurs more in women than men, it is not because of gender, but mainly behaviors associated with overconsumption of fluids.

Age   Individuals at both ends of the age spectrum may have problems exercising in the heat. The American Academy of Pediatrics (AAP) recognizes that when children and adolescents are engaging in sports and physical activity in the heat special considerations, preparations, modifications, and monitoring are essential. However, according to the most recent policy statement from the AAP "youth do not have less effective thermoregulatory ability, insufficient cardiovascular capacity or lower physical exertion tolerance compared with adults during exercise in the heat when adequate hydration is maintained." The American College of Sports Medicine, in a consensus statement, indicated that sports such as youth football may pose increased risks. The AAP recently outlined new recommendations for preventing heat illnesses in children, which are in accord with the recommendations provided in the next section. The ACSM also developed some guidelines that may be used to restrain physical activities for children under conditions of heat stress, which are presented in table 9.10.

At high levels of heat stress, tolerance to the heat is decreased in older individuals, possibly because they experience decreased blood flow to the skin and sweat less. Reduced heat toleration in the elderly may also be related to fitness levels. However, more and more people have become and remain physically active throughout middle age and advanced years. Larry Kenney, an expert in temperature regulation at Penn State University, has studied thermoregulation in the elderly. In a review, Baker and Kenney note that well-trained and heat-acclimated older athletes' regulation of body temperature is comparable to that of younger athletes. They also indicate that for healthy older men and women who maintain a high degree of aerobic fitness, the risk of heat-related illness is not significantly greater than that of young adults. However, they do report a decreased thirst sensation when exercising and therefore a need to focus on consuming adequate fluid intake when exercising in the heat. Sports drinks may help. Baker found that when exercising intermittently in the heat, older men and women consumed adequate fluids to rehydrate and consumed more when sports drinks were available compared to water.

Obesity   Obese individuals not only have high amounts of body fat to deter heat losses, but also generate more heat during exercise because of a low level of fitness; thus, they are more susceptible to heat injuries. In the Marine Corps study cited previously, another major predictor of exertional heat illness was a higher body weight in relation to height.

Previous Heat Illness   Individuals who have experienced previous heat injury may be less tolerant of exercise in the heat. Many individuals do regain heat tolerance 8–12 weeks after heat injury. Others lose some of the ability for the circulatory system to adjust to heat stress, possibly because temperature-regulating centers in the brain are irreversibly damaged. The transfer of heat from the core to the skin becomes impaired and the body temperature rises faster.

Acclimatization   One of the more important factors determining an individual's response to exercise in the heat is degree of acclimatization, which is discussed on the following pages. Although some individuals may be susceptible to heat illnesses, all individuals who exercise under warm or hot environmental conditions may benefit from the following recommendations.

How can I reduce the hazards associated with exercise in a hot environment?

In his review, Eichner indicated that the best treatment for heat illness is prevention. The following list represents a number of guidelines which, if followed, will reduce considerably your chances of suffering heat injury.

1. Check the temperature and humidity conditions before exercising. Even if the dry temperature is only 65–75°F, high humidity will increase the heat stress. Warm, humid conditions cause fatigue sooner, so slow your pace or shorten your exercise session. As noted previously, local news stations and several Websites may provide information on heat stress conditions.
2. Exercise in the cool of the morning or evening to avoid the heat of the day.
3. Exercise in the shade, if possible, to avoid radiation from the sun. If you run in the sun, wear an appropriate sunscreen to prevent sun damage to the skin.
4. Wear sports clothing designed for exercise in the heat, such as CoolMax type material. Clothing should be loose to allow air circulation, white or a light color to reflect radiant heat, and porous to permit evaporation. Do not wear a hat if running in the shade, but wear a loose hat if running in the sun.
5. If you are running and there is a breeze, plan your route so that you are running into the wind during the last part of your run. The breeze will help cool you more effectively at the time you need it most.
6. Hyperhydrate if you plan to perform prolonged, strenuous exercise in the heat. In general, drink about 16 ounces of fluid 30–60 minutes prior to exercising.
7. Drink cold fluids periodically. For a long training run, plan your route so that it passes some watering holes, such as gas stations or other sources of water. Alternatively, you may

TABLE 9.10	WBGT temperature guidelines to modify practice sessions for exercising children	
WBGT (°F)	**WBGT (°C)**	**Restraints on activities**
<75.0	<24.0	All activities allowed, but watch for symptoms of heat illnesses in prolonged events
75.0–78.6	24.0–25.9	Have longer rest periods in the shade; enforce fluid intake every 15 minutes
79.0–84.0	26.0–29.0	Stop activity for unacclimatized and high-risk children; limit activities of others; cancel long-distance races and cut the duration of other activities
>85.0	>29.0	Cancel all athletic activities

Modifications of the recommendations on climatic heat stress in exercising children and adolescents proposed by the American Academy of Pediatrics Committee on Sports Medicine and Fitness.

purchase a special water-bottle belt or backpack that will help you carry your own water supply. Take frequent water breaks, consuming about 6–8 ounces of water every 15 minutes or so. As a rough gauge, one mouthful of water is approximately one ounce of fluid.

8. Replenish your water daily. Keep a record of your body weight. For each pound you lose, drink about 20–24 ounces of fluid. Your body weight should be back to normal before your next workout.

9. Replenish lost electrolytes (salt) if you have sweated excessively. Put a little extra salt on your meals and eat foods high in potassium, such as bananas and citrus fruits.

10. Avoid excessive intake of protein, as extra heat is produced in the body when protein is metabolized. This may contribute slightly to the heat stress.

11. Avoid dietary supplements containing ephedrine. Ephedrine is a potent stimulant that can increase metabolism and heat production, leading to an increased body temperature during exercise in warm environmental conditions and predisposing to heat illness.

12. If you drink caffeinated beverages, check your responses. Current research indicates that caffeinated beverages may not affect hydration status or temperature regulation during exercise. However, some individuals may respond differently to caffeine intake. Caffeine can increase heat production at rest, which could raise the body temperature before exercise.

13. Because alcohol is a diuretic, excess amounts should be avoided the night before competition or prolonged exercise in the heat.

14. If you are sedentary, overweight, or aged, you are less likely to tolerate exercise in the heat and should therefore use extra caution.

15. Be aware of the signs and symptoms of heat exhaustion and heat stroke, as well as the treatment for each. Chills, goose pimples, tingling arms, dizziness, weakness, fatigue, mental disorientation, nausea, and headaches are some symptoms that may signify the onset of heat illness. Stop activity, get to a cool place, and consume some cool fluids.

16. Do not exercise if you have been ill or have had a fever within the last few days.

17. Check your medications. Some medications, such as antihistamines used to treat cold symptoms, may block sweat production. Drugs used to treat high blood pressure, such as beta-blockers and calcium-channel blockers, may impair skin blood flow and decrease heat loss from the body.

18. If you plan to compete in a sport held under hot environmental conditions, you must become acclimatized to exercise in the heat.

www.gssiweb.com   The Gatorade Sports Science Institute (GSSI) provides very useful information on a wide variety of topics in sports nutrition, especially information relative to proper hydration practices to help enhance performance and prevent heat illness when exercising in the heat.

How can I become acclimatized to exercise in the heat?

It is a well-established fact that **acclimatization** to the heat will help increase performance in warm environments as compared with an unacclimatized state. Simply living in a hot environment confers a small amount of acclimatization. Physical training, in and of itself, provides a significant amount of acclimatization, possibly up to 50 percent of that which can be expected, and also increases body-water levels. However, neither of these two adjustments, either singly or together, can prevent the deterioration of exercise performance in the heat by an unacclimatized individual. Thus, a period of active acclimatization is necessary to optimize performance when exercising in the heat.

The technique of acclimatization is relatively simple. Simply cut back on the intensity or duration of your normal activity when the hot weather begins. Do not avoid exercise in the heat completely, but after an initial reduction in your activity level, increase it gradually. For example, if you were running five miles a day, cut your distance back to two to three miles in the heat; if you need to do five a day, do the remaining miles in the evening. Eventually build up to three, four, and five miles. The acclimatization process usually takes about 10 to 14 days to complete. However, even when acclimatized, an athlete's endurance capacity in the heat, particularly with high humidity, still will be less than under cooler conditions.

If you live in a cool climate, like New England, and want to compete in a marathon in Florida in January, how do you become acclimatized? Exercising indoors at a warmer temperature will help. Extra layers of clothes can help prevent evaporation and build a hot, humid microclimate around your body. Research has shown that this technique can provide a degree of acclimatization. However, this is advisable only in cool weather and should not be attempted under hot conditions. Wearing a sweat suit or rubberized suit while exercising in the heat may precipitate heat illness. Moreover, even in a cool environment this technique may cause heat injury. Again, be wary of the symptoms of impending heat illness.

Repeated exposure to a high core temperature during exercise helps the body make the following important adjustments during acclimatization to the heat. The ACSM indicates 10–14 days of exercising in the heat will improve heat acclimatization in adults. Bar-Or notes that heat acclimatization in children takes several weeks. Here are some of the benefits of heat acclimatization that will help improve performance and reduce the risk of heat stroke and heat exhaustion.

1. Total body water increases considerably, which usually includes increased plasma volume. Blood vessels may conserve more sodium, which tends to hold plasma water. This occurs because the blood vessels conserve more protein and sodium, which tend to hold water.

2. The increased blood volume allows the heart to pump more blood per beat, so the stress on the heart is reduced.

3. When volume increases, more blood flows to the muscles and skin. The muscles receive more oxygen and skin cooling increases, improving endurance performance.

4. Less muscle glycogen may be used as an energy source at a given rate of exercise, sparing this energy source in endurance events.
5. The sweat glands hypertrophy and secrete about 30 percent more sweat, allowing for greater evaporative heat loss.
6. Body salt losses decrease. The amount of salt in the sweat decreases considerably; evaporation becomes more efficient and electrolytes are conserved. Sweat losses of calcium, magnesium, copper, zinc, and iron also decrease with acclimatization.
7. Sweating starts at a lower core temperature, leading to earlier cooling.
8. The core temperature will not rise as high or as rapidly as in the unacclimatized state.
9. The psychological feeling of stress is reduced at a given exercise rate.

In essence, as illustrated in figure 9.13, these changes increase the ability of the body to dissipate heat with less stress on the cardiovascular system. The end result is a more effective body-temperature control and improved performance when exercising in the heat. These adaptations may be maintained by exercising in the heat several days per week but are lost in about 7–10 days in a cool environment. If you are interested in learning more about acclimatization, consult the review by Sawka and Young.

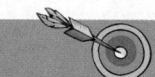

Key Concepts

▶ Heat injuries, of which heat stroke is potentially the most dangerous, may be due to increased body core temperature, loss of body fluids, or loss of electrolytes. Some individuals, such as the obese, are more susceptible to heat injury.

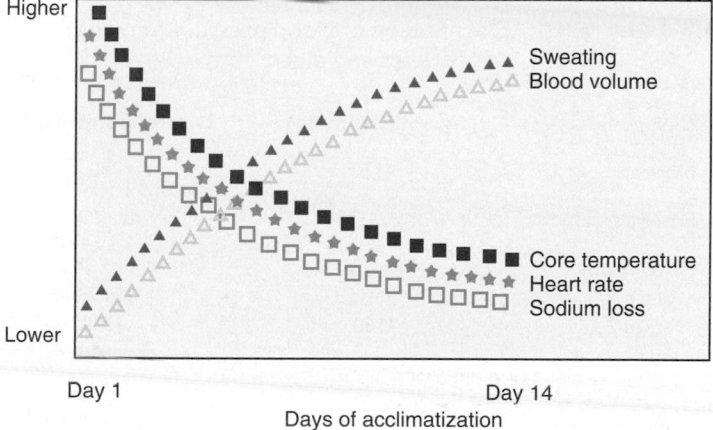

FIGURE 9.13 Changes with acclimatization. Acclimatization to the heat for 7 to 14 days will lead to an increase in the blood volume and the ability to sweat. For a standardized exercise task in the heat, these changes will lead to a lower heart rate, less sodium loss, and a lower core temperature. These changes will lead to improved exercise performance in the heat.

▶ The general treatment for heat-stress illnesses is to rest, drink cool liquids, and cool the body. Rapid body cooling is essential in cases of heat stroke.
▶ If you exercise in the heat, you should be aware of signs of impending heat injury, such as chills, dizziness, and weakness. You should also be aware of methods to reduce heat gain to the body and methods to facilitate heat loss.
▶ Acclimatization to exercise in the heat takes about 10–14 days, but endurance capacity in the heat is still limited somewhat even when one is fully acclimated.

Health Aspects: High Blood Pressure

What is high blood pressure, or hypertension?

Everybody has blood pressure. Without it we would not be able to sustain body metabolism. Simply speaking, blood pressure is the force that the blood exerts against the blood vessel walls. Although pressure is present in all types of blood vessels, the arterial blood pressure is the one most commonly measured and most important to our health. Blood pressure is usually measured by a sphygmomanometer, which records the pressure in millimeters of mercury (mmHg) (see figure 9.14). Blood pressure readings are given in two numbers, for example 120/80 mmHg. The higher number represents the *systolic* phase, when the heart is pumping blood through the arteries. The lower number represents the *diastolic* phase, when the heart is resting between beats and blood is flowing back into it. Two important determinants of blood pressure are the volume of blood in the circulation and the resistance to blood flow, known as peripheral vascular resistance.

High blood pressure, also known as **hypertension** (hyper = high; tension = pressure), is known as a silent disease. Israili and others noted that hypertension affects approximately 1 billion individuals worldwide. At least 65 million individuals in the United States have hypertension. Surprisingly, Hansen and others estimated that about 2 million American youth have high blood pressure, which they associated with rising levels of obesity in children. The Consumers Union referred to high blood pressure as an uncontrolled epidemic, noting that most individuals with hypertension do not have it under control. One reason is that nearly a third do not even know they are hypertensive, mainly because it has no outstanding symptoms. With younger people this is even higher, with estimates by Aglony and others of approximately 75 percent of the cases of hypertension and 90 percent of the prehypertensive cases in children and adolescents not yet diagnosed. Some general symptoms include headaches, dizziness, and fatigue, but because they can be caused by a multitude of other factors, they may not be recognized as symptoms of high blood pressure. Although a great deal of research about the cause of high blood pressure has been conducted, the exact cause is unknown in about 90 percent of all cases. In these cases, the condition is known as *essential hypertension,* which cannot be cured.

High blood pressure is dangerous for several reasons. The heart must work much harder to pump the extra blood volume or to overcome the peripheral vascular resistance. This normally leads to an

1. No sound is heard because there is no blood flow when the cuff pressure is high enough to keep the brachial artery closed.

2. **Systolic pressure** is the pressure at which a Korotkoff sound is first heard. When cuff pressure decreases and is no longer able to keep the brachial artery closed during systole, blood is pushed through the partially opened brachial artery to produce turbulent blood flow and a sound. The brachial artery remains closed during diastole.

3. As cuff pressure continues to decrease, the brachial artery opens even more during systole. At first, the artery is closed during diastole, but, as cuff pressure continues to decrease, the brachial artery partially opens during diastole. Turbulent blood flow during systole produces Korotkoff sounds, although the pitch of the sounds changes as the artery becomes more open.

4. **Diastolic pressure** is the pressure at which the sound disappears. Eventually, cuff pressure decreases below the pressure in the brachial artery and it remains open during systole and diastole. Nonturbulent flow is reestablished and no sounds are heard.

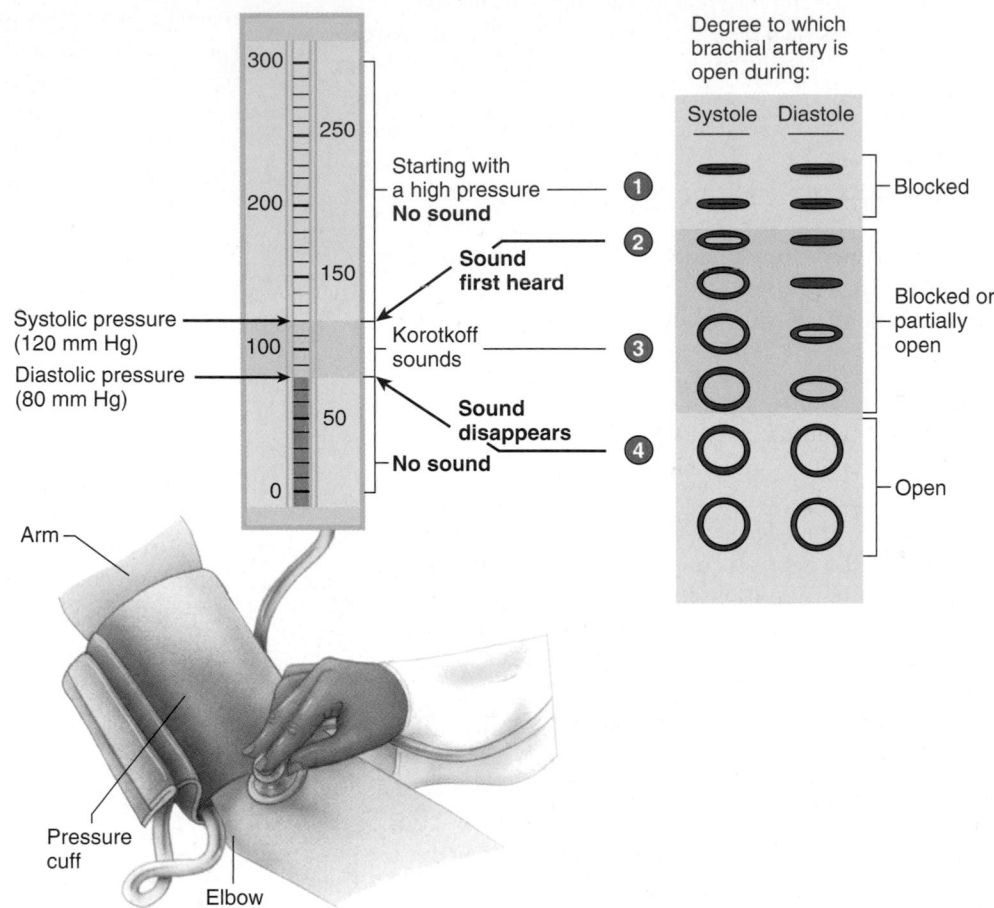

FIGURE 9.14 Blood pressure measurement

enlarged heart. Over time the increase in heart size becomes excessive and the efficiency of the heart actually decreases, making it more prone to a heart attack. Second, high blood pressure may directly damage the arterial walls. It is thought to be a major contributing factor in the development of atherosclerosis and a predisposing factor to coronary disease and stroke. High blood pressure is itself a disease and is also involved in the etiology of other diseases. It is one of the primary risk factors for heart disease and stroke.

The National Research Council has noted that any definition of high blood pressure is arbitrary. Traditionally, physicians have used elevations in diastolic blood pressure as the basis for their diagnosis, but the Joint National Committee on Detection, Evaluation, and Treatment of High Blood Pressure (JNCDET) of the National Institutes of Health, in its classification of blood pressure for adults age 18 years and older, includes both systolic and diastolic pressures. The classification system is presented in table 9.11.

www.americanheart.org Consult the American Heart Association Website for your personal risk factor assessment for high blood pressure.

TABLE 9.11 Classification of blood pressure for adults age 18 years and older

Category	Systolic (mmHg)	Diastolic (mmHg)
Normal	<120	<80
Pre-hypertension	120–139	80–89
Hypertension		
Stage 1	140–159	90–99
Stage 2	>160	>100

Source: National Heart, Lung, and Blood Institute.

How is high blood pressure treated?

Although essential hypertension is incurable, Israili and others suggest that gene therapy or the use of vaccines may be feasible to prevent its development, but are not likely to be available in the near future. Currently, many individuals with essential hypertension need to take medications to control their blood pressure. A variety of drugs are available to treat hypertension, including diuretics, beta-blockers, angiotensin-converting enzyme (ACE) inhibitors, and calcium-channel blockers. The Consumers Union recommends that if your blood pressure is elevated, you and your doctor need to take aggressive action. If drug therapy is recommended, you may need to experiment with your physician as to type and dose of medicine to use. This is especially important for athletic individuals. Oliveira and Lawless suggest using drugs that are less likely to have adverse effects on exercise performance. For example, diuretics and beta-blockers may impair aerobic endurance performance. Physicians should also be aware that use of beta-blockers is prohibited for competition in some sports. Tanji and Batt provide a detailed discussion of the pharmacological treatment of hypertension in physically active individuals.

Other than impairment of aerobic endurance capacity, blood-pressure drugs may cause other adverse health effects. Thus, a nonpharmacologic approach is often a first choice of treatment in cases of mild to moderate hypertension. The Canadian Hypertension Education Program emphasizes the point that lifestyle modifications are the cornerstone of antihypertensive therapy.

What dietary modifications may help reduce or prevent hypertension?

How much and what you eat may influence your blood pressure. The following are the key points to help reduce or prevent hypertension.

1. *Achieve and maintain a healthy body weight.* Numerous studies have shown that reducing body weight, even as little as 10 pounds, will reduce blood pressure in overweight, hypertensive individuals. Maintaining a healthy body weight may be one of the most effective preventive measures. Thus, restriction of caloric intake to either lose or maintain body weight may be a helpful dietary strategy. According to a review by Savica and others, obesity in adolescents seems to increase the sensitivity of blood pressure to salt intake. However, weight loss appears to decrease the sensitivity to salt in this younger population. Healthful methods of losing excess body fat are presented in chapter 11.

2. *Reduce or moderate sodium intake.* This remains one of the most controversial recommendations, but it may be a prudent behavior for most individuals. Some researchers, such as Alderman, indicate the available data provide no support for any universal recommendation for a particular level of sodium intake. In support of this viewpoint, Cohen and Alderman reported a "J shape" relationship between sodium intake and cardiovascular disease mortality, noting a direct association at high levels of average intake (over 4 g), an inverse association at lower levels (less than 2 g), and no measurable effect for the widely prevalent intakes in between. They suggest that both high and very low levels of sodium intake may be related to cardiovascular-related deaths. Others suggest that sodium restriction has only modest effects on blood pressure in normotensive individuals.

In contrast, others recommend a significant reduction in current sodium intake in industrialized societies. Cappuccio has noted that most prospective studies have shown that higher salt intake predicts the incidence of cardiovascular events, but the lack of large and long randomized trials on the effects of salt reduction has encouraged some people to argue against a policy of salt reduction in populations. However, Cook and others conducted such a study, the long-term Trials of Hypertension Prevention (TOHP) study. Adults with pre-hypertension reduced sodium intake by about 800 to 1,000 milligrams daily for 18 months and up to 4 years. In a follow-up assessment of 10–15 years, the sodium reduction resulted in a 25 percent lower risk of experiencing a cardiovascular event, such as a heart attack, stroke, or cardiovascular death. The investigators concluded that sodium reduction, previously shown to lower blood pressure, may also reduce long-term risk of cardiovascular events.

Most health governmental agencies and professional groups promote dietary sodium restriction. Penner and others noted that one in four Canadians have hypertension, and with the lifetime risk of developing hypertension being more than 90 percent in an average life span, the need for a population-based approach to reducing hypertension is clear. Thus, the 2010 Canadian Hypertension Education Program, as documented by Hackman and others, recommended restricting sodium intake to 1,500 milligrams/day for adults younger than 50 years of age, to 1,300 milligrams/day for adults 51–70 years of age, and to 1,200 milligrams/day for adults older than 70 years of age. The AI for Americans is 1,500 milligrams/day, whereas the UL is 2,300 milligrams/day. The American Medical Association (AMA) has developed a campaign to reduce sodium intake nationwide. The AMA has urged the FDA to remove salt from the GRAS (generally recognized as safe) list and also require high-salt foods to carry a distinctive label, such as pictures of salt shakers bearing the word *High*. Although some question the wisdom in recommending salt restriction in all individuals, many health professionals suggest that this is a good policy.

Why might it be prudent for most normotensive individuals to moderate salt intake? It is true that most individuals possess physiological control systems that effectively maintain a proper balance of sodium in the body. However, many individuals are sodium-sensitive, or salt-sensitive, in that their blood pressure may increase with excessive consumption of salt. Possibly because of a defect in excretion, sodium accumulates in the body and holds fluids, particularly blood, thereby raising the blood pressure. In their review, McCarron and Reusser report that salt sensitivity is present in about 30 percent of normotensive and 50 percent of hypertensive persons, and is more prevalent among African-Americans and older individuals. Franco and Oparil also note that salt sensitivity in both normotensive and hypertensive persons has been associated with increased cardiovascular disease events. That being so, and because many individuals do not know their blood pressure, millions of Americans may benefit from the recommendation to moderate salt intake. Moreover, the American Institute for Cancer Research report on nutrition and cancer indicates that high salt intake may damage the stomach lining and may have a synergistic interaction with gastric carcinogens. The research panel concluded that salted and salty foods are a probable cause of stomach cancer.

The current prudent medical recommendation for dietary prevention or treatment of hypertension is to decrease sodium consumption simply by eating a wide variety of foods in their natural state. Avoid highly salted foods, restrict intake of processed foods, and hide your salt shakers. The recommended upper limit is somewhat less than 6 grams of salt per day, just a little over 1 teaspoon, the equivalent of about 2.3 grams of sodium. The AI, based on potential healthful effects on blood pressure, is only 1.5 grams, or less than 4 grams of salt daily. Individuals who sweat during training most likely do not need to be concerned with the sodium content in sports drinks. Over the course of a month, Roberts reported no change in blood pressure in normotensive individuals who worked strenuously outside and consumed about 4.5 liters of a typical CES daily.

It should be noted that decreasing salt and sodium intake poses some practical difficulties. Most salt we eat comes from the packaged foods we buy. Even minimally processed foods, such as milk and bread, may contain significant amounts of sodium. Salt is also high in most restaurant foods; some single servings of fast food have more than 1,000 milligrams of sodium, some up to nearly 5,000 milligrams. Thus, one might have to buy most foods in their natural state and prepare and cook them at home, from scratch. For those with hypertension, it may be a challenge—but worth it.

3. *Consume a diet rich in fruits, vegetables, and low-fat, protein-rich foods and with reduced saturated and total fat.* McCarron and Reusser note that large-scale studies have shown that whereas manipulation of single nutrients may have beneficial health effects for some individuals, it is improving the total dietary profile that will consistently provide health benefits, such as reducing high blood pressure. The **DASH** (Dietary Approaches to Stop Hypertension) **diet** emphasizes fruits and vegetables, nuts, low-fat dairy foods, fish, and chicken instead of red meat, low-sugar and low-refined carbohydrate foods, and reduced saturated and total fat. The DASH eating plan for a 2,000-Calorie diet is presented in table 9.12. The number of servings may be modified to meet other caloric requirements. The DASH diet is rich in potassium, magnesium, calcium, and fiber, which have been suggested to help prevent high blood pressure. The JNCDET, in its seventh report, particularly recommends increased consumption of potassium, which is abundant in fruits and vegetables.

www.nhlbi.nih.gov For a detailed DASH eating plan, visit this website and type in DASH Eating Plan in the search box. This site also provides other detailed information on high blood pressure.

As noted in earlier chapters, Appel and others modified the DASH diet by replacing about 10 percent of the DASH's carbohydrates (mostly desserts and fruits) with either *good* proteins (fish, poultry, beans, tofu) or *good* fats (olive oil, canola oil, nuts). They found that such replacements resulted in additional decreases in blood pressure, and called it the OmniHeart diet. However, in a meta-analysis of randomized controlled trials, Shah and others concluded that although diets rich in carbohydrate may be associated with slightly higher blood pressure than diets rich in monounsaturated fat, the magnitude of the difference may not justify making recommendations to alter the carbohydrate and monounsaturated fat content of the diet to manage blood pressure. In a prospective study, Chen and others found that a reduction in sugar-sweetened beverage intake over an 18-month period resulted in reductions in both systolic and diastolic blood pressures. A reduction in sugar-sweetened beverage intake is one of the goals of the *Dietary Guidelines for Americans 2010*.

Both the DASH and OmniHeart diets are based on healthy concepts, being rich in fruits and vegetables, healthy protein, and phytonutrients, and low in bad fats, sweets, and salt. Both diet plans may help reduce blood pressure, and may also help reduce the risks of other risk factors associated with heart disease and stroke. For example, Azadbakht and others indicated that the DASH diet can likely produce multiple health benefits other than reduced blood pressure, including higher HDL-cholesterol and lower triglycerides, fasting blood glucose, and body weight. In a prospective cohort study, Fung and others assessed the association between adherence to a DASH-style diet and risk of coronary heart disease (CHD) and stroke in middle-aged women. They found, over the course of 24 years, that adherence to a DASH-style diet was associated with a lower risk of CHD and stroke.

For those with hypertension, and even normotensive individuals, some health professionals recommend the DASH or OmniHeart diet and the extra effort to cut back to 1,500 milligrams of sodium per day. In a randomized, controlled trial, Sacks and others found that the DASH diet for 30 days resulted in significant reductions in both systolic and diastolic blood pressure. All individuals in this study were also randomly assigned to three different levels of salt intake for a 30-day period, and the decrease in blood pressure was greatest when subjects consumed the diet with the lowest amount of salt, only 1,500 milligrams per day.

4. *Moderate alcohol consumption.* As noted in chapter 4, moderate alcohol consumption may actually confer some health benefits, particularly the prevention of cardiovascular disease. However, excess alcohol intake may increase the heart disease risk, possibly because it is linked to high blood pressure.

5. *Be cautious with dietary supplements.* Haddy and others report that potassium serves as a vasodilating substance, and indicate that potassium supplementation can lower blood pressure, but it is slow to appear, taking about 4 weeks. In a meta-analysis, Dickinson and others analyzed six randomly controlled trials and found that potassium supplementation resulted in a large but statistically

TABLE 9.12 The DASH Eating plan

Food group	Servings	Serving sizes	Examples and notes	Significance to the DASH eating plan
Grains	6–7 per day	1 slice bread 1 oz dry cereal ½ cup cooked rice, pasta, or cereal	Whole wheat bread, English muffin, pita bread, bagel, cereals, oatmeal, unsalted pretzels, popcorn	Major sources of energy and fiber
Vegetables	4–5 per day	1 cup raw leafy vegetable ½ cup cooked vegetable ½ cup vegetable juice	Tomatoes, potatoes, carrots, green peas, broccoli, kale, spinach, lima beans, sweet potatoes	Rich sources of potassium, magnesium, and fiber
Fruits	4–5 per day	½ cup fruit juice 1 medium fruit ¼ cup dried fruit	Apricots, bananas, dates, grapes, oranges, orange juice, melons, peaches pineapples, raisins, strawberries	Important sources of potassium, magnesium, and fiber
Low-fat or fat-free dairy foods	2–3 per day	1 cup milk 1 cup yogurt 1½ oz cheese	Fat-free (skim) milk, fat-free or low-fat regular or frozen yogurt, low-fat and fat-free cheese	Major sources of calcium and protein
Lean meats, poultry, and fish	6 or less per day	1 oz cooked meats, poultry, or fish 1 egg	Select only lean; trim away visible fats; broil, roast, or boil, instead of frying; remove skin from poultry	Rich sources of protein and magnesium
Nuts, seeds, and dry beans	4–5 per week	⅓ cup or 1½ oz nuts 2 Tbsp or ½ oz seeds ½ cup cooked dry beans or peas 2 Tbsp peanut butter	Almonds, mixed nuts, peanuts, walnuts, sunflower seeds, kidney beans	Rich sources of energy, magnesium, potassium, protein, and fiber
Fats and oils	2–3 per day	1 tsp soft margarine 1 Tbsp low-fat mayonnaise 2 Tbsp light salad dressing 1 tsp vegetable oil	Soft margarine, low-fat mayonnaise, light salad dressing, vegetable oil (olive, corn, canola)	DASH has 27 percent of Calories as fat, including fat in or added to foods 1 Tbsp fat-free dressing equals 0 servings
Sweets and added sugars	5 or less per week	1 Tbsp sugar 1 Tbsp jelly or jam ½ cup sorbet, gelatin 1 cup lemonade	Sugar, jelly, jam, jelly beans, hard candy, sorbet, ices	

Adapted from The DASH Eating Plan, National Heart, Lung, and Blood Institute. For more details, go to www.nhlbi.nih.gov/health/public/heart/hbp/dash/new_dash.pdf.

nonsignificant reduction in both systolic and diastolic blood pressure. They noted that given the data from these studies, the evidence about the effect of potassium supplementation on blood pressure is not conclusive, and additional research is needed. In their review, Savica and others concluded that there is significant controversy in the literature concerning whether high calcium and magnesium intakes lower blood pressure.

Given the potential health risks of potassium supplementation, as noted earlier, individuals considering such supplementation should do so only under the guidance of their physician.

As you probably noticed, all of these recommendations are in accord with the Prudent Healthy Diet. The more of these recommendations you follow, the better. In one study, subjects who lost weight, increased physical activity, and reduced sodium and alcohol intake experienced significant reductions in blood pressure, but subjects who also adhered to the DASH diet experienced the greatest reduction.

Can exercise help prevent or treat hypertension?

Regular mild- to moderate-intensity aerobic exercise, such as jogging, brisk walking, swimming, cycling, and aerobic dancing, has also been recommended to reduce high blood pressure. The exercise need not be continuous. Elley and others found that four 10-minute *exercise snacks* consisting of brisk walking, as compared to a single 40-minute continuous bout of brisk walking, done over the course of a day elicited similar reductions in both systolic and diastolic blood pressure. Individuals can work these exercise *snacks* into their daily schedule when they can't find a large block of free time.

Because exercise may be an effective means of losing excess body fat, it may exert a beneficial effect on blood pressure through this avenue. However, the exact role or mechanism of exercise as an independent factor in lowering blood pressure has not been totally resolved. Kramer and others theorize that exercise may exert favorable effects on the hypothalamus, inducing the sympathetic nervous system to decrease constriction of blood vessels and reduce vascular resistance, which is one factor contributing to elevated blood pressure.

Although a number of studies have shown that exercise training helps decrease resting systolic blood pressure in those who are hypertensive and may even elicit a slight decrease in those with normal blood pressure, not all studies are in agreement. Not all individuals will experience a decrease in blood pressure from an exercise program; they may be exercise-insensitive, or nonresponders. Nevertheless, most health professionals find the available information sufficient to justify an aerobic exercise program as a useful adjunct for the treatment of high blood pressure.

Most research has focused on the chronic effect of exercise training on blood pressure. Most recent reviews and meta-analyses report significant reductions in both diastolic and systolic blood pressure, more so in hypertensive than normotensive individuals. In a meta-analysis of 72 studies, Fagard concluded that aerobic endurance exercise training reduced blood pressure by about 3.0 mmHg, and the reduction was greater in subjects with hypertension (−6.9 mmHg) than those who were normotensive (−1.9 mmHg). Although the number of studies was limited, Fagard also noted that resistance training was able to reduce blood pressure. These overall reductions in blood pressure appear to be small, but Israili and others note that even small reductions in systolic blood pressure (for example, 3–5 mmHg) produce dramatic reduction in adverse cardiac events and stroke.

The American College of Sports Medicine, in its position stand on exercise and hypertension, stated that exercise is the cornerstone therapy for the primary prevention, treatment, and control of hypertension. These are some of the major points of the position stand.

- Exercise programs that involve endurance activities, such as walking, jogging, running, or cycling, coupled with resistance training, help to prevent the development of hypertension and to lower blood pressure in adults.
- Exercise should be done daily for 30 minutes or more at a moderate level.
- A higher level of physical activity and fitness resulting from long-term exercise training has a protective effect against hypertension; fitter people with hypertension will have lower blood pressure than those who are less fit.
- Even a single session (acute) exercise bout provides an immediate reduction in blood pressure, which can last for a major portion of the day. Promoting the benefits of lowering blood pressure through single bouts of exercise may help motivate people to exercise.

Special considerations for exercise with hypertension include the following:

- Individuals with controlled hypertension and no cardiovascular or kidney disease may participate in an exercise program.
- Overweight adults should use exercise to lose weight.
- People on medications, such as beta-blockers, should be cautious of developing heat illness when exercising.
- Adults with hypertension should extend the cool-down period of the workout; some medications may cause blood pressure to lower too much after abruptly ending exercise.

Individuals who have high blood pressure and who have concerns about exercising should consult with their physicians about mode and intensity of exercise. Although aerobic exercise may help reduce blood pressure at rest and may evoke a lessened blood pressure rise during exercise, a protective effect, other exercises may be harmful. For example, high-intensity anaerobic exercise and activities that require intense straining, lifting, or hanging, such as isometric exercises, weight lifting, or pull-ups might be inappropriate for some individuals. The use of hand-held weights in aerobic exercises may also be a concern. These activities may create a physiological response that rapidly raises the blood pressure to rather high levels. This increase may be hazardous to someone whose resting blood pressure is already at an elevated level. Thus, hypertensive individuals need to consult with their physicians regarding exercise indications and contraindications.

In summary, the more healthful behaviors one adopts, the greater will be the reduction in blood pressure. In a review, the JNCDET noted that a healthy lifestyle may be sufficient to avoid pharmacologic therapy for some patients and is a valuable adjunct to drug therapy for most. The JNCDET quantified the potential blood pressure lowering effects of various health behaviors, as follows:

- Weight reduction (5–20 mmHg/10 kg)
- DASH eating plan (8–14 mmHg)
- Dietary sodium reduction (2–8 mmHg)
- Increased physical activity (4–9 mmHg)
- Moderation of alcohol consumption (2–4 mmHg)

Key Concept
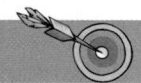

▶ Lifestyle practices to help prevent or treat high blood pressure include maintaining an optimal body weight, aerobic exercise, moderation in salt and sodium intake, moderation in alcohol consumption, and increased intake of fruits, vegetables, whole grains, and low-fat, high-protein foods.

Check for Yourself

▶ Have your blood pressure checked at rest. If possible, have it checked immediately after both an aerobic-type and resistance-type exercise.

Determine your body temperature response and sweating rate.

First, measure your body temperature accurately before exercise. An oral thermometer is acceptable, but keep your mouth closed tightly during all measurements. Also, weigh yourself exactly in dry, light clothes.

Second, exercise for about 30–60 minutes, preferably under warm environmental conditions, either indoors or outdoors. Record exactly the amount of fluid you consume during exercise.

Third, immediately after exercise, record your body temperature. Then, immediately towel dry and weigh yourself in the same dry set of clothes. Calculate your body temperature increase from the difference between the preexercise and postexercise recordings. Calculate your sweat loss by subtracting your postexercise weight from your initial weight and adding to this amount the number of ounces of fluid you consumed. This will provide you with your sweat rate for the time you exercised, which you can then calculate to sweat rate per hour.

If feasible, conduct this little self-experiment before and after acclimatization to exercise in the heat and compare the responses. What might you expect to find?

Body Temperature Response and Sweating Rate

Step 1		Step 2	Step 3	
Preexercise temperature		Fluid consumed during exercise	Postexercise temperature	
Preexercise weight			Postexercise weight	

Determination of body temperature response and sweating rate to exercise

Sweating rate

A. Enter your preexercise body weight (nearest 0.25 pound). _____

B. Enter your postexercise body weight in pounds (nearest 0.25 pound). _____

C. Subtract B from A. _____

D. Convert C to ounces (1 pound = 16 fluid ounces). _____

E. Enter the amount of fluid (in ounces) you consumed during the run. _____

F. Add E to D. _____

G. Divide F by the number of minutes of exercise to calculate sweat rate per minute. _____

H. Multiply G by 60 to obtain sweat rate per hour. _____

The final figure provides you with a guide to replenish fluids per hour. You need not fully replenish what you lose per hour, but replacing about 60 percent or more will help you prevent excessive dehydration.

Body temperature response

A. Enter your preexercise body temperature in degrees Fahrenheit or Celsius. _____

B. Enter your postexercise body temperature in degrees Fahrenheit or Celsius. _____

C. Subtract B from A. _____

The final figure represents your core body temperature increase for the intensity and duration of exercise and for the given environmental conditions (air temperature, humidity, solar radiation).

Review Questions—Multiple Choice

1. Which of the following blood pressure values for adults 18 years of age and older represents the minimal blood pressure for the first stage of hypertension (mild)? The values listed are systolic and diastolic, in that order.

   a. 130 and 80
   b. 130 and 90
   c. 140 and 90
   d. 160 and 100
   e. 210 and 120

2. Which of the following does *not* occur in acclimatization to exercise in the heat?

   a. increased sweat production during exercise

   b. increased blood volume
   c. a lower rise in the core temperature during exercise
   d. a lesser rise in the heart rate response to exercise
   e. an increased sodium loss in each liter of sweat

3. Which of the following statements is false?

   a. The maximal sweat rate appears to be about 2–3 liters per hour.
   b. Dehydration as low as 2 percent of the body weight may lead to a decrease in aerobic endurance performance.
   c. Sweat is mainly water.

   d. The major electrolytes found in sweat are calcium and potassium

4. Which of the following is most limited in the DASH diet?

   a. calcium
   b. fiber
   c. magnesium
   d. sodium
   e. potassium
   f. phytonutrients

5. Excessive loss of sweat during exercise in the heat will lead to a condition in the body known as

   a. hyperhydration
   b. hypohydration

c. homeostasis

d. normohydration

e. euhydration

6. Which of the following is not one of the physical means whereby heat is lost from the human body?

a. condensation

b. conduction

c. evaporation

d. convection

e. radiation

7. A high relative humidity and sunshine impose a heat stress during exercise by their adverse effects on the body, respectively, as:

a. increased condensation of sweat and decreased radiant heat to the body

b. increased convection heat loss and decreased radiant heat to the body

c. decreased evaporation of sweat and increased radiant heat to the body

d. decreased condensation of sweat and decreased convection of heat to the body

e. increased evaporation of sweat and increased convection of heat to the body

8. Calculate the increase in the body temperature, in degrees Celsius, that would occur if an individual was unable to dissipate heat and was exercising at an intensity of 3 liters of oxygen per minute for 20 minutes. The athlete weighs 60 kg, her mechanical efficiency is 20 percent, and the specific heat of her body is 0.83.

a. 2.2

b. 4.8

c. 10.2

d. 6.0

e. 9.4

9. Which of the following statements regarding bottled water is false?

a. Bottled water is normally much more expensive than municipal water supplies.

b. Bottled water must conform to the same safety standards as municipal water supplies.

c. Some bottled waters are simply municipal water that has undergone purification.

d. Bottled water normally contains more fluoride than fluoridated municipal water supplies.

10. During prolonged endurance exercise in the heat, excessive intake of water and inadequate intake of salt may lead to a dangerous health condition known as

a. hypercalcemia

b. hypotension

c. hypohydration

d. hyponatremia

e. hyperkalemia

Answers to multiple-choice questions:
1. c; 2. e; 3. d; 4. d; 5. b; 6. a; 7. c; 8. b; 9. d; 10. d.

Review Questions—Essay

1. Discuss the means whereby your body maintains normal water balance. Include in your discussion the role of the blood, hypothalamus, pituitary gland, antidiuretic hormone, and kidney.

2. Name the four components of heat stress that are recorded by the wet-bulb globe temperature (WBGT) thermometer, and discuss how each factor may contribute

to heat stress during exercise under warm environmental conditions.

3. Your friend is going to run a marathon. The projected weather forecast is sunny, warm, and humid. What advice would you offer regarding consumption of fluids, including carbohydrate and electrolytes, before and during the race?

4. List and discuss five strategies to help reduce the hazards associated with exercise in a hot environment.

5. What is high blood pressure? Why is it dangerous to your health? What lifestyle behaviors may help in its prevention or treatment?

References

Books

American Institute of Cancer Research. 2007. *Food, Nutrition, Physical Activity, and the Prevention of Cancer: A Global Perspective.* Washington, DC: AICR.

Armstrong, L. 2003. *Exertional Heat Illnesses.* Champaign, IL: Human Kinetics.

National Academy of Sciences, Institute of Medicine, Food and Nutrition Board. 2004. *Dietary Reference Intake for Water,*

Potassium, Sodium, Chloride, and Sulfate. Washington, DC: National Academy Press.

Noakes, T. 2003. *Lore of Running.* Champaign, IL: Human Kinetics.

Reviews

Aglony, M., et al. 2009. Hypertension in adolescents. *Expert Review of Cardiovascular Therapy* 7:1595–1603.

Alderman, M. 2006. Evidence relating dietary sodium to cardiovascular disease. *Journal*

of the American College of Nutrition 25:256S–61S.

American Academy of Pediatrics. 2000. Climatic heat stress and the exercising child and adolescent. *Pediatrics* 106:158–59.

American College of Sports Medicine. 2007. American College of Sports Medicine Position Stand: Exertional heat illness during training and competition. *Medicine & Science in Sports & Exercise* 39:556–72.

American College of Sports Medicine. 2007. Exercise and fluid replacement. *Medicine & Science in Sports & Exercise* 39:377–90.

American College of Sports Medicine. 2005. Youth football: Heat stress and injury risk. *Medicine & Science in Sports & Exercise* 37:1421–30.

American College of Sports Medicine. 2004. American College of Sports Medicine position stand: Exercise and hypertension. *Medicine & Science in Sports & Exercise* 36:533–53.

American Running and Fitness Association. 1996. Glycerol helps fluid balance. *FitNews* 14(6):1.

Armstrong, L., et al. 2007. Caffeine, fluid-electrolyte balance, temperature regulation, and exercise-heat tolerance. *Exercise and Sport Sciences Reviews* 35:135–40.

Baker, L., and Kenney, W. 2007. Exercising in the heat and sun. *President's Council on Physical Fitness and Sports Research Digest* 8(2):1–8.

Bar-Or, O. 1994. Children's responses to exercise in hot climates: Implications for performance and health. *Sports Science Exchange* 7(2):1–4.

Barr, S. I. 1999. Effects of dehydration on exercise performance. *Canadian Journal of Applied Physiology* 24:164–72.

Barrow, M., and Clark, K. 1998. Heat-related illnesses. *American Family Physician* 58:749–56.

Bergeron, M. 2002. Averting muscle cramps. *Physician and Sportsmedicine* 30(11):14.

Bonci, L. 2002. "Energy" drinks: Help, harm, or hype? *Sports Science Exchange* 15(1):1–4.

Burfoot, A. 2003. Drink to your health. *Runner's World.* 38 (7):52–59.

Burke, L. 2001. Nutritional needs for exercise in the heat. *Comparative Biochemistry and Physiology. Part A. Molecular & Integrative Physiology* 128:735–48.

Cappuccio, F. 2007. Salt and cardiovascular disease. *British Medical Journal* 334:859–60.

Carter, R., et al. 2006. Heat related illnesses. *Sports Science Exchange* 19(3):1–6.

Casa, D., et al. 2007. Cold water immersion: The gold standard for exertional heatstroke treatment. *Exercise and Sport Sciences Reviews* 35:141–49.

Center for Science in the Public Interest. 2007. *CSPI year-end report.* Washington, DC: CSPI.

Cheung, S., and Sleivert, G. 2004. Multiple triggers for hyperthermic fatigue and exhaustion. *Exercise and Sports Sciences Reviews* 32:100–6.

Cheuvront, S., and Sawka, M. 2005. Hydration assessment of athletes. *Sports Science Exchange* 18(2):1–6.

Cheuvront, S., et al. 2007. Fluid replacement and performance during the marathon. *Sports Medicine* 37:353–57.

Chorley, J. 2007. Hyponatremia: Identification and evaluation in the marathon medical area. *Sports Medicine* 37:451–54.

Cohen, H., and Alderman, M. 2007. Sodium, blood pressure, and cardiovascular disease. *Current Opinion in Cardiology* 22:306–10.

Consumers Union. 2006. A guide to the best and worst drinks. *Consumer Reports on Health* 18(7):8–9.

Consumers Union. 2003. Clear choices for clean drinking water. *Consumers Reports* 68(1):33–38.

Consumers Union. 2002. Blood-pressure perils. *Consumer Reports on Health* 14(9): 1, 4–6.

Consumers Union. 2002. High blood pressure: The uncontrolled epidemic. *Consumer Reports on Health* 14(10):6–8.

Consumers Union. 1999. Do you drink enough water? *Consumer Reports on Health* 11(11):8–10.

Coombes, J., and Hamilton, K. 2000. The effectiveness of commercially available sports drinks. *Sports Medicine* 29:181–209.

Costill, D. 1990. Gastric emptying of fluids during exercise. In *Perspectives in Exercise Science and Sports Medicine. Fluid Homeostasis During Exercise,* eds. C. Gisolfi and D. Lamb. Indianapolis, IN: Benchmark.

Costill, D. 1977. Sweating: Its composition and effects on body fluids. *Annals of the New York Academy of Sciences* 301: 160–74.

Council on sports medicine and fitness and council on school health. 2011. Policy Statement—Climatic Heat Stress and Exercising Children and Adolescents. *Pediatrics* Aug 8. [Epub ahead of print].

Coyle, E. 2004. Fluid and fuel intake during exercise. *Journal of Sports Sciences* 22:39–55.

Eichner, E. 2002. Heat stroke in sports: Causes, prevention, and treatment. *Sports Science Exchange* 15(3):1–4.

Eichner, E. 1998. Treatment of suspected heat illness. *International Journal of Sports Medicine* 19:S150–S153.

Eichner, R. 2007. The role of sodium in "heat cramping." *Sports Medicine* 37:368–70.

Fagard, R. 2006. Exercise is good for your blood pressure: Effects of endurance training and resistance training. *Clinical and Experimental Pharmacology & Physiology* 33:853–56.

Febbraio, M. 2001. Alterations in energy metabolism during exercise and heat stress. *Sports Medicine* 31:47–59.

Febbraio, M. 2000. Does muscle function and metabolism affect exercise performance in the heat? *Exercise and Sport Sciences Reviews* 28:171–76.

Franco, V., and Oparil, S. 2006. Salt sensitivity: A determinant of blood pressure, cardiovascular disease and survival. *Journal of the American College of Nutrition* 25:247S–55S.

Gardner, J. 2002. Death by water intoxication. *Military Medicine* 167:432–34.

Geerling, J., and Loewy, A. 2008. Central regulation of sodium appetite. *Experimental Physiology* 93:177–209.

Gisolfi, C. 1996. Fluid balance for optimal performance. *Nutrition Reviews* 54: S159–S168.

Gledhill, N. 1999. Haemoglobin, blood volume, cardiac function, and aerobic power. *Canadian Journal of Applied Physiology* 24:54–65.

Goulet, E., et al. 2007. A meta-analysis of the effects of glycerol-induced hyperhydration on fluid retention and endurance performance. *International Journal of Sport Nutrition and Exercise Metabolism* 17:391–410.

Hackman, D., et al. 2010. The 2010 Canadian hypertension education program recommendations for the management of hypertension: Part 2—Therapy. *Canadian Journal of Cardiology* 26:249–58.

Haddy, F., et al. 2006. Role of potassium in regulating blood flow and blood pressure. *American Journal of Physiology. Regulatory, Integrative and Comparative Physiology* 290:R546–52.

Hargreaves, M., and Febbraio, M. 1998. Limits to exercise performance in the heat. *International Journal of Sports Medicine* 19:S115–S116.

Hew-Butler, T., et al. 2005. Consensus statement of the 1st International Exercise-Associated Hyponatremia Consensus Development Conference. *Clinical Journal of Sports Medicine* 15:208–13.

Hiller, D. 1989. Dehydration and hyponatremia during triathlons. *Medicine & Science in Sports & Exercise* 21:S219–S221.

Hsieh, M. 2004. Recommendations for treatment of hyponatremia at endurance events. *Sports Medicine* 34:231–38.

Israili, Z., et al. 2007. The future of antihypertensive treatment. *American Journal of Therapeutics* 14:121–34.

Jeukendrup, A., and Martin, J. 2001. Improving cycling performance: How should we spend our time and money? *Sports Medicine* 31:559–69.

Johnson, A. 2007. The sensory psychobiology of thirst and salt appetite. *Medicine & Science in Sports & Exercise* 39:1388–1400.

Joint National Committee on Prevention, Detection, Evaluation and Treatment of High Blood Pressure. 2003. The Seventh Report of the Joint National Committee on Prevention, Detection, Evaluation and Treatment of High Blood Pressure. *Hypertension* 42:1206–52.

Kaplan, R. 2007. Beverage guidance system is not evidence-based. *American Journal of Clinical Nutrition* 84:1248–49.

Kenefick, R., and Sawka, M. 2007. Heat exhaustion and dehydration as causes of marathon collapse. *Sports Medicine* 37:378–81.

Kenefick, R., et al. 2007. Thermoregulatory function during the marathon. *Sports Medicine* 37:312–15.

Khan, N., et al. 2007. The 2007 Canadian Hypertension Education Program recommendations for the management of hypertension: Part 2—therapy. *Canadian Journal of Cardiology* 23:539–50.

Kramer, J., et al. 2002. Exercise and hypertension: A model for central neural plasticity. *Clinical and Experimental Pharmacology & Physiology* 29:122–26.

Lamb, D., and Shehata, A. 1999. Benefits and limitations to prehydration. *Sports Science Exchange* 12(2):1–6.

Latzka, W., and Sawka, M. 2000. Hyperhydration and glycerol: Thermoregulatory effects during exercise in hot environments. *Canadian Journal of Applied Physiology* 25:536–45.

Lefferts, L. 1990. Water: Treat it right. *Nutrition Action Health Letter* 17:5–7.

Liebman, B. 2006. Pour better or pour worse. How beverages stack up. *Nutrition Action Health Letter* 33(5):1–7.

Lien, Y., and Shapiro, J. 2007. Hyponatremia: Clinical diagnosis and management. *American Journal of Medicine* 120(8):653–58.

Luetkemeier, M., et al. 1997. Dietary sodium and plasma volume levels with exercise. *Sports Medicine* 23:279–86.

Luft, F. 1998. Salt and hypertension at the close of the millennium. *Wiener Klinische Wochenschrift* 110:459–66.

Macdonald, I. 1992. Food and drink in sport. *British Medical Journal* 48:605–14.

Mack, G. 2006. The body fluid and hemopoietic systems. In *ACSM's Advanced Exercise Physiology,* ed. C. Tipton. Philadelphia: Lippincott Williams & Wilkins.

Manz, F., et al. 2002. The most essential nutrient: Defining the adequate intake of water. *Journal of Pediatrics* 141:587–92.

Marino, F. 2002. Methods, advantages, and limitations of body cooling for exercise performance. *British Journal of Sports Medicine* 36:89–94.

Maughan, R., and Shirreffs, S. 2010. Development of hydration strategies to optimize performance for athletes in high-intensity sports and in sports with repeated intense efforts. *Scandinavian Journal of Medicine & Science in Sports* 20(Suppl 2):59–69.

Maughan, R. 2000. Water and electrolyte loss and replacement in exercise. In *Nutrition in Sport,* ed. R. Maughan. Oxford: Blackwell Science.

Maughan, R. 1999. Exercise in the heat: Limitations to performance and the impact of fluid replacement strategies. Introduction to the symposium. *Canadian Journal of Applied Physiology* 24;149–51.

Maughan, R. 1998. The sports drink as a functional food: Formulations for successful performance. *Proceedings of the Nutrition Society* 57:15–23.

Maughan, R., et al. 2007. Errors in the estimation of hydration status from changes in body mass. *Journal of Sports Sciences* 25:797–804.

McCann, D., and Adams, W. C. 1997. Wet bulb globe temperature index and performance in competitive distance runners. *Medicine & Science in Sports & Exercise* 29:955–61.

McCarron, D., and Reusser, M. 2000. The power of food to improve multiple cardiovascular risk factors. *Current Atherosclerosis Reports* 2:482–86.

Montain, S., et al. 2007. Marathon performance in thermally stressing conditions. *Sports Medicine* 37:320–23.

Murray, R. 2007. The role of salt and glucose replacement drinks in the marathon. *Sports Medicine* 37:358–60.

Murray, R., and Shi, X. 2006. The gastrointestinal system. In *ACSM's Advanced Exercise Physiology,* ed. C. Tipton. Philadelphia: Lippincott Williams & Wilkins.

Noakes, T. 2007. Drinking guidelines for exercise: What evidence is there that athletes should drink "as much as tolerable," "to replace the weight lost during exercise" or "ad libitum"? *Journal of Sports Sciences* 25:781–96.

Noakes, T. 2007. Hydration in the marathon. *Sports Medicine* 37:463–66.

Nybo, L. 2010. CNS fatigue provoked by prolonged exercise in the heat. *Frontiers in Bioscience* E2:779–92.

Nybo, L. 2008. Hyperthermia and fatigue. *Journal of Applied Physiology* 104:871–78.

Oliveira, L., and Lawless, C. 2010. Hypertension update and cardiovascular risk reduction in physically active individuals and athletes. *Physician and Sportsmedicine* 38:11–20.

Penner, S., et al. 2007. Dietary sodium and cardiovascular outcomes: a rational approach. *Canadian Journal of Cardiology* 23:567–72.

Peters, H., et al. 1995. Gastrointestinal symptoms during exercise: The effect of fluid supplementation. *Sports Medicine* 20:65–76.

Popkin, B., et al. 2006. A new proposed guidance system for beverage consumption in the United States. *American Journal of Clinical Nutrition* 83:529–42.

Quod, M., et al. 2006. Cooling athletes before competition in the heat: Comparison of techniques and practical considerations. *Sports Medicine* 36:671–82.

Rehrer, N. 2001. Fluid and electrolyte balance in ultra-endurance sport. *Sports Medicine* 31:701–15.

Roberts, W. 2007. Exercise-associated collapse care matrix in the marathon. *Sports Medicine* 37:431–33.

Roberts, W. 2007. Exertional heat stroke in the marathon. *Sports Medicine* 37:440–43.

Sallis, R. 2004. Collapse in the endurance athlete. *Sports Science Exchange* 17(4):1–6.

Savica, V., et al. 2010. The effect of nutrition on blood pressure. *Annual Review of Nutrition* 30:365–401.

Sawka, M., and Greenleaf, J. 1992. Current concepts concerning thirst, dehydration, and fluid replacement: Overview. *Medicine & Science in Sports & Exercise* 24:643–44.

Sawka, M., and Pandolf, K. 1990. Effects of body water loss on physiological function and exercise performance. In *Perspectives in Exercise Science and Sports Medicine. Fluid Homeostasis During Exercise,* eds. C. Gisolfi and D. Lamb. Indianapolis, IN: Benchmark.

Sawka, M., and Young, A. 2006. Physiological systems and their responses to conditions of heat and cold. In *ACSM's Advanced Exercise Physiology,* ed. C. Tipton. Philadelphia: Lippincott Williams & Wilkins.

Sawka, M., et al. 2001. Hydration effects on thermoregulation and performance in the heat. *Comparative Biochemistry and Physiology. Part A. Molecular and Integrative Physiology* 128:679–90.

Sawka, M., et al. 2000. Effects of dehydration and rehydration on performance. In *Nutrition in Sport,* ed. R. J. Maughan. Oxford: Blackwell Science.

Schwellnus, M., et al. 2008. Muscle cramping in athletes—risk factors, clinical assessment, and management. *Clinics in Sports Medicine* 27:183–94.

Schwellnus, M. 2007. Muscle cramping in the marathon. *Sports Medicine* 37:364–67.

Schwellnus, M. 1999. Skeletal muscle cramps during exercise. *Physician and Sportsmedicine* 27(12):109–15.

Shirreffs, S., and Maughan, R. 2000. Rehydration and recovery of fluid balance after exercise. *Exercise and Sport Sciences Reviews* 28:27–32.

Spickard, A. 1968. Heat stroke in college football and suggestions for prevention. *Southern Medical Journal* 61:791–96.

Tanji, J., and Batt, M. 1995. Management of hypertension: Adapting new guidelines for active patients. *Physician and Sportsmedicine* 23(2):47–55.

Tejada, T., et al. 2006. Nonpharmacologic therapy for hypertension: Does it really work? *Current Cardiology Reports* 8:418–24.

Tufts University. 2000. Purified bottled water . . . from public water supplies. *Health & Nutrition Letter* 18(1):1.

Valtin, H. 2008. In the drink. *Nutrition Action Health Letter* 35(5):12–13.

Valtin, H. 2002. "Drink at least eight glasses of water a day." Really? Is there scientific evidence for "8 × 8"? *American Journal of Physiology. Regulatory Integrative and Comparative Physiology* 283:R993–1004.

Van Rosendal, S., et al. 2010. Guidelines for glycerol use in hyperhydration and rehydration associated with exercise. *Sports Medicine* 40:113–39.

Young, A. 1990. Energy substrate utilization during exercise in extreme environments. *Exercise and Sport Sciences Reviews* 18:65–118.

Specific Studies

Almond, C., et al. 2005. Hyponatremia among runners in the Boston Marathon. *New England Journal of Medicine* 352:1550–56.

Anastasiou, C., et al. 2009. Sodium replacement and plasma sodium drop during exercise in the heat when fluid intake matches fluid loss. *Journal of Athletic Training* 44:117–23.

Anderson, M., et al. 2001. Effect of glycerol-induced hyperhydration on thermoregulation and metabolism during exercise in heat. *International Journal of Sport Nutrition and Exercise Metabolism* 11:315–33.

Appel, L., et al. 2005. Effects of protein, monounsaturated fat, and carbohydrate intake on blood pressure and serum lipids: Results of the OmniHeart randomized trial. *Journal of the American Medical Association* 294:2455–64.

Armstrong, L., et al. 2006. No effect of 5% hypohydration on running economy of competitive runners at 23 degrees C. *Medicine & Science in Sports & Exercise* 38:1762–69.

Armstrong, L., et al. 2005. Fluid, electrolyte, and renal indices of hydration during 11 days of controlled caffeine consumption. *International Journal of Sport Nutrition and Exercise Metabolism* 15:252–65.

Azadbakht, L., et al. 2005. Beneficial effects of a Dietary Approaches to Stop Hypertension eating plan on features of the metabolic syndrome. *Diabetes Care* 28:2823–31.

Baker, L., et al. 2007. Dehydration impairs vigilance-related attention in male basketball players. *Medicine & Science in Sports & Exercise* 39:976–83.

Baker, L., et al. 2007. Progressive dehydration causes a progressive decline in basketball skill performance. *Medicine & Science in Sports & Exercise* 39:1114–23.

Baker, L., et al. 2005. Sex differences in voluntary fluid intake by older adults during exercise. *Medicine & Science in Sports & Exercise* 37:789–96.

Barr, S., et al. 1991. Fluid replacement during prolonged exercise: Effects of water, saline, and no fluid. *Medicine & Science in Sports & Exercise* 23:811–17.

Below, P., et al. 1995. Fluid and carbohydrate ingestion independently improve performance during 1 h of intense exercise. *Medicine & Science in Sports & Exercise* 27:200–210.

Bilzon, J., et al. 2000. Short-term recovery from prolonged constant pace running in a warm environment: The effectiveness of a carbohydrate-electrolyte solution. *European Journal of Applied Physiology* 82:305–12.

Bird, S., et al. 2006. Liquid carbohydrate/protein amino acid ingestion during a short-term bout of resistance exercise suppresses myofibrillar protein degradation. *Metabolism* 55:570–77.

Byrne, C., et al. 2006. Continuous thermoregulatory responses to mass-participation distance running in heat. *Medicine & Science in Sports & Exercise* 38:803–10.

Castle, P., et al. 2006. Precooling leg muscle improves intermittent sprint exercise in hot, humid conditions. *Journal of Applied Physiology* 100:1377–84.

Chen, L., et al. 2010. Reducing consumption of sugar-sweetened beverages is associated with reduced blood pressure: A prospective study among United States adults. *Circulation* 121:2398–406.

Cheuvront, S., and Haymes, E. 2001. Ad libitum fluid intakes and thermoregulatory responses of female distance runners in three environments. *Journal of Sport Sciences* 19:845–54.

Cheuvront, S., et al. 2002. Comparison of sweat loss estimates for women during prolonged high-intensity running. *Medicine & Science in Sports & Exercise* 34:1344–50.

Clarke, N., et al. 2005. Strategies for hydration and energy provision during soccer-specific exercise. *International Journal of Sport Nutrition and Exercise Metabolism* 15:625–40.

Cook, N., et al. 2007. Long term effects of dietary sodium reduction on cardiovascular disease outcomes: Observational follow-up of the trials of hypertension prevention (TOHP). *British Medical Journal* 334:885.

Costill, D., et al. 1982. Dietary potassium and heavy exercise: Effects on muscle water and electrolytes. *American Journal of Clinical Nutrition* 36:266–75.

Coutts, A., et al. 2002. The effect of glycerol hyperhydration on Olympic distance triathlon performance in high ambient temperatures. *International Journal of Sport Nutrition and Exercise Metabolism* 12:105–19.

de Castro, J. 2005. Stomach filling may mediate the influence of dietary energy density on the food intake of free-living humans. *Physiology & Behavior* 86:32–45.

Dougherty, K., et al. 2006. Two percent dehydration impairs and six percent carbohydrate drink improves boy's basketball skills. *Medicine & Science in Sports & Exercise* 38:1650–58.

Drust, B., et al. 2005. Elevations in core and muscle temperature impairs repeated sprint performance. *Acta Physiologica Scandinavica* 183:181–90.

Edwards, A., et al. 2007. Influence of moderate dehydration on soccer performance: Physiological responses to 45 min of outdoor match-play and the immediate subsequent performance of sport-specific and mental concentration tests. *British Journal of Sports Medicine* 41:385–91.

Elley, R., et al. 2006. Do snacks of exercise lower blood pressure? A randomized crossover trial. *New Zealand Medical Journal* 113:2642–50.

Freund, B., et al. 1995. Glycerol hyperhydration: Hormonal, renal, and vascular fluid responses. *Journal of Applied Physiology* 79:2069–77.

Fritzsche, R., et al. 2000. Water and carbohydrate ingestion during prolonged exercise increase maximal neuromuscular power. *Journal of Applied Physiology* 88:730–37.

Fudge, B., et al. 2008. Elite Kenyan endurance runners are hydrated day-to-day with *ad libitum* fluid intake. *Medicine & Science in Sports & Exercise* 40:1171–79.

Fung, T., et al. 2008. Adherence to a DASH-style diet and risk of coronary heart disease and stroke in women. *Archives of Internal Medicine* 168:713–20

Gant, N., et al. 2007. Gastric emptying of fluids during variable-intensity running in the heat. *International Journal of Sport Nutrition and Exercise Metabolism* 17:270–83.

Gardner, J., et al. 1996. Risk factors predicting exertional heat illness in male Marine Corps recruits. *Medicine & Science in Sports & Exercise* 28:939–44.

Gisolfi, C., et al. 2001. Intestinal fluid absorption during exercise: Role of sport drink osmolality and [Na⁺]. *Medicine & Science in Sports & Exercise* 33:907–15.

Gisolfi, C., et al. 1998. Effect of beverage osmolality on intestinal fluid absorption during exercise. *Journal of Applied Physiology* 85:1941–48.

Godek, S., et al. 2005. Sweat rate and fluid turnover in American football players compared with runners in a hot and humid environment. *British Journal of Sports Medicine* 39:205–11.

Goulet, E., et al. 2006. Effect of glycerol-induced hyperhydration on thermoregulatory and cardiovascular functions and endurance performance during prolonged cycling in a 25 degrees C environment. *Applied Physiology, Nutrition and Metabolism* 31:101–9.

Greiwe, J., et al. 1998. Effect of dehydration on isometric muscular strength and endurance. *Medicine & Science in Sports & Exercise* 30:284–88.

Hampson, N., et al. 2003. Oxygenated water and athletic performance. *JAMA* 290: 2408–9.

Hansen, M., et al. 2007. Underdiagnosis of hypertension in children and adolescents. *Journal of the American Medical Association* 298:874–79.

Hargreaves, M., et al. 1996. Effect of fluid ingestion on muscle metabolism during prolonged exercise. *Journal of Applied Physiology* 80:363–66.

Hargreaves, M., et al. 1994. Influence of sodium on glucose bioavailability during exercise. *Medicine & Science in Sports & Exercise* 26:365–68.

Hew-Butler, T., et al. 2006. Sodium supplementation is not required to maintain serum sodium concentrations during an Ironman triathlon. *British Journal of Sports Medicine* 40:255–59.

Hitchins, S., et al. 1999. Glycerol hyperhydration improves cycle time trial performance in hot humid conditions. *European Journal of Applied Physiology* 80:494–501.

Hunter, I., et al. 2006. Warming up with an ice vest: Core body temperature before and after cross-country racing. *Journal of Athletic Training* 41:371–74.

Jentjens, R., et al. 2006. Exogenous carbohydrate oxidation rates are elevated after combined ingestion of glucose and fructose during exercise in the heat. *Journal of Applied Physiology* 100:807–16.

Judelson, D., et al. 2007. Effect of hydration state on strength, power, and resistance exercise performance. *Medicine & Science in Exercise & Sports* 39:1817–24.

Kavouras, S., et al. 2006. Rehydration with glycerol: Endocrine, cardiovascular, and thermoregulatory responses during exercise in the heat. *Journal of Applied Physiology* 100:442–50.

Kenefick, R., et al. 2007. Rehydration with fluid of varying tonicities: Effects on fluid regulatory hormones and exercise performance in the heat. *Journal of Applied Physiology* 102:1899–1905.

Kenefick, R., et al. 2002. Hypohydration adversely affects lactate threshold in endurance athletes. *Journal of Strength and Conditioning Research* 16:38–43.

Lalumandier, J., and Ayers, L. 2000. Flouride and bacterial content of bottled water vs tap water. *Archives of Family Medicine* 9:246–50.

Lambert, G., et al. 1993. Effects of carbonated and noncarbonated beverages at specific intervals during treadmill running in the heat. *International Journal of Sport Nutrition* 3:177–93.

Latzka, W., et al. 1998. Hyperhydration: Tolerance and cardiovascular effect during uncompensable exercise-heat stress. *Journal of Applied Physiology* 84:1858–64.

Latzka, W., et al. 1997. Hyperhydration: Thermoregulatory effects during compensable exercise-heat stress. *Journal of Applied Physiology* 83:860–66.

Lindeman, A. 1991. Nutrient intake of an ultraendurance cyclist. *International Journal of Sport Nutrition* 1:79–85.

Lyons, T., et al. 1990. Effects of glycerol-induced hyperhydration prior to exercise in the heat on sweating and core temperature. *Medicine & Science in Sports & Exercise* 22:477–83.

Magal, M., et al. 2003. Comparison of glycerol and water hydration regimens on tennis-related performance. *Medicine & Science in Sports & Exercise* 35:150–56.

Marino, F., et al. 2003. Glycerol hyperhydration fails to improve endurance performance and thermoregulation in humans in a warm humid environment. *Pflugers Archiv* 446:455–62.

Massicotte, D., et al. 2006. Metabolic fate of a large amount of 13C-glycerol ingested during prolonged exercise. *European Journal of Applied Physiology* 96:322–29.

Maughan, R., et al. 2007. Water balance and salt losses in competitive football. *International Journal of Sport Nutrition and Exercise Metabolism* 17:583–94.

Maughan, R., et al. 2005. Fluid and electrolyte balance in elite male football (soccer) players training in a cool environment. *Journal of Sports Sciences* 23:72–79.

Michaud, D., et al. 1999. Fluid intake and the risk of bladder cancer in men. *New England Journal of Medicine* 340:1390–97.

Millard-Stafford, M. 1997. Water versus carbohydrate-electrolyte ingestion before and during a 15-km run in the heat. *International Journal of Sport Nutrition* 7:26–38.

Millard-Stafford, M., et al. 2005. Should carbohydrate concentration of a sports drink be less than 8% during exercise in the heat? *International Journal of Sport Nutrition and Exercise Metabolism* 15:117–30.

Montain, S., et al. 1998. Hypohydration effects on skeletal muscle performance and metabolism: A 31P-MRS study. *Journal of Applied Physiology* 84:1889–94.

Montain, S., et al. 1998. Thermal and cardiovascular strain from hypohydration: Influence of exercise intensity. *International Journal of Sports Medicine* 19:87–91.

Montner, P., et al. 1996. Pre-exercise glycerol hydration improves cycling endurance time. *International Journal of Sports Medicine* 17:27–33.

Murray, R., et al. 1999. A comparison of the gastric emptying characteristics of selected sports drinks. *International Journal of Sport Nutrition* 9:263–74.

Osterberg, K., et al. 2010. Carbohydrate exerts a mild influence on fluid retention following exercise-induced dehydration. *Journal of Applied Physiology* 108:245–50.

Osterberg, K., et al. 2009. Pregame urine specific gravity and fluid intake by National Basketball Association players during competition. *Journal of Athletic Training* 44:53–57.

Parisi, A., et al. 2002. Complex ventricular arrhythmia induced by overuse of potassium supplementation in a young male football player. Case report. *Journal of Sports Medicine and Physical Fitness* 42:214–16.

Passe, D., et al. 2007. Voluntary dehydration in runners despite favorable conditions for fluid intake. *International Journal of Sport Nutrition and Exercise Metabolism* 17:284–95.

Passe, D., et al. 2004. Palatability and voluntary intake of sports beverages, diluted orange juice, and water during exercise. *International Journal of Sport Nutrition and Exercise Metabolism* 14:272–84.

Ray, M., et al. 1998. Effect of sodium in a rehydration beverage when consumed as a fluid or meal. *Journal of Applied Physiology* 85:1329–36.

Rehrer, N., et al. 1992. Gastrointestinal complaints in relation to dietary intake in triathletes. *International Journal of Sport Nutrition* 2:48–59.

Roberts, D. 2006. Blood pressure response to 1-month electrolyte-carbohydrate beverage consumption. *Journal of Occupational and Environmental Hygiene* 3:131–36.

Rogers, G., et al. 1997. Water budget during ultra-endurance exercise. *Medicine & Science in Sports & Exercise* 29:1477–81.

Rogers, I., and Hew-Butler, T. 2009. Exercise-associated hyponatremia: Overzealous fluid consumption. *Wilderness and Environmental Medicine* 20:139–43.

Rogers, J., et al. 2005. Gastric emptying and intestinal absorption of a low-carbohydrate sport drink during exercise. *International Journal of Sport Nutrition and Exercise Metabolism* 15:220–35.

Ronneberg, K., et al. 2008. Temporal artery temperature measurements do not detect hyperthermic marathon runners. *Medicine & Science in Sports & Exercise* 40:1373–75.

Roti, M., et al. 2006. Thermoregulatory responses to exercise in the heat: Chronic caffeine intake has no effect. *Aviation, Space, and Environmental Medicine* 77:124–29.

Rowland, T., et al. 2008. Exercise tolerance and thermoregulatory responses during cycling in boys and men. *Medicine & Science in Sports & Exercise* 40:282–87.

Ryan, A., et al. 1998. Effect of hypohydration on gastric emptying and intestinal absorption during exercise. *Journal of Applied Physiology* 84:1581–88.

Sacks, F., et al. 2001. Effects on blood pressure of reduced dietary sodium and the Dietary Approaches to Stop Hypertension (DASH) diet. *New England Journal of Medicine* 344:3–10.

Sanders, B., et al. 1999. Water and electrolyte shifts with partial fluid replacement during exercise. *European Journal of Applied Physiology* 80:318–23.

Scheett, T., et al. 2001. Effectiveness of glycerol as a rehydrating agent. *International Journal of Sport Nutrition and Exercise Metabolism* 11:63–71.

Schoffstall, J., et al. 2001. Effects of dehydration and rehydration on the one-repetition maximum bench press of weight-trained males. *Journal of Strength and Conditioning Research* 15:102–8.

Seifert, J., et al. 2006. Protein added to a sports drink improves fluid retention. *International Journal of Sport Nutrition and Exercise Metabolism* 16:420–29.

Shah, M., et al. 2007. Effect of high-carbohydrate or high-cis-monounsaturated fat diets on blood pressure: A meta-analysis of intervention trials. *American Journal of Clinical Nutrition* 85:1251–56.

Shirreffs, S., et al. 2007. Rehydration after exercise in the heat: A comparison of 4 commonly used drinks. *International Journal of Sport Nutrition and Exercise Metabolism* 17:244–58.

Sims, S., et al. 2007. Preexercise sodium loading aids fluid balance and endurance for women exercising in the heat. *Journal of Applied Physiology* 103:534–41.

Sims, S., et al. 2007. Sodium loading aids fluid balance and reduces physiological strain of trained men exercising in the heat. *Medicine & Science in Sports & Exercise* 39:123–30.

Speedy, D., et al. 2002. Oral salt supplementation during ultradistance exercise. *Clinical Journal of Sport Medicine* 12:279–84.

Speedy, D., et al. 2000. Exercise-induced hyponatremia in ultradistance triathletes is caused by inappropriate fluid retention. *Clinical Journal of Sport Medicine* 10:272–78.

Stofan, J., et al. 2005. Sweat and sodium losses in NCAA football players: A precursor to heat cramps. *International Journal of Sport Nutrition and Exercise Metabolism* 15:641–52.

Stookey, J. 1999. The diuretic effects of alcohol and caffeine and total water intake misclassification. *European Journal of Epidemiology* 15:181–88.

Sulzer, N., et al. 2005. Serum electrolytes in Ironman triathletes with exercise-associated muscle cramping. *Medicine & Science in Sports & Exercise* 37:1081–85.

Tucker, R., et al. 2004. Impaired exercise performance in the heat is associated with an anticipatory reduction in skeletal muscle recruitment. *Pflugers Archive* 448:422–30.

Twerenbold, R., et al. 2003. Effects of different sodium concentrations in replacement fluids during prolonged exercise in women. *British Journal of Sports Medicine* 37:300–3.

Uckert, S., and Joch, W. 2007. Effects of warm-up and precooling on endurance performance in the heat. *British Journal of Sports Medicine* 41:380–84.

Van Essen, M., and Gibala, M. 2006. Failure of protein to improve time trial performance when added to a sports drink. *Medicine & Science in Sports & Exercise* 38:1476–83.

Volpe, S., et al. Estimation of prepractice hydration status of National Collegiate Athletic Association Division I athletes. *Journal of Athletic Training* 44:624–29.

von Fraunhofer, J., and Rogers, M. 2005. Effects of sports drinks and other beverages on dental enamel. *General Dentistry* 53:28–31.

Watson, P., et al. 2005. Blood-brain barrier integrity may be threatened by exercise in a warm environment. *American Journal of Physiology. Regulatory, Integrative, and Comparative Physiology* 288:R1689–94.

Webster, J., et al. 2005. A light-weight vest enhances performance of athletes in the heat. *Ergonomics* 48:821–37.

Wharam, P., et al. 2006. NSAID use increases the risk of developing hyponatremia during an Ironman triathlon. *Medicine & Science in Sports & Exercise* 38:618–22.

White, J., et al. 1998. Fluid replacement needs of well-trained male and female athletes during indoor and outdoor steady state running. *Journal of Science and Medicine in Sport* 1:131–42.

Wing-Gaia, S., et al. 2005. Effects of purified oxygenated water on exercise performance during acute hypoxic exposure. *International Journal of Sport Nutrition and Exercise Metabolism* 15:680–88.

Wingo, J., et al. 2004. Influence of a pre-exercise glycerol hydration beverage on performance and physiologic function during mountain-bike races in the heat. *Journal of Athletic Training* 39:169–75.

Yaspelkis, B., et al. 1993. Carbohydrate metabolism during exercise in hot and thermoneutral environments. *International Journal of Sports Medicine* 14:13–19.

Yeargin, S., et al. 2006. Body cooling between two bouts of exercise in the heat enhances subsequent performance. *Journal of Strength and Conditioning Research* 20:383–89.

Zachwieja, J., et al. 1992. The effects of a carbonated carbohydrate drink on gastric emptying, gastrointestinal distress, and exercise performance. *International Journal of Sport Nutrition* 2:239–50.

the right composition, may be advantageous to other athletes.

At the other end of the body-weight continuum, weight losses leading to excessive thinness also may have an impact upon health and physical performance. Anorexia nervosa and bulimia are two serious health disorders associated with obsessive concern about body weight. Although losing excess body fat may improve performance in some sports, excessive weight losses may have a negative impact upon both health and athletic performance.

The major focus of this chapter is on the basic nature of body composition and its effect on health and physical performance. The following two chapters deal with weight-control methods used to maintain or modify body composition.

Body Weight and Composition

What is the ideal body weight?

We all have heard at one time or another that there is an ideal body weight for our particular height. But ideal in terms of what? Health? Appearance? Physical performance? There appears to be no sound evidence to suggest a specific ideal weight for a given individual, but some general guidelines have been proposed relative to health and physical performance, the major focus of this chapter.

Most of us have our own images of how we would like to look, and indeed most individuals who attempt to attain an ideal body weight do so to enhance their appearance. An enhanced physical appearance may improve one's body image and self-esteem, factors important to psychological health. An enhanced physical appearance may also influence performance in certain sports that involve judging of aesthetic movements, such as gymnastics and diving. Although society may create a perception of an ideal body weight for appearance, this perceived ideal body weight may or may not be in accord with optimal health and physical performance.

Most research efforts have attempted to find an ideal body weight for good health. For example, data collected during the past century, mainly by life insurance companies, have been compiled into normal or desirable ranges of body weight for a given height and age. These height-weight charts represent the ideal weights at which Americans can expect to live the longest. The terminology of ideal weight has changed over the years, today being referred to as a *healthy body weight*. Although height-weight charts have been used to screen for normal body weight in the past, the Body Mass Index (BMI) is the current standard, which is also based on a height-weight relationship.

The **Body Mass Index (BMI),** also known as *Quetelet's Index,* is a weight:height ratio. Using the metric system, the formula is

$$\frac{\text{Body weight in kilograms}}{(\text{Height in meters})^2}$$

An adult who weighs 70 kg (154 pounds) and is 1.78 meters (70 inches) in height would have a BMI of 22.1 ($70 \div [1.78^2]$). If you want to use pounds and inches, the formula is

$$\frac{(\text{Body weight in pounds}) \times 705}{(\text{Height in inches})^2}$$

For the same example using pounds and inches, the BMI is also 22.1 ($154 \times 705 \div [70^2]$). In general, a BMI range of 18.5–25 is considered to be normal for adults. You may calculate your BMI using method A in appendix D or at the following Website. *www.nhlbisupport.com/bmi*

Calculating the BMI for children and teens is somewhat more complex, and includes both age and gender. The BMI is used as a screening tool to identify possible weight problems for children, and both the Centers for Disease Control (CDC) and the American Academy of Pediatrics (AAP) recommend the use of BMI in children beginning at 2 years old. The CDC has developed BMI-for-age growth charts for girls and boys that can be consulted to provide a percentile for a child's or teen's sex and age. The percentile ranking places the child in one of four categories: Underweight; Healthy Weight; Overweight; Obese. The following Website provides detailed information on calculation and interpretation of the BMI for children and teens. *http://apps.nccd.cdc.gov/dnpabmi/*

What are the values and limitations of the BMI?

In relation to determining whether an individual possesses normal body weight for a given height, the BMI may be a useful screening device for health problems. The Consumers Union indicates that a low BMI may be a symptom of a serious disease, whereas a high BMI may be indicative of obesity. Specific BMI values related to potential health status are presented later.

However, for any given individual, the BMI reveals nothing about body composition. The BMI value does not represent percent body fat, as some mistakenly think. As illustrated in figure 10.1, two individuals may be exactly the same height and weight and have the same BMI, but the distribution of their body weight might be so different that one individual could possibly be considered obese while the other might be considered very muscular. For example, Ode and others compared the BMI of college athletes and nonathletes with body fat levels determined by body composition analysis (discussed later). They reported that because of a large muscle mass among male and female athletes, the BMI incorrectly classifies normal-fat athletes as overweight. Conversely, many female nonathletes were classified as normal weight by the BMI but actually were overfat; the authors noted that those who do not exercise, and yet are thin, may have excessive amounts of internal fat and thus may be thin on the outside but fat on the inside. They concluded that the BMI should be used cautiously when classifying fatness in college athletes and nonathletes.

Although the BMI is not perfect and may be inappropriate for use with very muscular individuals, it is a good guide that the average person may use to think about a healthier body weight. However, other methods are needed to evaluate actual body composition.

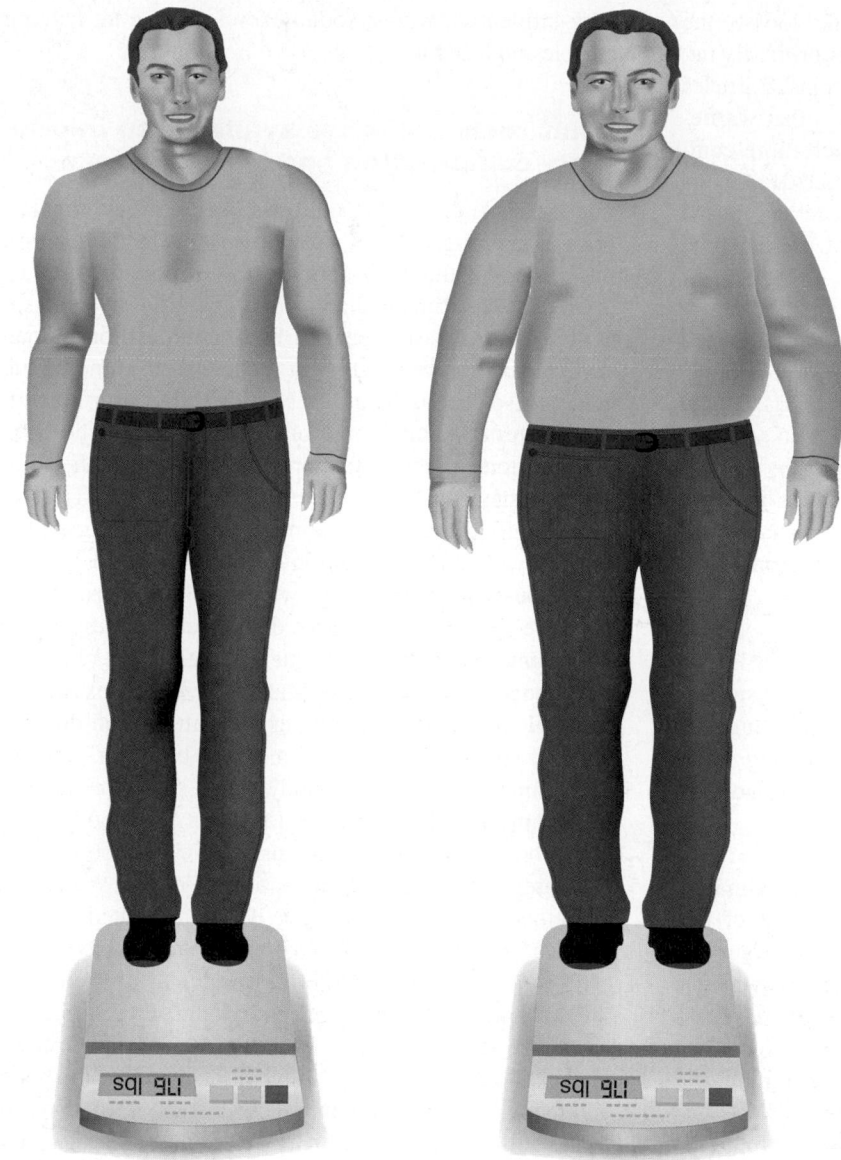

6'0"

176 lbs   176 lbs

FIGURE 10.1 The Body Mass Index (BMI), although a good general indicator of overweight and obesity, does not assess body composition in any given individual. Two individuals may have the same height and weight, but one may have excess body fat while the other may be very muscular with a low body-fat percentage.

and others noted that, depending on the purpose, body composition may be evaluated at five levels: atomic, molecular, cellular, tissue-system, and whole-body levels. Of major interest to body composition scientists are four major body components: total body fat, fat-free mass, bone mineral, and body water; the location of the body fat, either under the skin or deep in the body, is of particular interest in relationship to health status. Each of these components has a different density. Density represents mass divided by volume, and in body composition, analysis is usually expressed as grams per milliliter (g/ml) or grams per cubic centimeter (g/cc^3). The standard for comparison is water, which has a density of 1.0, or 1 g/ml. Corresponding densities for the other components are approximately 1.3–1.4 for bone, 1.1 for fat-free protein tissue, and 0.9 for fat. The density of the human body as a whole may have a wide range, approximately 1.020 to 1.100. The body-density value may be used to determine the body-fat percentage; a higher density represents a greater amount of fat-free mass and a lower amount of body fat. For example, an animal study using specific gravity, a measure of density, reported that rodents with a specific gravity of 1.08 possessed only 5 percent fat, whereas those with a specific gravity of 1.04 possessed 24 percent fat.

Depending on the purpose, body composition is usually analyzed as two, three, or all four components. The two components most commonly measured are total body fat and fat-free mass; bone mineral content and body water may be measured with more elaborate techniques. Wang and others also introduced a six-component model, which in addition to these four components adds measurement of soft-tissue minerals and glycogen.

What is the composition of the body?

The human body contains many of the elements of the earth, 25 of which appear to be essential for normal physiological functioning. Most of the human body, about 96 percent, consists of four elements (carbon, hydrogen, oxygen, and nitrogen) in various combinations. These four elements are the structural basis for body protein, carbohydrate, fat, and water. The remaining 4 percent of the body is composed of minerals, primarily calcium and phosphorus in the bones, but also including others, such as iron, potassium, sodium, chloride, and magnesium.

Because body composition may have a significant impact on health and physical performance, scientists have developed a variety of techniques to measure various body components. Wang

Total Body Fat The total body fat in the body consists of both essential fat and storage fat. **Essential fat** is necessary for proper functioning of certain body structures such as the brain, nerve tissue, bone marrow, heart tissue, and cell membranes. Essential fat in adult males represents about 3 percent of the body weight. Adult females also have additional essential fat associated with their reproductive processes. This additional 9–12 percent of sex-specific fat gives them a total of 12–15 percent essential fat, although this amount may vary considerably among individuals. **Storage fat** is simply a depot for excess energy, and the quantity of body fat in this form also may vary considerably.

Some storage fat is found around body organs for protection, but about 70–80 percent of total body fat is found just under the skin and is known as **subcutaneous fat.** When this latter type of fat is separated by connective tissue into small compartments that extrude into the dermis, it gives a dimpled, quilt-like look to the skin and is popularly known as **cellulite.** Cellulite is primarily fat, but may contain high concentrations of glycoproteins, particles that can attract water and possibly give cellulite skin that waffle-like appearance. The appearance of cellulite is much more common in women than in men. Other storage fat is located deep in the body, particularly in the abdominal area. This deep fat is referred to as **visceral fat,** which as noted later is associated with increased health risks.

Fat-Free Mass   **Fat-free mass** primarily consists of protein and water, with smaller amounts of minerals and glycogen. The tissue of skeletal muscles is the main component of fat-free mass, but the heart, liver, kidneys, and other organs are included also. A more common term often used interchangeably with fat-free mass is **lean body mass;** technically, however, lean body mass includes essential fat. In a two-component body composition analysis, fat-free or lean body mass complements total body fat. An individual who has 20 percent body fat has 80 percent fat-free mass.

Bone Mineral   Bone gives structure to the body, but it is also involved in a variety of metabolic processes. Bone consists of about 50 percent water and 50 percent solid matter, including protein and minerals. Although total bone weight, including water and protein, may be 12–15 percent of the total body weight, the mineral content is only 3–4 percent of total body weight.

Body Water   The average adult body weight is approximately 60 percent water, the remaining 40 percent consisting of dry weight materials that exist in this internal water environment. Some tissues, like the blood, have a high water content, whereas others, like adipose tissue, are relatively dry. The fat-free mass is about 70 percent water, while adipose fat tissue is less than 10 percent. Under normal conditions the water concentration of a given tissue is regulated quite nicely relative to its needs. When we look at the percentage of the body weight that may be attributed to a given body tissue, the weight of that tissue includes its normal water content.

Although the amount of fat, lean tissue, bone, and water may vary widely in individuals, the following might represent a normal distribution in a young, lean adult male: 60 percent body water and 40 percent solid matter subdivided into 14 percent fat, 22 percent protein, and 4 percent bone minerals.

Body composition may be influenced by a number of factors such as age, sex, diet, and level of physical activity. Age effects are significant during the developmental years as muscle and other body tissues are being formed. Also, during adulthood, muscle mass may decrease, probably because the level of physical activity declines. There are some minor differences in body composition between boys and girls up to the age of puberty, but at this age the differences become fairly great. In general, girls deposit more fat beginning with puberty, whereas boys develop more muscle tissue. Diet can affect body composition over the short haul, such as during acute water restriction and starvation, but the main effects are seen over the long haul. For example, chronic overeating may lead to increased body-fat stores. Physical activity may also be very influential, with a sound exercise program helping to build muscle and lose fat.

What techniques are available to measure body composition and how accurate are they?

The measurement of body fat has become very popular in recent years. Many high school and university athletic departments routinely analyze the body composition of their athletes in attempts to predict an optimal weight for competition. In some sports, such as wrestling, measurement of body composition is mandated by various state or national sport associations. Fitness and wellness centers also usually include a body-fat analysis as one of their services. Unfortunately, some of the individuals who analyze body composition in these situations are unaware of the limitations of the tests they employ.

The only direct, accurate method of analyzing body composition is by chemical extraction of all fat from body tissues, which is obviously not appropriate with living humans. Thus, a variety of indirect methods have been developed to assess body composition. Some are relatively simple, such as visual observation by an experienced judge, and others are rather complex, such as nuclear magnetic resonance imaging, using multimillion-dollar machines. Indirect methods are used to measure body fat, lean body mass, bone mineral content, and body water. Some techniques are also used to measure fat in specific locations of the body.

Before continuing this discussion, it must be emphasized that measurement of body composition is not an exact science. All techniques, even technologically sophisticated ones, currently used to predict body density or percentage of body fat are only estimates and are prone to error, particularly when used to determine the body fat of a given individual. Such errors usually are expressed statistically as standard errors of measurement or estimate, which can be used to show the accuracy of the body-fat measurement. Without going into the statistics of standard errors, look at the following example. Let us suppose that a formula using skinfold techniques predicts your body fat at 17 percent, yet the formula has a standard error of 3 percent. What this means is that your true body fat percentage is probably (about 70 percent probability) somewhere between one standard error of the predicted value, or somewhere between 14–20 percent. It may even be lower than 14 and higher than 20 percent, but less likely so. Thus, you should not think of body-fat determinations as precise measures, but consider them as a possible range associated with the error of measurement.

Most field methods used, such as skinfolds and bioelectrical impedance analysis (BIA), are two-component models, as are some laboratory methods, such as underwater weighing. Going indicates that methods based on two-component models are associated with greater errors than are methods based on multicomponent models, such as dual energy X-ray absorptiometry (DEXA). Three- and four-component models that combine measures of body density with body water and mineral content dramatically reduce the errors associated with the traditional two-compartment model (fat and fat-free mass). A number of body composition measurement techniques are highlighted in table 10.1, but only the

TABLE 10.1 Methods used to determine body composition using the two (2)- or three (3)-component models

Anthropometry (2)	Measures body segment girths to predict body fat
Bioelectrical impedance analysis (BIA) (2)	Measures resistance to electric current to predict body-water content, lean body mass, and body fat
Body plethysmography (2)	Whole-body plethysmograph measures air displacement and calculates body density; comparable to water displacement protocol used in underwater weighing
Computed tomography (CT) (3)	X-ray scanning technique to image body tissues; useful in determining subcutaneous and deep fat to predict body-fat percentage; used to calculate bone mass
Dual energy X-ray absorptiometry (DEXA; DXA) (3)	X-ray technique at two energy levels to image body fat; used to calculate bone mass
Dual photon absorptiometry (DPA) (3)	Beam of photons passes through tissues, differentiating soft tissues and bone tissues; used to predict body fat and calculate bone mass
Infrared interactance (2)	Infrared light passes through tissues, and interaction with tissue components used to predict body fat
Magnetic resonance imaging (MRI) (3)	Magnetic-field and radio-frequency waves are used to image body tissues similar to CT scan; very useful for imaging deep abdominal fat
Neutron activation analysis (3)	Beam of neutrons passes through the tissues, permitting analysis of nitrogen and other mineral content in the body; used to predict lean body mass
Skinfold thicknesses (2)	Measures subcutaneous fat folds to predict body-fat content and lean body mass
Total body potassium (2)	Measures total body potassium, the main intracellular ion, to predict lean body mass and body fat
Total body water (Hydrometry) (2)	Measures total body water by isotope dilution techniques to predict lean body mass and body fat
Ultrasound (2)	High frequency ultrasound waves pass through tissues to image subcutaneous fat and predict body-fat content
Underwater weighing (Hydrodensitometry) (2)	Underwater-weighing technique based on Archimedes' principle to predict body density, body fat, and lean body mass

more commonly used or promising techniques will be discussed. For more details on body composition analysis, the interested reader is referred to the review by Going. Consult the review by Malina for an assessment of body composition in athletes. The book by Heyward and Wagner provides an excellent review, and also provides available prediction formulae for athletic groups.

When determining changes in body composition of an individual over time, such as in a weight-loss program, it is important to use the same method throughout the testing to help minimize errors that may occur when using different methods. For example, if you select the skinfold procedure, it should be used consistently throughout, not interspersed with other techniques such as BIA. Moreover, Going suggests that when used, two-compartment estimates should employ population-specific equations if available. Population-specific equations include gender and age, and some may be specific to different ethnic and athletic groups. Going has provided a supplement to choosing the best equation for estimating body composition from skinfolds or BIA, which can be accessed at the Gatorade Sports Science Institute (GSSI) Website.

www.gssiweb.com Type Body Composition in the Search box, and click on SSE #101 *Optimizing Techniques for Determining Body Composition.*

Underwater Weighing One of the most common research techniques for determining body density is **underwater weighing,** also known as *hydrodensitometry.* The technique is based on Archimedes' principle that a body immersed in a fluid is acted upon by a buoyancy force in relation to the amount of fluid the body displaces (see figure 10.2). Because fat is less dense and bone and muscle tissue are more dense than water, a given weight of fat will displace a larger volume of water and exhibit a greater buoyant effect than the corresponding weight of bone and muscle tissue. Different formulas are recommended for determination of body density, depending upon the age and sex of the individual. Although this technique was once referred to as the "gold standard" in body-composition analysis, it is an indirect two-component model with associated weaknesses. For example, the assumption that the density of the fat-free protein tissue is 1.10 g/cc^3 may not be valid for all individuals, such as athletes and older persons. The standard error is still about 2–2.5 percent. Thus, Wagner and Heyward noted that underwater weighing should not be regarded as the "gold standard" because of these errors. Because the underwater-weighing technique is rather time-consuming and difficult for some individuals, other techniques have been developed either for research purposes or practical applications. The interested reader is referred to the review by Going and the book by Heyward and Wagner.

Air Displacement Plethysmography (ADP) Another technique is **air displacement plethysmography (ADP),** sometimes referred to as body plethysmography. Subjects enter a dual-chamber plethysmograph designed to measure the amount of air they displace, somewhat comparable to the water displacement technique of underwater weighing. One commercial product available is called the Bod Pod (see figure 10.3). It is portable, easy to operate, requires little time, and eliminates the necessity of going underwater, several clear advantages compared to underwater weighing. Several reviews, including one by Wagner and

Heyward, have noted that it may be more valid and reliable than hydrodensitometry for certain individuals, such as those who fear underwater submersion, but has similar limitations. In this regard, Fields noted that the ADP and underwater weighing agree within 1 percent of body fat for adults and children, but when compared to multicomponent models ADP generally underestimated body fat by 2–3 percent. Several studies compared the Bod Pod to DEXA and reached different conclusions. A study with men reported a 2.2 percent difference in body fat between the two methods, whereas a study with women reported no significant differences. Overall, Noreen and Lemon indicate that ADP appears to be a reliable method to use in tracking changes in body composition in individuals over time.

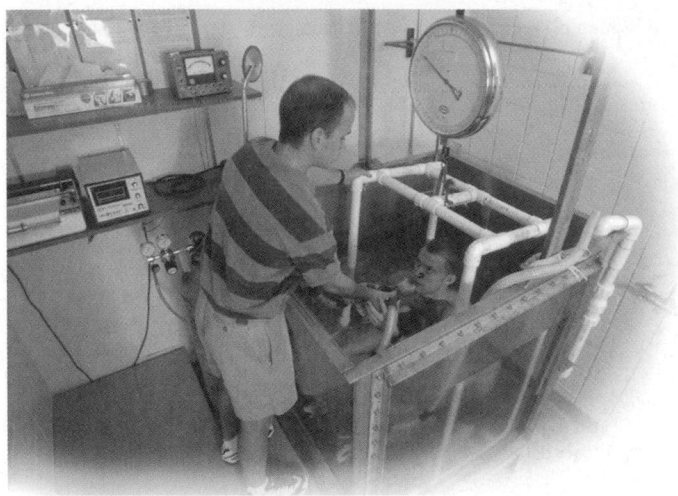

FIGURE 10.2 Underwater weighing is one of the more common laboratory means for determining body composition. However, all current techniques for estimating percent body fat are subject to error. See text for discussion.

FIGURE 10.3 The Bod Pod. An application of total body plethysmography, an air displacement technique, to evaluate body composition.

Photo courtesy of Life Measurement Instruments.

Skinfolds The **skinfold technique** is designed to measure the subcutaneous fat (see figure 10.4). It appears to be the most common procedure for nonresearch purposes. The values obtained are inserted into an appropriate formula to calculate the body-fat percentage. The formula chosen should be specific to the sex, age, and ethnicity of the individual. Some formulas also have been developed for specific athletic groups. To improve the accuracy of this technique, skinfold measures should be obtained from a variety of body sites, because using a single skinfold site may be unrepresentative of total storage fat. The test also should be administered with an acceptable pair of skinfold calipers by an experienced tester. Ultrasound techniques are also available to assess skinfold thicknesses, but these are more expensive than calipers. Orphanidou and others found that measurements of subcutaneous body fat with skinfold techniques were comparable to those obtained by ultrasound and computed tomography, suggesting that the use of skinfold calipers in the clinical setting is appropriate. In their study, Utter and Hager found that ultrasound

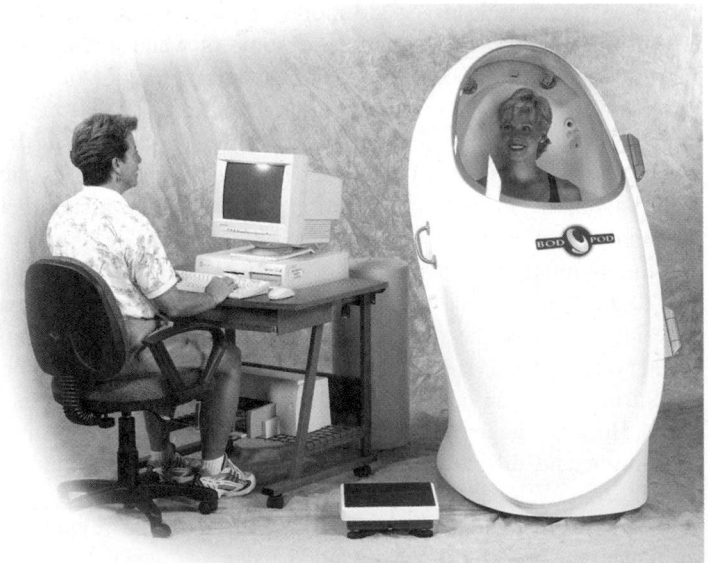

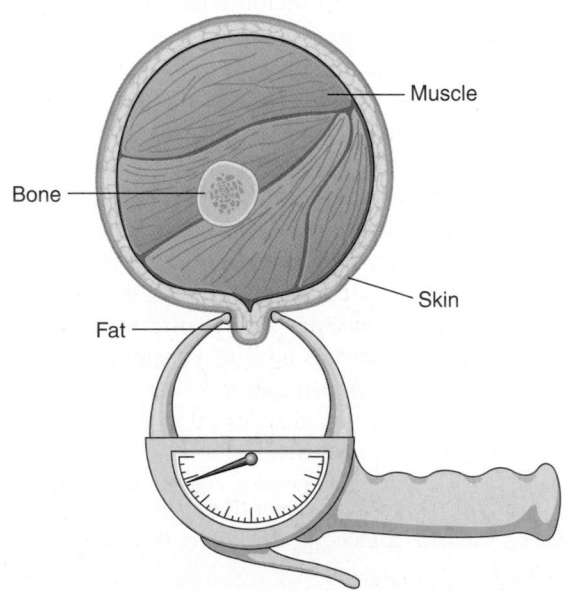

FIGURE 10.4 A schematic drawing showing the skinfold of fat that is pinched up away from the underlying muscle tissue.

Muscle

Bone

Skin

Fat

provided similar estimates of fat-free mass as hydrostatic weighing in high school wrestlers, and suggested it could be an alternative field-based method.

Because this method involves some measurement error, and because the formulas are usually based upon the underwater-weighing technique, the skinfold technique is actually a double-indirect method. Thus, the standard error for the skinfold technique is about 3–4 percent, which should be kept in mind when using this method to estimate body fat. Nevertheless, Lohman and others indicated that the skinfold technique is one of the best practical methods to measure body composition, and Wagner and Heyward noted that it can provide accurate results for lean subjects, such as athletes. Using a population-specific formula for gender, age, ethnicity, and sport, if available, will help reduce prediction errors. For example, Clark and others validated the NCAA skinfold technique as a means to predict minimal weight classes for wrestlers. Some sport organizations use the seven-site protocol promoted by the International Society for Advances in Kinanthropometry, the seven skinfolds being abdominal, biceps, front thigh, medial calf, subscapular, supraspinatus, and triceps. For those who have access to a good skinfold caliper, some generalized equations for the calculation of body fat may be found in appendix D for males and females of several ages. Moreover, as noted previously, the GSSI Website provides some skinfold formulae for specific populations, while O'Connor and others have developed equations for non-Hispanic White, Hispanic, and African-American adults with standard errors of estimate between 3–4 percent.

Bioelectrical Impedance Analysis (BIA) A more expensive, practical field technique is **bioelectrical impedance analysis (BIA).** BIA is based on the principle of resistance to an electrical current that is applied to the body. The less the recorded resistance, the greater the water content, and hence the greater the body density. Early research with BIA revealed large standard errors in predicting lean body mass, so it was not considered to be very valid. However, Jaffrin, in an update on BIA, reported that it has been compared with medical impedance meters and with dual X-ray absorptiometry measurements and found reasonably accurate, except for individuals with very low or high BMI. The BIA instrument may have preprogrammed prediction equations to use, which ideally should include age, gender, and ethnicity; most do not have athlete-specific equations. In its position stand on nutrition for the athlete, the American Dietetic Association, Dietitians of Canada, and American College of Sports Medicine indicated that the prediction accuracy of BIA is similar to that of skinfold assessment, but BIA may be preferable because it does not require the technical skill associated with skinfold measurements. As noted previously, the GSSI Website provides some BIA formulae for specific populations. Pichard and others reported valid BIA formulas for female runners, but recommended research to validate formulas for other athletes.

Dual Energy X-Ray Absorptiometry (DXA; DEXA) **Dual energy X-ray absorptiometry (DXA or DEXA)** is a computerized X-ray technique used to image body tissues and has been used to assess bone mineral content, fat-free mass, and body fat concurrently (see figure 10.5). DEXA may also be used to assess regional fat depots such as deep visceral fat, as can other sophisticated techniques, such as magnetic resonance imaging (MRI) and computed tomography (CT). Moreover, DEXA may measure bone density to detect the presence of osteoporosis.

Going notes that DEXA has emerged as a criterion method used to validate other methods. However, he also notes that different manufacturers' scanners and software give different results, which is the main limitation of DEXA.

Infrared Interactance Another device marketed commercially is based upon infrared interactance. In essence, infrared light passes through the tissues, and its interaction with tissue components is used to predict body fat. One commercial model is the Futrex 5000. Wagner and Heyward reported somewhat higher standard errors of measurement with infrared interactance, greater than 3.5 percent.

Anthropometry Anthropometry, or measurement of body parts, is an inexpensive, practical method to assess body composition. Body measurements include girths such as the neck and abdomen, and bone diameters such as the hip, shoulders, elbow, and wrist. Girth and bone diameter measurements may be incorporated into various formulas to predict body fat and lean body mass.

Girth measurements of the abdomen, hips, buttocks, thigh, and other body parts, may be important indicators of **regional fat distribution,** which is a concept representing the anatomical distribution of fat over the body. As discussed later, regional

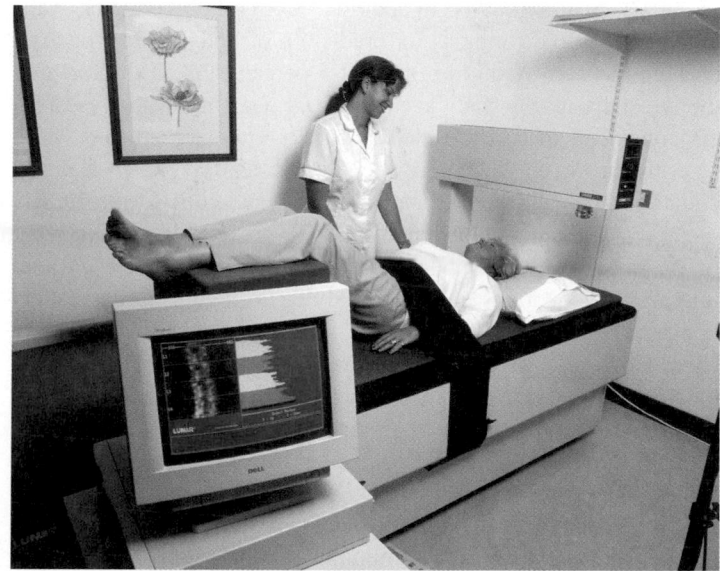

FIGURE 10.5 Dual energy X-ray absorptiometry (DEXA). This method measures body fat by releasing small doses of radiation through the body that a detector then quantifies as fat, lean tissue, or bone. The scanner arm moves from head to toe and in doing so can determine body fat as well as bone density. DEXA is currently considered the most accurate method for determining body fat as long as the person is not too obese to fit on the table and/or under the arm of the instrument. The radiation dose is minimal.

fat distribution may be associated with several major health problems. The principal measure of regional fat distribution is the **waist circumference,** the abdominal or waist girth measured by a flexible tape at the narrowest section of the waist as seen from the front. The waist circumference is a good screening technique for regional fat distribution, but does not provide an accurate measure of deep visceral fat, such as provided by CT or MRI techniques.

Multicomponent Models   The multicomponent model uses several methods, such as hydrodensitometry, total body water, and DEXA to reduce the errors associated with any single method and to provide information on body fat, body water, bone mass, and lean body mass. Lohman and Going recommend use of a multicomponent model when assessing body composition in children and youths, including waist circumference, selected skinfolds, and DEXA. Wagner and Heyward note that the multicomponent model is now regarded as the "gold standard" in body composition assessment and should be used when feasible.

What problems may be associated with rigid adherence to body fat percentages in sport?

Table 10.1 lists most of the methods used to estimate body composition. Several studies have attempted to validate these techniques, usually against the underwater-weighing method, and have shown some significant differences. In one study comparing four different methods, some individuals were estimated to have body-fat percentages that ranged as much as 10 percent depending on the method used, and another study using four different prediction equations with the BIA reported predicted body-fat percentages ranging from 12.2 to 22.8 in gymnasts. In addition, Stout and others cross-validated 16 skinfold formulas for prediction of body fat in wrestlers, and reported error values of almost 5 percent. Given the fact that the wrestlers in this study averaged 10.8 percent fat, the researchers concluded that this level of accuracy is not acceptable. More recently, however, Clark and others found that the NCAA skinfold equation is a valid predictor of body fat, and support the NCAA method of estimating body fat in college wrestlers for establishment of minimum weight. Oppliger and others developed new infrared interactance equations to predict body fat in high school wrestlers and noted that they are comparable to skinfold equations currently used. However, given the problems with assumptions underlying the various methods of body composition determination, estimates of body-fat percentages are approximations only.

The rigid use of body-fat percentages in weight-control sports, such as gymnastics and wrestling, may lead to excessive weight loss. For example, suppose you are a wrestler and your college coach requires you to reach the minimal permitted—5 percent body-fat level. Using a skinfold caliper technique, he finds that you are at 8 percent body fat and suggests that you lose 3 percent more body fat. However, given the standard error of 3–4 percent, you may already be at 5 percent. Losing extra weight may be very difficult because you are already near minimal body-fat levels, so additional weight loss may include muscle tissue that may lead to possible decreases in performance. In young athletes, such practices may also lead to disordered eating and, possibly, clinical eating disorders.

How much should I weigh or how much body fat should I have?

That is a complex question, and the response depends on whether you are concerned primarily about appearance, health, or physical performance. From the perspective of physical appearance, you are the best judge of how you wish to look. However, a distorted image may lead to serious health problems or impairment in physical performance. For example, many individuals do not recognize that they are overweight and may suffer adverse health consequences. Already thin individuals who desire to be even thinner may be prone to eating disorders. Muscular bodybuilders who perceive themselves as not sufficiently muscular may suffer psychologically.

The effect of body weight and body fat on physical performance is discussed in a later section, although some general guidelines are presented here. The effect of body weight and fat on health has received considerable research attention. Although being underweight may impair health, most of the focus has been on excess body weight and fat, particularly the relationship of obesity to health. By medical definition, **obesity** is simply an accumulation of fat in the adipose tissue. Obesity is also referred to as a disease or disorder and is the most common nutritional health problem in North America. The actual measurement and determination of clinical obesity is a controversial issue. Several approaches have been used to define the point at which a person is classified as clinically obese.

Unfortunately, our present level of knowledge does not provide us with the ability to predict precisely what the optimal weight or percent body fat should be for health in any given individual. However, some general guidelines have been developed by various professional and health organizations.

Body Mass Index   As a screening method for health, you may calculate your BMI to assess your body weight. See appendix D or Websites previously mentioned in this chapter for details. The following are some general guidelines presented by the National Institutes of Health regarding the relationship of BMI to health risks in adults. Keep in mind that these are BMI values, not body-fat percentages, which are discussed in the next section.

Below 18.5: May signal malnutrition or serious disease
18.5–24.9: Healthy weight range that carries little health risk
25–29.9: Overweight; at increased risk for health problems, especially if you have one or two weight-related medical conditions
Above 30: Obesity, more than 20 percent over healthy body weight; poses high risk to your health

These values are in accordance with figures presented by the National Academy of Sciences. Additionally, the Food and Agriculture Organization has proposed the use of a BMI less than 18.5 as a criterion for starvation. Other investigators indicate that a BMI greater than 35 or 40 is classified as severe, clinical, or

morbid obesity. An expanded BMI health risk table, in association with waist circumference, is presented later.

Body Fat Percentage As noted previously, the use of the BMI height-weight relationship does not evaluate body composition. Thus, health professionals note that there are exceptions to these BMI classifications, indicating that a low BMI may be a symptom of a serious disease, not a cause, and that muscular people may have a high BMI and not be obese.

For health purposes, the body has a need for the essential fat described previously. At a minimum, essential fat approximates 3 percent for males and 12–15 percent for females. Several authorities have included additional levels of storage fat and suggested that minimal levels of total body fat for health range from 5–10 percent for males and 15–18 percent for females.

Lower levels of body fat may be required for optimal performance in certain types of athletic events. Certain male athletes such as wrestlers and gymnasts may function effectively at 5–7 percent body fat. Recommendations have been made for females who compete in distance running to have no more than 10 percent body fat. However, some athletes have performed very successfully even though their body-fat percentage was higher than the recommended values.

Although different levels of body-fat percentages have been cited as the criterion for obesity, the American Dietetic Association and the National Research Council set the value at 25 percent for males and 30 percent for females. The National Academy of Sciences, in its new DRI on energy intake, also published criteria for obesity, setting the level at 25 percent body fat for males but 37 percent for females; the NAS noted that over 31 percent and 42 percent body fat in males and females, respectively, was indicative of clinical obesity.

One national fitness organization has proposed a rating scale, as presented in table 10.2, based on body-fat percentages ranging from essential fat to obesity. Keep several points in mind when using such tables. First, remember that all body-fat prediction methods contain a source of error. Second, the athletic category is associated with athletes competing in weight-control sports or sports where excess body fat may be a disadvantage. Third, as noted later, although obesity generally increases health risks, some individuals with higher body-fat percentages may not develop obesity-related health problems if they are otherwise physically fit and consume a healthful diet. Fourth, location of the fat in your body may have significant health consequences.

Waist Circumference It may not be how much fat you have that affects your health but where that fat is located. The health implications of regional fat distribution are discussed later, but you may use method C in appendix D to calculate your waist circumference and evaluate associated health risks. As a screening measure for deep visceral fat, increased health risks are associated with waist circumferences greater than 35 inches in females and 40 inches in males. However, as discussed later, lower waist circumferences may be associated with increased risks if accompanied by other conditions, such as high blood pressure. Table 10.3 highlights the risk of chronic disease associated with the BMI and waist size.

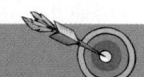

Key Concepts

▶ The Body Mass Index (BMI) does not measure body composition, but it may be useful as a screening device to determine whether one is overweight or obese. *Overweight* and *obese* are not synonymous terms.

▶ The body consists of four components: body fat, protein, minerals, and water. However, for practical purposes, body composition may be classified as consisting of two components: fat-free weight, which is about 70 percent water, and body fat.

▶ All techniques that are currently used to measure body composition, primarily body fat, are indirect and prone to error; even the underwater-weighing technique, once considered to be the most accurate, may be in error by 2.0–2.5 percent.

▶ Our present level of knowledge does not provide us with the ability to predict precisely what the optimal body composition should be for health or physical performance. However, BMI and body-fat levels higher than normal are associated with increased health risks.

Check for Yourself

Using appendix D, calculate both your Body Mass Index (BMI) and your waist circumference. Compare your findings to the rating scale in table 10.3.

TABLE 10.2	One proposed rating scale based on body-fat percentages	
Rating	**Males**	**Females**
Essential fat	2–5	12–15
Athletic	6–13	16–20
Fitness	14–17	21–24
Acceptable	18–25	25–31
Overweight/obese	25+	32+

Note: Keep in mind that these are approximate values. The essential category represents fat necessary to meet basic physiological needs. The athletic category may apply particularly to athletes who compete in events where excess body fat may be a disadvantage. See text for additional information.

Regulation of Body Weight and Composition

How does the human body normally control its own weight?

As noted previously, you may eat more than a ton of food—nearly a million Calories—a year and yet not gain one pound of body weight. For this to occur, your body must possess an intricate

TABLE 10.3 Risk of associated disease according to BMI and waist size

BMI		*Waist less than or equal to 40 in. (men) or 35 in. (women)	*Waist greater than 40 in. (men) or 35 in. (women)
18.5 or less	Underweight	—	N/A
18.5–24.9	Normal	—	N/A
25.0–29.9	Overweight	Increased	High
30.0–34.9	Obese	High	Very High
35.0–39.9	Obese	Very High	Very High
40 or greater	Extremely Obese	Extremely High	Extremely High

Source: http://www.nhlbi.nih.gov/health/public/heart/obesity/lose_wt/risk.htm

*Note: Research suggests that waist sizes greater than 37 inches in men and 31.5 inches in women may increase health risks when accompanied by other conditions, such as high blood pressure.

regulatory system that helps to balance energy intake and output both on a short-term and a long-term basis. The regulation of human energy balance is complex, involving numerous feedback loops to help control energy balance. At the present time we do not know all the exact physiological mechanisms whereby body weight is maintained relatively constant over short or long periods, but research suggests that a variety of specific interactions between the brain and peripheral tissues may be involved in the control of both energy intake and energy expenditure.

Energy Intake George Bray, an international authority on weight control, indicates that food intake is a regulated system. The central nervous system, the brain in particular, is the center for appetite control, either creating a sensation of satiety or stimulating food-seeking behavior. However, its activity is dependent upon a complex array of afferent signals from various body systems. The interaction of the brain with these afferent signals helps regulate the appetite on a short-term (daily) basis, or on a long-term basis, as in keeping the body weight constant for a year.

The forebrain (prefrontal cortex) is involved in the conscious selection of foods we eat, while the brainstem controls the motor aspects of eating, such as chewing and swallowing. Between these two structures lies the hypothala-

mus, a small substructure that appears to be the center for appetite control (see figure 10.6). You may recall from the last chapter that the hypothalamus is also involved in body-temperature control, involving neural receptors that function as a thermostat to either stimulate energy (heat) production or loss. In a similar fashion, the hypothalamus may contain neural centers that help regulate appetite, often referred to as an **appestat.** In general, the appestat may contain a **hunger center** that may stimulate eating behavior, and a **satiety center** which when stimulated will inhibit the hunger center. As a means of controlling energy intake, specific neural receptors within the appestat monitor various afferent stimuli that may stimulate or inhibit the appetite. These stimuli may come from the stomach, intestines, muscle, fat depots, pancreas, liver, and other body tissues and organs, and are integrated and interpreted by the hypothalamus and directed to other brain centers and body organs to help maintain energy balance. As discussed later, Woods suggests that one of these brain centers may involve receptors that induce sensations of pleasure, which may increase the desire to consume food.

As depicted in figure 10.7, various stimuli may influence the appetite, including blood levels of various nutrients, metabolites, hormones, neural stimuli from other parts of the body, and environmental cues. Some factors may function to control body weight on a short-term basis while others may exert long-term effects. The following afferent stimuli may be involved in body-weight control in one way or another.

- *Senses.* Stimulation of several senses like sight, sound, and smell may influence neural or hormonal activity to stimulate or depress our appetites, even before food is ingested. The sense of taste also has a significant impact on appetite and energy intake.

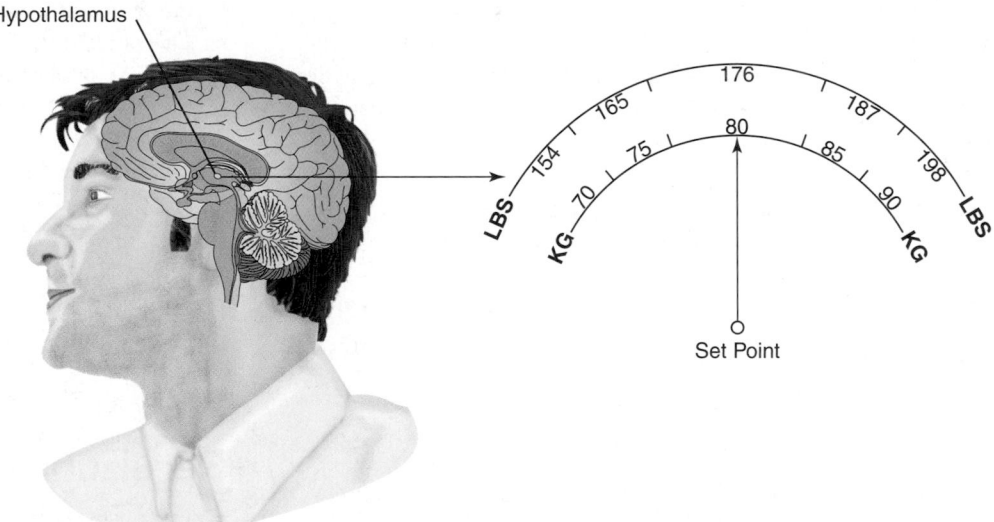

FIGURE 10.6 The hypothalamus. This site in the brain does most of the processing of signals regarding food intake. Some theorize that the hypothalamus regulates a set point for body weight, comparable to its role as a thermostat in regulating body temperature. Increases in the normal body weight would lead to compensations, such as decreased appetite or increased basal metabolic rate that would lead to weight loss and restoration of normal body weight. The opposite would occur with decreases in the normal body weight.

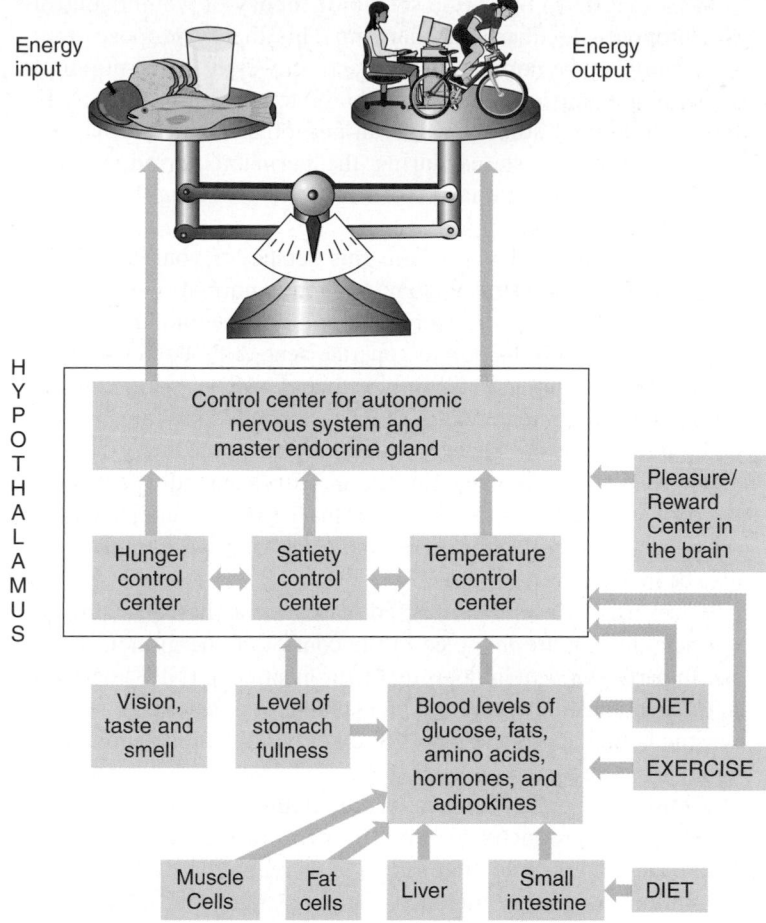

Energy input

Energy output

HYPOTHALAMUS

Control center for autonomic nervous system and master endocrine gland

Pleasure/ Reward Center in the brain

Hunger control center

Satiety control center

Temperature control center

Vision, taste and smell

Level of stomach fullness

Blood levels of glucose, fats, amino acids, hormones, and adipokines

DIET

EXERCISE

Muscle Cells

Fat cells

Liver

Small intestine

DIET

FIGURE 10.7 Theoretical control mechanisms for body weight. The control of food intake (energy intake) and resting metabolism (energy output) is governed primarily by the hypothalamus in the brain. The numerous control centers in the hypothalamus are influenced by feedback from the body, such as the blood concentration of glucose and other nutrients. Such nutrients may also affect the pleasure/reward center in the brain, which may influence the hypothalamus. Exercise may influence the hypothalamus in a variety of ways, such as stimulating the secretion of several hormones by endocrine glands in the body, stimulating the temperature control center, and modifying blood levels of several nutrients, all of which may affect energy intake and output. See the text for an expanded discussion of the various factors that may influence energy input and energy output.

- *Stomach fullness.* An empty or full stomach may influence mechanical stretch receptors in the stomach walls that generate neural activity. An empty stomach may stimulate the hunger center by various neural pathways, whereas a full stomach may stimulate the satiety center. The stomach may also release hormone-like substances that stimulate or diminish hunger.
- *Blood nutrient levels.* Nutrient levels in the blood may be able to influence receptors in the hypothalamus. Receptors in the hypothalamus, liver, or elsewhere may be able to monitor blood levels of various nutrients. In regard to this, three theories center on the three energy nutrients. The **glucostatic theory**

suggests that food intake is related to changes in the levels of blood glucose. Fehm and others indicated that a fall in blood glucose will stimulate glucose-sensitive neurons in the hypothalamus and increase appetite, whereas an increased blood glucose level will decrease appetite. The **lipostatic theory** suggests a similar mechanism for fats, as does the **aminostatic theory** for amino acids, or protein. In essence, by-products of carbohydrate, fat, and protein metabolism may influence production of neurotransmitters that influence appetite, such as serotonin and norepinephrine, in the hypothalamus.

- *Body temperature.* A thermostat in the hypothalamus may respond to changes in body temperature and influence the feeding center. For example, an increase in body temperature inhibits the appetite.
- *Hormones, cytokines, and neuropeptides.* A number of different hormones, cytokines, and neuropeptides (neurotransmitters) in the body have been shown to affect feeding behavior, including insulin, serotonin, norepinephrine, leptin, ghrelin, cortisol, and thyroxine. As discussed later, some hormones may function on a short-term basis to help control meal size, whereas other hormones may be involved in long-term regulation of body weight.

Energy Expenditure Although all of the above may be involved in the physiological regulation of food intake, the other side of the energy-balance equation is energy expenditure, or metabolism. Although exercise is one way to increase energy expenditure, the vast majority of the energy that is expended by the body on a daily basis is accounted for by the basal energy expenditure (BEE) or resting energy expenditure (REE), as was detailed in chapter 3. Changes in the REE may be involved in the regulation of body weight. Several mechanisms of body-weight regulation have been proposed.

- *Brown fat.* **Brown fat,** which is distinct from the white fat that comprises most fat tissue in the body, is found in small amounts around the neck, back, and chest areas. It has a high rate of metabolism and releases energy in the form of heat without ATP production. Basically, uncoupling proteins (UCP) in brown fat uncouple respiration from oxidative phosphorylation and convert fuel to heat without producing ATP. Activity of the brown fat tissue may be increased or decreased under certain conditions, such as after a meal or exposure to the cold. This activity is referred to as *nonshivering thermogenesis.* Research with rats has indicated that low levels of brown fat are associated with a higher incidence of dietary-induced obesity. The amount of brown fat in humans appears to be small (about 1 percent of body fat or less) but Stock indicates that as little as 50 grams (about 2 ounces) could make a contribution of 10–15 percent energy turnover in humans. The amount of brown fat in the body decreases with aging. Mattson reported data suggesting that individuals with low levels of brown fat are prone to obesity, insulin resistance, and cardiovascular disease, whereas those with higher levels maintain lower body weights and exhibit superior health as they age. Although this is an interesting finding, the role of brown fat in the etiology of human obesity is controversial and is being researched.

- *White fat tissue and muscle tissue.* UCP are also found in other tissues. In a review, Melby and others noted that both white adipose tissue and muscle tissue may also experience thermogenesis without ATP production under conditions of high energy intake, particularly as dietary fat. Such an effect could help prevent weight gain.
- *Hormones.* Levels of hormones from the thyroid and adrenal glands may rise or fall and affect energy metabolism accordingly. Triiodothyronine and thyroxine, hormones from the thyroid gland, may be involved in the stimulation of brown adipose tissue. Hormones, such as epinephrine, also may increase the activity of certain enzymes resulting in increased energy expenditure. Decreases in such hormonal activity may depress energy metabolism. Other hormones may stimulate or depress thermogenesis in adipose or muscle tissues.
- *Nonexercise activity thermogenesis (NEAT).* Levine indicates that nonexercise activity thermogenesis (NEAT) is the energy expended for everything we do that is not sleeping, eating, or sports-like exercise. Varying levels of NEAT could have a significant impact on daily energy expenditure.

Feedback Control of Energy Intake and Expenditure As noted in an earlier chapter, the human body has developed a number of physiological systems, called *feedback systems,* to regulate most body processes. Temperature control is a good example. Feedback systems controlling body weight may operate on both a short-term (daily) and long-term (yearly) basis.

Short-term control mechanisms may either decrease or increase food intake. For example, as the stomach expands while eating a meal, nerve impulses are sent from receptors in the stomach wall to the hypothalamus to help suppress food intake. Additionally, Moran notes that during and after a meal, the ingested nutrients alter the release of a variety of peptides from the stomach, intestines, and pancreas. Peptides such as cholecystokinen, pancreatic glucagon, obestatin, and amylin are released rapidly with eating and have short actions leading to meal termination. Body stores of carbohydrate, protein, and fat are also regulated on a short-term basis. The human body has a limited capacity to store excess carbohydrate and protein, so changes in blood glucose and amino acid levels help regulate carbohydrate and protein intake. Although the human body possesses a high capacity to store fat, blood lipids and other factors help maintain body-fat balance on a short-term basis. However, Stubbs indicated that although dietary protein and carbohydrate exert potent effects on satiety, dietary fat is less satiating and may lead to excess energy intake. Other short-term mechanisms increase food intake. For example, **ghrelin** is a peptide hormone released by the stomach, mainly before mealtime when the stomach is relatively empty. Ghrelin acts on the hypothalamus to stimulate the appetite. Abizaid indicates that ghrelin may also affect dopaminergic neurons in the brain, possibly increasing secretion of dopamine, which induces sensations of pleasure that may be involved in long-term regulation of body weight, as discussed later.

On a long-term basis, the **set-point theory** of weight control is a proposed feedback mechanism. This theory proposes that your body is programmed to be a certain weight, or a set point, something comparable to a set body temperature of 98.6°F. Based on animal studies, Sullivan and others indicate that the maternal nutrition status during the perinatal period, or just before and after birth, may be critical in establishing the child's body weight set point.

If you begin to deviate from this set point, your body will make metabolic adjustments to return you to normal. This is often referred to as *adaptive thermogenesis,* which can either increase or decrease energy production to generate heat. Although developed primarily with rats and still only a theory, the set-point concept does involve the interaction of those factors cited previously, particularly the lipostatic theory, which may influence energy intake and expenditure in humans. Keesey and Hirvonen indicate that the hypothalamus appears to play the primary role in establishing the set point for body weight; Fehm indicates the hippocampus may also be involved.

In several reviews, Levin noted that the brain has special sensing neurons that are involved in the control of energy homeostasis. In particular, Levin notes that neuropeptide Y (NPY) neurons in the hypothalamus represent an example of a neuron capable of sensing both glucose and a host of other peripheral metabolic signals, such as leptin.

Leptin, an adipokine, is a regulating peptide hormone encoded and produced by the OB gene in the adipose cells. Klok and others note that leptin is a mediator of long-term regulation of energy balance, suppressing food intake and thereby inducing weight loss. Leptin helps to decrease appetite. Long-term imbalances in body weight are usually reflected by changes in body-fat stores. The more body fat you have, the more leptin you produce; conversely, less leptin is produced when body-fat stores are low. When leptin is released into the blood, it circulates to the hypothalamus and is believed to inhibit the production of NPY (see figure 10.8). NPY is a potent stimulant of food intake and also acts to reduce energy expenditure by decreasing the REE. Thus, as you begin to accumulate body fat, your fat cells produce more leptin, which then circulates to the hypothalamus and depresses the formation of NPY. Because NPY stimulates food intake and depresses energy expenditure, decreased levels of NPY will suppress hunger and reduce voluntary food intake, and may also stimulate increases in REE by activating thermogenesis in adipose and muscle tissues. Thus, your body reacts to the increased body fat by decreasing energy intake and increasing energy expenditure. Conversely, if you decrease body fat rapidly via dieting, leptin production is decreased, reducing the inhibitory effect on NPY production. Increased levels of NPY stimulate hunger and reduce energy expenditure, thus resisting the effect of the diet and promoting restoration of the lost weight. Baile notes that leptin and its receptors provide the molecular basis for the lipostatic theory of energy-balance regulation proposed 40 years ago, namely that circulating factors generated in proportion to body-fat stores act as signals to the brain and elicit changes in energy intake and expenditure.

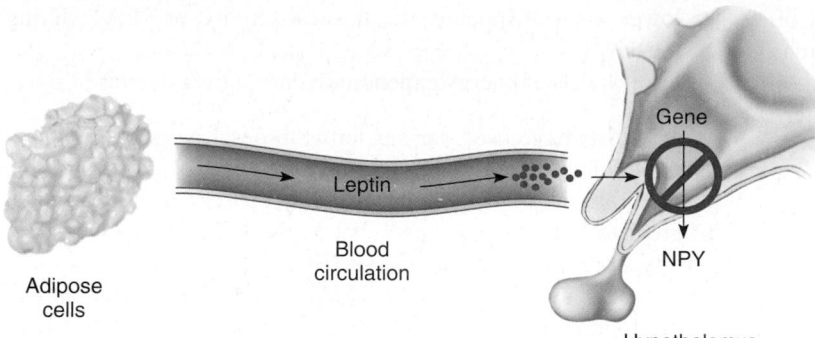

Adipose cells

Leptin

Blood circulation

Gene

NPY

Hypothalamus

FIGURE 10.8 One possible mechanism of the set-point theory. Leptin is produced in proportion to body-fat stores. When body fat increases, more leptin is released into the bloodstream, circulates to the hypothalamus, and inhibits the formation or release of neuropeptide Y (NPY). NPY is a potent stimulator of food intake and may also decrease energy expenditure.

Ghrelin may also be involved in long-term control of body weight. Abizaid notes that in addition to the hypothalamus, ghrelin may affect other parts of the brain that may stimulate eating behavior. In particular, ghrelin may stimulate the ventral tegmental area (VTA) in the brain. The VTA contains cells that secrete dopamine, a neurotransmitter. Dopamine may stimulate various pleasure centers in the brain, including the forebrain, a significant component of the brain's pleasure system. Thus, ghrelin not only stimulates the appetite, but concomitantly also the brain's pleasure center, helping to establish strong memories between eating certain foods and sensations of pleasure. Kessler and Liebman note that some food ingredients, such as sugar and fat, may stimulate the desire to eat more, possibly because of such stored memories. They note that such pleasurable memories may lead to becoming a *hypereater,* a condition that could lead to long-term weight gain.

Less research has been conducted relative to feedback control of physical activity, but Rowland proposed an **activity-stat,** a center in the brain that functions as a set point to increase or decrease physical activity. Increasing or decreasing the daily amounts of NEAT may be related to the activity-stat, but no studies have been uncovered to evaluate such a relationship. If substantiated, such a center could also support the set-point theory of body-weight control.

Although the set point is a theory, it may help explain why some people maintain a normal body weight throughout life, but when disrupted may lead to an excessive gain or loss of body mass. It is important to note that although the set-point theory is based on subconscious control mechanisms underlying energy intake and energy expenditure, the forebrain can consciously override these subconscious mechanisms and increase or decrease body mass if necessary.

How is fat deposited in the body?

The actual deposition of fat in the human body may occur in two ways: **hyperplasia** (an increase in the number of adipocytes, or fat cells), or **hypertrophy** (an increase in the amount of fat in each cell). Earlier research appeared to support the theory that hyperplasia is a major cause in the development of childhood obesity, whereas hypertrophy is the primary cause in adulthood. However, Avram and others noted that the development of obesity is dependent on the coordinated interplay of an increased fat cell size as well as an increased fat cell number, and evidence suggests that adipocyte hyperplasia occurs throughout life, both in response to normal cell turnover as well as in response to the need for additional fat mass stores that arises when caloric intake exceeds nutritional requirements. Existing fat cells apparently have a maximal size potential (about 1 microgram of fat per cell), which when exceeded stimulates the formation of new fat cells or the accumulation of fat in preadipocytes, small cells in the adipose tissue that have the potential to become adipocytes. Thus, although a genetic predisposition to inherit a greater number of fat cells, thereby facilitating the development of obesity, may exist, individuals without this genetic predisposition may still become obese with a positive energy balance stored as fat. Interestingly, Pi-Sunyer indicated that once fat cells are formed, the number seems to remain fixed even if weight is lost. To lose body fat, one must reduce the amount of fat in the adipose cells to normal, or even below normal.

What is the cause of obesity?

A National Geographic cover story asked the question, *Why are we so fat?* The answer is simple, but the devil is in the details. Energy processes in the human body, like those of other machines, are governed by the laws of thermodynamics. If the human body consumes less energy in the form of food Calories than it expends in metabolic processes, then a negative energy balance will occur and the individual will lose body weight. Conversely, a greater caloric intake in comparison to energy expenditure will result in a positive energy balance and a gain in body weight. In simple terms, obesity is caused by this latter condition of energy imbalance—more Calories in than out.

Although the first law of thermodynamics provides the basic answer as to how we get fat, it does not provide any insight relative to the specific mechanisms. Claude Bouchard, a prominent international authority on obesity and weight control, noted that at this time there is no common agreement on the specific determinants of obesity, stressing that numerous factors are correlated with body-fat content. In general, most leading obesity scientists, such as Grundy, support a multicausal theory involving the interaction of a number of genetic and environmental factors.

Genetic Factors   Heredity appears to be a very important factor in the etiology of obesity, particularly morbid obesity. For example, several genetic diseases result in clinical obesity. Also, studies of adopted children, including both fraternal and identical twins who were separated and adopted by different families, have shown a greater relationship of the body composition between the children and their biological parents as compared to the adoptive parents. For a review of two meticulous studies of the genetic role in obesity, the interested reader is referred to the reports by Bouchard and others on long-term overfeeding of identical twins, and by Stunkard and others on the Body Mass Index of twins who were raised apart. Based on his and others' research, Bouchard indicated that genetic heritability of obesity approximates 25–40 percent. It appears that heredity may determine those internal factors in the body that may predispose one to gain weight.

Research into the genetics of obesity has been progressing at a rapid pace. Hirsch and Leibel note that several obesity genes have already been identified, which in some persons may maintain an unhealthful set point. Levin cites one possibility, suggesting that individuals with a genetic susceptibility to obesity may be predisposed to abnormalities in neural function. They establish neural circuits that are not easily abolished, particularly circuits involving the brain's pleasure center. In essence, obesity genes influence appetite to increase energy intake or affect metabolism to decrease energy expenditure. For example, genes in the hypothalamus may decrease the number of protein receptors for leptin, causing *leptin resistance,* thus preventing leptin from inhibiting the formation of NPY. NPY may then stimulate the appetite. Also, as noted previously, a protein known as the uncoupling protein (UCP) is believed to activate thermogenesis; UCP1 activates thermogenesis in brown fat, whereas UCP2 activates thermogenesis in white fat and muscle tissue. Defects in UCP genes may decrease resting energy expenditure. In general, researchers indicate that genes affecting energy balance in the body appear to be very efficient as a means to promote energy intake and weight gain, but relatively inefficient to promote energy expenditure and weight loss.

More than 340 genes may be involved in weight control. One of the most prominent genes, according to Fawcett and Barroso, is the Fat Mass and Obesity-associated (FTO) gene, which plays a role in controlling both feeding behavior and energy expenditure. However, Hetherington and Cecil indicate that common obesity is polygenic, involving complex gene-gene and gene-environment interactions that increase energy intake. They also note that gene variants involved in pathways regulating addiction and reward behaviors may also play a role in predisposition to obesity. A 5-year study reported by Small and others identified a *master gene* that regulates numerous genes throughout the body associated with obesity. Rankinen and others have developed a human obesity gene map whose purpose is to identify loci on chromosomes associated with the development of obesity in humans; the map is updated annually. Genetic factors that have been implicated in the development of obesity include the following:

- a predisposed taste for sweet, high-fat foods
- impaired function of hormones such as insulin and cortisol
- decreased levels of human growth hormone
- low plasma leptin concentrations
- leptin resistance
- inability of nutrients or hormones in the blood to suppress the appetite control center
- a greater number of white fat cells
- lower body levels of brown fat
- an enhanced metabolic efficiency in storing fat
- a lower REE
- a decreased TEF
- low rates of fat oxidation

- lower levels of spontaneous physical activity, or NEAT, during the day
- lower levels of energy expenditure during light exercise

Scientists have used various terms to describe genes involved in the etiology of obesity. The *Thrifty Gene* is used to describe the high efficiency with which the body conserves energy, which in prehistoric times was beneficial as food was scarce and body energy stores had to be conserved. However, Wells indicates that such efficiency, or thrift, is maladaptive in today's environment where food is plentiful. The *Selfish Gene,* as described by Lutter and Nestler, involves the role that the pleasure center in the brain plays in controlling food intake, overriding the basic role of the hypothalamus by increasing the desire to consume foods that are highly palatable.

Environmental Factors   Although heredity may predispose one to obesity, environmental factors are also highly involved. Capturing the role of environmental factors in a nutshell, Wadden and others indicated that the marked increase in obesity worldwide appears to be attributable to a modern society that explicitly encourages the consumption of supersized portions of high-fat, high-sugar foods while implicitly discouraging physical activity. In particular, Mendoza and others concluded in their review that dietary energy density is a major predictor of obesity. Consuming a high-Calorie diet, either high or low in fat, may lead to excess caloric intake and weight gain. Moreover, Cohen and Farley contend that eating may be an automatic behavior over which the environment has more control than does the individual. The amount of food eaten is strongly influenced by factors such as portion size, food visibility, and the ease of obtaining food.

The following discussion highlights the variety of environmental factors that may contribute to excessive weight gain. The main contributors are excessive caloric intake and decreased physical activity, both of which may be influenced by other environmental factors.

High-fat, high-calorie foods   Excess Calories, or overfeeding, may lead to obesity. For example, Pearcey and de Castro evaluated eating behavior and activity levels of weight-gaining and weight-stable men and women, and found that the basic difference was that the weight-gaining individuals consumed about 400 more Calories per day during the period of active weight gain. Kelly Brownell, an expert on food policy and obesity, indicates that one of the main reasons most Americans are overweight is because the food industry is driving us to eat. Typical serving sizes are loaded with Calories, such as the small unbuttered popcorn at Regal Theaters at 670 Calories. He notes that access to unhealthy, fattening food choices is nearly ubiquitous.

Eating fast foods may be an important contributing factor. Ebbeling and others note that nutritional factors inherent to fast food, such as high palatability, high-fat content, high content of sugar in liquid form, and high energy density, promote excess energy intake. Additionally, fast foods are relatively inexpensive, mainly because fat and sugar are the cheapest source of Calories on earth, and thus are generally high in fat and Calories. Several longitudinal studies have linked fast-food consumption with weight gain. For example, in a 15-year prospective study, Pereira and others found that those who ate at fast-food restaurants more than two times a week gained about 10 pounds more than their peers who dined at such places less than once a week. The fast-food consumption had strong positive associations with weight gain and insulin resistance, suggesting that fast food increases the risk of obesity and type 2 diabetes.

Although an excess of caloric input over output will lead to a weight gain, researchers suggest that the main culprit in the diet that leads to obesity is dietary fat. For various reasons, the National Academy of Sciences concluded that higher fat intakes are accompanied with increased energy intake and therefore increased risk for weight gain in populations that are already disposed to being overweight and obese, such as that of North America. Obesity researchers have postulated several of these reasons. First, dietary fat is highly palatable to most individuals, stimulating hedonistic responses and encouraging overconsumption. Dietary fat contains more Calories per gram, and may not provide the same satiety as carbohydrate and protein. Gibbs noted that the body systems respond quickly to protein and carbohydrates but slowly to fat, too slowly to stop ingestion of a high-fat meal before the body has had too much. Green and Blundell also note that high-fat foods give rise to higher energy intake during a meal than do carbohydrate foods, and Calorie for Calorie are less effective in suppressing subsequent food intake. In support of this point, Shah and Garg reported that spontaneous energy intake is higher on an unrestricted high-fat diet compared to a high-carbohydrate diet. Second, dietary fat may be stored as fat more efficiently compared to carbohydrate and protein. It takes some energy to process fat and store it in the adipose tissue, but Dattilo noted that in comparison to dietary fat, it may cost up to three or four times more energy to convert carbohydrate and protein to body fat. Third, other investigators indicate that chronic intake of a high-fat diet will produce resistance in the hypothalamus to various factors that normally suppress appetite, such as leptin, the end result being increased energy intake and body-fat deposition. The interested student is referred to the reviews by Dattilo, Tso and Liu, and Rolls and Shide regarding the relationship of dietary fat to body weight.

Low-fat, large-portion size, high-calorie foods Although excess dietary fat, for reasons cited, may be a major culprit in the etiology of obesity, researchers such as Willett have noted that the prevalence of obesity in the United States has increased dramatically over the past two decades even though the energy derived from dietary fat has actually decreased, both in absolute terms and in percent of total dietary energy. One reason for this apparent inconsistency may be an increased daily Calorie intake. Fat-free does not mean Calorie-free. Appetizing low-fat, but high-Caloric food is everywhere, and in supersize proportions with significantly increased caloric content. At latest count, more than 300,000 packaged foods are available, and a large supermarket may carry 50,000 or more. Portion sizes have increased dramatically; what was once small is now large.

Liquid Calories appear to be involved in weight gain. Think about it. A 12-ounce sugar-sweetened soda contains the equivalent of 10 teaspoons of table sugar, or about 150 Calories. However, portion sizes have changed over the years. Today, the average soft drink is more than 50 percent larger compared to past years, containing more sugar and Calories. Geier and others report that people consume food on a "unit" basis. If you buy and consume a 20-ounce bottle of soda, which is one unit, rather than a 12-ounce bottle, you will consume about an additional 100 Calories. Flood and others reported that Americans drink about 22 percent of their total daily caloric intake, many from sweetened high-carbohydrate beverages, and do not compensate by eating less solid food at meals. In their review of 30 high-quality studies, Malik and others found that the weight of epidemiologic and experimental evidence indicates that a greater consumption of sugar-sweetened beverages is associated with weight gain and obesity. Consuming sugar-sweetened drinks *per se* may not be a cause of obesity, but it may be one avenue to exceed recommended caloric intake. For example, Johnson and others recently noted that Americans consume about 22 teaspoons of sugar daily, about 350 Calories, almost 75 more Calories per day than was consumed about 30 years ago. These additional daily Calories would increase body weight by 8 pounds over the course of a year, an example of creeping obesity as discussed later.

Physical inactivity and NEAT Although the epidemic of obesity development may be associated with excess consumption of energy-dense foods, Astrup suggests that it also may be explained by concomitantly decreasing levels of physical activity. Modern technology is wonderful, helping to make our lives more comfortable and enjoyable in numerous ways. However, technology may also exert a negative effect on our health, as the development of television, computers, and other labor-saving devices may decrease levels of physical activity. In a review, DiPietro noted that the influence of regular physical activity on body composition is complex. However, although there are some methodological problems with the epidemiological research, DiPietro indicated that several cross-sectional studies have reported an inverse relationship between physical activity and body weight; that is, those who were physically inactive weighed more. DiPietro and other reviewers, such as Saris, noted that physical activity and exercise are important factors in the prevention of overweight or obesity. Furthermore, de Groot and van Staveren indicate that once an individual becomes obese, physical activity decreases, setting up a vicious cycle of increasing body weight and even less physical activity.

Levine contends that the variability in total daily energy expenditure is attributed mainly to nonexercise activity thermogenesis (NEAT). Technology has decreased the amount of energy we normally expend via NEAT each day, such as walking, standing, and even fidgeting, which may lead to an energy imbalance and weight gain. Researchers followed lean and mildly obese people for 10 days, reporting those who were mildly obese stayed seated for about 2.5 hours longer per day than the lean individuals; they indicated that this could amount to 350 fewer Calories expended daily. Watching television and other such sedentary seated behaviors decrease NEAT, which Levine indicates may be of profound importance in the development of obesity. In their review, Levine and fish, may provide health benefits beyond those associated with weight loss. Chapters 4, 5, and 6 highlight healthful carbohydrates, fats, and protein, and chapter 9 discusses the DASH and OmniHeart diets.

Does being physically fit negate the adverse health effects associated with being overweight?

In general, research findings documenting increased health risks associated with obesity have been derived from the general population, and have been based primarily on BMI values. However, in an article titled *Hefty and Healthy,* the Consumers Union indicates that the BMI does not do a good job of assessing health, particularly for people who are moderately overweight, and also notes that there is some difference of opinion regarding the role of fitness and fatness in health.

As noted previously, the BMI does not evaluate body composition. Although it may be useful in determining health risks in the general population because a high BMI is usually associated with excess body fat, it does not apply to muscular individuals. A high BMI may be associated with the development of various chronic diseases if it does represent obesity and increases various risk factors, such as high serum cholesterol levels and high blood pressure. However, it is important to stress the point that the BMI does not measure fatness in all individuals.

The BMI also does not measure fitness, and a physically active lifestyle may be an important moderating factor in the association between fatness and health. However, whether or not fitness counteracts the adverse health effects of fatness is a matter of debate among exercise scientists.

Several studies suggest that fitness counteracts the adverse effects of fatness on heart health. Sui and others conducted a study to determine the association among cardiorespiratory fitness, adiposity, and mortality in older adults (> 60 years). In general, they found that being obese (BMI ≥ 30) or having a large waist circumference (34 inches, women; 40 inches, men) was significantly associated with increased mortality, but not when cardiorespiratory fitness was considered. High levels of fitness have been shown to be protective against premature mortality. Farrell and others investigated the association of cardiorespiratory fitness and adiposity on all-cause mortality in women. They found that across all levels of adiposity, higher levels of cardiorespiratory fitness were associated with lower incidence of mortality. They concluded that using adiposity measures as predictors of all-cause mortality in women may be misleading unless cardiorespiratory fitness is also considered. Some suggest that being overweight does not increase mortality unless it is associated with adverse effects on blood pressure, glucose tolerance, serum cholesterol levels, and other risk factors for chronic diseases. Physical activity may help to counteract such adverse effects.

The *Health at Any Size* movement, as advocated by Jonas, promotes physical activity for the obese individual, suggesting that exercise, even though it may not result in weight loss, may confer health benefits. In support of this contention, Miller and Dunstan found that physical activity intervention for the treatment of type 2 diabetes can lead to small but clinically meaningful improvements in glycemic control, even in the absence of weight loss. Borghouts and Keizer noted that both acute and chronic exercise may affect blood glucose and insulin activity favorably. Up to 2 hours after an acute bout of exercise, glucose uptake in active muscles is in part elevated due to insulin independent mechanisms, probably involving an increase in GLUT-4 receptors in the muscle cell membrane induced by exercise. Additionally, an exercise bout can increase insulin sensitivity for up to 16 hours afterwards. Chronic exercise training potentiates the effect of exercise on insulin sensitivity through multiple adaptations in glucose transport and metabolism. Gerson and Braun reported that when compared with lean fit women, estimated insulin sensitivity was only slightly lower in overweight women with equally high cardiovascular fitness levels. Overall, although exercise training may not help some individuals lose weight on the outside, they will improve their health on the inside.

Although fitness is important to counteract some of the adverse health effects of fatness, losing excess body fat may provide additional health benefits. Carroll and Dudfield indicated that exercise works best when coupled with weight loss. The combination of exercise and weight loss has been shown to produce numerous health effects, including decreased blood pressure, improved serum lipid status, reduced blood glucose, increased self-esteem, improved psychological health, and increased longevity.

Stevens and others examined the effects of both fitness (*fit, unfit*) and fatness (*fat, not fat*) on mortality from all causes and from cardiovascular disease. They found that *fit and not fat* individuals had the lowest mortality rates, those who were *fit and fat* or *unfit and not fat* had mortality rates about 30–40 percent higher, while *fat and unfit* individuals had the highest mortality rates. In a similar study, Kenchaiah and others studied the relationship between BMI and heart failure in men over the course of 20 years. The following hazard ratios were calculated for the corresponding categories based on BMI (lean, overweight, obese) and fitness (active, inactive) levels:

1.00—Lean, active
1.19—Lean, inactive
1.49—Overweight, active
1.78—Overweight, inactive
2.68—Obese, active
3.93—Obese, inactive

The lean, active men had the lowest hazard ratio (1.0) of heart failure, and the obese, inactive men had the highest (3.93). Heart failure risk increased with weight gain, but the risk was reduced somewhat by being physically active.

Weinstein and others, in a prospective study of nearly 39,000 women over the course of nearly 11 years, evaluated the interaction of physical activity and Body Mass Index on the risk of coronary heart disease (CHD). They found that the lowest risk for CHD was found in women who were of normal weight and physically active. Being overweight and physically inactive increased the risk, and women who were obese and inactive had the highest risk. The authors concluded that although the risk of CHD associated with elevated body mass index is considerably reduced by increased physical activity levels, the risk is not completely eliminated, reinforcing the importance of being lean and physically active. These investigators concluded that being fit does not reverse all of the increased health risks associated with excess adiposity. Although being *fit and fat* appears to be better healthwise than being *unfit and fat,* losing weight to become *fit and unfat* may confer some additional health benefits.

One should note that a normal BMI does not automatically connote good health. The Consumers Union indicates that individuals with a normal BMI but whose body composition is high in fat, recently referred to as *normal-weight obesity,* may have increased health risks. One may have a normal BMI but have relatively high amounts of abdominal fat and associated health risk.

Prevention of obesity is the key because once individuals become obese, treatment is difficult. When used in conjunction with appropriate dietary prescriptions and consistent behavior modification, exercise serves as a promising modality not only to prevent obesity in the first place, but perhaps also to help reverse it both during childhood and adulthood.

http://win.niddk.nih.gov/Publications/PDFs/ActiveatAnySize_04.pdf

Active at Any Size is a government program to encourage and help overweight individuals plan an exercise program. Access the Weight Control Information Network to access *Active at Any Size.*

Key Concepts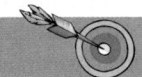

▶ Excessive body fat is associated with a variety of chronic diseases and impaired health conditions, including coronary heart disease, diabetes, high blood pressure, and arthritis.

▶ Although being obese increases health risks, the deposition of fat in the abdominal area exacerbates these risks. Referred to as android-type, or male-type, obesity, increased abdominal fat is associated with the metabolic syndrome and risk factors for heart disease and diabetes.

▶ For children and adolescents, the major adverse health effects of excessive body fat appear to be social and psychological. However, overweight and obese children are at high risk for type 2 diabetes even when young. Moreover, current research indicates that obese children are more prone to chronic diseases in adulthood than are their nonobese peers.

▶ Being physically fit and eating a healthful diet may help reduce some of the health risks associated with being overweight. One can be overweight, yet fit, but it appears the greatest health benefits may be associated with being fit and not fat.

Check for Yourself

▶ Conduct an observational study. Learn to use the "eyeball" technique to determine if a child is overweight. One afternoon sit outside a secondary public school in your community and as the students exit, make a check in a notebook as to how many out of the first 50 or 100 you would classify as being overweight. Compare your findings to the text discussion and to the findings of classmates who may also undertake this small observational study.

Excessive Weight Loss and Health

Losing excess body fat, even only 5–10 percent of body weight, and attaining a desirable body weight may confer some significant health benefits by counteracting the adverse effects of obesity. However, many individuals attempt to lose weight for other reasons. Slimness is currently very fashionable, particularly among females of all ages. It is desired not only for attractiveness but also for psychological undertones of independence, achievement, and self-control. Also, both male and female athletes, such as distance runners, gymnasts, wrestlers, jockeys, and dancers, practice weight control to improve their performance. Losing body weight for improved performance may also provide some health benefits, for Paul Williams theorized that the elevated HDL-cholesterol concentrations of long-distance runners are primarily a result of reduced adiposity. However, excessive weight loss may actually lead to deterioration of health.

What health problems are associated with improper weight-loss programs and practices?

As shall be noted in chapter 11, a well-designed diet and proper exercise are the cornerstones of a sound weight-control program. However, some individuals may establish unrealistically low body-weight goals, which may lead to pathogenic weight-control behaviors. Such techniques as complete starvation, self-induced vomiting, or the improper or excessive use of drugs, diet pills, laxatives, and diuretics may initially be employed to achieve rapid weight losses, but may evolve into serious medical disorders, even death, if prolonged. In their review of the association between BMI and all-cause mortality, Berrington and others reported that hazard ratio among women was 1.47 for a BMI of 15.0 to 18.4, which is classified as being underweight. The following discussion highlights some of the areas of concern in which weight-loss practices may be harmful if abused. The use, efficacy, and potential health risks of dietary supplements for weight loss are discussed in chapter 11.

Dehydration   Dehydration may be induced by exercise, exposure to the heat (as with a sauna), or the use of diuretics and laxatives. The effect of dehydration upon one's health, particularly in relation to heat illnesses, was detailed in chapter 9. The use of diuretics and laxatives may increase potassium losses from the body, which may lead to electrolyte imbalances and disturbed neurological function, including heart function. For example, in a case study Sturmi and Rutecki reported life-threatening hyperkalemia associated with ECG changes and indicators of muscle and kidney damage in a bodybuilder who used diuretics and potassium supplements, along with dietary restrictions, in preparation for competition. Vigorous potassium-lowering maneuvers helped resolve these problems, but the patient's symptoms resembled those of another professional bodybuilder who died after employing similar drug and diet strategies. Disturbed kidney function has also been observed following severe dehydration.

Weight-Loss Drugs   Various drugs have been developed to stimulate weight loss and generally are prescribed for the obese, not

▶ Although the average body-fat percentages for young men and women are, respectively, 15–20 percent and 23–30 percent, those involved in certain types of athletic competition may be advised to reduce those levels.

▶ Excessive loss of body weight may impair sport performance. For athletes in sports where weight loss may enhance performance, basic specific fitness tests may be used periodically to ascertain that performance is maintained or improved.

APPLICATION EXERCISE

Have your body-fat percentage measured with as wide a variety of techniques as possible, such as skinfolds, bioelectrical impedance analysis, air displacement plethysmography, and others. Compare the differences and relate to the text discussion.

If access to a variety of techniques is not available, have four or five individuals measure your skinfolds and calculate your body fat according to the directions in appendix D. Compare the differences and compare to the text discussion.

Body-Fat Percentage Measurements

	Skinfold analysis	Bioelectrical impedance	Air displacement plethysmography	Other	Other
Body-fat percentage					

Skinfold Measurements

	Measurement 1	Measurement 2	Measurement 3	Measurement 4	Measurement 5
Skinfold measurement					

Review Questions—Multiple Choice

1. Which of the following best describes the role of leptin in the human body?

   a. It is secreted by the hypothalamus and stimulates lipolysis in adipose cells.

   b. It is secreted by the liver and inhibits the digestion of fats.

   c. It is secreted by the adipose cells and inhibits hunger.

   d. It is secreted by the stomach and stimulates appetite.

   e. It is secreted by the intestines and stimulates appetite.

2. Which of the following statements regarding android/gynoid obesity is false?

   a. Gynoid obesity is associated with a higher incidence of certain diseases, such as hypertension.

   b. Android obesity is characterized by excess accumulation of fat deposits in the abdominal area.

   c. Android obesity is seen more often in men, while gynoid obesity is more prevalent in women.

   d. Gynoid-type fat deposits are more resistant to weight loss compared to android obesity.

   e. Development of both types of obesity is influenced by heredity.

3. If a skinfold technique for body composition has a standard error of estimate of 3 percent, you can have 70 percent confidence that for a person who has a predicted body fat of 18 percent, the actual value is within a range of

   a. 6–18 percent

   b. 18–21 percent

   c. 12–24 percent

   d. 15–21 percent

   e. 18–30 percent

4. Which of the following ranges of the Body Mass Index (BMI) is indicative of a normal height to weight relationship?

   a. 5–8

   b. 10–12

   c. 15–17

   d. 20–22

   e. 27–28

5. In which sports might the condition of anorexia athletica appear to be more prevalent?

   a. football and basketball

   b. swimming and baseball

   c. wrestling and field hockey

   d. ballet and gymnastics

   e. tennis and golf

6. The set-point theory of weight control is based upon a feedback system, suggesting that the individual is programmed to be a certain body weight and that the body will always attempt to maintain that weight by regulating

hunger and metabolism. What part of the body is believed to be the regulatory center for the control of the various feedback mechanisms?

a. liver receptors
b. stomach receptors
c. blood receptors in the kidney
d. receptors in the hypothalamus in the brain
e. receptors in the small intestine where absorption takes place

7. The disorder of bulimia, which is often characterized by the binge-purge syndrome, is found

a. only in those with anorexia nervosa
b. only in extremely underweight individuals
c. only in normal-weight individuals
d. only in moderately or morbidly obese individuals
e. in individuals across the body-weight spectrum

8. Which of the following is mainly an environmental rather than a possible hereditary factor in the multicausal etiology of obesity?

a. a sedentary lifestyle
b. hormonal imbalance
c. disorder in the brain's hunger and satiety centers
d. lower basal metabolic rate
e. a higher set point

9. Obesity has been associated as a potential risk factor in all the following diseases or health problems except which one?

a. coronary heart disease
b. anemia
c. hyperlidemia
d. diabetes
e. hypertension

10. Protein consumed during a starvation-type diet most likely will be:

a. used to rebuild muscle tissue
b. used to replace worn-out cells
c. converted to glucose for energy
d. used to stabilize fluid balance
e. stored as fat

Answers to multiple-choice questions:
1. c; 2. a; 3. d; 4. d; 5. d; 6. d; 7. e; 8. a; 9. b; 10. c.

1. List and describe five different techniques used to evaluate body composition, and highlight at least one value of each.
2. Discuss the set-point theory of body-weight control and relate it to body-fat levels, leptin, and neuropeptide Y.
3. List the various genetic and environmental factors that may be involved in the etiology of obesity. Highlight two of each and explain their possible role.
4. Explain the metabolic syndrome and associated health risks.
5. List the three components of the Female Athlete Triad. Discuss the underlying theories regarding its etiology, the potential effects on hormonal status, and subsequent serious health problems.

References

Books

Agatston, A. 2003. *The South Beach Diet.* Emmaus, PA: Rodale.

American Institute of Cancer Research. 2007. *Food, Nutrition, Physical Activity, and the Prevention of Cancer: A Global Perspective.* Washington, DC: AICR.

American Psychiatric Association. 2000. *Diagnostic and Statistical Manual of Mental Disorders DSM IRTB.* Washington, DC: American Psychiatric Association.

Heymsfield, S., et al. 2005. *Human Body Composition.* Champaign, IL: Human Kinetics.

Heyward, V., and Wagner, D. 2004. *Applied Body Composition Assessment.* Champaign, IL: Human Kinetics.

Houston, M. 2006. *Biochemistry Primer for Exercise Science* Champaign, IL: Human Kinetics.

National Academy of Sciences. 2002. *Dietary Reference Intakes for Energy, Carbohydrates, Fiber, Fat, Protein and Amino Acids (Macronutrients).* Washington, DC: National Academy Press.

National Research Council 1989. *Diet and Health: Implications for Reducing Chronic Disease Risk.* Washington, DC: National Academy Press.

Shils, M., et al., eds. 2006. *Modern Nutrition in Health and Disease.* Philadelphia: Lippincott Williams & Wilkins.

U.S. Department of Health and Human Services Public Health Service. 2010. *Healthy People 2020.* Washington, DC: U.S. Government Printing Office.

Reviews

Abizaid, A. 2009. Ghrelin and dopamine: New insights on the peripheral regulation of appetite. *Journal of Neuroendocrinology* 21:787–93.

Alberti, K., et al. 2005. The metabolic syndrome: A new worldwide definition. *Lancet* 366:1059–62.

American College of Sports Medicine. 2007. The Female Athlete Triad: Position stand. *Medicine & Science in Sports & Exercise* 39:1867–82.

American College of Sports Medicine. 2009. ACSM Position Stand on the Appropriate Intervention Strategies for Weight Loss and Prevention of Weight Regain for Adults. *Medicine & Science in Sports & Exercise* 41:459–71.

American College of Sports Medicine. 1996. American College of Sports Medicine Position Stand: Weight loss in wrestlers. *Medicine & Science in Sports & Exercise* 28(6):ix–xii.

American Dietetic Association. 2001. Position of the American Dietetic Association: Nutrition intervention in the treatment of anorexia nervosa, bulimia nervosa, and eating disorders not otherwise specified (EDNOS). *Journal of the American Dietetic Association* 101:810–19.

American Dietetic Association, Dietitians of Canada, American College of Sports Medicine, and Rodriguez, N., et al. 2009. American College of Sports Medicine position stand: Nutrition and athletic performance. *Medicine & Science in Sports & Exercise* 41:709–31.

Anderson, A. 1990. A proposed mechanism underlying eating disorders and other disorders of motivated behavior. In *Males with Eating Disorders,* ed. A. Anderson. New York: Brunners/Mazel.

Anderson, J. 2007. Orlistat for the management of overweight individuals and obesity: A review of potential for the 60-mg, over-the-counter dosage. *Expert Opinion on Pharmacotherapy* 8:1733–42.

Anderson, J., et al. 2001. Long-term weight-loss maintenance: A meta-analysis of US studies. *American Journal of Clinical Nutrition* 74:579–84.

Anderson, P., and Butcher, K. 2006. Childhood obesity: Trends and potential causes. *Future Child* 16:19–45.

Astrup, A. 2001. The role of dietary fat in the prevention and treatment of obesity. Efficacy and safety of low-fat diets. *International Journal of Obesity and Related Metabolic Disorders* 25:S46–S50.

Astrup, A., and Rossner, S. 2000. Lessons from obesity management programmes: Greater initial weight loss improves long-term maintenance. *Obesity Reviews* 1:17–19.

Astrup, A., et al. 2002. Low-fat diets and energy balance: How does the evidence stand in 2002? *Proceedings of the Nutrition Society* 61:299–309.

Atkinson, R. 1989. Low and very low calorie diets. *Medical Clinics of North America* 73:203–16.

Attila, E. 2010. Anorexia nervosa: Current status and future directions. *Annual Review of Medicine* 61:425–35.

Aucott, L. 2008. Influences of weight loss on long-term diabetes outcomes. *Proceeding of the Nutrition Society* 67:54–59.

Avram, M., et al. 2007. Subcutaneous fat in normal and diseased states 3. Adipogenesis: From stem cell to fat cell. *Journal of the American Academy of Dermatology* 56:472–92.

Badman, M., and Flier, J. 2005. The gut and energy balance: Visceral allies in the obesity war. *Science* 307:1909–14.

Baile, C. 2000. Regulation of metabolism and body mass by leptin. *Annual Reviews in Nutrition* 20:105–27.

Baker, S., et al. 2009. Effects and clinical potential of very-low-calorie diets (VLCDs) in type 2 diabetes. *Diabetes Research and Clinical Practice* 85:235–42.

Bar-Or, O. 2000. Juvenile obesity, physical activity, and lifestyle changes. *Physician and Sportsmedicine* 28(11):51–58.

Bays, H., et al. 2008. Pathogenic potential of adipose tissue and metabolic consequences of adipocyte hypertrophy and increased visceral adiposity. *Expert Review of Cardiovascular Therapy* 6:343–68.

Beals, K., and Meyer, N. 2007. Female Athlete Triad update. *Clinics in Sports Medicine* 26:69–89.

Bellisle, F., and Drewnowski, A. 2007. Intense sweeteners, energy intake and the control of body weight. *European Journal of Clinical Nutrition* 61:691–700.

Benardot, D. 2000. Gymnastics. In *Nutrition in Sport,* ed. R. J. Maughan. Oxford: Blackwell Science.

Benardot, D., and Thompson, W. R. 1999. Energy from food for physical activity: Enough and on time. *ACSM's Health & Fitness Journal* 3 (4):14–18.

Berkman, N., et al. 2007. Outcomes of eating disorders: A systematic review of the literature. *International Journal of Eating Disorders* 40:293–309.

Berrington de Gonzalez, A., et al. 2010. Body-mass index and mortality among 1.46 million white adults. *New England Journal of Medicine* 363:2211–9.

Bonci, C., et al. 2008. National Athletic Trainers' Association position statement: Preventing, detecting, and managing disordered eating in athletes. *Journal of Athletic Training* 43:80–108.

Borghouts, L., and Keizer, H. 2000. Exercise and insulin sensitivity: A review. *International Journal of Sports Medicine* 21:1–12.

Bouchard, C. 1997. Genetic determinants of regional fat distribution. *Human Reproduction* 12(Supplement 1):1–5.

Bouchard, C. 1991. Heredity and the path to overweight and obesity. *Medicine & Science in Sports & Exercise* 23:285–91.

Bray, G. 2004. How do we get fat? An epidemiologic and metabolic approach. *Clinics in Dermatology* 22:281–88.

Bray, G. 2004. Medical consequences of obesity. *Journal of Clinical Endocrinology and Metabolism* 89:2583–89.

Brownell, K. 1998. The pressure to eat. *Nutrition Action Health Letter* 25 (6):3–5.

Brownell, K., and Liebman, B. 2010. In your face: How the food industry drives us to eat. *Nutrition Action Health Letter* 37 (4):1–6.

Brownell, K., and Rodin, J. 1994. Medical, metabolic, and psychological effects of weight cycling. *Archives of Internal Medicine* 154:1325–29.

Bulik, C., et al. 2007. Anorexia nervosa treatment: A systematic review of randomized controlled trials. *International Journal of Eating Disorders* 40:310–20.

Burfoot, A. 2007. What's your ideal weight? *Runner's World* 42 (7):67–69.

Busetto, L. 2001. Visceral obesity and the metabolic syndrome: Effects of weight loss. *Nutrition, Metabolism and Cardiovascular Disease* 11:195–204.

Carmichael, A., and Bates, T. 2004. Obesity and breast cancer: A review of the literature. *Breast* 13:85–92.

Carroll, S., and Dudfield, M. 2004. What is the relationship between exercise and metabolic abnormalities? A review of the metabolic syndrome. *Sports Medicine* 34:371–78.

Catenacci, V., et al. 2009. The obesity epidemic. *Clinics in Chest Medicine* 30:415–44.

Chaput, J., et al. 2007. Currently available drugs for the treatment of obesity: Sibutramine and orlistat. *Mini Reviews in Medicinal Chemistry* 7:3–10.

Chu, S., et al. 2007. Maternal obesity and risk of stillbirth: A metaanalysis. *American Journal of Obstetrics and Gynecology* 197:223–8.

Cohen, D., and Farley, T. 2008. Eating as an automatic behavior. *Preventing Chronic Disease* 5:A23.

Consumers Union. 2008. Hefty and healthy. *Consumers Reports on Health* 20 (7):8–9.

Consumers Union. 2004. Outwitting your appetite. *Consumer Reports on Health* 16 (9):8–10.

Coughlin, J., and Guarda, A. 2006. Behavioral disorders affecting food intake: Eating disorders and other psychiatric conditions. In *Modern Nutrition in Health and Disease,* eds. M. Shils et al. Philadelphia: Lippincott Williams & Wilkins.

Currie, A., and Morse, E. 2005. Eating disorders in athletes: Managing the risks. *Clinics in Sports Medicine* 24:871–83.

Dallman, M., et al. 2004. Minireview: Glucocorticoids—food intake, abdominal obesity, and wealthy nations in 2004. *Endocrinology* 145:2633–38.

Daly, R., et al. 2002. Does training affect growth? *Physician and Sportsmedicine* 30 (10):21–29.

Daniels, S. 2006. The consequences of childhood overweight and obesity. *Future Child* 16:47–67.

Dattilo, A. 1992. Dietary fat and its relationship to body weight. *Nutrition Today* 27(January/February): 13–19.

Davey, R., 2004. The obesity epidemic: Too much food for thought? *British Journal of Sports Medicine* 38:360–63.

de Groot, L., and van Staveren, W. 1995. Reduced physical activity and its association with obesity. *Nutrition Reviews* 53:11–12.

Dham, S., and Banerji, M. 2006. The brain-gut axis in regulation of appetite and obesity. 34: *Pediatric Endocrinology Reviews* 3 (Supplement 4):544–54.

Dietz, W. 2006. Childhood obesity. In *Modern Nutrition in Health and Disease,* eds. M. Shils et al. Philadelphia: Lippincott Williams & Wilkins.

DiPietro, L. 1995. Physical activity, overweight, and adiposity: An epidemiologic perspective. *Exercise and Sport Sciences Reviews* 23:275–303.

Donnelly, J., et al. 2009. American College of Sports Medicine Position Stand: Appropriate physical activity intervention strategies for weight loss and prevention of weight regain for adults. *Medicine & Science in Sports & Exercise* 41:459–71.

Drewnowski, A., and Bellisle, F. 2007. Liquid calories, sugar, and body weight. *American Journal of Clinical Nutrition* 85:651–61.

Eckel, R., and Krauss, R. 1998. American Heart Association call to action: Obesity as a major risk factor for coronary heart disease. *Circulation* 97:2099–2100.

Ellis, K. 2001. Selected body composition methods can be used in field studies. *Journal of Nutrition* 131:1589S–95S.

Fantuzzi, G. and Mazzone, T. 2007. Adipose tissue and atherosclerosis: Exploring the connection. *Arteriosclerosis, Thrombosis, and Vascular Biology* 27:996 1003.

Fawcett, K., and Barroso, I. 2010. The genetics of obesity: FTO leads the way. *Trends in Genetics* 26:266–74.

Fehm, H., et al. 2006. The selfish brain: Competition for energy resources. *Progress in Brain Research* 153:129–40.

Fields, D., et al. 2002. Body-composition assessment via air-displacement plethysmography in adults and children: A review. *American Journal of Clinical Nutrition* 75:453–67.

Forbes, G. 2002. Perspectives on body composition. *Current Opinion in Clinical Nutrition and Metabolic Care* 5:25–30.

Froom, P., et al. 1998. Smoking cessation and weight gain. *Journal of Family Practice* 46:460–64.

Gaesser, G. 1999. Thinness and weight loss: Beneficial or detrimental to longevity? *Medicine & Science in Sports & Exercise* 31:1118–28.

Galassi, A., et al. 2006. Metabolic syndrome and the risk of cardiovascular disease: A meta-analysis. *American Journal of Medicine* 119:812–19.

Gami, A., et al. 2007. Metabolic syndrome and risk of incident cardiovascular events and death: A systematic review and meta-analysis of longitudinal studies. *Journal of the American College of Cardiology* 49:403–14.

Geier, A., et al. 2006. Unit bias. A new heuristic that helps explain the effect of portion size on food intake. *Psychological Science* 17:421–25.

Gerson, L., and Braun, B. 2006. Effect of high cardiorespiratory fitness and high body fat on insulin resistance. *Medicine & Science in Sports & Exercise* 38:1709–15.

Gibbs, W. 1996. Gaining on fat. *Scientific American* 275 (August):88–94.

Going, S. 2006. Optimizing techniques for determining body composition. *Sports Science Exchange* 19 (2):1–6.

Griffiths, L., et al. 2010. Self-esteem and quality of life in obese children and adolescents: A systematic review. *International Journal of Pediatric Obesity* 5:282–304.

Grodner, M. 1992. Forever dieting: Chronic dieting syndrome. *Journal of Nutrition Education* 24:207–10.

Grundy, S. 2007. Metabolic syndrome: A multiplex cardiovascular risk factor. *Journal of Clinical Endocrinology and Metabolism* 92:399–404.

Grundy, S. 1999. Hypertriglyceridemia, insulin resistance, and the metabolic syndrome. *American Journal of Cardiology* 83:25F–29F.

Grundy, S. 1998. Multifactorial causation of obesity: Implications for prevention. *American Journal of Clinical Nutrition* 67:563S–572S.

Gutin, B., and Humphries, M. 1998. Exercise, body composition, and health in children. In *Exercise, Nutrition, Weight Control,* eds. D. Lamb and R. Murray. Carmel, IN: Cooper Publishing Group.

Halford, J., et al. 2010. Pharmacological management of appetite expression in obesity. *Nature Reviews Endocrinology* 6:255–69.

Haller, E. 1992. Eating disorders: A review and update. *Western Journal of Medicine* 157:658–62.

Hansen, J., et al. 2010. Is thermogenesis a significant causal factor in preventing the "globesity" epidemic? *Medical Hypotheses* 75:250–6.

Hetherington, M., and Cecil, J. 2010. Gene-environment interactions in obesity. *Forum on Nutrition* 63:195–203.

Heymsfield, S., and Baumgartner, R. 2006. Body composition and anthropometry. In *Modern Nutrition in Health and Disease,* eds. M. Shils et al. Philadelphia: Lippincott Williams & Wilkins.

Hill, J., et al. 2006. Obesity: Etilogy. In *Modern Nutrition in Health and Disease,* eds. M. Shils et al. Philadelphia: Lippincott Williams & Wilkins.

Hills, A., et al. 2007. The contribution of physical activity and sedentary behaviours to the growth and development of children and adolescents: Implications for overweight and obesity. *Sports Medicine* 37:533–45.

Hirsch, J., and Leibel, R. 1998. The genetics of obesity. *Hospital Practice (Office Edition)* 33:55–70.

Jaffrin, M. 2009. Body composition determination by bioimpedance: An update. *Current Opinion in Clinical Nutrition & Metabolic Care* 12:482–6.

James, W., 2008. WHO recognition of the global obesity epidemic. *International Journal of Obesity* 32: Supplement 7: S120–6.

Johnson, R., et al. 2009. Dietary sugars intake and cardiovascular health: A scientific statement from the American Heart Association. *Circulation* 120:1011–20.

Jonas, S. 2001. Weighing in on the obesity epidemic: What do we do now? *ACSM's Health & Fitness Journal* 5 (5):710.

Keel, P., et al. 2007. Clinical features and physiological response to a test meal in purging disorder and bulimia nervosa. *Archives of General Psychiatry* 64: 1058–66.

Keesey, R., and Hirvonen, M. 1997. Body weight set-points: Determination and adjustment. *Journal of Nutrition* 127:1875S–1883S.

Kessler, D., and Liebman, B. 2009. Why we overeat. *Nutrition Action Health Letter* 16 (6):1–6.

King, B. 2006. The rise, fall, and resurrection of the ventromedial hypothalamus in the regulation of feeding behavior and body weight. *Physiology & Behavior* 87:221–44.

King, P. 2005. The hypothalamus and obesity. *Current Drug Targets* 6:225–40.

Klok, M., et al. 2007. The role of leptin and ghrelin in the regulation of food intake and body weight in humans: A review. *Obesity Reviews* 8:21–34.

Kojima, M., and Kangawa, K. 2005. Ghrelin: Structure and function. *Physiological Reviews* 85:495–522.

Kolotkin, R., et al. 2001. Quality of life and obesity. *Obesity Reviews* 2:219–29.

Kral, T., and Rauh, E. 2010. Eating behaviors of children in the context of their family environment. *Physiology & Behavior* 100:567–73.

Lafontan, M. 2005. Fat cells: Afferent and efferent messages define new approaches to treat obesity. *Annual Review of Pharmacology and Toxicology* 45:119–46.

Lamarche, B. 1998. Abdominal obesity and its metabolic complications: Implications for the risk of ischaemic heart disease. *Coronary Artery Disease* 9:473–81.

Lee, Y. 2009. The role of genes in the current obesity epidemic. *Annals Academy of Medicine Singapore* 38:45–3.

Levin, B. 2006. Metabolic sensing neurons and the control of energy homeostasis. *Physiology & Behavior* 89:486–89.

Levin, B. 2000. Metabolic imprinting on genetically predisposed neural circuits perpetuates obesity. *Nutrition* 16:909–15.

Levin, B. 2002. Metabolic sensors: Viewing glucosensing neurons from a broader perspective. *Physiology & Behavior* 76:387–401.

Levine, J. 2004. Non-exercise activity thermogenesis. *Nutrition Reviews* 62:S82–S97.

Levine, J., et al. 2006. Non-exercise activity thermogenesis: The crouching tiger hidden dragon of societal weight gain. *Arteriosclerosis, Thrombosis, and Vascular Biology* 26:729–36.

Lohman, T., and Going, S. 2006. Body composition assessment for development of an international growth standard for preadolescent and adolescent children. *Food and Nutrition Bulletin* 27:S314–25.

Lohman, T., et al. 1997. Body fat measurement goes high-tech: Not all are created equal. *ACSM's Health & Fitness Journal* 1 (1):30–35.

Loucks, A. 2006. The endocrine system: Integrated influences on metabolism, growth, and reproduction. In ACSM's *Advanced Exercise Physiology,* ed. C. M. Tipton. Philadelphia: Lippincott Williams & Wilkins.

Loucks, A. 2004. Energy balance and body composition in sports and exercise. *Journal of Sports Sciences* 22:1–14.

Loucks, A. 2003. Energy availability, not body fatness, regulates reproductive function in women. *Exercise and Sports Sciences Reviews* 31:144–48.

Lutter, M., and Nestler, E. 2009. Homeostatic and hedonic signals interact in the regulation of food intake. *Journal of Nutrition* 139:629–32.

Major, G., et al. 2007. Clinical significance of adaptive thermogenesis. *International Journal of Obesity* 31:204–12.

Malik, V., et al. 2006. Intake of sugar-sweetened beverages and weight gain: A systematic review. *American Journal of Clinical Nutrition* 84:274–88.

Malina, R. 2007. Body composition in athletes: Assessment and estimated fatness. *Clinics in Sports Medicine* 26:37–68.

Manore, M. 2002. Dietary recommendations and athletic menstrual dysfunction. *Sports Medicine* 32:887–901.

Manore, M. 2000. The overweight athlete. In *Nutrition in Sport,* ed. R. J. Maughan. Oxford: Blackwell Science.

Marshall, S., et al. 2004. Relationships between media use, body fatness and physical activity in children and youth: A meta-analysis. *International Journal of Obesity and Related Metabolic Disorders* 28:1238–46.

Mattson, M. 2010. Perspective: Does brown fat protect against diseases of aging? *Ageing Research Reviews* 9:69–76.

McGilley, B., and Pryor, T. 1998. Assessment and treatment of bulimia nervosa. *American Family Physician* 57:2743–50.

Melby, C., et al. 1998. Exercise, macronutrient balance, and weight control. In *Exercise, Nutrition, and Weight Control,* eds. D. Lamb and R. Murray. Carmel, IN: Cooper Publishing Group.

Miller, Y., and Dunstan, D. 2004. The effectiveness of physical activity interventions for the treatment of overweight and obesity and type 2 diabetes. *Journal of Science and Medicine in Sport* 7:52–59.

Mitra, A., and Clarke, K. 2010. Viral obesity: Fact or fiction? *Obesity Reviews* 11:289–96.

Moran, T. 2006. Gut peptide signaling in the control of food intake. *Obesity* 14:250S–53S.

Moreno, L., and Rodríguez, G. 2007. Dietary risk factors for development of childhood obesity. *Current Opinion in Clinical Nutrition and Metabolic Care* 10:336–41.

Mosca, L. 2007. Evidence-based recommendations for cardiovascular disease prevention in women: 2007 Update. *Circulation* 115:1481–1501.

Mottillo, S., et al. 2010. The metabolic syndrome and cardiovascular risk a systematic review and meta-analysis. *Journal of the American College of Cardiology* 56:1113–32.

National Task Force on the Prevention and Treatment of Obesity. 1996. Long-term pharmacotherapy in the management of obesity. *Journal of the American Medical Association* 276:1907–15.

National Task Force on the Prevention and Treatment of Obesity. 1994. Weight cycling. *Journal of the American Medical Association* 272:1196–1202.

National Task Force on the Prevention and Treatment of Obesity. 1993. Very-low-Calorie diets. *Journal of the American Medical Association* 270:967–74.

Nelson, R., and Bremer, A. 2010. Insulin resistance and metabolic syndrome in the pediatric population. *Metabolic Syndrome and Related Disorders* 8:1–14.

Newbold, R. 2010. Impact of environmental endocrine disrupting chemicals on the development of obesity. *Hormones* 9:206–17.

Newman, C. 2004. Why are we so fat? *National Geographic* 206 (2):48–61.

Owen, N., et al. 2010. Too much sitting: The population health science of sedentary behavior. *Exercise and Sport Sciences Reviews* 38:105–13.

Pate, R. 1993. Physical activity in children and youth: Relation to obesity. *Contemporary Nutrition* 18 (2):1–2.

Patel, S. 2009. Reduced sleep as an obesity risk factor. *Obesity Reviews* 10: Supplement 2:61–8.

Peters, J. 2006. Obesity prevention and social change: What will it take? *Exercise and Sport Sciences Reviews* 34:4–9.

Peters, J., et al. 2002. From instinct to intellect: The challenge of maintaining healthy weight in the modern world. *Obesity Reviews* 3:69–74.

Pi-Sunyer, F. 2007. How effective are lifestyle changes in the prevention of type 2 diabetes mellitus? *Nutrition Reviews* 65:101–10.

Pi-Sunyer, F. 2006. The relation of adipose tissue to cardiometabolic risk. *Clinical Cornerstone* 8 (Supplement 4):S14–23.

Pi-Sunyer, F. 2002. The medical risks of obesity. *Obesity Surgery* 12:6S–11S.

Pi-Sunyer, F. 1999. Obesity. In *Modern Nutrition in Health and Disease,* eds. M. Shils et al. Baltimore: Williams & Wilkins.

Pittler, M., et al. 2005. Adverse events of herbal food supplements for body weight reduction: Systematic review. *Obesity Reviews* 6:89–92.

Pronk, N. 2011. The problem with too much sitting. *ACSM's Health & Fitness Journal* 15 (1):41–3.

Putukian, M. 1998. The Female Athlete Triad. *Clinics in Sports Medicine* 17:675–96.

Rankinen, T., et al. 2006. The human obesity gene map: The 2005 update. *Obesity* 14:529–644.

Rask-Andersen, M., et al. 2010. Molecular mechanisms underlying anorexia nervosa: focus on human gene association studies and systems controlling food intake. *Brain Research Reviews* 62:147–64.

Ravussin, E., and Liebman, B. 2010. Fat chance: New clues to why we gain weight. *Nutrition Action Health Letter* 17 (10):1–9.

Reaven, G. 2006. The metabolic syndrome: Is this diagnosis necessary? *American Journal of Clinical Nutrition* 83:1237–47.

Reaven, G. 2006. Metabolic syndrome: Definition, relationship to insulin resistance, and clinical utility. In *Modern Nutrition in Health and Disease,* eds. M. Shils et al. Philadelphia: Lippincott Williams & Wilkins.

Renehan, A., et al. 2008. Body-mass index and incidence of cancer: A systematic review and meta-analysis of prospective observational studies. *The Lancet* 371:569–78.

Robinson, T. 2001. Television viewing and childhood obesity. *Pediatric Clinics of North America* 48:1017–25.

Rolls, B., and Shide, D. 1992. The influence of dietary fat on food intake and body weight. *Nutrition Reviews* 50:283–90.

Rondinone, C. 2006. Adipocyte-derived hormones, cytokines, and mediators. *Endocrine* 29:81–90.

Rowland, T. 1998. The biological basis of physical activity. *Medicine & Science in Sports & Exercise* 30:392–99.

Saris, W. 1998. Fit and fat free: The metabolic aspects of weight control. *International Journal of Obesity and Related Metabolic Disorders* 22:S15–S21.

Schnirring, L. 2005. NFHS finalizes weight cutting rules for wrestlers. *Physician and Sportsmedicine* 33 (7):9–12.

Sell, H., et al. 2004. The brown adipocyte: Update on its metabolic role. *International Journal of Biochemistry & Cell Biology* 36:2098–2104.

Shah, M., and Garg, A. 1996. High-fat and high-carbohydrate diets and energy balance. *Diabetes Care* 19:1142–52.

Shapiro, J., et al. 2007. Bulimia nervosa treatment: A systematic review of randomized controlled trials. *International Journal of Eating Disorders* 40:321–36.

Sodersen, P., et al. 2006. Understanding eating disorders. *Hormones and Behavior* 50:572–78.

Smith, G. 2006. Controls of food intake. In *Modern Nutrition Health and Disease,* eds. M. Shils et al. Philadephia: Lippincott Williams & Wilkins.

Smolak, L., et al. 2000. Female athletes and eating problems: A meta-analysis. *International Journal of Eating Disorders* 27:371–80.

Southern, M. 2001. Exercise as a modality in the treatment of childhood obesity. *Pediatric Clinics of North America* 48:995–1015.

Steinhausen, H. 2002. The outcome of anorexia nervosa in the 20th century. *American Journal of Psychiatry* 159:1284–93.

Steinhausen, H., and Weber, S. 2009. The outcome of bulimia nervosa: findings from one-quarter century of research. *American Journal of Psychiatry* 166:1331–41.

Stobbe, M. 2010. Obesity's impact on costs bigger than thought. *Associated Press*: October 17.

Stock, M. 1989. Thermogenesis and brown fat: Relevance to human obesity. *Infusiontherapie* 16:282–84.

Strecker, L. 2010. School nutrition and childhood obesity. *Update Plus* September/October: 4–5.

Stubbs, R. 1999. Peripheral signals affecting food intake. *Nutrition* 15:614–25.

Sullivan, E., et al. 2011. Perinatal exposure to high-fat diet programs energy balance, metabolism and behavior in adulthood. *Neuroendocrinology* 93:1–8.

Sundgot-Borgen, J. 2000. Eating disorders in athletes. In *Nutrition in Sport,* ed. R. J. Maughan. Oxford: Blackwell Science.

Swinburn, B., and Shelly, A. 2008. Effects of TV time and other sedentary pursuits. *International Journal of Obesity* 32: Supplement 7:S132–6.

Terán-García, M., and Bouchard, C. 2007. Genetics of the metabolic syndrome. *Applied Physiology, Nutrition, and Metabolism* 32:89–114.

Trayhurn, P., and Beattie, J. 2001. Physiological role of adipose tissue: White adipose tissue as an endocrine and secretory organ. *Proceedings of the Nutrition Society* 60:329–39.

Tsai, A., and Wadden, T. 2006. The evolution of very-low-calorie diets: An update and meta-analysis. *Obesity* 14:1283–93.

Tso, P., and Liu, M. 2004. Ingested fat and satiety. *Physiology & Behavior* 81:275–87.

Vella-Zarb, R., and Elgar, F. 2009. The "freshman 5": a meta-analysis of weight gain in the freshman year of college. *Journal of the American College of Health* 58:161–6.

Wadden, T., et al. 2006. Obesity: Management. In *Modern Nutrition in Health and Disease,* eds. M. Shils et al. Philadelphia: Lippincott Williams & Wilkins.

Wadden, T., et al. 2002. Obesity: Responding to the global epidemic. *Journal of Consulting and Clinical Psychology* 70:510–25.

Wagner, D., and Heyward, V. 1999. Techniques of body composition assessment: A review of laboratory and field methods. *Research Quarterly for Exercise and Sport* 70:135–49.

Wang, L., et al. 1992. The five-level model: A new approach to organizing body-composition research. *American Journal of Clinical Nutrition* 56.19–28.

Wang, Y., and Beydoun, M. 2007. The obesity epidemic in the United States—gender, age, socioeconomic, racial/ethnic, and geographic characteristics: a systematic review and meta-regression analysis. *Epidemiologic Reviews* 29:6–28.

Wells, J. 2006. The evolution of human fatness and susceptibility to obesity: An ethological approach. *Biological Reviews of the Cambridge Philosophical Society* 81:183–205.

Weinsier, R., et al. 1998. The etiology of obesity: Relative contribution of metabolic factors, diet, and physical activity. *American Journal of Medicine* 105:145–50.

Wilder, R., and Cicchetti, M. 2009. Common injuries in athletes with obesity and diabetes. *Clinics in Sports Medicine* 28:441–53.

Wildman, R. 2009. Healthy obesity. *Current Opinion in Clinical Nutrition & Metabolic Care* 12:438–43.

Willett, W. 2002. Dietary fat plays a major role in obesity: No. *Obesity Reviews* 3:59–68.

Wolin, K., et al. 2010. Obesity and cancer. *Oncologist* 15:556–65.

Woods, S. 2007. The endocannabinoid system: Mechanisms behind metabolic homeostasis and imbalance. *American Journal of Medicine* 120(Supplement 1):S9–S17.

Specific Studies

Adams, T., et al. 2007. Long-term mortality after gastric bypass surgery. *New England Journal of Medicine* 357:753–61.

Alderman, B., et al. 2004. Factors related to rapid weight-loss practices among international-style wrestlers. *Medicine & Science in Sports & Exercise* 36:249–52.

Andersen, R., et al. 1998. Relationship of physical activity and television watching with body weight and level of fatness among children. *Journal of the American Medical Association* 279:938–42.

Angelopoulos, T., et al. 2002. Significant enhancements in glucose tolerance and insulin action in centrally obese subjects following ten days of training. *Clinical Journal of Sport Medicine* 12:113–18.

Baker, J., et al. 2007. Childhood body-mass index and the risk of coronary heart disease in adulthood. *New England Journal of Medicine* 357:2329–37.

Ball, S., and Altena, T. 2004. Comparison of the Bod Pod and dual energy x-ray absorptiometry in men. *Physiological Measurement* 25:671–78.

Beals, K., and Manore, M. 2000. Behavioral, psychological, and physical characteristics of female athletes with subclinical eating disorders. *International Journal of Sport Nutrition and Exercise Metabolism* 10:128–43.

Benardot, D., and Czerwinski, C. 1991. Selected body composition and growth measures of junior elite gymnasts. *Journal of the American Dietetic Association* 91:29–33.

Bigaard, J., et al. 2005. Waist circumference and body composition in relation to all-cause mortality in middle-aged men and women. *International Journal of Obesity and Related Metabolic Disorders.* 29:778–84.

Bouchard, C., et al. 1990. The response to long-term overfeeding in identical twins. *New England Journal of Medicine* 322:1477–82.

Bowman, S., et al. 2004. Effects of fast-food consumption on energy intake and diet quality among children in a national household survey. *Pediatrics* 113:112–18.

Budd, G. 2007. Disordered eating: Young women's search for control and connection. *Journal of Child and Adolescent Psychiatric Nursing* 20:96–106.

Bulik, C., et al. 2006. Prevalence, heritability, and prospective risk factors for anorexia nervosa. *Archives of General Psychiatry* 63:305–12.

Calle, E., et al. 2003. Overweight, obesity, and mortality from cancer in a prospectively studied cohort of U.S. adults. *New England Journal of Medicine* 348:1625–38.

Christakis, N., and Fowler, J. 2007. The spread of obesity in a large social network over 32 years. *New England Journal of Medicine* 357:404–7.

Clark, R., et al. 2004. Minimum weight prediction methods cross-validated by the four-component model. *Medicine & Science in Sports & Exercise* 36:639–47.

Clark, R., et al. 2002. Cross-validation of the NCAA method to predict body fat for minimum weight in collegiate wrestlers. *Clinical Journal of Sport Medicine* 12:285–90.

Daly, R., et al. 2005. Growth of highly versus moderately trained competitive female artistic gymnasts. *Medicine & Science in Sports & Exercise* 37:1053–60.

Dick, R. 1993. Eating disorders in NCAA athletics programs: Replication of a 1990 study. *NCAA Sports Sciences* 3 (Spring).

Ebbeling, C., et al. 2007. Altering portion sizes and eating rate to attenuate gorging during a fast food meal: Effects on energy intake. *Pediatrics* 119:869–75.

Ebbeling, C., et al. 2006. Effects of decreasing sugar-sweetened beverage consumption on body weight in adolescents: A randomized, controlled pilot study. *Pediatrics* 117:673–80.

Elliot, D., et al. 2006. Definition and outcome of a curriculum to prevent disordered eating and body-shaping drug use. *Journal of School Health* 76:67–73.

Farrell, S., et al. 2010. Cardiorespiratory fitness, adiposity, and all-cause mortality in women. *Medicine & Science in Sports & Exercise* 42:2006–12.

Field, A., et al. 2004. Association of weight change, weight control practices, and weight cycling among women in the Nurses' Health Study II. *International Journal of Obesity and Related Metabolic Disorders* 28:1134–42.

Finucane, M., et al. 2011. National, regional, and global trends in body-mass index since 1980: systematic analysis of health examination surveys and epidemiological studies with 960 country-years and 9.1 million participants. *Lancet* 377:557–67.

Flood, J., et al. 2006. The effect of increased beverage portion size on energy intake at a meal. *Journal of the American Dietetic Association* 106:1984–90.

Fogelholm, G., et al. 1993. Gradual and rapid weight loss: Effects on nutrition and performance in male athletes. *Medicine & Science in Sports & Exercise* 25:371–77.

Fontaine, K., et al. 2003. Years of life lost due to obesity. *JAMA* 289:187–93.

Franks, P., et al. 2010. Childhood obesity, other cardiovascular risk factors, and premature death. *New England Journal of Medicine* 362:485–93.

Frisch, R., et al. 1989. Lower prevalence of nonreproductive system cancers among female former college athletes. *Medicine & Science in Sports & Exercise* 21:250–53.

Green, S., and Blundell, J. 1996. Effect of fat- and sucrose-containing foods on the size of eating episodes and energy intake in lean dietary restrained and unrestrained females: Potential for causing overconsumption. *European Journal of Clinical Nutrition* 50:625–35.

Harp, J., and Hecht, L. 2005. Obesity in the National Football League. *JAMA* 293:1061–62.

Hoch, A., et al. 2009. Prevalence of the female athlete triad in high school athletes and sedentary students. *Clinical Journal of Sport Medicine* 19:421–8.

Jacobs, E., et al. 2010. Waist circumference and all-cause mortality in a large US cohort. *Archives of Internal Medicine* 170:1293–301.

Jago, R., et al. 2010. Fatness, fitness, and cardiometabolic risk factors among sixth-grade youth. *Medicine & Science in Sports & Exercise* 42:1502–10.

Janssen, I., et al. 2002. Body mass index, waist circumference, and health risk: Evidence in support of current National Institutes of Health guidelines. *Archives of Internal Medicine* 162:2074–79.

Johnson, C., et al. 1999. Athletes and eating disorders: The National Collegiate Athletic Association Study. *International Journal of Eating Disorders* 26:179–88.

Kenchaiah, S., et al. 2009. Body mass index and vigorous physical activity and the risk of heart failure among men. *Circulation* 119:44–52.

Kiningham, R., and Gorenflo, W. 2001. Weight loss methods of high school wrestlers. *Medicine & Science in Sports & Exercise* 33:810–13.

Koral, J., and Dosseville, F. 2009. Combination of gradual and rapid weight loss: effects on physical performance and psychological state of elite judo athletes. *Journal of Sports Sciences* 27:115–20.

Larson-Meyer, D., et al. 2010. Caloric restriction with or without exercise: the fitness versus fatness debate. *Medicine & Science in Sports & Exercise* 42:152–9.

Lotti, T., et al. 1990. Proteoglycans in so-called cellulite. *International Journal of Dermatology* 29:272–74.

Mayer, L., et al. 2007. Does percent body fat predict outcome in anorexia nervosa? *American Journal of Psychiatry* 164:970–2.

McCargar, L., et al. 1996. Chronic dieting does not result in a sustained reduction in resting metabolic rate in overweight women. *Journal of the American Dietetic Association* 96:1175–77.

Mendoza, J., et al. 2007. Dietary energy density is associated with obesity and the metabolic syndrome in U.S. adults. *Diabetes Care* 30:974–79.

Nader, P., et al. 2006. Identifying risk for obesity in early childhood. *Pediatrics* 118:594–601.

Noreen, E., and Lemon, P. 2006. Reliability of air displacement plethysmography in a large, heterogeneous sample. *Medicine & Science in Sports & Exercise* 38:1505–509.

O'Brien, M., et al. 2007. The ecology of childhood overweight: A 12-year longitudinal analysis. *International Journal of Obesity* 31:1469–78.

O'Connor, D., et al. 2010. Generalized equations for estimating DXA percent body fat of diverse young women and men: The TIGER study. *Medicine & Science in Sports & Exercise* 42:1959–65.

Ode, J., et al. 2007. Body mass index as a predictor of percent fat in college athletes and nonathletes. *Medicine & Science in Sports & Exercise* 39:403–409.

Ogden, C., et al. 2006. Prevalence of overweight and obesity in the United States, 1999–2004. *Journal of the American Medical Association* 295:1549–55.

Oppliger, R., et al. 2006. NCAA rule change improves weight loss among National Championship wrestlers. *Medicine & Science in Sports & Exercise* 38:963–70.

Oppliger, R., et al. 2003. Weight loss practices of wrestlers. *International Journal of Sport Nutrition and Exercise Metabolism* 13:29–46.

Orphanidou, C., et al. 1994. Accuracy of subcutaneous fat measurement: Comparison of skinfold calipers, ultrasound, and computed tomography. *Journal of the American Dietetic Association* 94:855–58.

Pate, R., et al. 1989. Relationship between skinfold thickness and performance of health related fitness test items. *Research Quarterly for Exercise and Sport* 60:183–88.

Pearcey, S., and de Castro, J. 2002. Food intake and meal patterns of weight-stable and weight-gaining persons. *American Journal of Clinical Nutrition* 76:107–12.

Pereira, M., et al. 2005. Fast-food habits, weight gain, and insulin resistance (the CARDIA study): 15-year prospective analysis. *The Lancet* 365:36–42.

Pichard, C., et al. 1997. Body composition by x-ray absorptiometry and bioelectrical impedance in female runners. *Medicine & Science in Sports & Exercise* 29:1527–34.

Rodin, J., et al. 1990. Weight cycling and fat distribution. *International Journal of Obesity* 14:303–10.

Roemmich, J., and Sinning, W. 1996. Sport-seasonal changes in body composition, growth, power and strength of adolescent wrestlers. *International Journal of Sports Medicine* 17:92–99.

Romero-Corral, A., et al. 2010. Modest visceral fat gain causes endothelial dysfunction in healthy humans. *Journal of the American College of Cardiology* 56:662–6.

Rosenbaum, M., et al. 1998. An exploratory investigation of the morphology and biochemistry of cellulite. *Plastic and Reconstructive Surgery* 101;1934–39.

Salvy, S., et al. 2009. The presence of friends increases food intake in youth. *American Journal of Clinical Nutrition* 90:282–7.

Simkin-Silverman, L., et al. 1998. Lifetime weight cycling and psychological health in normal-weight and overweight women. *International Journal of Eating Disorders* 24:175–83.

Small, K., et al. 2011. Identification of an imprinted master trans regulator at the KLF14 locus related to multiple metabolic phenotypes. *Nature Genetics* 43:561–4.

Stevens, J., et al. 2002. Fitness and fatness as predictors of mortality from all causes and from cardiovascular disease in men and women in the Lipid Research Clinics Study. *American Journal of Epidemiology* 156:832–41.

Stout, J., et al. 1995. Validity of skinfold equations for estimating body density in youth wrestlers. *Medicine & Science in Sports & Exercise* 27:1321–25.

Stunkard, A., et al. 1990. The body-mass index of twins who have been reared apart. *New England Journal of Medicine* 322:1483–87.

Sturmi, J., and Rutecki, G. 1995. When competitive body builders collapse. *Physician and Sportsmedicine* 23 (11):49–53.

Sui, X., et al. 2007. Cardiorespiratory fitness and adiposity as mortality predictors in older adults. *Journal of the American Medical Association* 298:2507–16.

Theintz, G., et al. 1993. Evidence for a reduction of growth potential in adolescent female gymnasts. *Journal of Pediatrics* 122:306–13.

Torstveit, M., and Sundgot-Borgen, J. 2005. The Female Athlete Triad exists in both elite athletes and controls. *Medicine & Science in Sports & Exercise* 37:1449–59.

Torstveit, M., and Sundgot-Borgen, J. 2005. Participation in leanness sports but not training volume is associated with menstrual dysfunction: A national survey of 1276 elite athletes and controls. *British Journal of Sports Medicine* 39:141–47.

Torstveit, M., and Sundgot-Borgen, J. 2005. The Female Athlete Triad: Are elite athletes at increased risk? *Medicine & Science in Sports & Exercise* 37:184–93.

Tremblay, A., et al. 1995. Alcohol and a high-fat diet: A combination favoring overfeeding. *American Journal of Clinical Nutrition* 62:639–44.

Trevisan, M., et al. 1998. Syndrome X and mortality: A population-based study. *American Journal of Epidemiology* 148:958–66.

Utter, A., and Hager, M. 2008. Evaluation of ultrasound in assessing body composition of high school wrestlers. *Medicine & Science in Sports & Exercise* 40:943–49.

Vorona, R., et al. 2005. Overweight and obese patients in a primary care population report less sleep than patients with a normal body mass index. *Archives of Internal Medicine* 165:25–30.

Wadden, T., et al. 2005. Randomized trial of lifestyle modification and pharmacotherapy for obesity. *New England Journal of Medicine* 353:2111–20.

Wagner, D., et al. 2000. Validation of air displacement plethysmography for assessing body composition. *Medicine & Science in Sports & Exercise* 32:1339–44.

Wang, Y., et al. 2005. Comparison of abdominal adiposity and overall obesity in predicting risk of type 2 diabetes among men. *American Journal of Clinical Nutrition* 81:555–63.

Wang, Z., et al. 1998. Six-compartment body composition model: Inter-method comparisons of total body fat measurement. *International Journal of Obesity and Related Metabolic Disorders* 22:329–37.

Webster, B., and Barr, S. 1993. Body composition analysis of female adolescent athletes: Comparing six regression equations. *Medicine & Science in Sports & Exercise* 25:648–53.

Weinsier, R., et al. 2000. Do adaptive changes in metabolic rate favor weight regain in weight-reduced individuals? An examination of the set-point theory. *American Journal of Clinical Nutrition* 73:1088–94.

Weinstein, A., et al. 2008. The joint effects of physical activity and body mass index on coronary heart disease risk in women. *Archives of Internal Medicine* 168:884–90.

Wiecha, J., et al. 2006. When children eat what they watch: Impact of television viewing on dietary intake in youth. *Archives of Pediatrics & Adolescent Medicine* 160:436–42.

Williams, P. 1990. Weight set-point theory and the high-density lipoprotein concentrations of long-distance runners. *Metabolism* 39:460–67.

Yard, E., and Comstock, D. 2011. Injury patterns by body mass index in US high school athletes. *Journal of Physical Activity and Health* 8:182–91.

Yusuf, S., et al. 2005. Obesity and the risk of myocardial infarction in 27,000 participants from 52 countries: A case control study. *Lancet* 366:1640–49.

Zachwieja, J., et al. 2001. Short-term dietary energy restriction reduces lean body mass but not performance in physically active men and women. *International Journal of Sports Medicine* 22:310–16.

Zhang, C., et al. 2008. Abdominal obesity and the risk of all-cause, cardiovascular, and cancer mortality: Sixteen years of follow-up in US women. *Circulation* 117:1658–67.

Zhang, J., et al. 2005. Obestatin, a peptide encoded by the ghrelin gene, opposes effects on food intake. *Science* 310:996–99.

Weight Maintenance and Loss through Proper Nutrition and Exercise

CHAPTER ELEVEN

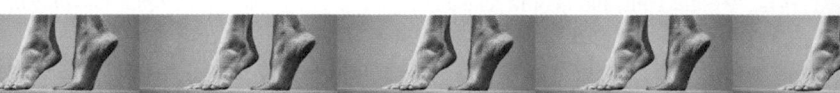

LEARNING OBJECTIVES

After studying this chapter, you should be able to:

1. Determine how many Calories per day are needed to maintain one's current body weight with either a sedentary or physically active lifestyle.

2. Calculate the amount of weight loss needed to attain a healthier BMI or body-fat percentage.

3. Identify behavior modification techniques that are appropriate to incorporate into a recommended weight-loss program.

4. Determine the number of daily Calories needed to lose body fat by diet alone, or with a combination diet-exercise program.

5. State the key principles underlying a weight-control diet designed to maintain a healthy body weight for a lifetime.

6. Use the Food Exchange System to plan a healthy, balanced diet containing sufficient Calories to meet one's daily energy needs for weight loss or weight maintenance.

7. Describe the value of exercise, including type, intensity, duration, and frequency, in a comprehensive weight-loss or weight-maintenance program.

8. Use heart rate responses as a guide to appropriate aerobic exercise intensity.

9. Design a progressive exercise program that will increase caloric expenditure to 300–500 Calories per day as part of a comprehensive weight-loss or weight-maintenance program.

10. Understand how diet and exercise complement each other to help lose or maintain body weight, citing the benefits of each that help compensate for the possible deficiencies of the other.

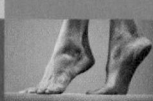

Given the obsession we have with slimness and the fact that millions of Americans and Canadians are overweight, it is no wonder that a multibillion-dollar weight-control industry has developed. Weight-loss centers and health and fitness spas cater to this obsession and promise us new bodies just in time for the swimsuit season. Pharmaceutical companies produce drugs, both prescription and over-the-counter types, to help us lose fat the easy way. Food manufacturers market convenient, low-Calorie, prepackaged—but expensive—meals. Exercise equipment manufacturers advertise devices that burn twice as many Calories as a treadmill. Newspaper and magazine advertisements claim you can "Lose weight while you sleep" or "Lose 30 pounds in just 30 days." Each year at least one diet book on the best-seller list is advertised as the last diet we will ever need.

A variety of techniques, some useful and some not, are used in attempts to stimulate weight loss. Dietary supplements are marketed to depress the appetite or increase metabolism. Creams are applied to specific body parts to shrink local fat deposits. Surgical techniques include intestinal bypasses, removal of or stapling part of the stomach, excision or suction removal of subcutaneous fat tissue, and wiring the jaw shut. Weight-loss diets involve almost every possible manipulation, including the high-fat diet, the high-protein diet, the chocolate diet, the grapefruit diet, the starvation diet, and even the "no diet" diet. Advertisements claim that specially designed clothing worn during exercise can help you lose inches of fat in hours. Psychological techniques such as hypnosis or behavior modification are designed to change your eating habits.

The Committee to Develop Criteria for Evaluating the Outcomes of Approaches to Prevent and Treat Obesity identified three types of programs and approaches to treat obesity or overweight: clinical programs, nonclinical programs, and do-it-yourself programs. No matter which program an individual selects to lose weight, the committee recommended consultation with one's primary health care provider before engaging in a weight-loss program.

In severe cases of clinical obesity, treatment usually is administered in a *clinical program* under medical supervision and may involve a combination of many techniques, including surgery, hormone therapy, drugs, and starvation-type diets. An individualized, medically supervised weight-control program is very important for the clinically obese because so many health risks are related to obesity. Surgery may be effective, and various techniques may be used, including gastric bypass surgery and insertion of a small, flexible gastric band around the top part of the stomach. Government regulations indicate that individuals who have a BMI greater than 40, or a lower BMI with a serious health condition, such as diabetes, may benefit from weight-loss surgery. In two studies, Adams and Sjöström reported that gastric bypass surgery in severely obese individuals decreased long-term mortality by 40 percent as compared with that in the control group, mainly attributed to lower death rates from coronary heart disease, diabetes, and cancer. Gastric band surgery in the morbidly obese has helped individuals lose 50 pounds or more. However, in a meta-analysis, Garb and others reported that gastric bypass surgery resulted in better weight-loss outcomes compared to gastric banding. Additionally, a stomach pacemaker, somewhat comparable to a cardiac pacemaker, was recently developed. The device consists of a sensor and a stimulator in the stomach that sends electrical impulses to the brain, helping to curb the appetite within a few minutes of commencing eating. Thus, total caloric intake at a meal is decreased. The device has been tested in Europe, is approved for use by the European Union, and the manufacturer hopes it will be available in the United States by 2014.

Unfortunately, however, clinical obesity is very resistant to other forms of treatment, particularly dieting: More than 95 percent of those individuals who lose weight regain it within 1–5 years, and they may do this repeatedly. As noted in chapter 10, these fluctuations in body weight, known as weight cycling, may not exert deleterious effects on metabolism and health and should not deter obese individuals from attempts to lose weight. The National Institute of Health notes that other groups may need medically supervised weight-loss programs, including children, pregnant women, persons over the age of 65, and individuals with medical conditions that could be exacerbated by weight loss.

Nonclinical programs for the treatment of obesity are primarily commercial franchises, using packaged materials provided by counselors who usually are not professional health care providers; an example is Weight Watchers.

Do-it-yourself programs include any effort by the individual to lose weight by himself or herself or through community-based and work-site programs. These treatment programs may be well suited for individuals who have accumulated excess body fat through environmental conditions, such as excessive eating and decreased physical activity. Such programs may be beneficial to the typical adult, for substantial amounts of body fat appear to accumulate between the ages of 25 and 35. The prevalence of overweight individuals, as measured by the Body Mass Index (BMI), in the United States has increased in the past quarter-century in both children and adults, and this weight gain has been associated with an increased incidence of health complications. However, Jones and others noted that weight losses as small as 5–10 percent of initial weight can improve health, such as reducing the risk of type 2 diabetes.

Because the majority of obese people who lose weight put it back on, most weight-control experts indicate that the focus should be on prevention and maintenance. Prevention of excess weight gain is more effective than treatment. Prevention should be a lifelong lifestyle, beginning in childhood and continuing through adulthood. Preventive techniques may be especially helpful during the first two years of college, when young females typically gain weight. As noted in a study of twins by Newman and others, prevention may also curtail the weight gain in those genetically predisposed. Many overweight individuals often note that the hard part is not losing weight, it's keeping it off, but that may not necessarily be so. Maintenance of a

healthy body weight is a simple form of prevention; preventing weight regain is comparable to preventing weight gain in the first place.

This chapter centers on some basic questions relative to the construction, implementation, and maintenance of a sound weight-control program using the *do-it-yourself* approach. The principles and suggestions advanced here apply to the overweight individual who wants to lose excess body fat, and also to the person with normal body weight who may want to maintain that weight level or even lose additional poundage in order to improve physical performance. Individuals who are already lean should consult with qualified health professionals before attempting to lose weight. As Fontana and Klein note, it is possible that even moderate caloric restriction may be harmful in some individuals, such as lean persons who have minimal amounts of body fat. One potential problem is the development of an eating disorder, as discussed in chapter 10. For individuals interested in participating in *nonclinical* or *clinical programs,* some guidelines are offered later in this chapter.

A comprehensive weight-control program involves three components: (1) a dietary regimen stressing balanced nutrition but with reduced caloric intake; (2) an aerobic and resistance exercise program to increase caloric expenditure and maintain lean body mass; and (3) a behavior modification program to facilitate the implementation of the first two components. These components are emphasized in this chapter.

Although proper dieting and exercise are the two keys to weight control, the

same diet and exercise plan may not be appropriate for all individuals. In a discussion of genotype-specific weight-loss treatment, Adamo and Tesson indicate that like obesity itself, weight loss is a complex phenomenon dependent on many environmental and genetic influences, and thus individual responses to weight-loss interventions are incredibly variable.

Weight loss is difficult, but it can be done. Haruki Murakami, in his book *What I Talk About When I Talk About Running,* cited a sign he saw in a Tokyo gym that read "Muscles are hard to get and easy to lose, fat is easy to get and hard to lose." There is a lot of truth in that statement, as many individuals find it very difficult to lose body fat and maintain that loss. For example, Nieman noted that only one in five overweight and obese individuals is able to lose 10 percent of body weight and keep it off for at least one year. However, some weight-loss strategies are effective. Nieman also notes that thousands of members of the National Weight Control Registry (NWCR) have lost more than 30 pounds and kept it off for more than a year. The diet and exercise strategies of the NWCR will be presented throughout this chapter.

However one does it, creating a negative energy balance in the body will lead to weight loss. As we shall see, a wide variety of diet and exercise programs may satisfy the criteria for a healthy weight-loss program and most individuals can find a program to meet their individual needs. The best diet and exercise strategy for weight loss is the one that works for you.

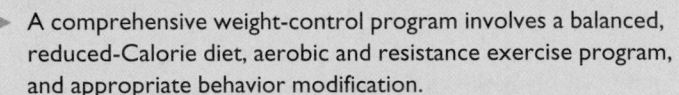

Key Concept

▶ A comprehensive weight-control program involves a balanced, reduced-Calorie diet, aerobic and resistance exercise program, and appropriate behavior modification.

Basics of Weight Control

How many Calories are in a pound of body fat?

One pound is equivalent to 454 grams. Because we know that 1 gram of fat is equal to 9 Calories, it would appear that a pound of body fat would equal about 4,086 Calories (9 × 454).

However, the fat stored in adipose tissue contains small amounts of protein, minerals, and water, which reduces the caloric content of 1 pound of body fat to approximately 3,500 Calories.

Is the caloric concept of weight control valid?

The caloric concept of weight control is relatively simple. As illustrated in figure 11.1, if you take in more Calories than you expend, you will gain weight, a positive energy balance. If you expend more than you take in, you lose weight, a negative energy balance. To maintain your body weight, caloric input and output must be equal. As far as we know, human energy systems are governed by the same laws of physics that rule all energy transformations. The First Law of Thermodynamics is as pertinent to us in the conservation and expenditure of our energy sources as it is to any other machine. Because a Calorie is a unit of energy, and because energy can neither be created nor destroyed, those Calories that we eat must either be expended in some way or conserved in the body. No substantial evidence is available to disprove the caloric theory. It is still the physical basis for body-weight control.

Keep in mind, however, that the total body weight is made up of different components, those notable in weight-control programs being body water, protein in the fat-free mass, small amounts of carbohydrate, and fat stores. Changes in these components may bring about daily body-weight fluctuations of 3–5 pounds that would appear to be contrary to the caloric concept because protein and carbohydrate contain only 4 Calories per gram and water contains no Calories. You may gain water weight by consuming a high-salt diet for a day, or by menstrual cycle changes. You may lose 5 pounds in an hour, but it will be mostly water weight lost through sweating. Starvation techniques may lead to rapid weight losses, but some of the weight loss will be in glycogen stores, body-protein stores such as muscle mass, and the water associated with glycogen and protein stores. In programs to lose body weight, we usually desire to lose excess body fat, and certain dietary and exercise techniques may help to maximize fat losses while minimizing protein losses.

The metabolism of human energy sources is complex, and although the caloric theory is valid relative to body-weight control, one must be aware that weight changes will not always be exactly in line with caloric input and output, and that weight losses may not be due to body fat loss alone. Also keep in mind one of the concepts advanced in the last chapter relative to individual variability in metabolic rates; two individuals with the same body weight may consume the same amount of Calories, yet one may gain while the other may maintain or even lose weight. Other than differences in metabolism, this possibility also may be related to the type of Calories in the diet; research has suggested that the body may store dietary fat Calories in the adipose tissue more efficiently than carbohydrate or protein Calories. In essence, compared to dietary fat, it may take more energy to convert dietary carbohydrate and protein into body fat. These concepts are explored further in this chapter.

How many Calories do I need per day to maintain my body weight?

This depends on a number of factors, notably age, body weight, gender, resting energy expenditure (REE), the thermic effect of feeding (TEF), and physical activity levels.

Age The caloric requirement per kilogram of body weight is very high during the early years of life when a child is developing and adding large amounts of body tissue. The Calorie/kilogram requirement decreases throughout the years from birth to old age, with exceptions during pregnancy and lactation.

Body Weight Body weight influences the total amount of daily Calories you need, but not the Calorie/kilogram level. The large individual simply needs more total Calories to maintain body weight. Body weight is the most significant factor determining daily caloric intake necessary to maintain weight, although body composition also may be important.

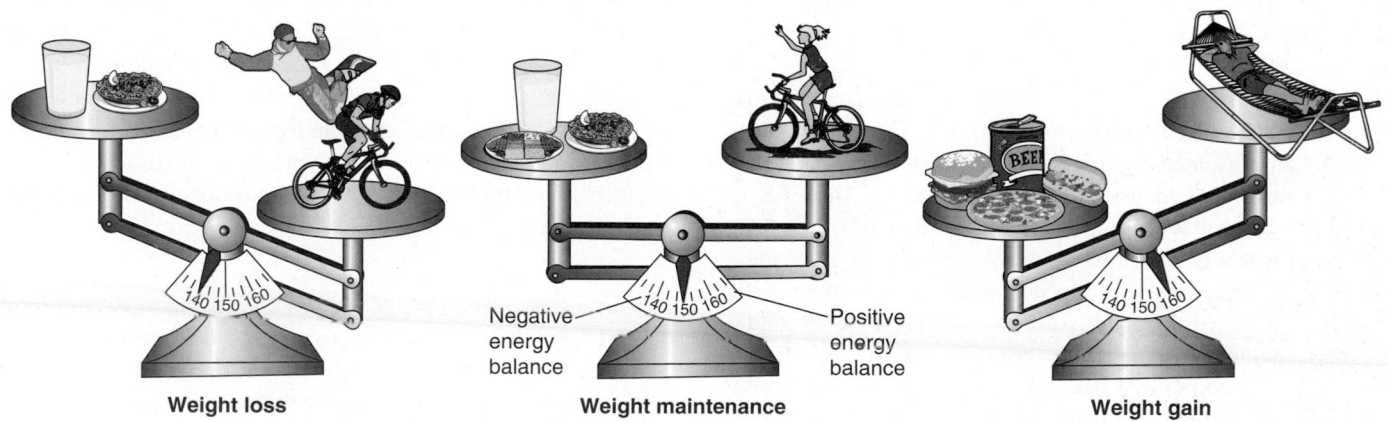

Weight loss   **Weight maintenance**   **Weight gain**

Negative energy balance   Positive energy balance

FIGURE 11.1 Weight control is based upon energy balance. Too much food input or too little exercise output can result in a positive energy balance or weight gain. Decreased food intake or increased physical activity can result in a negative caloric balance or weight loss.

Gender Up to the age of 11 or 12, the caloric needs of boys and girls are similar in terms of Calories/kilogram body weight. After puberty, however, males need slightly more Calories/kilogram, probably because of their greater percentage of muscle tissue in comparison to females.

REE Individual variations in REE may either increase or decrease daily caloric needs, depending on whether the REE is above or below normal. Individual variations may deviate 10–20 percent from normal. An extended discussion of the REE was presented in chapter 3.

TEF The TEF effect may also vary among individuals. The TEF is also covered in more detail in chapter 3.

Physical Activity Physical activity levels above resting may have a very significant impact on caloric needs. Some activities, like bowling, may increase energy needs only slightly, whereas others, such as running for an hour or more, may add 1,000–1,500 or more Calories to the daily energy requirement. You may wish to review chapter 3 regarding the caloric cost of exercise.

All of these factors make it difficult to make an exact recommendation relative to daily caloric needs. As noted in chapter 3, the doubly labeled water (DLW) technique may provide a fairly accurate measure of total daily energy expenditure (TDEE). However, it is rather expensive and not readily available to most individuals.

The following methods are available to help you determine the amount of Calories you need to consume daily to maintain a stable body weight. Some are more detailed than others. Calculating your daily energy needs by the Estimated Energy Requirement (EER) technique will provide you with an in-depth understanding of the role physical activity may play in daily caloric expenditure. It is a labor-intensive protocol, but provides you with more details about the physical activity quotient (PA) and the physical activity level (PAL) used in calculation of your daily energy needs. Using the following computer-based ChooseMyPlate method simplifies this process, and subsequent methods provide even more simplified approaches to estimating daily energy needs. However, keep in mind that all are estimates of daily energy needs and may contain some degree of error.

Estimated Energy Requirement (EER) Technique In chapter 3 we introduced the concept of Estimated Energy Requirement (EER) as presented by the National Academy of Sciences (NAS) in its document focusing on DRI for energy. The EER is defined as the dietary energy intake that is predicted to maintain energy balance in a healthy individual of a defined age, gender, weight, height, and level of physical activity consistent with good health. As you may recall, your total daily energy expenditure (TDEE) includes your resting energy expenditure (REE), the thermic effect of food (TEF), and the thermic effect of exercise (TEE). The EER formulae for gender and different age categories are presented in table 11.1. As noted, the formulae require age, height, weight, and physical activity quotient (PA). You can easily determine the first three criteria, which is all you need to obtain

---

TABLE 11.1 Estimated Energy Requirement (EER) formulae

Females age 19 and over:

EER = 354 − 6.91 × Age + [PA × (9.361 × Weight + 726 × Height)]

Males age 19 and over:

EER = 662 − 9.53 × Age + [PA × (15.91 × Weight + 539.6 × Height)]

Females age 9–18:

EER = 135.3 − 30.8 × Age + [PA × (10.0 × Weight + 934 × Height)] + 25 (Calories/day for energy deposition)

Males age 9–18:

EER = 88.5 − 61.9 × Age + [PA × (26.7 × Weight + 903 × Height)] + 25 (Calories/day for energy deposition)

Age: In years.
Weight: In kilograms (kg). To convert weight in pounds to kilograms, multiply by 0.454.
Height: In meters (m). To convert height in inches to meters, multiply by 0.0254.

Adapted from National Academy of Sciences. 2002. *Dietary Reference Intakes for Energy, Carbohydrates, Fiber, Fat, Protein and Amino Acids* (Macronutrients). Washington, DC. National Academy Press.

---

an estimate of your energy requirements if you are sedentary, but determination of your PA requires some effort.

To calculate your EER, you should first determine your energy needs for a sedentary lifestyle. Select the appropriate formula for your gender and age category from table 11.1 and use the value of 1.0 as the PA. For example, a 20-year-old sedentary male weighing 175 pounds (80 kilograms) who is 71 inches (1.8 meters) tall would have a daily EER of 2,715 Calories.

$$EER = 662 − 9.53 × 20 + [1.0 × (15.91 × 80 + 539.6 × 1.8)]$$
$$= 2,715$$

As you may recall from chapter 3, the PA is based on your physical activity level (PAL), which is the ratio of your TDEE to your BEE, or TDEE:BEE, over a 24-hour period. The NAS indicates that physical activity is the most variable component of TDEE, and also notes that the assessment of physical activity-induced increments in TDEE is fraught with considerable uncertainties. Nevertheless, the NAS has developed four categories of PAL: Sedentary, Low Active, Active, and Very Active.

> *www.nap.edu* If you would like to calculate your PAL and resultant PA based on the NAS protocol, type in Dietary Reference Intakes for Energy in the Search box, click on the book title, and then peruse chapters 5 and 12 for details of the procedure.

However, we will use a modified approach to estimate your EER based on your daily record of physical activities and associated caloric expenditure as calculated from appendix B. The correlation between the NAS procedure and our estimates of exercise caloric expenditure are not exact because different calculations are used. However, both provide reasonable values for the energy cost of daily physical activity.

The NAS bases the PAL on the amount of daily physical activity that is the equivalent of walking at a rate of 3–4 miles per hour. To reach a specific PAL category, you are required to expend the energy equivalent of walking a set number of miles. Although the NAS bases the PAL on an energy equivalent of walking, keep in mind that you do not need to walk the required miles to attain a specific PAL category. You may do a multitude of physical activities, such as golfing, swimming, and jogging, that add up to this energy equivalent. For your body weight, use appendix B to find the Calories you expend each minute for walking at a given pace, such as 3 to 4 miles per hour. Then locate other activities that expend similar amounts of Calories per minute. Engaging in such activities for 15–20 minutes is the equivalent of walking a mile.

Here is a brief summary of the amount of physical activity needed for each PAL category. Table 11.2 complements this discussion. Some guidelines based on the energy expenditure equivalents of walking (3–4 mph) or jogging are presented.

Sedentary category The energy expenditure of individuals in the Sedentary category represents their REE, including the TEF, plus various physical activities associated with independent living, such as walking from the house or work to the car, walking your dog, typing, daily household tasks, and other forms of very light activity. If you engage in no daily physical activity, your PAL will range from 1.00–1.39, but your PA for the formula is set at a baseline of 1.0. Individuals who walk less than 30 minutes daily generally fall in this category.

Low Active category In addition to the normal daily activities of independent living, you need to expend the physical activity equivalent of walking about 2.2 miles per day to be in the Low Active category. Your PAL for the Low Active category will range from 1.40–1.59, but the PA for the formula is set at 1.11–1.16 depending on gender and stage of life. Individuals who walk 30–40 minutes, or jog 10–15 minutes, daily generally fit this category.

Active category In addition to the normal daily activities of independent living, you need to expend the physical activity equivalent of walking about 7 miles per day to be in the Active category. Your PAL for the Active category will range from 1.60–1.89, but the PA for the formula is set at 1.25–1.31 depending on gender and stage of life. Individuals who walk 1.75 hours, or jog 40–45 minutes, daily generally fall in this category.

Very Active category In addition to the normal daily activities of independent living, you need to expend the physical activity equivalent of walking about 17 miles per day to be in the Very Active category. Your PAL for the Very Active category will range from 1.90–2.50, but the PA for the formula is set at

1.42–1.56 depending on gender and stage of life. Individuals who walk 4.25 hours, or jog 1.5 hours, daily generally fit this category.

Let us continue with the example of our 20-year-old male and determine the number of Calories he would need to expend to move from the Sedentary category (2,715 Calories) into each of the active categories. If we consult table 11.2, we see that the PAs for the Low Active, Active, and Very Active categories are, respectively, 1.11, 1.25, and 1.48.

Low Active:
$$EER = 662 - 9.53 \times 20 + [1.11 \times (15.91 \times 80 + 539.6 \times 1.8)]$$
$$= 2,962 \text{ Calories}$$

Active:
$$EER = 662 - 9.53 \times 20 + [1.25 \times (15.91 \times 80 + 539.6 \times 1.8)]$$
$$= 3,276 \text{ Calories}$$

Very Active:
$$EER = 662 - 9.53 \times 20 + [1.48 \times (15.91 \times 80 + 539.6 \times 1.8)]$$
$$= 3,793 \text{ Calories}$$

As his EER for the Sedentary category is 2,715 Calories, he would need to expend about 247, 561, or 1,078 Calories through physical activity to attain, respectively, the Low Active, Active, and Very Active PAL categories.

TABLE 11.2 The physical activity level categories

PAL category	Physical activity level (PAL)	Physical activity coefficient (PA)			
		Males	Females	Boys	Girls
Sedentary	≥1.0–<1.4	1.00	1.00	1.00	1.00
Low Active	≥1.4–<1.6	1.11	1.12	1.13	1.16
Active	≥1.6–<1.9	1.25	1.27	1.26	1.31
Very Active	≥1.9–<2.5	1.48	1.45	1.42	1.56

Adapted from National Academy of Sciences. 2002. *Dietary Reference Intakes for Energy, Carbohydrates, Fiber, Fat, Protein and Amino Acids (Macronutrients)*. Washington, DC. National Academy Press.

We will talk more about exercise later in this chapter. In chapter 3 we introduced you to appendix B and explained how you might calculate your daily energy expenditure through physical activity. You may wish to review that discussion on page 103. In brief, record the number of minutes of each type of physical activity you do daily. Then, consult appendix B, find your body weight in the top margin, and determine how many Calories you expend per minute doing each activity.

Let's apply this procedure and complete the example of our 20-year-old male. Let us assume that he has engaged in the following physical activities over the course of a week, has calculated his energy expenditure from appendix B, totaled his weekly energy expenditure, and then figured his daily average caloric expenditure.

Day	Physical activity	Duration	Calories/ min	Total calories
Monday	Tennis, singles	40 min	8.8	352
	Walking, 3 mph	20 min	4.8	96
Tuesday	Running, 7 mph	40 min	14.9	596
Wednesday	Tennis, singles	40 min	8.8	352
	Walking, 3 mph	20 min	4.8	96
Thursday	Running, 8 mph	30 min	17.1	513
Friday	Tennis, singles	40 min	8.8	352
	Bowling	30 min	4.9	147
Saturday	Golf, carry clubs	180 min	4.8	864
Sunday	Running, 7 mph	40 min	14.9	596
Total weekly Calories				3,964
Daily average caloric expenditure (3,700 Calories 7 days)				566

Thus, with an average daily energy expenditure through physical activity totaling 566 Calories, he is in the Active PAL category and can use that formula to calculate his EER. Alternatively, he may simply add the 566 Calories to his Sedentary EER to determine the number of Calories needed to maintain his body weight if it has been stable. Using the formula for the Active category, his EER as noted would total 3,276 Calories. Adding the 566 Calories to his Sedentary category EER of 2,715 would total 3,281 Calories. The difference between the two estimates is negligible in this case, but may vary some in other cases.

Using this same procedure, you may calculate your EER to maintain your normal body weight. Use the formula in table 11.1 that is appropriate for your gender and age and, using the appropriate PA values from table 11.2, calculate your EER for each of the four PAL categories. Next, as per the previous example, record the type and amount of time devoted to various physical activities over the course of a week and calculate your average daily physical activity energy expenditure; you may then either add this amount to your Sedentary EER or use the appropriate formula to estimate your total daily EER.

Estimated Energy Requirement (EER) ChooseMyPlate Technique You may more easily calculate your EER by using the program available in the *ChooseMyPlate* Website. When you join, you enter your age, height, and weight, which are used as part of the basis to calculate your EER and can be updated as needed. There are two options available. In brief, the *condensed option* is recommended for people with few leisure-time activities or for people who are not regularly physically active. Based on the age, gender, weight, and height information in your personal profile, an estimated Basal Energy Expenditure (BEE) is calculated and adjusted to include routine activities (i.e., personal hygiene, housework, light yard work, computer use, and driving a car) of estimated duration. You may also enter in some leisure-time activities. However, the Website notes that with or without additional leisure-time physical activity, the assessment of EER

using the condensed physical activity entry option may not be accurate. The *standard option* provides the most accurate assessment of your EER. You must enter all activities you performed in the past 24 hours, including sleeping, eating, sitting while reading or watching television, personal hygiene, housework, transportation, employment, leisure, and exercise. The total duration of these activities should add up to 1,440 minutes (24 hours).

www.ChooseMyPlate.gov The ChooseMyPlate program provides a means to calculate your Estimated Energy Requirement (EER). Click on Interactive Tools, then Food Tracker and Assess Your Physical Activity. The *standard option* is the most accurate. Helpful hints are presented in the text.

With the standard option, your level of physical activities over the course of a typical week will provide a good estimate of your EER. You can enter each day of the week separately. If you do, you may save your "Frequently Performed Activities" to ease data entry. You may also enter the data once, calculating an average amount of time for each activity beforehand. For example, if you jog 45 minutes four days per week, this totals 180 minutes per week, or an average 26 minutes daily. Calculate a daily average for other activities as well. Once you input the data, click on *Energy Balance*. Disregard the food input message, and you will be provided with your EER.

Mayo Clinic Calorie Calculator The prestigious Mayo Clinic provides a computerized estimate of daily energy needs based on age, gender, height, weight, and level of physical activity ranging from sedentary to very active. The estimated daily energy needs may be found at the Mayo Clinic Website, http://www .mayoclinic.com/health/calorie-calculator/NU00598.

Calorie Counting Technique If your body weight has been stable, keeping track of the Calories you eat for 3–7 days may provide you with a good estimate of your daily energy requirement. Eat your normal diet, but record everything you consume. Some guidelines for measuring, recording, and calculating your daily caloric intake are presented on pages 476–478. Computerized dietary analysis programs are available to facilitate this task. For example, the MyTracker program also has a dietary analysis program to assess your daily caloric intake.

Simplified Technique The National Institutes of Health, in its MedlinePlus Website, has provided some guidelines for the approximate daily caloric intake needed to maintain current body weight. The guidelines are presented in table 11.3. For example, if you are moderately active and weigh 170 pounds, you will need about 2,550 Calories (170 × 15) to maintain a desirable body weight.

Keep in mind that no matter which procedure you follow, your actual daily caloric needs may vary somewhat from the estimate obtained. In the section of this chapter on dietary modifications, we will discuss how many Calories you may need in your diet if you desire to lose weight. If that is the case, you may wish to estimate your daily energy needs by several techniques and use the lowest value obtained to optimize the caloric deficit needed for

TABLE 11.3	Approximate daily caloric intake needed to maintain desirable body weight	
Activity level	Calories per pound	Calories per kilogram
1. Sedentary or very obese	10	22
2. Low activity level, or over age 55	13	28.5
3. Regular moderate activity	15	33
4. Regular strenuous activity	18	39.5

- Low activity: No planned, regular physical activity; occasional weekend or weekly activity (such as golf or recreational tennis) is the only type of physical activity
- Moderate activity: Participating in physical activities such as swimming, jogging, or fast walking for 30–60 minutes at a time
- Strenuous activity: Participating in vigorous physical activity for 60 minutes or more at least 4–5 days per week

Source: http://www.nlm.nih.gov/medlineplus/ency/article/001943.htm

weight loss, as long as it meets the recommendations presented for safe weight loss.

How much weight can I lose safely per week?

If you decide to lose weight without medical supervision, keep in mind that the recommended maximal weight loss is 2 pounds per week. Because there are 3,500 Calories in a pound of body fat, this would necessitate a deficit of 7,000 Calories for the week, or 1,000 Calories per day. For growing children who carry excess fat, the general recommendation is about 1 pound per week, or a daily 500-Calorie deficit. Keep in mind that these are *maximal* recommended weight-loss values for medically unsupervised programs. Lower weight-loss goals, such as 1 pound per week for adults and one-half pound per week for children and adolescents, may be more appropriate, realizable goals. These recommendations are in line with guidelines presented by health professionals, such as the American College of Sports Medicine.

As we shall see later in this chapter, weight losses may not parallel the caloric deficit we incur during early stages of a weight-reduction program, and the 2-pound limit may be adjusted during this time period. In addition, as mentioned previously, we want our weight loss to be body-fat tissue, not lean body mass. A loss of 10 pounds of body weight may help improve physical performance, but if 5 pounds is muscle tissue, then performance could possibly deteriorate. Thus, you should monitor your weight loss not only with a scale but also with skinfolds and girth measures, or other body-composition procedures, to help ensure that you are losing body fat, and in the right places.

How can I determine the amount of body weight I need to lose?

As noted chapter 10, individuals desire to lose weight for one of three reasons—to improve appearance, health, or physical performance. As for your appearance, you are the judge, but consult with your physician or other health professional. You do not want your weight-loss program to induce an eating disorder. Losing excess body fat for health is a good reason. Check with your physician, who can also monitor health risks, such as blood pressure, serum lipids, blood glucose, and regional adiposity, associated with excess body weight. A loss of 5–10 percent body weight or 2–4 inches off the waist, easily achieved in 3–4 months, may help reduce several health risk factors. Losing weight in attempts to enhance physical performance should involve interactions between the athlete, coach, and team physician; in the case of young athletes, parents should also be involved. Janet Walberg-Rankin noted that body-weight goals for athletes should be based on current body composition, time remaining until the competitive season, body-weight history, and sport-specific rules.

In their review, Brownell and Rodin indicated that weight-loss goals should account for how much weight an individual can reasonably lose and should not be determined solely by health standards. The same reasoning applies for appearance and physical performance standards. They note that pursuit of an unrealistic ideal may lead to various health problems.

Several procedures may be used to estimate desired weight loss. Using the Body Mass Index (BMI) as a guide, you will need to calculate your current BMI and determine your target BMI. Calculation of the BMI was presented on page 404 and a healthy BMI range is approximately 18.5–25. The formula to calculate your desired body weight in kilograms is

Target body weight (kg) = Target BMI × height in meters^2

As an example, if you are 5'7" (1.70 meters) tall and weigh 170 pounds (77.2 kilograms), then you have a BMI of 26.7 (77.2/1.70^2). If you want to achieve a healthier BMI of 24, simply multiply 24 by 1.70^2 to determine your body-weight goal; 24 by 2.89 equals 69.4 kilograms, or 153 pounds. The desired weight loss would be 17 pounds (170 − 153), which represents a 10 percent reduction in total body weight (17/170 = 0.10; 0.10 × 100% = 10%).

If you want to use body-fat percentage as the guide to weight loss, you will need to measure your current body-fat percentage and determine your target goal. Methods of determining body-fat percentage are presented in appendix D. If you are an athlete with 20 percent body fat who desires to get down to 15 percent, you may use the following formula:

$$\text{Target body weight} = \frac{\text{Lean body mass in pounds}}{1.00 - \text{desired body-fat percentage}}$$

As an example, an athlete who weighs 150 pounds and is 20 percent body fat has 30 pounds of body fat, and the remaining 120 pounds (150 − 30) is lean body mass. Substituting in the formula provides the following data:

$$\frac{120}{1.00 - 0.15} = \frac{120}{0.85} = 141 \text{pounds}$$

Thus, this athlete would need to lose 9 pounds of body fat (150 − 141) to achieve a 15 percent body-fat percentage. If proper methods of weight loss are used as discussed later in this chapter, the losses will be in body fat, not lean body mass.

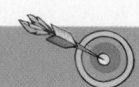
Behavior Modification

What is behavior modification?

In his excellent book, *Mindless Eating: Why We Eat More Than We Think,* Brian Wansink, a food psychologist at Cornell University, indicates that we make numerous food-related decisions every day. Most of these decisions are made at the subconscious level, many triggered by cues in the food environment that modify our behavior and encourage us to eat more.

One of the key components of a successful weight-control program is the need to identify and modify those behaviors that contribute to the weight problem. The subject of human behavior development and change is very complex, but psychologists note that three factors are generally involved: the physical environment, the social environment, and the personal environment. For the person with a weight problem, a refrigerator brimming with food (physical environment), a family that consumes high-Calorie snack foods around the house (social environment), and an acquired taste for high-fat or sweet foods (personal environment) may trigger behaviors that make it very difficult to maintain a proper body weight.

A model often used to explain the development or modification of health behaviors, such as a proper diet and exercise program for weight control, involves three steps: knowledge, values, and behavior. First, proper knowledge is essential. A considerable amount of misinformation relative to the roles of nutrition and exercise in weight control exists, so you need to possess accurate information. Second, the health implications of this knowledge may help you develop a set of personal values, or attitudes, toward a specific health behavior. If you perceive excess body fat as a threat to your personal physical or psychological health, you are more likely to initiate behavioral changes. Third, your health behavior should then reflect the knowledge you acquired and the values you developed.

Behavior modification is a technique often used in psychological therapy to elicit desirable behavioral changes. The rationale underlying behavior modification is that many behavioral patterns are learned via stimulus-response conditioning; for example, a stimulus in your environment such as a commercial break in a television program elicits a response of a mad dash to the refrigerator. Because such responses are learned, they also may be unlearned. For a discussion of a comprehensive program conducted by a behavioral psychologist, the reader is referred to the review by Brownell and Kramer.

Relative to a self-designed program of weight control, behavior modification is used primarily to reduce or eliminate physical or social stimuli that may lead to excessive caloric intake or decreased physical activity. George Bray, an international authority on obesity treatment, noted that the most important component of any weight-control program is the associated behavior modification through which the individual learns new ways to deal with old problems. In a study stressing the importance of behavior modification, Haus and others recommended that potential weight-program participants learn and practice the weight-maintenance behavior of reduced dietary fat and regular exercise, independent of and before any weight-reduction attempts. The Consumers Union notes that exercising more and switching to a leaner, healthier diet will yield innumerable health benefits even if you don't lose a single pound.

How do I apply behavior-modification techniques in my weight-control program?

When breaking any well-established habit, self-discipline, or will power, is the key. The most important component of a weight-control program is you. You must want to lose weight, and you must take the major responsibility for achieving your goals. You need to face the fact that being overweight and sedentary is dangerous to your health. You must be convinced that reduced body weight will enhance your life, and you must establish this goal as a high priority. You must be able to tolerate some discomfort as you make lifestyle changes. Data from the National Weight Control Registry, which consists of people who have lost at least 30 pounds and kept it off, indicate that the key factor is to do it for yourself. Your desire to lose weight must become more important than the desire to overeat or to not exercise. Your cerebrum, the higher cognitive control center of the brain, must learn to control the hypothalamus, the subconscious appetite center.

Both long-range and short-range realistic goals should be established. Several experts in weight control, such as Tremblay and Wadden, indicated that for overweight individuals, a 10–15 percent weight loss is a reasonable goal over 4–6 months. Thus, a long-range goal may be to lose 30 pounds over 6 months, whereas a short-range goal would be to lose about 1–2 pounds per week. Losing 30 pounds may seem like a daunting task, but setting small goals, a few pounds at a time, is one of the keys to success indicated by the National Weight Control Registry. A long-range goal may also include a large number of behavioral changes to achieve the 30-pound weight loss, but the number of changes would be phased in gradually on a short-term basis. Do not expect to make all recommended behavioral changes overnight. (See figure 11.2.)

As the saying goes, nothing breeds success like success, so it is extremely important to set short-term goals that may be attainable in a reasonable length of time so that you may experience multiple successes in pursuit of your long-term goal. When you achieve your first short-term goal, a new short-term goal should be established as you progress toward your long-term goal. It is also important to remember that no initial short-term goal is too small, nor is any new short-term goal too small in the progress toward your long-term goal. The U.S. Department of Health and Human Services has developed a Website focusing on many small steps that may help individuals achieve diet and exercise goals in a weight-loss program. Appendix H lists 120 small steps to a healthier diet and increased physical activity. As you achieve each short-term goal, you should reward yourself with something appropriate to the occasion; a reward will provide you with positive feedback to your commitment to your weight-loss program. One example might be to purchase a new pair of designer jeans with your lower waist measurement to encourage you to continue with your program.

www.smallstep.gov This Website provides numerous small steps relative to diet, cooking, drinking, and exercise that help promote weight loss. One set of small steps is for children and another for teens and adults.

One of the first steps in a behavior modification program is to identify those physical and social environmental factors that may lead to problem behaviors. Keeping a diary of your daily activities in your daily planner for a week or two may help you identify some behavioral patterns that may contribute to overeating

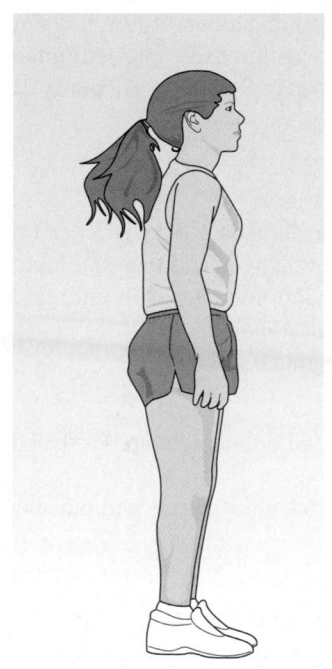
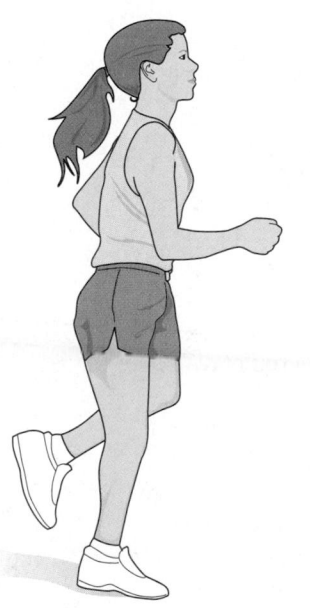
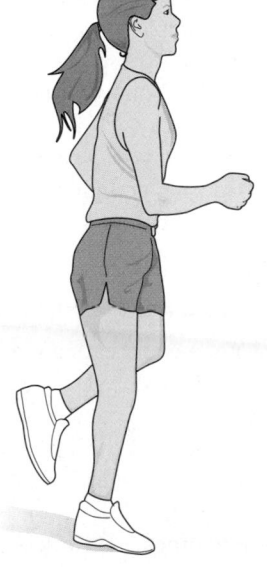

	Short-term goals	Long-term goals
Time	1 month	6 months
Running	1 mile nonstop	5 miles nonstop
Weight	Lose 6 pounds	Lose 30 pounds

FIGURE 11.2 Goal setting is an important factor in an exercise program.

Record of 24-hour diet and physical activity

Time of day	Activity	Total minutes	Meal or snack	Degree of hunger*	Activity while eating	Place of eating	Food and quantity	Others present	Reason for choice

Note: Record time, activity such as sleeping, sitting, watching TV, and exercise, and minutes of activity. For meals, fill in the other columns. You may also use these columns for comments regarding activities other than eating. You can expand this table to incorporate a 24-hour period of time. Entering the data into a computer, such as in a Microsoft Excel format, may be helpful.
*Degree of Hunger: 0 = none; 1 = little; 2 = moderate; 3 = high

and extra body weight. The following are some of the factors that might be recorded each time you eat, along with a brief explanation of their possible importance. You should also record your daily physical activity. You may use the record of 24-hour activity form as a guide, which also may help in the calculation of your EER in the MyTracker program.

Type of food and amount   This may be related to the other factors. For example, do you eat a high-Calorie food during your snacks?

Meal or snack   You may find yourself snacking four or five times a day.

Time of day   Do you eat at regular hours or have a full meal just before retiring at night?

Degree of hunger   How hungry were you when you ate—very hungry or not hungry at all? You may be snacking when not hungry.

Activity   What were you doing while eating? You may find that TV watching and eating snack foods are related.

Location   Where do you eat? The office or school cafeteria may be the place you eat a high-Calorie meal.

Persons involved   With whom do you eat? Do you eat more when alone or with others? Being with certain people may trigger overeating.

Emotional feelings   How do you feel when eating? You might eat more when depressed than when happy, or vice versa.

Exercise   How much walking, stair climbing, or regular aerobic exercise do you get? Do you ride when you could possibly walk? How much time do you just sit?

Recording this information may make you more aware of the physical and social circumstances under which you tend to overeat or be physically inactive. This awareness may be useful to help implement behavioral changes that may make weight control easier. The following suggestions are often helpful:

Self-discipline and self-control, and advanced planning:

1. Establish realistic weight-loss goals. A loss of 10 percent can produce significant health benefits.
2. Establish weight loss as a high priority; commit to permanent lifestyle changes.
3. Think about this priority before eating.
4. Take small helpings deliberately as a means to control your weight.
5. Plan for a modest daily energy deficit, about 300–500 Calories, which will result in a gradual weight loss.
6. Check your body weight and shape on a regular basis, either daily or 2 to 3 times a week. Use this as a motivational tool.

Foods to eat:
1. Use low-Calorie healthful foods for snacks.
2. Plan low-Calorie, high-nutrient meals.
3. Plan your food intake for the entire day.
4. Eat only foods that have had minimal or no processing.
5. Allow yourself very small amounts of high-Calorie foods that you like, but stay within daily caloric limitations.
6. Know the Food Exchange System, particularly serving size and high-fat foods.

Food purchasing:
1. Do not shop when hungry.
2. Prepare a shopping list and do not deviate from it.
3. Buy only foods that are low in Calories and high in nutrient value. Read and compare food labels to limit fat and sugar content.
4. Buy natural foods as much as possible.

Food storage:
1. Keep high-Calorie food out of sight and in sealed containers or cupboards.
2. Have low-Calorie snacks like carrots and radishes readily available.

Food preparation and serving:
1. Buy only foods that need preparation of some type.
2. Do not add fats or sugar in preparation, if possible.
3. Prepare only small amounts. Be able to visualize one serving size for any given food.
4. Do not use serving bowls on the table.
5. Put the food on the plate, preferably a small one.

Location:
1. Eat in only one place, such as the kitchen or dining area.
2. Avoid food areas such as the kitchen or snack table at a party.
3. Avoid restaurants where you are most likely to buy high-Calorie items.

Restaurant eating:
1. When eating out, select the low-Calorie items.
2. Request that your meals be prepared without fat.
3. Have condiments like butter, mayonnaise, and salad dressing served on the side; use sparingly.
4. Order water, not a high-Calorie beverage.
5. Be wary of portion sizes, as most restaurant servings contain 2–3 normal servings. Ask for a take-home box before you eat and put half of your meal in the box.

Methods of eating:
1. Eat slowly; chew food thoroughly or drink water between bites.
2. Eat with someone, for conversation can slow down the eating process.
3. Cut food into small pieces.
4. Do not do anything else while eating, such as watching TV.
5. Relax and enjoy the meal.
6. Eat only at specified times.
7. Eat only until pleasantly satisfied, not stuffed.
8. Spread your Calories over the day, eating small amounts more often.

Activity:
1. Decrease the amount of time spent in sedentary activities. Increase the amount of nonexercise activity thermogenesis (NEAT) by moving more and sitting less.
2. Walk more. Park the car or get off the bus some distance from work. Briskly walk the dog.
3. Use the stairs instead of the elevator when possible.
4. Do *exercise snacks*. Take a brisk 10-minute walk instead of a coffee-donut break. Do this several times a day.
5. Get involved in activities with other people, preferably physical activities that will burn Calories.
6. Avoid sedentary night routines.
7. Start a regular exercise program, including both aerobic and resistance exercises.
8. Schedule exercise as an appointment in your daily planner.

Sleep and stress reduction:
1. Try to get 7 to 8 hours of sleep each night.
2. Reduce emotional stress; try yoga or other stress-reduction techniques.

Mental attitude:
1. Recognize that you are not perfect and lapses may occur.
2. Deal positively with your lapse; put it behind you and get back on your program.
3. Put reminders on the refrigerator door at home or on your telephone at work.
4. Reward yourself for sticking to your plans.

For the interested reader, the books by Dusek and Miller provide an in-depth coverage of behavior modification for weight-control purposes. Many of the commercial, medically oriented weight-loss centers, as well as organizations such as Weight Watchers International also may be sources of information.

Self-taught, self-administered weight-loss programs may also be very effective, as indicated in the study by Wayne Miller and his associates.

Stress-reduction techniques may also be important in a weight-control program. Dallman indicates that emotional stress can hinder weight control by triggering the release of cortisol into the blood, which conserves fat and increases hunger. Dallman also notes that emotional stressors may degrade executive function, replacing thoughtful responses with formed habits, such as overeating. Exercise in itself may help reduce emotional stress, as may various relaxation techniques such as meditation and yoga.

Lack of adequate sleep may contribute to weight gain. In a study with more than a thousand subjects, Taheri and others concluded that getting less than 7 to 8 hours of sleep per night, such as only 4 to 5 hours, may decrease serum leptin and increase serum ghrelin levels, leading to an increased appetite and possible weight gain.

Individuals with clinical obesity may need professional assistance from health counselors to implement a behavior modification program for weight control. However, others with less severe weight problems may be able to initiate their own program if they have adequate accurate information.

Research has shown that most individuals initiating a weight-loss program do use acceptable strategies, such as exercising and eating a low-fat, low-Calorie diet, but use of these strategies becomes inconsistent in subsequent years, resulting in weight regain.

In a position statement, the American Dietetic Association resolved that successful weight management requires a lifelong commitment to healthful lifestyle behaviors, emphasizing eating practices and daily physical activities that are attainable and enjoyable. The remainder of this chapter focuses on the development of a proper lifelong diet and exercise program for losing weight safely and keeping it off. What usually happens is that individuals suffer a lapse in the weight-loss program, such as an injury that prevents participation in their normal exercise program. If they do not have an alternative exercise program, some weight gain may occur until they can resume exercising. Kelly Brownell, in the LEARN (Lifestyle, Exercise, Attitudes, Relationships, Nutrition) program for weight control, indicates that one of the keys in weight control is to prevent a lapse from becoming a relapse, or a resumption of old behaviors and total weight regain. When a lapse occurs, Brownell recommends that you stay calm, analyze the lapse, and renew your diet and exercise commitment. By analyzing your lapse, you should be able to find a solution to help you get back on track. If unable to do so, seek some assistance from a qualified health professional.

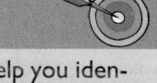

Key Concepts

▶ Keeping a record of your daily eating habits will help you identify behavioral patterns relative to overeating and may be used as a basis for the elimination of cues that trigger eating.

▶ Behavior modification is a very important part of a weight-control program. For weight control to be effective over a lifetime, you may need to adjust dietary and exercise behaviors to curtail caloric intake and increase energy expenditure.

Dietary Modifications

Numerous weight-loss dietary plans are available and each is based on some combination of macronutrient—carbohydrate, fat, protein—content. To achieve weight loss, the key to each diet plan is to consume fewer Calories than expended. Most diet plans do so. For example, the Consumers Union rated 15 different diet books and plans varying in macronutrient content; the daily range was 1,340 to 1,910 Calories and most averaged about 1,500 Calories, an energy intake that would lead to weight loss in most individuals.

As we shall see, there are high-carbohydrate, high-fat, and high-protein diets, and supporters for each. For example, in a recent interview, Taubes, author of *Good Calories, Bad Calories,* indicates that the key to weight loss is to eat fewer carbohydrates. He recommends the original Atkins diet, which is basically a high-fat diet. In contrast, Dean Ornish, in his book *Eat More, Weigh Less,* recommends a diet containing 70 percent or more carbohydrate with no more than 10 percent fat. Barry Sears, who developed *The Zone* diet, stresses the importance of a high-protein diet.

As noted earlier, and as supported by numerous studies, a key concept of weight-loss diets is to consume fewer Calories than are expended. Moreover, as far as Calories are concerned, the macronutrient content of the diet is irrelevant. For example, in one study, Sacks and others assigned more than 800 subjects to one of four diets with an equal amount of Calories but varying percentages derived from carbohydrate (35 to 65 percent), fat (20 to 40 percent), and protein (15 to 25 percent). They reported that all diets resulted in meaningful weight loss, with no differences among them. To stress this point, Albers cites a case study of a professor of human nutrition who ate what was referred to as the *Twinkie Diet.* Sixty percent of his caloric intake consisted of such items as cookies, chips, sugar cereal, snack cakes, and other sugary, processed foods, while the remaining 40 percent was healthier, such as vegetable snacks. However, total daily intake was limited to 1,600 Calories, much less than his total daily energy expenditure, and he lost 27 pounds in 10 weeks. Although not a recommended healthy diet for weight loss, it does support the point was trying to make: It does not matter what you eat as long as your caloric intake is less than your daily caloric expenditure.

However, Foreyt and others note that although this *A Calorie is a Calorie* concept of weight control is valid as a metabolic unit, its interpretation may be much more complex in the free-living situation. They note that the different diet-related factors that condition energy balance, including total energy intake, satiety and hunger sensory triggers, and palatability, must be considered when assessing the efficacy of weight-reducing diets of different macronutrient composition. These points are discussed later.

Sufficient evidence is available to provide prudent dietary guidelines for not only weight loss and maintenance, but also to promote health. For example, Ma and others compared the dietary quality of popular weight-loss plans for their capacity to prevent cardiovascular disease, and we discussed the concepts of healthful sources of carbohydrate, fat, and protein in the DASH and Omni-Heart diets in chapter 9. In general, healthful weight-control diets are based on selecting *good* carbohydrates, *good* fats, and *good* proteins. You can use the *ChooseMyPlate* food guide as a means to plan a healthful diet to achieve your desired body weight goal. In addition, the American Dietetic Association Website provides sound advice on a number of weight-control topics.

> *www.ChooseMyPlate.gov* Look under the column entitled *I want to* and click on an item of interest, such as Get a Personalized Plan, Get Weight Loss Information, Plan a Healthy Menu, or Analyze My Diet.
>
> *www.eatright.org* For weight control, click on *For the Public* and then *Healthy Weight Loss.*

How can I determine the number of Calories needed in a diet to lose weight?

To answer this question you need to provide two figures. First, you need to provide an estimate of how many Calories you need to consume daily to maintain your current body weight. As noted previously on pages 461–465, several techniques are available, so you should select one to provide an estimate of the number of Calories you may need to consume daily to maintain your current body weight. Second, you need to provide an estimate of the amount of weight that you want to lose, as discussed on page 465, and then determine how much you want to lose per week. One pound is the preferable goal, but you may lose up to 2 pounds safely. Some computerized dietary analysis programs will calculate your estimated energy intake needed to lose about 1–2 pounds per week.

> *http://caloriecount.about.com/cc/calories-goal.php* Consult this Website to provide a calculation of your daily caloric intake needed to achieve a given weight loss over a specified amount of time.

For our purposes, we will use the value of 3,500 Calories to represent 1 pound of body-fat, or body-weight, loss. To lose 1 pound of body fat, you must create a 3,500-Calorie deficit. To lose 1 pound per week, your daily caloric deficit should be 500 (3,500/7). To lose 2 pounds per week, the recommended maximum unless under medical supervision, the daily caloric deficit should be 1,000 (7,000/7).

Once you calculate your daily energy needs to maintain your current body weight, simply subtract your daily caloric deficit from it; the result will be your recommended daily caloric intake. An example is presented below:

Example: 35-year-old woman with low physical activity levels who weighs 140 pounds desires to lose 1 pound per week.

1. From table 11.3, Calories/lb needed to maintain body weight: 13
2. Predicted total number of Calories to maintain body weight:

$$13 \times 140 = 1,820 \text{ Calories/day}$$

3. Recommended daily caloric deficit = 500 Calories/day
4. Recommended daily caloric intake = 1,320 Calories

$$(1,820 - 500 = 1,320 \text{ Calories/day})$$

However, it is important to note that most health professionals do not recommend weight-loss diets lower than 1,000 Calories unless medically supervised.

How can I predict my body-weight loss through dieting alone?

As mentioned in chapter 10, the human body is composed of different components, most commonly compartmentalized into body fat and lean body mass; lean body mass is about 70 percent water. On a dietary program, weight loss may reflect decreases in body fat, body water, or muscle mass, all of which present different caloric values. For example, 1 pound of body fat equals about 3,500 Calories, whereas an equivalent weight of water contains no Calories. Because of this fact, it is difficult to predict exactly how much body weight one will lose on any given diet, but an approximate value of the time it will take to lose excess body fat may be obtained.

The key point is the caloric deficit. The number of days it takes for this daily deficit to reach 3,500 is how long it will take you to lose 1 pound.

Table 11.4 illustrates the importance of the caloric deficit in determining the rapidity of weight loss by dieting. This table is based upon the value of 3,500 Calories for a pound of body fat. The higher the deficit, the faster you lose weight. However, rapid weight-loss programs are not usually desirable, and the dieter should realize that a moderate caloric deficit, say 500 Calories/day, may effectively reduce weight in time and yet provide a satisfying diet. As noted later, however, as body weight is lost the caloric intake must be reduced slightly if one wants to maintain a standard daily caloric deficit.

Although these prediction methods are good for the long run, daily body-weight changes may not coincide with daily caloric deficits.

It is very important to note that although we are discussing dieting alone to create a daily caloric deficit, exercise also may be used to increase this deficit. When starting a weight-loss program, the National Institutes of Health recommends that most of the 500–1,000 daily Calorie deficit be achieved by eating less food. However, 100–200 Calories of this deficit is achievable through daily exercise, such as walking for 30 minutes

or so. Using exercise to contribute to your daily caloric deficit means your food caloric deficit may be reduced accordingly.

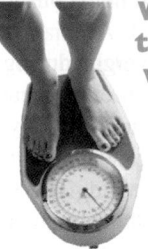

Why does a person usually lose the most weight during the first week on a reducing diet?

The principal objective of a diet is to lose body fat, not just body weight. If you start a diet with a significant caloric deficit, say 1,000 Calories/day, it would normally take you about 3.5 days to lose 1 pound of body fat. However, body-weight loss would be more rapid than this during the first several days, possibly totaling as much as 3–4 pounds. A large percentage of this weight loss would be due to a decrease in body carbohydrate and associated water stores. When you restrict your food intake, the body would then draw on its reserves to meet its energy needs. These reserves consist of both fat and carbohydrate stores, but much of the carbohydrate, stored as liver and muscle glycogen, could be used up in several days, particularly with low-carbohydrate intake, such as the Atkins diet. Because 1 gram of glycogen is stored with about 3 grams of water, a significant weight loss could occur. For example, 300 grams of glycogen, along with 900 grams of water stored with it, would account for a loss of 1,200 grams, or 1.2 kilograms; this would equal more than 2.5 pounds alone. About 70 percent of the weight loss during the first few days of a reduced-Calorie diet may be due to body-water losses. About 25 percent comes from body-fat stores and 5 percent from protein tissue. As body protein is used for energy, the excess

TABLE 11.4 Approximate number of days required to lose weight for a given caloric deficit

Daily caloric deficit	To lose 5 pounds	To lose 10 pounds	To lose 15 pounds	To lose 20 pounds	To lose 25 pounds
100	175	350	525	700	875
200	87	175	262	350	438
300	58	116	175	232	292
400	44	88	131	176	219
500	35	70	105	140	175
600	29	58	87	116	146
700	25	50	75	100	125
800	22	44	66	88	109
900	19	39	58	78	97
1,000	17	35	52	70	88
1,250*	14	28	42	56	70
1,500*	12	23	35	46	58

See text for explanation.

*Note: Weight loss more than 2 pounds per week generally not recommended.

other stages with increasing amounts of carbohydrates, but much lower than AMDR levels. Such diets are also referred to as low-carbohydrate, high-fat, and high-protein weight-loss diets. The South Beach Diet, by Agatston, limits saturated fats and focuses on healthier carbohydrates, which health professionals indicated appears to be a healthier version of the Atkins diet.

Research suggests that such diets may be effective. Liebman indicated that the Atkins diet may work because it virtually eliminates a whole category of food (carbohydrates), whereas a Tufts University report indicates that individuals who adopt the Atkins diet generally cut an average of 1,000 Calories per day from their diet, which is most likely the reason underlying its success. Correspondingly, Bravata and others reviewed 109 studies involving the use of low-carbohydrate diets and concluded that participant weight loss was principally associated with decreased caloric intake.

One of the criticisms of the Atkins diet was the possible adverse effects on the serum lipid profile and predisposition to cardiovascular disease. However, reviewers such as Volek and Sharman also noted that low-carbohydrate diets had no significant adverse effect on serum lipids, fasting serum glucose, fasting serum insulin levels, or blood pressure. Wylie-Rosett and Davis reported current research suggesting that low-carbohydrate diets can be a viable option for achieving weight loss and may have beneficial effects on glycemic control, triglyceride levels, and high-density lipoprotein cholesterol levels in some patients. The Consumers Union notes that if you have a healthy serum lipid profile, you most likely will do no harm to your health by adopting the Atkins diet plan for 12 weeks to jump-start your weight-loss program.

Based on their comprehensive review, Bravata and others concluded that there is insufficient evidence to make recommendations for or against the use of low-carbohydrate diets. However, although low-carbohydrate diets such as the Atkins diet may be successful, they are not well represented among those in the National Weight Control Registry. Only 8 percent of registry members adhered to a diet containing 90 grams or less of carbohydrate per day.

Moderation in dietary fat intake may be the key. As noted, individuals in the National Weight Control Registry consume about 30 percent of daily energy from fat, which is considered moderate. In a 14-month study, Azadbakht and others reported significantly greater reductions in body weight, waist circumference, and cardiovascular risk factors in subjects consuming a moderate-fat (30 percent) versus a low-fat (20 percent) diet. The authors suggested that better dietary adherence with the moderate-fat diet may be the reason for its successful effects. Shai and others also suggested that the Mediterranean diet, which is a moderate-fat diet, may be an effective alternative to low-fat diets.

High-Protein Weight-Loss Diets Some diets, such as the *Zone* diet, recommend that protein should account for 30 percent or more of energy, and are marketed as high-protein diets. Although this recommendation falls within the AMDR for protein (10–35 percent), it is generally regarded as high because it may be twice the typical protein intake of 12–15 percent. However, other diets such as Atkins and South Beach also may be regarded as somewhat high in protein.

High-protein weight-loss diets have been recommended for several reasons. For example, reports by Westerterp-Plantenga and Leidy, along with their associates, cited several possible benefits from increased protein intake.

- Increased satiety; increased oxidation of excess amino acids and decrease in ghrelin may help suppress the appetite.
- Increased thermogenesis; increased body temperature suppresses appetite.
- Decreased energy efficiency; more energy is used to process protein, such as in gluconeogenesis.
- Maintenance of lean body mass; muscle is the main protein reservoir in the body.

Some recommend that weight-loss diets contain 20–30 percent of energy content from protein. In a study with normal-weight individuals who were not on a weight-loss diet, Weigle and others found that increasing dietary protein content from 15 to 30 percent of energy intake, while keeping carbohydrate content constant, produced a sustained decrease in caloric intake. In another study involving high-protein diets (30 percent), Leidy and others reported improved perceptions of satiety and pleasure during dietary energy restriction, and the diet helped women preserve lean body mass. Mettler and others also reported that a high-protein (35 percent) diet, as compared to normal protein (15 percent) intake, was significantly superior for maintenance of lean body mass during a short-term weight loss program.

In a review of clinical trials, Hu concluded that short-term, high-protein diets induce weight loss and improve blood lipids, but also noted that long-term data are missing; the evidence suggests partially replacing refined carbohydrates with protein sources that are low in saturated fat. In this regard, Layman and others indicated that high-protein, low-carbohydrate diets have been found to have some positive health effects, such as reducing serum triglycerides and blood pressure, increasing HDL-cholesterol, and improving glycemic control, factors that could reduce risk for heart disease and diabetes.

St. Jeor and others, representing the Nutrition Committee of the American Heart Association, noted that high-protein diets may not be harmful for most healthy people for a short period of time, but as Hu notes, there are no long-term scientific studies to support their overall efficacy and safety. Friedman indicated no clear kidney-related contraindication to high-protein diets in individuals with healthy kidney function, but individuals at risk for chronic kidney disease should be screened for serum creatinine and proteinuria before the initiation of such a diet. Another health concern with high-protein diets is increased calcium losses, but Johnston and others reported no adverse effects of such diets on calcium balance. Although diets containing 25–30 percent protein may be marketed as high-protein, such diets are actually within the AMDR of 10–35 percent of energy from protein. Nevertheless, individuals who have any health concerns should check with their health professionals before initiating such dietary changes.

Balanced Weight-Loss Diets   In the middle of Riley's continuum of popular weight-loss diets are mainly those recommended by most professional health organizations, such as the American Heart Association and the American Dietetic and American Diabetes Associations' Food Exchange System Diet, which is the basis of the diet plan advocated in this text.

Highly recommended diets are based upon sound nutritional principles and also are designed to satisfy the individual's personal food tastes. Research with dieters has shown that any weight-reduction diet, to be safe, effective, and realistic, should adhere to the following principles:

1. It should be reduced in Calories and yet supply all nutrients essential to normal body functions. It is important to stress the importance of dietary Calories. Dich and others purposely overfed normal young men, about 1,200 additional Calories per day, with either a carbohydrate-rich or a fat-rich diet for 21 days. They found that the increase in body weight and fat mass was no different between the two diets. Excess dietary Calories lead to weight gain and this study indicates that it does not matter if they come from carbohydrate or fat. As far as energy is concerned, a Calorie from a banana is the same as a Calorie from a brownie.
2. It should contain a wide variety of foods that appeal to your taste and help prevent hunger sensations between meals. Low-glycemic-index diets with dietary fiber and moderate amounts of protein and fat may help to suppress the appetite. With respect to weight control, Kris-Etherton and others suggest that a moderate-fat diet can be as, or even more, effective than a lower-fat diet, because of advantages with long-term adherence and potentially favorable effects on lipids and lipoproteins. However, they also note that because fat is energy dense, moderation in fat intake is essential for weight control.
3. It should be suited to your current lifestyle and personal preferences, being easily obtainable whether you eat most of your meals at home or you dine out frequently.
4. It should provide for a slow rate of weight loss, about 1–2 pounds per week.
5. It should be a lifelong diet, one that will satisfy the first three principles once you attain your desired weight.

In any diet plan, foods should be selected that adhere to the principles of healthful eating. This information was summarized in chapter 2, and 20 guidelines you can use in the selection and preparation of foods to reduce caloric intake are presented later in this chapter. As proper knowledge is a key to behavioral modification, learning the caloric and nutrient content of a wide variety of foods may be a very important strategy in a weight-control program.

Is it a good idea to count Calories when attempting to lose body weight?

There are both pros and cons to counting Calories. On the con side, counting Calories may not be practical for many who are too busy to plan a daily menu designed around a caloric limit. How many Calories are in the lunch or dinner you eat out daily? And how about serving sizes? Can you picture 3 ounces of roast beef or an ounce of cheese? Also, it may be difficult to calculate the exact amount of Calories consumed, as the caloric content in foods may vary somewhat. For example, certain slices of bread are larger than others and may have a correspondingly higher caloric content. Although these problems are not difficult to solve, it does take some effort.

On the pro side, counting Calories may be very helpful during the early stages of a diet. Knowledge of the food exchange lists and use of Nutrition Facts on food labels will enable you to substitute one low-Calorie food for another in your daily menu. Additionally, research suggests that recording everything you eat when you start dieting, including the caloric content, can help you stick with your weight-loss program. As you become familiar with the caloric content of various foods, it becomes easier to select those that are low in Calories but high in nutrient value, and to avoid those foods just the opposite, high in Calories and low in nutrients. It will require a little effort in the beginning phases of a diet to learn the Calories in a given quantity of a certain food, but once learned and incorporated into your lifestyle, this knowledge is a valuable asset to possess not only when trying to lose weight but also when maintaining a healthy weight over a lifetime. As you incorporate low-Calorie, high-nutrient foods into your diet, it will eventually become second nature to you, and you may eliminate the need to count Calories.

The key to keeping track of Calories is to keep track of dietary fat and sugar and portion sizes. With knowledge of the Food Exchange System and the new food labels, you should be able to determine the grams of fat that you consume daily. Less than 30 percent of your dietary Calories should be derived from fat. On a diet of 1,800 Calories per day, fewer than 540 Calories should come from fat ($1,800 \times 0.30$), which is the equivalent of 60 grams of fat because 1 gram of fat contains 9 Calories (540/9). Diets containing only 20 percent fat Calories may also be recommended. Less than 10 percent of your dietary Calories should come from sugar. On this 1,800-Calorie diet, that would be fewer than 180 Calories (45 grams) from sugar. As noted later, reducing the amount of fat and sugar in the daily diet may be a very effective means to reduce daily energy intake and lose excess body fat.

How often should i weigh myself?

Once you have attained your desired weight, a good set of scales would be most helpful. Keeping track of your weight on a day-to-day or weekly basis will enable you to decrease your caloric intake for several days once you notice your weight beginning to increase again. Most individuals in the National Weight Control Registry who have lost weight and kept it off weigh themselves daily once their weight goal is reached, noting that it is easier to deal with a gain of a few pounds rather than 10 or 20. Short-term prevention is more effective than long-term treatment. The dietary habits you acquire during the Calorie-counting phase of your diet will help you during these short-term prevention periods.

What is the food exchange system?

At this time it is important to expand our discussion of the Food Exchange System, which was introduced in chapter 2. The Food Exchange System was developed by a group of health organizations, including the American Diabetes Association and the American Dietetic Association, as a means of advising patients about healthy eating. In essence, six food groups were established, and foods were assigned to these groups on the basis of similar caloric content and nutritional value. For our purposes at this time, we will concentrate upon the caloric value, but you may also want to refresh your memory on the grams of fat per food exchange.

The six food exchange lists may be found in appendix E. You should study these lists and get an idea of the types and amounts of foods in each that constitute one exchange. Memorizing the caloric value of each food exchange is instrumental in determining the number of Calories you consume daily and also in planning a healthful, low-Calorie diet. In their study, Benezra and others found that the intake of most nutrients can remain at recommended levels when the Food Exchange System is used to plan a weight-loss program. The caloric content and grams of fat of one serving from each of the six exchanges are listed below and expressed in figure 11.3.

1 vegetable exchange	=	25 Calories; 0 g fat
1 fruit exchange	=	60 Calories; 0 g fat
1 fat exchange	=	45 Calories; 5 g fat
1 starch exchange	=	80 Calories; 0–1 g fat
1 meat exchange	=	35–100 Calories
Very lean	=	35 Calories; 0–1 g fat
Lean	=	55 Calories; 3 g fat
Medium fat	=	75 Calories; 5 g fat
High fat	=	100 Calories; 8 g fat
1 milk exchange	=	90–150 Calories
Skim	=	90 Calories; 0–3 g fat
Low fat	=	120 Calories; 5 g fat
Whole	=	150 Calories; 8 g fat

Table 11.6 presents a breakdown of the carbohydrate, fat, protein, and Calorie content of each food exchange.

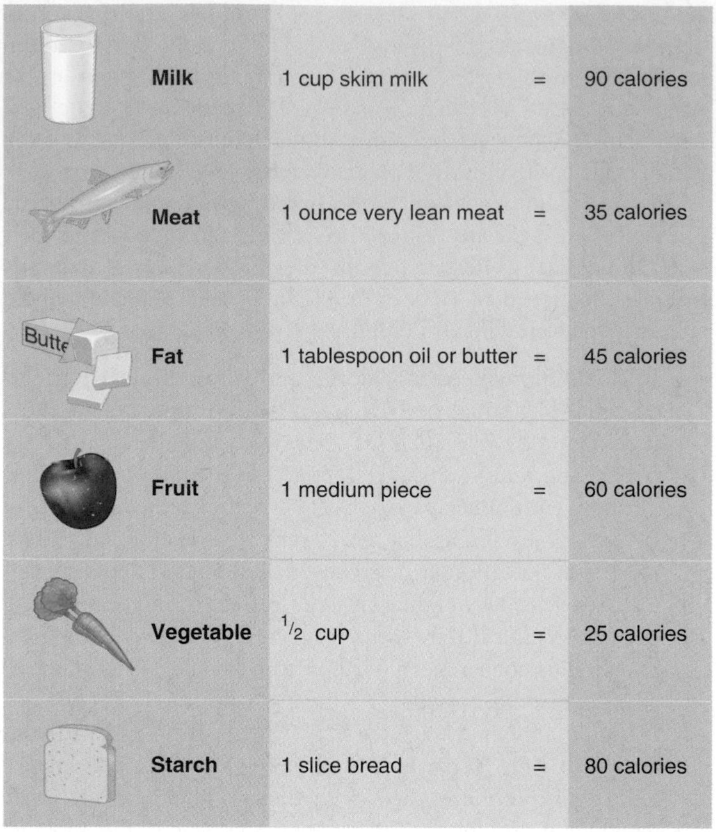

How can I determine the number of Calories I eat daily?

You may use the guide presented earlier in this chapter to record your daily physical activity, including what you eat and drink. Carry a small notebook with you along with some reminder, such as a rubber band around your wrist, to record your activity and food intake in detail. One suggestion to document your food intake is to take a photo of what you eat with your cell phone, which provides you with a daily record. To calculate your caloric intake, you can use information provided by food labels or from the Food Exchange System in appendix E. Food intake should be recorded over a 3–7 day period, as one single day may give a biased value. Experiments have shown that this method may provide relatively accurate accounts of caloric intake if the amounts of food ingested are measured accurately. The main problem for most people is determining what and how

Milk	1 cup skim milk	=	90 calories
Meat	1 ounce very lean meat	=	35 calories
Fat	1 tablespoon oil or butter	=	45 calories
Fruit	1 medium piece	=	60 calories
Vegetable	½ cup	=	25 calories
Starch	1 slice bread	=	80 calories

FIGURE 11.3 Knowledge of the various food exchanges and their caloric values can be very helpful in planning a diet. With a little effort, you can learn to estimate the caloric value of most basic foods. See appendix E for other food examples and serving sizes.

much has been eaten. An 8-ounce glass of skim milk may be easy to record, and the caloric value from the food label or from appendix E is rather precise. However, how many Calories are in a slice of pizza at your favorite Italian restaurant? How big was the piece? What is the caloric content of the cheese, green peppers, pepperoni, and mushrooms? When we deal with complex food combinations such as this, our estimates of caloric content are not as precise. However, some estimates are presented in appendix E in the section on combination foods. For example, one-quarter of a 10-inch cheese pizza with thin crust contains two starch, two medium-fat meat, and one fat exchange, or the equivalent of 355 Calories.

Although you may wish to use a ruler, a small measuring scale, and a measuring cup at home to accurately record the amount of food you eat, they are not practical for many dining situations. Lisa Young, in her book *The Portion Teller Plan: The No-Diet Reality Guide to Eating, Cheating and Losing Weight Permanently,* states that learning how to eyeball portion sizes accurately is an important skill. Some common objects in everyday life may serve as representative portion sizes for various foods, and some examples are presented in figure 11.4. The

TABLE 11.6 Carbohydrate, fat, protein, and Calories in the six food exchanges

Food exchange	Carbohydrate	Fat	Protein	Calories	Average serving size*
Vegetables	5	0	2	25	½ cup cooked; 1 cup raw
Fruits	15	0	0	60	½ cup fresh fruit or juice
Fat	0	5	0	45	1 teaspoon (5 grams)
Meat and meat substitutes					1 ounce
Very lean	0	0–1	7	35	
Lean	0	3	7	55	
Medium fat	0	5	7	75	
High fat	0	8	7	100	
Starch	15	0–1	3	80	⅓–½ cup cereal or pasta; 1 slice of bread
Milk					1 cup (8 fluid ounces)
Skim and very low fat	12	0–3	8	90–110	
Low fat	12	5	8	120	
Whole	12	8	8	150	

Carbohydrate, fat, and protein in grams.
1 g carbohydrate = 4 Calories
1 g fat = 9 Calories
1 g protein = 4 Calories

*See appendix E for specific foods.

Source: *Exchange Lists for Meal Planning*, American Diabetes Association and American Dietetic Association, Chicago, ADA, 1995.

following may serve as guidelines for you to record the type and amount of food you eat:

1. In your notebook, record the foods you have eaten as soon as possible, noting the kind of food and the amount. Keep in mind that many servings today are supersized so that one of these servings may actually contain the Calories of 2–3 regular servings. Learn to visualize proper portion sizes and the associated Calorie content in various foods.

2. Check the labels of the foods you eat. Most commercial products today have nutritional information listed, including the number of Calories per serving. Record these data when available.

3. Calories for most fluids are given in relationship to ounces. For fluids, remember that 1 cup or regular glass is about 8 ounces, but many glasses now hold 12–16 ounces. Most regular canned drinks contain 12 ounces, although smaller and larger sizes are available; 20-ounce bottles are becoming increasingly popular.

4. Calories for meat, poultry, fish, and other related products are usually given by ounces. To get an idea of how many ounces are in these products, you could purchase a set weight of meat, say 16 ounces, and cut it into four equal pieces. Each would weigh approximately 4 ounces, or about the visual size of a deck of playing cards. For cheese, one ounce is about the size of a ping pong ball. Get a mental picture of these sizes and use them as a guide to portion sizes.

5. For fruits and vegetables the caloric values are usually expressed relative to ½ cup or a small-sized piece. At home, measure ½ cup of vegetables or fruit and place it in a bowl or on a plate. Again, make a mental picture of this serving size and use it as a reference. Compare the sizes of different fruits and notice the difference between a small, medium, and large piece. A medium piece of fruit is about the size of a tennis ball, while a medium potato is about the size of a computer mouse.

6. For starch products, the Calories are most often expressed per serving, such as an average-size slice of bread or a dinner roll. In these cases it is relatively easy to determine quantity, but one slice of bread may contain 50 to 150 Calories or more, depending on its size and density. Depending on the type of cereal, pasta, grain, or starchy vegetable, the measure for one exchange is usually ⅓ or ½ cup, but some serving sizes are larger, such as those of puffed cereals. See appendix E. Use a measuring cup and the mental-picture concept again to estimate quantities. A cup of cold cereal is about the size of a large handful, whereas ½ cup of hot cereal is about the size of a tennis ball. A 2-ounce bagel is the size of a yo-yo.

7. For substances such as sugar, jams, jellies, nondairy creamers, and related products, make a mental picture of a teaspoon and tablespoon. These are common means whereby Calories are given. A teaspoon of butter or margarine is about the size of the tip of your thumb. One level teaspoon of sugar is

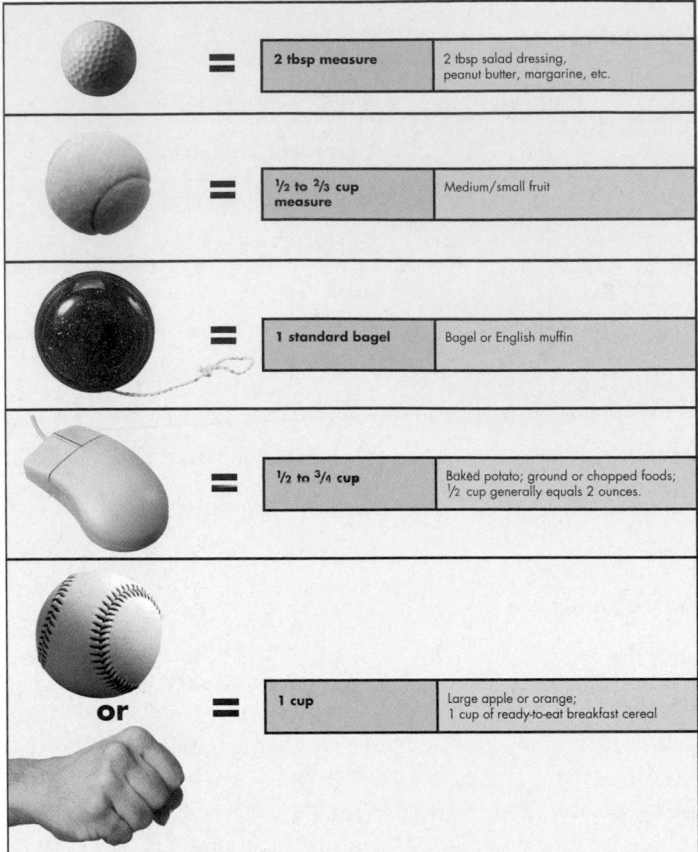

		2 tbsp measure	2 tbsp salad dressing, peanut butter, margarine, etc.
		½ to ⅔ cup measure	Medium/small fruit
		1 standard bagel	Bagel or English muffin
		½ to ¾ cup	Baked potato; ground or chopped foods; ½ cup generally equals 2 ounces.
or		1 cup	Large apple or orange; 1 cup of ready-to-eat breakfast cereal

FIGURE 11.4 A golf ball, tennis ball, large yo-yo, computer mouse, baseball, and fist make convenient guides to judge MyPyramid serving sizes. Additional handy guides include:

thumb = 1 oz of cheese;
4 stacked dice = 1 oz cheese;
thumb tip to first joint = 1 tsp;
matchbox = 1 oz meat;
bar of soap or deck of
cards = 3 oz meat;

palm of hand = 3 oz
1 ice cream scoop = 1/2 cup
handful = 1 or 2 oz of a
snack food; and
ping-pong ball = 2 tbsp.

about 20 Calories; jams and jellies contain similar amounts. Caloric values of other products may be obtained from nutrition labels.

8. Some combination foods, such as a homemade casserole, are included in appendix E. However, for combination foods not listed, you will need to list the ingredients separately to calculate the caloric content. Labels on most food products list caloric content per serving.

9. Caloric values for some national chain and fast-food restaurant items may be found in appendix F. Most fast-food restaurants provide fact sheets detailing information on the nutrient content of their products. The FDA proposed that national restaurant chains, as well as other businesses, such as convenience stores that sell prepared food, be required to display Calorie counts for menu items so the consumer may make an informed judgment when ordering. Some national chains, such as Chili's and Olive Garden, are currently marketing low-Calorie (400–500 Calories) meals. If caloric

values are not displayed, you may access them at various Websites. If nutrition fact sheets are not available when dining out in restaurants, you may obtain the caloric value of food items via e-mail.

www.CalorieKing.com Check the caloric content of numerous food items in national chain and fast-food restaurants.

Working with the Food Exchange System helps you learn the portion size and caloric content of various foods. Through experience you should be able to readily identify, within a small error range, the quantities of food you eat. This is not only helpful for determining your caloric intake but may also serve as a motivational device to restrict portion sizes when you are on a weight-loss diet.

The following represents an example of how you might record one meal and calculate the caloric intake from appendix E or food labels.

Breakfast Food	Quantity	Calories
Milk, skim	1 glass, 8 ounces	90
Eggs	2, poached	150
Toast, whole wheat	2 slices	160
with butter	2 pats	90
with jelly	1 tablespoon	60
Orange juice	1 glass, 8 ounces	120
Coffee	1 cup, 8 ounces	0
with sugar	1 teaspoon	20
TOTAL		690

Reading food labels and consulting the Food Exchange System helps you learn the caloric and nutrient value of various foods, and is recommended as a learning tool. You can then use computer programs to assess your diet on a daily basis. The Choose-MyPlate Website, discussed previously, gives you the opportunity to keep a detailed history of your caloric and nutrient intake, and you can use the *Energy Balance* option to plan a weight-control diet. Appropriate dietary analysis software is also provided with your purchase of this textbook.

www.mhhe.com/williams Access the McGraw-Hill Website to obtain dietary software available with the purchase of this book.

What are some general guidelines I can use in the selection and preparation of foods to promote weight loss or maintain a healthy body weight?

A *Consumer Reports* survey of more than 32,000 dieters found that more than 80 percent who successfully lost weight and kept it off did so without following a specific plan. Instead, they used sensible strategies such as cutting portion size and staying away from sweets and junk food. The following 20 guidelines for weight control and healthy eating are based on several reputable sources of information, including the Food Exchange System, the National

Weight Control Registry, and the DASH and OmniHeart diets. In essence, the four key points are:

- Eat fewer Calories from fat and sugar
- Eat healthier carbohydrates
- Eat healthier fats
- Eat healthier proteins

1. *Eat more nutrient-dense foods and fewer energy-dense foods.* You need to decrease the number of Calories you consume daily. The key principle is to select foods, in appropriate portion sizes, and with high-nutrient density from across the six food exchanges or the food groups in the MyPlate approach. Avoid energy-dense foods and drinks, such as bagels, soft pretzels, energy bars, smoothies, special coffees, and cocktails, all of which may be loaded with Calories. If you do buy convenience meals, select those that are low in Calories and fat. Check the label for total fat and total Calories from fat and sugar. This you can easily do by reading the label. Check figure 11.5.

2. *Eat foods that make you feel full.* Barbara Rolls, a renowned diet expert at Penn State University, based her excellent book, *The Volumetrics Eating Plan,* on this principle, as did Dean Ornish with his book, *Eat More, Weigh Less.* Research from Rolls's laboratory reported that reducing dietary energy density is associated with weight loss in overweight individuals. High-volume, low-Calorie foods, such as salads, soups, vegetables, and whole grains, are rich in dietary fiber and water, and help provide a sensation of fullness that curbs hunger.

3. *Restrict portion sizes.* Although the intake of high-volume, low-Calorie foods like vegetables will help curtail hunger and promote weight loss, one of the major problems contributing to the increasing obesity in the United States is the consumption of large volumes of high-Calorie foods. Most fast-food eateries and convenience stores have increased portion sizes dramatically to give customers their *money's worth.* As examples, years ago a *family* bottle of cola soda was 32 ounces, and now single servings of cola drinks may total up to 64 ounces, with free refills; a McDonald's meal of a single hamburger, small fries, and cola had totalled 600 Calories, but today a larger meal with the same basic foods may total 1,800 Calories; a small bagel that once contained 200 Calories has been supersized to 500–600 Calories or more. Even manufacturers of "healthy" foods for dieters advertise "heartier" portions that weigh 50 percent more than the original version and contain more Calories. In contrast, some food manufacturers are now marketing 100-Calorie healthful snacks, such as almonds, and some restaurants, such as TGIFriday's, are offering smaller portion sizes with reduced Calories and prices. Decreasing the volume of high-Calorie foods is one of the most important dietary means to reduced body fat.

4. *Eat less fat.* Although restricting dietary Calories is most important, and some research indicates that the source of caloric intake is irrelevant to weight gain, according to Jequier dietary fat appears to play several roles in the development and maintenance of obesity. First, it is rich in Calories—more than double the amount of Calories per gram as compared to carbohydrate and protein. In their study, Rolls and Bell found that when individuals were fed diets varying in caloric density (fat content) and could eat as much as they liked, they ate the same amount of food by weight, so the caloric intake varied directly with the caloric density of the food. Second, dietary fat is appetizing and does not appear to rapidly suppress the appetite, leading to a greater intake of Calories, as suggested by Blundell and Green. Third, dietary fat has a lower TEF, or higher metabolic efficiency, than carbohydrate and protein. Melby and Hill indicated that dietary fat appears to be stored as fat more efficiently than either carbohydrate or protein, even if the caloric intake is similar; this is especially true in individuals who have lost weight and may be one of the most important reasons why they regain weight so readily. Fourth, dietary fat may also be stored preferentially in the abdominal region, which may increase health risks. In a major 7-year study of more than 48,000 women, Howard and others reported that weight loss was greatest among women who decreased their percentage of energy intake from fat.

To reduce the amount of fat in your diet, you may wish to count the total grams of fat you eat each day. As mentioned previously, a general recommendation is to keep your daily total fat intake to 30 percent or less of your total caloric intake. To calculate the total grams of fat you may eat per day, simply multiply your caloric intake by 30 percent and divide by 9 (the Calories per gram of fat). You may wish to get the fat content to a lower percentage, such as 20 percent. Table 11.7 presents the formula and some calculations for

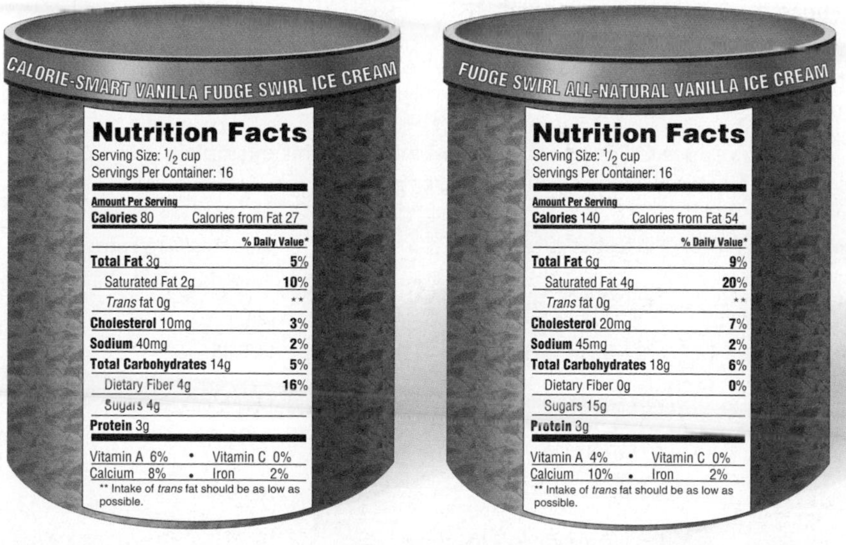

CALORIE-SMART VANILLA FUDGE SWIRL ICE CREAM

Nutrition Facts
Serving Size: 1/2 cup
Servings Per Container: 16

Amount Per Serving
Calories 80   Calories from Fat 27

                   % Daily Value*

Total Fat 3g   5%
   Saturated Fat 2g   10%
   Trans fat 0g   **
Cholesterol 10mg   3%
Sodium 40mg   2%
Total Carbohydrates 14g   5%
   Dietary Fiber 4g   16%
   Sugars 4g
Protein 3g

Vitamin A 6%   •   Vitamin C 0%
Calcium 8%   •   Iron 2%
** Intake of *trans* fat should be as low as possible.

FUDGE SWIRL ALL-NATURAL VANILLA ICE CREAM

Nutrition Facts
Serving Size: 1/2 cup
Servings Per Container: 16

Amount Per Serving
Calories 140   Calories from Fat 54

                   % Daily Value*

Total Fat 6g   9%
   Saturated Fat 4g   20%
   Trans fat 0g   **
Cholesterol 20mg   7%
Sodium 45mg   2%
Total Carbohydrates 18g   6%
   Dietary Fiber 0g   0%
   Sugars 15g
Protein 3g

Vitamin A 4%   •   Vitamin C 0%
Calcium 10%   •   Iron 2%
** Intake of *trans* fat should be as low as possible.

FIGURE 11.5 Reading labels helps you choose foods with less fat, sugar, and Calorie content.

TABLE 11.7 Calculation of daily fat intake in grams

To use this table, determine the number of Calories per day in your diet and the percent of dietary Calories you want from fat, and then find the grams of fat you may consume daily. For example, if your diet contains 2,200 Calories and you desire to consume only 20 percent of your daily Calories as fat, then you could consume 49 grams of fat. The formula is:
% fat × Daily Calories ÷ 9 Calories per fat gram = Daily fat grams
[0.20 × 2,200 ÷ 9 = 49]

Daily caloric intake	30% fat Calories (maximal grams)	20% fat Calories (maximal grams)	10% fat Calories (maximal grams)
1,000	33	22	11
1,200	40	26	13
1,500	50	33	16
1,800	60	40	20
2,000	66	44	22
2,200	73	49	24
2,500	83	55	28

different caloric intake levels and percentages of dietary fat intake.

The development of fat substitutes may be helpful in reducing fat intake. Many fat-free products are currently available and may decrease total fat and caloric intake if used judiciously within a healthful diet. The American Dietetic Association, in its position statement on fat replacers authored by Mattes, indicated that they can be used effectively to reduce fat and Calorie intake. The American Heart Association also noted that use of fat substitutes may be associated with reduced fat and Calorie intake compared with nonuse of any fat-modified products, and also noted that when used appropriately, fat substitutes may provide some flexibility with diet planning. However, Miller and Groziak noted that although fat substitutes may help decrease dietary fat intake and percentage of caloric intake from fat, many individuals will compensate by increasing their consumption of other macronutrients, primarily carbohydrate. Research by Shide and Rolls supports this point, indicating that individuals eat more food at a given meal if they know some of the meal consists of low-fat items. Additionally, fat-free does not mean Calorie-free, and Manore indicated that some fat-free foods may have similar amounts of Calories as the original. Again, check the food label. Cotton and others suggest that you gradually blend fat substitutes into your diet; making many changes at one time may lead to overconsumption of other foods, and hence your overall caloric intake may remain the same, or even increase. Fat substitutes can be part of an overall healthful diet for weight loss, provided you do not compensate for the saved Calories by ingesting other Calorie-rich foods.

Remember that you need some fat in your diet for essential fatty acids and fat-soluble vitamins, which you may be able to obtain in a diet containing 10 percent fat Calories. An example of grams of fat and Calories saved by using fat substitutes for a luncheon meal is presented in table 11.8. In this example, using fat substitutes reduced the energy density of the lunch by about 350 Calories.

Several modified fats have been proposed to facilitate weight loss. Diglycerides are components of a new oil to replace the traditional triglycerides. Although the caloric content of the two oils is the same, diglycerides are theorized to increase fat oxidation and not be stored as body fat as readily as triglycerides. However, research with this new oil is limited and health professionals currently recommend that its potential minor effects on weight loss do not justify its price; they recommend olive or canola oils, while limiting intake of other fats and oils.

TABLE 11.8 Using foods with fat substitutes may help reduce Calories and fat from meals. In this example, the fat-substitute lunch contains about 350 fewer Calories and 40 fewer grams of fat.

Regular lunch	Calories/fat grams	Fat-substitute lunch	Calories/fat grams
Sandwich		Sandwich	
2 slices whole wheat bread	140/2	2 slices whole wheat bread	140/2
2 oz bologna	180/16	2 oz fat-free bologna	44/0.35
1 oz cheese	85/6.4	1 oz fat-free cheese	43/0
2 Tbsp mayonnaise	114/10	2 Tbsp fat-free mayonnaise	26/1.0
Banana, medium	105/0.4	Banana	105/0.4
1 cup ice cream	265/14	1 cup fat/sugar-free ice cream	182/0
Totals	889/43.8	Totals	540/3.75

Other suggestions for reducing dietary fat are included in the following guidelines, but you may wish to review chapter 5 for additional information. Once individuals adapt to a low-fat diet, they may prefer it because high-fat meals are digested more slowly, possibly leading to indigestion and some gastro-intestinal distress.

5. *Eat fewer and smaller amounts of refined sugar.* This may be accomplished by restricting the amount of sugar added directly to foods and limiting the consumption of highly processed foods that may add substantial amounts of sweeteners, particularly sugar-sweetened beverages. A report in the Tufts University *Health & Nutrition Letter* indicated that Americans consume about 475 Calories daily from added sugars.

   Artificial sweeteners may be helpful. For example, Raben and others found that overweight individuals who consumed large amounts of sucrose in their daily diets, mostly as beverages, had increased energy intake, body weight, and fat mass after 10 weeks, but these effects were not seen in a similar group that consumed artificial sweeteners. Pi-Sunyer noted that substitution of artificial sweeteners, such as aspartame, for sugar has been shown to reduce caloric intake without leading to an increased consumption of other foods. Drewnowski also reported that some short-term studies and one long-term study have shown that artificial sweeteners could decrease caloric intake and increase weight loss, but more long-term research is recommended. Again, like fat substitutes, sugar substitutes may be an effective part of a healthful weight-loss diet, but individuals must be cautious not to compensate and eat more food later.

6. *Reduce the intake of both added fat and sugar.* In many cases, simply reducing the fat and sugar content in the diet will save substantial numbers of Calories and may be all that is needed. Did you know that fat and sugar together account for nearly 50 percent of the Calories in the average American diet? That represents 5 out of every 10 Calories. Table 11.9 provides some examples of how to save Calories via simple substitutions for comparable foods containing fat or sugar. We often unwittingly consume high-fat, high-sugar items when we dine out. Did you know that a glass of iced tea may contain 10 percent of your daily caloric needs? A large glass of sweet tea at McDonalds contains nearly 60 grams of sugar and 230 Calories. Did you know that some appetizers may contain several thousand Calories? For example, a fried whole onion with dipping sauce contains about 2,100 Calories. Even supposedly healthy fast foods, such as salads, can contain as much fat and Calories as the burgers on the menu, mainly because large amounts of fat are added with the dressing; one popular salad contains more than 800 Calories, with more than 70 percent fat Calories. As noted earlier, most national restaurant chains can provide you with the caloric content of their meal items.

7. *Eat more low-fat dairy products.* As noted previously, increased protein intake may help suppress the appetite more than equivalent amounts of carbohydrate or fat. In chapter 8 we discussed the hypothesis that a dairy-rich diet could promote weight loss but as noted, in general, research findings do not support this hypothesis. Nevertheless, milk exchange

TABLE 11.9	Simple food substitutions to save Calories	
Instead of	**Select**	**To save this many Calories by reducing sugar and fat**
1 croissant	1 whole wheat bagel	80
1 whole egg	2 egg whites	50
1 ounce cheddar chesse	1 ounce mozzarella (skim)	30
1 ounce regular bacon	1 ounce Canadian bacon	100
3 ounces tuna in oil	3 ounces tuna in water	60
Cream of mushroom soup	Black bean soup	90
1 cup regular ice cream	1 cup fat-free frozen dessert	150
1 ounce turkey bologna	1 ounce turkey breast	50
1 McDonald's Big Mac	1 McDonald's grilled chicken	120
1 cup whole milk	1 cup skim milk	60
French fried potatoes	Baked potato	100
1 ounce potato chips	1 ounce pretzels	90
1 tablespoon mayonnaise	1 tablespoon fat-free mayonnaise	90
1 can regular cola	1 can diet cola	150

products are excellent sources of high-quality protein and other essential vitamins and minerals. The key is to select the healthier, low-fat versions, which are healthier protein foods. Use skim milk, low-fat cottage cheese, low-fat yogurt, and nonfat dried milk instead of their high-fat counterparts like whole milk, sour cream, and powdered creamers.

8. *Eat more low-fat meat and meat substitutes.* The meat and meat substitute exchange products also are sources of high-quality protein and many other nutrients but also may contain excessive fat Calories. To eat healthier proteins, select very lean and lean meat exchanges, including meat substitutes such as legumes. Per one ounce serving, very lean meat and meat substitutes contain only 35 Calories and less than 1 gram of fat. Examples include the white meat of chicken and turkey, 99 percent fat-free ground turkey, tuna fresh or canned in water, shrimp, fat free cheese, egg whites, and egg substitutes. See appendix E for other sources. If you enjoy beef and pork, use leaner cuts such as beef eye of round, flank steak, pork tenderloin, and 96 percent fat-free hamburger. Trim away excess fat; broil or bake your meats to let the fat drip away. If you eat in national chain and fast-food restaurants, select

foods that are low in fat, such as grilled chicken, lean meats, and salads. Avoid the high-fat foods, which normally contain 40–60 percent fat Calories. Also be aware that serving sizes have increased dramatically in recent years. That large hamburger deluxe may have triple or more the Calories of a regular hamburger. Select legumes as an excellent meat substitute.

9. *Eat more whole, unprocessed carbohydrates.* The starch exchange contains healthy carbohydrates and is high in vitamins, minerals, and fiber. Eating a low-glycemic, high-fiber diet increases the gastric volume, which might help suppress appetite. Use whole-grain breads and cereals, brown rice, oatmeal, beans, bran products, and starchy vegetables for dietary fiber. Limit the use of processed grain products that add fat and sugar. Substitute products low in fat, such as standard-size whole wheat bagels, for those high in fat, like croissants.

10. *Eat more fruits.* Foods in the fruit exchange are high in vitamins and fiber. Select fresh, whole fruits or those canned or frozen in their own juices. Avoid those in heavy sugar syrups. Limit the intake of dried fruits, which are high in Calories. Eat at least one citrus fruit daily. Limit intake of fruit juices, which are rich in Calories.

11. *Eat more veggies.* The vegetable exchange foods are low in Calories yet high in vitamins, minerals, and fiber. Select dark-green leafy and yellow-orange vegetables daily. Low-Calorie items like carrots, radishes, and celery are highly nutritious snacks for munching. Many of these vegetables are listed as free exchanges in appendix E because they contain fewer than 20 Calories per serving. Fruits and vegetables may provide bulk to the diet and a sensation of fullness without excessive amounts of Calories.

12. *Consume fewer high-Calorie fat exchanges.* Use smaller amounts of high-Calorie fat exchanges. Many salad dressings, butter, margarine, and cooking oils are pure fat. If necessary, substitute low-Calorie or fat-free dietary versions instead. Fat-free mayonnaise tastes good and has 90 fewer Calories than a serving of regular mayonnaise. Do not prepare foods in fats, such as with frying. Use nonstick cooking utensils or nonfat cooking sprays.

13. *Reduce liquid Calories.* Beverages other than milk and fruit juice should have no Calories. High-Calorie liquids, such as sodas and alcoholic beverages, may be especially harmful in weight-loss programs because they not only add Calories to the diet, but also do not appear to suppress the appetite as well as similar amounts of Calories in solid foods. In a review of 30 high-quality studies, Malik and others found that the weight of epidemiologic and experimental evidence indicates that a greater consumption of sugar-sweetened beverages is associated with weight gain and obesity, and that sufficient evidence exists for public health strategies to discourage consumption of sugary drinks as part of a healthy lifestyle. Popkin suggests that about half of the daily Calories that contribute to weight gain are consumed as sugary beverages. Other beverages may also contain excess Calories. For example, the Consumers Union notes that a 24-ounce Starbucks Vanilla Bean Frappuccino (without whipped cream) contains about as many Calories as a McDonald's Big Mac.

However, fluid intake should remain high, for it helps create a sensation of satiety during a meal. Concerned with the increase in obesity in the United States, Popkin assembled a Beverage Guidance Panel to provide guidance on the relative health and nutritional benefits and risks of various beverage categories. Plain drinking water was ranked as the preferred beverage to fulfill daily water needs, whereas calorically sweetened, nutrient-poor beverages were ranked as least preferred. The panel recommends that the consumption of beverages with no or few calories should take precedence over the consumption of beverages with more Calories.

14. *Limit your intake of alcohol.* It is high in Calories and zero in nutrient value. One gram of alcohol is equal to 7 Calories, almost twice the value of protein and carbohydrate. For 100 Calories in a shot of gin you receive zero nutrient value, but for the same amount of Calories in approximately 2 ounces of chicken breast you get nearly one-third of your RDA in protein plus substantial amounts of iron, zinc, niacin, and other vitamins. Research indicates that consuming alcohol with a meal does not substitute for other foods, so the total caloric intake of the meal is increased. Additionally, excess alcohol Calories are stored as body fat. If you desire alcohol, select the light varieties of wine and beer. Substitution of a light beer for a regular beer will save about 50 Calories. You may wish to try the nonalcoholic wines and beers, which may contain even fewer Calories. Additional information is presented in chapter 13.

15. *Limit salt intake.* Salt intake should be limited to that which occurs naturally in foods. Try to use dry herbs, spices, and other nonsalt seasonings as substitutes to flavor your food. Salt may increase the appetite or thirst for Calorie-containing beverages.

16. *Eat slowly.* Slowing down the process of eating, by taking time to smell the aromas from your food and chewing slowly, will provide time to help curb your appetite. The Consumers Union notes that it takes about 20–25 minutes for your brain to receive signals from your stomach and intestines that you are satisfied. Eat a salad or soup as an appetizer, which may help curb your appetite for the main course.

17. *Eat at least three meals a day.* In their review, Leidy and Campbell reported that eating fewer than three meals daily could negatively affect appetite control. They noted several studies that have found an increase in appetite and reduction in perceived satiety when a meal or two was eliminated from the daily diet. Individuals who want to graze, or eat 5–6 smaller meals a day instead of the traditional 3 meals, may find that it helps curb the appetite. In particular, low-Calorie but high-protein and moderate fat snacks, such as a hard-boiled egg or a handful of nuts with a total of 100 Calories, may be rather satiating. Nevertheless, current research suggests that grazing may not be more effective than a traditional meal pattern if total daily caloric intake is the same.

18. *Eat breakfast.* About 80 percent of individuals in the National Weight Control Registry eat breakfast. A hearty breakfast may help curb hunger throughout the morning hours. One study has shown that when more Calories were

eaten in the morning, caloric intake for the entire day was less as compared to eating most daily Calories in the evening; researchers suggested that the appetite may be suppressed more easily in the morning than in the evening. In this regard, a high-protein breakfast may be important. Vander Wal and others found that eating eggs for breakfast can curb appetite at lunch and for the remainder of the day, reducing total daily intake by about 250 fewer Calories. Egg substitutes (egg whites) may be used, as can other high-protein, high-fiber breakfasts, such as whole-grain cereals with skim milk or whole wheat toast with smoked salmon. Conversely, Giovannini and others reported that breakfast skipping may lead to up-regulation of appetite throughout the day, possibly leading to weight gain over time.

19. *Learn to cook!* Microwaves and electric grills make cooking easy. Microwave cooking needs no fat for preparation, and electric grilling helps remove fat from meats. Cook and serve small portions of food for meals. The temptation to overeat may be removed.

20. *Learn low-Calorie foods.* Learn what foods are low in Calories in each of the six food exchanges and incorporate those palatable to you in your diet. Learn to substitute low-Calorie foods for high-Calorie ones. The key to a lifelong weight-maintenance diet is your knowledge of sound nutritional principles and the application of this knowledge to the design of your personal diet. Knowledge, however, is not the total answer; your behavior should reflect your knowledge. You may know that whole milk contains about 60 more Calories per glass than skim milk, but if you cannot switch, then the advantage of your knowledge is lost in this instance. Sometimes making changes in small steps helps, such as first switching from whole to low-fat milk, and then to skim milk. Appendix H contains many *Small Steps* that may help facilitate various healthful dietary transitions.

How can I plan a nutritionally balanced, low-Calorie diet?

The key to a sound diet for weight loss is nutrient density, or the selection of low-Calorie, high-nutrient foods. The 20 points addressed in the previous section represent important guidelines to implement such a diet. Table 11.10 presents a suggested meal pattern based on the Food Exchange System. The foods should be selected from the food exchange lists found in appendix E. You may use the form shown in the next column as a guide.

The total caloric values are close approximations for a three-meal pattern. If you decide to include snacks in your diet, such as a fruit or vegetable, then remove each snack from one of the main meals. The salads should contain vegetables with negligible Calories, such as lettuce and radishes. Note that under the exchange system, starchy vegetables such as potatoes are included in the starch group because their caloric content is similar. The beverages, other than milk and fruit juice, should contain no Calories. Although you may drink as many noncaloric beverages as you wish over the course of the day, drinking at least one at each

Calories: _____

Meal	Number of servings	Calories per serving	Total Calories	Foods selected
Breakfast				
Milk, skim		90		
Meat, very lean		35		
Fruit		60		
Vegetable		25		
Starch		80		
Fat		45		
Beverage		0		
Lunch				
Milk, skim		90		
Meat, very lean		35		
Fruit		60		
Vegetable		25		
Salad		20		
Starch		80		
Fat		45		
Beverage		0		
Dinner				
Milk, skim		90		
Meat, very lean		35		
Fruit		60		
Vegetable		25		
Salad		20		
Starch		80		
Fat		45		
Beverage		0		

meal will help provide a feeling of satiation and may help suppress the appetite somewhat.

Although only seven levels of caloric intake are presented in table 11.10, you may adjust it according to your needs by simply adding or subtracting appropriate food exchanges. For example, if you wanted a 1,700-Calorie diet, you could subtract one starch exchange and one-half fat exchange (about 100 Calories) from the 1,800-Calorie diet.

After you have determined the number of Calories you need daily, select the appropriate diet plan from table 11.10. To help implement your diet plan and to keep day-to-day track of the food exchanges you eat, you should design a 3″ × 5″ card similar to the model below for the number of food exchanges in your daily diet. As you consume an exchange at each meal, simply cross it off on the card. Make a new card for each day. The model shown is for 1,500 Calories. The total exchanges are summed from table 11.10.

TABLE 11.10 Suggested daily meal pattern based on the Food Exchange System

	Approximate daily caloric intake						
	1,000	1,200	1,500	1,800	2,000	2,200	2,500
Breakfast							
Milk, skim	1	1	1	1	1	1	1
Meat, very lean	1	1	2	2	2	3	3
Starch	1	2	2	3	3	3	3
Fruit	1	1	1	1	2	2	2
Fat	0	0	1	1	1	2	2
Beverage	1	1	1	1	1	1	1
Lunch							
Milk, skim	1	1	1	1	1	1	2
Meat, very lean	2	2	2	3	3	3	4
Starch	2	2	2	2	2	3	3
Vegetable	1	1	2	2	2	2	2
Salad	1	1	1	1	1	1	1
Fruit	1	2	2	2	2	2	2
Fat	½	½	1	2	2	2	2
Beverage	1	1	1	1	1	1	1
Dinner							
Milk, skim	0	0	0	1	1	1	1
Meat, very lean	2	2	3	3	3	4	4
Starch	2	2	3	3	4	4	5
Vegetable	1	2	2	2	2	2	3
Salad	1	1	1	1	1	1	1
Fruit	0	0	1	2	2	2	3
Fat	½	1	1	1	2	2	2
Beverage	1	1	1	1	1	1	1
Totals							
Milk, skim	2	2	2	3	3	3	4
Meat, very lean	5	5	7	8	8	10	11
Starch	5	6	7	8	9	10	11
Vegetable	2	3	4	4	4	4	5
Salad	2	2	2	2	2	2	2
Fruit	2	3	4	5	6	6	7
Fat	1	2	3	4	5	6	6
Beverage	3	3	3	3	3	3	3

Key points
1. Caloric values:
    Milk exchange, skim = 90
    Meat exchange, very lean = 35
    Fruit exchange = 60
    Vegetable exchange = 25
    Starch exchange = 80
    Fat exchange = 45
    Beverage = 0
    Salad = 20
2. See appendix E for a listing of foods in each exchange. Note the following:
    a. Foods other than milk, such as yogurt, are included in the milk exchange.
    b. The meat list includes foods such as eggs, cheese, fish, and poultry; low-fat legumes, like beans and peas, may be considered as meat substitutes.
    c. Some starchy vegetables are included in the bread list.
3. Foods should not be fried or prepared in fat unless you count the added fat as a fat exchange. Broil or bake foods instead.
4. Low-Calorie vegetables like lettuce and radishes should be used in the salads. Use only small amounts of very-low-Calorie salad dressing.
5. Beverages should contain no Calories.

Daily meal plan   **1,500 Calories**

Milk exchange, skim	(2)	1 2
Meat exchange, very lean	(7)	1 2 3 4 5 6 7
Starch exchange	(6)	1 2 3 4 5 6 7
Vegetable exchange	(3)	1 2 3 4
Salads	(2)	1 2
Fruit exchange	(4)	1 2 3 4
Fat exchange	(2)	1 2 3
Beverages	(3)	1 2 3

Keep in mind that this is not a rigid diet plan. At a minimum you should have 2 skim milk exchanges, 5 very lean meat exchanges, 5 starch exchanges, 2–3 vegetable exchanges, and 2–3 fruit exchanges. Once you have guaranteed these minimum requirements, you may do some substitution between the various exchanges so long as you keep the total caloric content within range of your goals. For example, you may delete 2 starch exchanges (160 Calories) in the model and substitute 1 skim milk and 2 very lean meat exchanges (160 Calories). You may also shift a limited number of the exchanges from one meal to another.

If you prefer a more substantial breakfast and a lighter lunch, simply shift some of the exchanges from lunch to breakfast.

It may be a good idea to take a little time and construct a diet for yourself, using the following guidelines for your calculations. Use the form on page 483. Table 11.11 presents an example of a 1,500-Calorie diet based on the Food Exchange System.

1. Calculate the number of Calories you want per day. See pages 470–471 for guidelines.
2. Use table 11.10 to determine how many servings you need from each food exchange.
3. Multiply the number of servings by the Calories per serving to get the total Calories. Add the total Calories column to get total daily intake.
4. Select appropriate foods from the exchange list in appendix E.

One final point: If your diet contains less than 1,600 Calories, it would be wise to take a daily vitamin/mineral supplement with the RDA for all essential vitamins and key minerals.

The purpose of planning your own diet plan is to familiarize yourself with the caloric and nutrient content of the majority of

TABLE 11.11 A 1,500-Calorie diet based on the Food Exchange System

Exchange	Number of servings	Calories per exchange	Total calories	Foods selected
Breakfast				
Meat, very lean	2	35	70	1 ounce very lean ham and
Fat	1	45	45	1 ounce low-fat cheese melted on
Starch	2	80	160	2 pieces whole-grain toasted bread
Fruit	1	60	60	4 ounces orange juice
Beverage	1	0	0	1 cup coffee with noncaloric sweetener
Lunch				
Milk, low-fat	1	120	120	8 ounces plain, low-fat yogurt
Fruit	1	60	60	with cut-up fresh fruit (1/2 banana)
Meat, very lean	2	35	70	2 ounces turkey breast on
Starch	2	80	160	whole-grain bun
Vegetable	1	25	25	1 carrot
Salad	1	20	20	lettuce with
Fat	1	45	45	low-Calorie dressing
Beverage	1	0	0	diet cola
Dinner				
Milk, skim	1	90	90	1/2 cup ice milk
Meat, very lean	3	35	105	3 ounces broiled fish
Starch	3	80	240	1 baked potato and 1 slice whole wheat bread
Vegetable	3	25	75	1 1/2 cups steamed broccoli and cauliflower
Salad	1	20	20	cucumbers
Fat	1	45	45	small amount of margarine for potato and low-Calorie dressing for salad
Fruit	2	60	120	1 banana cut up on ice milk
Beverage	1	0	0	iced tea
TOTAL			1,530	

foods that constitute your diet. You can plan your diet manually, or with computer-based programs if preferred. For example, the ChooseMyPlate program permits you to develop a personalized diet; an example of a 2,000-Calorie diet is presented in appendix I. Other computerized diet plans are available, such as the following:

www.shapeup.org This program from Shape Up America provides you with a diet plan, labeled the Cyberkitchen, to balance your diet and physical activity to lose weight. Moreover, various diet plans are compatible for use with your cell phone. Simply *Google* the terms *diet plan cell phone* to review those applications (apps) available.

Are very-low-Calorie diets effective and desirable as a means to lose body weight?

As noted in chapter 10, very-low-Calorie diets (VLCDs) are defined technically as containing less than 800 Calories per day and are often referred to as modified fasts. In some medical institutions, total fasting programs are used. Under proper medical supervision, such diets are generally regarded as safe and have been effective in inducing rapid weight losses in very obese patients. However, VLCD are not recommended for the individual who wants to lose 10–20 pounds or for the individual who is not under medical supervision, not only because of the possible adverse health consequences as noted in chapter 10, but also because VLCD may be counterproductive to the ultimate goal of long-term weight loss. They do not satisfy the criteria for a recommended weight-loss program for individuals who are not medically supervised and they often lead to weight cycling.

It is recommended that any individual contemplating the use of VLCD should consult a physician and a dietitian.

Are weight-loss dietary supplements effective and safe?

Numerous over-the-counter and Internet-sales dietary supplements are marketed as weight-loss agents, using marketing ploys such as *Lose 30 Pounds in 30 Days Without Dieting or Exercising* or *Lose Belly Fat and Gain Muscle While You Sleep*. Some weight-loss dietary supplements consist of essential nutrients, such as carnitine and chromium. However, as noted in chapters 5 and 8, research does not support the efficacy of either carnitine or chromium supplementation as a means to lose body fat or gain muscle mass. Most weight-loss supplements are herbals, extracts, or metabolites, such as caffeine, synephrine, green tea catechins, guarana, conjugated linoleic acid, and others. Such products are classified as dietary supplements rather than drugs and thus need not undergo extensive clinical testing to document efficacy before they can appear in the marketplace.

Weight-loss dietary supplements are theorized to induce weight loss by several mechanisms. One is to induce a sensation of satiety and suppress the appetite, another is to stimulate fat oxidation and thermogenesis. For example, yohimbine is thought to suppress appetite by blocking receptors in the brain, whereas caffeine may stimulate thermogenesis through fat oxidation. Most research has focused on herbals or other supplements that promote thermogenesis. In their review, Hursel and Westerterp-Plantenga indicated that caffeine, capsaicin, and green tea may increase energy expenditure by 4 to 5 percent and fat oxidation by 10 to 16 percent, and thus may help in preventing weight gain.

Caffeine, which is covered in detail in chapter 13, is a stimulant drug found in many popular beverages, particularly coffee and tea. Caffeine is also found in many weight-loss dietary supplements and is found naturally in guarana and yerba mate, two herbals marketed for weight loss. Green tea contains a combination of caffeine and catechins, a combination marketed for weight control. As noted in chapter 13, caffeine use may stimulate metabolism and may play a small beneficial role in weight control. Heckman and others also reported a link between caffeine use and weight loss, with a consequent reduction of the overall risks for developing the metabolic syndrome. In addition, Rains and others noted that green tea catechins, like caffeine, may influence the sympathetic nervous system, increasing energy expenditure and fat oxidation. However, in a meta-analysis of 15 studies, Phung and others concluded that although green tea catechins with caffeine did reduce body weight and waist circumference, the clinical significance of these reductions was modest at best. Moreover, they also noted that the data do not suggest an independent effect of catechins. In general, research supports a modest effect of caffeine, either alone or combined with catechins, on weight loss, but additional research is warranted.

Other related herbal stimulants have been studied as a means to induce weight loss. Ma huang, or *Ephedra sinica,* contains ephedrine, a stimulant drug. Ephedrine is also covered in detail in chapter 13. Although ephedrine was marketed as a weight-loss dietary supplement, it was removed from the marketplace in 2006 because its use was associated with serious health problems. Ephedrine-based products have since been replaced with synephrine, also known as *bitter orange,* which is also a stimulant chemically similar to ephedrine. However, as noted in chapter 13, research does not appear to support a beneficial effect of synephrine supplementation on weight loss. Moreover, as noted later, use of synephrine may be associated with health risks.

Numerous other herbals and extracts, such as ginseng, yohimbine, and *Garcinia cambogia* have been studied for their effect on weight loss, but research that evaluates their efficacy is very limited. Rader and others noted that the U.S. market for botanical dietary supplements has grown so rapidly that use of new botanical ingredients has often outpaced an adequate scientific understanding of the ingredients themselves. However, Egras and others, in a review of such dietary supplements used for weight loss, concluded that to date there is little clinical evidence to support their use, and also indicated that more data are necessary to determine the efficacy and safety of these supplements.

The safety of weight-loss dietary supplements has been a concern. Although Heckman and others indicate that moderate caffeine consumption is considered safe and its use as a food ingredient has been approved, within certain limits, by numerous regulatory agencies around the world, its use may increase health risks for some, such as individuals with hypertension or women who are pregnant, as discussed in chapter 13.

Other stimulant supplements may pose significant health risks. As noted earlier, ephedrine was once a very popular weight-loss supplement, but its use was associated with numerous health problems. More recently, Rossato and others reported that the growing use of synephrine has raised concerns, as it has been accompanied by reports of adverse cardiac effects, including hypertension, angina, ventricular fibrillation, myocardial infarction, and sudden death. They note that the mechanisms involved in synephrine-induced cardiotoxicity are still unknown, because studies related to its safety are scarce. In a related vein, Kearney and others reported a substantial increase in the prevalence of adverse effects associated with herbal products containing yohimbine, and questioned whether yohimbine should continue to be considered a safe dietary supplement. Moreover, in 2009 the FDA removed Hydroxycut products—popular weight-loss dietary supplements—from the market because their use was associated with serious liver damage.

Contamination of dietary supplements may contribute to such health problems. As noted in chapter 2, dietary supplements are not subject to the same quality control as drugs and food. For example, Meadows indicates that some products made overseas and sold on the Internet may contain prescription drug ingredients; some diet pills contain the active ingredients found in antidepressant or anxiolytic drugs, such as Prozac and Librium, or stimulants comparable to amphetamine. Such potent drugs may increase health risks. Moreover, athletes who use weight-loss supplements in conjunction with their sport may consume products containing drugs whose use is prohibited in competition or training, and may be suspended from competition for a positive drug test.

www.fda.gov Type "Weight loss products" in the search box for updated information on dietary supplements for weight loss.

www.ods.od.nih.gov Click on *Dietary Supplement Fact Sheets* to get information on a specific dietary supplement.

Some organizations, such as U.S. Pharmacopeia (USP) may place a seal on the supplement label indicating that the product has been treated for purity and quality. However, the seal does not guarantee that the product will be effective as advertised.

Is it harmful to overeat occasionally?

Most of us occasionally overindulge in food, particularly on holidays and other festive occasions or when we dine at all-you-can-eat restaurants. Eating is a pleasurable activity, and an occasional pig-out is not harmful, as long as it does not become a habit. As noted in chapter 5, try to avoid high-fat meals if you are prone to cardiovascular disease, because such meals may increase the risk of heart attacks. After a very large meal, you may step on the scale the next day and find that you have gained 5 pounds or more. Not to worry. Most of that weight is water, which may be bound to the increased carbohydrate (glycogen stores) in your body. Additionally, if the meal was high in sodium, your extracellular water stores will also increase. Going back to your regular diet and exercise program will reduce these water stores in a day or so, and your body weight will return to normal.

It is important to recognize that occasional overeating may be a lapse in your diet and that you treat it as such. Renew your commitment to your weight-loss plan and prevent the occasional lapse from becoming a relapse.

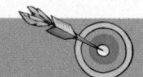

Key Concepts

▶ Rapid loss of body weight, which may occur during the early stages of dieting, is due primarily to body-water changes. The rate at which weight loss occurs will slow down as your body weight decreases, for then body-fat stores are the prime source of weight loss and necessitate a greater caloric deficit.

▶ Numerous weight-loss diet plans are available, including low-fat diets, low-carbohydrate diets, and high-protein diets. All may be effective and safe if the daily caloric energy intake is less than the daily caloric energy expenditure. The DASH and Omni-Heart diets may be highly recommended for weight control, as may a healthful Mediterranean diet.

▶ Counting Calories and grams of fat may be a useful technique during the early stages of a diet, for the more knowledge you have about the caloric and nutrient content of foods, the better equipped you are to make wise selections.

▶ The key principle of dieting is to select from among the six food exchanges low-Calorie, high-nutrient foods that appeal to your taste and are easily incorporated into your daily lifestyle.

▶ Very-low-Calorie diets (VLCD) may be effective for weight loss under strict medical supervision, but are not recommended for the average individual trying to lose some excess fat.

▶ In general, weight-loss dietary supplements do not appear to be effective, and their use may be associated with adverse health effects.

Check for Yourself

▶ Using the Food Exchange System, plan a balanced, healthy diet of 1,600 Calories for an individual who needs to consume this much to lose excess body fat.

▶ Go to a local health food store and ask the clerk for weight-loss products. Check those available and determine the active ingredient in each. How many contain various herbals or caffeine? Alternatively, ask only for those with herbals or herbals with caffeine (guarana), and inquire about the safety of each. Compare your findings to the text discussion.

Exercise Programs

In their review of interactions between genes and physical activity, Rankinen and Bouchard noted considerable research indicating that the level of physical activity plays a role in the risk of excessive weight gain, in weight-loss programs, and particularly in the prevention of weight regain. This section highlights the development of an exercise program to help prevent weight gain, promote weight loss, and maintain a healthy body weight. The following government Websites provide information on exercise and weight loss for Canadians and Americans.

What role does exercise play in weight reduction and weight maintenance?

Humans are meticulously designed for physical activity, and yet our modern mechanical age has eliminated many of the opportunities that our ancient ancestors had to incorporate moderate physical activity as a natural part of daily living. The regulation of our food intake has not adapted to the highly mechanized conditions in today's society. As discussed in chapter 10, physical inactivity may be one of the major contributing factors to the development and maintenance of obesity. For example, a sedentary lifestyle, principally TV watching, has been significantly associated with obesity in adolescents and adults. Indeed, the late Dr. Jean Mayer, an international authority on weight control, reported that no single factor is more frequently responsible for obesity than lack of physical exercise.

There are basically two ways you can become more physically active and increase your total daily energy expenditure. First, decrease the amount of time that you are physically inactive, particularly time watching television. Robinson noted that most studies support the suggestion that reducing television viewing may help to reduce the risk for obesity or help promote weight loss in obese children. The same thinking applies to adults as well. In general, you want to increase your level of nonexercise activity themogenesis (NEAT). Keep moving throughout the day; walk rather than ride, don't sit when you can stand; and keep moving, or fidget, when you have to sit. In one study, researchers followed lean and mildly obese people for 10 days, and found that the obese subjects remained seated for about 2.5 hours longer per day than the lean individuals, which could result in more than 300 fewer Calories expended daily.

Second, start a planned exercise program. The Consumers Union noted that to slim down permanently, you need to make a lifelong commitment to regular exercise, including not only aerobic exercise to burn Calories, but also strength (resistance) training to build or at least preserve muscle.

Resistance Exercise Training   Resistance-training, or weight-training, programs are detailed in chapter 12 in relation to gaining body weight as muscle mass, but such programs may also be very helpful during weight-loss programs. One possibility, as suggested by the American College of Sports Medicine, is that increased strength through resistance training may lead to a more active lifestyle in sedentary overweight and obese individuals, thus leading to health benefits that may include weight loss and prevention of weight regain. Another possibility is maintenance of REE during weight loss. Poehlman and Melby noted that although resistance training may increase the metabolic rate during exercise, its effects on regulation of body weight appear to be mediated primarily by its effects on body composition rather than by the direct energy costs of the resistance exercise. Recall that protein tissue, primarily muscle, may be lost along with body fat during a weight-reduction program. However, resistance training may stimulate muscular development and help prevent significant decreases in lean body mass. Such an effect may also help prevent decreases in the REE. Additionally, as is noted in chapter 12 the typical resistance-training workout does not burn many Calories, mainly because of frequent recovery periods; however, dynamic circuit-type resistance-training programs may also be used to burn additional Calories.

Aerobic Exercise   Exercise burns Calories (figure 11.6). The primary function of aerobic exercise in a weight-control program is simply to increase the level of energy expenditure and help tip the caloric equation so that energy output is greater than energy input. As mentioned in chapter 3, the metabolic rate may be increased tremendously during aerobic exercise. For example, while the average person may expend only 60–70 Calories per hour during rest, this value may approach 1,000 Calories per hour during a sustained high-level activity such as rapid walking, running, swimming, or bicycling. Athletes involved in extreme endurance events, such as the Tour de France, and ultradistance runners, such as Yannis Kouros, have been reported to consume between 6,000 and 13,000 Calories per day.

If you are overweight, the same amount of aerobic weight-bearing exercise will cost you more Calories than your leaner counterpart. Because you have more weight to move, you will expend more energy and lose more body fat in the long run. For example, the energy cost of jogging 1 mile would be about 70 Calories for the 100-pound individual and about 140 Calories for someone twice that weight. Figure 11.7 depicts this concept graphically for one type of exercise—walking.

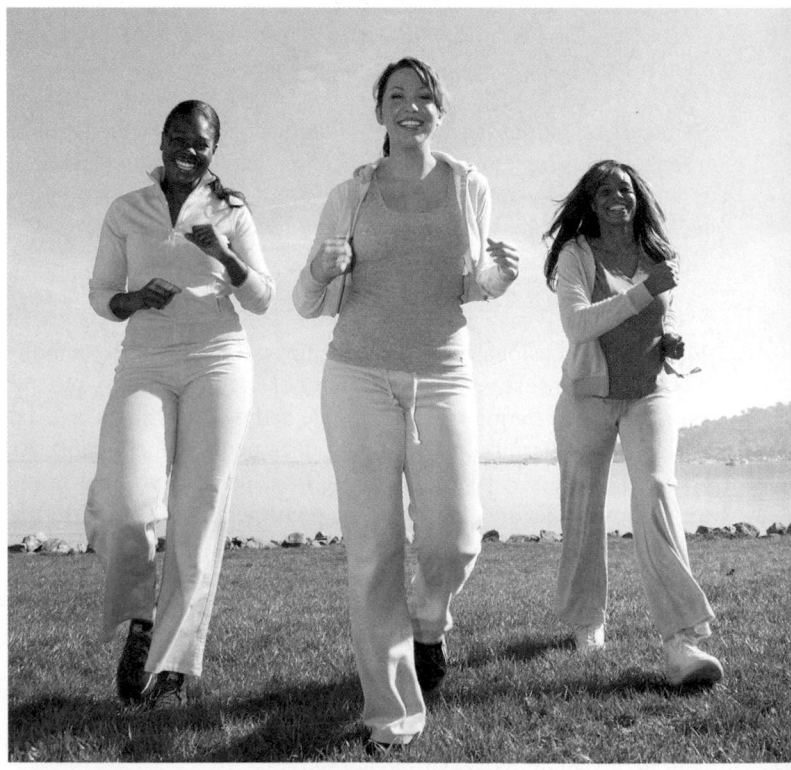

FIGURE 11.6   Exercise can be an effective means of increasing energy expenditure and losing excess Calories.

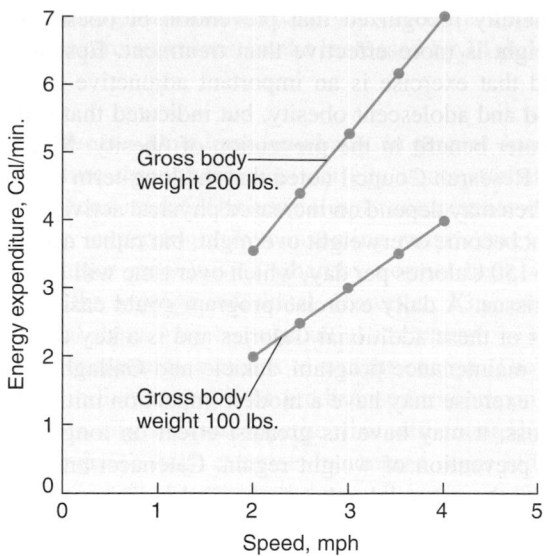

FIGURE 11.7 Effect of speed (mph) and gross body weight (lbs) on energy expenditure (Calories/minute) of walking. The heavier the individual, the greater the expenditure of Calories for any given speed of walking. The same would be true for running and other physical activities in which the body must be moved by foot.

From *Textbook of Work Physiology* by P. O. Astrand and K. Rodahl. Copyright © 1977 McGraw-Hill Book Company. Used with the permission of McGraw-Hill Book Company.

One major misconception may deter many individuals from initiating an exercise program for weight control. They believe that exercise is a poor means to lose body weight because it expends so few Calories. For example, they have heard that you have to jog about 35 miles to lose a pound of body fat. Because the average-sized male uses approximately 100 Calories per mile of jogging, and because 1 pound of body fat contains about 3,500 Calories, there is some truth to that statement. However, you must look at the **long-haul concept** of weight control (figure 11.8). Jogging about 2 miles a day will expend about 6,000 Calories in a month, accounting for almost 2 pounds of body fat. Over 6 to 8 months or longer, the weight loss may be substantial provided the individual does not compensate by consuming more Calories.

In addition to the direct effect of increased energy output during exercise, exercise has been theorized to facilitate weight loss by other means. As noted in chapter 3, aerobic exercise may increase the REE during the period immediately following the exercise bout and may also increase the thermic effect of food (TEF) if you exercise after eating a meal. Unfortunately, the magnitude of this increased REE or TEF is relatively minor and not considered to be of any practical importance in a weight-loss program. Related to the TEF, it does not matter if you exercise before or after a light meal, although as noted in the following text, exercise before a meal may help curb the appetite.

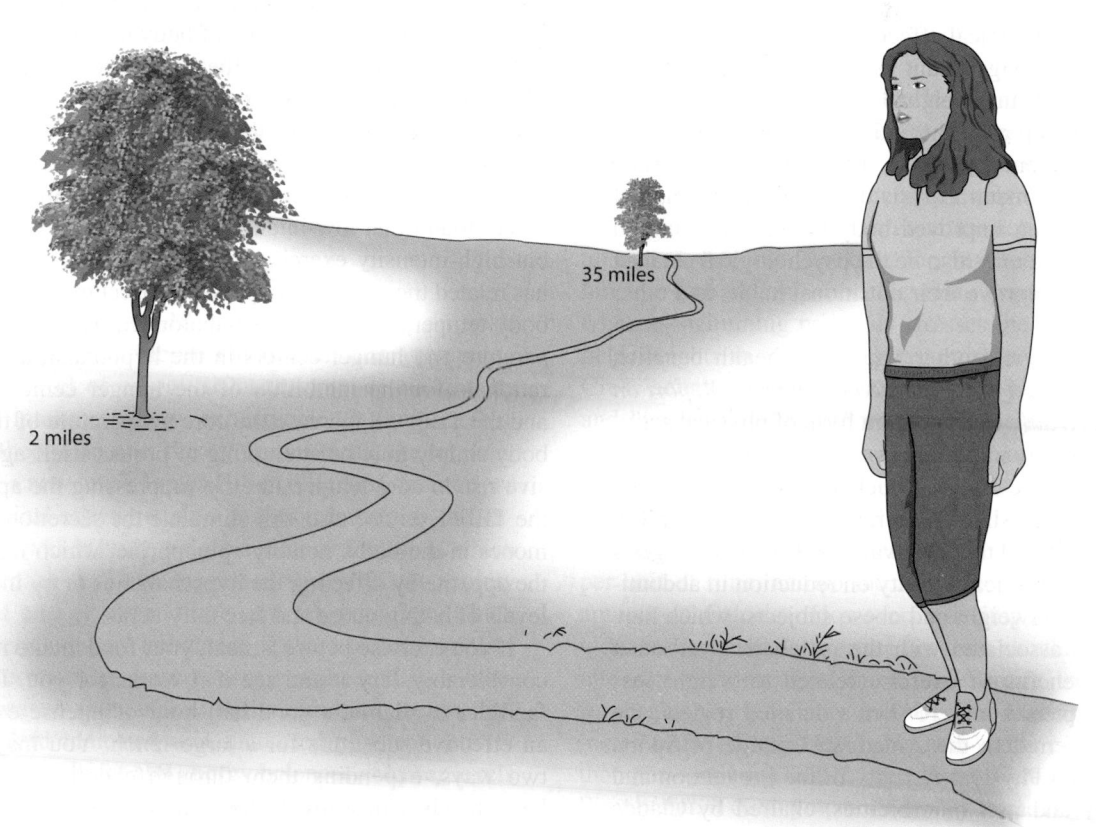

FIGURE 11.8 To lose body fat by exercising, you must look at the long-haul concept of weight control. The average-weight individual needs to jog about 35 miles to burn off 1 pound of body fat. This would be nearly impossible for most of us to do in 1 day. At 2 miles per day, however, it could be done in about 2 1/2 weeks—and at 5 miles per day, in only 1 week. Even though it takes time, an exercise program is a very effective approach to reducing excess body fat.

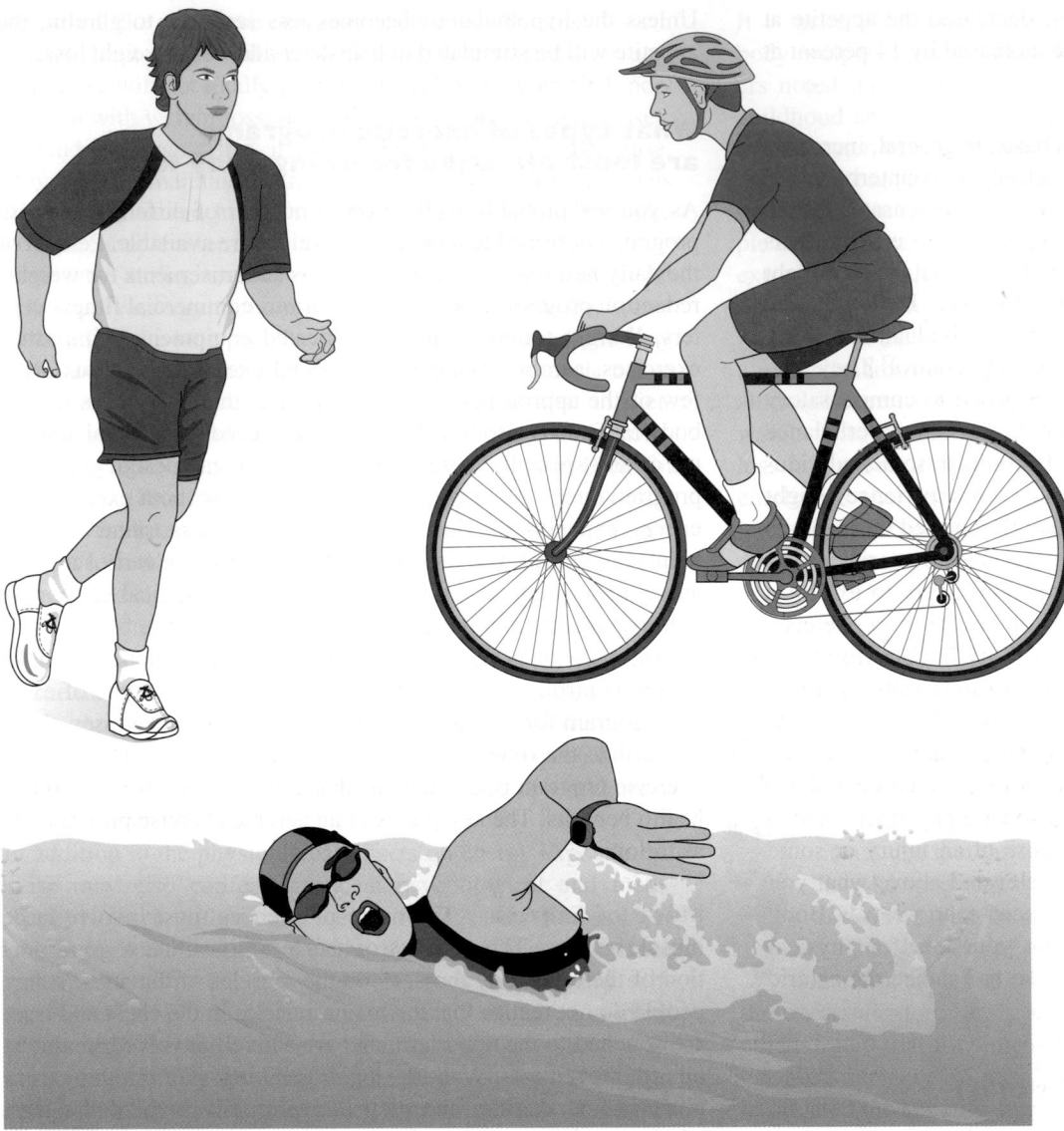

2. The figures in the table are only for the time you are performing the activity. For example, in an hour of basketball, you may exercise strenuously only for 35–40 minutes, as you may take time-outs and may rest during foul shots. In general, record only the amount of time that you are actually moving during the activity.

3. The figures may give you some guidelines to total energy expenditure, but actual caloric costs might vary somewhat according to such factors as skill level, environmental factors (running against the wind or up hills), and so forth.

4. Not all body weights could be listed, but you can approximate by going to the closest weight listed.

5. There may be small differences between men and women, but not enough to make a marked difference in the total caloric value for most exercises.

Appendix B or table 3.6 on page 108 may be useful to determine which types of activities may be of the appropriate intensity for your weight-control program. Listing those activities with higher caloric expenditure per minute may suggest several that you could blend into your lifestyle. Several Websites can provide you with an estimate of caloric expenditure in a wide variety of physical activities.

FIGURE 11.9 Aerobic-mode exercises—such as running, bicycling, or swimming—must involve large muscle groups.

are interrelated, but for burning the most total Calories, duration becomes more important, and the intensity must be adapted for the amount of time you plan to exercise.

To get an idea of exercises with high intensity, check appendix B for Calorie cost per minute relative to your body weight. It is a composite table of a wide variety of individual reports in the literature. When using this appendix, keep these points in mind.

1. The figures are approximate and include the resting metabolic rate. Thus, the total cost of the exercise includes not only the energy expended by the exercise itself, but also the amount you would have used anyway during the same period. Suppose you ran for 1 hour and the calculated energy cost was 800 Calories. During that same time at rest you may have expended 75 Calories, so the net cost of the exercise is 725 Calories.

http://www.primusweb.com/fitnesspartner Enter your body weight and the amount of time you exercise and this program will provide you with your caloric expenditure for more than 200 physical activities.

http://sites.google.com/site/compendiumofphysicalactities
The Compendium of Physical Activities, revised by Barbara Ainsworth and her associates in 2011, provides energy expenditure for more than 800 physical activities. The intensity of the activity is provided in MET values, and you may recall that one MET is your resting energy expenditure. You may review chapter 3 to convert METS to caloric expenditure.

Duration of Exercise Probably the most important factor in total energy expenditure is the duration of the exercise. In swimming, bicycling, running, or walking, distance is the key. For example, running a mile will cost the average-sized individual about 100 Calories. Five miles would approximate 500 Calories. An individual running 1 mile a day would take more than 1 month to expend the caloric equivalent of 1 pound of fat, whereas running 5 miles a day would shorten the time span to about 1 week. Thus, if the purpose of the exercise program is to lose weight, the individual should stress the **duration concept.** In their review, Catenacci and Wyatt reported that subjects lost substantially more weight in studies that prescribed greater amounts of exercise. For example, Tate and others found that over the course of 18 months, subjects who were encouraged to expend 2,500 Calories or more weekly lost significantly more weight than those who were encouraged to expend the standard 1,000 Calories weekly. At the end of 30 months, subjects who continued to expend 2,500 Calories or more weekly lost approximately 25 more pounds than those who exercised less.

One of the key points about the duration concept is the notion of distance traveled rather than time. For example, tennis and running are both good exercises. However, the runner will expend considerably more Calories in an hour than the tennis player because the activity involved in running is continuous. The tennis player has a number of rest periods in which the energy expenditure is lower. Consequently, at the end of an hour's activity, the runner may have expended two to three times as many Calories as the tennis player. A similar comparison can be made between runners and walkers.

If you cannot find a big block of time, such as 40 minutes, to do your exercise, then try to incorporate more frequent short bouts of exercise throughout the day. Do more *exercise snacks.* Several studies by Jakicic and Murphy and their associates reported that exercising in multiple short bouts per day, such as four 10-minute bouts, was just as effective as a single 40-minute bout in producing weight loss and improving cardiovascular fitness over a 20-week period. If your day is filled with other activities, try to squeeze in some short exercise bouts such as brisk walking, possibly before breakfast, during morning and afternoon work breaks, and before or after lunch and dinner. This strategy may increase adherence to your exercise program, and it may also help your study or work productivity by providing a psychological pick-me-up during the day.

A major reason many adults do not use exercise as a weight-loss mechanism is that their level of physical fitness is so low they cannot sustain a moderate level of exercise intensity for very long. However, keep in mind that as you continue to train, your body will begin to adapt so that in time you will be able to exercise for longer and longer periods.

Additionally, intensity and duration are interrelated, and if balanced, will result in equal weight losses. Melanson and others found that compared to a sedentary day, expending 400 Calories during exercise intensities of 40 and 70 percent of VO_2 max increased 24-hour energy expenditure, but there was no difference attributed to exercise intensity. Grediagin and others also found no significant difference in body-fat losses when women engaged in either high-intensity or low-intensity exercise, provided the total caloric expenditure per exercise session was the same. In both cases, it simply took the low-intensity exercise group longer to expend the same amount of Calories. However, in a study controlling total exercise energy expenditure in both exercise tasks, Irving and others reported that high-intensity exercise was more effective than low-intensity exercise as a means to reduce total abdominal fat. As you improve your fitness level, Hunter recommends incorporating some higher-intensity exercise in your program, not only because it burns Calories more rapidly, but also because it will make your moderate-intensity workouts seem much easier. Additionally, as noted in chapter 1 and later in this chapter, additional health benefits may be associated with higher-intensity exercise.

Frequency of Exercise **Exercise frequency** complements duration and intensity. Frequency of exercise refers to how often each week you participate. As would appear obvious, the more often you exercise, the greater the total weekly caloric expenditure. In general, three to four times per week would be satisfactory, provided duration and intensity were adequate, but six to seven times would just about double your caloric output. A daily exercise program is recommended if weight control is the primary goal.

Enjoyment of Exercise An important factor is enjoyment of the exercise. For an activity to be effective in the long run, it should be one that you enjoy, yet one that will help expend Calories because it has a recommended intensity level, can be performed for a long time, or both. For example, you may not enjoy jogging or running, so other activities may be substituted. Fast walking with vigorous arm action, golf (pulling a cart), swimming, bicycling, tennis, handball, racquetball, aerobic dancing, and a variety of other activities may produce a greater feeling of enjoyment and still burn a considerable number of Calories. Even leisure activities and home chores done vigorously, such as gardening, yard work, washing the car, and home repairs, may be useful in burning Calories and developing fitness. Exercise need not be unpleasant. Enjoy your exercise. Try to make it a lifelong habit by viewing it as play. Next time you vacuum the house or mow the lawn, try to think about it as a good workout rather than work.

Practicality of Exercise Practicality is another important factor. You may enjoy swimming, tennis, racquetball, soccer, and a variety of other sports, but lack of facilities, poor weather conditions, no playing partners, or high costs may limit your ability to participate. For the active person who travels, this may be a major concern. You probably have noticed by now that an underlying bias toward walking and running exists throughout this book. It is probably because, to the authors, they satisfy all the previously mentioned criteria necessary for maintaining proper body weight. Moreover, they are very practical activities. All you need is a good pair of shoes and proper clothes for the weather, so nothing short of an injury should deter you from your daily exercise routine. Walking, jogging, or running can be very practical substitutes on those days when you cannot participate in your regular physical activity. The late Peter Wood, an esteemed researcher at Stanford University, indicated that brisk walking is perhaps the best single exercise in regard to energy expenditure, feasibility, and acceptability to a large proportion of the population; for those who are physically unfit, overweight, or elderly, it is probably the best choice of exercise. Some guidelines to an effective walking program are presented later.

Indoor exercise equipment is also very practical for a number of reasons. For example, it can be used while watching children, avoiding inclement weather, or doing two things at one time, such as reading or watching television news. This is a highly recommended way to watch television. Numerous types of aerobic indoor exercise equipment are available, such as bicycling apparatus, cross-country skiing simulators, rowing machines, stair-steppers, and treadmills. Computerized fitness programs, such as Wii Fit, can provide a strenuous indoor workout. All can provide an aerobic workout, but in their study Zeni and others reported that the treadmill is the optimal indoor exercise machine for enhancing energy expenditure at a set rating of perceived exertion. Resistance- or strength-training indoor equipment is also available. *Consumer Reports* magazine offers periodic analyses of various types of indoor exercise equipment. Indoor exercise equipment can be expensive. If expense is a concern, a total of about $100 may purchase an array of inexpensive equipment, such as elastic bands, dumbbells, an exercise mat, a stability ball, and DVDs with various aerobic exercise routines.

Versatility of Exercise Versatility is also an important factor. Learn and engage in a variety of physical activities, such as running, cycling, swimming, rowing on stationary machines, stair climbing, striding on elliptical trainers, aerobic dancing, and aerobic walking. By cross-training, such as running 3 days per week, cycling 2 days, and swimming 2 days, you are less likely to become bored with exercise or to sustain overuse injuries. Also, if you plan to exercise for an hour daily, one-half hour each of running and cycling, or some other combination of exercises, is also an effective way to cross-train. Moreover, if you become injured and cannot do your favorite type of exercise, you may be able to expend Calories and maintain fitness by using alternative exercises until you heal. For example, if weight-bearing activities such as jogging bother you, do nonweight-bearing activities such as cycling or swimming, or water-jogging wearing a buoyancy vest.

If I am inactive now, should I see a physician before I initiate an exercise program?

Various medical groups, such as the American College of Sports Medicine and the American Heart Association, have developed guidelines to determine who should receive a medical exam prior to initiating an exercise program. A thorough review of these guidelines is not presented here because they are extensive and beyond the scope of this text. However, the following points represent a synthesis of these guidelines.

1. Before initiating any exercise program, you should be aware of any personal medical problems that possibly could be aggravated. If you have concern about any facet of your health, check with your physician before starting an exercise program. This is especially important in weight-reduction exercise programs where the main stress is placed on the heart and blood vessels, the cardiovascular system.
2. No matter what your age, if you have any of the coronary heart disease risk factors noted in table 11.12, you should have a medical examination. You may also wish to assess your cardiac risk profile at the American Heart Association's Website.
3. If you are young (twenties or early thirties), healthy, and have no risk factors, it is probably safe to initiate an exercise program.
4. The older you are, the better the idea to get a medical examination. In fact, it is prudent for those over 40 to have an examination.

www.amhrt.org To determine your cardiac risk profile at the American Heart Association Website, type *Heart Attack Risk Assessment* in the search box.

What other precautions would be advisable before I start an exercise program?

Your initial level of physical fitness is an important determinant of the intensity of exercise during the early stages of the program. If you are completely unconditioned, you should start at a lower intensity level—walk before you jog, for example. Keep in mind that it took time for you to gain weight and become unconditioned, so it will also take time to reverse the process. A gradual progression is the key point. Examples are presented later.

Other general precautions involve safety factors, timing of meals, environmental hazards, and equipment. The individual should adhere to safety principles for the activity selected, particularly swimming, bicycling, and pedestrian safety. Strenuous

TABLE 11.12 Major and predisposing risk factors associated with coronary heart disease
1. High blood pressure
2. Cigarette smoking
3. Dyslipidaemia (High LDL-cholesterol; Low HDL-cholesterol)
4. Impaired fasting blood glucose
5. Obesity
6. Family history of coronary heart disease
7. Sedentary lifestyle/physical inactivity

Sources: Data from American College of Sports Medicine, ACSM's *Guidelines for Exercise Testing and Prescription*, 7th ed., 2005.

Note: Normal serum cholesterol or normal blood pressure may still be counted as a risk factor if medications are taken for its control.

exercise should not be undertaken within 2 or 3 hours of a heavy meal, but may be done earlier with a light meal or just liquids. As noted in chapter 9, a hot environment poses the most serious threat to the person in training. Be aware of signs of heat stress such as dizziness, nausea, and weakness. If these occur, stop exercising and find a means to help cool your body. Proper equipment should be selected for the chosen activity. For example, of critical importance to the jogger or walker is a well-designed pair of shoes. They may help prevent certain medical problems, such as tendinitis and shin splints, which may occur during the early stages of training. Bicycling with a helmet is a must.

What is the general design of exercise programs for weight reduction?

Both resistance- and aerobic-exercise training are recommended components of a weight-loss program. Resistance training is covered in chapter 12. The basic principles of exercise training were discussed in chapter 1.

In essence, aerobic-exercise programs to reduce body fat or to help maintain an optimal weight are based on the same principles that underlie exercise programs to improve the efficiency of the cardiovascular system. The total exercise program is based on a balance of exercise intensity, duration, and frequency. However, each daily exercise bout is usually subdivided into three phases—warm-up, stimulus, and warm-down, in that order (figure 11.10). A proper warm-up and warm-down are important components of the aerobic-exercise prescription. Both may help prevent excessive strain on the heart and may also be helpful in the prevention of muscular soreness or injuries.

The **warm-up** precedes the stimulus period and may be done in several ways. It may be general in nature, such as calisthenics, or specific to the type of exercise you plan to do, such as initially exercising at a lower level of intensity of the actual mode of exercise. Some gentle static stretching exercises are also helpful in the warm-up period.

For most aerobic-type exercise, it is probably better to warm up the specific muscles to be used. For example, if you plan to use jogging as your mode of aerobic exercise, you should stretch your leg muscles gently at first and then jog at a slower than normal pace for several minutes. Breaking into a sweat is a good external sign that you have sufficiently elevated your body temperature;

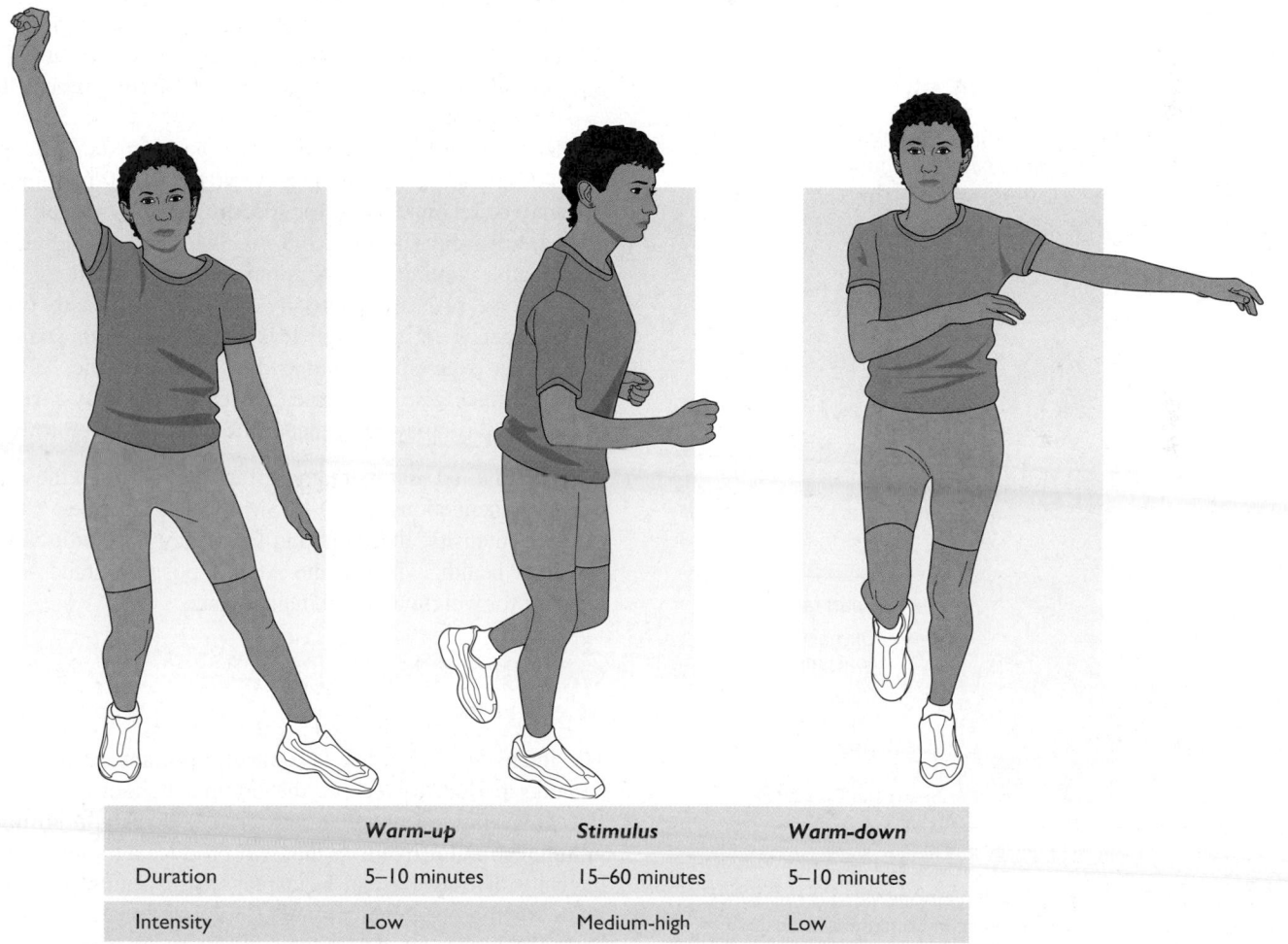

	Warm-up	Stimulus	Warm-down
Duration	5–10 minutes	15–60 minutes	5–10 minutes
Intensity	Low	Medium-high	Low

FIGURE 11.10 The exercise prescription. The exercise prescription is divided into three phases: warm-up period, stimulus period, and warm-down period. The stimulus period is the key to burning Calories.

by using a specific type of warm-up, the temperature of your exercising muscles will also be increased.

The **warm-down** phase follows the stimulus period and is designed primarily to help restore the cardiovascular system to normal. If one stops exercising abruptly, blood may possibly pool in the exercised body parts, thereby decreasing return of blood to the heart. With less blood to the heart, the heart rate will increase rapidly in attempts to maintain blood flow. Research also indicates that abrupt cessation of exercise may increase certain blood hormone levels that may cause abnormal rhythm of the heart. These factors increase stress on the heart, which may induce a heart attack in individuals at risk. Decreased blood flow to the brain may also cause dizziness and may be a cause of *exercise-associated collapse,* discussed in chapter 9. When the warm-down occurs gradually after strenuous exercise—by walking or jogging after a strenuous run, for example—the muscles help massage the blood through the veins back to the heart. These points emphasize the importance of a gradual warm-down. Complete your warm-down by stretching. Because the muscles are now warm from the exercise they are easier to stretch, which may help prevent muscle stiffness.

The warm-up and warm-down are important components of the daily exercise bout, but most of the Calories are expended during the stimulus period.

What is the stimulus period of exercise?

The **stimulus period** is the most important phase of the daily exercise bout. By modifying the intensity and duration of the exercise, the individual achieves the level of stimulus necessary to elicit a conditioning effect. As illustrated in figure 11.11, several

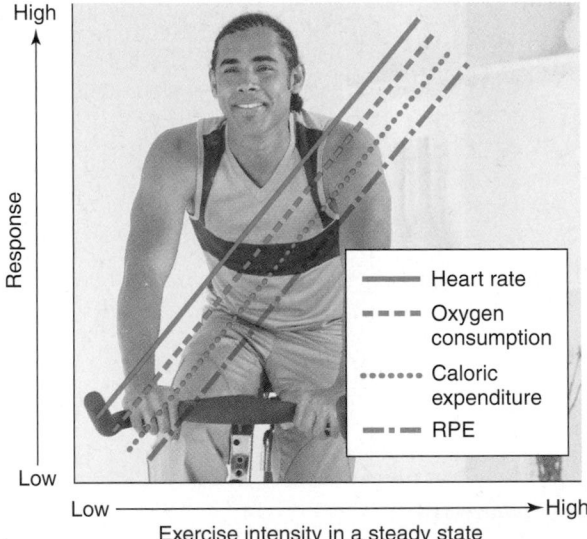

FIGURE 11.11 The relationship among various measures of energy expenditure. Heart rate, oxygen consumption, caloric expenditure, and RPE are, in general, directly related to the intensity of the exercise under steady-state conditions, i.e., when the oxygen supply is adequate for the energy cost of the exercise.

important physiological and psychological measures increase in proportion to the exercise intensity.

The two major components of the stimulus period are intensity and duration of exercise. In any exercise session, these two components are usually inversely related. In other words, if intensity is high, duration is short, and if intensity is low, duration is long. Frequency (the number of exercise sessions per week) is also an important part of the exercise prescription. As discussed in detail in chapter 1, two joint reports from the American College of Sports Medicine and the American Heart Association, authored by Haskell and Nelson and their colleagues, provided recommendations on exercise for adults (age 18–65) and older adults (over age 65) as a means to help prevent chronic diseases. More recently, the American College of Sports Medicine, under the guidance of Donnelly and others, revised its position stand on appropriate physical activity intervention strategies for weight loss and prevention of weight regain for adults, and this position stand will be used as the basis for developing the aerobic exercise program here. However, some of the ACSM/AHA guidelines will be incorporated as deemed appropriate.

1. Intensity of training: For aerobic exercise, the ACSM position stand recommends moderate-intensity exercise, whereas the ACSM/AHA recommends both moderate- and vigorous-intensity exercise. Several techniques, such as heart rate measurement, to determine exercise intensity are discussed below. Intensity levels are based on the fitness level of the individual.
2. Duration of training: The ACSM position stand recommends a minimum of 150 minutes weekly, but 250 minutes or more may be recommended for specific weight-loss outcomes. For cardiovascular health, the ACSM/AHA guidelines recommend a minimum of 30 minutes daily for moderate-intensity exercise, or 20 minutes daily of vigorous-intensity exercise.
3. Frequency of training: The ACSM position stand recommends exercising about 5 days a week. The ACSM/AHA guidelines also recommend exercising 5 days weekly, but only 3 days may be needed if the exercise is vigorous.

Keep in mind that there are differences between these two sets of recommendations. The ACSM/AHA guidelines recommend exercise intensity, duration, and frequency for cardiovascular fitness and health, whereas the ACSM position stand focuses on exercise for weight loss and maintenance.

What is an appropriate level of exercise intensity?

The intensity of exercise is a very important component of the stimulus period; to receive the optimal benefits from the exercise program, you must attain a certain **threshold stimulus,** the minimal stimulus intensity that will produce a training effect. The intensity of exercise can be expressed in a number of different ways, such as percentage of VO_2 max and Calories/minute, but these techniques are not suitable for everyday exercise. However, other easily measured variables may provide you with a good estimate of your exercise intensity, including your heart rate, your perception of how strenuous the exercise is, and your ability to carry on a conversation.

Heart Rate   As noted in figure 11.11, the heart rate is linearly related to oxygen consumption, which is the major measure of energy expenditure. Because the heart rate is easily obtained, it is usually used to determine the threshold level of exercise intensity.

To obtain the heart rate, press lightly with the index and middle fingers on the carotid artery, located just under the jawbone and beside the Adam's apple. Do not use the thumb as it also has a pulse, and do not press hard on the carotid artery, for it may cause a reflex slowing of the beat in some persons. The radial artery pulse is obtained by placing your fingers on the inside of the wrist on the thumb side. These are the two most common locations for monitoring pulse rate, but other locations (the temple, inside the upper arm, and directly over the heart) may be used (see figure 11.12).

To obtain the heart rate per minute, simply count the pulse rate for 6 seconds and add a zero. Resting and recovery heart rates are easily obtainable, as they may be taken while you are motionless, but it is difficult to manually monitor the heart rate while exercising. Research has shown that the exercise heart rate correlates very highly with the heart rate during the early stages of recovery. Hence, to monitor exercise heart rate, secure the pulse *immediately* upon cessation of exercise and count the beats for 6 seconds. This provides a reliable measure of exercise heart rate, although it may be slightly lower due to the beginning of the recovery effect. If it is difficult for you to monitor your heart rate for 6 seconds, then use a 10-second period and multiply the count by six to obtain your heart rate per minute. You probably should use 30 seconds to determine your resting heart rate; multiply your results by two. It may also be better to measure your resting pulse early in the morning, just after rising. Additionally, for the calculations to follow, you should take your resting heart rate in the position in which you will exercise; for example, lying down if you swim, seated if you cycle, or standing if you walk or run.

If you become serious about heart rate monitoring as the basis for your exercise training, you may want to invest in a device that monitors your heart rate while you exercise. Such devices usually use a comfortable chest band that transmits your heart rate to a wrist band so you can easily see your heart rate response during any phase of exercise.

One of the most prevalent techniques to determine the threshold stimulus for exercise is based upon the **maximal heart rate reserve (HR max reserve),** the difference between the resting heart rate and the maximum heart rate. You may determine your resting heart rate shortly after you arise in the morning. If you have not been physically active in some time, it may not be advisable for you to engage in strenuous physical activity in order to determine your actual maximal heart rate (HR max), but there are ways to predict it based upon your age. Although there are individual variations, the traditional formula (A) for the prediction of HR max in women and untrained men is 220 minus the person's age. Gellish and others, using longitudinal data, indicated that the 220 – age formula is biased as it overestimates measured HR max for men and women under the age of 40 years, and underestimates HR max of those older than 40. They suggested a more relevant formula (B), 207 minus 0.7 × age. Others suggest that for physically trained men, the formula (C) 205 minus one-half the person's age may be more appropriate, whereas for obese

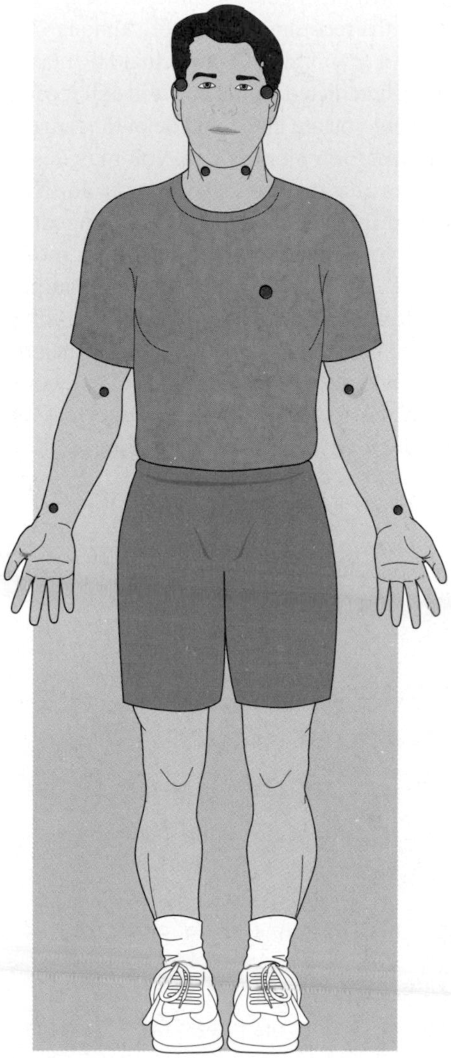

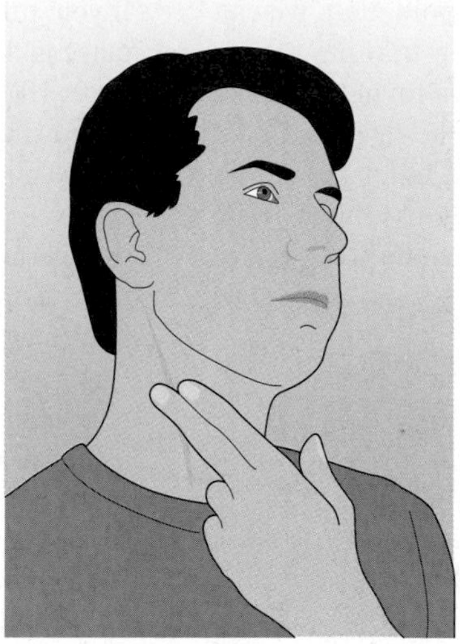

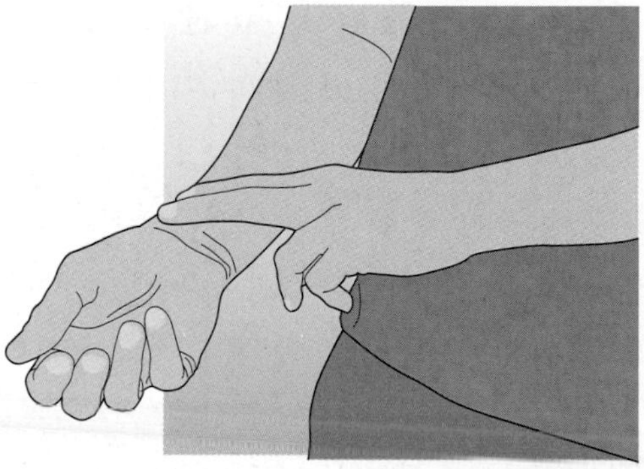

FIGURE 11.12   Palpation of the heart rate. The pulse rate may be taken at a variety of body locations *(a)*, but the two most common locations are *(b)* the neck (carotid artery) and *(c)* the wrist (radial artery).

individuals, the formula (D) 200 minus one-half the person's age may be best.

Based upon the traditional formula A, a 40-year-old untrained individual would have a predicted HR max of 180, which is about the same value predicted by the formula B. Using the formula C, a trained 40-year-old male would have a predicted HR max of 185, whereas an obese individual would have a predicted HR max of 180. Keep in mind, however, that there is considerable individual variation relative to predicted HR max no matter which formula is used. For example, a 40-year-old man may predict a HR max of 180, yet it may be 200, 160, or much lower if he was a victim of coronary heart disease.

There is rather widespread general agreement that in order to obtain a training effect, the heart rate response should be increased above the resting level by about 50–85 percent of the HR max reserve. Research has revealed that lower levels, 40–45 percent, may also be effective, particularly in individuals with poor levels of physical fitness.

Continuing with our example of the 40-year-old man, we can calculate the heart rate range needed to elicit a training effect. This is called the **target heart rate range, or target HR.** To complete the calculations, we need to know the age-predicted HR max and the resting heart rate (RHR); the latter should be determined under relaxed circumstances. If we assume a RHR of 70 and a HR max of 180, the following formula would give us the target range:

$$\text{Target HR} = X\% \, (\text{HR max} - \text{RHR}) + \text{RHR}$$

For the 50 percent threshold level, the target heart rate for our example would be calculated as follows:

$$0.5 \, (180 - 70) + 70 =$$
$$0.5(110) + 70 = 55 + 70 = 125$$

For the 85 percent level, the target heart rate would be

$$0.85(180 - 70) + 70 =$$
$$0.85(110) + 70 = 93 + 70 = 163$$

Thus, to achieve a training effect, our 40-year-old man needs to train within a target HR range of 125–163.

If you wish to bypass the calculations, table 11.13 presents the target HR ranges for various age groups with RHR between 45 and 90 beats/minute. Simply find your age group and RHR in the headings and locate your target HR range. The table is based on a predicted HR max of 220 – age. If you prefer to use one of the other formulae to predict HR max, you may calculate your target HR range using the formula presented.

In general, this table is a useful guide to the threshold heart rate and target HR range. However, there is considerable variability in HR max among individuals, particularly in the older age groups. If your true HR max is below the predicted value (220 – age), the target HR range in the table would be higher than the recommended level. If your true HR max is higher than the predicted value, the target HR range in the table is lower than the recommended level. Although the target HR range might vary by a few beats, if your actual HR max is slightly higher or lower than the predicted value, you will still receive a good training effect—assuming you are in the middle of the range.

Once you have been training for a month or so, you may desire to determine your HR max in the specific activity you do. You may use the procedures described below, that is, running on a track at different speeds until you reach your maximal level, modifying the test dependent upon your aerobic exercise. For example, research has revealed that HR max is lower in swimming, possibly as much as ten to fifteen beats per minute, so the target heart rate may be slightly lower if this mode of exercise is used. One recommendation states that use of the formula 205 minus age may be appropriate to predict maximal heart rate while swimming.

TABLE 11.13 Target heart rate zones

RHR	Age											
	15–19	20–24	25–29	30–34	35–39	40–44	45–49	50–54	55–59	60–64	65–69	70–74
45–49	125–180	123–175	120–171	118–167	115–163	113–158	110–154	108–150	105–146	103–141	100–137	98–133
50–54	127–181	125–176	122–172	120–168	117–164	115–159	112–155	110–151	107–147	105–142	102–138	100–134
55–59	130–181	128–176	125–172	123–168	120–164	118–159	115–155	113–151	110–147	108–142	105–138	103–134
60–64	132–182	130–177	127–173	125–169	122–165	120–160	117–156	115–152	112–148	110–143	107–139	105–135
65–69	135–183	133–178	130–174	128–170	125–166	123–161	120–157	118–153	115–149	113–144	110–140	107–136
70–74	137–184	135–179	132–175	130–171	127–167	125–162	122–158	120–154	117–150	115–145	112–141	110–137
75–79	140–184	138–180	135–176	133–172	130–168	128–163	125–159	123–155	120–151	118–146	115–142	113–138
80–84	142–185	140–181	137–177	135–173	132–169	130–164	127–160	125–156	122–152	120–147	117–143	115–139
85–89	145–186	143–181	140–177	138–173	135–169	133–164	130–160	128–156	125–152	123–147	120–143	118–139

The target zone (50–85 percent threshold) is based upon the median figure for each age range and resting heart rate range.

As you can see, the range for the target heart rate may span about 30–50 beats. For example, a 36-year-old individual with a resting heart rate of 72 beats per minute has a target heart rate range of 127–167, or a span of 40 beats per minute. Exercising at the lower end of this range, about 127–147 beats per minute, may be considered moderate-intensity exercise, while exercising at about 148–167 beats may be considered vigorous-intensity exercise. However, for an untrained individual just starting a fitness program, a heart rate of 127–147 may appear to be vigorous at first, but as she continues to exercise and improves her physical fitness this same heart rate response may become less taxing and be perceived as moderate intensity. Moreover, as her fitness improves, her resting heart rate may decrease over time, possibly by 10 or more beats per minute, which will necessitate recalculation of the target heart rate range.

Rating of Perceived Exertion (RPE)   Although the target heart rate approach is a sound means for monitoring exercise intensity, you may also wish to use other methods. One popular method is the **rating of perceived exertion (RPE),** which is basically your perception of how hard you feel your body is working during exercise. Developed by Gunnar Borg, this scale was originally designed to reflect heart rate responses by adding a zero to the rating. You simply rate the perceived difficulty or strenuousness of the exercise task according to the column A scale in table 11.14. If you are running, how do your legs feel? Do they feel light and easy to move, or are they heavy, or possibly beginning to ache or burn? How is your breathing? Are you breathing easily and able to carry on a conversation, or are your sentences shortened to a few words? In general, how does your total body feel? Is the exercise too easy, or are you working too hard?

Borg also developed an abbreviated RPE scale with 0–10 points, which is depicted in Column B in table 11.14B. The OMNI-RPE scale uses a 0–10 pictorial version of runners or cyclists displaying varying degrees of exertion, and Utter and others validated its use as comparable to the Borg RPE scale.

When you determine your exercise heart rate, it is a good idea to associate an appropriate RPE value with it, so that you individualize the RPE to your specific exercise program. For example, at an exercise heart rate of 150 you might make a mental note of the exercise difficulty and assign a value of 15, or hard, to that level of exercise intensity. Research has shown that the RPE can be an effective means to measure exercise intensity in healthy individuals, particularly at heart rates above 150 beats/minute.

Talk Test   Another possible way to monitor your exercise effort, validated by Persinger and others, is associated with breathing and is often referred to as the *talk test.* David Swain, an expert on exercise intensity from Old Dominion University, provided some guidelines to determine moderate and vigorous levels of exercise intensity. If you are breathing harder but still able to carry on a conversation in complete sentences, you are probably exercising at a moderate intensity. However, if it is difficult for you to speak in complete sentences, you are probably exercising at a vigorous intensity. Another general rule of thumb is: If you cannot maintain a conversation while exercising, you are probably exercising too hard, unless you are training for sports competition.

How can I determine the exercise intensity needed to achieve my target HR range?

To determine the exercise intensity necessary to reach your target HR range, all you need is a stopwatch. You may record your heart rate manually as explained previously, but use of a heart rate monitor would facilitate this task and probably increase the accuracy. Where distances are involved, such as with running, swimming, or cycling, an accurate measure is needed. An ideal situation for walking or running would be a quarter-mile (400 meters) high school or college track.

A steady-state HR response may be obtained in 3 to 5 minutes of evenly paced activity. A sound method for walking, jogging, or running follows, but this system may be adapted easily to other activities such as swimming, cycling, calisthenics, and aerobic dance.

Mark a one-half mile course. Two laps on a quarter-mile track would be ideal, but you can pace out a quarter-mile on the sidewalks near your home. Measure your resting HR. Walk until you have an even pace and then time yourself for the one-half mile. Immediately record your HR at the conclusion of the exercise. During your walk, mentally record the RPE. Did you reach the target HR? Was your RPE related to your HR? If the HR response was in the target range or the RPE was not too strenuous, you are at a level to begin your training program. If the HR response was not in the target range, rest until your HR returns close to normal and then take the test at a faster pace. Repeat this procedure until

TABLE 11.14	The RPE scales	
A	**B**
6 Sitting, relaxing	0 Extremely easy
7 Very, very light	1
8	2 Easy
9 Very light	3
10	4 Somewhat easy
11 Light	5
12	6 Somewhat hard
13 Somewhat hard	7
14	8 Hard
15 Hard	9
16	10 Extremely hard
17 Very hard	
18	
19 Very, very hard	
20 Maximal effort	

Table 11.16 presents an exercise program with a rapid progression to jogging, using an interval-training approach. **Interval training** alternates periods of rest and exercise. Again, the target HR method should be used during this exercise program. As compared to walking, jogging or running may expend 2–3 times the amount of Calories per unit of time. Thus, it may be worthwhile to interject short bouts of more intense exercise into a workout, such as jogging one block out of every three or four

TABLE 11.16 Sample aerobic jogging program (interval training)

	Warm-up	Target zone exercising	Warm-down	Total time
Week 1*	Stretch and limber up 5 minutes	Walk (nonstop) 10 minutes	Walk slowly 3 minutes; stretch 2 minutes	20 minutes
Week 2	Stretch and limber up 5 minutes	Walk 5 minutes; jog 1 minute; walk 5 minutes; jog 1 minute	Walk slowly 3 minutes; stretch 2 minutes	22 minutes
Week 3	Stretch and limber up 5 minutes	Walk 5 minutes; jog 3 minutes; walk 5 minutes; jog 3 minutes	Walk slowly 3 minutes; stretch 2 minutes	26 minutes
Week 4	Stretch and limber up 5 minutes	Walk 5 minutes; jog 5 minutes; walk 5 minutes; jog 5 minutes	Walk slowly 3 minutes; stretch 2 minutes	30 minutes
Week 5	Stretch and limber up 5 minutes	Walk 4 minutes; jog 6 minutes; walk 4 minutes; jog 6 minutes	Walk slowly 3 minutes; stretch 2 minutes	30 minutes
Week 6	Stretch and limber up 5 minutes	Walk 4 minutes; jog 7 minutes; walk 4 minutes; jog 7 minutes	Walk slowly 3 minutes; stretch 2 minutes	32 minutes
Week 7	Stretch and limber up 5 minutes	Walk 4 minutes; jog 8 minutes; walk 4 minutes; jog 8 minutes	Walk slowly 3 minutes; stretch 2 minutes	34 minutes
Week 8	Stretch and limber up 5 minutes	Walk 4 minutes; jog 9 minutes; walk 4 minutes; jog 9 minutes	Walk slowly 3 minutes; stretch 2 minutes	36 minutes
Week 9	Stretch and limber up 5 minutes	Walk 4 minutes; jog 10 minutes; walk 4 minutes; jog 10 minutes	Walk slowly 3 minutes; stretch 2 minutes	38 minutes
Week 10	Stretch and limber up 5 minutes	Walk 4 minutes; jog 11 minutes Walk 4 minutes; jog 11 minutes	Walk slowly 3 minutes; stretch 2 minutes	40 minutes
Week 11	Stretch and limber up 5 minutes	Walk 4 minutes; jog 12 minutes Walk 4 minutes; jog 12 minutes	Walk slowly 3 minutes; stretch 2 minutes	42 minutes
Week 12	Stretch and limber up 5 minutes	Walk 4 minutes; jog 14 minutes Walk 4 minutes; jog 14 minutes	Walk slowly 3 minutes; stretch 2 minutes	46 minutes
Week 13	Stretch and limber up 5 minutes	Walk 2 minutes; jog slowly 2 minutes; jog 15 minutes Walk 2 minutes; jog slowly 2 minutes; jog 15 minutes	Walk slowly 3 minutes; stretch 2 minutes	48 minutes
Week 14	Stretch and limber up 5 minutes	Walk 1 minute; jog slowly 3 minutes; jog 15 minutes Walk 1 minute; jog slowly 3 minutes; jog 15 minutes	Walk slowly 3 minutes; stretch 2 minutes	48 minutes
Week 15	Stretch and limber up 5 minutes	Jog slowly 3 minutes; jog 17 minutes Jog slowly 3 minutes; jog 17 minutes	Walk slowly 3 minutes; stretch 2 minutes	50 minutes

From week 16 on, check your pulse periodically to see if you are exercising within your target zone. As you become more fit, try exercising within the upper range of your target zone. For weight loss, exercise 5 days or more per week. Daily exercise may be needed to achieve 250 minutes of aerobic exercise per week, because some of the total time consists of stretching.

Note: If you find a particular week's pattern tiring, repeat it before going on to the next pattern. *You do not have to complete the jogging program in 15 weeks.* Remember that your goal is to continue getting the benefits you are seeking—and to enjoy your activity.

Source: U.S. Department of Health and Human Services, modified to include recent American College of Sports Medicine guidelines for weight loss.

when walking. Moreover, research has indicated that more intense exercise may confer additional health benefits. Swain and Franklin concluded that exercise performed at a vigorous intensity appears to convey greater cardioprotective benefits than exercise of moderate intensity.

Whatever mode of exercise you select, the target HR should be maintained for 30 minutes or more. This may be continuous or intermittent. If 30 minutes is the allotted time, the target HR should be achieved for 30 continuous minutes or three 10-minute intervals of exercise with several minutes of rest in between.

The frequency of exercise should be daily or at least five times per week. During the early stages, however, it may be advisable to exercise daily in order to form sound habits. The exercise intensity at this time may not be too severe, such as walking, and hence daily exercise bouts may be undertaken without serious muscle soreness or related injury patterns. If you switch to jogging or running, decrease the frequency to three or four times per week to avoid overuse injuries. The frequency per week may be increased as you become better physically conditioned. To increase weekly energy expenditure and help prevent overuse injuries, engage in cross-training exercises on days you do not jog or run.

For weight-control purposes, duration and frequency of exercise are key elements. The longer and more often you exercise, the greater will be the total amount of energy expended. Aerobic walking for 5 miles on a daily basis is the equivalent of approximately 1 pound of body fat per week.

There are a number of other excellent conditioning programs available for the unconditioned individual. Probably the most popular is the aerobics program developed by Dr. Kenneth Cooper. Although dated, his programs may be found in *The Aerobics Program for Total Well Being,* a highly recommended paperback found in most bookstores. Also, books on initiating walking and other aerobic exercise programs are available at your library or local bookstores, and various Websites provide very helpful information.

www.americaonthemove.org

www.walking.org   These Websites provide detailed information on beginning and maintaining a fitness walking program and associated health benefits, including weight loss.

www.10000steps.org.au   This Australian Website provides advice on how to walk 10,000 steps daily, with a link on how to convert other activities into steps.

www.gmap-pedometer.com   This program permits you to calculate distances of walking or jogging routes in your neighborhood or anywhere in the country.

Numerous fitness applications are also available for cell phones. Google "fitness apps" to review recommended programs.

How much exercise is needed to lose weight?

Although a properly planned exercise program may produce significant health benefits even without weight loss, many individuals use exercise to decrease body fat. Although weight loss depends on both a balance of energy expenditure through exercise and energy intake through your diet, some guidelines on recommended amounts of exercise for weight loss are available from professional and governmental health organizations.

The ACSM/AHA minimum recommendation (30 minutes of moderate-intensity exercise, 5 days per week) for cardiovascular health benefits totals 2.5 hours per week, which would approximate 1,000–1,200 Calories energy expenditure. However, the ACSM/AHA notes that this is a minimum, and *more exercise is better.* This is particularly so for weight loss and maintenance. Increasing exercise duration and frequency is the key.

The American College of Sports Medicine, under the guidance of Donnelly and others, has revised its position stand on appropriate physical activity intervention strategies for weight loss and prevention of weight regain for adults. The following represent the key exercise recommendations emanating from this position stand, expressed in weekly minutes of moderate physical activity.

- 150–250 minutes
  - Prevent weight gain
  - Produce modest weight loss
  - Improve weight loss with moderate diet restriction
- 250 minutes or more
  - Produce clinically significant weight loss
  - Maintain weight after weight loss

The ACSM position stand recommends moderate-intensity exercise, which is appropriate for overweight individuals. For example, Nybo and others found that moderate-intensity running was more effective than high-intensity exercise as a means to lose body fat, although the high-intensity exercise was more effective in promoting cardiorespiratory fitness. As weight loss increases, some vigorous exercise may be incorporated into the exercise regimen as a means to enhance cardiovascular fitness in addition to the weight loss.

Several other groups have also provided recommendations. Wing and Phelan noted that successful weight losers in the National Weight Control Registry exercised about 1 hour or more per day. Walking is their number one exercise, but they also engage in resistance training and other physical activities. Collectively, this amount of physical activity would approximate 1,500–2,000 Calories weekly. Finally, the Institute of Medicine of the National Academy of Sciences indicates that 30 minutes per day of regular activity is insufficient to maintain body weight within the recommended Body Mass Index range, and hence recommends 60 minutes of daily moderate-intensity physical activity. Walking or jogging at 4–5 miles per hour (mph) is recommended, in addition to the activities required by a sedentary lifestyle. This amount of physical activity leads to an active lifestyle, corresponding to physical activity levels (PAL) greater than 1.6, and is appropriate for both children and adults. Such an activity level for 6–7 days a week would approximate 2,000 Calories or more of energy expenditure.

Collectively, the optimal exercise energy-expenditure goal appears to be 1,500–2,000 Calories per week, or about 200–300 Calories per day. For walkers, this approximates 10,000 steps daily. The average person walks about 5,000 steps a day, and studies have shown that such individuals are overweight as compared to those who walk 10,000 or more steps daily. Gradually adding about 5,000 or 6,000 steps of brisk walking per day to a sedentary routine would approximate 200–300 additional Calories expended, or about 1,500–2,000 per week. Use of a good pedometer will help you keep track of daily steps, and will also serve as a motivation device to encourage you to walk. The average person takes about 2,000 steps per mile. Walking 100 steps per minute, about 3 miles per hour, may be a moderate-intensity pace. Walking about 130 steps per minute approximates 4 miles per hour, which is definitely a brisk pace and may be a recommended long-term goal. Walking even faster may approach the energy equivalency of jogging at the same pace. As noted previously, the step rate may be modified based on the height of the individual, with shorter persons taking more steps per minute than taller persons.

As related to the PAL presented earlier in this chapter, Tudor-Locke and others proposed similar guidelines relative to walking and level of daily physical activity:

Sedentary	<5,000 steps
Low active	5,000–7,499 steps
Somewhat active	7,500–9,999 steps
Active	10,000–12,499 steps
Highly active	>12,500 steps

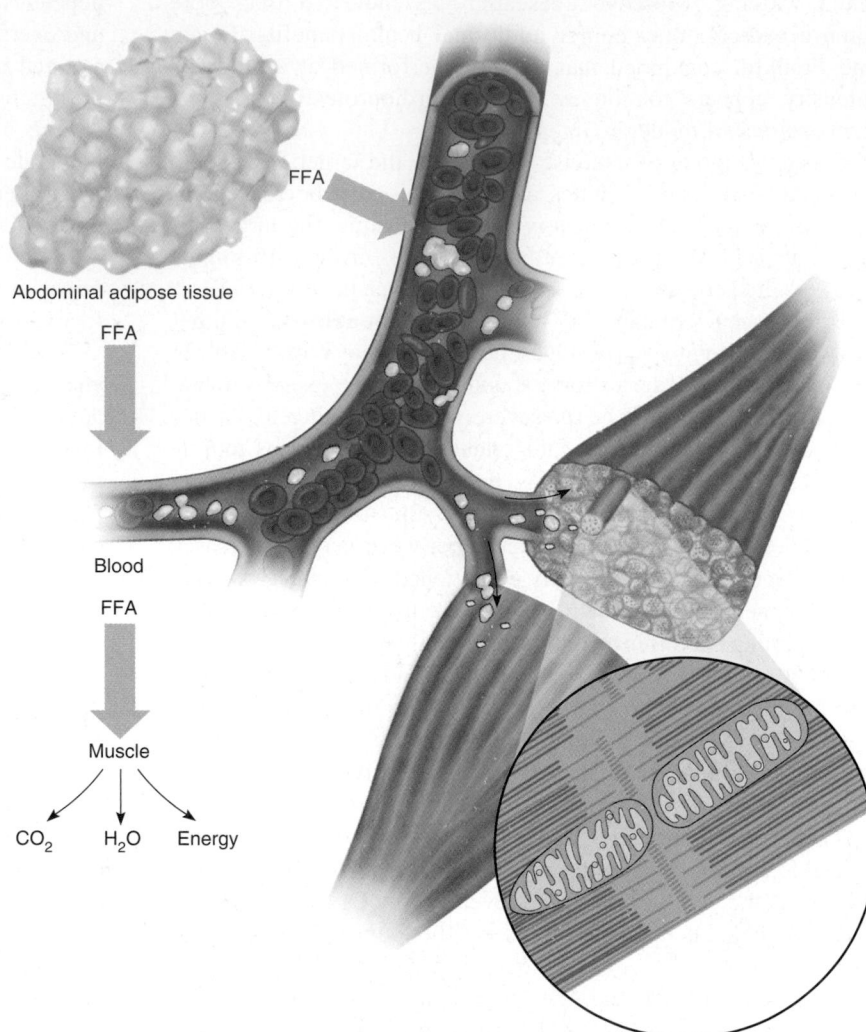

FIGURE 11.14 Exercise helps to release fat (free fatty acids) from the adipose tissues, particularly abdominal fat cells. The fat then travels by way of the bloodstream to the muscles where the free fatty acids are oxidized to provide the energy for exercise. Thus, exercise is an effective measure of reducing body fat.

From what parts of the body does the weight loss occur during an exercise weight-reduction program?

As mentioned previously, weight loss may come from any one of three body sources: body water, lean tissue such as muscle, and body-fat stores. A diet program, especially one very low in Calories, will cause a rapid weight loss due to decreases in body water and lean tissue. Body-fat losses are moderate at first but may increase in later stages of the diet. In contrast, weight lost through an exercise program alone is lost at a much slower rate. Body water levels remain relatively normal after replacement of water lost through exercise. The lean tissues, particularly muscle, might actually increase in amount from the stimulating effect of exercise on muscle development. Because a good proportion of the energy demand for exercise is met by the oxidation of fat, most of the body-weight reduction comes from the body-fat stores, particularly in the abdominal area (figure 11.14). As we learned previously, the caloric cost of 1 pound of fat is much higher than that of water or lean muscle tissue. Thus, loss of body fat through exercise takes time, highlighting the importance of the long-haul concept and long-term weight loss goals.

Should I do low-intensity exercises to burn more fat?

A myth that is circulating contends that in order to burn fat, you must exercise at a lower percentage of your VO_2 max. As noted in chapters 3, 4, and 5, it is true that the *percentage* of energy obtained from fat is greater at lower exercise intensities (e.g., 50 percent VO_2 max) than at higher exercise intensities (e.g., 70 percent VO_2 max). However, at the higher energy intensity you will derive a lower percentage of your energy output from fat, but the total energy expenditure will be greater and you will still burn about the same amount of fat Calories as you would exercising at the lower intensity, providing you are exercising for the same amount of time. If you want to burn Calories to lose body fat, your objective should be to burn the greatest total Calories possible within the time frame you have to exercise. As an example, suppose a female had 30 minutes to exercise and exercised at 50 percent VO_2 max, running 10-minute miles and deriving

50 percent of her energy from fat. She would cover 3 miles, expending 300 total Calories at an energy cost of about 100 Calories per mile, 150 (0.50 × 300) of which would be fat Calories. If she was able to run at 75 percent VO₂ max, running 7.5-minute miles and deriving 33 percent of her energy from fat, she would cover 4.5 miles, expending 450 total Calories, of which 150 (0.33 × 450) would still be fat Calories. However, she has expended a total of 450 versus 300 Calories at the higher exercise intensity, which will lead to a greater weight loss or permit her to consume an additional 150 Calories in her daily diet. But, if she has unlimited time, she may be able to exercise longer at the lower exercise intensity and eventually burn more total Calories including more fat Calories. Keep in mind, as noted in chapters 4 and 5, as you become highly trained in aerobic endurance exercise, you become a better fat burner and will be able to oxidize fat at higher exercise intensities. For example, Romijn and others have found that in endurance-trained men and women, the highest rate of fat oxidation was during exercise at 65 percent of maximal oxygen uptake. If you want to burn 500 Calories per day by running 5 miles, it does not matter how fast you run. For weight-control purposes, the total distance covered, which translates into total Calories expended, is the key point. As noted in chapter 3, you may estimate the energy it costs you to run 1 mile by simply multiplying your body weight in pounds by 0.73 Calories.

Is spot reducing effective?

Spot reducing uses isolated exercises in an attempt to deplete local fat deposits in specific body areas. These techniques do not appear to be effective. In one study the fat tissue was biopsied to determine whether sit-ups would reduce fat in the abdominal area. Subjects did a total of 5,000 sit-ups over a 27-day period, but this localized exercise did not preferentially reduce the adipose cell size in the abdominal area. In another study, magnetic resonance imaging (MRI) was used to quantify the subcutaneous fat tissue in the upper arm. Kostek and others reported no changes in men and women engaged in resistance training of one arm for 12 weeks.

In their review, Smith and Zachwieja indicated that the current view suggests that the reduction of fat in body areas is most likely to occur where fat deposits are the most conspicuous (usually the abdominal area), regardless of the weight-loss format, including exercise. However, some areas of the body are somewhat resistant to change, particularly the gynoid-type fat distribution around the hips and thighs. Although both large-muscle activities and local isolated-muscle exercises may be beneficial in reducing fat stores, the former are recommended because the total caloric expenditure will be larger.

Is it possible to exercise and still not lose body weight?

Many individuals are disappointed during the early stages of an exercise program because they do not lose weight very rapidly. Unless they understand what is happening in their bodies, the results on the scale may

convince them that exercise is not an effective means of reducing weight, and they may quit exercising altogether. There are several reasons why an individual may not lose weight during the early stages of a weight-reduction program, and also why losing weight becomes more difficult after weight loss has occurred.

One reason may involve a compensation effect, such as increasing the amount of caloric intake or reducing the amount of other daily physical activities. For example, in a study involving the effects of exercise on weight loss, Manthou and others reported that nearly one-third of the subjects were responders, and lost body weight as expected. The remaining two-thirds were nonresponders who did not lose and actually gained weight. Further analysis revealed that the nonresponders reduced their daily physical activities outside of their exercise sessions.

Another reason involves changes in body composition, but changes that are actually favorable to health. When a sedentary individual begins a daily exercise program, the body reacts to the exercise stress and changes so it can more easily handle the demands of exercise (figure 11.15):

1. The muscles may increase in size because of hypertrophy of the muscle cells. The increased protein will hold water.
2. Certain structures within the muscle cell that process oxygen, along with numerous enzymes involved in oxygen use, will increase in quantity.

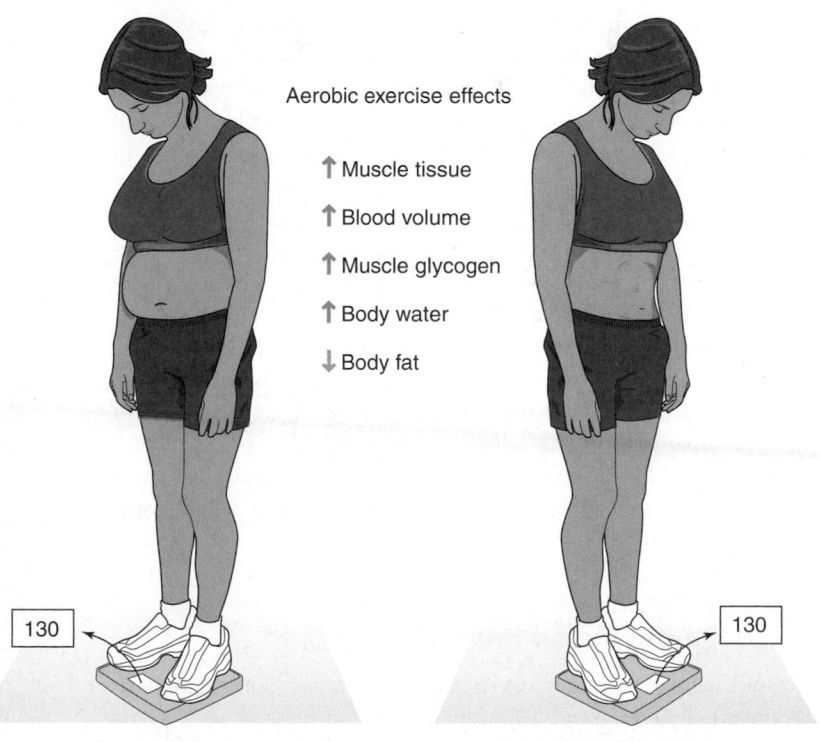

Aerobic exercise effects

↑ Muscle tissue

↑ Blood volume

↑ Muscle glycogen

↑ Body water

↓ Body fat

130

Start exercise program

130

One month later

FIGURE 11.15 Body weight may not change much during the beginning phases of an aerobic exercise program. However, body composition may change. The exercise stimulates an increase in muscle tissue, blood volume, and muscle glycogen stores, which tend to increase weight. Body fat is reduced, but the increases in the other components can balance out the fat losses with no net loss of body weight. Eventually, body weight, particularly abdominal fat, begins to drop as the exercise program is continued.

3. Energy substances in the cell will increase, particularly glycogen, which binds water.
4. The connective tissue will toughen and thicken.
5. The total blood volume may increase. An increase of approximately 500 milliliters, or about a pound, has been recorded in 1 week.

At the same time, however, body-fat stores will begin to diminish somewhat as fat is used as a source of energy for exercise. Overall, there may be an increase in body water and lean body mass, particularly the muscle tissues, and a decrease in body fat. These changes may counterbalance each other, and the individual may not lose any weight. However, although little or no weight is lost during those early phases, the body composition changes are favorable. Body fat is being lost, particularly from the abdominal fat depots.

Once these adaptive changes have occurred, which may take about a month, body weight should decrease in relationship to the number of Calories lost through exercise. Keep in mind that weight loss will be slow on an exercise program, but if you can build up to an exercise energy expenditure of about 300 Calories per day, then about 2.5 pounds per month will be exercised away provided you do not compensate by eating more.

After several months you may begin to notice that your body weight has stabilized even though you continue to exercise and have not reached your weight goal. Part of the reason may be your lower body weight. If you look at appendix B, you can see that the less you weigh, the fewer Calories you burn for any given exercise. If you have been doing the same amount of exercise all along, you may now be at the body weight where your energy output is matched by your energy input in food and your body weight has stabilized. In theory, you have reached your settling point. In addition, you may become more skilled, and hence more efficient, in your physical activity. Fewer Calories may then be expended for any given amount of time. However, this is usually true only of activities that involve a skill factor. It can be highly significant in swimming, but not as great in jogging.

In summary, your body weight may not change during the early stages of an exercise program; it may then begin to drop during a second stage, and then plateau at the third stage. If you are aware of these possible stages, your adherence to an exercise program may be enhanced. Also, during the third stage, if you desire to lose more weight by exercise, the amount of exercise will have to be increased.

What about the five or six pounds a person may lose during an hour of exercise?

A rapid weight loss may occur during exercise. Some individuals have lost as much as 10–12 pounds in an hour or so. As you probably suspect, this weight loss may be attributed to body-water losses. This is particularly evident while exercising in warm or hot weather. The weight loss is temporary, and under normal food and water intake the body-water content will return to normal. Each pound of weight lost this way is 1 pint of fluid, or 16 ounces. A 2.2-pound weight loss would be the equivalent of 1 liter.

In the heat of summer, you may occasionally see an individual training with heavy sweat clothes or a rubberized suit. The reason often given is to lose more body weight. The individual will lose more body weight, but again it will be body water which will be regained as soon as he or she drinks fluids. In this regard, the technique is worthless. Moreover, it may predispose the individual to an unusually high heat stress, causing severe medical problems. Remember, only sweat that actually evaporates will help reduce the heat stress on the body.

Any water lost through dehydration should be replaced before the next exercise session, especially when exercising in warm environments. The importance of rehydration and problems associated with exercise in the heat were covered in chapter 9.

Key Concepts
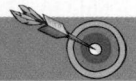

▶ Aerobic exercise can increase energy expenditure considerably, but in order to lose body fat through exercise one should think in terms of months, not days.

▶ To be aerobic, weight-reduction exercises must involve large muscle masses, such as the legs in jogging or bicycling or the arms and legs in swimming. Brisk walking is a highly recommended exercise program.

▶ The general design of the aerobic weight-reduction exercise programs involves three phases: warm-up, exercise stimulus, and warm-down.

▶ An effective means of monitoring aerobic exercise intensity is the exercise heart rate (HR). The exercise target HR varies depending upon age and level of conditioning. Ratings of perceived exertion (RPE) and the talk test may also be used to gauge exercise intensity.

▶ Walking is one of the recommended exercises for health and weight control. Here are a few historical quotes relative to the benefits of walking.

   Walking is our best medicine. *Hippocrates*
   Before supper take a little walk. After supper do the same. *Erasmus*
   I have two doctors, my left leg and my right leg. *Sir George Trevelyan*

▶ A slow, steady progression in exercise intensity is important in preventing excess stress and injuries.

▶ Duration and frequency of exercise are important considerations for weight loss. A weekly expenditure of 1,500–2,000 Calories from exercise appears to be a reasonable and effective means to induce and maintain weight loss.

▶ For several reasons, weight loss may not occur in the early stages of an exercise program; however, the body composition changes are favorable, that is, a decrease in body fat and increase in fat-free mass. A resistance-exercise program may be very helpful to maintain or increase fat-free mass.

▶ The rapid weight loss observed after a single bout of exercise is due to water loss through sweating.

Check for Yourself

▶ Using several different types of physical activity that you enjoy, use appendix B and calculate how much time you would need to allocate to each in order to burn 500 Calories per day.

Comprehensive Weight Control Programs

Although numerous studies with well-planned diet or diet-and-exercise programs have provided evidence of significant weight loss during the course of the research, many have also shown a high rate of relapse once the study ended. Accordingly, in a conference relative to methods for voluntary weight loss and control, the National Institutes of Health indicated that the most important feature of a successful weight-loss or weight-control program is maintenance of the stable or reduced body weight. The NIH noted that the fundamental principle of weight loss and control is a commitment to a change in lifestyle, a viewpoint shared by the American Dietetic Association in its most recent position statement on weight management. Behavioral modification incorporating properly designed diets and exercise programs, as detailed in this chapter, is the key to a comprehensive weight-control program not only to take off excess body fat, but to keep it off.

Which is more effective for weight control—dieting or exercise?

Dieting alone or exercise alone may be an effective means to reduce body fat, but each technique has certain advantages and disadvantages. However, it appears that the advantages of one technique help counterbalance the disadvantages of the other. Dieting will contribute to a negative caloric balance and may help bring about a rapid weight reduction early in the program.

Dieting alone may be an effective means to lose excess body fat. In a 6-month study, Redman and others found that dieting alone (25% reduction in caloric intake) induced similar total body fat and abdominal fat losses compared to subjects who created a similar energy deficit by both diet and aerobic exercise (12.5% reduction in caloric energy intake plus 12.5% increase in exercise energy expenditure). Both weight-loss programs induced similar changes in body composition. Several studies indicate that increasing the proportion of caloric intake from protein may also help maintain lean body mass on a weight-loss diet.

Aerobic exercise alone may also be an effective means to lose excess body fat. Stiegler and Cunliffe note that exercise training is associated with an increase in energy expenditure, thus promoting changes in body weight and composition provided that dietary intake remains constant. Moreover, adding resistance exercise may provide additional benefits.

Contrary to the results of the study by Redman and others, in their review Stiegler and Cunliffe stated that research to date suggests that the addition of exercise programs to dietary restriction can promote more favorable changes in body composition than diet on its own. For example, Hansen and others note that adding exercise to a diet program may prevent decreases in lean body mass, which could help maintain resting energy expenditure. Exercise may confer other benefits. Hansen and others also contend that exercise may improve dietary compliance. Once the body weight goal has been attained, expending 400–500 Calories daily through physical activity allows one to consume that many additional Calories. Instead of a 2,000-Calorie diet, one may consume 2,400 to 2,500 Calories. Hill notes that dieting alone to maintain weight is designed to fail in the long run. Although some can do it, they are few in number. Exercise enables one to eat more during the maintenance phase. Finally, Larson-Meyer and others note that despite similar effects of dieting or exercise on fat losses, combining caloric restriction with exercise increases aerobic fitness in parallel with improved insulin sensitivity, LDL-cholesterol, and diastolic blood pressure.

Some of the most meaningful data regarding long-term weight maintenance have been obtained by studying the habits of members of the National Weight Control Registry. The average member has lost about 70 pounds and has kept it off for more than 6 years. Nieman noted that almost all members modified their food intake and increased their physical activity to lose weight. Some of their key behaviors include the following:

- Eat a low-Calorie diet, low in fat and high in carbohydrate
- Eat breakfast; reduce hunger later in the day
- Watch only a limited amount of television
- Do about 60 minutes or more of physical activity daily; walking is the favorite exercise, but also engage in aerobic classes, resistance training, cycling, and swimming. They expend 2,000 or more Calories weekly through physical activity.
- Weigh themselves frequently; daily or several times a week; helps prevent a lapse from becoming a relapse

Resistance training (covered in chapter 12) added to a weight-reduction program may also be very effective in helping to maintain lean body mass. Preferably, both aerobic and resistance exercise should be part of a comprehensive weight-control program. A study by Kraemer and others found that the combination of aerobic endurance training and resistance training, compared to dieting alone, exerted more favorable effects on body composition and health-related fitness measures. Sillanpää and others compared the effects of strength and endurance training, both separately and combined, on body composition of men from age 40 to 65. Over the course of 21 weeks, they found that the combination of strength and endurance exercise optimized body composition compared to either exercise done separately. Combining aerobic and resistance exercise appears to provide the beneficial effects of both types of exercise.

Consider the following. A dietary reduction of 500 Calories per day, along with an exercise energy expenditure of 500 Calories per day, could lead to approximately 2 pounds of weight loss per week, about the maximal amount recommended unless under medical supervision. The removal of 500 Calories from the diet could be done immediately by simply reducing the amount of sugar and fat in the daily diet and using some of the behavioral modification techniques cited earlier. You should review those suggestions given earlier relative to the substitution of nutrient-dense foods for high-Caloric ones. Relative to exercise, it may take a month or more before you may be able to use 500 Calories daily, but by following the progressive plans outlined earlier in this chapter you should be able to reach that level safely. In the meantime, increase your level of NEAT by climbing stairs and walking more to add to your daily caloric expenditure.

A comprehensive weight-reduction program involving both a dietary and an exercise regimen, along with supportive behavioral modification techniques, is highly recommended by major health-related organizations such as the American Dietetic Association and the American College of Sports Medicine. Three reviews and meta-analyses by Södlerlund, Brown, and Sweet, along with their associates, concluded that the most effective weight-loss programs included multiple components—diet, exercise, and behavior modification. The principles of developing such a program have been presented in the preceding three sections of this chapter.

If I want to lose weight through a national or local weight-loss program, what should I look for?

The weight-loss industry is a multibillion-dollar business. National programs, such as NutriSystem, Weight Watchers, Jenny Craig, the South Beach Diet, and the Atkins Diet, may provide three flash-frozen meals daily, along with two snacks. Costs can range up to $10,000 per year, per person. Unfortunately, there is little governmental control over many of these programs, and although the national programs may be well designed, others may not provide appropriate programs for safe and effective long-term weight loss.

What do authorities recommend you should receive for your money if you want to enroll in a commercial weight-loss program? The following points are adapted and summarized from the report of a task force to establish weight-loss guidelines for the state of Michigan, and from other health professional sources, such as Partnership for Healthy Weight Management.

1. The staff should be well trained in their specialty, preferably having appropriate educational backgrounds, such as a physician, nurse, dietitian, or exercise physiologist.
2. You should receive a medical screening, verifying that you have no medical or psychological condition that might be exacerbated by weight loss through dieting or exercise.
3. A reasonable weight goal should be established given your weight history.
4. The rate of weight loss, after the first 2 weeks, should not exceed 2 pounds per week.
5. You should receive an individualized treatment plan based on your weight-loss goal. You should also obtain an itemized list of costs.
6. The program should disclose in writing all health risks and benefits associated with the program, and you should have the opportunity to read them and sign an informed consent form.
7. The diet should be one that
   a. contains no less than 1,000–1,500 Calories per day
   b. has at least 100 grams of carbohydrate per day
   c. provides at least 100 percent of the RDA; supplements, if used, should not exceed 100 percent of the RDA
   d. if under medical supervision, contains at least 600 Calories and 50 grams of carbohydrate per day
8. The program should have a nutrition-education component that stresses permanent lifestyle changes in your eating habits.

9. Both aerobic and resistance exercise should be a component in the program. The focus should be on aerobic exercise, following the standards relative to mode, intensity, duration, and frequency discussed earlier in this chapter. It should be an exercise program you can live with for a lifetime. Guidelines for resistance exercise are presented in the next chapter.
10. Behavior-modification techniques should be individualized to help you incorporate sound dietary and exercise habits into your personal lifestyle.
11. There should be a weight-maintenance phase in the program once you have achieved your weight-loss goal. This should be a high priority to help you maintain your healthy body weight.

Tsai and Wadden conducted a systematic review of major commercial weight-loss programs in the United States, and indicated that all programs can work to induce weight loss. For example, Furlow and Anderson reported that individuals who completed supervised, commercial weight-loss programs involving meal replacement lost an average of about one kilogram per week over the course of about 18 weeks. The major problem is getting people to stick with the program. The greater the compliance, such as in programs like Weight Watchers, the greater the success. In a *Consumer Reports* review, Jenny Craig, Slim-Fast, and Weight-Watchers were the three top-rated commercial weight-loss programs.

Guidelines similar to those just given should be used if you want to join a health or fitness club facility, particularly the qualifications of the staff and the availability of a variety of safe exercise equipment. Personal trainers should be certified by reputable professional organizations. The Consumers Union indicates that anyone can become a certified personal trainer, as there are no national standards for certification. Some Websites offer certification for minimal effort and several hundred dollars. The Consumers Union indicates that the best certification is provided by:

- The American College of Sports Medicine
- The American Council on Exercise
- The National Strength and Conditioning Association

Additionally, a Certified Specialist in Sports Dietetics (CSSD) would be a well-qualified contact for weight control, not only for the general population but also for athletes.

A personal trainer may help you plan an effective exercise program, including both aerobic and resistance exercise, to help you lose excess body weight. You can check with local fitness-oriented organizations, such as the YMCA, for a list of personal trainers, their certification, and their fees.

www.acefitness.org;

www.acsm.org;

www.nsca-lift.org   The Consumers Union indicates that the best certification programs for personal trainers are presented by the American Council on Exercise, the American College of Sports Medicine, and the National Strength and Conditioning Association. You can use the Website to obtain a list of certified trainers in your vicinity.

www.eatright.org   The American Dietetic Association Website provides a list of local registered dietitians (RD) with specialty in sports nutrition and weight control.

Although some individuals may need the structure of such programs, many successful individuals, including about half the members in the National Weight Control Registry, have lost excess body fat and kept it off with programs they designed by themselves.

www.nwcr.ws Access the National Weight Control Registry to review research findings as to how individuals lost weight and kept it off. Several success stories highlight methods used by individual members.

What type of weight-reduction program is advisable for young athletes?

The American Academy of Pediatrics notes that weight control is perceived to be advantageous for youths involved in sports such as bodybuilding, cheerleading, dancing, distance running, cross-country skiing, diving, figure skating, gymnastics, martial arts, rowing, swimming, weight-class football, and wrestling, which emphasize thinness, leanness, and/or competing at the lowest possible weight for aesthetic appeal or economy of movement. Such athletes may want to maintain or lose body weight, but weight lost should be fat, not muscle.

In general, athletes who desire to lose weight to enhance performance must rely primarily on dietary modifications because they are already exercising intensely. Excessive weight loss, especially in young athletes, is a major concern in sports.

As noted in chapter 10, use of improper weight-loss methods such as starvation, diuretics, laxatives, appetite-suppressing drugs, and dehydration may predispose young athletes to various health problems and impaired performance. Of particular concern are young female athletes in leanness sports who may develop long-term health problems associated with the female athlete triad, such as osteoporosis.

The American Academy of Pediatrics has recommended healthy weight-maintenance or weight-loss practices for young athletes. Some of its key points for young athletes are:

- To start early to permit a gradual weight loss over a realistic time period.
- To eat enough to cover the energy costs of daily living, growth, building and repairing muscle tissue, and participating in sports.
- To lose excess fat without reducing lean muscle mass or causing dehydration, both of which can impair performance.
- To exceed no more than 1.5 percent of the total body weight, or 1 to 2 pounds per week.
- To lose excess weight by both diet and extra exercise.
- To obtain from the diet approximately 55–65 percent of energy from carbohydrate, 15–20 percent from protein, and 20–30 percent from fat.
- To maintain the desired body weight, once attained, rather than cycling up and down.
- To discuss any desired weight loss with a health care professional and the family.

Other sports-related organizations, such as the National Collegiate Athletic Association, and the National Federation of State High School Associations, have made regulations and recommendations specific to the sport of wrestling, including the following:

- Dehydration techniques such as rubber suits, saunas, steam baths, hot rooms, laxatives, and diuretics should be prohibited.
- Have the weigh-in immediately prior to performance to discourage rapid dehydration and weight-gain techniques.
- Encourage methods to predict a minimum body-fat percentage or body weight.

Additionally, athletes on weight-loss programs should also increase the proportion of their energy intake from protein. Mettler and others reported that young athletes who consumed 35 percent of their energy intake as protein, as compared to others consuming 15 percent from protein, were better able to maintain lean body mass on a short-term weight-loss diet.

What is the importance of prevention in a weight control program?

Health practices designed to prevent the development of chronic diseases currently are being promoted heavily by several major health organizations, and many have focused on the adverse health effects of obesity. For example, the Canadian Task Force on Preventive Health Care has recommended that obesity prevention be a high priority for health professionals. Changing your diet by reducing caloric intake, saturated fats, and cholesterol, and eating more nutritious foods (quality Calories), and concurrently initiating and continuing a good aerobic- and resistance-type exercise program are considered to be two steps toward positive health and the prevention of obesity. James Hill, founder of the obesity-prevention program *America on the Move,* indicated that walking an extra 2,000 steps a day and eating 100 fewer Calories will help prevent the average weight gain of 1–3 pounds per year. If you like to eat, additional exercise may help you burn these Calories and maintain your body weight (figure 11.16).

Although most of this chapter has focused on treatment programs for the reduction of excess body fat, the same guidelines may be applied to a prevention program. Obesity in our society is a serious medical problem of epidemic proportions. Although treatment programs for the clinically obese may be successful on a short-term basis, unfortunately much of the weight loss is regained by the vast majority of those treated. As noted by Levin, the formation of neural circuits in the brain that help perpetuate maintenance of excess body weight are not easily abolished. We need to have strong prevention programs, particularly for children and adolescents, for this appears to be the time of life when chronic cases of obesity develop.

Prevention of obesity on a large scale necessitates a multi-pronged effort involving various groups. Some examples are listed.

- Government can set standards for food advertisements to children.
- Food manufacturers could produce healthier products. One example is Fun Fruits, containing a variety of fruits and marketed specifically to kids.

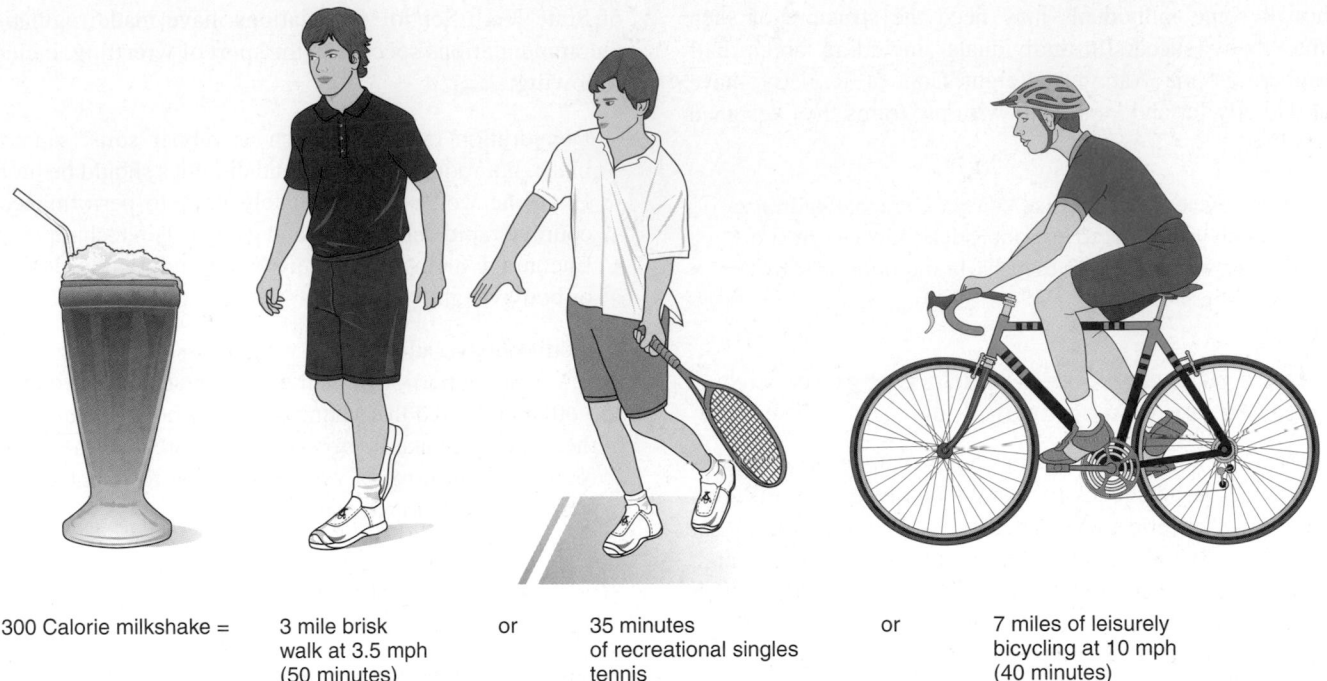

| 300 Calorie milkshake = | 3 mile brisk walk at 3.5 mph (50 minutes) | or | 35 minutes of recreational singles tennis | or | 7 miles of leisurely bicycling at 10 mph (40 minutes) |

FIGURE 11.16 It is very easy to consume 300 additional Calories per day, which can lead to an increase of about 2.5 pounds of body fat per month. However, increased physical activity may help to expend these Calories (170-pound individual).

- Communities could plan more bike paths, playgrounds, and recreation centers.
- Schools could schedule daily physical education classes and provide opportunities for students to participate in intramural sports and physical activity clubs after school. Schools could also provide healthier products in vending machines.
- Parents could provide healthy foods and limit sedentary behaviors such as TV and computer time.

Various Websites to obtain helpful information relative to the prevention of obesity have been listed throughout this chapter, several of which have been recommended by the Consumers Union.

It is incumbent upon those involved with the food habits and physical activity of our youth, notably parents and health and physical educators, to instruct and motivate them toward sound health habits. According to the American Medical Association, prevention is the treatment of choice in dealing with obesity. The bottom line is, *we need to eat less and move more.*

www.win.niddk.nih.gov An excellent source of information is the Weight-Control Information Network (WIN).

http://www.healthfinder.gov/prevention/ Free information and plans to help prevent excess weight gain in children. Click on *Nutrition and Fitness* and then *Help Your Child Stay at a Healthy Weight.*

Key Concepts

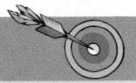

▶ Although diet and exercise may each be effective in losing body weight, a combination of the two would be even more beneficial, particularly when coupled with behavior modification techniques.
▶ Prevention of obesity is more effective than treatment, and appropriate programs should be developed early for children and adolescents.

Albert's Weight Status

	Weight	Calorie intake	Maintenance calories
Current status			
Goal status			

Albert's Weight-Loss Plan

1. Desired weight loss per week:
2. Caloric energy intake reduction:
3. Caloric energy expenditure increase:
4. Total daily caloric deficit:
5. Maintenance Calories at goal weight:

Albert is overweight by 25 pounds and is very serious about reducing his body weight from 200 pounds down to 175 and a healthier BMI of 22. He is currently sedentary, is consuming an average 3,600 Calories per day, and is still gaining weight. You may assume that he needs 15 Calories per pound body weight to maintain his current weight. Using information presented in the text, develop a weight-loss program for Albert. Calculate an appropriate rate of weight loss per week. Based on your calculation, determine the daily caloric deficit needed to achieve his goal. The caloric deficit should incorporate reduced caloric energy intake and increased caloric energy expenditure through your recommended energy program. Once Albert is at his desired body weight and is involved in your exercise program, how many Calories may he consume daily to maintain that weight?

1. If you were to design an aerobic training program for a 30-year-old individual and wanted that person to maintain an exercise intensity of 60–80 percent of the predicted HR max (traditional method) as the target heart rate range, what exercise heart rate range would you recommend?

   a. 114–152
   b. 132–176
   c. 140–180
   d. 154–198
   e. 180–220

2. Which of the following statements relative to an exercise program for weight maintenance or loss is true?

   a. The mode of exercise should involve large muscle groups that are activated in rhythmic, continuous-type movement.
   b. The higher the intensity of aerobic exercise that the individual can sustain, the better, because the greater the intensity, the greater the number of Calories burned per minute.
   c. The greater the duration of activity, the better.
   d. The more frequent the exercise during the week, the better.
   e. All statements are true.

3. Which of the following has the least amount of Calories as per the Food Exchange System developed by the American Dietetic Association and the American Diabetes Association?

   a. three servings of skim milk
   b. four servings of lean meat such as turkey
   c. five servings of vegetables
   d. four servings of fruit
   e. one serving of whole milk

4. Aerobic-type exercise may be an effective part of a comprehensive weight-control program for all of the following reasons except which one?

   a. It increases the metabolic rate.
   b. It mobilizes and utilizes free fatty acids from the adipose tissues.
   c. It helps reduce body water stores.
   d. It will increase the resting metabolic rate for 30 minutes or so after the exercise period.
   e. It may help to curb the appetite in some individuals if done prior to mealtime.

5. Suppose a young sedentary woman wanted to lose 5 pounds of body fat in a period of 5 weeks. She now weighs 150 pounds and her activity level is so low that she needs only 13 Calories per pound of body weight to maintain her weight. Calculate the number of Calories she may consume daily in order to lose the 5 pounds by diet only.

   a. 800
   b. 1,250
   c. 1,450
   d. 1,750
   e. 1,950

6. In the exchange lists, high-fat foods are usually found in which two exchanges?

   a. fruit and vegetables
   b. starch/bread and lean meat
   c. whole milk and starch/bread
   d. fat and vegetable
   e. medium fat meat and whole milk

7. Research with effective dieters has shown that, to be successful, a diet should follow all the following principles except which?

   a. be low in Calories
   b. supply all essential nutrients
   c. contain bland foods to curb the intake of Calories
   d. be able to be accommodated within one's current lifestyle
   e. be a lifelong diet

8. The rate of weight loss on an appropriate low-Calorie diet may be rapid at first, but then may slow down. This decreased rate of weight loss is most likely due to:

a. an increased BMR and increased use of body-protein stores

b. a decrease in body weight and increased use of body-fat stores

c. an increased use of carbohydrate stores and retention of body water

d. a decreased BMR and an increased loss of body-water stores

e. an increased BMR and decreased use of body-fat stores

9. Which of the following substitutes would not save Calories in a diet plan?

a. skim milk in place of whole milk

b. regular hard-stick margarine in place of butter

c. plain yogurt in place of sour cream on a baked potato

d. nonalcoholic beer in place of regular beer

e. air-popped popcorn in place of potato chips

10. An example of a behavior-modification program for a weight-loss program is

a. Feel guilty after you overeat.

b. Eat fast so there is no visible food to tempt you to eat more.

c. Keep a record of your eating habits so you can see what situations cause you to overeat.

d. Always clean your plate when you eat.

e. Always wait until you are hungry to go food shopping.

Answers to multiple-choice questions: 1. a; 2. e; 3. c; 4. c; 5. c; 6. e; 7. c; 8. b; 9. b; 10. c.

Review Questions—Essay

1. Melinda wants to lose 30 pounds by summer, which is 20 weeks away. She currently weighs 150 pounds and is maintaining her body weight with an energy intake of 14 Calories per pound body weight. Based on dietary changes only, calculate her daily energy needs during the first week of the diet if she wants to lose weight at a steady level over the 20-week period.

2. Explain the concept of behavior modification in a weight-loss program, and describe some of the strategies one might employ to help change undesirable behaviors.

3. Discuss the potential positives and negatives of the high-carbohydrate, low-fat diet and the high-protein, high-fat, low-carbohydrate diet. What appears to be the key factor underlying the potential success of each on a short-term basis?

4. Discuss the importance of mode, intensity, duration, and frequency of exercise in a weight-loss program, and provide an example of an appropriate program incorporating each for a physically fit individual who wanted to lose one pound per week through exercise alone.

5. Both dieting and exercise may be helpful in a weight-loss program, but each may possess some drawbacks. Explain how the benefits of exercise may help counteract the possible drawbacks of dieting, and vice versa.

References

Books

Agatston, A. 2003. *The South Beach Diet.* Emmaus, PA: Rodale Press.

American Diabetes Association and American Dietetic Association. 1995. *Exchange Lists for Meal Planning.* Chicago: American Dietetic Association and American Diabetes Association.

Atkins, R. 1999. *Dr. Atkins' New Diet Revolution: Revised and Updated.* New York: M. Evans.

Brownell, K. 2004. *The LEARN Program for Weight Management.* Dallas, TX: American Health Publishing Company.

Cooper, K. 1982. *The Aerobics Program for Total Well-Being.* New York: M. Evans.

Dusek, D. 1989. *Weight Management: The Fitness Way.* Boston: Jones and Bartlett.

Katzen, M., and Willett, W. 2006. *Eat, Drink, & Weigh Less.* New York: Hyperion.

Mayer, J. 1968. *Overweight: Causes, Cost and Control.* Englewood Cliffs, NJ: Prentice-Hall.

Miller, W. 1998. *Negotiated Peace: How to Win the War Over Weight.* Boston: Allyn and Bacon.

Murakami, Haruki. 2008. *What I Talk About When I Talk About Running.* London: Harvill Secker.

Ornish, D. 2001. *Eat More, Weigh Less: Dr. Dean Ornish's Life Choice Program for Losing Weight Safely While Eating Abundantly.* New York: HarperCollins Publishers.

Rolls, B. 2005. *The Volumetrics Eating Plan.* New York: HarperCollins.

Sears, B. 1995. *The Zone.* New York: Regan Books.

Shils, M., et al. 2006. *Modern Nutrition in Health and Disease.* Philadelphia: Lippincott Williams & Wilkins.

Taubes, G. 2007. *Good Calories, Bad Calories: Challenging the Conventional Wisdom on Diet, Weight Control, and Disease.* New York: Alfred A. Knopf.

Wansink, B. 2007. *Mindless Eating: Why We Eat More Than We Think.* New York: Bantam Books.

Young, L. 2006. *The Portion Teller Plan: The No-Diet Reality Guide to Eating, Cheating and Losing Weight Permanently.* New York: Morgan Road Books.

Reviews

Adamo, K., and Tesson, F. 2007. Genotype-specific weight loss treatment advice: How close are we? *Applied Physiology, Nutrition, and Metabolism* 32:351–66.

Ainsworth, B., et al. 2011. 2011 Compendium of physical activities: A second update of codes and MET values. *Medicine & Science in Sports & Exercise* 43:1575–81.

American Academy of Pediatrics. 2005. Promotion of healthy weight-control practices in young athletes. *Pediatrics* 116:1557–64.

American Diabetes Association. 2000. Role of fat replacers in diabetes medical nutrition therapy. *Diabetes Care* 23:S96–S97.

American Dietetic Association. 2002. Position of the American Dietetic Association: Weight management. *Journal of the American Dietetic Association* 102:1145–545.

American Heart Association. 2006. Diet and lifestyle recommendations. *Circulation* 114:82–96.

Arciero, P., et al. 2006. Increased dietary protein and combined high intensity aerobic and resistance exercise improves body fat distribution and cardiovascular risk factors. *International Journal of Sport Nutrition and Exercise Metabolism* 16:373–92.

Astrup, A. 2006. How to maintain a healthy body weight. *International Journal for Vitamin and Nutrition Research* 76:208–15.

Astrup, A., et al. 2002. Low-fat diets and energy balance: How does the evidence stand in 2002? *Proceedings of the Nutrition Society* 61:299–309.

Bellisle, F., et al. 1997. Meal frequency and energy balance. *British Journal of Nutrition* 77 (Supplement): S57–S70.

Blundell, J., and Green, S. 1997. Effect of sucrose and sweeteners on appetite and energy intake. *International Journal of Obesity and Related Metabolic Disorders* 20 (Supplement 2): S12–S17.

Borg, G. 1973. Perceived exertion: A note on "history" and methods. *Medicine & Science in Sports* 5:90–93.

Bouchard, C., and Blair, S. 1999. Introductory comments for the consensus on physical activity and obesity. *Medicine & Science in Sports & Exercise* 31:S498–S501.

Bravata, D., et al. 2003. Efficacy and safety of low-carbohydrate diets: A systematic review. *JAMA* 289:1837–50.

Bray, G. 1990. Exercise and obesity. In *Exercise, Fitness and Health,* eds. C. Bouchard, et al. Champaign, IL: Human Kinetics.

Brehm, B., and D'Alessio, D. 2008. Weight loss and metabolic benefits with diets of varying fat and carbohydrate content: Separating the wheat from the chaff. *Nature Clinical Practice. Endocrinology & Metabolism* 4;140–46.

Brown, T., et al. 2009. Systematic review of long-term lifestyle interventions to prevent weight gain and morbidity in adults. *Obesity Reviews* 10:627–38.

Brownell, K., and Kramer, F. 1989. Behavioral management of obesity. *Medical Clinics of North America* 73:185–202.

Brownell, K., and Rodin, J. 1994. The dieting maelstrom: Is it possible and advisable to lose weight? *American Psychologist* 49:781–91.

Campbell, A., and Hausenblas, H. 2009. Effects of exercise interventions on body image: A meta-analysis. *Journal of Health Psychology* 14:780–93.

Catenacci, V., and Wyatt, H. 2007. The role of physical activity in producing and maintaining weight loss. *Nature Clinical Practice. Endocrinology & Metabolism* 3:518–29.

Consumers Union. 2011. Pick your ideal diet. *Consumer Reports* 76 (6):14–16.

Consumers Union. 2007. A truce in the diet wars. *Consumer Reports on Health* 19 (5):8–9.

Consumers Union. 2007. Gym traps—and solutions. *Consumer Reports on Health* 19 (2):7.

Consumers Union. 2007. New diet winners. *Consumer Reports* 72 (6):12–17.

Consumers Union. 2006. 10 ways to make exercise a lasting part of your life. *Consumer Reports on Health* 18 (5):1, 4–6.

Consumers Union. 2005. Rating the diets. *Consumer Reports* 70 (6):1818–22.

Consumers Union. 2003. Eat more without gaining weight. *Consumer Reports on Health* 15 (6):8–9.

Convertino, V. 1991. Blood volume: Its adaptation to endurance training. *Medicine & Science in Sports & Exercise* 23:1338–48.

Dallman, M. 2010. Stress-induced obesity and the emotional nervous system. *Trends in Endocrinology and Metabolism* 21:159–65.

Donnelly, J., and Smith, B. 2005. Is exercise effective for weight loss with ad libitum diet? Energy balance, compensation, and gender differences. *Exercise and Sport Sciences Reviews* 33:169–74.

Donnelly, J., et al. 2009. American College of Sports Medicine Position Stand: Appropriate physical activity intervention strategies for weight loss and prevention of weight regain for adults. *Medicine & Science in Sports & Exercise* 41:459–71.

Drewnowski, A. 1995. Intense sweeteners and the control of appetite. *Nutrition Reviews* 53:1–7.

Egras, A., et al. 2011. An evidence-based review of fat modifying supplemental weight loss products. *Journal of Obesity* pii: 297315.

Elder, S., and Roberts, S. 2007. The effects of exercise on food intake and body fatness: A summary of published studies. *Nutrition Reviews* 65:1–19.

Epstein, L., et al. 1996. Exercise in treating obesity in children and adolescents. *Medicine & Science in Sports & Exercise* 28:428–35.

Fontana, L., and Klein, S. 2007. Aging, adiposity, and calorie restriction. *Journal of the American Medical Association* 297:986–94.

Ford, H., and Frost, G. 2010. Glycaemic index, appetite and body weight. *Proceedings of the Nutrition Society* 69:199–203.

Foreyt, J., et al. 2009. Weight-reducing diets: Are there any differences? *Nutrition Reviews* 67 Suppl 1:S99–101.

Forman, A. 2011. Boosting metabolism: What works, what doesn't. *Environmental Nutrition* 33g:1, 4.

Friedman, A. 2004. High protein diets: Potential effects on the kidney in renal health and disease. *American Journal of Kidney Disease* 44:950–62.

Garb, J., et al. 2009. Bariatric surgery for the treatment of morbid obesity: A meta-analysis of weight loss outcomes for laparoscopic adjustable gastric banding and laparoscopic gastric bypass. *Obesity Surgery* 19:1447–55.

Gellish, R., et al. 2006. Longitudinal modeling of the relationship between age and maximal heart rate. *Medicine & Science in Sports & Exercise* 38:822–29.

Giovannini, M., et al. 2010. Symposium overview: Do we all eat breakfast and is it important? *Critical Reviews in Food Science and Nutrition* 50:97–9.

Haskell, W., et al. 2007. Physical activity and public health: Updated recommendation for adults from the American College of Sports Medicine and the American Heart Association. *Medicine & Science in Sports & Exercise* 39:1423–34.

Heckman, M., et al. 2010. Caffeine (1, 3, 7-trimethylxanthine) in foods: A comprehensive review on consumption, functionality, safety, and regulatory matters. *Journal of Food Science* 75:R77–87.

Hill, J., and Commerford, R. 1996. Physical activity, fat balance, and energy balance. *International Journal of Sport Nutrition* 6:80–92.

Hill, J., et al. 1994. Physical activity, fitness, and moderate obesity. In *Physical Activity, Fitness, and Health,* eds. C. Bouchard, et al. Champaign, IL: Human Kinetics.

Howarth, N., et al. 2001. Dietary fiber and weight regulation. *Nutrition Reviews* 59:129–39.

Hu, F. 2005. Protein, body weight, and cardiovascular health. *American Journal of Clinical Nutrition* 82:242S–47S.

Hunter, G., et al. 1998. A role for high intensity exercise on energy balance and weight control. *International Journal of Obesity and Related Metabolic Disorders* 22:489–93.

Hursel, R., and Westerterp-Plantenga, M. 2010. Thermogenic ingredients and body weight regulation. *International Journal of Obesity* 34:659–69.

Jakicic, J., and Gallagher, K. 2003. Exercise considerations for the sedentary, overweight adult. *Exercise and Sport Sciences Reviews* 31:91–95.

Jakicic, J., and Otto, A. 2006. Treatment and prevention of obesity: What is the role of exercise? *Nutrition Reviews* 64:S57–S61.

Jequier, E. 2000. Pathways to obesity. *International Journal of Obesity and Related Metabolic Disorders* 26:S12–S17.

Jeukendrup, A., and Aldred, S. 2004. Fat supplementation, health, and endurance performance. *Nutrition* 20:678–88.

Jones, L., et al. 2007. Lifestyle modification in the treatment of obesity: An educational challenge and opportunity. *Clinical Pharmacology and Therapeutics* 81:776–79.

Kay, S., and Fiatarone Singh, M. 2006. The influence of physical activity on abdominal fat: A systematic review of the literature. *Obesity Reviews* 7:183 200.

Kearney, T., et al. 2010. Adverse drug events associated with yohimbine-containing products: A retrospective review of the California Poison Control System reported cases. *Annals of Pharmacotherapy* 44:1022–9.

King, N. 1999. What processes are involved in the appetite response to moderate increases in exercise-induced energy expenditure? *Proceedings of the Nutrition Society* 58:107–13.

King, N., et al. 2007. Metabolic and behavioral compensatory responses to exercise interventions: Barriers to weight loss. *Obesity* 15:1373–83.

Kris-Etherton, P., et al. 2002. Dietary fat: Assessing the evidence in support of a moderate-fat diet; The benchmark based on lipoprotein metabolism. *Proceedings of the Nutrition Society* 61:287–98.

Larson-Meyer, D., et al. 2010. Caloric restriction with or without exercise: The fitness versus fatness debate. *Medicine & Science in Sports & Exercise* 42:152–9.

Layman, D., et al. 2008. Protein in optimal health: Heart disease and type 2 diabetes. *American Journal of Clinical Nutrition* 87:1571S–75S.

Leidy, H., and Campbell, W. 2011. The effect of eating frequency on appetite control and food intake: Brief synopsis of controlled feeding studies. *Journal of Nutrition* 141:154–7.

Levin, B. 2002. Metabolic sensors: Viewing glucosensing neurons from a broader perspective. *Physiology & Behavior* 76:387–401.

Levine, J., and Kotz, C. 2005. NEAT—nonexercise activity thermogenesis—egocentric & geocentric environmental factors vs. biological regulation. *Acta Physiologica Scandinavica* 184:309–18.

Liebman, B. 2005. Bigger meals: Smaller waists. *Nutrition Action Health Letter* 32 (5):1–7.

Liebman, B. 2004. Weighing the diet books. *Nutrition Action Health Letter* 31 (1):3–8.

Lohman, T., et al. 2004. Seeing ourselves through the obesity epidemic. *President's Council on Physical Fitness and Sports Research Digest* 5 (3):1–8.

Malik, V., and Hu, F. 2007. Popular weight-loss diets: From evidence to practice. *Nature Clinical Practice. Cardiovascular Medicine* 4:34–41.

Malik, V., et al. 2006. Intake of sugar-sweetened beverages and weight gain: A systematic review. *American Journal of Clinical Nutrition* 84:274–88.

Manore, M. 1999. Low-fat foods and weight loss. *ACSM's Health & Fitness Journal* 3 (3):37–39.

Mattes, R. 1998. Position of the American Dietetic Association: Fat replacers. *Journal of the American Dietetic Association* 98:463–68.

Melby, C., and Hickey, M. 2005. Energy balance and body weight regulation. *Sports Science Exchange* 18 (4):1–6.

Melby, C., and Hill, J. 1999. Exercise, macronutrient balance, and body weight regulation. *Sports Science Exchange* 12 (1):1–6.

Miller, G., and Groziak, S. 1996. Impact of fat substitutes on fat intake. *Lipids* 31:S293–S296.

Murphy, M., et al. 2007. The effect of walking on fitness, fatness and resting blood pressure: A meta-analysis of randomized, controlled trials. *Preventive Medicine* 44:377–85.

National Institutes of Health. 1992. Methods for voluntary weight loss and control: Technology Assessment Conference Statement. *Nutrition Today* 50 (July/August):27–33.

Nelson, M., et al. 2007. Physical activity and public health in older adults: Recommendation from the American College of Sports Medicine and the American Heart Association. *Medicine & Science in Sports & Exercise* 39:1435–45.

Nieman, D. 2010. You asked for it. *ACSM's Health & Fitness Journal* 14 (3):5–6.

Nordmann, A., et al. 2006. Effects of low-carbohydrate vs low-fat diets on weight loss and cardiovascular risk factors: A meta-analysis of randomized controlled trials. *Archives of Internal Medicine* 166:285–93.

Phung, O., et al. 2010. Effect of green tea catechins with or without caffeine on anthropometric measures: A systematic review and meta-analysis. *American Journal of Clinical Nutrition* 91:73–81.

Pi-Sunyer, F. 1990. Effect of the composition of the diet on energy intake. *Nutrition Reviews* 48:94–105.

Pittas, A., and Roberts, S. 2006. Dietary composition and weight loss: Can we individualize dietary prescriptions according to insulin sensitivity or secretion status? *Nutrition Reviews* 64:435–48.

Poehlman, E., and Melby, C. 1998. Resistance training and energy balance. *International Journal of Sport Nutrition* 8:143–59.

Popkin, B., et al. 2006. A new proposed guidance system for beverage consumption in the United States. *American Journal of Clinical Nutrition* 83:529–42.

Rains, T., et al. 2011. Antiobesity effects of green tea catechins: A mechanistic review. *Journal of Nutritional Biochemistry* 22:1–7.

Rankinen, T., and Bouchard, C. 2008. Gene-physical activity interactions: Overview of human studies. *Obesity* 16 Suppl 3:S47–50.

Riley, R. 1999. Popular weight loss diets. *Clinics in Sports Medicine* 18:691–701.

Roberts, S. 2000. High-glycemic index foods, hunger, and obesity: Is there a connection? *Nutrition Reviews* 58:163–69.

Robinson, T. 2001. Television viewing and childhood obesity. *Pediatric Clinics of North America* 48:1017–25.

Rolls, B., and Bell, E. 1999. Intake of fat and carbohydrate: Role of energy density. *European Journal of Clinical Nutrition* 53:S166–S173.

Rossato, L., et al. 2011. Synephrine: From trace concentrations to massive consumption in weight-loss. *Food and Chemical Toxicology* 49:8–16.

Smith, S., and Zachwieja, J. 1999. Visceral adipose tissue: A critical review of intervention strategies. *International Journal of Obesity and Related Metabolic Disorders* 23:329–35.

Södlerlund, A., et al. 2009. Physical activity, diet and behaviour modification in the treatment of overweight and obese adults: A systematic review. *Perspectives in Public Health* 129:132–42.

Stiegler, P., and Cunliffe, A. 2006. The role of diet and exercise for the maintenance of fat-free mass and resting metabolic rate. *Sports Medicine* 36:239–62.

St. Jeor, S., et al. 2001. Dietary protein and weight reduction: A statement for health-care professionals from the Nutrition Committee of the Council on Nutrition, Physical Activity, and Metabolism of the American Heart Association. *Circulation* 104:1869–74.

Swain, D., and Franklin, B. 2006. Comparison of cardioprotective benefits of vigorous versus moderate intensity aerobic exercise. *American Journal of Cardiology* 97:141–47.

Sweet, S., and Fortier, M. 2010. Improving physical activity and dietary behaviours with single or multiple health behaviour interventions: A synthesis of meta-analyses and reviews. *International Journal of Environmental Research and Public Health* 7:1720–43.

Tremblay, A., and Doucet, E. 1999. Influence of intense physical activity on energy balance and body fatness. *Proceedings of the Nutrition Society* 58:99–105.

Tremblay, A., et al. 1999. Physical activity and weight maintenance. *International Journal of Obesity and Related Metabolic Disorders* 23 (Supplement 3):S50–S54.

Tsai, A., and Wadden, T. 2006. The evolution of very-low-calorie diets: An update and meta-analysis. *Obesity* 14:1283–93.

Tsai, A., and Wadden, T. 2005. Systematic review: An evaluation of major commercial weight loss programs in the United States. *Annals of Internal Medicine* 142:56–66.

Tudor-Locke, C., and Bassett, D. 2004. How many steps/day are enough? Preliminary pedometer indices for public health. *Sports Medicine* 34:1–8.

Tudor-Locke, C., et al. 2008. Revisiting "How many steps are enough?" *Medicine & Science in Sports & Exercise* 40:S537–S543.

Tufts University. 2011. Extra sugar adds 475 calories a day. *Tufts University Health & Nutrition Letter* 28 (12):3.

Volek, J., and Sharman, M. 2004. Cardiovascular and hormonal aspects of very-low-carbohydrate ketogenic diets. *Obesity Research* 12:115S–23S.

Volek, J., et al. 2005. Diet and exercise for weight loss: A review of current issues. *Sports Medicine* 35:1–9.

Wadden, T., et al. 2004. Efficacy of lifestyle modification for long-term weight control. *Obesity Research* 12:151S–62S.

Walberg-Rankin, J. 2000. Forfeit the fat, leave the lean: Optimizing weight loss for athletes. *Sports Science Exchange* 13 (1):1–4.

Weigle, D., et al. 2005. A high-protein diet induces sustained reductions in appetite, ad libitum caloric intake, and body weight despite compensatory changes in diurnal plasma leptin and ghrelin concentrations. *American Journal of Clinical Nutrition* 82:41–48.

Wells, K., and Wells, T. 2007. Preventing relapse after weight loss. *Journal of the American Medical Athletic Association* 20 (1):5–8, 16.

Westerterp-Plantenga, M., et al. 2009. Dietary protein, weight loss, and weight maintenance. *Annual Review of Nutrition* 29:21–41.

Whigham, L., et al. 2007. Efficacy of conjugated linoleic acid for reducing fat mass: A meta-analysis in humans. *American Journal of Clinical Nutrition* 85:1203–11.

Williams, M. 2008. Nutrition for the school aged child athlete. In *The Young Athlete,* eds. H. Hebestreit and O. Bar-Or. Oxford: Blackwell Publishing.

Wing, R., and Phelan, S. 2005. Long-term weight maintenance. *American Journal of Clinical Nutrition* 82:222S–25S.

Wood, P. 1996. Clinical applications of diet and physical activity in weight loss. *Nutrition Reviews* 54:S131–S135.

Wylie-Rosett, J., and Davis, N. 2009. Low-carbohydrate diets: An update on current research. *Current Diabetes Reports* 9:396–404.

Wylie-Rosett, J., et al. 2004. Carbohydrates and increases in obesity: Does the type of carbohydrate make a difference? *Obesity Research* 12:124S–29S.

Specific Studies

Adams, T., et al. 2007. Long-term mortality after gastric bypass surgery. *New England Journal of Medicine* 357:753–61.

Albers, S. 2010. The Twinkie diet. www.psychologytoday.com. November 10.

Arciero, P., et al. 2006. Increased dietary protein and combined high intensity aerobic and resistance exercise improves body fat distribution and cardiovascular risk factors. *International Journal of Sport Nutrition and Exercise Metabolism* 16:373–92.

Azadbakht, L., et al. 2007. Better dietary adherence and weight maintenance achieved by a long-term moderate-fat diet. *British Journal of Nutrition* 97:399–404.

Benezra, L., et al. 2001. Intakes of most nutrients remain at acceptable levels during a weight management program using the food exchange system. *Journal of the American Dietetic Association* 101:554–61.

Browning, R., and Kram, R. 2007. Effects of obesity on the biomechanics of walking at different speeds. *Medicine & Science in Sports & Exercise* 39:1632–41.

Church, T., et al. 2010. Effects of aerobic and resistance training on hemoglobin A1c levels in patients with type 2 diabetes: A randomized controlled trial. *JAMA* 304:2253–62.

Cotton, J., et al. 1996. Replacement of dietary fat with sucrose polyester: Effects on energy intake and appetite control in non-obese males. *American Journal of Clinical Nutrition* 63:891–96.

Dansinger, M., et al. 2005. Comparison of the Atkins, Ornish, Watchers, and Zone diets for weight loss and heart disease risk reduction: A randomized trial. *JAMA* 293:43–53.

Das, S., et al. 2007. Long-term effects of 2 energy-restricted diets differing in glycemic load on dietary adherence, body composition, and metabolism in CALERIE: A 1-y randomized controlled trial. *American Journal of Clinical Nutrition* 85:1023–30.

Dich, J., et al. 2000. Effects of excessive isocaloric intake of either carbohydrate or fat on body composition, fat mass, de novo lipogenesis and energy expenditure in normal young men. *Ugeskrift for Laeger* 162:4794–99.

Ebbeling, C., et al. 2007. Effects of a low-glycemic load vs low-fat diet in obese young adults: A randomized trial. *Journal of the American Medical Association* 297:2092–102.

Ello-Martin, J., et al. 2007. Dietary energy density in the treatment of obesity: A year-long trial comparing 2 weight-loss diets. *American Journal of Clinical Nutrition* 85:1465–77.

Foster-Schubert, K., et al. 2005. Human plasma ghrelin levels increase during a one-year exercise program. *Journal of Clinical Endocrinology and Metabolism* 90:820–25.

Furlow, E., and Anderson, J. 2009. A systematic review of targeted outcomes associated with a medically supervised commercial weight-loss program. *Journal of the American Dietetic Association* 109:1417–21.

Grediagin, M., et al. 1995. Exercise intensity does not effect body composition change in untrained, moderately overfat women. *Journal of the American Dietetic Association* 95:661–65.

Hall, C., et al. 2004. Energy expenditure of walking and running: Comparison with prediction equations. *Medicine & Science in Sports & Exercise* 36:2128–34.

Hansen, D., et al. 2007. The effects of exercise training on fat-mass loss in obese patients during energy intake restriction. *Sports Medicine* 37:31–46.

Haus, G., et al. 1994. Key modifiable factors in weight maintenance: Fat intake, exercise, and weight cycling. *Journal of the American Diebetic* Association 94:409–13.

Howard, B., et al. 2006. Low-fat dietary pattern and weight change over 7 years: The Women's Health Initiative Dietary Modification Trial. *Journal of the American Medical Association* 295:39–49.

Hultquist, C., et al. 2005. Comparison of walking recommendations in previously inactive women. *Medicine & Science in Sports & Exercise* 37:676–83.

Irving, B., et al. 2008. Effect of exercise training intensity on abdominal visceral fat and body composition. *Medicine & Science in Sports & Exercise* 40:1863–72.

Jakicic, J., et al. 1995. Prescribing exercise in multiple short bouts versus one continuous bout: Effects on adherence, cardiorespiratory fitness, and weight loss in overweight women. *International Journal of Obesity and Related Metabolic Disorders* 19:893–901.

Johnston, C., et al. 2004. High-protein, low-fat diets are effective for weight loss and favorably alter biomarkers in healthy adults. *Journal of Nutrition* 134:586–91.

Johnston, C., et al. 2002. Postprandial thermogenesis is increased 100% on high-protein, low-fat diet versus a high-carbohydrate, low-fat diet in healthy, young women. *Journal of the American College of Nutrition* 21:55–61.

Kostek, M., et al. 2007. Subcutaneous fat alterations resulting from an upper-body resistance training program. *Medicine & Science in Sports & Exercise* 39:1177–85.

Kraemer, W., et al. 1999. Influence of exercise training on physiological and performance changes with weight loss in men. *Medicine & Science in Sports & Exercise* 31:1320–29.

Laan, D., et al. 2010. Effects and reproducibility of aerobic and resistance exercise on appetite and energy intake in young, physically active adults. *Applied Physiology, Nutrition, and Metabolism* 35:842–7.

Layman, D., et al. 2005. Dietary protein and exercise have additive effects on body composition during weight loss in adult women. *Journal of Nutrition* 135:1903–10.

Leidy, H., et al. 2011. The effects of consuming frequent, higher protein meals on appetite and satiety during weight loss in overweight/obese men. *Obesity* 19:818–24.

Leidy, H., et al. 2007. Effects of acute and chronic protein intake on metabolism, appetite, and ghrelin during weight loss. *Obesity* 15:1215–25.

Leidy, H., et al. 2007. Higher protein intake preserves lean mass and satiety with weight loss in pre-obese and obese women. *Obesity* 15:421–29.

Linde, J., et al. 2005. Self-weighing in weight gain prevention and weight loss trials. *Annals of Behavioral Medicine* 7:1–14.

Ludwig, D., et al. 2001. Relation between consumption of sugar-sweetened drinks and childhood obesity: A prospective, observational analysis. *Lancet* 357:505–8.

Ma, Y., et al. 2007. A dietary quality comparison of popular weight-loss plans. *Journal of the American Dietetic Association* 107:1786–91.

Manthou, E., et al. 2010. Behavioral compensatory adjustments to exercise training in overweight women. *Medicine & Science in Sports & Exercise* 42:1221–8.

Martins, C., et al. 2007. Effects of exercise on gut peptides, energy intake and appetite. *Journal of Endocrinology* 193:251–58.

Melanson, E., et al. 2002. Effect of exercise intensity on 24-h energy expenditure and nutrient oxidation. *Journal of Applied Physiology* 92:1045–52.

Mettler, S., et al. 2010. Increased protein intake reduces lean body mass loss during weight loss in athletes. *Medicine & Science in Sports & Exercise* 42:326–37.

Moloney, F., et al. 2004. Conjugated linoleic acid supplementation, insulin sensitivity, and lipoprotein metabolism in patients with type 2 diabetes mellitus. *American Journal of Clinical Nutrition* 80:887–95.

Murphy, M., et al. 2002. Accumulating brisk walking for fitness, cardiovascular risk, and psychological health. *Medicine & Science in Sports & Exercise* 34:1468–74.

Newman, B., et al. 1990. Nongenetic influences of obesity on other cardiovascular disease risk factors: An analysis of identical twins. *American Journal of Public Health* 80:675–78.

Nybo, L., et al. 2010. High-intensity training versus traditional exercise interventions for promoting health. *Medicine & Science in Sports & Exercise* 42:1951–58.

Persinger, R., et al. 2004. Consistency of the Talk Test for exercise prescription. *Medicine & Science in Sports & Exercise* 36:1632–36.

Pritchard, J., et al. 1997. A worksite program for overweight middle-aged men achieves lesser weight loss with exercise than with dietary change. *Journal of the American Dietetic Association* 97:37–42.

Puthoff, M., et al. 2006. The effect of weighted vest walking on metabolic responses and ground reaction forces. *Medicine & Science in Sports & Exercise* 38:746–52.

Raben, A., et al. 2002. Sucrose compared with artificial sweeteners: Different effects on ad libitum food intake and body weight after 10 wk of supplementation in overweight subjects. *American Journal of Clinical Nutrition* 76:721–29.

Redman, L., et al. 2007. Effect of calorie restriction with or without exercise on body composition and fat distribution. *Journal of Clinical Endocrinology & Metabolism* 92:865–72.

Romijn, J., et al. 2000. Substrate metabolism during different exercise intensities in endurance-trained women. *Journal of Applied Physiology* 88:1707–14.

Rowe, D., et al. 2011. Stride rate recommendations for moderate-intensity walking. *Medicine & Science in Sports & Exercise* 43:312–18.

Sacks, F., et al. 2009. Comparison of weight-loss diets with different compositions of fat, protein, and carbohydrates. *New England Journal of Medicine* 360:859–73.

Sedlock, D., et al. 1989. Effect of exercise intensity and duration on postexercise energy expenditure. *Medicine & Science in Sports & Exercise* 21:662–66.

Shai, I., et al. 2008. Weight loss with a low-carbohydrate, Mediterranean, or low-fat diet. *New England Journal of Medicine* 359:229–41.

Shide, D., and Rolls, B. 1995. Information about the fat content of preloads influences energy intake in healthy women. *Journal of the American Dietetic Association* 95:993–98.

Sillanpää, E., et al. 2008. Body composition and fitness during strength and/or endurance training in older men. *Medicine & Science in Sports & Exercise* 40:950–58.

Sjodin, A., et al. 1996. The influence of physical activity on BMR. *Medicine & Science in Sports & Exercise* 28:85–91.

Sjöström, L., et al. 2007. Effects of bariatric surgery on mortality in Swedish obese subjects. *New England Journal of Medicine* 357:741–52.

Stubbs, R., et al. 2004. A decrease in physical activity affects appetite, energy, and nutrient balance in lean men feeding ad libitum. *American Journal of Clinical Nutrition* 79:62–69.

Taheri, S., et al. 2004. Short sleep duration is associated with reduced leptin, elevated ghrelin, and increased body mass index. *PLoS Medicine* 1 (3):e62.

Tate, D., et al. 2007. Long-term weight losses associated with prescription of higher physical activity goals. Are higher levels of physical activity protective against weight regain? *American Journal of Clinical Nutrition* 85:954–59.

Thompson, D., et al. 2004. Relationship between accumulated walking and body composition in middle-aged women. *Medicine & Science in Sports & Exercise* 36:911–14.

Thompson, D., et al. 1988. Acute effects of exercise intensity on appetite in young men. *Medicine & Science in Sports & Exercise* 20:222–27.

Truby, H., et al. 2006. Randomized controlled trial of four commercial weight loss programmes in the UK: Initial findings from the BBC "diet trials." *British Medical Journal* 332:1309–14.

Utter, A., et al. 2006. Validation of Omni Scale of Perceived exertion during prolonged cycling. *Medicine & Science in Sport & Exercise* 38:780–86.

Vander Wal, J., et al. 2005. Short-term effect of eggs on satiety in overweight and obese subjects. *Journal of the American College of Nutrition* 4:510–15.

Weigle, D., et al. 2005. A high-protein diet induces sustained reductions in appetite, ad libitum caloric intake, and body weight despite compensatory changes in diurnal plasma leptin and ghrelin concentrations. *American Journal of Clinical Nutrition* 82:41–48.

Zeni, A., et al. 1996. Energy expenditure with indoor exercise machines. *Journal of the American Medical Association* 275:1424–27.

Weight Gaining through Proper Nutrition and Exercise

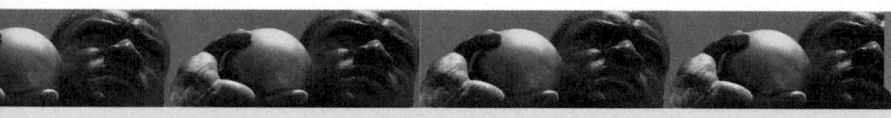

CHAPTER TWELVE

LEARNING OBJECTIVES

After studying this chapter, you should be able to:

1. Describe the steps an individual might take to gain body weight, mainly as muscle mass.

2. Plan a diet for an individual who desires to gain muscle mass in concert with a resistance-training program, focusing on recommended caloric intake and foods compatible with the Prudent Healthy Diet.

3. Identify dietary supplements used by physically active individuals to stimulate muscle building and body-fat loss, and list those, if any, that may be effective.

4. List and explain the principles of resistance training.

5. Understand the basic differences among resistance-training programs for muscular hypertrophy, muscular strength and power, and muscular endurance.

6. Design a total-body resistance-training program for an individual who desires to gain body weight as muscle mass.

7. Identify the potential health benefits of resistance exercise and compare them to the health benefits associated with aerobic endurance exercise, noting similarities and differences.

Introduction

As noted in chapter 11, there are basically three reasons why individuals attempt to lose excess body weight—to improve appearance, health, or athletic performance. Some individuals may also wish to gain weight for the same three reasons, and may use resistance training, also known as weight training or strength training, as a means to stimulate weight gain.

For those who wish to improve appearance, resistance training will increase muscularity, a desired physical attribute among many males. Resistance training is becoming increasingly popular, particularly among women. According to the U.S. Centers for Disease Control and Prevention (CDC), approximately 20 percent of adults engage in resistance training, including about 21.5 percent of males and 17.5 percent of females. In the previous CDC report, only 14.5 percent of females did strength training.

Gaining weight, particularly muscle mass stimulated by resistance training, may also be associated with some health benefits. An increased muscularity that improves physical appearance and body image may help elevate self-esteem, contributing to positive psychological health. Additionally, resistance training, done alone even without weight gain, is recommended for several other health benefits, such as increased bone mineral density. The American Heart Association and the American College of Sports Medicine, in their reports on physical activity and health, recommend resistance exercise as an effective means to promote overall good health. Resistance training is particularly recommended for older adults to help prevent the muscle wasting, and associated health problems, seen with aging, as documented by Nelson and others. A popular book, *Dr. David Reuben's Quick Weight-Gain Program,* has been designed to provide sound medical advice for the 26 million Americans who need to gain weight for a variety of medical and cosmetic reasons.

Increased body weight, particularly increased muscle mass, may be associated with improvements in strength and power, two performance factors important for a wide variety of sports. Enhanced muscularity also may influence performance in judged aesthetic sports, such as diving and gymnastics. Most colleges and universities, as well as many high schools, have strength-training programs for their athletes, both males and females. At the elite level, sport-specific resistance-training programs are tailored to the individual athlete.

No matter what the reason for gaining body weight, you should be concerned about where the extra pounds will be stored. The energy-balance equation works as well for gaining weight as it does for losing weight, but excess body fat in general will not improve physical appearance, health, or athletic performance. On the contrary, it may detract from all three. To put on body weight, you have to concentrate on means to increase the fat-free mass, particularly muscle tissue, with little or no increase in body-fat stores.

Rasmussen and Phillips note that resistance exercise and nutritional provision are two independent and major stimuli of muscle protein synthesis and overall muscle growth, and numerous related approaches have been employed to increase muscle mass. Specialized exercise equipment or exercise techniques are advertised as the most effective methods available to build muscles. Protein supplements have been a favorite among weight lifters for years, but today athletes can buy numerous dietary supplements that are advertised to produce an anabolic, or muscle-building, effect. Some athletes and nonathletes even use drugs to gain weight for enhanced performance or appearance, a topic that is discussed in chapter 13. Although resistance training may confer significant health benefits, Pope indicated that some very muscular individuals have a distorted body image, perceiving themselves as too thin or not sufficiently muscular, which he labeled muscle dysmorphia or the Adonis Complex. Grieve noted that muscle dysmorphia is most prevalent in males, but has characteristics, such as low self-esteem, body dissatisfaction, and perfectionism, similar to those observed in females with eating disorders. Muscle dysmorphia may lead to unhealthful practices, such as the use of drugs, to enhance muscularity. Interestingly, Pickett and others reported that muscle dysmorphia is not confined to competitive bodybuilders, but is also found in noncompetitive weight trainers and even physically active men who do not train with weights.

Like weight-loss programs, weight-gaining programs may be safe and effective or they can be potentially harmful to your health. Gaining weight, particularly as muscle mass, is difficult for some individuals; the purpose of this chapter is to present basic information on the type of diet and exercise program that is most likely to be effective as a means to put on weight without compromising your health.

Although some basic information regarding advanced resistance-training programs will be provided, detailed coverage of such programs is beyond the scope of this text. References to advanced resistance-training programs will be provided for the interested reader.

Basic Considerations

Why are some individuals underweight?

Being significantly under a healthy body weight may be due to several factors. Heredity may be an important factor, as genetic factors may predispose some individuals to leanness. For example, a lean body frame or high basal metabolic rate may have been acquired from your parents. Medical problems such as heartburn, infections, or cancer could adversely affect food intake and digestion, so a physician should be consulted to rule out nutritional problems caused by organic disease, hormonal imbalance, or inadequate absorption of nutrients. Social pressures, such as the strong desire of a teenage girl to have a slender body, could lead to undernutrition; an extreme example is anorexia nervosa, discussed in chapter 10. Emotional problems also may affect food intake. In many cases, food intake is increased during periods of emotional crisis, but the appetite may also be depressed in some individuals for long periods. Economic hardship may reduce food purchasing power, so some individuals simply may sacrifice food intake for other life necessities.

Being considerably underweight, such as a Body Mass Index below 18.5, may be considered a symptom of malnutrition or undernutrition. It is important to determine the cause before prescribing a treatment. Our concern here is the individual who does not have any of these medical, psychological, social, or economic problems but who simply cannot create a positive energy balance because of excess energy expenditure or insufficient energy (Calorie) intake. Caloric intake has to be increased, and the output has to be modified somewhat.

What steps should I take if I want to gain weight?

The following guidelines may help you develop an effective program to maximize your gains in muscle mass and keep body-fat increases relatively low.

1. Have an acceptable purpose for the weight gain. The desire for an improved physical appearance and body image may be reason enough. For athletes, increased muscle mass may be important for a variety of sports, particularly if strength and power are improved. However, you do not want to gain weight at the expense of speed if speed is important to your sport.

2. Calculate your average energy needs daily, as discussed in chapter 11. For a weight-gain program, you may wish to use several techniques to estimate your daily energy needs and select the highest value.

3. Keep a 3- to 7-day record of what you normally eat. See pages 476–478 for guidelines to determine your average daily caloric intake. If the obtained value is less than your energy needs calculated under item 2 in this list, this may be a reason why you are not gaining weight.

4. Check your living habits. Do you get enough rest and sleep? If not, you may be burning more energy than the estimate in item 2 of this list. Smoking increases your metabolic rate almost 10 percent and may account for approximately 200 Calories per day. Caffeine in coffee and soft drinks also increases the metabolic rate for several hours. Getting enough rest and sleep and eliminating smoking and caffeine will help decrease your energy output.

5. Set a reasonable goal within a certain time period. Weight gain may be rapid at first but then tapers off as you near your genetic potential. Peter Lemon, an expert in resistance training and protein metabolism, indicated that someone starting a resistance-training program may increase body mass by 20 percent in the first year. After that, gains are somewhat less, possibly only 1–3 percent per year. In general, about 0.5–1 pound per week is a sound approach for a novice, but weight gaining is difficult for some individuals and may occur at a slower rate. Specific goals may also include muscular hypertrophy in various parts of the body.

6. Increase your caloric and protein intake. A properly designed diet should include adequate Calories and protein and not violate the principles of healthful nutrition.

7. Start a resistance-training exercise program. This type of exercise program will serve as a stimulus to build muscle tissue. Guidelines for developing a resistance-training program are presented later in this chapter.

8. Use a good cloth or steel tape to take body measurements before and during your weight-gaining program. Be sure you measure at the same points about once a week. Those body parts measured should include the neck, upper and lower arm, chest, abdomen, hips, thigh, and calf. This is to ensure that body-weight gains are proportionately distributed. You should look for good gains in the chest and limbs; the abdominal and hip girth increase should be kept low because that is where fat is more likely to be stored. If available, skinfold calipers may be used to measure subcutaneous fat skinfolds at multiple sites over the body. Fat skinfold thicknesses should remain the same or decrease to ensure that the weight gain is muscle rather than fat.

In summary, adequate rest, increased caloric intake, and a proper resistance-training program may be very effective as a means to gain the right kind of body weight.

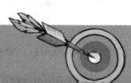

Key Concepts

▶ There may be a variety of reasons why an individual is underweight, and the cause should be determined before a treatment is recommended.

▶ For those who want to gain weight, a weekly increase of 0.5–1.0 pound is a sound approach, but the desired weight gain should be muscle tissue and not body fat. In essence, adequate rest and sleep, increased caloric intake, and a proper resistance-training program should be effective in helping to increase lean body mass.

Nutritional Considerations

In the last chapter we discussed nutritional considerations for losing body weight, particularly body fat. In general, the recommendation consists of a healthy diet but with reduced caloric intake.

In this chapter we consider nutritional considerations for gaining body weight, particularly lean body mass as muscle. In this case the recommendation still is to eat a healthy diet, but with increased caloric intake.

Gaining weight as muscle mass may be difficult for some. Remember the quote from chapter 11: *"Muscles are hard to get and easy to lose, fat is easy to get and hard to lose."* Resistance training, discussed later in this chapter, is important to help stimulate muscle growth so extra Calories are used to develop muscle, not fat. As noted, gaining about 0.5–1.0 pound per week is a reasonable goal, although some may be able to gain more, while some may gain less.

How many Calories are needed to form one pound of muscle?

Muscle tissue consists of about 70 percent water, 22 percent protein, and the remainder is fat, carbohydrate, and minerals. Because the vast majority of muscle tissue is water, which has no caloric value, the total caloric value is only about 700–800 Calories per pound. However, extra energy is needed to help synthesize the muscle tissue.

It is not known exactly how many additional Calories are necessary to form 1 pound of muscle tissue in human beings, nor is it known in what form these Calories have to be consumed. The National Research Council notes that 5 Calories are needed to support the addition of 1 gram of tissue during growth, while Forbes cites a value of 8 Calories per gram in adults. Because 1 pound equals 454 grams, a range of 2,300–3,500 additional Calories appears to be a reasonable amount. With a recommended weight gain of 1 pound per week, about 400–500 Calories above your daily needs would provide an amount in the suggested range, 2,800–3,500 Calories per week. A study by Robert Bartels and his associates at Ohio State University revealed that an additional 500 Calories per day resulted in nearly a 1-pound increase in lean body weight per week during a resistance-training program. For our purposes, we shall consider 3,500 Calories as the weekly excess energy intake necessary to support an increase in 1 pound of muscle tissue.

How can I determine the amount of Calories I need daily to gain one pound per week?

First, review the techniques presented in chapter 11 to determine the number of Calories needed simply to maintain your current body weight. Then add the Calories that you expend during exercise and the additional amount needed to synthesize the muscle tissue. Table 12.1 presents an example of a 154-pound 18-year-old male who desires to gain a pound per week. You may modify the figures according to your own needs. You can use the ChooseMyPlate Website to plan a weight-gain diet as well as a weight-loss diet. Other methods presented in chapter 11, such as the Mayo Clinic Calorie Calculator, may also be used. Remember, a weight gain of 0.5–1.0 pound muscle mass per week is a reasonable goal during the early stages of resistance training. If you are maintaining your weight with your current dietary intake, adding 500 Calories per day may also be an acceptable approach.

Increased caloric intake is the key dietary principle, along with adequate protein intake, to gain mass during resistance training, as

TABLE 12.1 Caloric intake needed for a 154-pound, 18-year-old male to gain one pound per week

Energy expenditure	Daily Calories needed
Recommended caloric intake to maintain current weight 19 Calories/pound	2,468
Resistance training 200 Calories per session 4 sessions per week 800/7	115
Aerobic exercise 300 Calories per session 4 sessions per week 1,200/7	170
Muscle tissue synthesis 3,500 Calories per pound 3,500/7	500
Total daily caloric intake	3,253

noted in a Gatorade Sports Science Institute review of weight-gain strategies in athletes by leading experts in the area, Gail Butterfield, Susan Kleiner, Peter Lemon, and Michael Stone.

Is protein supplementation necessary during a weight-gaining program?

One of the most researched areas in sports nutrition is the recommended protein intake for individuals who are attempting to increase muscle mass with resistance training. Topics of interest include amount, quality, timing, co-ingestion with carbohydrate, and cost.

Amount   From a mathematical viewpoint, adding a pound of muscle protein per week does not require a substantial increase in daily protein intake. Consider the following! Muscle tissue is about 22 percent protein and 70 percent water, with the remainder composed of carbohydrate and fat and trace amounts of vitamins and minerals. One pound of muscle is equal to 454 grams, but only about 100 grams (0.22 × 454 grams) is protein. If we divide 100 grams by 7 days, we would need approximately 14 grams of protein per day above our normal protein requirements to support the growth of one pound of muscle per week—if we are in protein balance. Incidentally, 14 grams of protein could be obtained in such small amounts of food as 2 glasses of milk; 2 ounces of meat, fish, or poultry; 2 eggs; or various combinations (see figure 12.1).

As you may recall, the Acceptable Macronutrient Distribution Range (AMDR) for protein is 10 to 35 percent of daily caloric intake. In an earlier review, Phillips indicated that strength-trained athletes should consume protein consistent with general population guidelines, or about 12–15 percent of energy from protein. As noted in table 12.1, our 70-kilogram (154-pound) male needs a daily intake approximating 3,250 Calories to add a pound of

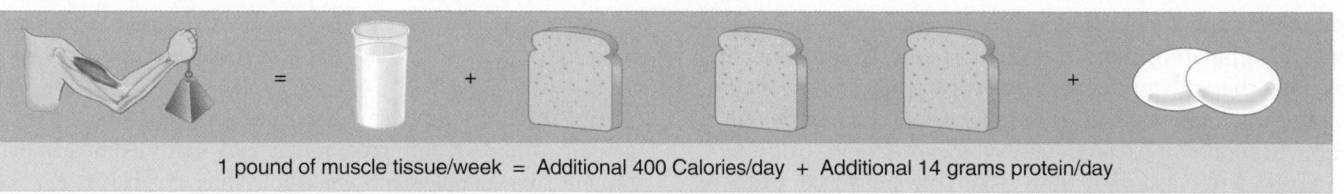

1 pound of muscle tissue/week = Additional 400 Calories/day + Additional 14 grams protein/day

FIGURE 12.1 To add a pound of muscle tissue per week, you need to consume approximately 400 additional Calories and 14 grams of additional protein per day. A weight-training program is an essential part of a muscle-building program. One glass of skim milk, three slices of whole wheat bread, and two hard-boiled egg whites provide the necessary Calories and about 23 grams of protein.

muscle per week. If he consumed a diet containing 12 to 15 percent of energy from protein, his daily protein intake would approximate 98 (3,250 × 0.12 ÷ 4) to 122 (3,250 × 0.15 ÷ 4) grams.

As noted in chapter 6, there is a difference of opinion as to whether individuals need more protein than the RDA (0.8 gram per kilogram body weight) to gain muscle mass with resistance training. Some contend that because the RDA has a built-in safety factor, it provides adequate protein to support gains in muscle mass, whereas others believe that additional protein is necessary, and suggest that intake be increased to 1.6 grams or more per kilogram body weight. The RDA for our 70-kilogram male is 56 grams (0.8 × 70 kg) daily; adding 14 grams, as calculated above, totals 70 grams, which is less than would be consumed on a diet with 12–15 percent protein. If our young male consumed 1.6 grams per kilogram as recommended by some, his daily protein intake would total 112 grams, still within the 12–15 percent range. Protein intake could be increased even more and still remain within the AMDR of 10–35 percent.

For individuals attempting to lose weight but maintain lean body mass, increasing the percentage of energy intake from protein may be recommended. Mettler and others reported that a low-Calorie diet containing 35 percent protein (2.3 grams/kg), as compared to a diet containing 15 percent protein (1.0 gram/kg), was significantly superior for maintenance of lean body mass in resistance-trained athletes who were undergoing short-term weight loss.

Timing Timing of protein intake is an important consideration. Hulmi and others indicated that protein intake close to a resistance exercise workout may alter messenger-RNA expression in a manner that may promote muscle hypertrophy. This may be the mechanism underlying the contention of Beelen and others that postexercise protein administration is warranted to stimulate muscle protein synthesis, inhibit protein breakdown, and allow net muscle protein accretion. In support of these viewpoints, Stuart Phillips from McMaster University in Canada reviewed the scientific literature and concluded that evidence increasingly supports the conclusion that consumption of protein in close temporal proximity to the performance of resistance exercise promotes greater muscular hypertrophy.

In a review by several sport nutrition experts, Beelen and others quantified this recommendation, suggesting that the consumption of about 20 grams intact protein, or an equivalent of about 9 grams essential amino acids, has been reported to maximize muscle protein-synthesis rates during the first hours of

postexercise recovery. They also suggested that ingestion of such small amounts of dietary protein 5 or 6 times daily (a total of about 100 to 120 grams), might support maximal muscle protein-synthesis rates throughout the day.

Although consuming protein within a short time of completing a resistance training workout appears to be beneficial to maximize muscle hypertrophy, and possibly strength and power, some have contended there would be little difference if the total amount of protein consumed throughout the day was similar, in essence hypothesizing that timing is not an important consideration. Several studies have tested this hypothesis. In general, the study protocol provided protein supplements to some subjects immediately before and/or after exercise, while other subjects consumed the supplements at different times of the day, either several hours after the workout or in the morning and evening. Both groups consumed the same total amount of protein daily.

Results from studies support both viewpoints. For example, Cribb and Hayes reported that consuming a protein/carbohydrate supplement, which also contained creatine, immediately before and after a resistance-training workout, as contrasted to consuming the same supplement in the morning and evening, resulted in greater increases in lean body mass and strength testing. In contrast, Hoffman and others conducted a similar study with resistance-trained men and concluded that the time of protein-supplement ingestion in resistance-trained athletes during a 10-week training program does not make any difference in strength, power, or body-composition changes. Studies with older subjects, men in their seventies, show a similar disparity. Esmarck and others concluded that oral protein supplement immediately after resistance training, as contrasted to 2 hours later, resulted in greater muscle hypertrophy in skeletal muscle of elderly men in response to resistance training. Conversely, Verdijk and others, in a similar 12-week study, concluded that timed protein supplementation immediately before and after exercise does not further augment the increase in skeletal muscle mass and strength after prolonged resistance-type exercise training in healthy elderly men who habitually consume adequate amounts of dietary protein.

Given the available research, consuming protein after resistance training appears to be prudent, as it may do some good and is unlikely to do any harm.

Quality Current research suggests that the quality of the ingested protein may also be an important consideration. In his most recent review on the science of muscle hypertrophy, Phillips indicated that certain types of proteins, particularly those that are digested rapidly and are high in leucine content, appear to be more efficient at stimulating muscle protein synthesis. In particular, Phillips notes that milk proteins, specifically whey and casein proteins, are of the highest quality. He indicates that whey protein is better able to support muscle protein synthesis than is soy protein, and the practice of consuming high-quality proteins after exercise should lead to greater hypertrophy.

Carbohydrate As noted in chapter 4, consuming carbohydrate after exercise is recommended to replace muscle glycogen, a key energy source for exercise, but Phillips notes that carbohydrate alone is not sufficient for muscle protein synthesis. However, ingesting a protein and carbohydrate mixture immediately following resistance exercise, as well as following aerobic endurance exercise, may be recommended. Both the carbohydrate and the protein will stimulate insulin secretion, which will help move both glucose and amino acids into the muscle to facilitate recovery and support muscle protein synthesis.

Ivy and Portman recommend a tasty postworkout carbohydrate/protein drink, with a ratio of about 3–4 grams of carbohydrate for each gram of protein. One simple choice is chocolate milk; an 8-ounce glass contains about 32 grams of carbohydrate and 8 grams of protein, a 4:1 ratio (see figure 12.2). Approximately 82 percent of cow's milk is casein protein and about 18 percent is whey protein. Some of the carbohydrate in chocolate milk is lactose, but most is glucose in the added chocolate syrup. Lactose-free chocolate milk is available for those with lactose intolerance. Several studies have shown that chocolate milk is an effective postexercise recovery fluid. Additionally, research by Josse, from Phillip's laboratory,

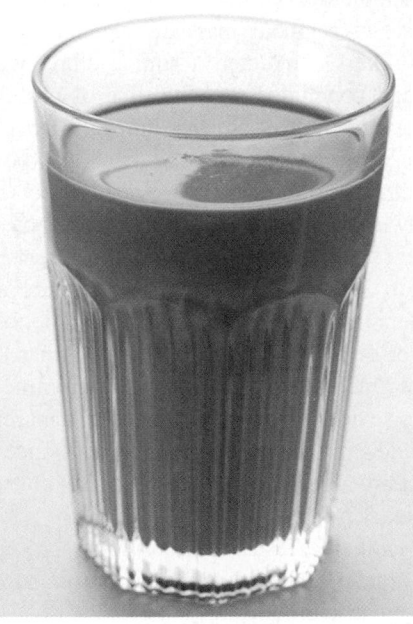

FIGURE 12.2 Chocolate milk may be an excellent source of nutrients before or after a resistance-training workout. One glass provides about 32 grams of carbohydrate and 8 grams of protein, a 4:1 ratio. Chocolate milk also provides important minerals and vitamins as well.

found that fat-free milk is also an effective drink to support favorable body composition changes with resistance training.

Cost As noted in table 6.8 on page 235 the cost for a standard amount of high-quality protein may vary considerably. In particular, protein sport supplements may be rather expensive. For example, Goldman noted that one popular product providing about 25 grams of protein cost $3 to $4 per bottle. A comparable amount of high-quality protein from fat-free milk would cost approximately 60 cents.

Are dietary supplements necessary during a weight-gaining program?

Dietary supplements appear to be very popular among athletes and others attempting to increase muscle mass and strength, if we can use advertisements as evidence to support this contention. For example, in a survey of only five magazines targeted to bodybuilding athletes, Grunewald and Bailey reported more than 800 performance claims made for 624 commercially available supplements. This survey was conducted nearly 20 years ago, but such marketing practices continue unabated. Numerous products are marketed not only to increase muscle mass, strength, and power, but also to help prevent injuries during resistance training. Bloomer notes that marketing of nutritional supplements for the purposes of attenuating muscle injury associated with strength training is rampant within the popular fitness media and athletic world, largely without scientific support.

Although there may be some truth underlying the alleged performance-enhancing mechanisms of these supplements, the effectiveness of most has not been evaluated by scientific research. In a review of nutritional supplements for strength-trained athletes, Williams indicated that there is little or no scientific evidence supporting positive effects on muscle growth, body-fat reduction, or strength enhancement in strength-trained athletes for most products. The effects of many of these supplements, such as specific individual amino acids, vitamins, minerals, and other individual nutrients, have been discussed in previous chapters, and in general have not been found to be effective as performance-enhancing agents. Research has found that many are ineffective, whereas other supplements are inadequately researched.

Some supplements may be helpful. As noted previously, high-quality protein, such as whey, may help maximize the anabolic process associated with resistance training. Also, as noted in chapter 6, creatine monohydrate supplementation does appear to increase muscle mass, and numerous studies have reported gains in strength, particularly in high-intensity resistance exercises with short-term recovery. Although early increases in body weight may be primarily water, an increased resistance-training capacity may lead to muscle gains over time. Numerous studies support this finding. You may wish to review the discussion of creatine supplementation on pages 246–252. As shall be noted in the next section, resistance training is a very important consideration to help prevent or reduce loss of muscle mass in the elderly. Creatine supplementation may help augment the anabolic effects of resistance training in the elderly, increasing muscle mass and strength, according to reviews by Candow and Rawson and Venezia.

Several other dietary supplements marketed to athletes are patterned after anabolic/androgenic steroids. Some herbal products are marketed for their supposed anabolic potential. In general, as noted in chapter 13, research indicates that such supplements do not increase muscle mass and may cause adverse health effects.

In a symposium sponsored by the Gatorade Sports Science Institute, five experts on muscle-building supplements provided this advice:

- Train hard
- Follow a sound diet with adequate energy, protein, and carbohydrate
- Don't rely on dietary supplements

If you do use supplements, be sure to consult with an expert, such as a sports-oriented dietitan or physician, not the clerk at a health food store.

What is an example of a balanced diet that will help me gain weight?

As with losing weight, the Food Exchange System may serve as the basis for a sound weight-gaining diet. Foods must be selected for high nutrient value as well as additional Calories to support the weight gain.

The following suggestions may be helpful for those trying to gain weight as muscle. In general, the focus is on healthy dietary sources of carbohydrates, protein, and fats.

Milk exchange—Drink 1% or 2% milk instead of skim milk, which will add 15–30 Calories per glass. Chocolate milk provides both carbohydrate and high-quality protein. If you want to decrease caloric intake from fat, fat-free chocolate milk is available. Prepare milk shakes with dry milk powder and supplement with fruit. Add low-fat cheeses to sandwiches or snacks. Eat yogurt supplemented with fruit. The milk exchange is rich in high-quality protein.

Meat and meat substitute exchange—Increase your intake of lean meats, poultry, and fish, which are also sources of high-quality protein. Legumes such as beans and dried peas are high in protein, carbohydrate, and Calories and low in fat. Use nuts, seeds, and limited amounts of peanut butter for snacks. The meat exchange is also high in protein.

Starch exchange—Increase your consumption of whole-grain products. Pasta and rice are nutritious side dishes that provide adequate Calories. Starchy vegetables like potatoes are also nutritious sources of Calories. Breads and muffins can possibly be supplemented with fruits and nuts. Whole-grain breakfast cereals can provide substantial Calories and even make a tasty dessert or snack with added fruit. The starch exchange is high in complex carbohydrates but also contains about 15 percent of its Calories as protein.

Fruit exchange—Add fruit to other food exchanges. Drink more fruit juices, which are high in both Calories and nutrients. Dried fruits such as apricots, pineapple, dates, and raisins are high in Calories and make excellent snacks.

Vegetable exchange—Use fresh vegetables like broccoli and cauliflower as snacks with melted low-fat cheese or a nutritious dip.

Fat exchange—Try to minimize the intake of saturated fats, using monounsaturated and polyunsaturated fats instead, particularly olive and canola oils. Nuts and seeds are good sources of monounsaturated fats. Salad dressings and soft margarine added to vegetables can increase their caloric content.

Beverages—Milk and juices are nutritious and high in Calories. Those who drink alcohol should obtain only limited amounts of Calories in this way. Some liquid supplements are available commercially and may contain 300–400 Calories with substantial amounts of protein. However, check the label for fat and sugar content.

Snacks—Eat three balanced meals per day supplemented with two or three snacks. Dried fruits, nuts, and seeds are excellent snacks. Some of the high-Calorie, high-protein, high-nutrient liquid meals and sports bars on the market also make good snacks.

Table 12.2 presents an example of a high-Calorie diet plan based upon the Food Exchange System. It consists of three main meals and three snacks and totals about 4,000 Calories, with 160 grams of protein, which is 16 percent of the Calories. It is also high in carbohydrate, which may increase insulin release, facilitating amino acid transport into the muscle to help promote protein synthesis. Carbohydrate also spares the use of protein as an energy source. Alternative foods may be substituted from the food exchange list presented in appendix E. This suggested diet provides the necessary nutrients, Calories, and protein essential for increased development of muscle mass, and yet fewer than 30 percent of the Calories are derived from fat. The total number of Calories can be adjusted to meet individual needs. You may plan your weight-gain diet on the ChooseMyPlate Website.

Meal plans may be adjusted to the energy needs of individual athletes. For example, Lambert and others note that competitive bodybuilders should consume a diet that contains about 55–60 percent carbohydrate, 25–30 percent protein, and 15–20 percent fat for both the off-season and pre-contest phases. However, during the off-season the diet should be slightly hyperenergetic (approximately 15 percent increase in energy intake) and during the pre-contest phase the diet should be hypoenergetic (approximately 15 percent decrease in energy intake). As noted previously, for 6–12 weeks prior to competition, bodybuilders attempt to retain muscle mass and reduce body fat to low levels, so they need to be in negative energy balance to facilitate oxidation of body fat. Lambert and others recommend that the diet contain 30 percent protein at this time to help prevent loss of muscle mass and possibly also provide a thermic effect to help burn fat.

For more detailed meal plans, the interested reader is referred to *Nutrient Timing* by John Ivy and Robert Portman.

Would such a high-Calorie diet be ill advised for some individuals?

As noted in chapter 5, one of the general recommendations for an improved diet is to reduce the consumption of fats, particularly saturated fats. Unfortunately, many high-Calorie diets are also high in fats. If there is a history of heart disease in the family or if

TABLE 12.2	A high-Calorie diet based on the Food Exchange System	
Exchange		**Calories**
Breakfast		
Milk	8 ounces 2% milk	120
Meat	1 poached egg	80
	2 ounces lean ham	110
Starch	2 slices whole wheat toast	160
Fruit	8 ounces orange juice	120
Other	1 tablespoon jelly	50
Mid-morning snack		
Fruit	8 ounces apricot nectar	160
Starch	2 slices whole wheat bread	160
Meat	1 tablespoon peanut butter	100
Lunch		
Milk	8 ounces 2% milk	120
Meat	4 ounces lean sandwich meat	220
Starch	2 slices whole wheat bread	160
	2 granola cookies	100
Fruit	1 banana	120
Vegetable, starchy	1 order French fries	300
Afternoon snack		
Fruit	1/4 cup raisins	120
Dinner		
Milk	8 ounces 2% milk	120
Meat	5 ounces salmon	275
Starch	2 slices whole wheat bread	160
Fruit	1 piece apple pie	350
Vegetable, starchy	1 cup peas	160
	1 sweet potato, candied	300
Evening snack		
Fruit	1/2 cup dried peaches	210
Milk	8 ounces 2% milk with banana	240
Total		4,015

an individual is known to have high blood lipid levels, then high-fat diets may be contraindicated. Individuals with kidney problems also may have difficulty processing high-protein diets because of the increased need to excrete urea. Any person initiating such a weight-gaining program as advised here should be aware of his or her medical history.

Selection of food for a weight-gaining diet, if done wisely, can satisfy the criteria for healthful nutrition. Foods high in complex carbohydrates with moderate amounts of protein and a moderate fat content are able to provide substantial amounts of Calories and nutrients, and yet minimize health risks that have been associated with the typical American and Canadian diet. To gain weight wisely, you need to continue to eat healthful foods, but just more of them.

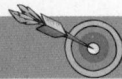

Key Concepts

▶ The individual attempting to gain body weight should obtain necessary protein for muscle synthesis through a well-balanced diet, rather than by consuming expensive protein supplements.
▶ Although creatine supplementation may help increase muscle mass during resistance training, most dietary supplements marketed to strength-trained individuals are not effective or have not been evaluated by scientific research.
▶ The Food Exchange System can serve as the basis for increasing caloric intake to gain body weight if the aspirant eats greater quantities of nutritious foods from each of the six lists, in three balanced meals plus several high-Calorie, high-nutrient snacks.

Check for Yourself

▶ Using the information presented in the text, calculate the additional number of Calories you would need in your daily diet to accumulate a weight gain of 0.5 pound per week. What foods could you add to your daily diet to provide these Calories?

Exercise Considerations

In chapter 11 we discussed the design of an aerobic exercise program for the loss of excess body fat, but also mentioned that a resistance-training program could be helpful, for it might help prevent the loss of lean body mass and maintain normal resting-energy expenditure. In this chapter the focus is upon resistance training, sometimes called weight training or strength training, as a means to increase lean body mass and body weight. Before we discuss the principles underlying the design of a proper resistance-training program, let us introduce some basic terminology.

Repetition simply means the number of times you do a specific exercise. *Intensity* is determined by the weight, or resistance, that is lifted. A term used to describe the interrelationship between repetitions and intensity in weight training is **repetition maximum (RM).** If you perform an exercise such as a bench press and lift 150 pounds once, but you cannot do a second repetition, you have done one repetition maximum, or 1RM. Individual workouts are generally based on a percentage of the RM, such as 80 percent of 1RM. For example, if your 1RM for the bench press is 150 pounds, 80 percent would be 120 pounds (0.8×150). If you bench press 120 pounds for five repetitions but cannot do a sixth, you have done five repetition maximum, or 5RM. A *set* is any particular number of repetitions, such as five or ten. The total volume of work you do in a single workout is the product of sets, repetitions, and resistance. For example, if you bench press three sets of five repetitions with a resistance of 100 pounds, your total volume of work is 1,500 pounds ($3 \times 5 \times 100$). The *recovery period* may represent the rest intervals between sets in a single workout or the rest interval between workouts during the week.

What are the primary purposes of resistance training?

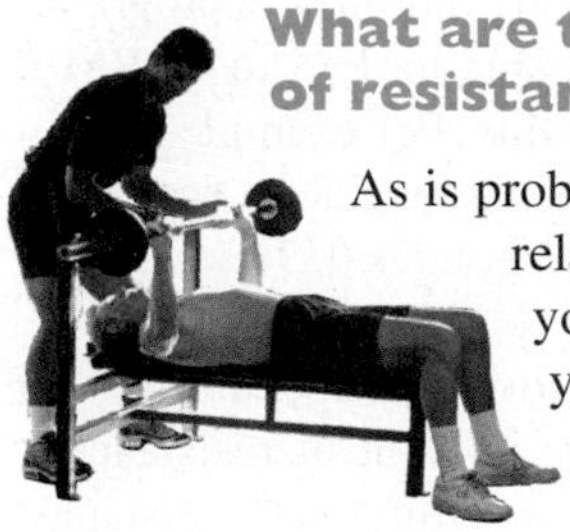

As is probably obvious to you, there is an inverse relationship between the amount of weight you can lift and the number of repetitions you can do. If your 1RM in the bench press is 150 pounds, you can do more repetitions with 100 pounds than you can with 140. The **strength-endurance continuum** is a training concept that focuses upon the inter-relationship between resistance and repetitions. As depicted in figure 12.3, to train for muscular strength you must combine high resistance with a low number of repetitions. Conversely, to train for muscular endurance, you must combine a low resistance with a high number of repetitions.

Resistance-training programs may be designed to train all three of the human energy systems. The ATP-PCr energy system predominates in strength and power activities, the lactic acid energy system is primarily involved in anaerobic endurance, and the oxygen system is involved in aerobic endurance

activities. Thus, resistance-training programs may be developed for various purposes. One purpose may be to improve health, as discussed below. Another purpose may be to enhance sports performance, including improved strength and power for such sports as weightlifting and aesthetic appearance for sports such as bodybuilding.

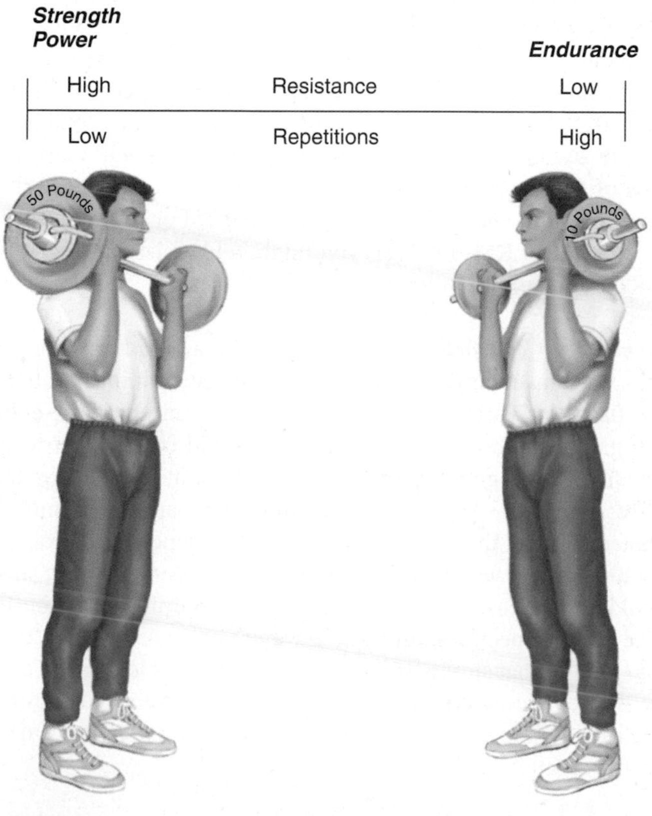

The American College of Sports Medicine (ACSM) and the American Heart Association (AHA), both separately and collectively, have provided recommendations for participation in resistance-training programs. The recommendations from the ACSM/AHA committee, chaired by Haskell, focus on resistance training as a component of an overall exercise program to improve muscular strength and endurance in healthy young adults, whereas those from the ACSM/AHA committee, chaired by Nelson, focus on programs for the elderly. The AHA scientific statement, developed by Williams and others, provides recommendations on resistance training for individuals with and without cardiovascular disease. The ACSM also developed a set of recommendations dealing with progression, or the gradual increase in overload placed on the body during training, and is more appropriate for the individual training to maximize muscular size and strength for bodybuilding or sport competition. Overall, these four sets of recommendations highlight the following purposes of resistance training, along with the recommended type of program.

Training for Muscular Hypertrophy   Higher-volume, multiple-set programs are recommended for maximizing muscle hypertrophy. Emphasize a range of 6–12 RM per set.

Training for Strength and Power   Multiple sets with fewer repetitions are recommended to maximize strength and power. Emphasize a range of 4–6 RM per set. Also, incorporate multiple sets of light loads (30–60 percent of 1 RM) at a fast contraction velocity.

Training for Local Muscular Endurance   Multiple sets with more repetitions and light to moderate loads, such as 15 or more repetitions at 40–60 percent of 1 RM, are recommended. Use a short recovery period between sets.

Training for Health-Related Benefits   Single sets are sufficient, approximating 8–12 RM. Include a variety of exercises that stress the major muscle groups of the body.

What are the basic principles of resistance training?

Given the different purposes for which individuals may do resistance training, the design of the individual training program will vary accordingly. Athletes training to maximize muscle mass, strength, and power for their sport will engage in a more rigorous training program compared to someone doing resistance training for health benefits. Although the design of the resistance-training program may vary, the underlying principles are the same. The following discussion will highlight recommendations to gain muscle mass.

Strength Power		Endurance
High	Resistance	Low
Low	Repetitions	High

FIGURE 12.3   The strength-endurance continuum. To gain strength, you need to train on the strength end of the continuum; to gain endurance, you need to train on the endurance end of the continuum.

As noted in chapter 1, the following principles are not restricted to resistance training but apply to all forms of exercise training. For example, intensity of exercise is simply another way of phrasing the overload principle.

Overload   The *principle of overload* is the most important principle in all resistance-training programs. The use of weights places a greater than normal stress on the muscle cell. This overload stress stimulates the muscle to grow—to become stronger—in effect to overcome the increased resistance imposed by the weights (see figure 12.4).

To overload the muscle, you must increase the volume of work it must do. There are basically two ways to do this. One is to increase the amount of resistance or weight that you use; the other way is to increase the number of repetitions and sets you do. For beginners, a single set of 8 to 10 exercises will help increase

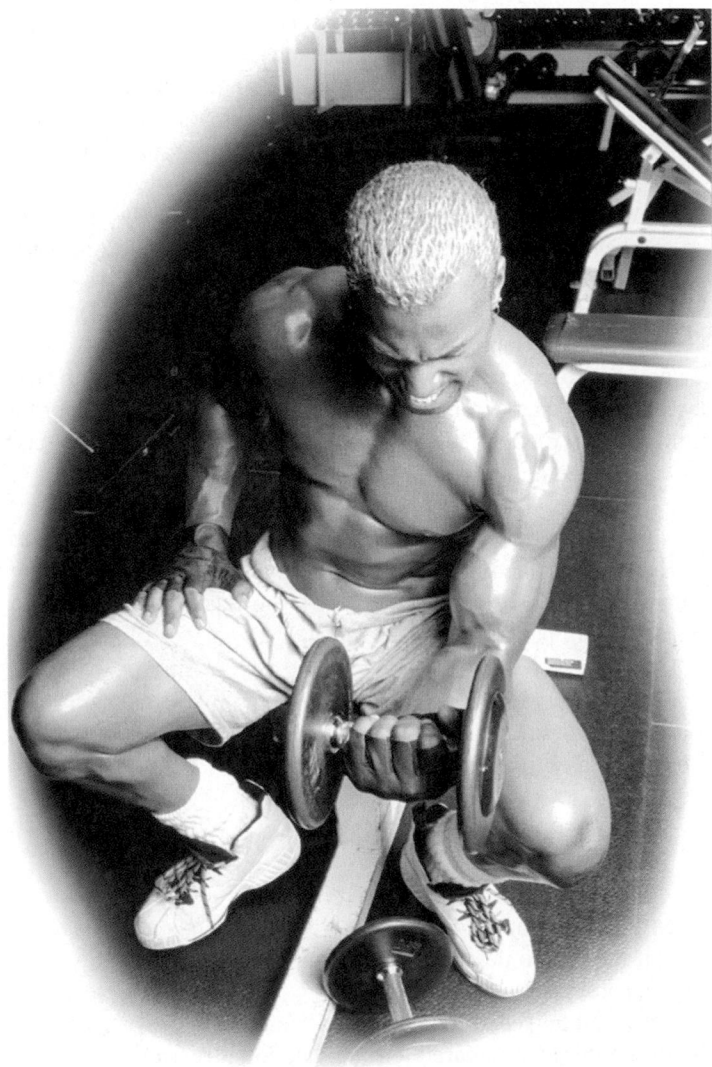

FIGURE 12.4 Lifting heavy weights illustrates the principle of overload in action with weight training. If improvement in strength is to continue, weights must be increased.

muscle mass and strength gains. Wolfe and others conducted a meta-analysis of available studies, and reported that single-set programs for an initial short training period in untrained individuals result in strength gains similar to those from multiple-set programs. If you know your 1 RM, you should be able to do 8 to 12 RM if you use 60 to 80 percent of your 1 RM value. For example, if your bench press 1 RM is 150 pounds, you should be able to do at least 8 RM with 70 percent of that value, or 105 pounds (0.70 × 150).

Progression   As the muscle continues to get stronger during your training program, you must increase the amount of resistance—the overload—to continue to get the proper stimulus for sustained muscle growth. This is known as the *principle of progressive resistance exercise (PRE),* another basic principle of resistance training.

The ACSM provides guidelines on progression as the individual advances in weight lifting skill and strength, from novice to intermediate and advanced. As progression occurs and higher gains are desired, multiple-set programs are more effective. Following a learning period, a recommended program for beginners is three to five sets using loads corresponding to 8–12 RM. The first step is to determine the maximum amount of weight that you can lift for eight repetitions. If you can do more than eight repetitions, the weight is too light and you need to add more poundage. As you get stronger during the succeeding weeks, you will be able to lift the original weight more easily. When you can perform 12 repetitions, add more weight to force you back down to eight repetitions; this is the progressive resistance principle. Over several months' time, the weight will probably have to be increased several times as you continue to get stronger. Such a transition is illustrated in figure 12.5. The ACSM recommends that as you become an intermediate or advanced lifter, you should emphasize loads of 1–6 RM and progress when you can do about 1–2 more repetitions than the upper limit of the range. For example, if you are using the 6 RM protocol, you might add resistance when you can do 8 repetitions.

Specificity   The *principle of specificity* is a broad training principle with many implications for resistance training, including specificity for various sports movements, strength gains, endurance gains, and body-weight gains. Frost and others suggest that to facilitate the greatest improvements to athletic performance, the resistance-training program employed by an athlete must be adapted to meet the specific demands of the sport. For example, a swimmer who wants to gain strength and endurance for a stroke should attempt to find a resistance-weight training program that exercises the specific muscles in a way as close as possible to the form used in that stroke. If you want to gain muscle mass in a certain part of the body, those muscles must be exercised. Strength coaches can help athletes develop resistance-training programs for specific sports.

Exercise Sequence   Your exercise routine should be based upon the *principle of exercise sequence.* This means that if you have ten exercises in your routine, they should be arranged in logical order so that fatigue does not limit your lifting ability. For

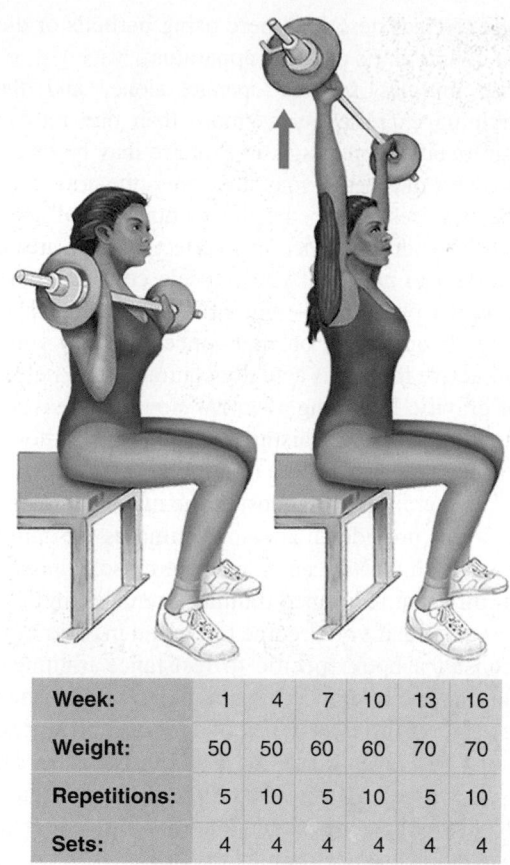

Week:	1	4	7	10	13	16
Weight:	50	50	60	60	70	70
Repetitions:	5	10	5	10	5	10
Sets:	4	4	4	4	4	4

FIGURE 12.5 The principle of progressive resistance exercise (PRE) states that as you get stronger, you need to progressively increase the resistance to continue to gain strength and muscle. In this example, the individual increases the resistance when she can complete ten repetitions with a given weight, but then does only five repetitions with the increased weight.

example, the first exercise in a sequence of ten might stress the biceps muscle, the second the abdominals, the third the quadriceps, and so forth. After you perform one full set of each of the ten exercises, you then do a complete second set, followed by the third set. This approach may be best for beginners and is the sequence for the eight exercises presented in this chapter.

Another popular option is to do three sets of the same exercise with a rest between sets; then do three sets of the second exercise, and so on. This approach may be a little more fatiguing because you are using the same muscle group in three successive sets, but it appears to be very effective. The time spent in recovery will also lengthen the total time for the workout. The ACSM also provides some guidelines on exercise sequence, recommending the following:

- Do multiple-joint exercises before single-joint exercises.
- Do large-muscle-group exercises before small-muscle-group exercises.
- Do higher-intensity exercises before lower-intensity exercises.

Recuperation Resistance training, if done properly to achieve the greatest gains, imposes a rather severe stress on the muscles,

requiring a period of recovery both during the workout and between workouts. Research has shown that high-intensity resistance exercise can lead to rapid depletion of ATP and PCr, the high-energy phosphates stored in the muscles; however, most of these high-energy compounds may be restored in about 2 to 3 minutes of recovery. This is the *principle of recuperation.* Thus, several minutes should intervene between sets if you are using the same exercise. Taking adequate rest between sets may help maintain the quality of the workout. Ratamess and others studied the effect of varying rest intervals between five sets of the bench press. A rest interval of only 30–60 seconds resulted in a significant decrease in lifting volume in each subsequent set, whereas resting for 5 minutes impaired lifting capacity only in the fifth set. Resting for 2–3 minutes helped maintain lifting volume during the first 2–3 sets, but not in the latter sets. If the goal is muscular endurance, the ACSM recommends that rest periods be shortened to less than 90 seconds.

Additionally, for beginners, resistance training should generally be done about 3 days per week, with a rest or recuperation day in between. This day of rest allows sufficient time for your muscle to repair itself and to synthesize new protein as it continues to grow, for research has shown that muscle protein synthesis occurs for up to 24 hours after a single bout of heavy resistance exercise. The ACSM indicates that advanced lifters could train 4–5 days per week. For health benefits, the ACSM and AHA recommended resistance exercise at least twice a week on nonconsecutive days.

Periodization **Periodization** is a technique applied to resistance training, as well as other forms of exercise training, that modifies the amount of exercise stress placed on the individual over the course of time. Periodization of training is primarily applicable to athletes. In general, periodization is based on Hans Selye's theory on adaptation to stress. The body will adapt to exercise stress in ways beneficial to performance enhancement, but as noted in chapter 3, excessive exercise may predispose athletes to overreaching and overtraining, which may contribute to impaired performance. Periodization establishes the amount and intensity of training in various time cycles. A *microcycle* is about a week, whereas a *macrocycle* may be a year or more. A *mesocycle* is any intermediate time frame, and may involve phases in preparation for competition and peaking for championship-type events. A detailed discussion of periodization is beyond the scope of this book. An excellent summarization has been provided by Kraemer and Ratamess. Periodization programs are available in most resistance-training texts, such as *Principles and Practices of Resistance Training*, by Michael Stone and others, and are the major focus in the text *Periodization Training for Sports*, by Bompa and Carrera.

With the exception of periodization, these general principles should serve as guidelines during the beginning phase of your resistance-training program and should be used to guide your progress during the first 3 months of the basic resistance-training program described next. If you become serious about resistance training, additional reading is advised. Personal trainers may also be helpful.

What is an example of a resistance-training program that may help me to gain body weight as lean muscle mass?

If your goal is to gain significant amounts of muscle mass, you may wish to exercise on the strength end of the strength-endurance continuum, using six to ten different exercises that stress the major muscle groups of the body. About three to five sets of each exercise are done. For those with limited time, one set may also provide significant increases in strength and muscle mass, as documented by Starkey and others. You should work up to 10–12 repetitions. You may modify this range, either using 6–10 or 8–12 as the repetition base. We will use the 8–12 model below and in the illustrations. The PRE concept is used, starting with resistance you can handle for eight repetitions and progressively increasing the repetitions to twelve. After you reach twelve repetitions, increase the resistance until you must come back to eight repetitions.

Numerous resistance-training exercises are available to stress the major muscle groups in the body. The following exercises provide a sound basic resistance-training program for the adolescent and adult beginner.

1. Learn the proper technique for each exercise with a light weight, possibly only the bar itself, for 2 weeks. Do eight to twelve repetitions of each exercise to develop form. Do not strain during this initial learning phase. Concentrate on lowering the weight slowly.
2. For each exercise, determine the maximum weight that you can lift for eight repetitions after the 2-week learning phase.
3. A weekly record form, similar to the one presented in table 12.3, should be used to keep track of your progress.
4. Do one set of the eight exercises shown in figures 12.6 to 12.13. The sequence of exercises should be
   a. Bench press: chest muscles
   b. Lat machine pulldown or bent-arm pullover: back muscles
   c. Half squat: thigh muscles
   d. Standing lateral raise: shoulder muscles
   e. Heel raise: calf muscles
   f. Standing curl: front upper arm muscles
   g. Seated overhead press: back upper arm muscles
   h. Curl-up: abdominal muscles
5. Because the exercise sequence is designed to stress different muscle groups in order, not much recuperation is necessary between exercises—possibly only 30 seconds or so.
6. Do three to five complete sets. You may wish to rest 2 to 3 minutes between sets.
7. Exercise 3 days per week; in each succeeding day try to do as many repetitions as possible for each exercise in each set. When you can do twelve repetitions each after a month or so, add more weight so you can do only eight repetitions.
8. Repeat step 7 as you progressively increase your strength.

Because barbells and dumbbells appear to be the most common means of doing resistance training, this is the method utilized. However, other apparatus, such as the Nautilus, Hammer, and others, can also be used effectively to gain weight and strength.

Most of the exercises described here using barbells or dumbbells have similar counterparts on other apparatus.

Note that muscles seldom operate alone, and that most resistance-training exercises stress more than one muscle group. Thus, keep in mind that although an exercise may be listed specifically for the chest muscles, it may also stress the arm and shoulder muscles. The exercises described in this section generally stress more than one body area, although their main effect is on the area noted.

It is important to note that your muscle contracts during both the up and down phase of weight lifting. As noted later, some training methods are based on this concept. When you lower a weight, your active muscle is actually contracting to help decrease the force of gravity. Lowering a weight slowly increases the time your muscle must contract. Raising the weight takes more force as you are working against the force of gravity.

These eight exercises stress most of the major muscle groups in the body and thus provide an adequate stimulus for gaining body weight and strength through an increase in muscle mass. Literally hundreds of different resistance-training exercises and techniques to train are available; if you become interested in diversifying your program, consult a book specific to resistance training. Several may be found in the reference list at the end of this chapter. For example, nearly 30 different types of programs are presented in the classic text by Steven Fleck and William Kraemer, *Designing Resistance Training Programs*. Some professional organizations, such as the National Strength and Conditioning Association, also provide excellent resistance-training exercises.

Individuality in responses to resistance-training programs is an important consideration. In a review, Hayes and others indicated that optimal adaptations to resistance training may vary among different individuals. They noted that some participants experienced greater hypertrophy and strength increases in response to strength protocols, whereas others respond preferentially to strength/endurance protocols. It appears that, depending on the individual, one protocol may be more effective than another as a means to increase serum testosterone levels, the male anabolic hormone discussed in chapter 13.

www.nsca-lift.org For detailed illustrations of a wide variety of resistance-training exercises, either in video or slide format, click on *For the Public* and then *Free Training Videos*. The muscles involved in each exercise and safety tips are also provided.

www.nia.nih.gov/exercise Strength-training exercises for the elderly are presented using various types of equipment. Click on Chapter 4: Sample Exercises—Strength.

Are there any safety concerns associated with resistance training?

As noted later, several health problems may contradict participation in a strenuous resistance-training program. However, resistance training is generally regarded as a relatively safe sport, particularly if appropriate safety precautions are taken. The following guidelines should be incorporated into all resistance-training programs.

TABLE 12.3 Weekly resistance-training record, basic eight exercises

	Chest	Back	Thigh	Shoulder	Calf	Front arm	Back arm	Abdominal area
	(Bench Press)	(Lat Pulldown)	(Half Squat)	(Lateral Raise)	(Heel Raise)	(Curls)	(Seated Press)	(Curl-ups)
	Wt / Reps	Wt / Reps	Wt / Reps	Wt / Reps	Wt / Reps	Wt / Reps	Wt / Reps	Wt / Reps
Date _____								
Set 1								
Set 2								
Set 3								
Set 4								
Set 5								
Date _____								
Set 1								
Set 2								
Set 3								
Set 4								
Set 5								
Date _____								
Set 1								
Set 2								
Set 3								
Set 4								
Set 5								
Date _____								
Set 1								
Set 2								
Set 3								
Set 4								
Set 5								

1. *Learn to breathe properly.* During the most strenuous part of the exercise, you are likely to hold your breath. This is a natural response; it helps to stabilize your chest cavity to provide a more stable base for your muscles to function. Usually the breath hold is short and no problems occur. However, if prolonged, it may increase the chances of suffering some of the problems noted previously, such as a hernia.

Also associated with prolonged breath holding is a response known as the **Valsalva phenomenon** (Valsalva maneuver), which may lead to a possible blackout. Here is what happens. As you reach a sticking point in your lift and strain to overcome it, you normally hold your breath; this causes your glottis to close over your windpipe and the pressure in your chest and abdominal area to rise rapidly. The pressure creates resistance to blood flow, reducing the return

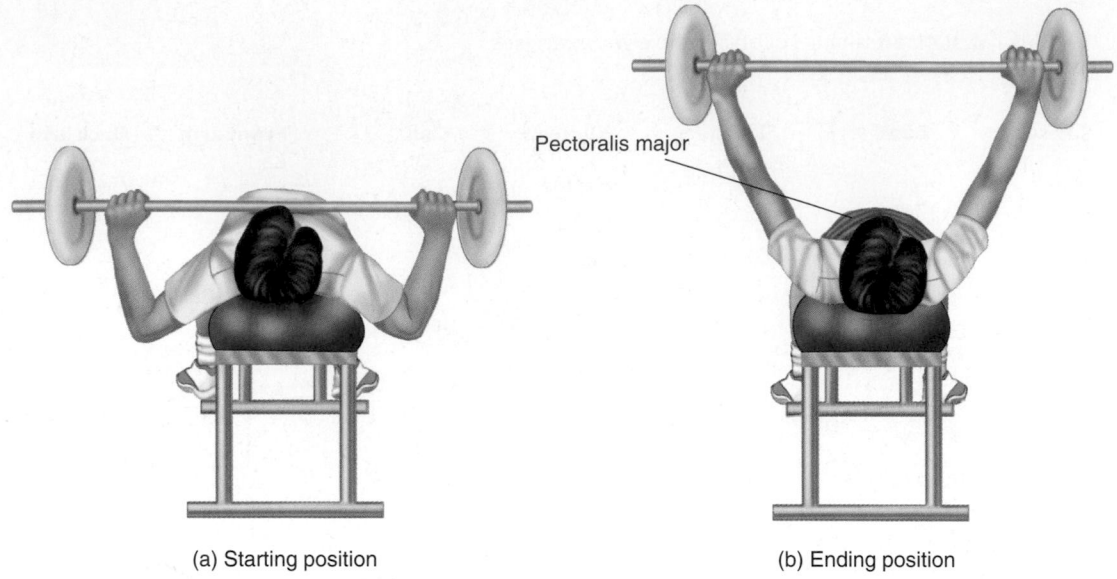

Pectoralis major

(a) Starting position   (b) Ending position

Chest	
Exercise	Bench press
Chest muscles	Pectoralis major
Other muscles	Deltoid, triceps
Sets	3–5
Repetitions	8–12, PRE concept
Safety	Have spotter stand behind bar to assist as fatigue sets in.
Equipment	Bench with support for weight, or two spotters to hand weight to you.
Description	Lie supine on bench. Use wide grip for chest development. Secure bar and lower *slowly* to chest. Press bar straight up to full extension. Do not arch back.

FIGURE 12.6 The bench press. The bench press primarily develops the pectoralis major muscle group in the chest; it also develops the deltoids in the shoulder and the triceps at the back of the arm.

Note: For safety reasons, a spotter should be present to assist in case of difficulty. The spotter is not depicted for purposes of illustration clarity.

of blood to the heart, and eventually leading to decreased blood flow to the brain and a possible blackout. Additionally, the Valsalva maneuver exaggerates the increase in blood pressure during resistance exercises, and although a brief Valsalva maneuver is unavoidable when doing near-maximal exercises, its effect may be minimized by proper breathing.

A recommended breathing pattern that will help minimize these adverse effects is to breathe out while lifting the weight and breathe in while lowering it. You should breathe through both your mouth and nose while exercising. Practice proper breathing when you learn new resistance-training exercises.
2. *Use spotters.* When using free weights, use spotters when doing exercises that may be potentially dangerous, such as the bench press. If you are doing a bench press alone and reach a sticking point in your lift, the Valsalva phenomenon may

lead to serious consequences if you lose control of the weight directly above your head. The use of machines such as Nautilus helps eliminate the need for spotters.
3. *Use safety equipment.* If using free weights, place lock collars on the bar ends so the plates do not fall off and cause injury to the feet. Again, the use of machines eliminates this safety hazard. However, do not attempt to change weight plates on machines while they are being used. Your fingers may get caught between the weights.
4. *Warm up.* Warm up with proper stretching exercises. Gently stretch the muscles to be used during exercise. Slow, static methods are recommended for cold muscles. Incidentally, Kokkonen and others found that if, for some reason, you are unable to participate in traditional resistance training, you may be able to increase strength by stretching. They found

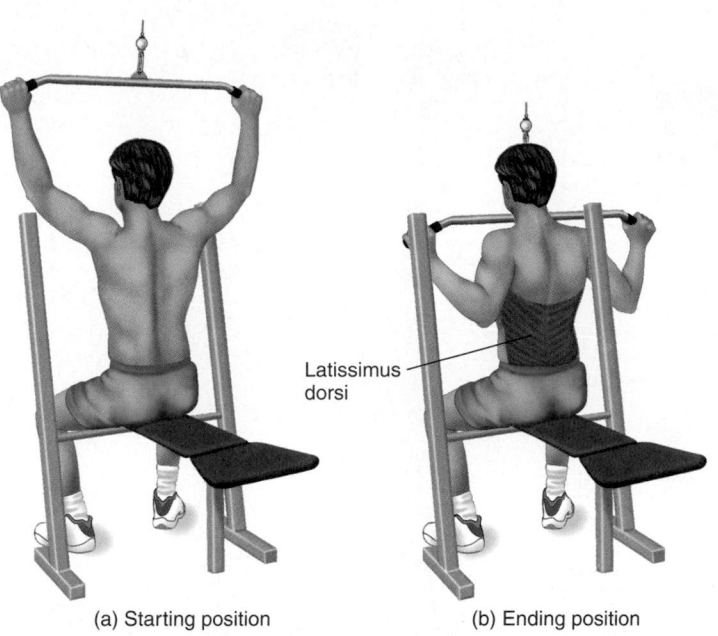

Latissimus
dorsi

(a) Starting position   (b) Ending position

Back	
Exercise	Lat machine pulldown
Back muscles	Latissimus dorsi
Other muscles	Biceps, pectoralis major
Sets	3–5
Repetitions	8–12, PRE concept
Safety	A very safe exercise
Equipment	Lat machine
Description	From seated or kneeling position, take a wide grip at arm's length on the bar overhead. Pull bar down until it reaches your chest. Return slowly to starting position.

Note: If a lat machine is not available, the bent-arm pullover may be substituted.

FIGURE 12.7A The lat machine pull-down. The lat machine pull-down trains the latissimus dorsi in the back and side of the upper body, and it also develops the biceps on the front of the upper arm and the pectoralis major in the chest.

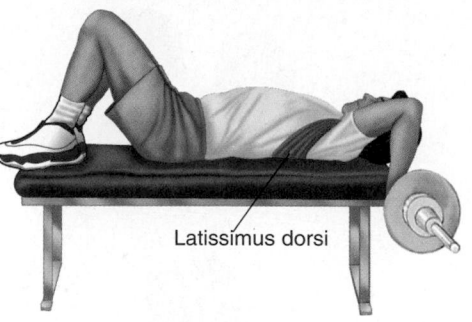

Latissimus dorsi

(a) Starting position

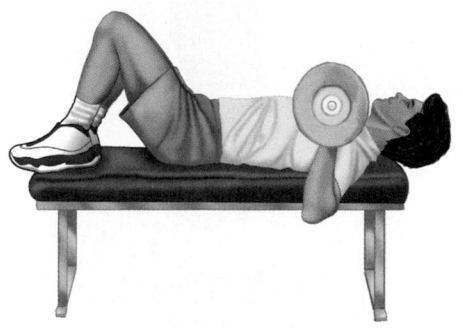

(b) Ending position

Back	
Alternate exercise	Bent-arm pullover
Back muscles	Latissimus dorsi
Other muscles	Pectoralis major
Sets	3–5
Repetitions	8–12, PRE concept
Safety	Do not arch back. Start with light weights when learning the technique.
Equipment	Bench
Description	Lie supine on bench, entire back in contact with the bench, feet on the bench, knees bent. Hold weight on chest with elbows bent. Swing weight over head, just brushing hair, and lower as far as possible without taking back off the bench. Keeping elbows in, return the weight to the chest.

FIGURE 12.7B The bent-arm pullover. The bent-arm pullover trains the latissimus dorsi and develops the pectoralis major.

Note: For safety reasons, a spotter should be present to assist in case of difficulty. The spotter is not depicted for purposes of illustration clarity.

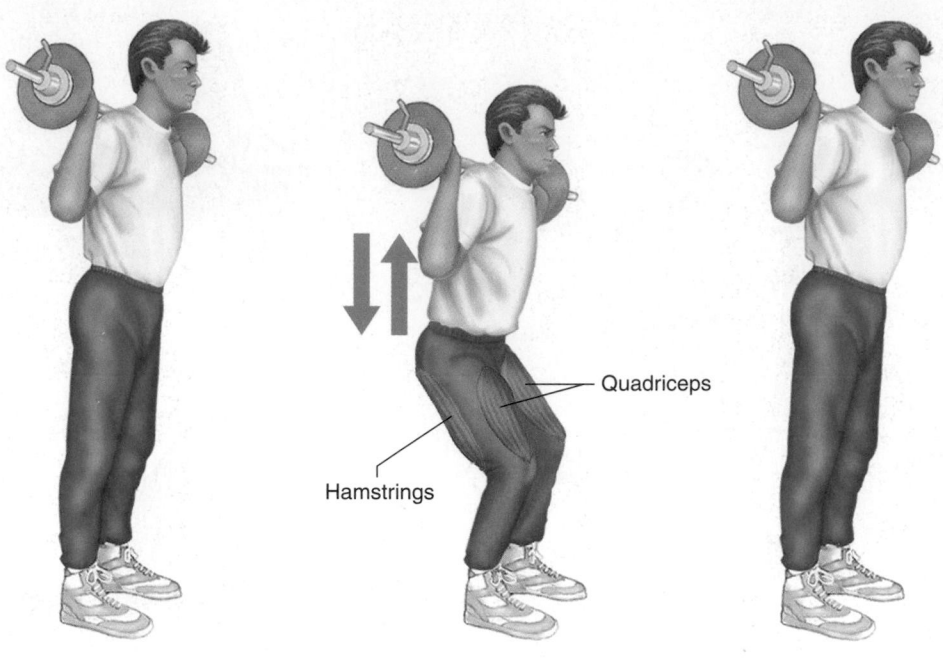

(a) Starting position   (b) Ending position

Thigh	
Exercise	Half squat or parallel squat
Thigh muscles	Quadriceps (front), hamstrings (back)
Other muscles	Gluteus maximus
Sets	3–5
Repetitions	8–12, PRE concept
Safety	Have two spotters to assist if using free weights. Keep back straight. Drop weight behind you if you lose balance. Do not squat more than halfway down.
Equipment	Squat rack if available. Pad the bar with towels if necessary.
Description	In standing position, take bar from squat rack or spotters and rest on the shoulders behind the head. Squat until thighs are parallel to ground or until buttocks touch a chair at this parallel position. Do not squat beyond halfway. Keep back as straight as possible. Return to standing position, but do not lock your knees. This will maximize stress on your thighs.

FIGURE 12.8 The half squat or parallel squat. The half squat develops the quadriceps muscle group on the front of the thigh and the hamstrings on the back of the thigh.

Note: For safety reasons, spotters should be present to assist in case of difficulty. The spotters are not depicted for purposes of illustration clarity.

that 10 weeks of static stretching, 40 minutes for 3 days per week, of all the major muscle groups in the lower extremity improved knee flexion and extension strength, and may facilitate the transition back to regular training.

5. *Use proper technique.* Use light weights to learn the proper technique of a given exercise so that you do not strain yourself if you do the exercise incorrectly. Learn to lift smoothly. Do not use jerking motions. When the proper technique is mas-

tered, the weights may be increased. Using proper technique ensures that the desired muscle group is being exercised.

6. *Protect your lower back.* Avoid exercises that may cause or aggravate low back problems. Try to prevent an excessive forward motion or stress in the lower back region. Figure 12.14 illustrates some positions that should be avoided.

7. *Lower weights slowly.* If you lower them rapidly, your muscles have to contract rapidly to slow the weights down as you

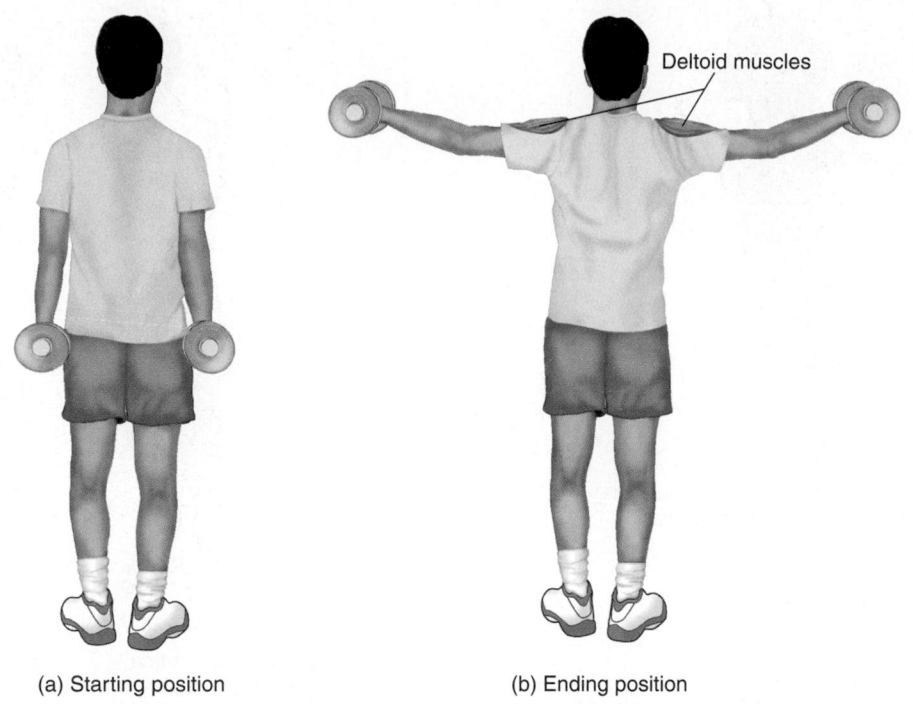

Deltoid muscles

(a) Starting position   (b) Ending position

Shoulders	
Exercise	Standing lateral raise
Shoulder muscles	Deltoid
Other muscles	Trapezius
Sets	3–5
Repetitions	8–12, PRE concept
Safety	Do not arch back.
Equipment	Dumbbells
Description	Stand with dumbbells in hands at sides. With palms down, raise straight arms sideways to shoulder level. Bend elbows slightly. Return slowly to starting position.

FIGURE 12.9 Standing lateral raise. The standing lateral raise primarily develops the deltoid muscles in the shoulder; the trapezius in the upper back and neck area is also trained.

reach the starting position. This necessitates the development of a large amount of force that may tear some muscle fibers or connective tissue and cause muscle soreness.

How does the body gain weight with a resistance-training program?

Muscle hypertrophy simply means increased muscle size. Figure 12.15 depicts the microstructure of muscle tissue. Resistance-training exercises place a heavy overload on the muscle cell, in some way stimulating the DNA within the multiple nuclei found in muscle cells. Carson indicated that the first stage of muscle hypertrophy, at the onset of overload, is associated with increased RNA activity and protein synthesis. Various hormones whose secretion is increased during exercise play important roles in stimulating muscle growth. In particular, Vingren and others state that testosterone is considered the major promoter of muscle growth and subsequent increase in muscle strength in response to resistance training in men. Human growth hormone and insulin-like growth factor are also involved. These hormones are discussed in more detail in chapter 13.

Over time, the muscle cell tends to adapt to such stress by increasing its size. It may do so in several possible ways. First, the individual muscle cells and myofibrils may simply increase their size by incorporating more protein. Second, the myofibrils in each cell may multiply, which will increase the size of each muscle fiber. Third, the amount of connective tissue around each muscle fiber and around each bundle of muscle may increase and thicken,

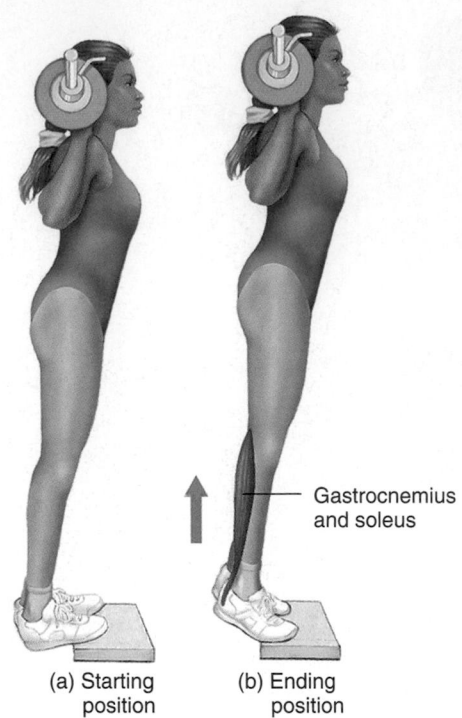

Gastrocnemius
and soleus

(a) Starting
position

(b) Ending
position

Calf	
Exercise	Heel raise
Calf muscles	Gastrocnemius, soleus
Other muscles	Deep calf muscles
Sets	3–5
Repetitions	8–12, PRE concept
Safety	Have two spotters if you use free weights.
Equipment	Squat rack if available. Pad the bar with a towel if necessary.
Description	Place bar on back of shoulders as in squat exercise. Raise up on your toes as high as possible and then return to standing position. Place the toes on a board so heels can drop down lower than normal. Point toes in, out, and straight ahead during different sets to work the muscles from different angles.

FIGURE 12.10 Heel raise. The heel raise develops the two major calf muscles—the gastrocnemius and the soleus.

Note: For safety reasons spotters should be present to assist in case of difficulty. The spotters are not depicted for purposes of illustration clarity.

leading to an overall increase in the size of the total muscle. Fourth, the cell may increase its content of enzymes and energy storage, particularly ATP and glycogen. The increased muscle glycogen, along with increased muscle protein, binds additional water, which contributes to an increased body weight. Finally, the muscle fibers themselves may increase in number (hyperplasia), but current evidence suggests that this is much less likely

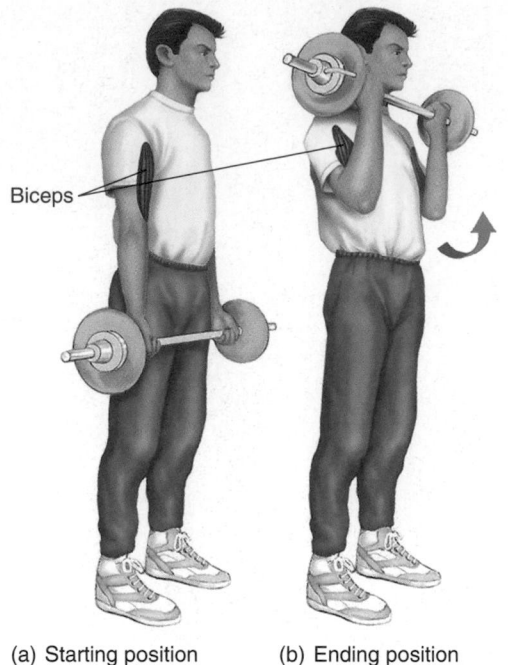

Biceps

(a) Starting position

(b) Ending position

Front of arm	
Exercise	Standing curl
Arm muscle	Biceps
Other muscles	Several elbow flexors
Sets	3–5
Repetitions	8–12, PRE concept
Safety	Do not arch back. Place back against wall to control arching motion.
Equipment	Curl bar if available
Description	Stand with weight held in front of body, palms forward. Place back against wall. Bend the elbows and bring the weight to the chest. Lower it slowly.

FIGURE 12.11 The standing curl. The standing curl strengthens the biceps muscle in the front of the upper arm as well as several other muscles in the region that bend the elbow.

to occur compared with the other four means to induce muscle hypertrophy. In their review, Folland and Williams noted that the primary factor contributing to increased overall muscle size is the increase in the size and number of the myofibrils. In addition to the effects on the muscle cell, although not all studies are in agreement, research data indicate that resistance-training exercises may increase bone mineral content, possibly owing to increased muscle tension effects on the bone, which might provide a slight increase in total body weight.

Resistance training may be an effective means to increase muscle size and mass. Such increases help improve muscular strength and endurance and may be important components

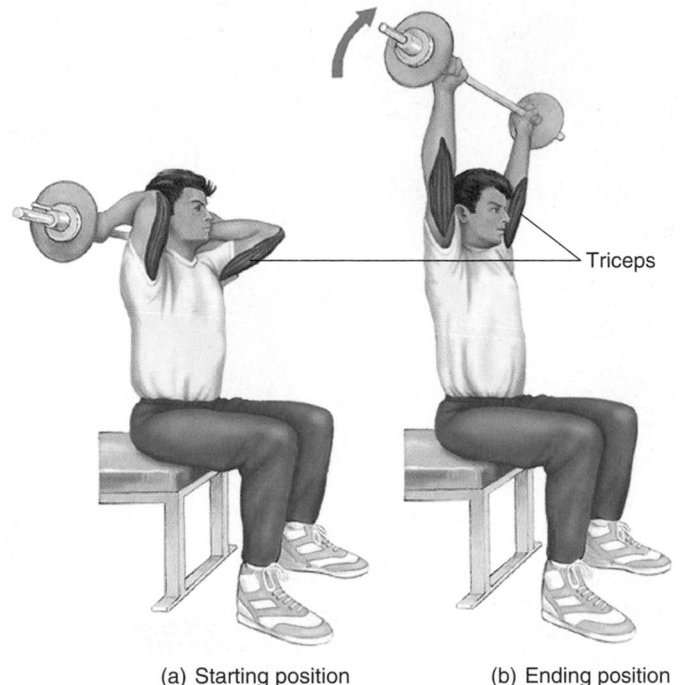

Triceps

(a) Starting position   (b) Ending position

Back of arm	
Exercise	Seated overhead press (triceps extension)
Arm muscle	Triceps
Other muscles	Trapezius, deltoids
Sets	3–5
Repetitions	8–12, PRE concept
Safety	Do not arch back excessively. Have spotter available as fatigue sets in.
Equipment	Bench or chair
Description	Sit on bench with weight held behind the head near the neck. Hands should be close together, elbows bent. Keep elbows in. Straighten elbows and press weight over head to arm's length. Lower weight slowly to starting position.

FIGURE 12.12 The seated overhead press. The seated overhead press primarily develops the triceps muscle on the back of the upper arm; the exercise also trains the trapezius in the upper back and neck and the deltoids in the shoulder.

Note: For safety reasons spotters should be present to assist in case of difficulty. The spotters are not depicted for purposes of illustration clarity.

Rectus abdominis

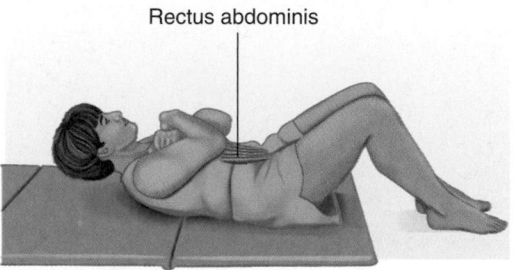

(a) Starting position

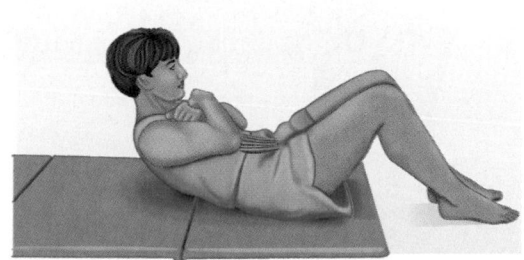

(b) Ending position

Abdominal area	
Exercise	Curl-up
Abdominal muscles	Rectus abdominis
Other muscles	Oblique abdominis muscles
Sets	3–5
Repetitions	8–12, PRE concept
Safety	Develop sufficient abdominal strength before using weights with this exercise. Do not arch back when exercising.
Equipment	Free-weight plates; incline sit-up bench if available.
Description	Lie on back, knees bent with heels close to buttocks. Hands should hold weights on chest. Curl up about a third to halfway. Return to starting position slowly.

Note: This exercise may be done without weights but with an increased number of repetitions.

FIGURE 12.13 The curl-up. The curl-up trains the rectus abdominis and the oblique abdominis muscles.

in weight-control programs. Traditionally, in research studies females did not normally experience the same amount of hypertrophy that males did, although they did experience proportional gains in muscular strength and endurance. However, more recent research revealed a significant increase in muscle cell size when women engaged in an intense, concentrated resistance-training program. Moreover, O'Hagan and others found that when exposed

to the same short-term resistance-training program, muscle size increased similarly in women and men.

Muscular hypertrophy associated with resistance training may be reduced in the elderly. Vingren and others report decreased secretion of testosterone in older men and women during exercise, which would mitigate the anabolic effect. Nevertheless, Peterson and others, in a meta-analysis of 49 studies, concluded that resistance

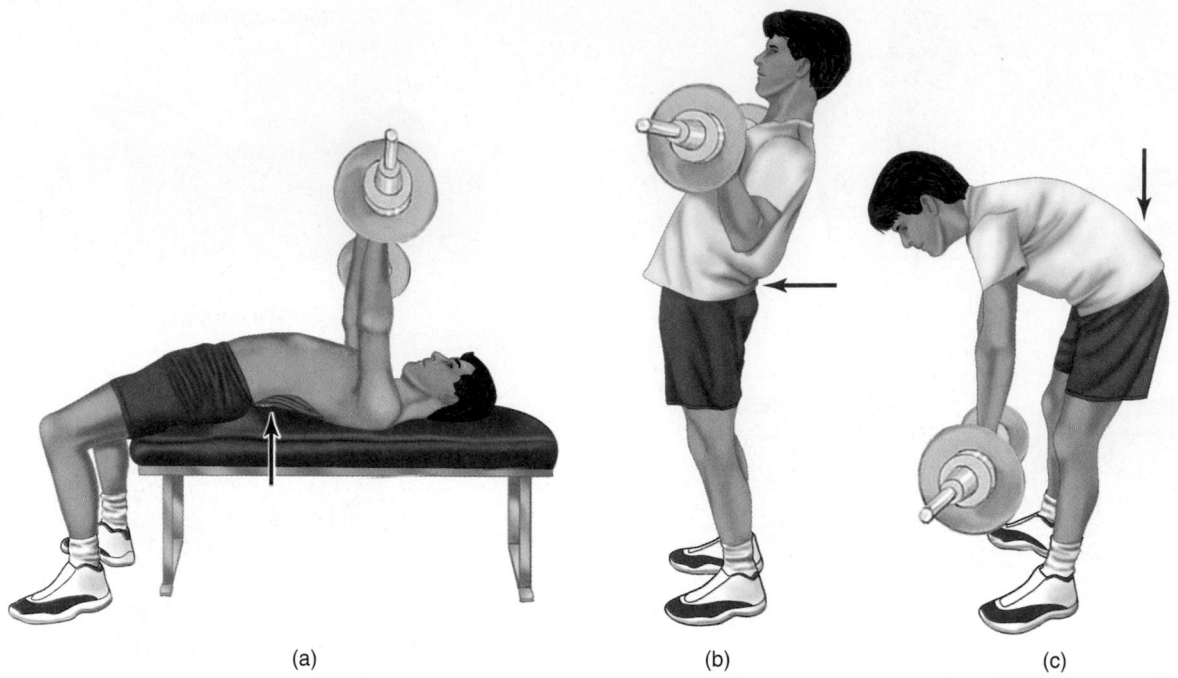

FIGURE 12.14 Avoid exercises or body positions that place excessive stress on the low-back region. Poor form in exercises like (a) the bench press and (b) the curl exaggerates the lumbar curve. Be sure to keep the lower back as flat as possible. Exercises similar to (c) the bent-over row place tremendous forces on the lower back because the weight or resistance is so far in front of the body.

training, particularly with higher-volume programs, is effective for gaining lean body mass in aging adults.

Is any one type of resistance-training program or equipment more effective than others for gaining body weight?

There are a variety of methods for resistance training. **Isometric methods** involve a muscle contraction against an immovable object, such as trying to pull a telephone pole out of the ground. However, if you succeed in moving the object, then you are doing an isotonic exercise. **Isotonic methods** are of two types. The **concentric method** means the muscle is shortening, as the biceps does in the up phase of a pull-up. The **eccentric method** means the muscle is lengthening even though it is trying to shorten. In the down phase of the pull-up the biceps is now contracting eccentrically as it slows your rate of descent. Gravity is attempting to pull you down, but your biceps is resisting it. Finally, the **isokinetic method** uses machines or other devices to regulate the speed at which you can shorten your muscles. For example, you may try to move your arm as fast as possible, but you will be able to move only as fast as the setting on the isokinetic machine. Isokinetic exercise is also known as accommodating-resistance exercise because the resistance automatically adjusts to the force exerted, thus controlling the speed of movement.

Several different resistance-training apparatuses are available, such as Atlantis, Nautilus, Hammer, Cybex, Hydra-Gym, Soloflex, and other similar machines. Depending upon the model, they are designed to utilize one or more of the training methods cited previously.

A number of research studies have been conducted to determine which of these methods or machines is best, particularly in relation to strength and power gains. Research suggests that at present it is probably safe to say that the various training methods are comparable in their ability to produce gains in muscle size and strength. For example, in a comprehensive review comparing the effects of dynamic exercise (including free weights and weight machines), accommodating resistance (isokinetic and semi-isokinetic devices), and isometric resistance, Wernbom and others concluded that there is insufficient evidence for the superiority of any mode and/or type of muscle action over other modes and types of training.

In a study comparing the effects of concentric and eccentric muscle training in women, Nickols-Richardson and others reported no significant differences between the methods for improvements in muscular strength, fat-free body mass, or bone mineral content and density. However, Roig and others, in a meta-analysis of 20 studies, concluded that when eccentric exercise was performed at higher intensities compared with concentric training, total strength and eccentric strength increased more significantly. They suggested that the superiority of eccentric training to increase muscle strength and mass appears to be related to the higher loads developed during eccentric contractions. However, such training programs should be used with caution at least until the muscle adapts to a program of progression in intensity, because high-intensity eccentric exercise may be more likely to cause muscle tissue damage and muscle soreness. Such programs would appear to be of interest primarily to highly trained athletes.

scope of this text, so the interested reader is referred to more detailed resources, such as the texts cited in the reference list at the end of this chapter.

If exercise burns Calories, won't I lose weight on a resistance-training program?

Although exercise does cost Calories, the amount expended during resistance training is relatively small compared to more active aerobic exercise. Resistance training can be a high-intensity exercise, but the time spent actually lifting during a typical workout is usually short, therefore limiting the number of Calories used. For example, in an hour workout, only about 15 minutes may be involved in actual exercise, the remaining time being recovery between each exercise. Based upon metabolic data collected in research studies, the average-sized male uses about 200 Calories in a typical workout, while the average-sized female uses about 150 (see figure 12.16). Resistance training appears to have a small effect on postexercise energy expenditure.

In one study, Ormsbee and others reported that energy expenditure, mostly from fat, was increased following a 40–45 minute intense resistance-training workout. The increased caloric expenditure was only about 10 Calories over a 45–minute recovery period, not a very significant amount. However, Melanson and others indicated that circuit resistance training, as discussed later, may lead to a total daily energy expenditure comparable to aerobic cycling exercise.

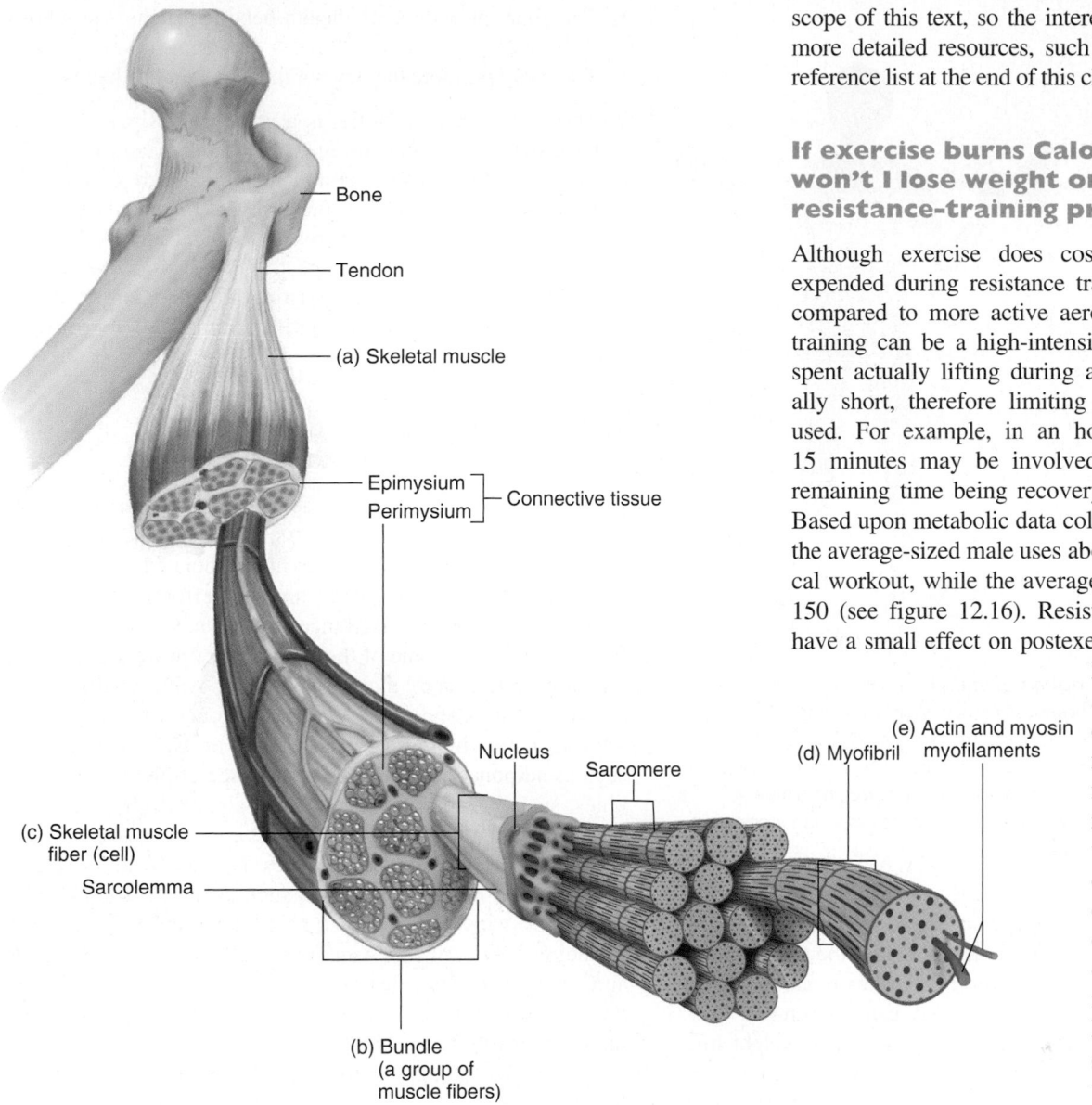

FIGURE 12.15 Muscle structure. The whole muscle is composed of separate bundles of individual muscle fibers. Each fiber is composed of numerous myofibrils, each of which contains thin protein filaments arranged so that they can slide by each other to cause muscle shortening or lengthening. Several layers of connective tissue surround the muscle fibers, bundles, and whole muscles, which eventually band together to form the tendon.

Bone
Tendon
(a) Skeletal muscle
Epimysium
Perimysium
Connective tissue
Nucleus
Sarcomere
(e) Actin and myosin myofilaments
(d) Myofibril
(c) Skeletal muscle fiber (cell)
Sarcolemma
(b) Bundle (a group of muscle fibers)

All methods may be effective in increasing body weight provided the basic principles of resistance training, particularly the principle of overload, are followed. The ACSM recommends that your exercise program include both concentric and eccentric exercise, which are incorporated in most machines and free weights. If you use machines, be sure to exercise all major muscle area. Free weights are relatively inexpensive and can be used for a wide variety of exercises. They also may be constructed at home, using pipe or solid broomstick handles for the bar and different-sized tin cans filled with cement for the weights.

There may be some specific training programs that are better suited for specific purposes, such as specific sport performance enhancement or injury rehabilitation. These topics are beyond the

Are there any contraindications to resistance training?

Several health conditions may be aggravated by resistance training, primarily by the increased pressures that occur within the body when you strain to lift heavy weights and hold your breath at the same time. Because the blood pressure can increase rapidly and excessively during weight lifting, to 300 mmHg or higher, individuals with resting blood pressures over 90 mmHg diastolic and 140 mmHg systolic should refrain from heavy lifting, for they may be exposed to an increased risk of blood vessel rupture and a possible stroke. Lifting with the arms and straining exercises also increase the stress on the heart and thus should be

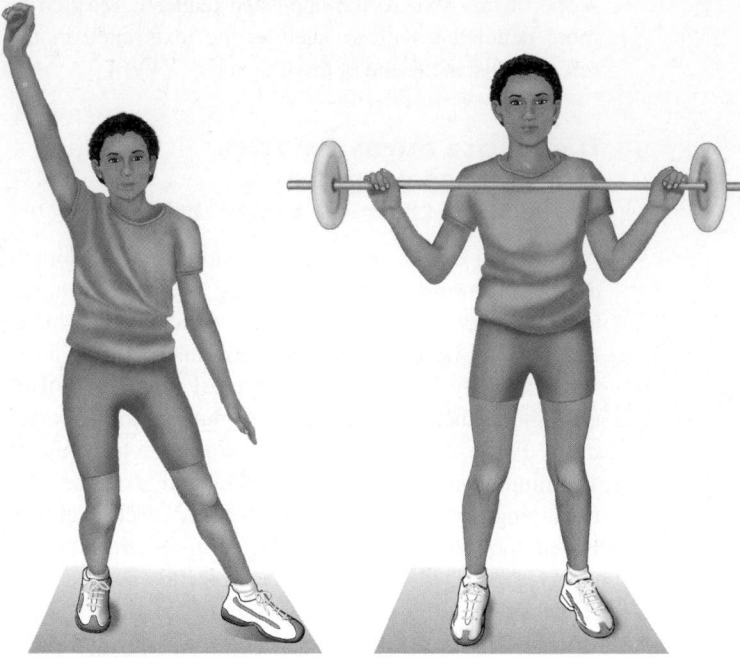

1 hour = 600–800 Calories   1 hour = 150–200 Calories

FIGURE 12.16 All models of exercise increase caloric expenditure. However, an hour of regular weight training expends only about one-third to one-fourth as many Calories as vigorous aerobic activity. Combining aerobic exercises with weight training (circuit aerobics) helps burn more Calories than weight training alone; it also provides cardiovascular health benefits while increasing muscular strength and endurance.

avoided by individuals who have heart problems, such as arrhythmias. Individuals with a hernia (a weakness in the musculature of the abdominal wall) also should refrain from strenuous weight lifting, because the increased pressure may cause a rupture. Low back problems also may be aggravated by improper weight lifting techniques. Improper technique may also contribute to muscle strain and joint pain, particularly in the shoulder. Some individuals may suffer peripheral nerve injuries, such as carpal tunnel syndrome, involving weakness and numbness in the hand due to compressed nerves from improper lifting techniques. Individuals with these types of health problems should seek medical advice and be cleared by a physician before initiating or continuing with a resistance-training program.

There has been some concern about the advisability of prepubescent youth lifting weights. However, two recently updated policy and position statements, by the American Academy of Pediatrics (AAP) and by Faigenbaum and others for the National Strength and Conditioning Association (NSCA), provided an analysis of resistance-training programs for youngsters. The AAP and NSCA indicate the following benefits from participation in programs that are properly designed and supervised specifically for youth:

- They are safe.
- They can enhance muscular strength and power.
- They can help increase resistance to sports-related injuries.

- They may provide some health benefits, such as psychosocial well-being.
- They may promote the development of exercise habits.

The key to these benefits is a properly designed and supervised program. Gradual progression is important, as it is with adults. The AAP also recommends that both preadolescents and adolescents should avoid power lifting, bodybuilding, and maximal lifts until they reach physical and skeletal maturity. Moreover, the AAP suggested that caution be used with young athletes who have preexisting hypertension or other cardiovascular problems, as strength training may aggravate such conditions.

Are there any health benefits associated with resistance training?

Although resistance training has been recommended mainly as a means of gaining muscle mass, body weight, and strength, in the past its use normally was not associated with any health benefits. However, increasing research efforts focusing on the health implications of resistance training have suggested several favorable effects. Some of the health benefits are associated with increases in lean body mass and strength. Additionally, de Salles and others, in a review of 17 studies, concluded that resistance training could increase the secretion of beneficial cytokines, such as adiponectin, and decrease the secretion of harmful cytokines, such as tumor necrosis factor-alpha. Both an increase in muscle mass and beneficial cytokines could increase insulin sensitivity and protect against diabetes. Direct effects of resistance exercise on other body systems, such as the neuromuscular and skeletal systems, may produce health benefits. Various reviews, including those by the American College of Sports Medicine and American Diabetes Association, Deschenes and Kraemer, Phillips, Strasser and others, and Williams, have reported multiple health benefits associated with resistance training—benefits which, along with those cited in other reports, include the following:

1. Increased lean body mass to help prevent the development of **sarcopenia** (loss of muscle mass) as one ages; a major health benefit
2. Decreased risk of the metabolic syndrome and its comorbidities, such as high blood pressure
3. Increased strength and improved gait, to prevent falls and injury as one ages
4. Decreased pain in chronic low-back-pain patients to improve mobility
5. Increased bone mineral density to help prevent osteoporosis, particularly in females
6. Improved glucose metabolism and insulin sensitivity to help prevent diabetes or improve glucose control in diabetics
7. Improved serum lipid profiles, such as increased HDL-cholesterol and decreased LDL-cholesterol, to help prevent atherosclerosis and coronary heart disease
8. Improved ability to complete activities of daily living and enhance the quality of life in older individuals

9. Improved mood, body image, self-concept, and psychological health in children, adolescents, and adults
10. Improve rate of recovery from some types of surgery, such as hip replacement surgery

These findings are contrary to the belief that resistance training does not confer any health benefits comparable to aerobic exercise. It is also notable that many cardiac rehabilitation programs now incorporate resistance-training exercises.

Nevertheless, it still appears to be prudent health behavior to incorporate some aerobic exercise into your lifestyle, even when trying to gain body weight. Although the ACSM and AHA have incorporated resistance training in their recommended exercise program for healthy adults, it is designed to complement aerobic exercise, not to substitute for it. The American Academy of Pediatrics also noted that if long-term health benefits for children and adolescents are the goal, then strength training should be combined with an aerobic training program. Aerobic exercise programs do consume more Calories, so you would have to balance the expenditure with increased food intake if you want to gain weight. However, the energy expenditure need not be excessive to provide a beneficial training effect. For example, running 2 to 3 miles about 4 days per week would provide you with an adequate aerobic-exercise training effect for your heart, but it would cost you only about 200–300 Calories a day. This 200- to 300-Calorie expenditure could be replaced easily by consuming two glasses of orange juice or similar small amounts of food.

Doing both resistance and aerobics exercise may provide additional health benefits. For example, Pitsavos and others, in a large study involving more than 3,000 subjects, suggested that combining aerobic and resistance-type activities may confer a better effect on lipoprotein profile in healthy individuals than aerobic activities alone.

Can I combine aerobic and resistance-training exercises into one program?

Although the principles underlying the development of an aerobic-training program and a resistance-training program are similar, the purposes of the two programs are rather different. An aerobic exercise program is designed to improve the efficiency of the cardiovascular system; the basic purpose of a resistance-training program is to increase muscle size, strength, and body weight.

One form of resistance training that has been used to provide some moderate benefits to the cardiovascular system is **circuit weight training,** a method in which the individual moves rapidly from one exercise to the next. Generally, this type of program uses lighter weights with greater numbers of repetitions, thus increasing the aerobic component of training. Research reported energy expenditure of approximately 10 Calories per minute for males and 7 Calories per minute for females. Circuit weight training can improve strength, but Harber and others indicated that strength gains are attributed more to neural adaptations because the relatively low resistance loads do not induce appreciable muscle hypertrophy.

A newer version of this method is **circuit aerobics.** Circuit aerobics may be done in a variety of ways, but basically it involves an integration of aerobic and resistance-training exercises. It is actually a form of interval aerobic training, but instead of resting or doing a lower level of aerobic activity during the recovery interval, you do resistance-training exercises. Circuit aerobics may offer multiple health and performance benefits, such as improved cardiovascular fitness, increased caloric expenditure for loss of body fat, improved muscular strength and endurance, and increased muscle tone in body areas not normally stressed by aerobic exercise alone. Curves, the largest fitness franchise in the world, has developed a 30-minute exercise program specifically for women using this concept.

However, if the main purpose of your resistance-training program is to gain body weight as muscle mass, then you need to train near the strength end of the strength-endurance continuum. For athletes who need to maximize gains in lean body mass, strength, and especially power, some sports scientists suggest that aerobic training should be markedly reduced if not eliminated. For example, Malisoux and others, reviewing studies involving single muscle fibers to help understand the effects of different forms of exercise training, reported that muscle fiber peak power is increased after resistance training, but over time is decreased with endurance training. Elliott and others indicate that cardiovascular endurance-training programs are detrimental for the performance of power athletes, suggesting contributing factors such as inappropriate neuromuscular adaptations, a catabolic hormonal profile, or ineffective motor learning environment. They note that there are unequivocal drawbacks to distance training in the power athlete.

http://growingstronger.nutrition.tufts.edu **This Tufts University** Website presents an evidence-based exercise program designed to increase muscle strength, maintain bone health, and improve balance, coordination, and mobility in older adults.

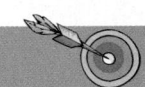

Key Concepts

▶ A basic principle underlying all resistance-training programs is the overload principle, which simply means the muscle should be stressed beyond normal daily levels.

▶ Progressive resistance is also a basic principle of resistance training, for as you get stronger through use of the overload principle, you must progressively increase the resistance.

▶ To increase muscle mass and body weight, you should exercise near the strength end of the strength-endurance continuum.

▶ Your resistance-training program should exercise all major muscles groups in the body.

▶ A variety of methods and apparatuses are available for resistance training, but research suggests that they are equally effective as a means of gaining strength and muscle mass if the basic principles of resistance training are followed.

▶ Resistance training is generally regarded as a safe form of exercise, but it may be contraindicated in some individuals, for example, those with high blood pressure and hernias.

▶ Although resistance-training programs may confer some significant health benefits, it is also highly recommended that one add an aerobic exercise program to help condition the cardiovascular system.

Do this after 2–3 weeks of resistance training. Using free weights or an appropriate weight-training machine, such as Nautilus, determine your one repetition maximum (1RM) for a given exercise, such as the bench press. Start out with a light weight that you know you can easily lift one time, and then gradually add on amounts until you reach your limit. You should need only 3–4 attempts. Record the weight of the last successful attempt.

APPLICATION EXERCISE

If you have time and are interested, start a resistance-training program, using the principles in the text. Record your 1 RM for an exercise (such as the bench press) initially and every two weeks for several months. Use a tape measure to determine body girth changes in the upper arm, chest, waist, and upper thigh. If you have access to skinfold calipers or other measures of body composition, keep similar records. Use a model comparable to those presented, (adjusting the numbers in the vertical column to represent weight lifted for 1 RM, millimeters for skinfold measurement, and centimeters or inches for girth measurement), graph the results, and compare to the text discussion.

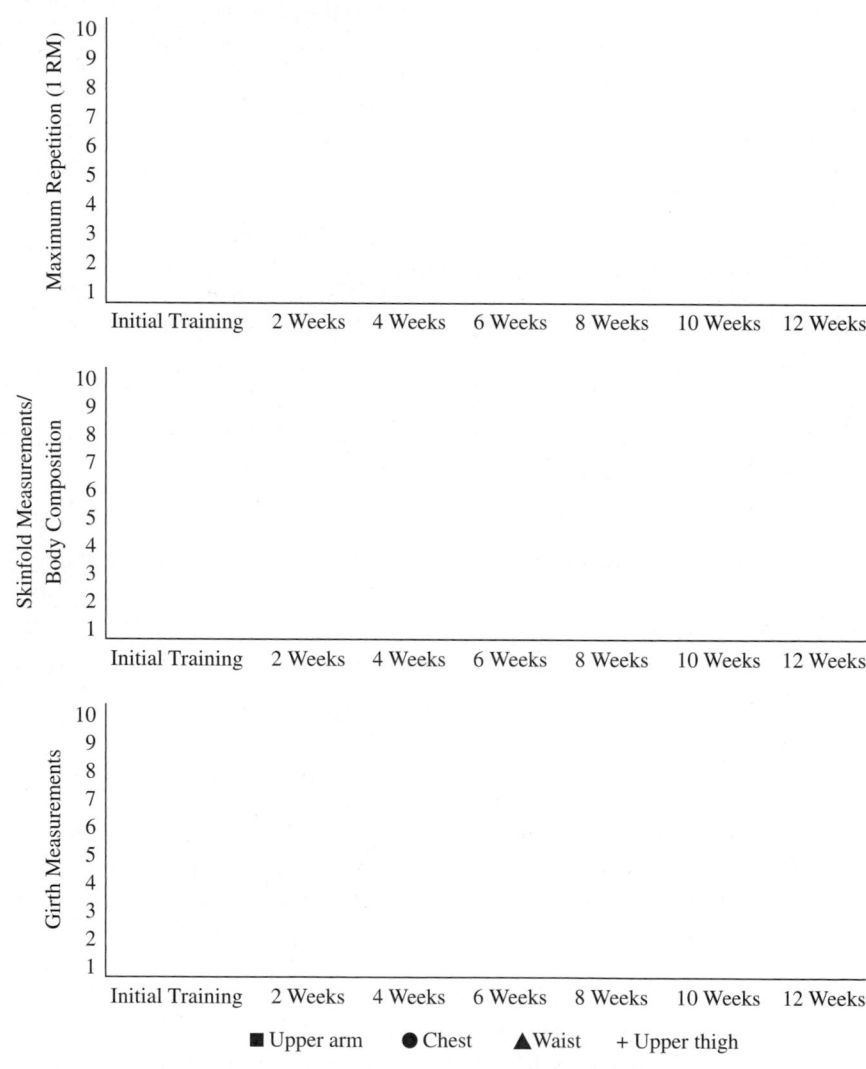

1. Which of the following would be least recommended for someone who wants to gain weight healthfully?

   a. stop smoking
   b. set a goal of about 0.5 pound per week
   c. get enough rest and sleep
   d. start a resistance-training program
   e. drink more caffeinated beverages

2. Which of the following is not one of the basic principles of resistance training?

   a. overload
   b. specificity
   c. progressive resistance
   d. aerobic
   e. sequence

3. The bench press exercise is designed to have the greatest effect on which group of muscles?

   a. calf
   b. thigh
   c. back
   d. chest
   e. abdominal

4. The standing lateral raise is designed to have the greatest effect on which group of muscles?

   a. shoulder
   b. thigh
   c. calf
   d. chest
   e. abdominal

5. Resistance training will stimulate muscle hypertrophy by a variety of mechanisms. Which of the following is considered to be least likely, according to the text discussion?

   a. Individual muscle cells and myofibrils increase in size.
   b. Myofibrils in each cell may multiply.
   c. Connective tissue in muscle may increase and thicken.
   d. Muscle cells will increase water content by binding to increased glycogen.
   e. Muscle fibers themselves increase rapidly in number.

6. For the purpose of gaining weight, which type of resistance-training equipment is best according to research findings, provided equal amounts of resistance work are done on each?

   a. isokinetic concentric machines
   b. isometric devices
   c. isotonic eccentric free weights
   d. isotonic concentric free weights
   e. no equipment is better than any other

7. Which dietary supplement has the most research supporting its potential to help increase muscle mass and weight gain during a resistance-training program?

   a. HMB
   b. chromium
   c. creatine
   d. ginseng
   e. carnitine

8. Research suggests that proper resistance training may confer some significant health benefits. Which of the following is least likely?

   a. increased strength to prevent falls and injury as one ages
   b. increased bone mineral density to help prevent osteoporosis
   c. increased testosterone levels to help reduce serum HDL-cholesterol
   d. improved muscle mass and insulin sensitivity to help prevent type 2 diabetes
   e. improved body image and psychological health

9. Which of the following would be the least likely dietary recommendation for someone trying to gain weight in lean mass?

   a. Wait at least 4 hours after exercise before eating some protein and carbohydrate.
   b. Increase the intake of high-Calorie, high nutrient foods.
   c. Keep the intake of saturated fats to a minimum.
   d. Eat three balanced meals a day supplemented with snacks.
   e. Supplement the diet with high-Calorie, high nutrient liquids.

10. To gain one pound of muscle weight per week on a weight-training program, an individual might need an additional 14 grams of protein per day above the RDA, in addition to increased Calories. Which of the following would not supply that amount of protein daily?

    a. 2 glasses of skim milk
    b. 1 glass of orange juice and 2 eggs
    c. 1 slice of toast, 1 egg, and 1 ounce of ham
    d. 1 glass of orange juice, 2 slices of toast, and 1 banana
    e. 2 ounces of cheese

Answers to multiple choice questions:
1. e; 2. d; 3. d; 4. a; 5. e; 6. e;
7. c; 8. c; 9. a; 10. d.

1. Explain the strength-endurance continuum as a training concept.
2. List the five basic principles of resistance training and provide an example of each.
3. Discuss the physiological means whereby resistance training leads to increases in muscle growth.
4. Describe at least five of the potential health benefits associated with resistance training.
5. Discuss the importance of protein in a weight-gaining diet and provide some recommendations for amounts of protein and types of protein-rich foods in the diet.

Books

Bompa, T., and Carrera, M. 2005. *Periodization Training for Sports.* Champaign, IL: Human Kinetics.

Fleck, S., and Kraemer, W. 2004. *Designing Resistance Training Programs.* Champaign, IL: Human Kinetics.

Ivy, J., and Portman, R. 2004. *Nutrient Timing: The Future of Sports Nutrition.* North Bergen, NJ: Basic Health Publications.

National Academy of Sciences. 2002. *Dietary Reference Intakes for Energy, Carbohydrate, Fiber, Fat, Protein and Amino Acids.* Washington, DC: National Academy Press.

Pope, H., et al. 2000. *The Adonis Complex.* New York: Free Press.

Reuben, D. 1996. *Dr. David Reuben's Quick Weight-Gain Program.* New York: Crown Publishers.

Stone, M., et al. 2007. *Principles and Practices of Resistance Training.* Champaign, IL: Human Kinetics.

U.S. Department of Health and Human Services. 2010. *Healthy People 2020.* Washington, DC: U.S. Government Printing Office.

Reviews

American Academy of Pediatrics Council on Sports Medicine and Fitness. 2008. Strength training by children and adolescents. *Pediatrics* 121:835–40.

American College of Sports Medicine. 2009. American College of Sports Medicine position stand: Progression models in resistance training for healthy adults. *Medicine & Science in Sports & Exercise* 41:687–708.

American College of Sports Medicine; American Diabetes Association. 2010. American College of Sports Medicine and the American Diabetes Association joint position statement: Exercise and type 2 diabetes. *Medicine & Science in Sports & Exercise* 42:2282–303.

Beelen, M., et al. 2010. Nutritional strategies to promote postexercise recovery. *International Journal of Sport Nutrition and Exercise Metabolism* 20:515–32.

Bloomer, R. 2007. The role of nutritional supplements in the prevention and treatment of resistance exercise-induced skeletal muscle injury. *Sports Medicine* 37:519–32.

Candow, D. 2011. Sarcopenia: Current theories and the potential beneficial effect of creatine application strategies. *Biogerontology* 12:273–81.

Candow, D., and Chilibeck, P. 2007. Effect of creatine supplementation during resistance training on muscle accretion in the elderly. *Journal of Nutrition, Health & Aging* 11:185–88.

Carson, J. 1997. The regulation of gene expression in hypertrophying skeletal muscle. *Exercise and Sport Sciences Reviews* 25:301–20.

Clarkson, P., and Rawson, E. 1999. Nutritional supplements to increase muscle mass. *Critical Reviews in Food Science and Nutrition* 39:317–28.

Coleman, E., et al. 2002. Herbal supplements and sport performance. *Sports Science Exchange Roundtable* 13 (4):1–4.

Consumers Union. 2000. A 12-step program for safe exercise. *Consumer Reports on Health* 12 (4):8–9.

de Salles, B., et al. 2010. Effects or resistance training on cytokines. *International Journal of Sports Medicine* 31:441–50.

Deschenes, M., and Kraemer, W. 2002. Performance and physiologic adaptations to resistance training. *American Journal of Physical and Medical Rehabilitation* 81:S3–S16.

Elliott, M., et al. 2007. Power athletes and distance training: Physiological and biomechanical rationale for change. *Sports Medicine* 37:47–57.

Faigenbaum, A., et al. 2009. Youth resistance training: Updated position statement paper from the National Strength and Conditioning Association. *Journal of Strength and Conditioning Research* 23 Suppl:S60–79.

Faigenbaum, A. 2003. Youth resistance training. *President's Council on Physical Fitness and Sports Research Digest* 4 (3):1–8.

Folland, J., and Williams, A. 2007. The adaptations to strength training: Morphological and neurological contributions to increased strength. *Sports Medicine* 37:145–68.

Foran, B. 1985. Advantages and disadvantages of isokinetics, variable resistance, and free weights. *National Strength and Conditioning Association Journal* 7:24–25.

Frost, D., et al. 2010. A biomechanical evaluation of resistance: Fundamental concepts for training and sports performance. *Sports Medicine* 40:303–26.

Gatorade Sports Science Institute. 1995. Methods of weight gain in athletes. *Sports Science Exchange Roundtable* 6 (3):1–4.

Goldman, M. 2011. Much ado about Muscle Milk. *University of California Berkeley Wellness Letter* 27 (4):2.

Grieve, F. 2007. A conceptual model of factors contributing to the development of muscle dysmorphia. *Eating Disorders* 15:63–80.

Haskell, W., et al. 2007. Physical activity and public health: Updated recommendation for adults from the American College of Sports Medicine and the American Heart Association. *Medicine & Science in Sports & Exercise* 39:1423–34.

Hayes, L., et al. 2010. Interactions of cortisol, testosterone, and resistance training: Influence of circadian rhythms. *Chronobiology International* 27:675–705.

Kraemer, W., et al. 2003. Strength training basics. *Physician and Sportsmedicine* 31 (8):39–45.

Kraemer, W., et al. 1998. Resistance training and elite athletes: Adaptations and program considerations. *Journal of Orthopaedic and Sports Physical Therapy* 28:110–19.

Kraemer, W., et al. 1996. Strength and power training: Physiological mechanisms of adaptation. *Exercise and Sport Sciences Reviews* 24:363–97.

Kreider, R. 1999. Dietary supplements and the promotion of muscle growth with resistance exercise. *Sports Medicine* 27:97–110.

Lambert, C., et al. 2004. Macronutrient considerations for the sport of bodybuilding. *Sports Medicine* 34:317–27.

Lemon, P. 1996. Is increased dietary protein necessary or beneficial for individuals with a physically active lifestyle? *Nutrition Reviews* 54:S169–S175.

Lodhia, K., et al. 2005. Peripheral nerve injuries in weight training. *Physician and Sportsmedicine* 33 (7):24–37.

Malisoux, L., et al. 2007. What do single-fiber studies tell us about exercise training? *Medicine & Science in Sports & Exercise* 39:1051–60.

National Strength and Conditioning Association. 1987. Breathing during weight training. *National Strength and Conditioning Association Journal* 9:17–24.

Nelson, M., et al. 2007. Physical activity and public health in older adults: Recommendation from the American College of Sports Medicine and the American Heart Association. *Medicine & Science in Sports & Exercise* 39:1435–45.

Paddon-Jones, D., and Rasmussen, B. 2009. Dietary protein recommendations and the prevention of sarcopenia. *Current Opinion in Clinical Nutrition and Metabolic Care* 12:86–90.

Peterson, M., et al. 2011. Influence of resistance exercise on lean body mass in aging adults: A meta-analysis. *Medicine & Science in Sports & Exercise* 43:249–58.

Phillips, S. 2011. The science of muscle hypertrophy: Making dietary protein count. *Proceedings of the Nutrition Society* 70:100–3.

Phillips, S. 2009. Physiologic and molecular bases of muscle hypertrophy and atrophy: Impact of resistance exercise on human skeletal muscle (protein and exercise dose effects). *Applied Physiology, Nutrition, and Metabolism* 34:403–10.

Phillips, S. 2006. Dietary protein for athletes: From requirements to metabolic advantage. *Applied Physiology, Nutrition and Metabolism* 31:647–54.

Rasmussen, B., and Phillips, S. 2003. Contractile and nutritional regulation of human muscle growth. *Exercise and Sport Sciences Reviews* 31:127–31.

Rawson, E., and Venezia, A. 2011. Use of creatine in the elderly and evidence for effects on cognitive function in young and old. *Amino Acids* 40:1349–62.

Roig, M., et al. 2009. The effects of eccentric versus concentric resistance training on muscle strength and mass in healthy adults: A systematic review with meta-analysis. *British Journal of Sports Medicine* 43:556–68.

Schardt, D. 2007. Saving muscle: How to stay strong and healthy as you age. *Nutrition Action Health Letter* 34 (3):1, 3–8.

Strasser, B., et al. 2010. Resistance training in the treatment of the metabolic syndrome: A systematic review and meta-analysis of the effect of resistance training on metabolic clustering in patients with abnormal glucose metabolism. *Sports Medicine* 40:397–415.

Tsika, R. 2006. The muscular system: The control of muscle mass. In *ACSM's Advanced Exercise Physiology,* ed. C. Tipton. Philadelphia: Lippincott Williams & Wilkins.

Vingren, J., et al. 2010. Testosterone physiology in resistance exercise and training: The up-stream regulatory elements. *Sports Medicine* 40:1037–53.

Volek, J., et al. 2006. Nutritional aspects of women strength athletes. *British Journal of Sports Medicine* 40:742–48.

Wernbom, M., et al. 2007. The influence of frequency, intensity, volume and mode of strength training on whole muscle cross-sectional area in humans. *Sports Medicine* 37:225–64.

Williams, M. 1993. Nutritional supplements for strength trained athletes. *Sports Science Exchange* 6 (47):1–6.

Williams, M., et al. 2007. Resistance exercise in individuals with and without cardiovascular disease: 2007 update: A scientific statement from the American Heart Association Council on Clinical Cardiology and Council on Nutrition, Physical Activity, and Metabolism. *Circulation* 116:572–84.

Wolfe, B., et al. 2004. Quantitative analysis of single- versus multiple-set programs in resistance training. *Journal of Strength and Conditioning Research* 18:35–47.

Yaspelkis, B. 2006. Resistance training improves insulin signaling and action in skeletal muscle. *Exercise and Sport Sciences Reviews* 34:42–46.

Specific Studies

Bartels, R., et al. 1989. Effect of chronically increased consumption of energy and carbohydrate on anabolic adaptations to strenuous weight training. In *Report of the Ross Symposium on the Theory and Practice of Athletic Nutrition: Bridging the Gap,* eds. J. Storlie and A. Grandjean. Columbus, OH: Ross Laboratories.

Cribb, P., and Hayes, A. 2006. Effect of supplement timing and resistance training on skeletal muscle hypertrophy. *Medicine & Science in Sports & Exercise* 38:1918–25.

Depcik, E., and Williams, L. 2004. Weight training and body satisfaction of body-image-disturbed women. *Journal of Applied Sport Psychology* 16:287–99.

Esmarck, B., et al. 2001. Timing of postexercise protein intake is important for muscle hypertrophy with resistance training in elderly humans. *Journal of Physiology* 535:301–11.

Grunewald, K., and Bailey, R. 1993. Commercially marketed supplements for bodybuilding athletes. *Sports Medicine* 15:90–103.

Harber, M., et al. 2004. Skeletal muscle and hormonal adaptations to circuit weight training in untrained men. *Scandinavian Journal of Medicine and Science in Sports* 14:176–85.

Hoffman, J., et al. 2009. Effect of protein-supplement timing on strength, power, and body-composition changes in resistance-trained men. *International Journal of Sport Nutrition and Exercise Metabolism* 19:172–85.

Hulmi, J., et al. 2009. Acute and long-term effects of resistance exercise with or without protein ingestion on muscle hypertrophy and gene expression. *Amino Acids* 37:297–308.

Josse, A., et al. 2010. Body composition and strength changes in women with milk and resistance exercise. *Medicine & Science in Sports & Exercise* 42:1122–30.

Kokkonen, J., et al. 2007. Chronic static stretching improves exercise performance. *Medicine & Science in Sports & Exercise* 39:1825–31.

Kraemer, W., and Ratamess, N. 2005. Progression and resistance training. *President's Council on Physical Fitness and Sports Research Digest* 6 (3):1–8.

MacDougall, J., et al. 1992. Factors affecting blood pressure during heavy weight lifting and static contractions. *Journal of Applied Physiology* 73.1590–97.

McLafferty, C., et al. 2004. Resistance training is associated with improved mood in healthy older adults. *Perceptual and Motor Skills* 98:947–57.

Melanson, E., et al. 2002. Resistance and aerobic exercise have similar effects on 24-h nutrient oxidation. *Medicine & Science in Sports & Exercise* 34:1783–1800.

Mettler, S., et al. 2010. Increased protein intake reduces lean body mass loss during weight loss in athletes. *Medicine & Science in Sports & Exercise* 42:326–37.

Nickols-Richardson, S., et al. 2007. Concentric and eccentric isokinetic resistance training similarly increases muscular strength, fat-free soft tissue mass, and specific bone mineral measurements in young women. *Osteoporosis International* 18:789–96.

O'Hagan, F., et al. 1995. Response to resistance training in young women and men. *International Journal of Sports Medicine* 16:314–21.

Ormsbee, M., et al. 2007. Fat metabolism and acute resistance exercise in trained men. *Journal of Applied Physiology* 102:1767–72.

Pickett, T., et al. 2005. Men, muscles, and body image: Comparisons of competitive bodybuilders, weight trainers, and athletically active controls. *British Journal of Sports Medicine* 39:217–22.

Pitsavos, C., et al. 2009. Resistance exercise plus to aerobic activities is associated with better lipids' profile among healthy individuals: the ATTICA study. *QJM* 102:609–16.

Ratamess, N., et al. 2007. The effect of rest interval length on metabolic responses to the bench press exercise. *European Journal of Applied Physiology* 100:1–17.

Starkey, D., et al. 1996. Effect of resistance training volume on strength and muscle thickness. *Medicine & Science in Sports & Exercise* 28:1311–20.

Staron, R., et al. 1989. Effects of heavy resistance weight training on muscle fiber size and composition in females. *Medicine & Science in Sports & Exercise* 21:S71.

Verdijk, L., et al. 2009. Protein supplementation before and after exercise does not further augment skeletal muscle hypertrophy after resistance training in elderly men. *American Journal of Clinical Nutrition* 89:608–16.

Whipple, T., et al. 2004. Acute effects of moderate intensity resistance exercise on bone cell activity. *International Journal of Sports Medicine* 25:496–501.

Food Drugs and Related Supplements

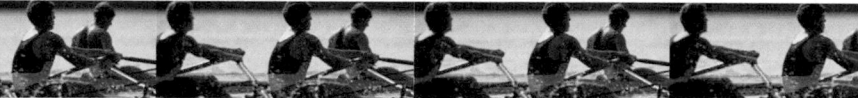

CHAPTER THIRTEEN

L E A R N I N G   O B J E C T I V E S

After studying this chapter, you should be able to:

1. Explain the metabolic, physiological, and psychological effects of alcohol in the body, and evaluate its efficacy as an ergogenic acid.

2. Explain the possible beneficial and detrimental effects of alcohol consumption on health.

3. List and explain the several theories whereby caffeine supplementation is proposed to be an effective ergogenic aid, and summarize its effect on exercise performance.

4. Explain the possible beneficial and detrimental health-related effects of caffeine in the body, and cite current recommendations for coffee consumption.

5. Understand the potential health problems associated with dietary supplements containing stimulants such as ephedra.

6. Describe the theory underlying the use of sodium bicarbonate as an ergogenic aid, and understand the current research findings regarding its efficacy to enhance exercise performance.

7. Identify drugs and related dietary supplements used by physically active individuals to stimulate muscle building and summarize the effects on exercise performance and potential health risks associated with their use.

8. Explain the theory as to how ginseng may enhance sport performance, and highlight the research findings regarding its ergogenic efficacy.

9. List those drugs or dietary supplements discussed in this chapter whose use is prohibited in sports.

10. Describe the four different recommendation levels for dietary supplements regarding their efficacy, safety, and permissibility as ergogenic aids for athletes, and cite examples of each.

Introduction

As noted in chapter 1, winning in sports is dependent not only on genetic endowment with physiological, psychological, and biomechanical attributes inherent to success in any given sport, but also on optimal training of those attributes. However, over the years athletes have attempted to go beyond training to gain a competitive edge on their opponents, and have used a wide variety of ergogenic aids in the process.

The most historic and popular international sporting event is the Olympic Games. The first Olympics were held in Greece, starting in 776 BC and continuing for more than 1,000 years, being cancelled in 393 AD because they were regarded as a pagan ritual. Similar to today, athletes who were successful in these ancient Olympics achieved fame and fortune.

Most elite Grecian athletes had personal trainers, called *paidotribes,* to plan their exercise program and their diet to prepare them for competition. In a sense, paidotribes were the first sport scientists and sport nutritionists. Several famous Greek scientists, including Galen and Pythagoras, were paidotribes who advocated specific, but different, diets for their athletes; Galen promoted beans as a staple of the athlete's diet, whereas Pythagoras prohibited them. During these early Olympic Games various plants served as sources of ergogenic drugs. For example, certain mushrooms contained hallucinogens and *Strychnos nux vamica* was the source of strychnine; in small doses, both could serve as a stimulant. Athletes in the ancient Olympics were reported to consume such plants for their potential ergogenic effect.

The modern Olympic Games were resurrected in 1896 and continue today with competition among thousands of athletes in dozens of sports. As in the ancient Olympics, athletes in the modern Olympics have been reported to use drugs in attempts to obtain that competitive edge. As several of these drugs are found in some common foods or beverages that we may consume, they have been referred to as *food drugs.* Additionally, some plant extracts, or phytochemicals, may be marketed as dietary supplements designed to imitate ergogenic drugs. Others, particularly herbals, may be used for their pharmaceutical effects by practitioners of alternative medicine.

In this chapter, we will evaluate the effects of several food drugs and related dietary supplements on exercise performance and health. Two very common food drugs, alcohol and caffeine, have been studied for their ergogenic effects for more than 100 years, and have been used by athletes as a means to enhance performance since the early 1900s. Each has also been studied extensively for possible health effects, both positive and negative.

The dietary supplement ma huang contains ephedra, or ephedrine, a stimulant theorized to enhance exercise performance, particularly when combined with caffeine. Ephedrine has also been studied for its potential health effects.

Sodium bicarbonate, or baking soda, is used in many food products, and has been studied for 80 years as a means to enhance performance; it also has been marketed as part of a dietary supplement for athletes.

Several anabolic hormones, and related steroid drugs, are used to increase muscle mass and have been popular with strength/power athletes for more than 50 years. Because the use of such drugs has been controlled and illegal for sport competition for many years, companies have marketed prohormones, or precursors to these hormones, as dietary supplements to avoid drug regulations. However, now these prohormones have also been classified as controlled drugs and their use is illegal in sports. Use of these anabolic agents may also pose serious health risks.

Finally, several herbals and other phytochemicals, most notably ginseng, are used in alternative medicine for various purposes, one being enhancement of physical performance. Collectively, with the exception of alcohol and anabolic hormones, most of these performance-enhancing substances are marketed as dietary supplements, or sports supplements when targeted to athletes. The sports supplements industry has become a multibillion-dollar business. Some reports indicate that approximately 90 percent of elite athletes use sports supplements, while Greydanus and Patel note that the drive toward success in sport has driven many adolescents to use such products.

Some of the dietary supplements discussed in this chapter have been banned by the World Anti-Doping Agency (WADA) for use in sports competition, and others are being monitored by WADA. Specific details will be provided where warranted.

www.wada-ama.org The World Anti-Doping Agency (WADA) provides the complete list of drugs and doping techniques whose use is prohibited or monitored in sports competition. Click on *Prohibited List.* The list is updated annually.

Alcohol: Ergogenic Effects and Health Implications

The alcohol produced for human consumption is ethyl alcohol, or **ethanol.** Ethanol may be classified as a psychoactive drug, a toxin, or a nutrient.

The use of alcohol as a means to enhance exercise or sport performance has a long history. Ancient Greek athletes drank wine or brandy prior to competition, thinking that these alcoholic beverages enhanced performance. In more modern times, Olympic marathon runners in the Paris (1900) and London (1908) games drank brandy or cognac to enhance performance, while in the Paris Olympics in 1924 wine was served at fluid replacement stations in the marathon. In 1939, Boje noted that in cases of extreme athletic exertion or in events of brief maximal effort, alcohol has been given to athletes to serve as a stimulant by releasing inhibitions and lessening the sense of fatigue. Today, WADA prohibits use of alcohol in about a half-dozen sports.

The use of alcohol as a social, psychoactive drug also has a long history, and its effects on human health have been studied extensively. In general, most research has focused on the numerous adverse health effects of excessive alcohol consumption. However, within the last quarter-century some research has revealed some possible health benefits associated with light or moderate drinking. Nevertheless, abstinence may be the best strategy for some individuals.

What is the alcohol and nutrient content of typical alcoholic beverages?

Alcohol is a transparent, colorless liquid derived from the fermentation of sugars in fruits, vegetables, and grains. Although classified legally as a drug, alcohol is a component of many common beverages served throughout the world. In the United States, alcohol is consumed mainly as a natural ingredient of beer, wine, and liquors. Although the alcohol content may vary in different types, in general, beer is about 4–5 percent alcohol, wine is about 12–14 percent alcohol, and typical bar liquor (whiskey, rum, gin, vodka) is about 40–45 percent alcohol (figure 13.1). Other alcoholic beverages are also available, such as wine coolers and *energy* drinks, normally containing about 5–7 percent alcohol; some alcoholic malt energy drinks contain up to 10–12 percent alcohol, about twice the content of regular beer. The term **proof** is a measure of the alcohol content in a beverage and is double the percentage; an 86-proof bottle of whiskey is 43 percent alcohol, while a 150-proof bottle of Caribbean rum is 75 percent alcohol.

One drink of alcohol is the equivalent of one-half ounce of pure ethyl alcohol or the equivalent of about 13–14 grams of alcohol. The following amounts of beer, wine, and liquor contain approximately equal amounts of alcohol and are classified as one drink:

12 ounces (one bottle) of beer
4 ounces (one wine glass) of wine
1.25 ounces (one jigger or shot glass) of liquor

However, some beers may contain more than10 percent alcohol, some wines are fortified to 18–24 percent, and some liquors are 50–75 percent. Such beverages would provide significantly more alcohol per standard drink. Technically, alcohol may be classified as a nutrient because it provides energy, one of the major functions of food. Alcohol contains about 7 Calories per gram, almost twice the value of an equal amount of carbohydrate or protein. Beer and wine also contain some carbohydrate, a source of additional Calories. In general, a bottle of regular beer has about 150 Calories, while a 4-ounce glass of wine or a shot glass of liquor contains about 100 Calories. Table 13.1 provides an approximate analysis of the caloric content of common alcoholic beverages and nonalcoholic beer.

In general, the alcohol Calories found in beer, wine, and liquor are empty Calories. Although wine and beer contain trace amounts of protein, vitamins, minerals, and phytochemicals, liquor is void of any nutrient value.

What is the metabolic fate of alcohol in the body?

About 20 percent of the alcohol ingested may be absorbed by the stomach; the remainder passes on to the intestine for absorption. The absorption is rapid, particularly if the digestive tract is empty. The alcohol enters the blood and is distributed to the various tissues, being diluted by the water content of the body. A small portion of the alcohol, about 3–10 percent, is excreted from the body through the breath, urine, or sweat, but the majority is metabolized by the liver, the organ that metabolizes other drugs. As the blood circulates, the liver of an average adult male will metabolize about one-third ounce (8–10 grams) of alcohol per hour, or somewhat less than the amount of alcohol in one drink.

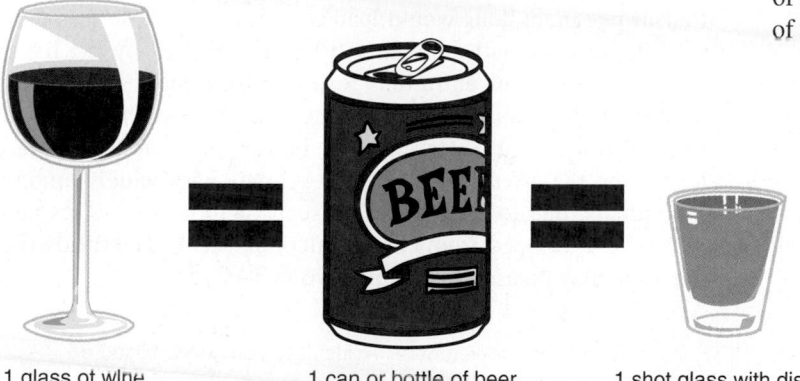

1 glass of wine	1 can or bottle of beer	1 shot glass with distilled spirits
4 oz. of table wine	12 oz. of beer	1.25 oz. of whiskey or other hard liquor
12% alcohol by volume	4% alcohol by volume	40% alcohol by volume or 80 proof
4 × 0.12 = 0.48 oz. of ethyl alcohol per serving	12 × 0.04 = 0.48 oz. of ethyl alcohol per serving	1.25 × 0.40 = 0.50 oz. of ethyl alcohol per serving

FIGURE 13.1 Alcohol equivalencies in typical beverages.

TABLE 13.1   Caloric content of typical alcoholic beverages

Beverage	Amount	Carbohydrate		Alcohol		Total
		Grams	Calories	Grams	Calories	Calories
Beer, regular	12 ounces	13	52	13	91	150
Beer, light	12 ounces	7	28	11	77	109
Beer, nonalcoholic	12 ounces	12	48	1	7	55
Beer, alcohol-free	12 ounces	12	48	0	0	48
Wine, table	4 ounces	4	16	12	84	100
Liquor, 80 proof	1.25 ounces	0	0	14	98	100
Energy drink, alcoholic	12 ounces	32	128	15	105	233

The small discrepancies in the calculation of total Calories for beer and liquor may be attributed to a small protein content in beer and trace amounts of carbohydrate in liquor.

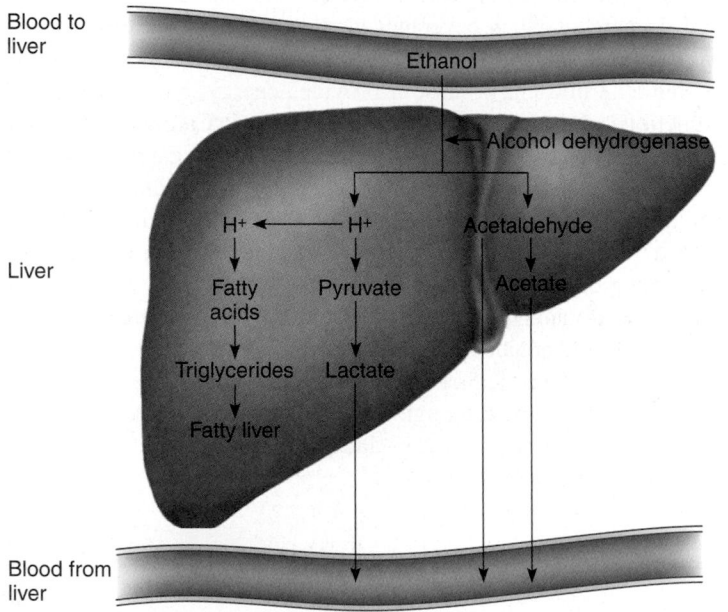

FIGURE 13.2 Simplified metabolic pathways of ethanol (alcohol) in the liver. Hydrogen ions are removed from ethanol as it is converted to acetaldehyde, which may be released into the blood for transport to other tissues. The excess hydrogen ions may combine with fatty acids to form triglycerides or with pyruvate to form lactate. Excessive accumulation of triglycerides may lead to the development of a fatty liver and eventually to cirrhosis.

Although alcohol is derived from the fermentation of carbohydrates, it is metabolized in the body like fat. The liver helps convert the metabolic by-products of alcohol into fatty acids, which may be stored in the liver or transported into the blood. Several other compounds, such as lactate, acetate, and acetaldehyde, may also be released into the blood. These products may eventually be utilized for energy and converted into carbon dioxide and water. A schematic of alcohol metabolism is presented in figure 13.2.

As noted, the liver of a 150-pound male can metabolize only about one-third ounce of alcohol, or less than one drink, per hour. The rate is lower in smaller individuals and higher in larger individuals. Thus, consumption of alcohol at a rate greater than one drink per hour will result in an accumulation of alcohol in the blood; this is measured as the **blood alcohol concentration (BAC)** in grams per 100 milliliters of blood. The ingested alcohol is diluted throughout the total body water, both inside and outside body cells, including the blood. For the average male, one drink will result in a BAC of about 0.025, or 0.025 gram (25 milligrams) per 100 milliliters of blood; four drinks in an hour would lead to a BAC of a little less than 0.10 because a small amount will be metabolized by the liver. However, BAC concentrations resulting from the same amount of drinks may vary widely among individuals, due to food intake, gender, and differences in body weight and body fat. Moreover, the effects of a given BAC may vary widely among individuals, due to differences in such factors as genetics and tolerance developed from chronic alcohol intake. The following Web site may be used to calculate your BAC.

www.bloodalcoholcalculator.org   Calculate your BAC based on your gender, body weight, number of drinks, and amount of time over which drinks were consumed.

Is alcohol an effective ergogenic aid?

For more than a century, athletes have consumed alcohol just prior to or during competition in attempts to improve performance. Alcohol has been alleged to alter energy metabolism, improve physiological processes, or modify psychological factors so as to benefit the athlete. Let us look at the available research to evaluate the truth of these allegations.

Use as an energy source Although alcohol contains a relatively large number of Calories and its metabolic pathways in the body are short, the available evidence suggests that it is not utilized to any significant extent during exercise. First, the major sources of energy for exercise are carbohydrates and fats, which are in ample supply in most individuals. Alcohol may help form fats, but there is no evidence that it can substitute for other fat sources in the body. Even if it could, this would be of no benefit because the body has more than enough fat to supply energy during prolonged exercise. Second, the by-products of alcohol metabolism that are released by the liver into the blood may enter the skeletal muscles but appear to be of little importance to exercising muscle. Third, even if the energy from alcohol could be used, it would represent an uneconomical source. The amount of oxygen needed to release the Calories from alcohol is greater than for an equivalent amount of carbohydrate and fat. And lastly, the rate at which the liver metabolizes alcohol limits its use as an energy source during exercise, particularly in an individual working at a high level of intensity. In summary, these four factors suggest alcohol is not a key energy source during exercise, and even if it were, it would not offer any advantages over natural supplies of carbohydrate and fat. Research with carbon labeling revealed that alcohol did not significantly modify endogenous carbohydrate and fat utilization during exercise.

Effect on exercise metabolism and performance Numerous studies have evaluated the potential ergogenic effect of alcohol intake, both in small and large amounts, just prior to various exercise protocols. In general, the resultant effects depend on the alcohol dose and the type of exercise performance.

Research supports the finding that alcohol in small amounts (one to two drinks) neither improves nor deteriorates physiological processes associated with maximal aerobic exercise. For example, Coiro and others found that consuming small or moderate doses of alcohol before a 15-minute exercise test to exhaustion had no effect on heart rate, blood pressure, ventilation, oxygen consumption, or respiratory exchange ratio. Other studies indicate that alcohol does not affect other indicators of maximal aerobic performance such as exercise tests to exhaustion. For example, one study reported an apparent trend toward a deterioration in performance with increased alcohol intake, but there was no adverse effect on 5-mile (8 km) treadmill run time. Moreover, tests of anaerobic performance, such as strength and local muscular endurance, also are not affected.

However, a few studies have reported some potential adverse effects of consuming alcohol before or during submaximal exercise. Most of the studies alluded to earlier were conducted on males. A recent study reported some adverse acute effects of moderate alcohol consumption on cardiovascular and metabolic responses in females. In a submaximal cycling exercise task for 30 minutes, ingestion of alcohol increased the heart rate, oxygen consumption, blood pressure, and blood lactate, which the

investigators indicated were negative effects. Earlier studies also showed similar effects in males, including decreased pumping capacity of the heart with high BACs. Moreover, some research reported a significant decrease in aerobic endurance when alcohol was ingested before and during a treadmill run at about 80–85 percent VO_2 max, which may have been associated with impaired glucose metabolism. Impaired performance has also been reported in both an 800-meter and 1,500-meter run following alcohol consumption, and the detrimental effect was greater with increasing BACs from 0.01 to 0.10.

Several metabolic effects of alcohol intake could impair endurance performance. In their review, El Sayed and others noted studies suggesting that alcohol consumption decreases the use of glucose and amino acids by skeletal muscles, adversely affects energy supply, and impairs the metabolic process during exercise. Alcohol reduces gluconeogenesis by the liver and glucose uptake by the legs during the latter stages of exercise. In prolonged exercise, such as marathons, these effects could lead to an earlier onset of hypoglycemia or muscle glycogen depletion and a subsequent decrease in performance.

Alcohol intake during training could be counterproductive. Some studies have reported reduced absorption of vitamin B_1 associated with moderate intakes of alcohol. Theoretically, this could impair physical performance of an endurance nature because vitamin B_1 is involved in the aerobic metabolism of carbohydrate.

In its position statement on fluid replacement, the ACSM indicated that alcohol consumption can increase urine output and delay full rehydration. Alcohol ingestion may also increase urine production by decreasing release of the anti-diuretic hormone. This effect could possibly impair temperature regulation during exercise under warm/hot environmental conditions. Starting a prolonged endurance event under warm/hot conditions in a dehydrated state could certainly impair performance. As a rehydration fluid after dehydration, drinks containing 4 percent alcohol or more, such as beer, tend to delay the recovery process as measured by restoration of blood and plasma volume. Moreover, Hobson and Maughan reported that when dehydrated, as compared to euhydrated, after exercise, alcohol intake will lead to a higher BAC mainly because there are fewer body fluids to dilute the alcohol content. As noted later, a higher BAC could contribute to some adverse effects.

Additional research is merited to document any adverse effects of alcohol on cardiovascular or metabolic processes during exercise, but at this time it appears that alcohol intake before or during aerobic and anaerobic endurance exercise is not ergogenic and may be **ergolytic,** impairing exercise performance.

Effect on psychological processes Alcohol also has been used as an ergogenic aid primarily for its psychological effects. It is a narcotic, a depressant, that affects the brain. As a depressant of brain functions, alcohol would not be advocated as a means to improve sport performance. However, although classified as a depressant, some of alcohol's effects are euphoric. Alcohol is thought to bind with receptors in the brain that may cause the release of dopamine, a neurotransmitter associated with the pleasure center of the brain. Normal inhibitory control centers in the brain may be suppressed. Some have contended that increased feelings of self-confidence, reduced anxiety levels, and a perceived decrease in sensitivity to pain may offset any depressant effects and possibly benefit performance. Moreover, alcohol in small doses may exert a paradoxical stimulation effect. Parts of the brain that normally inhibit behavior may be depressed by alcohol, leading to a transitory sensation of excitement.

Although these effects may occur, research does not support the use of alcohol in sports involving psychological processes such as perceptual-motor abilities. Perceptual-motor activities involve the perception of a stimulus, integration of this stimulus by the brain, and an appropriate motor response (movement). The evidence overwhelmingly supports the conclusion that alcohol adversely affects psychomotor performance skills, such as reaction time, balance, hand/eye coordination, and visual perception. These are important in events with rapidly changing stimuli, such as tennis.

Nevertheless, by reducing anxiety and related hand muscle tremor, alcohol could enhance performance in certain forms of athletic competition, such as riflery, pistol shooting, dart throwing, and archery. Although research generally is not supportive of improved performance, one study with archers revealed a tendency toward reduced tremor with low blood alcohol levels, resulting in a smoother release. However, no actual performance data were revealed. Throwing accuracy improved in darts at a BAC of 0.02, but was impaired at a BAC of 0.05. This area of study merits additional research.

Social drinking and sports Only a limited number of studies have been conducted relative to the effect of social drinking upon physical performance, but there is rather general agreement that light social drinking will not impair performance on the following day. Tests of reaction time, strength, power, and cardiovascular performance were not adversely affected following the consumption of one drink the night before. In contrast, heavy drinking may impair performance on the following day owing to hangover effects, involuntary eye movement, or dehydration.

Permissibility The use of alcohol *in competition* by Olympic athletes had been banned previously by the IOC, but because wine and beer are commonly consumed as a part of many traditional European meals it was removed from the banned list prior to the 1972 Olympics. However, individual sports federations within the IOC still may consider alcohol use in competition as grounds for disqualification. At present, only several sports federations, such as archery and the pentathlon, which involve shooting competition, ban the use of alcohol.

In his review, Williams noted that although alcohol consumption is not prohibited for use by athletes *out of competition,* there are no data supporting an ergogenic effect, and some data to suggest an ergolytic effect. This viewpoint was supported by Burke and Maughan in their review. Athletes who drink socially should do so in moderation, and possibly abstain 24 hours prior to a prolonged endurance contest.

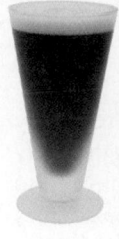

What effect can drinking alcohol have upon my health?

Consumption of alcoholic beverages is a popular pastime worldwide. People drink mainly for social reasons, but when and how much they drink may have a significant impact on their health and the health of others. As Klatsky noted, the basic disparity underlying all alcohol-health relations is between the effects of lighter and heavier drinking.

Alcohol's effect on health appears to be a mixed bag. Although many of the effects of alcohol may negatively affect health status, some effects may be positive. Both the negative and the positive effects are detailed in the National Institute on Alcohol Abuse and Alcoholism (NIAAA) state-of-the-science report on the effects of moderate drinking. Relative to its adverse health effects, the World Health Organization, in its *Global Status Report on Alcohol and Health,* reported that the harmful use of alcohol results in the death of 2.5 million people annually, causes illness and injury to many more, and increasingly affects younger generations and drinkers in developing countries.

Although both men and women may incur health problems from drinking alcohol, Epstein and others recently noted that due to differences in metabolism of alcohol, women of all ages compared to men are at higher risk for negative physical, medical, and psychological consequences associated with at-risk and higher levels of alcohol consumption. For several reasons, women may reach higher BAC levels than men for any given amount of alcohol intake. For one, women have lower levels of total body water, and thus the alcohol is less diluted. For another, some alcohol is metabolized in the stomach by one form of alcohol dehydrogenase, but the amount metabolized appears to be less in women than men. A higher BAC, either acutely or periodically over time, is associated with greater risk to health.

Negative Effects Alcohol affects all cells in the body, and many of these effects may have significant health implications. Room and others noted that alcohol is causally related to more than 60 different medical conditions, and is a major challenge to public health. Alcohol and its metabolite, acetaldehyde, can have direct toxic effects on cells, possibly damaging DNA. Alcohol may adversely affect functions of major body organs, particularly the liver and brain, and other metabolic functions important to good health.

Many of the adverse health effects of alcohol consumption are associated with heavy, or binge, drinking. Binge drinking in men is defined as consuming five or more drinks in one occasion, while the corresponding amount for women is four or more drinks.

Liver disease The liver is the only organ in the body that metabolizes alcohol, and alcohol may affect liver function in several ways. It may interfere with the metabolism of other drugs, increasing the effect of some and lessening the effects of others. Even with a balanced diet high in protein, consuming six drinks a day for less than a month has been shown to cause significant accumulation of fat in the liver. If continued for five years or more, the liver cells degenerate. Eventually the damaged liver cells are replaced by nonfunctioning scar tissue, a condition known as **cirrhosis.** As liver function deteriorates, fat, carbohydrate, and protein metabolism are not regulated properly; this has possible pathological consequences for other body organs such as the kidney, pancreas, and heart.

Nutrients, such as specific lipids from soybeans, are being studied as a means to help prevent this liver degeneration. Klatsky and others reported that epidemiological research suggests that drinking coffee, up to four cups daily, decreased the risk of developing alcoholic cirrhosis, suggesting some protective ingredient in coffee. Some scientists theorize that wine, because it contains antioxidants, may help prevent oxidative stress and subsequent liver damage, and may thus be the alcoholic beverage with less damaging effects. However, liver damage is one of the most consistent adverse effects of excess alcohol intake, and Reuben noted that safe and effective therapies for alcoholic cirrhosis have yet to be discovered.

Psychological problems Many of the adverse health effects of alcohol consumption are associated with disturbed mental functions. Although alcohol is a depressant, as mentioned previously, a small amount often provides pleasurable effects. For the most part, however, alcohol acts as a depressant, and its effects on the brain are dose-dependent. The effects occur in a hierarchical fashion related to the development of the brain. In general, alcohol first affects the higher brain centers. With increasing dosages, lower levels of brain function become depressed with subsequent disturbance of normal functions. This hierarchy of brain functions, from higher levels to lower levels, and some of the functions affected by alcohol may be generalized as follows:

Thinking and reasoning—Judgment
Perceptual-motor responses—Reaction time
Fine motor coordination—Muscles of speech
Gross motor coordination—Walking
Visual processes—Double vision
Alertness—Sleep, coma
Respiratory control—Respiratory failure, death

An overview of the effects of increasing BAC on mental and physical functions is presented in table 13.2.

As noted in table 13.2, a BAC of 0.06–0.09 may impair judgment, fine motor ability, and coordination—three factors that are extremely important in the safe operation of an automobile and other modes of transportation. In the United States, a BAC of 0.08 is the level normally associated with *driving under the influence* (DUI). At the least, being arrested for drunk driving may have serious social and personal consequences. At the worst, DUI may cause death. Although the number of alcohol-impaired driving fatalities has decreased by more than 32 percent in the past 20 years, estimates indicate that 30 percent of all automobile-crash fatalities are alcohol related, contributing to the deaths of about 11,000 Americans annually. As the saying goes, "Don't drink and drive!"

In recent years alcoholic energy drinks have become increasingly popular among the young. Some believe that the caffeine and other possible stimulants in these drinks may counteract the depressant effects of alcohol. Cloud notes research showning that

TABLE 13.2 Typical effects of increasing blood alcohol content

Number of drinks* consumed in 2 hours	Blood** alcohol content	Typical effects
2–3	.02–.04	Reduced tension, relaxed feeling, relief from daily stress
4–5	.06–.09	Legally drunk (0.08) in all states; impaired judgment, a high feeling, impaired fine motor ability and coordination
6–8	.11–.16	Slurred speech, impaired gross motor coordination, staggering gait
9–12	.18–.25	Loss of control of voluntary activity, erratic behavior, impaired vision
13–18	.27–.39	Stuporous, total loss of coordination
19 and above	>.40	Coma, depression of respiratory centers, death

*One drink = 12 ounces regular beer
4 ounces wine
1.25 ounces liquor
**BAC based on body weight of 160 pounds (72.6 Kg). The BAC will increase proportionally for individuals weighing less (such as a 120-pound female) and will decrease proportionally for individuals weighing more (such as a 200-pound football player). For example, four to five drinks in 2 hours could lead to a BAC of 0.08–0.12 in a 120-pound individual.

individuals who consume alcoholic energy drinks perceive their motor coordination to be better—but it is not. Energy drinks are discussed in more detail in the next section on caffeine.

Alcohol usage also is correlated highly with aggressive tendencies. Laboratory studies have indicated that aggressive behavior is directly related to the quantity of alcohol consumed. In a meta-analysis investigating the role of alcohol in fatal nontraffic injuries, Smith and others concluded that alcohol was an important factor in homicides and unintentional injury deaths. Alcohol abuse is also associated with sexual abuse.

Alcohol usage may also lead to depression and suicide. Galaif and others noted that alcohol use remains extremely widespread among today's youth and is related to both depression and suicidality, the occurrence of suicidal thoughts or suicidal behaviors. They note that suicide is currently the third leading cause of death for teenagers and young adults between the ages of 15 and 24 years. Monti and others reported that heavy drinking during the teenage years may cause permanent brain damage, which may be a related factor.

Most of these adverse psychological effects are associated with excessive alcohol intake, particularly as practiced in binge drinking. College students are known to engage in hazardous drinking, and not only in the United States and Canada. Karam and others noted that the prevalence of hazardous drinking among college students in Australia, Europe, and South America appears similar to that in North America. Recent surveys indicate that almost half of college students binge, and one of the most significant factors underlying alcohol-related behavior problems is the amount of alcohol consumed; the greater the amount of alcohol consumed, the more serious the problem. But even low drinking levels can cause problems. In their study, Gruenewald and others concluded that many problems among college students are associated with drinking relatively small amounts of alcohol (two to four drinks). According to the NIAAA, nationally there are more than 1,400 alcohol-related deaths each year among college students, most due to automobile accidents, but several attributed to heavy binge drinking with resultant respiratory failure.

Many physically active individuals, including competitive athletes, consume alcohol on a regular basis. In their periodic study of NCAA athletes, Green and others noted that alcohol was the most widely used drug, with more than 80 percent of athletes using alcohol within the past year. In their review, El Sayed and others reported that alcohol continues to be the most frequently consumed drug among athletes and habitual exercisers and alcohol-related problems appear to be more common in these individuals, which O'Brien and Lyons indicated may be due to their risk-taking mentality. Sports participation may, in some way, be associated with increased alcohol use. In their study, the Wichstrøms found that sports participation in adolescence, and participation in team sports in particular, may increase the growth in alcohol intoxication during late adolescent and early adult years. Martens and others have developed an Athlete Drinking Scale to explore the reasons athletes drink alcohol.

Cardiovascular disease Heavy drinking may increase the risk of heart disease and stroke. Klatsky noted that heavier drinking may increase some of the possible risks to heart and vascular health, including the following:

- Alcoholic cardiomyopathy, or impaired heart function
- Increased blood pressure
- Increased risk of hemorrhagic (bleeding) stroke
- Increased risk of certain heart rate arrhythmias

As we shall see, drinking alcohol in moderation may help to prevent cardiovascular disease, but Cargiulo concludes that heavy drinking is associated with increased risk of coronary heart disease and stroke. Individuals susceptible to cardiovascular disease may be prone to a heart attack with heavy drinking. For example, the *holiday heart syndrome,* an arrhythmia commonly resulting in a rapid heartbeat, may occur with binge drinking around vacations and holidays. Although not normally dangerous, it may be in individuals with underlying heart problems. George and Figueredo, in a comprehensive review, reported that numerous investigators have noted a causal relationship between alcohol and arrhythmias, as well as sudden cardiac death.

Cancer Laboratory research has shown that *in vitro* (that is, in a test tube), alcohol and acetaldehyde cause changes in DNA (the genetic material in body cells) comparable to changes elicited by carcinogens. This DNA damage may occur at an alcohol concentration equivalent to one to two drinks. In those who drink, this finding could be related to the increased risk of certain forms of cancer, including pharyngeal and esophageal cancer, whose tissues have direct contact with ingested alcohol, and also breast and colon cancer. Based on the carcinogenicity of acetaldehyde in animals, the Environmental Protective Agency has concluded that acetaldehyde is a probable human carcinogen.

One of the most debated issues is the risk of breast cancer. Possible mechanisms have been identified; in addition to potential DNA damage, alcohol ingestion may also increase estrogen levels, a factor that increases breast cancer risk. Research associating increased incidence of breast cancer with alcohol consumption is epidemiological in nature. The NIAAA indicated that the effect of alcohol intake on the risk for breast cancer remains controversial. In summary, the NIAAA noted that the overall evidence from epidemiologic data seems to indicate that alcohol may be associated with an increase in the risk of breast cancer in the population overall, but the relative effect of moderate consumption is small at the individual level. Reviews and studies support these general findings. Zhang and others, in the Women's Health Study, found that higher alcohol consumption, greater than 30 grams daily, or about two drinks, was associated with a modest increase in breast cancer risk, a relative risk (RR) of 1.32. Gonzalez and Riboli, in a review of studies by the European Prospective Investigation into Cancer and Nutrition, also reported that high alcohol intake increases the risk of breast cancer. Michels and others evaluated the role of more than 15 dietary variables of interest in the context of breast cancer, and found that alcohol intake was one of the few whose association with breast cancer was consistent, strong, and statistically significant. In a 7.2-year study of more than a million women from the United Kingdom, Allen and others found that low to moderate alcohol intake was associated with a significant increase in several cancers, including breast, oral cavity, larynx, and esophagus; there was a total excess of about 15 cancers per 1,000 women. The NIAAA reported that the increase in risk is most clearly evident for women with a family history of breast cancer and those using estrogen replacement therapy, and recommends that women, in conjunction with their health care provider, should weigh their potential increased risk for breast cancer against their potential reduced risk for cardiovascular disease in determining whether alcohol consumption should be reduced.

Fetal alcohol spectrum disorders Women who drink should abstain during pregnancy because even moderate consumption of alcohol, or even a single drinking binge, may affect DNA in the embryo and fetus. Haycock indicates that ethanol is a classic teratogen capable of inducing a wide range of developmental abnormalities, particularly during peak periods of epigenetic reprogramming in the fetus. In a review of 66 studies, Burd and others reported that alcohol intake during pregnancy may have numerous adverse effects on the placenta, including placental dysfunction and decreased placental size. Given these effects, alcohol may cause health problems in the newborn, which Green identifies as *Fetal Alcohol Spectrum Disorder (FASD).* FASD is the term used to describe birth anomalies associated with the mother's drinking alcohol while pregnant, and refers to several conditions involving alcohol-related neurodevelopment disorders, birth defects, and other abnormalities in normal development.

Fetal alcohol syndrome (FAS) is the most severe of the FASDs. The Centers for Disease Control and Prevention National Center on Birth Defects and Developmental Disabilities indicates that FAS is one of the leading known causes of mental retardation and birth defects. The incidence rate of FAS is very high in the United States, and FAS is currently the major cause of mental retardation in the Western world. The child may experience retardation in growth and mental development as well as facial birth defects (figure 13.3).

Fetal alcohol effects (FAE) may be observed in children when full-blown FAS is not present. Children with FAE are easily distracted and have poor attention spans, but do not have the facial features of FAS. Both FAS and FAE are associated with learning disorders in children. The Institute of Medicine has used more specific terms for FAE, including alcohol-related neurodevelopmental disorder and alcohol-related birth defects. Although a study from England, by Kelly and others, indicated that children of women who were classified as light drinkers (no more than 1–2 drinks a week) during pregnancy were not at increased risk for emotional or cognitive problems compared with children whose mothers did not drink while pregnant, abstinence still appears to be the safest approach. No "safe" amount of alcohol during pregnancy has been determined. Thus, the U.S. Surgeon General indicated that the safest approach is abstinence.

Obesity Alcohol is a significant source of Calories, about 7 per gram, somewhat comparable to the caloric content of fat. Research has indicated that if small amounts of alcohol (5 percent of daily caloric intake) are interchanged for an equivalent caloric intake from carbohydrates, there is no effect on daily energy expenditure. In other words, alcohol Calories themselves will not increase body fat as long as total daily caloric intake matches daily caloric expenditure. In general, the NIAAA indicates that the relationship between moderate alcohol consumption and obesity remains inconclusive. In their study, Beulens and others reported that moderate alcohol consumption (40 grams daily for four weeks)

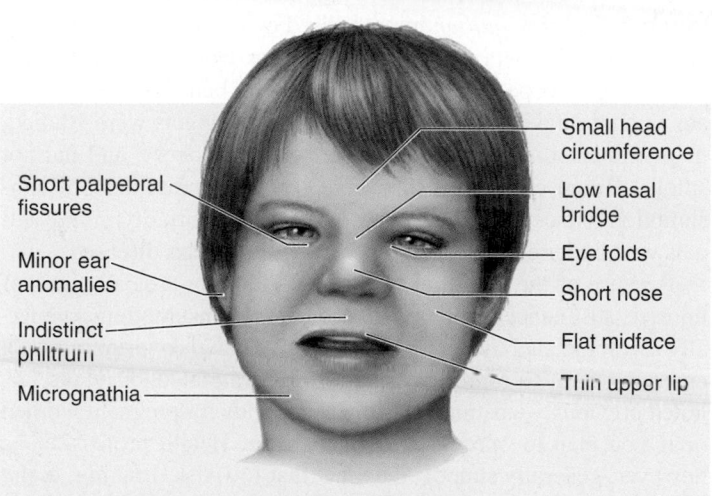

FIGURE 13.3 Common facial characteristics of children with fetal alcohol syndrome (FAS).

was not associated with increased adiposity or increased weight circumference.

However, Yeomans noted that alcohol may increase energy intake in several ways. Alcohol stimulates the appetite, increasing food intake, and alcohol contains energy. Angelo Tremblay, an esteemed scientist in weight control, and his colleagues found that alcohol has no inhibitory effect on food intake and its energy content, and when consumed in conjunction with a high-fat diet promotes overfeeding, a primary determinant of obesity. Additionally, Jequier notes that alcohol ingestion reduces fat oxidation and favors a positive fat balance. These points may underlie the conclusion of the study by Wannamethee and others, mainly that higher alcohol consumption is positively associated with both overall and abdominal adiposity, irrespective of the type of drink or whether the alcohol is drunk with meals or not. As noted in chapter 11, reducing alcoholic intake may be an important component of an effective weight control program.

Alcohol dependence Alcohol abuse, or excessive intake of alcohol, is the major drug problem in the United States, posing a problem for one in seven males and one in sixteen females, or about one out of every ten drinkers. Over time, alcohol abuse may lead to alcohol dependency, a disorder more commonly known as **alcoholism.** In a review, Cargiulo details many of the adverse health consequences of alcohol dependency, most of which have been discussed previously.

The etiology of alcoholism is unknown but probably is related to a variety of physiological, psychological, and sociological factors. Söderpalm and others indicate that alcohol activates the dopamine system, an important part of the brain reward system, and the positive psychological effects may reinforce the desire to continue to consume alcohol. Many genes are likely to be involved in increasing an individual's risk for alcoholism, and Gordis indicates that heavy, long-term use of alcohol modifies brain cells in such a way that certain individuals continue to drink despite growing difficulties. The National Council on Alcoholism suggests that there is no pat definition for alcoholism; it may be evidenced by a variety of behaviors. A deficiency of vitamin B may contribute to many of the neuropsychiatric problems seen in alcoholism. The number of behaviors exhibited by the drinker may be related to various stages in the progression toward alcoholism. Appendix C, a questionnaire developed by the National Council on Alcoholism, helps you perform an assessment of these behaviors. A shorter, online version known as the Alcohol Use Disorders Identification Test (AUDIT) is available at the following Web site: *http://www.testandcalc.com/etc/tests/audit.asp*

Positive Effects On the positive side, most recent epidemiological research and reviews have shown that light to moderate consumption of alcohol is associated with lessened mortality. For example, in a meta-analysis of the relationship of alcohol consumption to all-cause mortality, Holman and others noted that light drinking (less than 2 drinks per day in males; less than 1 drink per day in females) was associated with a lower relative risk for all-cause mortality compared to abstainers, but that the relative risk returned to normal with moderate alcohol intake and increased to 1.37 for heavy drinkers, those taking six or more drinks daily.

Alzheimer's disease and dementia Antonio and others theorize that moderate amounts of alcohol may improve brain blood flow and help delay the onset of certain brain diseases, such as Alzheimer's and Parkinson's. In a meta-analysis of 15 prospective studies, Anstey and others found that *drinkers,* when compared with *nondrinkers,* had a reduced risk of Alzheimer's disease (RR = 0.66) and any dementia (RR = 0.53), but not cognitive decline. Their results suggested that alcohol drinkers in late life have reduced risk of dementia. However, it was not clear whether the results reflected a protective effect of alcohol consumption throughout adulthood or a specific benefit of alcohol in late life. Additional research is merited to explore this possible positive health effect of alcohol consumption.

Cardiovascular disease Most research on the possible health benefits of alcohol consumption has focused on heart health. Research suggests that light to moderate alcohol intake reduces risk of coronary heart disease and stroke, a major factor in reducing risk for all-cause mortality. The mechanism is not known, but several have been proposed based on epidemiological and experimental studies.

One theory suggests small amounts of alcohol induce a relaxation effect, which may reduce emotional stress, a risk factor associated with CHD. Another theory suggests alcohol decreases platelet aggregability (clotting ability) by increasing the activity of a clot-dissolving enzyme in the blood. Still another theory involves an increased brain blood flow, noted previously by Antonio and others, which might help prevent certain forms of stroke. Other mechanisms may be working as well, such as an enhanced insulin sensitivity, which may help in the prevention of the metabolic syndrome and diabetes, both risk factors for CHD.

The most prevalent theory involves the effect of alcohol to raise levels of HDL-cholesterol, the form of cholesterol that protects against the development of CHD (see discussion on pages 191–194). A significant number of studies have supported this effect, although the mechanisms have not been determined. Some studies have shown an increase in one form of cholesterol, HDL_2, which is believed to be protective. Other studies note an increase in HDL_3, which may also elicit a protective effect. Gaziano and others noted that alcohol may reduce the risk of heart disease by raising the levels of both HDL_2 and HDL_3. However, Hines and others noted that individuals with a specific genetic predisposition may benefit more from alcohol intake, as they may produce a form of alcohol dehydrogenase that metabolizes alcohol more slowly, leading to greater increases in HDL-cholesterol.

Some investigators have theorized that the consumption of certain types of alcoholic beverages, most notably red wine, is responsible for the reported health benefits. Pigments in red wine contain polyphenols and other phytochemicals that may help prevent coronary heart disease by favorable actions on various processes. For example, de Lorimier indicates that phenolic compounds in wine can also increase HDL, have antioxidant activity, decrease platelet aggregation, and promote vasodilation—all potentially beneficial. Others suggest that wine components may reduce inflammation in arteries. Chopra and others noted also that alcohol-free red wine may provide some similar health benefits. However, Denke

indicates that there is no evidence to support endorsement of one type of alcoholic beverage over another, noting that beer has its own nutritional value. Compared to wine, beer contains more protein and B vitamins, is rich in flavonoids, and has an equivalent antioxidant content, but of different specific antioxidants derived from barley and hops. In one study, Mukamal and others found that men who consumed alcohol 3–4 days per week experienced a reduced risk of myocardial infarction, but the type of beverage consumed did not substantially alter this effect.

Although these factors may be important, Naimi and others contend that individuals who drink moderately may practice other lifestyle behaviors that reduce the risk for CHD. For example, Smothers and Bertolucci reported that people who moderate their alcohol intake also engage in more leisure-time activity, which may play an explanatory role in the alcohol-heart disease relationship. As noted in chapter 1, exercise itself may reduce the risk of CHD. However, Mukamal and others, reporting data from more than 50,000 males in the Health Professionals Follow-up Study over the course of 16 years, found that moderate alcohol intake, up to two drinks daily, is associated with lower risk for experiencing a heart attack even in men already at low risk for heart disease on the basis of Body Mass Index, physical activity, smoking, and diet. Nevertheless, data from the National Runners' Health Study, as reported by Williams, reveals that men's blood pressure increases in association with the amount of alcohol intake, regardless of running level. Thus, it should be reemphasized that although there appear to be some positive health effects associated with light to moderate alcohol intake, or at least no detrimental effects, heavier drinking is another matter.

Others have challenged the health benefits of alcohol from another perspective. Fillmore and others proposed that there may be a systematic error in prospective epidemiological mortality studies that have reported moderate regular use of alcohol to be protective against coronary heart disease. They suggest that people classified as abstainers may include those who have decreased or stopped drinking because of illness and thus their illness, and not the lack of alcohol intake, contributed to their increased rate of mortality. Some have classified such individuals as *sick quitters.* However, Rimm and Moats note that there is substantial evidence to refute this *sick quitter* hypothesis. For example, the study by Mukamal and others cited previously was from Rimm's laboratory, a large prospective study showing heart benefits from moderate alcohol intake even when only healthy subjects were studied, men who exercised, ate a good diet, were not obese, and did not smoke. Rimm and Moats also noted that moderate alcohol consumption reduces cardiovascular disease and mortality in individuals with hypertension, diabetes, and existing heart disease.

Because of the potential for abuse, addiction, and all types of injuries, abstinence from alcohol or prudent consumption is generally recommended by health authorities. "Low risk" drinking is an emerging term to represent light to moderate alcohol intake. As noted previously, abstinence is the best policy for pregnant women or if you plan to operate a motor vehicle. Health professionals, however, generally support the view that low-risk drinking, along with a balanced diet, should not pose any health problem to the average healthy individual. The definition of moderation varies, though. For example, in the United Kingdom and Denmark sensible drinking limits are established at 3 drinks a day for men and 2 for women. In the United States, the NIAAA indicates that except for individuals at particular risk, consumption of 2 drinks a day for men and 1 for women is unlikely to increase health risks. As risks for some conditions and diseases do increase at higher levels of consumption, men should be cautioned not to exceed 4 drinks on any day and women not to exceed 3 on any day.

Nevertheless, although there are actually some possible health benefits associated with alcohol consumption in moderation, health authorities caution that these potential benefits are not sufficient cause to start drinking if you currently abstain. The NIAAA stipulates that *moderate alcohol use* should not be construed as *healthy alcohol use,* because numerous individual differences, such as age, genetics, and metabolic rate, may affect the response to alcohol. You should consult with your physician if you are considering drinking for its possible health benefits.

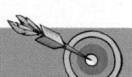

Key Concepts

▶ One drink of alcohol contains approximately 13–14 grams of alcohol, or about one-half ounce. One drink is typically the equivalent of 12 ounces of beer, 4 ounces of wine, and 1.25 ounces of 40-proof whiskey. However, the alcohol content in some beverages may be substantially greater.

▶ Alcohol is not an effective ergogenic aid; in fact, it may actually impair athletic performance, that is, it is ergolytic.

▶ Consumption of alcohol in moderation appears to cause no major health problems for the normal, healthy adult, and may actually confer some health benefits. However, alcohol may be contraindicated for some, such as women during pregnancy. Heavy drinking is associated with numerous health problems.

Check for Yourself

▶ Visit a local beer/wine store that carries a wide variety of products, including microbrews and fortified wines. Check the labels for percentage alcohol content, listing those from lowest to highest. Calculate how much alcohol would be in a standard drink from each.

www.niaaa.nih.gov This Website provides detailed information on a wide variety of alcohol-related topics. For example, if you want to decrease the amount of alcohol you drink, click on Publications and then on Pamphlet in the For the Public section to access the pamphlet, *How to Cut Down on Your Drinking.*

Caffeine: Ergogenic Effects and Health Implications

Coffee is one of the most widely consumed beverages throughout the world. The coffee bean, a plant product, contains caffeine, which has been theorized to enhance exercise performance. Indeed, Tunnicliffe and others noted that the majority of high-level Canadian athletes consume dietary caffeine, primarily in the form of coffee. Besides caffeine, coffee also contains numerous other biologically active phytonutrients, such as antioxidants, and has also been studied for its possible beneficial or adverse effects on health.

What is caffeine, and in what food products is it found?

Caffeine is an odorless, bitter, white alkaloid that appears naturally in many plants. Technically, caffeine may be classified as a food ingredient, a dietary supplement, or a drug.

As a food ingredient, caffeine is found in many of the foods and beverages that we consume every day, not only coffee but tea, colas, caffeinated waters, juices, energy drinks, sports drinks and sports bars, and chocolate. Some approximate amounts in the beverages we consume are 80–135 mg in a cup of perked coffee, 40–60 mg in a cup of tea, 35–45 mg in a can of cola, and 80–120 mg or more in an 8-ounce serving of an energy drink. Gupta indicates that up to 90 percent of Americans consume caffeine daily. Caffeine is also found in various dietary supplements, such as kola nuts and guarana, and even some over-the-counter stimulant supplements targeted to athletes; most recently, caffeine has been marketed as *performance candy,* such as Jolt Caffeine-Energy Gum and Buzz Bites, a chocolate chew candy. Such products may be construed to be sports supplements.

Caffeine is also legally classified as a drug and has some powerful physiological effects on the human body. A normal therapeutic dose of caffeine may range from 100–300 milligrams. As noted in table 13.3, some food products and supplements provide a therapeutic dose and meet the standards for classification as a drug. Indeed, caffeine has been identified as the most popular social drug in the United States (figure 13.4).

What effects does caffeine have on the body that may benefit exercise performance?

One of the primary effects of caffeine is to block the neurotransmitter adenosine, and thus influence a wide variety of metabolic processes throughout the body. Additionally, caffeine may stimulate the adrenal gland to release epinephrine (adrenaline) into the circulation. Caffeine, in conjunction with epinephrine, stimulates a wide variety of tissues. Together, they stimulate the central nervous system, potentiate muscle contraction, raise the rate of muscle and liver glycogen breakdown, increase release of free fatty acids (FFAs) from adipose tissue, and increase use of muscle triglycerides. One of the most observed effects at rest is an increase in blood levels of FFAs.

Caffeine has been studied for its potential ergogenic effects for more than 100 years. Early research focused on improvements in strength, power, and psychomotor parameters such as reaction time. However, in the late 1970s, researchers from David Costill's laboratory hypothesized caffeine could enhance performance of aerobic endurance athletes, such as marathoners, by increasing fat oxidation and sparing the use of muscle glycogen. Numerous investigators tested this hypothesis over the years, particularly

Product	Serving size	Caffeine (milligrams)
Coffee, brewed	8 ounce cup	80–135
Coffee, instant	8 ounce cup	65–100
Coffee, decaffeinated	8 ounce cup	3–4
Coffee, Starbucks	16 ounce cup	330
Tea, black or green	8 ounce cup	30–50
Hot cocoa	8 ounce cup	15
Sodas, cola	12 ounce can	35–45
Sodas, high caffeine	12 ounce can	55–70
POWERade Advance	16 ounce bottle	95
Energy drinks	8 ounce can	80–120
Performance candy	1 Buzz Bite	100
Stimulants	1 Vivarin tablet	200
Dietary supplements	5 grams guarana	250

TABLE 13.3 Caffeine content in selected products

Note: Check labels of over-the-counter stimulants and dietary supplements for caffeine content.

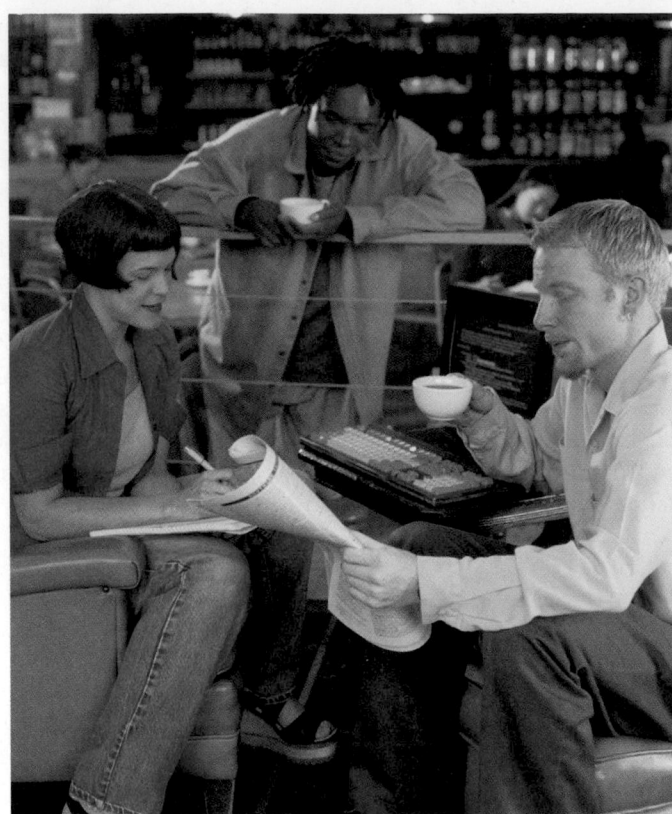

FIGURE 13.4 Caffeine is the most popular social drug in the United States. About 90 percent of all adults consume caffeine in one form or another, mainly as coffee.

Terry Graham and his colleagues from Guelph University. In one review, they concluded that there is very little evidence to support the hypothesis that caffeine has ergogenic effects as a result of enhanced fat oxidation and sparing of muscle glycogen use during prolonged aerobic endurance exercise.

In his review of the potential ergogenic effects of caffeine, Mark Tarnopolsky, a renowned exercise scientist from McMaster University in Canada, concluded that the ergogenic effect of caffeine on endurance exercise performance is multifactorial. For one, caffeine may stimulate the central nervous system, accelerating nerve cell activity in both the brain and spinal cord, and reduce the sensation of perceived effort (rating of perceived exertion or RPE) during exercise. In a meta-analysis of 21 studies, Doherty and Smith concluded that in comparison to a placebo, caffeine reduced the RPE during exercise by 5.6 percent while improving exercise performance by 11.2 percent; the authors concluded that the effect of caffeine on the RPE could account for approximately 29 percent of the improvement in performance. The effect of caffeine to reduce the psychological effort of exercise appears to be an important factor underlying its ergogenic effect. For another, caffeine may increase the force of muscle contraction. In her review, Jayne Kalmar from York University in Canada indicated that caffeine may influence muscle performance by stimulating the nervous system at various points along the motor pathway to the muscle. Caffeine may also increase the release of calcium from the sarcoplasmic reticulum in the muscle, possibly increasing the force of muscle contraction. Research by Tarnopolsky and Cupido, using electrical stimulation of the muscle, supports the hypothesis that some of the ergogenic effect of caffeine in endurance exercise performance occurs directly at the skeletal muscle level.

Overall, caffeine may influence central and peripheral metabolic processes, as well as psychological processes, to help delay the onset of fatigue, and has been theorized to enhance performance in many types of exercise, including endurance, strength, speed, and power.

Does caffeine enhance exercise performance?

Literally hundreds of studies have been conducted to test the ergogenic effectiveness of caffeine. Considerable differences exist in the experimental designs of caffeine studies in such aspects as caffeine delivery system (caffeine in coffee or capsule form), caffeine dosage (3–15 mg per kg body weight), the type of exercise task (power, strength, reaction time, short-term endurance, prolonged endurance), the intensity of the exercise (submaximal exercise, maximal exercise), the training status of the subject (trained, untrained), the preexercise diet (high-carbohydrate, mixed), the subjects' caffeine status (user, abstainer), and individual variability (reactor, nonreactor). These differences complicate interpretation of the results. Additionally, some investigators have combined caffeine with other related stimulants, such as ephedrine.

Use by Athletes Caffeine appears to be a popular ergogenic aid among athletes. In one study, Dascombe and others reported that a large majority of elite athletes at a national sports institute used caffeine as a sports supplement. In other reports Desbrow and Leveritt noted that almost 90 percent of athletes competing in the World Championship Ironman Triathlon competition used caffeine supplements, ranging from coffee before and caffeinated gels and energy drinks during the race; 75 percent believed that caffeine was ergogenic to their performance. Overall, caffeine is one of the most popular sports supplements used worldwide by a wide variety of athletes.

Effect on Psychomotor Responses Caffeine may affect a number of psychomotor responses that may enhance performance in some sports. Caffeine can increase alertness, which may improve simple reaction time. Doses of 200 milligrams have been effective, particularly when subjects are mentally fatigued. In several studies, Hogervorst and others have found that caffeine, as part of a carbohydrate-electrolyte solution or performance bar, improved cognitive function in trained athletes following an endurance cycling task. Maintaining cognitive function in many endurance activities may enhance performance. Stevenson and others theorized that a round of golf that lasts approximately four hours could be fatiguing from the prolonged walking, and may result in impaired motor skill or cognitive performance. In their study with experienced golfers, they found that the consumption of a caffeinated sports drink prior to and during a round of golf improved putting performance and increased feelings of alertness. In its position statement on caffeine and exercise performance, the International Society of Sports Nutrition indicated that caffeine can enhance vigilance during bouts of extended exhaustive exercise, as well as periods of sustained sleep deprivation.

However, larger doses, above 400 milligrams, may increase nervousness and anxiety in some individuals, and thus may adversely affect performance in events characterized by fine motor skills and control of hand steadiness, such as pistol shooting. Also, although caffeine may enhance visual attention, Hespel and others noted that in sports involving rapid visual stimuli, such as soccer, care must be taken not to overdose because visual information processing might be impaired.

Effect on Aerobic Endurance Performance Most research on the ergogenic effects of caffeine has focused on aerobic endurance performance, and numerous studies, reviews, meta-analyses, and position statements by sports-related associations support its efficacy as an ergogenic aid (Figure 13.5). For example, recent studies have found that caffeine enhances performance in the following:

- 15-minute cycling performance following 135 minutes of sustained cycling
- Cycling to exhaustion at 80 percent VO_2 max
- 2000-meter rowing time
- Run time to exhaustion at 85 percent VO_2 max (by 44 percent)
- 8-kilometer run time (by 23 seconds)

In their most recent review, Ganio and others restricted their analysis to studies that used only a time-trial endurance test, which has high reproducibility and is more applicable to sport. A total of 21 high-quality studies using time trials of 5 minutes or more were reviewed. Although the amount of improvement varied among

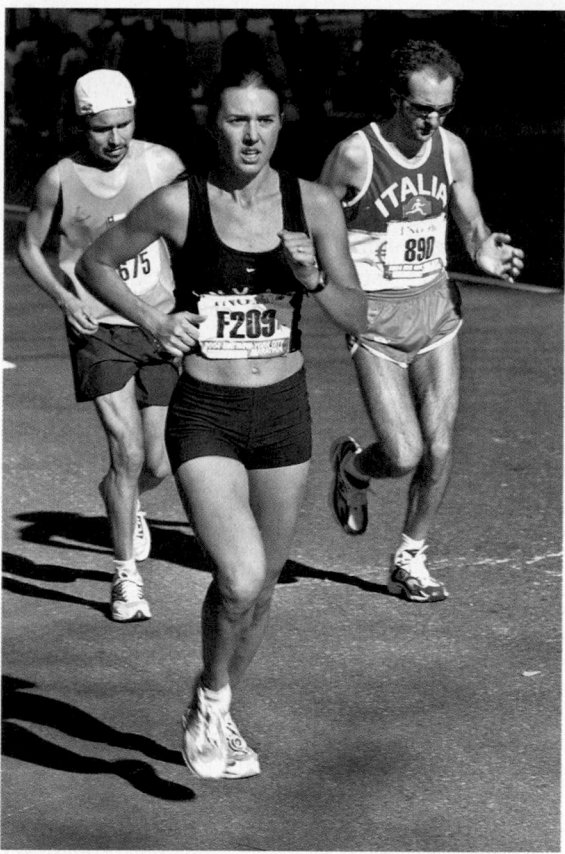

FIGURE 13.5 Caffeine may enhance performance in a wide variety of exercise endeavors, particularly events involving aerobic endurance.

studies, the mean improvement in performance with caffeine ingestion was 3.2 percent. As previously noted, in their meta-analysis of 21 studies Doherty and Smith reported that caffeine improved exercise performance by 11.2 percent. Jeukendrup and Martin, in their review on how to improve cycling performance, suggested that low doses of caffeine would improve 40-kilometer time by 55–84 seconds.

In its position stand on caffeine and exercise performance, the International Society of Sports Nutrition concluded that caffeine is ergogenic for sustained maximal endurance exercise, and has been shown to be highly effective for time-trial performance, as noted earlier. The American College of Sports Medicine, in its position statement on fluid replacement during exercise, also noted that caffeine intake may help sustain performance. Given these overall findings, it is no wonder caffeine is so popular among endurance athletes.

Effect on High-Intensity Anaerobic Exercise Davis and Green noted that the effect of caffeine on endurance performance is well founded, but comparatively less research has been conducted on the ergogenic potential of caffeine on anaerobic performance. For purposes of this discussion, high-intensity anaerobic exercise involves maximum exercise for 10–180 seconds, or intermittent high-intensity exercise in sports such as soccer, lacrosse, and field hockey.

In his review from more than 20 years ago, Williams reached a general conclusion that caffeine did not enhance performance in high-intensity anaerobic exercise tasks. However, Davis and Green noted that older studies often used untrained subjects and designs often not conducive to observation of an ergogenic effect, whereas more recent studies have incorporated trained subjects and more appropriate sport-specific research designs. In their review, they concluded that caffeine is ergogenic to an extent with anaerobic exercise. They note that caffeine seems highly ergogenic for speed-endurance exercise ranging in duration from 60–180 seconds. However, other traditional models examining power output (i.e., 30-second Wingate test) have shown minimal effect of caffeine on performance. Conversely, studies employing sport-specific methodologies (i.e., hockey, rugby, soccer) with shorter duration (4–6 seconds) show caffeine to be ergogenic during high-intensity intermittent exercise. In another recent review, Astorino and Roberson reported that 11 of 17 studies found significant improvements in team sports exercise and power-based sports with caffeine ingestion, but most commonly in elite athletes who do not regularly ingest caffeine. In its position stand on caffeine and exercise performance, the International Society of Sports Nutrition indicated that caffeine supplementation is beneficial for high-intensity exercise, including team sports such as soccer and rugby.

Caffeine appears to be an effective ergogenic for high-intensity, intermittent exercise, particularly within a period of prolonged duration, such as a soccer match.

Effect on Muscular Strength and Endurance   Research findings relative to the effect of caffeine supplementation on muscular strength and endurance are somewhat equivocal. In their review, David and Green note that research is somewhat limited regarding the effect of caffeine on resistance training and muscular strength and endurance. They also note recent studies showing that caffeine affects isometric maximal force and offers some evidence for enhanced muscle endurance for lower body musculature. However, the effects of caffeine on isokinetic peak torque, one-repetition maximum, and muscular endurance for upper body musculature are less clear. In their review, Astorino and Robinson indicate that 6 or 11 studies show that caffeine elicits significant benefits in resistance training. In their meta-analysis, Warren and others concluded that, overall, caffeine ingestion results in a small beneficial effect on maximal voluntary contraction strength, but primarily in the knee extensors and not in other muscle groups. The average increase in strength was about 7 percent. They also reported that caffeine exerted a small beneficial effect on muscular endurance, but only in some specific test protocols. However, Davis and Green conclude that because relatively few studies exist concerning caffeine and resistance training, a definite conclusion cannot be reached on the extent to which caffeine affects performance in this regard. The International Society of Sports Nutrition, in its position statement on caffeine and exercise performance, supports this viewpoint, concluding that

the scientific literature is equivocal relative to the effects of caffeine supplementation on strength-power performance.

Effect of Dietary Carbohydrate   As noted in chapter 4, carbohydrate is the main energy source for aerobic endurance exercise, and sport scientists have studied both carbohydrates and caffeine to see if there could be a synergistic effect on performance. Yeo and others reported that consuming caffeine with carbohydrate during prolonged aerobic exercise will significantly increase the oxidation of exogenous carbohydrate; exogenous carbohydrate oxidation was 0.72 gram per minute with glucose/caffeine intake, but only 0.57 gram per minute with glucose alone. In a meta-analysis of 21 studies, Conger and others concluded that supplementation with carbohydrate and caffeine provides a small, but significant, effect to improve endurance exercise performance when compared to carbohydrate alone. Additionally, Gant and others reported that when compared to a standard carbohydrate-electrolyte solution, a caffeinated version improved performance in a 90-minute intermittent shuttle-running trial designed to mimic a soccer match, suggesting that such a caffeine/carbohydrate combination also may be useful in prolonged intermittent high-intensity sports.

Effect of Caffeine Status   One possible factor determining whether caffeine is an effective ergogenic aid is the caffeine status of the subjects. In many of the studies that report an ergogenic effect, subjects abstained from caffeine use for 2–4 days prior to the experiment; they became caffeine-free for several days to possibly heighten the caffeine effect when taken. This abstention period was based on some research reporting no effects of caffeine on epinephrine or FFA levels if subjects abstained for less than 1 day. Other research documented a decreased sensitivity to caffeine following 6 weeks of increased caffeine ingestion; that is, the epinephrine level was decreased during exercise following this period of increased caffeine intake. In their review, Ganio and others recommended abstaining from caffeine for at least 7 days before use to give the greatest chance of optimizing the ergogenic effect.

However, in their earlier review, Graham and Spriet, two experts on the ergogenic effects of caffeine, suggested that caffeine withdrawal may have little effect on actual performance, and that subjects may consume caffeine products up to the day of the event. A study by Irwin and others supports this viewpoint. They found that a 3 mg/kg dose of caffeine significantly improves exercise performance irrespective of whether a 4-day withdrawal period is imposed on habitual caffeine users. As noted later, this issue may be related to the particular individual's sensitivity to caffeine.

Effect of Delivery System   Another factor influencing caffeine's effectiveness may be how it is consumed. Graham and others compared the effects of consuming the same dose of caffeine in coffee or as a capsule in water. In a well-designed, double-blind, repeated-measures study with 5 trials (3 caffeine and 2 placebo), they found that although the plasma epinephrine increased with the coffee, the increase was significantly greater with the caffeine capsule. Additionally, the caffeine capsule was the only treatment that improved exercise performance, a treadmill run to exhaustion at 85 percent VO_2 max. They suggested that some component or components in coffee may moderate the effect of caffeine. However, other studies have reported significant ergogenic effects when coffee was used to deliver caffeine. Nevertheless, in its position stand, the International Society of Sports Nutrition notes that caffeine exerts a greater ergogenic effect when consumed in an anhydrous, or pill, form as compared to coffee. For those who enjoy their coffee the morning of an event, McLellan and Bell reported that consuming coffee 30 minutes prior to taking capsulated caffeine did not negate its beneficial ergogenic effect on cycling endurance performance. Thus, drinking coffee would not seem to impair the potential ergogenic effect of caffeine tablets.

Effect of Exercise in the Heat Caffeine has been classified as a diuretic and also stimulates metabolism. Theoretically, increased water losses and an elevated metabolism before competition could impair exercise performance under warm, humid environmental conditions, possibly because of retarded sweat losses and excessive increases in body temperature. However, research has shown no changes in sweat loss, plasma volume, or body temperature following caffeine ingestion. For example, Del Coso and others reported that caffeine, whether consumed alone or in combination with water or a sports drink, did not alter heat production, forearm skin blood flow, or sweat rate, and did not impair heat dissipation when exercising for 120 minutes in a hot environment. Moreover, Cohen and others reported that caffeine ingestion did not impair performance in a 13.1-mile (21.1 km) half-marathon run outdoors under hot, humid conditions.

Lawrence Armstrong, from the University of Connecticut, is an international scholar on caffeine and thermoregulation during exercise. In their most recent review, Armstrong and others concluded that, in contrast to popular beliefs, caffeine consumption does not result in hypohydration, water-electrolyte imbalances, hyperthermia, or impaired exercise-heat tolerance. This viewpoint is supported by both the ACSM, which notes that caffeine consumption will not markedly alter daily urine output or hydration status, and the ISSN, which notes that the scientific literature does not support caffeine-induced diuresis during exercise or any harmful change in fluid balance that would negatively affect performance.

Athletes will not incur detrimental fluid-electrolyte imbalances if they consume caffeinated beverages in moderation and eat a typical diet. Additionally, Armstrong and others reported that consuming caffeine, either 3 or 6 milligrams per kilogram body weight for five days, did not cause hypohydration, and questioned the widely accepted notion that caffeine consumption acts chronically as a diuretic.

The Placebo Effect As mentioned in chapter 1, subjects in a study may experience a placebo effect if they think they received an effective ergogenic, such as caffeine. In a unique study, Beedie and others told subjects they would receive either a placebo, moderate, or high dose of caffeine before performing a 10-kilometer cycle time trial. Actually, in all trials the subjects received only a placebo; no caffeine was provided. Afterward the subjects were asked which treatment they received, and when they thought they had received caffeine, their performance was better, and even more so when they thought they received the high dose. Although this study provides evidence of a clear placebo effect Foad and others have shown there may also be clear pharmacological effects of caffeine on exercise performance. In a meticulous study with male competitive cyclists, six separate tests were used to establish a baseline for 40-kilometer cycling time-trial performance. The cyclists then performed eight more trials, two each under four experimental conditions (AA, BA, AB, BB) involving the interaction of receiving (A) or not receiving (B) caffeine and being informed they had (A) or had not (B) received caffeine. They found that caffeine exerted a pharmacological ergogenic effect, but also noted a possible beneficial psychological placebo effect, as the subjects performed somewhat better when informed they were given caffeine but were not. There was also a possible negative placebo (nocebo) effect when subjects were correctly informed that they received no caffeine. Their data support the ergogenic efficacy of caffeine but suggest that both positive and negative expectations may affect performance.

Effect of Dosage: Permissibility Because caffeine is a drug (a stimulant), its use as an ergogenic in sports has been regulated by the International Olympic Committee and the WADA. The ISSN notes that caffeine is effective for enhancing sport performance in trained athletes when consumed in low to moderate dosages, about 3 to 6 mg/kg, and overall does not result in further enhancement in performance when consumed in higher dosages, such as greater than 9 mg/kg. However, the amount of caffeine Olympic and international-class athletes have been permitted to use has varied over the years. The International Olympic Committee (IOC) banned the use of caffeine as a drug prior to the 1972 Olympics, removed it from the doping list from 1972 to 1982, banned the use of large amounts (8–10 mg/kg) for the 1984 Olympics, possibly for its ergogenic effects; and under the recommendation of the WADA, removed it from the banned list effective January 1, 2004. The WADA felt that the doping list should be adjusted to reflect changing times. The removal of caffeine from the prohibited list may be a reflection of the increased prevalence of caffeinated beverages, such as specialty coffees, fortified colas, energy drinks, and even sport drinks. These drinks, which may be larger and contain more caffeine, may be consumed in quantity by athletes. As noted earlier, caffeine is also found in a wide variety of other food products.

Currently, the WADA has caffeine in its monitoring list, meaning that caffeine levels in international-class athletes are tested and if caffeine abuse increases, it may be returned to the prohibited list. Some athletic governing organizations, such as the National Collegiate Athletic Association (NCAA), may test urine samples for caffeine concentration, and a level of 15 micrograms/milliliter is considered to be evidence of doping. Research by Bruce and others found that subjects consuming about 9 mg/kg body weight exceeded this limit. However, athletes need not use such large doses, as they are no more effective than smaller ones. About 5 mg/kg body weight has been shown by multiple studies to be an effective dose.

Individuality In general, studies have not reported a decrease in performance following caffeine ingestion. However, it should be noted that individuals vary in their responses to any drug. In two recent, well-designed caffeine studies, Jenkins and others reported a significant ergogenic effect overall on cycling performance, though Skinner and others reported no significant effect on rowing performance. However, both authors commented that large interindividual responses to caffeine suggest that individual characteristics should be considered when administering caffeine for performance enhancement. In several of the studies the investigators reported that some subjects had adverse reactions to the caffeine and thus had an impaired performance.

Caffeine appears to be an effective ergogenic aid in doses that are both safe and legal. However, some athletes believe that taking caffeine may be considered unethical because it is an artificial means of enhancing performance. Given its safety and legality, the decision to use caffeine as a performance enhancer rests with the ethical standards of the individual athlete. Although combining ephedrine with caffeine (as discussed in the next section) may increase the ergogenic effect of caffeine alone, ephedrine use may be illegal—so its use to increase sports performance is unethical.

Self-Experimentation If you are considering using caffeine as a potential ergogenic aid, it is wise to experiment with its use in training prior to use in competition. You might start by taking 200–400 milligrams of caffeine about an hour prior to some of your workouts. For example, if you are a distance runner, do your long runs periodically with and without the coffee or other caffeine source, and judge for yourself if it works for you. To make it a more valid case study, have someone randomly give you, blinded, a placebo (vitamin capsule) or caffeine capsule before the runs, but without informing you which until you have done each several times. Try this procedure also after abstaining from caffeine for 4–5 days. Keep a record of your feelings and times after the runs so you can compare differences.

Does drinking coffee, tea, or other caffeinated beverages provide any health benefits or pose any significant health risks?

The health effects of caffeine have been studied for nearly half a century. Early epidemiological research linked coffee or caffeine consumption with the development of a variety of health problems, including cancer, heart disease, osteoporosis, and birth defects. However, in an interview with Bonnie Liebman from the Center for Science in the Public Interest, Walter Willett, a renowned authority in nutrition and health, indicated that coffee is now considered to be a health-producing beverage. That appears to be the case given current research findings, but there are some possible exceptions.

Current research involving the health effects of caffeine has used a variety of techniques, including epidemiological prospective cohort studies, randomized clinical trials, and animal models. Investigators have looked at a variety of factors, including different sources of caffeine, such as coffee versus tea, regular versus decaffeinated coffee, and even the method of preparing coffee, such as filtered versus boiled. Investigators suggest that some of the potential health benefits of coffee and tea may be attributed to substances other than the caffeine found in these beverages. For example, green tea contains caffeine and has been studied for its health benefits. However, green tea also contains an antioxidant, epigallocatechin gallate (EGCG), which has been found in some animal studies to reduce the risk of several chronic diseases.

The following sections highlight some of the key findings relative the effect of caffeine on various health conditions. Most research involves the consumption of caffeinated beverages, but some involves caffeine in dietary supplements. A current hot topic involves the health effects of caffeinated energy drinks, particularly alcoholic energy drinks, and this is addressed separately from the other health conditions.

Energy Drinks Of special interest in recent years has been the increasing popularity of caffeinated energy drinks, particularly among youngsters and college-age adults. Temple noted that caffeine-containing drinks are now consumed regularly by children, with some specifically marketed to children as young as 4 years of age. Red Bull was the first energy drink, appearing in Austria in 1987 and in the United States in 1997; current sales in the United States alone exceed $5 billion annually. Hundreds of energy drinks are currently available, and the caffeine content in energy drinks varies tremendously, ranging from 2.5–35.7 milligrams per fluid ounce or about 50–500 milligrams per serving.

In their review, Arria and O'Brien indicated that energy-drink consumption is potentially harmful for various reasons, such as increased blood pressure in adolescents, and carries various risks for pregnant women, as discussed later. Additional research is needed to document the possible health effects of excessive caffeine intake on the young.

In particular, Arria and O'Brien note that the practice of mixing energy drinks with alcohol—a very common practice—has been consistently linked to drinking high volumes of alcohol per drinking session and subsequent serious alcohol-related consequences, such as driving while intoxicated. They also indicated that although consumers might be under the impression that caffeine counteracts the adverse effects of alcohol, research has demonstrated that individuals who combine energy drinks with alcohol underestimate their true level of impairment. This state of being less likely to accurately appraise the true level of impairment has been labeled "wide-awake drunkenness" and can lead to engaging in risky behavior.

Scientists indicate that additional research is needed to ascertain the potential health risks of energy-drink consumption, but also suggest that the government should be proactive in protecting the public. For example, current FDA regulations limit the amount of caffeine in cola-type sodas to approximately 48 milligrams per 8-ounce serving, but a similar serving of one highly caffeinated energy drink may contain about 285 milligrams of caffeine. Some question why this FDA regulation does not apply to energy drinks. The FDA did undertake some action relative to energy drinks containing both caffeine and alcohol, announcing in November 2010 that caffeine is an unsafe food additive to alcoholic beverages. This action will prohibit the sale of caffeine/alcohol energy drinks in the United States.

Cardiovascular Disease and Associated Risk Factors Caffeine has been studied for its effect on various risk factors associated with cardiovascular disease. One of the more important risk factors is an adverse serum lipid profile, a leading cause of atherosclerosis. Earlier studies investigating the relationship between coffee consumption and serum lipid levels have revealed inconsistent findings, some reporting elevated serum cholesterol levels and others reporting no effect. One possible cause of the different findings was the method of coffee preparation, which may vary in different countries. In parts of Europe where coffee is boiled, several cholesterol-raising compounds could remain in the coffee, whereas they are removed if a filtering process is used, as is most typical in Canada and the United States. Although research findings are inconsistent regarding the effects of coffee on the serum lipid profile, one study provides strong evidence that chronic coffee consumption does not cause atherosclerosis. In the CARDIA study, Reis and others followed more than 5,000 adults over the course of 20 years, and observed no substantial association between coffee or caffeine intake and coronary and carotid atherosclerosis.

Another important risk factor is high blood pressure, and caffeine may acutely increase blood pressure in individuals who are caffeine sensitive and also in individuals who are under stress. As noted, caffeine blocks the effect of adenosine, which may impair vasodilation and increase arterial stiffness, increasing blood pressure. Nevertheless, not all studies have shown that increased caffeine use is associated with high blood pressure. For example, Schardt cited one study that followed more than 150,000 women for 10 years and found that those who drank regular or decaffeinated coffee had no higher risk of hypertension than non-coffee drinkers. However, in a critical review of dietary caffeine and blood pressure, James concluded that findings from experimental and epidemiologic studies converge to show that blood pressure remains reactive to the pressor effects of caffeine in the diet; overall, the impact of dietary caffeine on population blood pressure levels is likely to be modest, probably increasing blood pressure by about 4 and 2 mmHg for systolic and diastolic blood pressure, respectively. As noted in chapter 9, individuals with high blood pressure should consult with their health care professionals for exercise recommendations, particularly resistance exercise. Todd and others reported that caffeine (6 mg/kg) consumed one hour prior to resistance training elevated systolic blood pressure by 8–10 mmHg. An excessive increase in blood pressure could induce a heart attack or stroke.

Some at-risk individuals should be cautious about caffeine use before exercise. Caffeine has also been found to cause a slight arrhythmia, or irregular heartbeat, in some caffeine-sensitive individuals, although Frost and Vestergaard reported that low to moderate consumption of caffeine, as coffee, does not cause the most common type of serious arrhythmia, known as atrial fibrillation. However, individuals known to be caffeine-sensitive, particularly those with high blood pressure, may be advised to use caution when exercising, as suggested in chapter 9. Although exercise is generally recommended in rehabilitation programs for those with coronary heart disease (CHD), caffeine consumption may pose a risk. Namdar and others reported that caffeine consumed before exercising (a dose corresponding to 2 cups of coffee) may reduce blood flow to the heart during exercise in older individuals (ages 58–61), and to a much greater degree in patients with CHD.

Although caffeine may affect some of the risk factors associated with heart disease, reviews suggest that the risk of developing coronary heart disease or having a heart attack from caffeine use is rather low. For example, in a meta-analysis of 21 prospective cohort studies, Wu and others reported that their findings do not support the hypothesis that coffee consumption increases the long-term risk of CHD. Actually, habitual moderate coffee drinking was associated with a lower risk of CHD in women.

Based on contemporary research, most health professional groups, such as the American Heart Association, recommend that moderate coffee consumption, about 1–2 cups daily, is safe and not associated with heart disease. However, the effects of consuming greater amounts of coffee are not as well known. James indicated that the effect of caffeine to increase blood pressure could account for premature deaths in the region of 14 percent for coronary heart disease and 20 percent for stroke, and indicates that strategies for encouraging reduced dietary levels of caffeine deserve serious consideration. Individuals who are hypertensive, or who are under stress, or who may have other risk factors for heart disease, should consult their physician regarding the use of caffeine.

Type 2 Diabetes Over the course of the past 10 years, several longitudinal studies and extensive reviews have indicated that consumption of caffeinated beverages, such as coffee and tea, was associated with a reduced risk of type 2 diabetes. In a more recent meta-analysis of 18 studies, Huxley and others found an inverse linear relationship between coffee consumption and subsequent risk of type 2 diabetes, such that every additional cup of coffee consumed in a day was associated with a 7 percent reduction in the excess risk of diabetes. However, they also reported similar beneficial effects with decaffeinated coffee and tea, concluding that high intakes of coffee, decaffeinated coffee, and tea are associated with reduced risk of diabetes. Such a finding suggests that other components in coffee and tea, such as magnesium, chromium, lignans, and chlorogenic acid, may be involved. For example, chlorogenic acid can delay glucose absorption. Researchers recommend randomized clinical trials as a means to determine active ingredients, which may reveal a combination effect of multiple substances.

Cancer The American Cancer Society, after reviewing the available scientific evidence, indicated that there is no known association between the consumption of coffee, tea, or other caffeinated beverages and the development of any type of cancer. In support of this viewpoint, Michels and others presented data from two large epidemiological studies involving men and women, and reported that the consumption of caffeinated coffee, tea with caffeine, or caffeine was not associated with incidence of colon or rectal cancer. Also, Schardt noted that a review of 66 studies of coffee and pancreatic cancer and 25 studies with kidney cancer concluded that coffee was unlikely to pose a substantial risk.

In one of the largest studies, a 22-year follow-up study of more than 85,000 women in the Nurses' Health Study, Ganmaa and others observed no substantial association between caffeinated and decaffeinated coffee and tea consumption and risk of breast cancer. However, in a meta-analysis of 18 epidemiological studies, Tang and others reported a possible influence of high coffee consumption on the risk of breast cancer. They reported a borderline risk (RR = 0.95) of breast cancer in women in the United States and Europe who consumed the highest amounts of caffeine.

Cognitive Functions   The extensive use of caffeine as a social drug is most likely attributable to its stimulating effect on cognitive functions. In one review, Lara stated that caffeine intake enhances mental energy and in effect, elevates mood and increases alertness, attention, and cognitive function (more evident in longer or more difficult tasks or situations of low arousal); accordingly, moderate caffeine intake (<6 cups/day) has been associated with fewer depressive symptoms, fewer cognitive failures, and lower risk of suicide.

Caffeine intake may also be associated with less aging-related cognitive decline, including later onset of Alzheimer's disease (AD) and Parkinson's disease (PD). Chen and others note that one mechanism implicated in the pathogenesis of AD and PD is blood-brain barrier (BBB) dysfunction, and they reported that caffeine exerts protective effects against AD and PD at least in part by keeping the BBB intact. Other theories suggest that caffeine may help prevent the decline in dopamine-secreting neurons that often occurs during aging. Research using animal models, according to Cunha and Agostinho, indicates that caffeine alleviates mental dysfunction in AD and PD. Research with humans also appears promising. In a meta-analysis of 11 studies quantifying the relationship between caffeine intake and cognitive decline or dementia, Santos and others reported a trend toward a protective effect of caffeine, but noted that the limited number of studies and different methodologies used preclude a more definitive statement. Additionally, in a review of available studies, Prediger concluded that caffeine is a promising therapeutic tool for the treatment of both motor and nonmotor symptoms in PD. Overall, research findings suggest habitual caffeine intake may be associated with less cognitive decline with aging.

Asthma   According to Chapman and Mickleborough, one of the often-overlooked effects of caffeine is its role as a very potent respiratory stimulant. Such an effect could be beneficial to individuals with various respiratory disorders. For example, Welsh and others, in a meta-analysis of 7 randomized clinical trials, concluded that caffeine, either as oral caffeine or coffee, appears to improve airway function modestly, for up to 4 hours, in people with asthma. Exercise-induce asthma may occur in some individuals during physical activity, and caffeine may possibly help reduce the symptoms.

Osteoporosis   Factors underlying the development of osteoporosis are discussed in detail in chapter 8. Essentially, calcium loss may lead to osteoporosis. For now, we may note that caffeine tends to accelerate the loss of calcium from bones and lead to its excretion in the urine. However, the amount is very small, approximating only 5 milligrams of calcium loss for every cup of coffee. Using 2 tablespoons of milk in the coffee would replace the amount of lost calcium. In one report, the National Institutes of Health indicated that caffeine use does not cause significant losses of calcium. However, drinking milk or eating calcium-rich foods is highly recommended if you drink caffeinated beverages. Individuals with osteoporosis should consult with their physician about the use of calcium supplements.

Pregnancy-Related Health Problems   Animal research has suggested that very high doses of caffeine could cause various problems during pregnancy, including low birth weight, miscarriage, or birth defects, whereas consumption of moderate amounts did not produce such effects. Similar findings are reported in research with humans.

Relative to low birth weight, a large prospective observational study by the CARE Study Group reported that caffeine consumption throughout pregnancy was associated with an increased risk of fetal growth restriction—the more caffeine consumed, the greater the risk.

Relative to miscarriage, Weng and others, in a prospective study of more than 1,000 pregnant women, reported that caffeine intake, particularly more than 200 milligrams daily, increased the risk of miscarriage. Women who consumed no caffeine were at the lowest risk for miscarriage. Moreover, Savitz and others studied 2,400 women who were relatively light coffee drinkers, with the heaviest drinkers consuming only about two cups daily, over the course of their pregnancies and found little indication of possible harmful effects of caffeine on miscarriage risk.

Regarding birth defects, Browne conducted a systematic review of studies involving the effect of caffeine and indicated that there is no evidence to support a teratogenic effect of caffeine in humans. In a more recent study using data from the National Birth Defects Prevention Study, Browne and others did not find convincing evidence of an association between maternal caffeine intake and birth defects. However, Schardt postulates that the data are not strong enough to say there is absolutely no increase in risk.

To be on the safe side, the Food and Drug Administration and the American Dietetic Association recommend that pregnant women consider abstaining from caffeine use, or, if they do drink caffeinated beverages, to do so in moderation. In its report, the Consumers Union recommended that they drink no more than two cups of coffee a day to avoid the possible risk of miscarriage.

Drinking caffeine beverages when breast feeding may make the child jittery, as caffeine gets into breast milk.

Weight Control   Caffeine use may stimulate metabolism, increasing the resting metabolic rate about 10 percent for several hours, an effect that theoretically could facilitate weight loss. Greenway notes that caffeine has a long history of safe, non-prescription use as a weight-loss supplement, and that the benefits of treating obesity appear to outweigh the small associated risk. In a metabolic ward study, Rudelle and others reported that a beverage containing caffeine, green tea catechins, and calcium increased 24-hour energy expenditure by 4.6 percent, but the contribution of the individual ingredients cannot be distinguished. Although the increase in energy expenditure was modest, they indicated that such modifications are sufficient to prevent weight gain and concluded that such a beverage may provide benefits for weight control. Lopez-Garcia and others studied the effect of caffeine intake over the course of 12 years and its effect on body weight in men and women. They found that increased caffeine consumption was associated with decreased weight gain, but the differences were very small, being less than one pound difference. Regular consumption of coffee or caffeine would appear to make a very minor contribution to weight control as contrasted to proper diet and exercise. Excessive amounts may cause adverse effects in some individuals using it for weight loss, especially when combined with ephedrine as discussed in the following text. Proper weight-control procedures are discussed in chapters 10 and 11.

Sleeplessness Caffeine use, particularly before retiring for the night, may delay the onset of sleep because of its stimulant effects. Inadequate sleep could be detrimental to cognitive functions the following day, and, as noted in chapter 10, could be a contributing factor to weight gain. Individuals who want to improve the quality of their sleep may want to consider caffeine abstinence. Sin and others reported that abstaining from caffeine for a whole day improves sleep quality.

In contrast, preventing sleepiness may be beneficial in some situations. For example, decreased drowsiness and increased alertness may contribute to safer automobile operation under certain conditions. Philip and others found that drinking coffee with about 200 milligrams of caffeine helped improve the quality of nighttime driving. Horne and Reyner reported that coffee intake is one of the few techniques useful to prevent vehicle accidents related to sleepiness.

Gastric Distress Some individuals experience stomach irritation due to increased secretion of gastric acids following ingestion of caffeinated beverages. In such cases, individuals should consult their physician or avoid caffeine.

Caffeine Naivete Abstainers or those who consume little caffeine may experience nervousness, irritability, headaches, or insomnia with moderate doses, although long-term consumption of coffee leads to development of tolerance and reduction of these "coffee nerves" symptoms. Youngstedt and others reported that moderate aerobic exercise may reduce the anxiety sometimes associated with caffeine intake.

Caffeine Dependence In a cover story for *National Geographic,* coffee was labeled the world's most popular psychoactive drug—buzzing our brains, fraying our nerves, and robbing our sleep. Yet we simply refuse to survive without it. Although not classified as an addictive drug, some individuals may develop caffeine dependence, often referred to as *caffeinism.* Various health organizations differ on their classification of caffeine dependence. The World Health Organization does recognize caffeine dependence in its *Classification of Mental and Behavioral Disorders,* whereas the American Psychiatric Association does not list it in the *Diagnostic and Statistical Manual of Mental Disorders,* although the APA does list caffeine-induced anxiety disorder. Juliano and Griffiths noted that caffeine-dependent individuals may experience various symptoms upon caffeine withdrawal, including headaches and nervousness, fatigue or drowsiness, depression, irritability, and difficulty concentrating. However, caffeine dependence is not considered a serious form of drug abuse.

Mortality In their study of health professionals spanning about 20 years, Lopez-Garcia and others reported that regular coffee consumption was not associated with increased mortality rate in either men or women. However, Kerrigan and Lindsey indicated that in large doses, caffeine can be profoundly toxic, resulting in arrhythmia, tachycardia, vomiting, convulsions, coma, and death. Although rare, death may result from caffeine abuse, usually from overdoses of caffeine-containing diet or stimulant pills. Fatal caffeine overdoses in adults are typically in excess of 5g. Individuals who take several different over-the-counter dietary supplements may be taking substantial amounts of caffeine along with other drugs. Such combinations, in excess, may be fatal.

Summary In general, most professional health organizations note that caffeine is regarded as a safe drug. If you are healthy and are not on medications, several cups of coffee or caffeinated beverages should pose no health problems. Where moderation is recommended, the dosage is the equivalent of about 200 to 300 milligrams of caffeine per day, or about 2 cups of coffee. And we are talking 6-ounce cups of coffee or so, not the supersize 20-ounce cups or higher from local convenience stores. Women who are pregnant may want to consider abstention, similar to the recommendations for alcohol intake during pregnancy. Moreover, keep in mind that individuals, based on their genetic variations, may respond differently to caffeine intake; some may be more prone to its possible adverse effects as a potent stimulant.

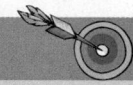

Key Concepts

▶ Caffeine is a stimulant drug and can affect a variety of metabolic and psychological processes in the body that may affect exercise performance and health.

▶ Research suggests that caffeine may improve performance in a variety of athletic endeavors, particularly prolonged aerobic endurance exercise. An effective dose is approximately 5 milligrams per kilogram body weight.

▶ In general, caffeine is regarded to be a safe drug, but physicians may recommend abstinence or use in moderation for some individuals. Various health professionals define moderation as the daily caffeine equivalent of 1–2 cups of coffee.

Ephedra (ephedrine): Ergogenic Effects and Health Implications

What is ephedra (ephedrine)?

Ephedra sinica, a plant most commonly referred to as **ephedra,** contains a variety of naturally occurring alkaloids, including **ephedrine** and pseudoephedrine. The Chinese version of ephedra is known as **ma huang** (see figure 13.6). Ephedrine is considered the most active alkaloid, and its synthetic version is ephedrine hydrochloride. Pure ephedrine is regulated as a drug, and the FDA allows only very small amounts in over-the-counter drugs such as cold medications.

Like caffeine, ephedrine is a stimulant and, because it is derived from the plant ma huang, in the United States it had been classified as a dietary supplement. Ephedra or ephedrine-containing dietary supplements were marketed to promote weight loss,

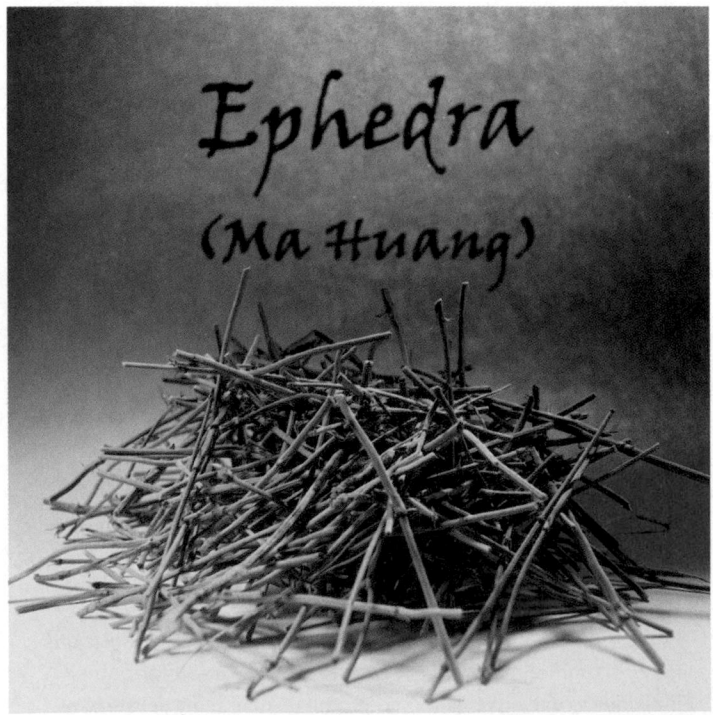

FIGURE 13.6 Seeds of *Ephedra sinica,* or ma huang. The seeds may be processed into tablets for sale as a dietary supplement.

increase energy, and enhance sports performance, with such names as Xtream Lean and Ripped Force. These products were popular with some athletes. For example, Bents and Marsh found that almost half of the ice hockey players in one collegiate conference reported having used ephedra at least once in attempts to improve athletic performance.

In 2004, the FDA prohibited the sale of ephedra or ephedrine-containing dietary supplements, mainly because such products may pose some serious health threats, as noted later. Although banned by the FDA in the United States in 2004, several Internet sites still market ephedra. However, most of these products may be extracts from species of ephedra with little or no ephedrine, the active ingredient. It is legal to sell ephedra products that do not contain ephedrine. They are not believed to be harmful, but they also will not induce the pharmacological effects of ephedrine. Ephedra-free products are also marketed to physically active individuals, but they contain other stimulants, such as caffeine, discussed previously, and pseudoephedrine and synephrine, discussed later.

Does ephedrine enhance exercise performance?

In general, although a powerful stimulant, ephedrine by itself has not been shown to consistently enhance exercise performance. In their review, Rawson and Clarkson concluded that although there are few studies of the efficacy of ephedrine in improving exercise performance, these studies are consistent in their findings of no ergogenic effects. Shekelle and others, in a meta-analysis, supported this viewpoint, as did Magkos and Kavouras in their review, indicating that ephedrine and related alkaloids have not been shown, *as yet,* to result in any significant performance improvements. However, subsequent research has supported an ergogenic effect of ephedrine. Jacobs and others reported that the acute ingestion of caffeine and ephedrine, as well as ephedrine alone, increases local muscular endurance during the first set of traditional resistance-training exercise; however, the performance enhancement was attributed primarily to the effects of ephedrine as there was no additive effect of caffeine.

Ephedrine with caffeine Graham indicated that the combination of ephedrine with caffeine has been suggested to be more potent than caffeine alone. Several studies by Bell and associates, working with Ira Jacobs at the Defence and Civil Institute of Environmental Medicine in Canada, have shown that caffeine/ephedrine combinations may enhance exercise performance in various exercise performance tasks, many of a military nature. Using pharmaceutical-grade caffeine and ephedrine doses approximating 4–5 mg/kg and 0.8–1.0 kg, respectively, they reported significant improvements in exercise tasks such as a 30-second Wingate test of anaerobic capacity, a maximal cycle ergometer performance about 12.5 minutes in duration, the Canadian Forces Warrior Test (3.2-kilometer run wearing combat gear weighing about 11 kilograms), and a 10-kilometer run wearing similar gear. In their review, Magkos and Kavouras indicated that caffeine/ephedrine combinations have been reported in several instances to confer a greater ergogenic benefit than either drug by itself. Research appears to support an ergogenic effect of caffeine/ephedrine supplementation in a number of studies, several involving exercise tasks of a military nature that may be applicable to enhancement of sports performance.

Pseudoephedrine Herbal pseudoephedrine may be found in some dietary supplements, but is most commonly found in over-the-counter cold medications. One Sudafed capsule contains 30 milligrams of pseudoephedrine.

Although research is limited, several studies have evaluated the ergogenic effect of pseudoephedrine supplementation and reported performance-enhancing effects on aerobic endurance. Hodges and others, in a well-controlled, double-blind, placebo, crossover study with seven male athletes, reported that pseudoephedrine (2.5 mg/kg body weight), taken 90 minutes prior to a 1,500-meter run, improved performance by 2.1 percent, or about 6 seconds. There were no changes in measured blood parameters, so they assumed it was a central effect. Additionally, Pritchard-Peschek and others, in a well-designed crossover study with well-trained athletes, reported that the ingestion of 180 milligrams of pseudoephedrine 60 minutes before a cycling time trial improved performance by 5.1 percent. They suggested that possible changes in metabolism or an increase in central nervous system stimulation is responsible for the observed ergogenic effect of pseudoephedrine. Although these two studies provide supportive evidence of an ergogenic effect of pseudoephedrine, additional research is recommended.

Permissibility in sports Use of ephedrine, ephedra, and ma huang in competition is prohibited by the WADA and the IOC. However, pseudoephedrine, like caffeine, has been removed from the WADA doping list and is now in the monitoring program. As ephedra is banned in competition only, athletes may use it in training. Magkos and Kavouras suggested that caffeine/ephedra mixtures may become one of the most popular ergogenic aids that athletes use in training. Given the research findings with pseudoephedrine, its use in sports competition may also increase.

Do dietary supplements containing ephedra pose any health risks?

Of all dietary supplements, the Consumers Union noted that the herbal supplement ephedra may be the most hazardous. Bent and others noted that ephedra use is associated with a greatly increased risk for adverse reactions compared with other herbs; they indicated that ephedra products accounted for 64 percent of all adverse reactions to herbs in the United States even though these products represented less than 1 percent of herbal product sales.

Use of ephedra has been associated with numerous health problems. Maglione and others reported adverse psychiatric effects of ephedra use, including psychosis, severe depression, mania or agitation, hallucinations, sleep disturbance, and suicidal ideation. Haller and others implicated ephedra in risk of seizures. Naik and Freudenberger indicated that ephedra was associated with heart arrhythmias, myocardial infarction, cardiac arrest, and even

sudden death. Haller and others reported that although ephedra alone may be dangerous, ephedra combined with caffeine exaggerates the potential adverse risks.

The Ephedra Education Council notes that 100 milligrams of ephedrine per day is safe, and may be useful for individuals on a weight-loss program mainly by increasing the resting metabolic rate. However, this dose may cause problems in individuals with existing disease, such as high blood pressure or heart disease, who are attempting to lose weight. Moreover, some individuals may exceed the recommended dosage. Indeed, Haller and Benowitz noted that ephedrine misuse may be associated with significant health risks.

In recent years, the deaths of several prominent collegiate and professional athletes made headlines when it was discovered they were using ephedra-containing supplements during training under warm environmental conditions. Ephedrine may increase the risk of heat stroke. The risk-taking behavior associated with sports participants is well known, so athletes taking more than the recommended dose is one of the major problems. Additionally, the purity and amount of ephedra in a product are not well controlled, particularly in products marketed on the Internet. Given these possibilities, and given its physiological effects, ephedrine could be involved in such tragedies.

Synephrine Ephedra-free dietary supplements have been marketed for weight loss (see figure 13.7). These products may contain synephrine, along with other stimulants such as caffeine. Synephrine is an extract from the Seville orange, or bitter, or sour orange. Neo-synephrine is also known as phenylephrine. Synephrine is a dietary supplement in the United States, but classified as a drug in Europe. Synephrine is structurally similar to ephedrine, and has been marketed as a safe alternative to ephedra.

There is little evidence to support weight loss with synephrine. Bent and others reported that synephrine was of no statistically significant benefit for weight loss. Greenway and others,

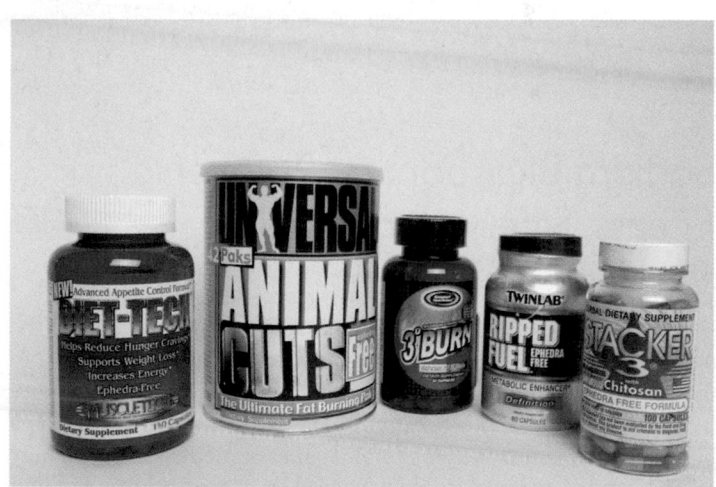

FIGURE 13.7 Ephedra-free dietary supplements are marketed for weight loss; many contain synephrine, a compound similar to ephedrine (see text for discussion).

in two studies, also found that phenylephrine is not efficacious for weight loss.

The Consumers Union also indicates that there is little evidence showing that synephrine is safe, and experts suspect it could cause the same kinds of problems that ephedra does, particularly when it is combined with caffeine. For example, Bui and others found that supplementation with a synephrine dietary supplement (900 milligrams standardized to 6 percent synephrine) increased both systolic and diastolic blood pressure for 5 hours after taken. Such supplements may increase risks for individuals with hypertension. Bouchard and others reported a case study indicating that synephrine may be associated with ischemic stroke.

For individuals interested in weight loss, safer approaches are available, as detailed in chapter 11.

Key Concepts

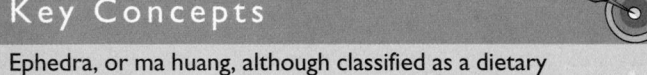

▶ Ephedra, or ma huang, although classified as a dietary supplement, contains a potent stimulant drug, ephedrine.

▶ In general, research suggests that ephedra or ephedrine supplementation does not enhance exercise or sport performance. However, supplementation with caffeine/ephedrine compounds has been shown to enhance performance in various exercise tasks.

▶ Use of ephedra or ephedra-containing supplements has been associated with serious health problems, including psychiatric disorders, increased cardiovascular risk factors, and heat stroke in athletes that could be fatal.

Check for Yourself

Visit a local health food store that primarily sells dietary supplements, including sports supplements. Ask the clerk to show you products containing ephedra-related supplements for weight loss and enhanced sport performance, and also ask if there are any health risks related to their use. Record the response for class discussion.

Sodium Bicarbonate: Ergogenic Effects, Safety, and Legality

What is sodium bicarbonate?

Sodium bicarbonate is an alkaline salt found naturally in the human body. It is the major component of the alkaline reserve in the blood, whose major function is to help control excess acidity by buffering acids. Thus, sodium bicarbonate is also known as a buffer salt. Its action is comparable to that of medications you may take to control an upset stomach caused by gastric acidity. Sodium bicarbonate may be purchased in a supermarket as baking soda (see figure 13.8), and it also has been marketed to athletes as part of a sports supplement.

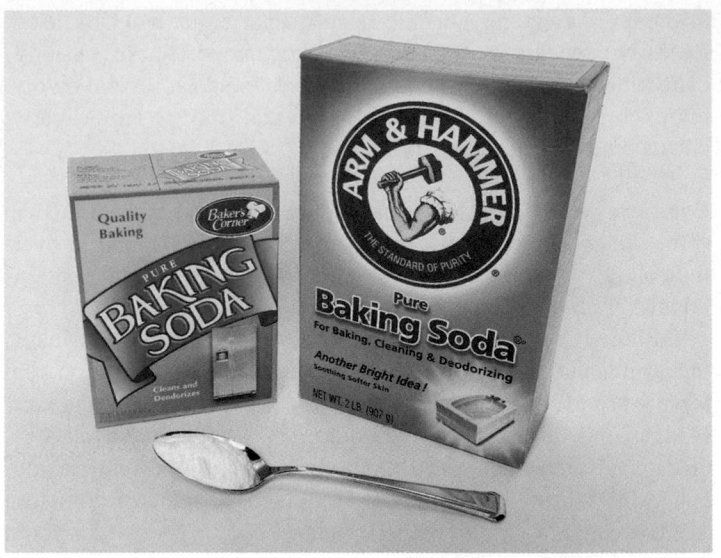

FIGURE 13.8 Baking soda is a commercial version of sodium bicarbonate.

Does sodium bicarbonate, or soda loading, enhance physical performance?

During high-intensity anaerobic exercise, sodium bicarbonate helps buffer the lactic acid that is produced when the lactic acid energy system is utilized. You may recall from chapter 3 that the accumulation of excess hydrogen ions from lactic acid in the muscle cell may interfere with the optimal functioning of various enzymes and thus lead to fatigue. The natural supply of sodium bicarbonate that you have in your blood can help delay the onset of fatigue during anaerobic exercise. It may facilitate the removal of the hydrogen ions associated with lactic acid from the muscle cell, thereby mitigating the adverse effects of the increased acidity (see figure 13.9). However, fatigue is inevitable if the rate of lactic acid production exceeds the capacity of your sodium bicarbonate supply to buffer it. Theoretically, an increase in the alkaline reserve could delay the onset of fatigue.

Alkaline salt supplementation has been studied for its ergogenic potential on all three human energy systems, but mainly the

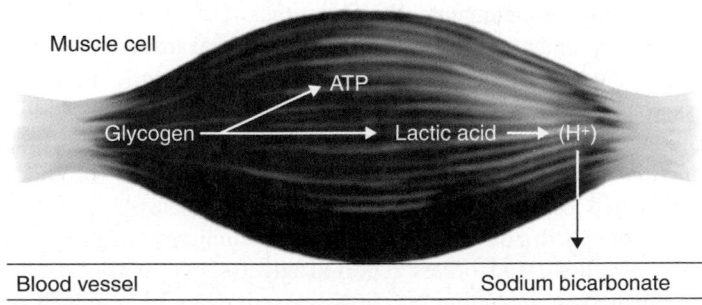

FIGURE 13.9 Alkaline salts, such as sodium bicarbonate, are theorized to reduce the acidity in the muscle cell by facilitating the efflux of hydrogen ions from the cell interior, promoting a more homeostatic environment for continued muscle contraction.

lactic acid energy system. Most studies have used a double-blind placebo design in which all subjects took all treatments. In the popular literature, sodium bicarbonate supplementation has been referred to as *soda loading,* from baking soda, or *buffer boosting,* for increasing the natural blood buffer content.

Supplementation Protocol and Exercise Tasks A relatively standard supplementation protocol has been used, but variations also have been studied. As noted later, the lactic acid energy system has been studied extensively, but research has also studied the effect of sodium bicarbonate supplementation on the ATP-PCr and oxygen energy systems.

The usual experimental protocol has been to have subjects ingest the dose about 1–3 hours before the test. However, other protocols supplemented over the course of 5 days and up to 8 weeks. A typical dosage was 0.15–0.30 grams of sodium bicarbonate per kilogram body weight. Research by McNaughton has indicated that 0.30 grams per kilogram body weight appears to be the optimum dose, with higher dosages providing no additional benefits. This amount totals less than 1 ounce for the average adult. Some studies have used sodium citrate in similar dosages, because it has been shown to increase the alkaline reserve. The exercise task selected was normally one that stressed the lactic acid energy system, or about 1–3 minutes of maximal exercise. Often these exercise tasks were classified as supramaximal, because they used workloads greater than 100 percent VO_2 max. Repeated bouts of intense exercise interspersed with short rest periods have also been used, such as five 100-yard swims with a 2-minute rest between each.

Lactic Acid Energy System More than 70 years ago, German scientists reported that the ingestion of sodium bicarbonate and other alkaline salts could help improve anaerobic work capacity. Since then, many studies have failed to support this finding, but now a substantial number of well-controlled experiments by highly respected investigators in sport nutrition research have provided supportive data, not only for the underlying ergogenic mechanism but also for the performance-enhancing effects.

A study by Raymer and others, using magnetic resonance spectroscopy, provided support for the main theory underlying the ergogenic efficacy of sodium bicarbonate supplementation. They reported that sodium bicarbonate ingestion delayed the onset of intracellular acidification during incremental exercise, which would help maintain a more homeostatic cellular environment to delay the onset of fatigue.

Based on the available scientific evidence, sodium bicarbonate supplementation does appear to enhance performance in exercise tasks dependent upon the lactic acid energy system (see figure 13.10). A consistent finding is an increased serum pH following sodium bicarbonate supplementation, the desired effect to induce buffering of lactic acid. Regarding other factors that have been investigated, approximately half of the well-controlled laboratory studies suggest that ingestion of sodium bicarbonate will reduce acidosis in the muscle cell, decrease the psychological sensation of fatigue at a standardized level of exercise, and increase performance in high-intensity anaerobic exercise tasks to exhaustion.

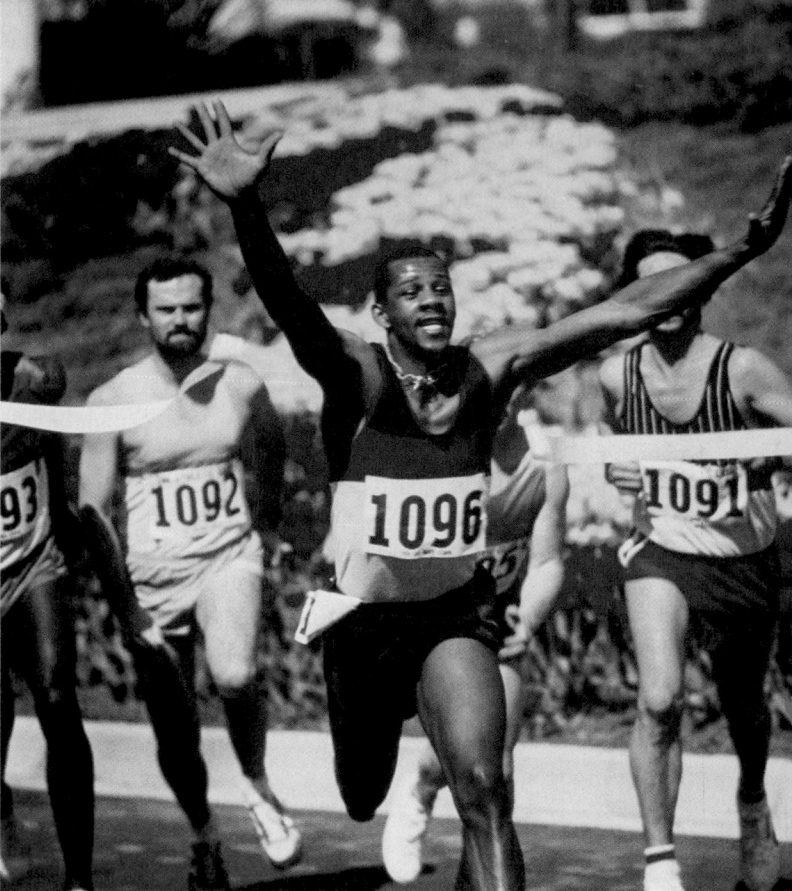

FIGURE 13.10 Sodium bicarbonate may enhance sports performance in a variety of events dependent primarily upon the lactic acid energy system (anaerobic glycolysis), such as the 400-meter sprint in track.

Various field studies have reported significant improvements in events that primarily use the lactic acid energy system, such as 400 or 800 meters in highly trained track athletes, 100-meter swims in experienced swimmers, and 5-kilometer bicycle races in trained cyclists. In support of these field studies showing improved performance following sodium bicarbonate supplementation, a laboratory study by Van Montfoort and others, comparing different sodium mixtures, reported that sodium bicarbonate improved run time to exhaustion in a test designed to evaluate the lactic acid energy system; the run to exhaustion approximated 77–82 seconds. Artioli and others reported a potential benefit of sodium bicarbonate supplementation in sports with multiple high-intensity bouts separated by brief periods of recovery. They reported that a standard bicarbonate-loading protocol (0.3 grams/kg 2 hours before testing) significantly improved performance in the latter phases of both a specific judo test and a Wingate test for anaerobic capacity of the upper arms. In a related study involving boxing, Siegler and Hirscher reported that sodium bicarbonate supplementation significantly increased the number of punches landed, or punch efficiency, during four 3-minute rounds, each separated by 1-minute seated recovery.

However, as with most research with nutritional ergogenic aids, not all studies find positive effects. For example, Kozak-Collins and her associates reported that sodium bicarbonate supplementation taken at moderate altitude did not improve the performance of competitive female cyclists on repeated 1-minute interval cycle tasks at 95 percent VO_2 max, nor did van Someren and others find any benefits on repeated 45-second high-intensity cycling bouts. Other more recent studies reported no ergogenic effects of sodium bicarbonate supplementation on anaerobic exercise tasks such as swim time performance in a simulated water polo match, run time to exhaustion at 120 percent VO_2max following multiple sprints, and total power output in 3 minutes of all-out cycling.

Although not all studies show ergogenic effects, reviews by Matson and Tran, Requena, and most recently McNaughton and others, have all concluded that sodium bicarbonate is an effective ergogenic aid in events that depend primarily on the lactic acid energy system. Matson and Tran provided the most convincing analysis, using the meta-analytic technique to statistically compare the effects reported in 29 of the best studies. In general, they noted that the ingestion of sodium bicarbonate enhanced performance, and in studies that measured exercise time to exhaustion, there was a mean improvement of 27 percent. The majority of the studies conducted subsequent to these reviews have indicated that sodium bicarbonate or sodium citrate supplementation was an effective ergogenic aid.

ATP-PCr Energy System Based on the available scientific data, alkaline salt supplementation does not appear to be an effective ergogenic aid for exercise tasks dependent primarily upon the ATP-PCr energy system; most studies have reported no beneficial effects on performance in exercise bouts lasting less than 30 seconds or in resistive exercise tasks stressing strength, power, or short-term local muscle endurance. For example, McNaughton and Cedaro reported no ergogenic effect on maximal cycle ergometer performance in either 10-second or 30-second trials. This lack of an ergogenic effect is most likely because such exercise tasks do not maximally stress the normal alkaline reserve. However, Price and others reported that ingestion of sodium bicarbonate improved performance in multiple, intermittent 14-second maximal sprints (one sprint every 3 minutes) during a 30-minute cycle ergometer trial. Moreover, Bishop and Claudius reported that sodium bicarbonate ingestion can improve intermittent-sprint performance. The test protocol involved two 36-minute halves with sprints interspersed with lesser-intensity exercise tasks, and the investigators suggested that sodium bicarbonate may be a useful supplement for team-sport athletes. Performance in these multiple sprints may have been somewhat dependent on the lactic acid energy system.

Oxygen Energy System Although sodium bicarbonate has been studied mainly for its buffering effects, the sodium content could theoretically expand blood volume and benefit aerobic endurance performance, as suggested in chapter 9. The effect of alkaline salt supplementation on performance in events that depend increasingly on the oxygen energy system, such as events approximating 4 minutes or more in duration, are equivocal.

Several studies have shown ergogenic effects. McNaughton and Cedaro reported an increased cycle ergometer work output in a 4-minute trial, as did Linossier and others in an exhausting exercise task at 120 percent of VO_2 peak lasting 4–5 minutes. Bird and others found that sodium bicarbonate supplementation improved 1,500-meter run performance, while Shave and others found that sodium citrate, as compared to a sodium chloride placebo, improved performance in a 3,000-meter run by almost 11 seconds. Using well-trained male college runners as subjects, Oopik and others found that sodium citrate supplementation improved performance in a simulated 5-kilometer treadmill run by 30 seconds. Although primarily aerobic in nature, such exercise tasks may still depend somewhat on the lactic acid energy system. However, several studies have shown ergogenic effects of alkaline salt supplementation on exercise tasks that depend primarily on oxidative metabolism. Potteiger and others reported that sodium citrate supplementation significantly improved performance by 1.7 minutes in 30-kilometer cycling performance, and McNaughton and others reported that sodium bicarbonate supplementation, compared to the placebo trial, produced a 13 percent improvement in maximal cycle ergometer work over 60 minutes.

Conversely, other studies report no ergogenic effect of alkaline salt supplementation. Potteiger and others reported no beneficial effect of sodium bicarbonate supplementation to male runners on performance in a run to exhaustion at 110 percent of the lactate threshold following 30 minutes of running at the lactate threshold. Schabort and others also found no effect of varying doses of sodium citrate (0.2, 0.4, and 0.6 g/kg) on cycling endurance. The laboratory cycling protocol was designed to compare with an actual 40-kilometer road race, with 10 sets of sprints within the 40-kilometer distance. Although the sodium citrate produced dose-dependent changes in blood alkalinity, there was no significant effect on total 40-kilometer time or on the various sprint performance times. Other studies have shown no ergogenic effects on 1,500-meter run performance or a cycling time trial lasting about 30 minutes. Additional research is needed to clarify this equivocality.

Stephens and others indicated that sodium bicarbonate ingestion has been shown to increase both muscle glycogenolysis and glycolysis during brief submaximal exercise, which could be detrimental to performance during more prolonged, exhaustive exercise. However, no studies have evaluated this potential ergolytic effect.

Is sodium bicarbonate supplementation safe and legal?

The dosage of sodium bicarbonate used in most of these studies, about 300 milligrams per kilogram body weight, appears to be effective yet medically safe. Relative to possible disadvantages, several investigators have noted that some subjects developed gastrointestinal distress, including nausea and diarrhea. Shave and others noted a high potential for gastrointestinal distress in their study that used 0.5 grams of sodium citrate per kilogram body weight, and suggested that this may limit the use of this strategy by athletes in competition. Excessive doses could lead to alkalosis, with symptoms of apathy, irritability, and possible muscle spasms.

Given the potential gastrointestinal distress often associated with an acute high dose of sodium bicarbonate, research by McNaughton and Thompson suggests that a chronic loading protocol, or taking the same total amount of sodium bicarbonate spread over a 6-day period, may be just as effective.

Use of sodium bicarbonate currently is not prohibited by the WADA. As noted, sodium bicarbonate (baking soda) use by athletes has been dubbed *soda loading,* possibly to liken it to *carbohydrate loading.* As you may recall, the purpose of carbohydrate loading is to increase the storage of muscle and liver glycogen as a means to prevent fatigue in prolonged endurance events. Soda loading is viewed by some in a similar context, an attempt to increase the supply of a natural body ingredient helpful in delaying fatigue. However, because sodium bicarbonate may be regarded as a drug, it remains to be seen whether this technique will be deemed illegal. Tim Noakes, in the newest edition of his classic text *Lore of Running,* indicated that the use of sodium bicarbonate may be prohibited by the International Olympic Committee in the near future. Currently there is no test to detect its use, except for urinary pH, which can also be affected by some antacids, and at present sodium bicarbonate is considered to be legal for use in sports.

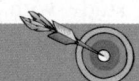

Key Concepts

▶ Sodium bicarbonate supplementation appears to be an effective ergogenic aid in exercise tasks that depend primarily upon the lactic acid energy system (anaerobic glycolysis), such as a 400-meter dash in track.

▶ Ingestion of sodium bicarbonate is generally regarded as safe, but may cause acute gastrointestinal distress and diarrhea. Supplementation over a longer time frame may be effective and less likely to cause intestinal problems.

Anabolic Hormones and Dietary Supplements: Ergogenic Effects and Health Implications

Several natural hormones in the body may exert significant anabolic effects on body composition by stimulating protein synthesis, particularly human growth hormone (HGH), insulin, insulin-like growth factors (IGF-1), and testosterone. As noted in previous chapters, several nutrient supplements, such as specific amino acids, have been utilized in attempts to increase the secretion of these hormones for anabolic purposes. Two of these hormones, HGH and testosterone, as well as drugs patterned after testosterone, have been used directly to increase muscle mass. Additionally, several prohormones that may be converted into testosterone have been marketed as dietary supplements, and some herbal supplements are marketed for their potential to stimulate testosterone production.

It should be noted that the WADA prohibits the use of the anabolic hormones discussed in this section, including human growth hormone, anabolic/androgenic steroids, and anabolic prohormone dietary supplements.

Is human growth hormone (HGH) an effective, safe, and legal ergogenic aid?

HGH is a natural hormone, which is secreted by the anterior pituitary gland and then circulates via the bloodstream to affect most cells in the body. HGH increases insulin-like growth factor (IGF-1) secretion from the liver, and within other tissues, such as muscle, which may function as an autocrine and work directly in the muscle. IGF-1 mediates the various metabolic effects of HGH. Exercise stimulates release of HGH, which, according to Widdowson and others, may persist over 24 hours and potentially contribute to the physiologic changes induced by exercise training.

HGH is an anabolic hormone that stimulates bone growth and the development of muscle tissue through its effects on protein, carbohydrate, and fat metabolism. A detailed discussion of the role of HGH is beyond the scope of this text. It is important to note, however, that extensive research into its effects began only when genetically engineered versions (recombinant HGH or rHGH) of the natural body hormone became available in the early 1990s. rHGH was developed for medical applications, primarily for children and older adults with HGH deficiency. rHGH may optimize growth in young children and may confer some health benefits on aging adults. Available data suggest that in elderly men, who normally have reduced levels of HGH, injections of the hormone may help improve body composition and functional capacity. Meta-analyses and reviews, such as those by Rubeck and others, Widdowson and Gibney, and Widdowson and others, reported that rHGH therapy in individuals who suffered from HGH deficiency helped to improve body composition, such as decreases in body fat and increases in lean body mass, and increase aerobic exercise capacity, including VO₂max. However, these investigators noted that rHGH therapy failed to increase muscle strength, possibly because some studies have found that the increase in lean body mass was primarily water, not muscle tissue.

Whether or not rHGH injections enhance exercise performance is a subject of debate. In general, the available research does not support an anabolic or ergogenic effect of rHGH supplementation in younger individuals. For example, Yarasheski and others studied the effect of rHGH versus a placebo on adult males who weight-trained for 12 weeks. They reported significant increases in lean body mass in the group receiving rHGH, but there were no significant increases in skeletal muscle protein synthesis and size, as measured by magnetic resonance imaging, or in muscular strength, over the effects produced by weight training alone in the placebo group. Other studies have supported this general finding with resistance-trained athletes. In her review, Anne Loucks concluded that supraphysiological doses of rHGH have only increased total body water, lean body mass, and whole-body protein synthesis in general without specifically increasing skeletal muscle protein synthesis or skeletal muscle mass, strength, or power in untrained young men or experienced young weight lifters. The review by Dean also concludes that there is no evidence of increased muscle strength with rHGH use in trained athletes.

However, a few studies have suggested that short-term rHGH use may benefit physical performance. For example, using recreationally trained young male and female athletes as subjects, Meinhardt and others found that rHGH injected subcutaneously (2 milligrams daily for 8 weeks) significantly reduced fat mass and significantly increased sprint capacity. However, the increase in sprint capacity was not maintained 6 weeks after discontinuation of the injections.

In a baseball scandal in the United States, some professional athletes admitted using rHGH to train harder and recover more rapidly, and anecdotal reports suggest that it may work for these intended purposes. In his review of rHGH as an ergogenic aid, Holt notes that although most scientific studies have not shown a performance-enhancing effect, athletes continue to use it. Based on his review, he believes the scientists are wrong. Time will tell.

Although athletes may continue to use rHGH, that may not be a wise idea based on its potential health risks and permissibility in sports. The potential adverse health effects of rHGH are substantial, including insulin resistance, high blood pressure, and increased risk of congestive heart failure. Liu and others indicated that because rHGH therapy is associated with increased rates of adverse events, it cannot be recommended as an antiaging therapy. Tentori and Graziani suggest that growth hormone or its mediator, IGF-1, have been associated with colon, breast, and prostate cancers. Most researchers caution that other long-term health risks of HGH administration are unknown. This is particularly distressing as one report indicated that approximately 5 percent of high school students have used HGH.

Use of rHGH is prohibited by the WADA. Although Guha and others noted that although detection of the application of rHGH is difficult, possibly because of its rapid half-life, some tests are available. They also note that as the tests for detection of rHGH doping become more sophisticated, athletes may turn to doping with recombinant rHIGF-1. Research is underway to develop tests for IGF-1 abuse in athletes. Currently, supplements are marketed as IGF on the Internet.

Some dietary supplements are marketed as HGH products, such as HGH Surge™, but they contain only nutrients, such as amino acids and chromium, that are theorized to be ergogenic. However, as noted in previous chapters, such nutrients have not been shown to have anabolic effects and some may be contaminated with illegal drugs that may lead to a positive doping test.

Are testosterone and anabolic/androgenic steroids (AAS) effective, safe, and legal ergogenic aids?

Testosterone, the male steroid sex hormone produced by the testes, was one of the first anabolic agents used in attempts to enhance physical performance, possibly as early as the 1936 Berlin Olympic Games. As documented in the study by Bhasin and the review by Evans, testosterone is a very effective ergogenic aid, increasing lean muscle mass, decreasing body fat, and increasing strength even without resistance training; these anabolic effects were augmented in subjects who also trained. Rogerson and others reported that testosterone injection once per week to resistance-trained individuals increased muscular strength and 10-second cycle sprint performance in 3–6 weeks. Testosterone must be injected because ingested testosterone will be catabolized by digestive enzymes. Although injected testosterone use is still prevalent among various athletic groups, oral drug forms of testosterone have been developed, as noted here.

Testosterone therapy has been studied for its health potential as well. Testosterone levels decrease in the aging male, accompanied by a host of physiological function changes that may be related to impaired health. In a review, Bain cited numerous adverse symptoms, such as frailty, fatigue, decreased energy, decreased motivation, cognitive impairment, decreased self-confidence, depression, and irritability, as well as increased risk for the metabolic syndrome, type 2 diabetes, anemia, stroke, and coronary heart disease. However, Bain also noted that treament of the aging male with testosterone therapy is controversial, as its use also may be associated with a number of possible health problems, similar to those associated with use of anabolic/androgenic steroids, as discussed later. Nevertheless, Bain suggests that short-term (4–6 months) therapeutic trial may be justified for some older men, particularly those at low risk for prostate cancer, which may be aggravated by excess testosterone. Moreover, Basaria and others noted that a study with testosterone supplementation to older men had to be canceled early because there was a significantly higher rate of adverse cardiovascular events in the testosterone group than in the placebo group. Nevertheless, the authors noted that several limitations in the study prevented the drawing of broader inferences about the safety of testosterone therapy.

Anabolic/androgenic steroids (AAS) represent a class of synthetic drugs designed to mimic the effects of testosterone. The chemical structure of testosterone may be modified in attempts to maximize the anabolic muscle-building effects and minimize the androgenic male secondary sex characteristics; both oral and injectable AAS have been developed.

In the United States, AAS are classified as Schedule III drugs under the Controlled Substances Act, and may be used in testosterone therapy for aging adults, as noted earlier.

AAS are the drugs of choice for many strength athletes and bodybuilders to improve performance and appearance. AAS have been used by professional athletes for years, as documented in the revealing book, *Wild Times, Rampant 'Roids, Smash Hits, and How Baseball Got Big,* written by a former professional baseball player. Congress and the FBI have investigated anabolic steroid use among prominent baseball players.

Bahrke and others noted surveys indicating that the use of AAS is also prevalent among adolescent athletes, particularly boys in strength-related sports. Their use is even common among young male nonathletes, and increasing numbers of teenage girls, according to Yesalis and others, who desire to increase muscle mass for an enhanced self-image; some may possess muscle dysmorphia, a condition discussed in chapter 12. Faigenbaum and others reported AAS use by middle-school students, ages 9–13, in the belief that they improved sports performance and physical appearance. In general, surveys indicate that approximately 4–6 percent of boys and 1–2 percent of girls have used AAS.

Although resistance training does not cause drug use, DuRant and others noted that adolescent AAS users in the United States, both athletes and nonathletes, are more likely to engage in strength training. AAS use is also associated with use of other recreational drugs. Thus, young adolescent athletes and nonathletes engaged in strength training should be educated about the health risks associated with AAS use.

The effects of AAS on body composition and strength have been studied rather extensively, and although there may be some flaws in the experimental designs used, most reviewers agree that AAS use may increase muscle mass and strength and decrease total body fat, a judgment supported by reviews of laboratory studies that included meta-analysis as part of the evaluative criteria. Schroeder and others found that AAS supplementation was also effective with healthy older men, significantly increasing muscle mass and strength after only 6 weeks. The increased muscle mass may be attributed to hypertrophy and the formation of new muscle fibers, in which key roles are played by the androgen receptors, as depicted in figure 13.11.

Baume and others note that although AAS are used mainly by strength athletes, endurance athletes have also used AAS because they are theorized to facilitate a better recovery and thus permit a higher training load. However, they found that compared to a placebo, two different anabolic steroids administered 12 times during a month of hard endurance training had no effect on standardized treadmill running performance test or blood markers for recovery from exercise. Research with AAS and endurance performance in young athletes is limited, but that which is available does not support an ergogenic effect. However, Sattler and others reported that supplemental testosterone increased aerobic endurance in older men, which may have been associated with the accompanying significant reduction in body fat.

AAS use has been associated with a number of medical problems, as documented in reviews by Hartgens and Kuipers, Talih and others, and Yesalis and Bahrke. Some are relatively minor, such as acne and loss of hair. AAS may also adversely affect psychological processes, leading to increased aggression, hostility, depression, and possible suicide attempts, and an increased tendency to commit violent crimes, including homicide. Continued use may predispose

adults to coronary heart disease by inducing structural changes in the heart muscle, decreasing HDL-cholesterol, and increasing blood pressure, as documented in both epidemiological and experimental studies and reviewed by Nnakwe. Prolonged steroid use may possibly lead to impaired development of tendons, decreasing their strength and contributing to a potential for rupture. Prolonged use has resulted in severe liver diseases, including cancer. Anabolic steroids may cause premature cessation of bone growth in children and adolescents and may result in the appearance of several male secondary sex characteristics in females, some of which may be irreversible, such as deepening of the voice. Table 13.4 highlights many of the health problems associated with abuse of AAS.

TABLE 13.4 Possible health risks associated with use of anabolic/androgenic steroids (AAS)

Cosmetic-related effects

Facial and body acne
Female-like breast enlargement in males (gynecomastia)
Premature baldness
Masculinization in females
Facial and body hair growth in females
Premature closure of growth centers in adolescents, leading to stunted growth
Deepening of the voice in females

Psychological effects

Increased aggressiveness and possible violent behavior

Reproductive effects

Reduction of testicular size
Reduction of sperm production
Decreased libido
Impotence in males
Enlargement of the prostate gland
Enlargement of the clitoris

Cardiovascular risk factors and diseases

Atherosclerotic serum lipid profile
    Decreased HDL-cholesterol
    Increased LDL-cholesterol
High blood pressure
Impaired glucose tolerance
Increased size of left ventricle
Stroke
Heart disease

Liver function

Jaundice
Peliosis hepatis (blood-filled cysts)
Liver tumors

Athletic injuries

Tendon rupture

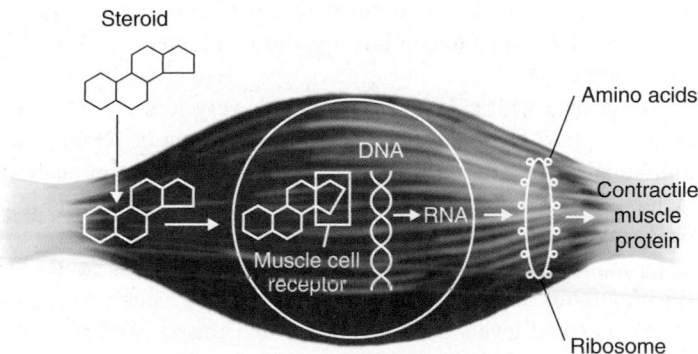

FIGURE 13.11 Anabolic steroids picked up by androgen in the cell nucleus initiate the process of protein formation in cells such as muscle fibers, leading to muscle hypertrophy.

However, many of the adverse health effects of AAS use appear to be reversible. For example, Hartgens and others found that bodybuilders who cycled off AAS steroids for 3 months had similar lipoprotein profiles and liver enzymes as their non-drug-using counterparts. Moreover, earlier reviews noted that although the short-term health effects of AAS have been increasingly studied and reviewed, and while AAS use has been associated with adverse and even fatal effects, the incidence of serious effects thus far reported has been extremely low. In a review, van Amsterdam and others indicated that severe side effects of AAS use appear only following prolonged use at high doses, and their occurrence is limited. They conclude that, based on the scores for acute and chronic adverse health effects, the prevalence of use, social harm, and criminality, AAS were ranked a group of drugs with a relatively low harm. Nevertheless, Urhausen and others reported that several years after discontinuation of anabolic steroid abuse, strength athletes (bodybuilders and powerlifters) who used AAS showed a slight concentric left ventricular hypertrophy in comparison with AAS-free strength athletes; left ventricular hypertrophy increases the risk of heart attack.

Because of the potential health risks, one of the risk-reduction objectives in *Healthy People 2020* is the reduction of AAS use among students in eighth through twelfth grades, where current use ranges from 1.3 to 2.2 percent. Moreover, the U.S. Congress has passed legislation to classify AAS as controlled substances, thus limiting their production and distribution by pharmaceutical companies. Penalties may be severe. According to Melnik and others, some AAS users obtain illegal prescriptions from physicians. However, many obtain these drugs illegally on the black market where quality is not controlled, and chemical analysis has revealed some potentially hazardous constituents in these "homemade" drugs. AAS users are known to use other illicit drugs as well, each carrying independent health risks. As is obvious, the use of testosterone or AAS for the purpose of gaining body weight and strength is not recommended.

The WADA prohibits the use of AAS in training and competition. The American College of Sports Medicine (ACSM) and the National Strength and Conditioning Association (NSCA) have developed position stands regarding the use of AAS in sports. Both groups condemn their use on the basis of ethics, the ideals of fair play in competition, and concerns for the athlete's health. The NSCA indicates that optimizing nutritional strategies for athletes is a key to preventing AAS use and abuse, and such strategies for strength/power athletes have been presented in chapter 12. Although an extensive discussion of AAS is beyond the scope of this text, the ACSM and NSCA reports provide detailed reviews for the interested reader, as does the most recent review by Yesalis and Bahrke.

Are anabolic prohormone dietary supplements effective, safe, and legal ergogenic aids?

Several dietary supplements marketed to athletes as potent anabolic agents are of special interest, particularly dehydroepiandrosterone (DHEA), androstenedione, and related compounds.

These supplements are classified as prohormones because they are precursors for testosterone and are thus theorized to increase muscle mass and decrease body fat. They may be derived from certain plants, such as wild yams. Although these prohormones have been marketed as dietary supplements, in 2005 the FDA classified them as controlled drugs, similar to anabolic steroids.

Dehydroepiandrosterone (DHEA) and its sulfated metabolite (DHEAS) are produced in the body by the adrenal and gonadal glands, and may be converted into androstenedione with subsequent conversion to testosterone in peripheral tissues, including fat and muscle tissue. Body levels of DHEA are high in young adulthood and gradually decrease to low levels with aging. Although Abbasi and others reported a low, but significant, inverse relationship between natural DHEA levels and body fat in men aged 60–80 years, there are few data supporting beneficial effects of DHEA supplementation. Using well-controlled experimental designs, studies by Wallace and Brown and their associates revealed no significant effects of DHEA supplementation (50–100 milligrams/day for 8–12 weeks) on serum testosterone levels, lean body mass, or muscular strength in either healthy middle-aged or young men involved in resistance training. In a more prolonged 2-year study, Nair and others reported no effect on body composition, physical performance, insulin sensitivity, or quality of life in elderly men and women who received DHEA supplementation.

DHEA has also been marketed as an anti-aging agent to help prevent the development of chronic diseases, but in one review, Sirrs and Bebb indicated that no good scientific data support this speculation. They caution against use of DHEA supplements, as high serum DHEA levels have been associated with several health risks, including several forms of cancer. Nevertheless, a study by Villareal and others provided some preliminary data supporting positive effects of DHEA supplementation on bone mineral density, body fat, and lean body mass in elderly subjects with very low levels of natural DHEA. Kenny and others reported that DHEA supplementation (50 milligrams daily for 6 months) improved muscle strength and physical function in frail older women who participated in 90-minute twice-weekly exercise sessions, but had no effect on bone mineral density, even though calcium and vitamin D supplements were also provided. Although such effects may help prevent falls and fractures in the elderly, these research groups indicated that more defined and specific research is needed before DHEA supplementation may be recommended as a standard treatment.

These data with elderly subjects with very low DHEA levels do not support DHEA supplementation to young or middle-aged individuals. For example, Conrad Earnest, an expert in anabolic dietary supplements, reported that DHEA supplementation at relatively low doses (50–150 milligrams) does not enhance serum testosterone in young men. Moreover, Acacio and others found that six months of supplementation with DHEA to young men aged 18–42 elevated levels of a metabolite that raised concerns about the potential negative impact of DHEA supplementation on the prostate gland. The Consumers Union advised that individuals avoid DHEA supplementation, as there is not enough evidence concerning its effectiveness or safety.

Androstenedione and related compounds, such as androstenediol and norandrostenediol, are potent anabolic agents, one step removed from the formation of testosterone. Androstenedione received considerable notoriety during the 1998 baseball season when Mark McGwire, who established a home run record at that time, acknowledged using the dietary supplement. Subsequently, androstenedione-related products flooded the marketplace for resistance-trained individuals, even though no reputable research was available supporting beneficial effects.

Doses of androstenedione and related androgens used in studies varied, usually between 100 to 300 milligrams per day. Studies using the higher doses generally showed an increase in serum testosterone. Leder and others, although finding no significant effects of a 100-milligram dose, reported significant increases in serum testosterone in adult men following a 300-milligram dose, but no exercise performance was measured. Earnest and others also reported significant, but small, increases in total testosterone with a 200-milligram dose of androstenedione, but not androstenediol, supplementation. In a study with young women, Brown and others reported that androstenedione intake (100 or 300 milligrams) significantly increased serum testosterone concentrations.

In general, most studies that have evaluated the ergogenic effects of androstenedione supplementation have shown no beneficial effects. In a short-term study, Rasmussen and others found no effect of oral androstenedione supplementation (100 milligrams/day for 5 days) on serum testosterone or muscle protein anabolism in young men. In a more prolonged study, Wallace and others reported no significant effects of androstenedione supplementation (100 milligrams/day for 12 weeks) on serum testosterone levels, lean body mass, or muscular strength in resistance-trained middle-aged men. Using three individual 100-milligram and rostenedione doses daily (total 300 milligrams/day), King and others reported no significant effects on serum testosterone, body fat, lean body mass, muscle fiber diameter, or muscular strength in young men during 8 weeks of resistance training.

More recent reviews also do not support an ergogenic effect of androstenedione and its congeners. Earnest noted that even though increases in testosterone following androstenedione ingestion have been found to be statistically significant, they have not been accompanied by favorable changes in protein synthesis or metabolism, muscle mass or lean body mass, or strength. Brown and others also concluded that the use of prohormone nutritional supplements does not produce either anabolic or ergogenic effects in men. These findings have also been supported in reviews by Ziegenfuss and Maughan.

Use of androstenedione and its congeners may be associated with increased health risks. Earnest indicated that androstenedione supplementation has been associated with impaired lipid metabolism, such as decreased HDL-cholesterol and increased LDL-cholesterol, which might increase risk for cardiovascular disease. Several studies have reported significant increases in estrogen hormones (estradiol or estrone), which could exert feminizing effects in males, such as gynecomastia (breast enlargement). Other adverse effects on gonadal hormones may be associated with testicular shrinkage and infertility. Leder also notes that women and children who use such supplements may be at risk. Unfortunately, given the recency of such supplements, no long-term safety data are available.

For athletes who may be tested for doping, the use of DHEA or androstenedione and related prohormones has been banned by the WADA and the International Olympic Committee; their use has also been banned by other sports organizations, including the National Collegiate Athletic Association and the National Football League. Although anabolic metabolic prohormones are currently banned for sale in the United States, a number of substitutes for these products are being marketed on the Internet. For example, Testosterone Factors™ is a blend of vitamins, amino acids, and herbal ingredients, none of which is banned. However, Maughan notes that some apparently legitimate dietary supplements on sale contain ingredients that are not declared on the label but that are prohibited by the doping regulations of the WADA and the International Olympic Committee. For example, Epstein and Dohrmann noted that in one study, 25 percent of 58 sports supplements tested contained steroids or stimulants. Geyer and others secured 634 nutritional supplements from 13 countries, and 14.8 percent contained anabolic androgenic steroids not declared on the label. The administration of some of the supplements resulted in positive doping tests.

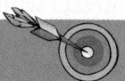

Key Concepts

▶ The use of anabolic drugs or hormones to increase body weight may be effective but may also lead to a variety of health problems. The WADA prohibits the use of anabolic hormones in sports training or competition.

▶ Research has shown that prohormone dietary supplements marketed as anabolic agents, such as androstenedione, do not effectively increase muscle mass or strength. Moreover, such prohormones have been classified as controlled anabolic steroids and their use is illegal and banned by the WADA.

Check for Yourself

▶ Go to the Internet search engine www.google.com, type in anabolic steroids, and check the advertisements and information related to laws and use of such products. Share the information with your classmates. Now that androstenediol products are illegal, check advertisements for various replacements, such as androstenetrione, the "Testosterone Booster."

Ginseng, Herbals, and Exercise and Sports Performance

Herbs contain various nutrients and phytonutrients, such as vitamins, minerals, and antioxidants, that may be part of a healthful diet. Additionally, herbal products have been used for centuries for their purported health benefits; St. John's wort has been used to treat depression, kava kava to reduce stress and anxiety, echinacea to reduce symptoms of the common cold, and numerous herbals to promote weight loss. In some countries, many herbals are regulated as drugs, but in the United States most are regulated as dietary supplements. A detailed discussion of the health effects of herbals is beyond the scope of this text. In general, however, well-controlled research with most herbal supplements and health outcomes is limited. Some may be effective and others not, and in many cases the research findings are equivocal. For example, Shah and others, in a meta-analysis, found that echinacea decreased the odds of developing the common cold by 58 percent and the duration of a cold by 1.4 days and concluded that the published evidence supports echinacea's benefit in decreasing the incidence and duration of the common cold. In contrast, Barrett and others, in their meta-analysis, reported that the research results are inconsistent and that although the preventive effects of echinacea might exist, they have not been shown in rigorous randomized trials.

Numerous herbal supplements are marketed for weight control, but the Consumers Union indicated that there is no good clinical evidence for various supplements, including herbals such as Hoodia, promoted for weight loss. Chitturi and Farrell noted that some herbal remedies marketed for weight reduction have been causally associated with significant liver injury. Moreover, the Consumers Union also notes that herbal supplements can interact dangerously with medications. For example, echinacea may interact with various drugs, including those for allergies, anxiety, asthma, diabetes, and high serum cholesterol. Individuals using herbal products for health purposes should consult with their physicians. Also recall that ephedra, an herbal supplement, may be dangerous in and of itself.

Herbals have also been marketed as ergogenic aids for athletes. Unfortunately, with the exception of ginseng and related products, limited research has evaluated their ability to enhance exercise or sport performance.

Do ginseng or ciwujia enhance exercise or sport performance?

Ginseng and ciwujia are comparable herbs, and both have been studied for their potential effects on exercise or sport performance.

Ginseng Extracts derived from the plant family Araliaceae contain numerous chemicals that may influence human physiology, the most important being the glycosides, or ginsenosides. Collectively, these extracts are referred to as **ginseng,** and their physiologic effects vary depending on the plant species, the part of the plant used, and the place of origin. The most common forms of ginseng include Chinese or Korean (*Panax ginseng*), American (*Panax quinquefolium*), Japanese (*Panax japonicum*), and Russian/Siberian (*Eleutherococcus senticosus*). *Eleutherococcus senticosus* is a totally different plant from Araliaceae, but it is recognized by some as a legitimate form of ginseng and its ginsenosides are also referred to as eleutherosides. The type and amount of ginsenosides present vary greatly among the different forms of ginseng.

Using such labels as Ginseng Energy, ginseng has been marketed in various forms as a means of enhancing health and physical performance (see figure 13.12). Although the underlying mechanisms are unknown, ginseng is believed to influence neural

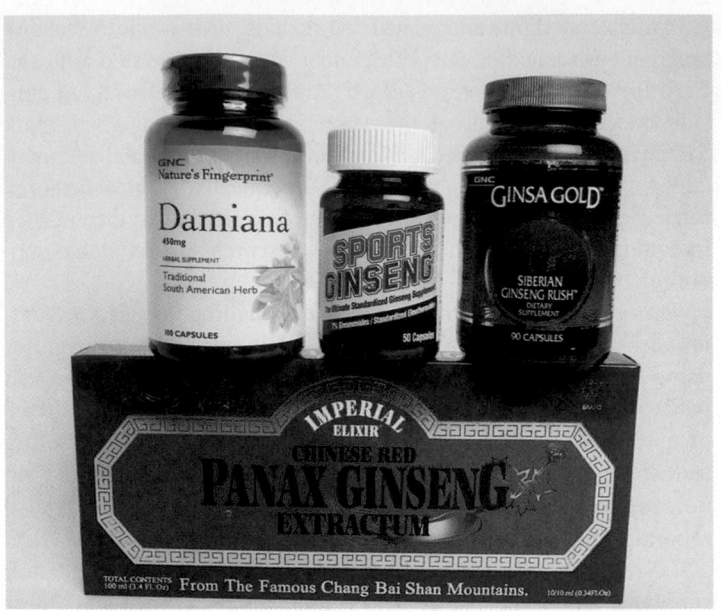

FIGURE 13.12 Various ginseng products are available as dietary supplements, some being marketed directly to athletes.

and hormonal activity in the body and has also been theorized to enhance the immune system. The most prevalent theory suggests that ginseng may stimulate the hypothalamus, the part of the brain that controls the pituitary gland, an endocrine gland often referred to as the master gland. The pituitary gland releases hormones that influence other endocrine glands in the body, such as the adrenal gland. The adrenal gland releases cortisol, a hormone involved in the response to stress. Russian sports scientists conducted much of the early exercise-related research with ginseng, and used the term "adaptogens" to characterize its ability to increase resistance to the catabolic effects of stress.

The Russians believed that ginseng helped develop resistance not only to mental stress but also to the physical stress of intense exercise training. Other theories suggest that ginseng supplementation may influence physical performance in other ways as well, such as increased cardiac function, blood flow, and oxygen transport during exercise; increased oxygen utilization and decreased lactic acid levels during exercise; enhanced muscle glycogen synthesis after exercise; and a positive effect on nitrogen or protein balance. In essence, given these theorized antistress effects, restorative effects, and metabolic effects, ginseng supplementation is theorized to enhance sport performance by allowing athletes to train more intensely and by influencing physiological processes associated with an antifatiguing effect that increase stamina during competition. It should be noted that although numerous theories have been advanced in attempts to explain the alleged ergogenic effects of ginseng supplementation, an underlying mechanism has yet to be determined.

Although numerous studies investigated the ergogenic possibilities of ginseng supplementation, few were well controlled. Research design flaws included no control or placebo group, no double-blind protocol, no randomization of order of treatment, and no statistical analysis. Highlighting these methodological problems in an extensive 1994 review of the ergogenic effect of ginseng supplementation, Michael Bahrke and William Morgan concluded that there is a lack of controlled research demonstrating the ability of ginseng to improve or prolong performance.

Subsequent to the review by Bahrke and Morgan, several well-controlled studies evaluated the ergogenic effects of both standardized ginseng extracts and commercial products and reported no significant effects. For example, Dowling and others reported no effect of *Eleutherococcus senticosus* on metabolic (oxygen uptake and lactic acid accumulation), physiologic (heart rate and ventilation), or psychologic (ratings of perceived exertion) responses to submaximal and maximal running. Using a similar research protocol but with cycling, Engels and Wirth reported no ergogenic effect of *Panax ginseng*. Other well-controlled studies by Engels and his associates have found no ergogenic effect of *Panax ginseng* on high-intensity, interval anaerobic exercise protocols. However, Ziemba and others reported that although *Panax ginseng* did not influence exercise capacity in soccer players, it did improve multiple-choice reaction time before and during a cycling exercise task. Such an effect may be of benefit to athletes who must react quickly in sports. This finding merits additional research.

Overall, in a 2009 update of their previous review, Bahrke and others noted that although more well-controlled research is needed, they again concluded that there is an absence of compelling research evidence regarding the efficacy of ginseng use to improve physical performance in humans. Goulet and Dionne reviewed studies evaluating the effect of *Eleutherococcus senticosus* on exercise performance, and concluded that it offers no advantage during exercise endurance tests ranging in duration from 6 to 120 minutes. Most recently, Palisin and Stacy concluded that ginsengs cannot be recommended to improve athletic performance.

Most commercial ginseng preparations appear to have relatively low acute or chronic toxicity when taken in dosages recommended by the manufacturer. Coon and Ernst noted that the most commonly experienced adverse effects of *Panax ginseng* are headache and sleep and gastrointestinal disorders. These effects may be attributed to the postulated stimulant effect of ginseng, or possibly to additional substances in the commercial preparation, such as the stimulant ephedrine. In general, however, they found that *Panax ginseng,* when taken alone and not combined with other substances, is rarely associated with adverse effects. For athletes involved in sports that may use drug testing, the use of ginseng products containing ephedrine could lead to disqualification.

Some research suggests that long-term ginseng supplementation may prevent some adverse effects of stress on the immune system. Although not studied extensively in athletes, a healthier immune system could help prevent illness or some of the symptoms of the overtraining syndrome during high-intensity training. However, Engels and others reported that *Panax ginseng* had no significant effect on immune functions during recovery from intense anaerobic exercise.

Given the available scientific evidence, ginseng supplements cannot be recommended. The consumer should also be aware that commercial ginseng products may suffer from quality control. An assay of 50 commercial ginseng preparations indicated that more than 10 percent of the products contained no detectable ginsenosides, and the amount in the remaining products varied from 1.9–9.0 percent. Many commercial products contain alcohol.

Individuals who desire to experiment with long-term ginseng supplementation should consult with their physicians, because ginseng use may exacerbate various health problems, such as high blood pressure.

Ciwujia **Ciwujia,** a Chinese herb, is similar to ginseng. Cheuvront and others indicate that ciwujia is extracted from Araliaceae, the same plant family as *Panax ginseng*. Along with Plowman and others, they also note that it may be derived from the leaves of *Eleutherococcus senticosus*. Ciwujia was first marketed as the commercial sports supplement, Endurox™. Currently it is marketed as Endurox Excel, whose advertisements suggest that it can increase fat oxidation (possibly sparing muscle glycogen), reduce lactate accumulation, raise the anaerobic threshold, lower the heart rate while maintaining the same level of workout intensity, and speed workout recovery. However, most of the claims for ciwujia are based on clinical trials with poor experimental designs. Plowman and others noted that none of the studies followed a randomized crossover or double-blind protocol, nor was the use of a placebo mentioned. None have been published in peer-reviewed journals.

Studies by Plowman, Cheuvront, and their associates, using double-blind, placebo-controlled, crossover experimental designs and published in peer-reviewed journals, reported that supplementation with Endurox™ (800 mg for 7–10 days) had no significant effect on heart rate, oxygen consumption, respiratory exchange ratio (a measure of fat oxidation), lactic acid accumulation, or ratings of perceived exertion during either cycle ergometer or stair-climbing exercise. The investigators indicated that their studies did not verify the claims made for Endurox™.

Based on the available evidence, products containing ciwujia do not appear to enhance exercise performance, and thus are not recommended for use by endurance athletes.

What herbals are effective ergogenic aids?

As noted earlier, caffeine may be derived from various herbals, such as guarana and the kola nut, whereas ephedra is a constituent of ma huang. Other than these and ginseng, athletes have experimented with a variety of other herbals, including cayenne for energy and gamma-oryzanol to increase muscle mass.

Kundrat, in a report on herbs and athletes, indicated that double-blind, placebo-controlled human research on herb use by athletes is limited or nonexistent. One reason may be that, at least in the United States, herbs are regulated as dietary supplements and are not required to be standardized, so there is little consistency among different brands. Moreover, herbal sport supplements may often contain several herbals and other substances in a commercial product, so it is difficult to isolate the potential ergogenic effect of a single ingredient. Studies conducted with such commercial herbal-based sports supplements, such as the study by Earnest and others, generally report no significant ergogenic effects.

Nevertheless, several reviews of herbal supplementation and exercise performance are available. In their review, Williams and Branch noted that much of what we know about the efficacy of herbal supplements as ergogenics is based on anecdotal data and poorly controlled studies. However, based on their analysis, they concluded that none of the following herbals have sufficient research support as a means of enhancing exercise or sport performance: bee pollen, capsicum, gamma-oryzanol, ginkgo biloba, kava kava, St. John's wort, *Tribulus terrestris,* and yohimbine. Recent studies support this viewpoint. For example, Neychev and Mitev found no effect of *Tribulus terrestris* supplementation for 4 weeks on testosterone or androstenedione production in young men, its theorized mechanism of action. Moreover, Rogerson and others reported no effects of *Tribulus terrestris* supplementation (450 mg/day for 5 weeks) on lean muscle mass and strength in Australian elite male rugby league players. Ostojic studied the effect of yohimbine in professional soccer players, who consumed 20 milligrams per day for 21 days. There was no significant effect on body mass, muscle mass, or performance indicators (bench and leg press, vertical jump, dribble and power test results, shuttle run) in these elite athletes.

Several other herbals have been studied for their purported ergogenic potential. The herb *Cordyceps sinensis* is a health tonic from China; although it is rare, a synthetic version is now available; one version is CordyMax Cs-4. *Cordyceps sinensis* is theorized to have favorable effects on the heart and circulation to improve oxidative capacity and endurance performance. However, Parcell and others reported that 5 weeks of CordyMax Cs-4 supplementation had no effect on aerobic capacity of endurance-trained male cyclists.

Rhodiola rosea, like ginseng, is categorized as an adaptogen, and has been theorized to enhance endurance performance through a stimulating effect. Walker and others also noted that the herb is purported to enhance physical performance by improving adenosine triphosphate (ATP) turnover. In a preliminary study, De Bock and others found that an acute dose (200 milligrams) of *Rhodiola rosea* improved time to exhaustion by 3 percent on a cycle ergometer, but there was no significant effect following 4 weeks of supplementation with 200 milligrams daily. Colson and others reported that *Rhodiola rosea,* in a product that also contained *Cordyceps sinensis,* had no effect on muscle-tissue oxygen saturation or on cycling time to exhaustion. In their study, De Bock and others reported no effect on maximal strength or various measures of reaction time or movement time. Walker and others, using nuclear magnetic resonance spectroscopy, reported no significant effects of *Rhodiola rosea* supplementation on ATP turnover during a wrist flexion test to exhaustion, nor were ratings of perceived exertion (RPE) or time to exhaustion different between the placebo and experimental sessions. Skarpanska-Stejnborn and others, using members of the Polish rowing team as subjects, noted that

although 4 weeks of *Rhodiola rosea* supplementation increased plasma antioxidant levels, there was no effect on oxidative damage induced by exhaustive exercise. Overall, research findings do not support an ergogenic effect of *Rhodiola rosea* supplementation to trained athletes.

Epigallocatechin-3-gallate (EGCG) is an extract from green tea, a flavonol that functions as an antioxidant and has been theorized by some to enhance exercise performance by reducing oxidative stress. Richards and others reported a significant increase in maximal oxygen uptake following consumption of seven separate doses (135 mg each) over the course of 2 days. However, there were no significant changes in maximal work rate, maximal heart rate, or maximal respiratory exchange ratio, nor any differences in maximal cardiac output in a subgroup of subjects. Given the nonsignificant effects on most study variables, the increase in maximal oxygen uptake may have been a chance finding. Moreover, several other studies reported no significant effect on endurance exercise. Dean and others, in a well-designed crossover study, reported no significant effect of EGCG supplementation (270 milligrams daily) over the course of 6 days on a self-paced, 40-kilometer cycling time trial following 60 minutes of moderate-intensity cycling. In a similar study, Eichenberger and others also reported no significant effect of 3 weeks of green tea extract supplementation on a 30-minute cycling time trial following 2 hours of moderate-intensity cycling, nor was there any effect on markers of energy metabolism. Overall, current research does not support an ergogenic effect of EGCG supplementation.

Cytoseira canariensis has been marketed as a new sports supplement designed to increase muscle mass and decrease body fat by inhibiting myostatin. Myostatin is a protein known as a growth and differentiation factor, and its role is to inhibit (not promote) the growth of muscles. Theoretically, by inhibiting the effects of myostatin, muscle growth may be increased. However, Darryn Willoughby, an exercise scientist at Baylor University, reported that 1,200 milligrams/day of *Cystoseira canariensis* supplementation during 12 weeks of resistance training had no effect on serum myostatin levels, nor did it have any effect on muscle mass, muscle strength, or body fat.

As noted in chapter 8, increasing erythropoietin (EPO) levels by living at altitude may confer a beneficial effect on oxygen transport during exercise by increasing production of red blood cells. In one study, Whitehead and others found that subjects receiving 8,000 mg of echinacea daily for 28 days significantly increased their serum erythropoietin levels. However, there was no change in red blood cells or hemoglobin concentrations. This is an interesting finding, and more research is recommended to evaluate the ergogenicity of echinacea supplementation.

Kundrat indicated that athletes should be concerned about the safety of herbals, as there may be some side effects or herb-drug interactions. For athletes using herbals for weight loss, Pittler concluded that the potential health risks argue against such use due to an increased risk relative to benefit. Athletes contemplating using herbals should consult with their health care professional.

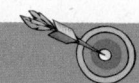

Key Concepts

▶ Results from well-controlled research indicate that ginseng and related adaptogens, such as ciwujia, are not effective ergogenic aids.

▶ There is limited well-controlled research regarding the effect of herbals on exercise or sport performance, and that which is available suggests that herbal sports supplements are not effective ergogenic aids.

Sports Supplements: Efficacy, Safety, and Permissibility

What sports supplements are considered to be effective, safe, and permissible?

Throughout this text we have discussed the role of a wide variety of dietary supplements relative to their efficacy, safety, and permissibility as ergogenic aids, namely their potential to enhance sport or exercise performance. Metabolites of carbohydrate and fat, special forms of protein, numerous amino acids, vitamins, and minerals, as well as food drugs and herbal supplements, have all been studied for their ergogenic potential. In their position stand on nutrition and athletic performance, the American College of Sports Medicine, the American Dietetic Association, and the Dietitians of Canada classified sports supplements into four categories; the Australian Institute of Sport developed similar guidelines. The four categories are described in the following text and, based on the currently available research presented in this text, include a list of those sports supplements that best fit that category. Listing in a specific category is based primarily on the ability of the supplement to enhance performance or promote training as a means to performance enhancement when added to a healthful diet that already provides adequate Calories and essential nutrients. The ergogenic effect of the supplement may also be limited to a specific type of athletic endeavor, such as sodium bicarbonate and high-intensity anaerobic exercise dependent primarily on anaerobic glycolysis. Individual needs also may dictate the inclusion of a specific dietary supplement for any given athlete. For example, females in weight-control sports may benefit from iron supplements to help prevent iron deficiency and anemia, and from calcium supplements to help maintain bone mass. Some supplements may be considered unsafe and not recommended if that is the research-based opinion of various health organizations.

• Sports supplements that are effective, safe, and permissible. The efficacy of these supplements is supported by quality research, they are considered safe to use, and they are not prohibited for use by sport-governing organizations. Although research indicates that they are effective ergogenics, responses of individual athletes may vary.

Caffeine
Carbohydrate (Sports bars/gels)
Creatine
Sodium bicarbonate
Water

• Sports supplements that *may be* effective, are safe, and are permissible. Preliminary research may suggest some ergogenic effects, but the data are too limited to make a robust recommendation. Additional research is needed to confirm or refute preliminary findings. These supplements are safe and permissible.

Aspartate salts
Beta-arginine
Colostrum
Glycerol
Phosphate salts
Protein/essential amino acids
Pseudoephedrine
Whey protein

• Sports supplements that are not effective. Research indicates that these supplements do not enhance exercise performance. However, athletes in weight-control sports consuming a reduced-Calorie diet may help prevent vitamin and mineral deficiencies by consuming a multivitamin/mineral supplement.

Antioxidant vitamins
Arginine
B vitamin complex
BCAA
Bee pollen
Boron
Calcium
Carnitine (L-carnitine)
Choline
Chondroitin
Chromium
Ciwujia
Conjugated linoleic acid
CoQ10
Cordyceps sinensis
Fat loading
Gamma oryzanol
Ginseng
Glucosamine
Glutamine
Glycine
HMB
Hydroxycitrate
Inosine
Iron
Magnesium
Medium-chain triglycerides
Niacin
Octacosanol
Omega-3 fatty acids
Ornithine
Pyruvate
Rhodiola rosea
Ribose
Selenium

Tribulus terrestris
Tryptophan
Vanadium
Vitamin A
Vitamin C
Vitamin D
Vitamin E
Wheat germ oil
Yohimbine
Zinc

Androstenediol
Androstenedione
DHEA
Ephedra/ephedrine
Synephrine
Yohimbine

- Sports supplements that should not be used because they are either not safe or not permissible. The WADA prohibits use of some of these supplements, and others may also cause various health problems. Note also that some dietary supplements, such as herbal testosterone precursors like *Tribulus terrestris,* may be contaminated with anabolic agents that may result in a positive doping test.

Keep in mind that numerous supplements are marketed to athletes included claims to promote testosterone production, maximize muscle mass, strength, and power, and enhance training and performance in competition. With few exceptions, research does not support the efficacy of most commercial sports supplements. Moreover, some supplements may be contaminated, intentionally or unintentionally, with substances that could lead to a positive doping test. In most cases athletes can meet their nutritional needs through consumption of a well-planned, healthful diet.

APPLICATION EXERCISE

If you or one of your colleagues is physically trained or an athlete, you might want to conduct a small case study with caffeine. Either of you should be physically trained to run a mile, swim 500 meters, or some comparable exercise task of 5–10 minutes of high-intensity exercise. Other exercise tasks of shorter duration may be selected. The activity is best done indoors to control environmental conditions. One of you can serve as the investigator and the other as the subject. A third colleague will administer the treatment on a double-blind basis. Randomly, over a 5-week period, the subject will participate in five trials, each involving maximal performance for the selected activity. Thirty minutes before the test, the subject should consume either two caffeine tablets, each containing 200 milligrams of caffeine (Vivarin or comparable over-the-counter tablet) or a comparable placebo (two multivitamin tablets) with some water. The subject's eyes should be closed while taking the tablets. Here is the weekly protocol.

Week 1—Learning protocol; no placebo or caffeine
Week 2—Placebo or caffeine
Week 3—Caffeine or placebo (opposite of week 2)
Week 4—Placebo or caffeine
Week 5—Caffeine or placebo (opposite of week 4)

Record the performance times (minutes: seconds) for each, average the two placebo and two caffeine trials, and compare the results for improvement, if any.

Caffeine Trial

	Week 1 (no placebo or caffeine)	Week 2 (placebo or caffeine)	Week 3 (opposite of week 2)	Week 4 (placebo or caffeine)	Week 5 (opposite of week 4)
Performance Time (minutes:seconds)	:	:	:	:	:

Review Questions—Multiple Choice

1. Of the drugs and supplements discussed in this chapter, which have the most research supporting their ability to enhance exercise or sports performance?

   a. caffeine and androstenedione
   b. ginseng and ephedrine
   c. alcohol and DHEA
   d. androstenedione and ephedrine
   e. sodium bicarbonate and caffeine

2. About how many milligrams of caffeine are in a 6-ounce cup of perked coffee?

   a. 25–30
   b. 100–125

c. 300–400
d. 500–600
e. 1,000

3. Which of the following is not a physiological effect of caffeine?

   a. decreases the metabolic rate
   b. stimulates the central nervous system
   c. increases the secretion of epinephrine
   d. increases heart rate and force of contraction
   e. increases force of skeletal muscle contractility

4. For an average-size male adult (150 pounds), the consumption of four drinks within a very short period of time would elevate the blood alcohol concentration (BAC) to about what level?

   a. 0.01
   b. 0.02
   c. 0.05
   d. 0.10
   e. 0.15

5. As a potential ergogenic aid, sodium bicarbonate would be most likely suited to which type of athlete?

   a. marathon runner (26.2 miles)
   b. 100-meter sprinter (track)
   c. 400-meter sprinter (track)
   d. pole vaulter (field)
   e. discus thrower (field)

6. Increasing research suggests that moderate alcohol consumption, or "low risk" drinking, may reduce the risk of CHD and all-cause mortality. All of the following, except which, are hypothesized to contribute to this reduced risk?

   a. a relaxation effect and reduced anxiety
   b. decreased platelet aggregability (decreased possibility of blood clots)
   c. increased blood flow to the brain
   d. reduced caloric intake, induced weight loss, and prevented metabolic syndrome
   e. an increase in HDL-cholesterol

7. Research generally supports the theory that caffeine may enhance performance in long-distance endurance events. Which of the following is the *least* likely hypothesis?

   a. It may exert a psychological stimulating effect.
   b. It stimulates the release of epinephrine from the adrenal gland.
   c. It decreases the use of both free fatty acids and muscle glycogen.
   d. It may decrease the perception of effort during exercise.
   e. It may exert a direct effect on the muscles to increase muscle contractile force.

8. Anabolic/androgenic steroids (AAS) are drugs popular with individuals with muscle dysmorphia, or those who desire to increase muscle mass even though already very muscular. AAS are designed to mimic mainly the anabolic effects of which natural hormone in the body?

   a. insulin
   b. human growth hormone (HGH)
   c. testosterone
   d. androsterone
   e. estrogen

9. Which of the following dietary supplements marketed to strength-trained individuals are precursors, or prohormones, for testosterone?

   a. creatine and conjugated linoleic acid
   b. gamma oryzanol and ginseng
   c. *Cordyceps sinensis* and *Cytoseira canariensis*
   d. HMB and *Tribulus terrestris*
   e. androstenedione and DHEA

10. Which of the following ergogenic aids are currently permitted for use by athletes in all sports competitions according to the doping list created by the World Anti-Doping Agency?

    a. caffeine and ephedrine
    b. sodium bicarbonate and caffeine
    c. caffeine and alcohol
    d. androstenedione and DHEA
    e. ginseng and ephedrine

Answers to multiple-choice questions:
1. e; 2. b; 3. a; 4. d; 5. c; 6. d; 7. c; 8. c; 9. e; 10. b.

Review Questions—Essay

1. Discuss both the potential beneficial and adverse health effects of consuming various amounts of alcohol.

2. Discuss the efficacy, safety, and legality of caffeine supplementation as an ergogenic aid for aerobic endurance athletes.

3. Discuss the efficacy, safety, and legality of sodium bicarbonate supplementation as an ergogenic aid. In which types of sports would it appear to be most effective?

4. Compare and contrast the effects of testosterone, versus its congeners DHEA and androstenedione, as ergogenic aids for the development of muscle mass and strength. Discuss possible health risks associated with use of each.

5. What is ginseng, why is it purported to be an ergogenic aid, and does research support its efficacy as an ergogenic?

References

Books

Bahrke, M., and Yesalis, C. 2002. *Performance-Enhancing Substances in Sport and Exercise.* Champaign, IL: Human Kinetics.

Noakes, T. 2003. *Love of Running.* Champaign, IL: Human Kinetics.

Reviews

Allen, D., et al. 2008. Impaired calcium release during fatigue. *Journal of Applied Physiology* 104:296–305.

American College of Sports Medicine. 2007. Exercise and fluid replacement. *Medicine & Science in Sports & Exercise* 39:377–90.

American College of Sports Medicine. 1987. American College of Sports Medicine position stand on use of anabolic-androgenic steroids in sports. *Medicine & Science in Sports & Exercise* 19:534–39.

Anstey, K., et al. 2009. Alcohol consumption as a risk factor for dementia and cognitive decline: Meta-analysis of prospective studies. *American Journal of Geriatric Psychiatry* 17:542–55.

Armstrong, L., et al. 2007. Caffeine, fluid-electrolyte balance, temperature regulation, and exercise-heat tolerance. *Exercise and Sport Sciences Reviews* 35:135–40.

Arria, M., and O'Brien, M. 2011. The "high" risk of energy drinks. *JAMA* Published online January 25, doi:10.1001/jama.2011.109

Astorino, T., and Roberson, D. 2010. Efficacy of acute caffeine ingestion for short-term high-intensity exercise performance: A systematic review. *Journal of Strength and Conditioning Research* 24:257–65.

Bahrke, M., and Morgan, W. 1994. Evaluation of the ergogenic properties of ginseng. *Sports Medicine* 18:229–48.

Bahrke, M., et al. 2009. Is ginseng an ergogenic aid? *International Journal of Sport Nutrition and Exercise Metabolism* 19:298–322.

Bain, J. 2010. Testosterone and the aging male: To treat or not to treat? *Maturitas* 66:16–22.

Basaria, S., et al. 2010. Adverse events associated with testosterone administration. *New England Journal of Medicine* 363:109–22.

Bent, S., et al. 2004. Safety and efficacy of citrus aurantium for weight loss. *American Journal of Cardiology* 94:1359–61.

Boje, O. 1939. Doping. *Bulletin of the Health Organization of the League of Nations* 8:439–69.

Brown, G., et al. 2006. Testosterone prohormone supplements. *Medicine & Science in Sports & Exercise* 38:1451–61.

Browne, M. 2006. Maternal exposure to caffeine and risk of congenital anomalies: A systematic review. *Epidemiology* 17:324–31.

Burd, L., et al. 2007. Ethanol and the placenta: A review. *Journal of Maternal-Fetal & Neonatal Medicine* 20:361–75.

Burke, L., and Maughan, R. 2000. Alcohol in sport. In *Nutrition in Sport,* ed. R. J. Maughan. Oxford: Blackwell Scientific.

Cargiulo, T. 2007. Understanding the health impact of alcohol dependence. *American Journal of Health-Systems Pharmacy* 64:S5–S11.

Chapman, R., and Mickleborough, T. 2009. The effects of caffeine on ventilation and pulmonary function during exercise: An often-overlooked response. *Physician and Sportsmedicine* 37:97–103.

Chen, X., et al. 2010. Caffeine protects against disruptions of the blood-brain barrier in animal models of Alzheimer's and Parkinson's diseases. *Journal of Alzheimer's Disease* 20:S127–41.

Chitturi, S., and Farrell, G. 2008. Hepatotoxic slimming aids and other herbal hepatotoxins. *Journal of Gastroenterology and Hepatology* 23:366–73.

Cloud, J. 2008. Libations: This ain't no wine cooler. *Time* July 28: 51–52.

Conger, S., et al. 2011. Does caffeine added to carbohydrate provide additional ergogenic benefits for endurance? *International Journal of Sport Nutrition and Exercise Metabolism* 21:71–84.

Consumers Union. 2008. Deflating the claims about DHEA. *Consumer Reports on Health* 20 (7):10.

Consumers Union. 2007. New diet winners. *Consumer Reports* 72 (6):12–17.

Consumers Union. 2007. Risky herb-drug combos. *Consumer Reports on Health* 19 (1):10.

Consumers Union. 2004. Coffee or tea? Battle of the brews. *Consumer Reports on Health* 17 (2):6.

Consumers Union. 2004. Ephedra: Heart dangers in disguise. *Consumer Reports* 69 (1):22–23.

Consumers Union. 2001. Coffee: How much is too much? *Consumer Reports* 66 (5): 64–65.

Coon, J., and Ernst, E. 2002. Panax ginseng: A systematic review of adverse effects and drug interactions. *Drug Safety* 25:323–44.

Cunha, R., and Agostinho, P. 2010. Chronic caffeine consumption prevents memory disturbance in different animal models of memory decline. *Journal of Alzheimer's Disease* 20:S95–116.

Daly, J., and Fredholm, B. 1998. Caffeine: An atypical drug of dependence. *Drug and Alcohol Dependence* 51:199–206.

Davis, J., and Green, J. 2009. Caffeine and anaerobic performance: Ergogenic value and mechanisms of action. *Sports Medicine* 39:813–32.

Dean, H. 2002. Does exogenous growth hormone improve athletic performance? *Clinical Journal of Sport Medicine* 12:250–53.

de Lorimier, A. 2000. Alcohol, wine, and health. *American Journal of Surgery* 180:357–61.

Denke, M. 2000. Nutritional and health benefits of beer. *American Journal of the Medical Sciences* 320:320–26.

Doherty, M., and Smith, P. 2005. Effects of caffeine ingestion on rating of perceived exertion during and after exercise: A meta-analysis. *Scandinavian Journal of Medicine & Science in Sports* 15:69–78.

Doherty, M., and Smith, P. 2004. Effect of caffeine ingestion on exercise testing: A meta-analysis. *International Journal of Sport Nutrition and Exercise Metabolism* 14:626–46.

Earnest, C. 2001. Dietary androgen supplements: Separating substance from hype. *Physician and Sportsmedicine* 29 (5): 63–79.

El Sayed, M., et al. 2005. Interaction between alcohol and exercise: Physiological and haematological implications. *Sports Medicine* 35:257–69.

Epstein, D., and Dohrmann, G. 2009. What you don't know might kill you. *Sports Illustrated* 110(30):54–63.

Epstein, E., et al. 2007. Women, aging, and alcohol use disorders. *Journal of Women & Aging* 19 (1–2):31–48.

Evans, N. 2004. Current concepts in anabolic-androgenic steroids. *American Journal of Sports Medicine* 32:534–42.

Fillmore, K., et al. 2007. Moderate alcohol use and reduced mortality risk: Systematic error in prospective studies and new hypotheses. *Annals of Epidemiology* 17:S16–S23.

Galaif, E., et al. 2007. Suicidality, depression, and alcohol use among adolescents: A review of empirical findings. *International Journal of Adolescent Medicine and Health* 19:27–35.

Ganio, M., et al. 2009. Effect of caffeine on sport-specific endurance performance: A systematic review. *Journal of Strength and Conditioning Research* 23:315–24.

George, A., and Figueredo, V. 2010. Alcohol and arrhythmias: A comprehensive review. *Journal of Cardiovascular Medicine* 11:221–8.

Gonzalez, C., and Riboli, E. 2006. Diet and cancer prevention: Where we are, where we are going. *Nutrition and Cancer* 56:225–31.

Gordis, E. 1999. Research on alcohol problems. *Kappa Phi Journal* 79 (4):24–27, 37.

Goulet, E., and Dionne, I. 2005. Assessment of the effects of eleutherococcus senticosus on endurance performance. *International Journal of Sport Nutrition and Exercise Metabolism* 15:75–83.

Graham, T. 2001. Caffeine, coffee, and ephedrine: Impact on exercise performance and metabolism. *Canadian Journal of Applied Physiology* 26:S103–19.

Graham, T., and Spriet, L. 1996. Caffeine and exercise performance. *Sports Science Exchange* 9 (1):1–5.

Graham, T., et al. 2008. Does caffeine alter muscle carbohydrate and fat metabolism during exercise? *Applied Physiology, Nutrition, and Metabolism* 33:1311–8.

Green, J. 2007. Fetal Alcohol Spectrum Disorders: Understanding the effects of prenatal alcohol exposure and supporting students. *Journal of School Health* 77:103–8.

Greenberg, J., et al. 2006. Coffee, diabetes, and weight control. *American Journal of Clinical Nutrition* 84:682–93.

Greenway, F. 2001. The safety and efficacy of pharmaceutical and herbal caffeine and ephedrine use as a weight loss agent. *Obesity Reviews* 2:199–211.

Greydanus, D., and Patel, D. 2010. Sports doping in the adolescent: The Faustian conundrum of Hors de Combat. *Pediatric Clinics of North America* 57:729–50.

Guha, N., et al. 2009. IGF-I abuse in sport: Current knowledge and future prospects for detection. *Growth Hormone & IGF Research* 19:408–11.

Gupta, S. 2007. The caffeine habit. *Time* 170 (17):62.

Haller, C., and Benowitz, N. 2000. Adverse cardiovascular and central nervous system events associated with dietary supplements containing ephedra alkaloids. *New England Journal of Medicine* 343:1833–38.

Hartgens, F., and Kuipers, H. 2004. Effects of androgenic-anabolic steroids in athletes. *Sports Medicine* 34:513–54.

Haycock, P. 2009. Fetal alcohol spectrum disorders: The epigenetic perspective. *Biology of Reproduction* 81:607–17.

Hespel, P., et al. 2006. Dietary supplements for football. *Journal of Sports Sciences* 24:749–61.

Hobson, R., and Maughan, R. 2010. Hydration status and the diuretic action of a small dose of alcohol. *Alcohol and Alcoholism* 45:366–73.

Holman, C. D., et al. 1996. Meta-analysis of alcohol and all-cause mortality. *Medical Journal of Australia* 164:141–45.

Holt, R. 2009. Is human growth hormone an ergogenic aid? *Drug Testing and Analysis* 1:412–8.

Horne, J., and Reyner, L. 1999. Vehicle accidents related to sleep: A review. *Occupational and Environmental Medicine* 56:289–94.

Huxley, R., et al. 2009. Coffee, decaffeinated coffee, and tea consumption in relation to incident type 2 diabetes mellitus: A systematic review with meta-analysis. *Archives of Internal Medicine* 169:2053–63.

International Society of Sports Nutrition; Graves, B., et al. 2010. International Society of Sports nutrition position stand: Caffeine and performance. *Journal of the International Society of Nutrition* 7(1):5.

James, J. 2004. Critical review of dietary caffeine and blood pressure: A relationship that should be taken more seriously. *Psychosomatic Medicine* 66:63–71.

Jequier, E. 1999. Alcohol intake and body weight: A paradox. *American Journal of Clinical Nutrition* 69:173–74.

Jeukendrup, A., and Martin, J. 2001. Improving cycling performance: How should we spend our time and money? *Sports Medicine* 31:559–69.

Juliano, L., and Griffiths, R. 2004. A critical review of caffeine withdrawal: Empirical validation of symptoms and signs, incidence, severity, and associated features. *Psychopharmacology* 176:1–29.

Kalmar, J. 2005. The influence of caffeine on voluntary muscle activation. *Medicine & Science in Sports & Exercise* 37:2113–19.

Karam, E., et al. 2007. Alcohol use among college students: An international perspective. *Current Opinion in Psychiatry* 20:213–21.

Kerrigan, S., and Lindsey, T. 2005. Fatal caffeine overdose: Two case reports. *Forensic Science International* 153:67–69.

Klatsky, A. 2007. Alcohol, cardiovascular diseases and diabetes mellitus. *Pharmacological Research* 55:237–47.

Klatsky, A. 2002. Alcohol and cardiovascular disease: A historical review. *New York Academy of Sciences* 957:7–15.

Koppes, L., et al. 2005. Moderate alcohol consumption lowers the risk of type 2 diabetes: A meta-analysis of prospective observational studies. *Diabetes Care* 28:719–25.

Kraemer, W., et al. 2002. Growth hormone: Physiological effects of exogenous administration. In *Performance-Enhancing Substances in Sport and Exercise,* eds. M. Bahrke and C. Yesalis. Champaign, IL: Human Kinetics.

Kundrat, S. 2005. Herbs and athletes. *Sports Science Exchange* 18 (1):1–6.

Lara, D. 2010. Caffeine, mental health, and psychiatric disorders. *Journal of Alzheimer's Disease* 20:S239–48.

Liebman, B. 2011. Unexpected surprising findings from the last 40 years. *Nutrition Action Health Letter* 38 (1):3–9.

Linde, K., et al. 2006. Echinacea for preventing and treating the common cold. *Cochrane Database of Systematic Reviews* 25:CD000530.

Liu, H., et al. 2007. Systematic review: The safety and efficacy of growth hormone in the healthy elderly. *Annals of Internal Medicine* 146:104–15.

Loucks, A. 2006. The endocrine system: Integrated influences on metabolism, growth, and reproduction. In ACSM's *Advanced Exercise Physiology,* ed. C. Tipton. Philadelphia: Lippincott Williams & Wilkins.

Magkos, F., and Kavouras, S. 2004. Caffeine and ephedrine: Physiological, metabolic and performance-enhancing effects. *Sports Medicine* 34:971–89.

Maglione, M., et al. 2005. Psychiatric effects of ephedra use: An analysis of Food and Drug Administration reports of adverse events. *American Journal of Psychiatry* 162:189–91.

Martens, M., et al. 2005. Development of the athlete drinking scale. *Psychology of Addictive Behaviors* 19:158–64.

Matson, L., and Tran, Z. 1993. Effects of sodium bicarbonate ingestion on anaerobic performance: A meta-analytic review. *International Journal of Sport Nutrition* 3:2–28.

Maughan, R. 2005. Contamination of dietary supplements and positive drug tests in sport. *Journal of Sports Sciences* 23:883–89.

Maughan, R., et al. 2004. Dietary supplements. *Journal of Sports Sciences* 22:95–113.

McNaughton, L., et al. 2008. Ergogenic effects of sodium bicarbonate. *Current Sports Medicine Reports* 7:230–36.

Melnik, B., et al. 2007. Abuse of anabolic-androgenic steroids and bodybuilding acne: An underestimated health problem.

Journal der Deutschen Dermatologischen Gesellschaft 5:110–7.

Michels, K., et al. 2007. Diet and breast cancer. A review of the prospective observational studies. *Cancer* 109 (Supplement 12):2712–49.

Monti, P., et al. 2005. Adolescence: Booze, brains, and behavior. Alcoholism: *Clinical & Experimental Research* 29:207–20.

National Institute on Alcohol Abuse and Alcoholism. 2003. *State of the science report on the effects of moderate drinking.* National Institutes of Health. December 19, 2003.

National Strength and Conditioning Association; Hoffman, J., et al. 2009. Position stand on androgen and human growth hormone use. *Journal of Strength and Conditioning Research* 23:S1–S59.

Nnakwe, N. 1996. Anabolic steroids and cardiovascular risk in athletes. *Nutrition Today* 31 (5): 206–8.

O'Brien, C., and Lyons, F. 2000. Alcohol and the athlete. *Sports Medicine* 29:295–300.

Palisin, T., and Stacy, J. 2006. Ginseng: Is it in the root? *Current Sports Medicine Reports* 5:210–14.

Pittler, M., et al. 2005. Adverse events of herbal food supplements for body weight reduction: Systematic review. *Obesity Reviews* 6:93–111.

Prediger, R. 2010. Effects of caffeine in Parkinson's disease: From neuroprotection to the management of motor and non-motor symptoms. *Journal of Alzheimer's Disease* 20:S205–20.

Rawson, E., and Clarkson, P. 2002. Ephedrine as an ergogenic aid. In *Performance-Enhancing Substances in Sport and Exercise,* eds. M. Bahrke and C. Yesalis. Champaign, IL: Human Kinetics.

Reid, T. 2005. Caffeine. *National Geographic* 207 (1):2–33.

Reissig, C., et al. 2009. Caffeinated energy drinks—a growing problem. *Drug and Alcohol Dependence* 99:1–10.

Requena, B., et al. 2005. Sodium bicarbonate and sodium citrate: Ergogenic aids. *Journal of Strength and Conditioning Research* 19:213–24.

Reuben, A. 2008. Alcohol and the liver. *Current Opinion in Gastroenterology* 24:328–38.

Rimm, E., and Moats, C. 2007. Alcohol and coronary heart disease: Drinking patterns and mediators of effect. *Annals of Epidemiology* 17:S3–S7.

Room, R., et al. 2005. Alcohol and public health. *Lancet* 365:519–30.

Rubeck, K., et al. 2009. Impact of growth hormone (GH) substitution on exercise capacity and muscle strength in GH-deficient adults: A meta-analysis of blinded,

placebo-controlled trials. *Clinical Endocrinology* 71:860–66.

Santos, C., et al. 2010. Caffeine intake and dementia: Systematic review and meta-analysis. *Journal of Alzheimer's Disease* 20:S187–204.

Schardt, D. 2008. Caffeine: The good, the bad, and the maybe. *Nutrition Action Health Letter* 35 (2):1, 3–7.

Shah, S., et al. 2007. Evaluation of echinacea for the prevention and treatment of the common cold: A meta-analysis. *The Lancet Infectious Diseases* 7:473–80.

Shekelle, P., et al. 2003. Efficacy and safety of ephedra and ephedrine for weight loss and athletic performance: A meta-analysis. *JAMA* 289:1537–45.

Sin, C., et al. 2009. Systematic review on the effectiveness of caffeine abstinence on the quality of sleep. *Journal of Clinical Nursing* 18:13–21.

Sirrs, S., and Bebb, R. 1999. DHEA: Panacea or snake oil? *Canadian Family Physician* 45:1723–28.

Smith, G., et al. 1999. Fatal nontraffic injuries involving alcohol: A meta-analysis. *Annals of Emergency Medicine* 33:699, 701.

Söderpalm, B., et al. 2009. Mechanistic studies of ethanol's interaction with the mesolimbic dopamine reward system. *Pharmacopsychiatry* 42:S87–94.

Talih, F., et al. 2007. Anabolic steroid abuse: Psychiatric and physical costs. *Cleveland Clinic Journal of Medicine* 74:341–4, 346, 349–52.

Tang, N., et al. 2009. Coffee consumption and risk of breast cancer: A meta-analysis. *American Journal of Obstetrics and Gynecology* 200:290.e1–9.

Tarnopolsky, M. 2008. Effect of caffeine on the neuromuscular system—Potential as an ergogenic aid. *Applied Physiology, Nutrition, and Metabolism* 33:1284–9.

Tarnopolsky, M. 1993. Protein, caffeine, and sports. *Physician and Sportsmedicine* 21 (March): 137–49.

Temple, J. 2009. Caffeine use in children: What we know, what we have left to learn, and why we should worry. *Neuroscience and Biobehavioral Reviews* 33:793–806.

Tentori, L., and Graziani, G. 2007. Doping with growth hormone/IGF-1, anabolic steroids or erythropoietin: Is there a cancer risk? *Pharmacological Research* 55:359–69.

van Amsterdam, J., et al. 2010. Adverse health effects of anabolic-androgenic steroids. *Regulatory Toxicology and Pharmacology* 57:117–23.

van Dam, R. 2006. Coffee and type 2 diabetes: From beans to beta-cells. *Nutrition,*

Metabolism and Cardiovascular Diseases 16:69–77.

Warren, G., et al. 2010. Effect of caffeine ingestion on muscular strength and endurance: A meta-analysis. *Medicine & Science in Sports & Exercise* 42:1375–87.

Welsh, E., et al. 2010. Caffeine for asthma. *Cochrane Database of Systematic Reviews* 20;(1):CD001112.

Widdowson, W., and Gibney, J. 2010. The effect of growth hormone (GH) replacement on muscle strength in patients with GH-deficiency: A meta-analysis. *Clinical Endocrinology* 72:787–92.

Widdowson, W., et al. 2009. The physiology of growth hormone and sport. *Growth Hormone & IGF Research* 19:308–19.

Williams, J. 1991. Caffeine, neuromuscular function and high-intensity exercise performance. *Journal of Sports Medicine and Physical Fitness* 31:481–89.

Williams, M. 2000. Smoking, alcohol, ergogenic aids, doping and the endurance performer. In *Endurance in Sport,* eds. R. Shephard and P. Astrand. Oxford: Blackwell Science.

Williams, M., and Branch, J. 2002. Herbals as ergogenic aids. In *Performance Enhancing Substances in Sports and Exercise,* eds. M. Bahrke and C. Yesalis. Champaign, IL: Human Kinetics.

Wu, J., et al. 2009. Coffee consumption and risk of coronary heart diseases: A meta-analysis of 21 prospective cohort studies. *International Journal of Cardiology* 137:216–25.

Yeomans, M. 2004. Effects of alcohol on food and energy intake in human subjects: Evidence for passive and active overconsumption of energy. *British Journal of Nutrition* 92:S31–S34.

Yesalis, C., and Bahrke, M. 2005. Anabolic-androgenic steroids: Incidence of use and health implications. *President's Council on Physical Fitness and Sports Research Digest* 5 (5):1–8.

Ziegenfuss, T., et al. 2002. Effects of pro-hormones supplementation in humans: A review. *Canadian Journal of Applied Physiology* 27:628–46.

Specific Studies

Abbasi, A., et al. 1998. Association of dehydroepiandrosterone sulfate, body composition, and physical fitness in independent community-dwelling older men and women. *Journal of the American Geriatric Society* 46:263–73.

Acacio, B., et al. 2004. Pharmacokinetics of dehydroepiandrosterone and its metabolites after long-term daily oral administration to healthy young men. *Fertility and Sterility* 81:595–604.

Ahrens, J., et al. 2007. The physiological effects of caffeine in women during treadmill walking. *Journal of Strength and Conditioning Research* 21:164–8.

Allen, N., et al. 2009. Moderate alcohol intake and cancer incidence in women. *Journal of the National Cancer Institute* 101: 296–305.

Artioli, G., et al. 2007. Does sodium-bicarbonate ingestion improve simulated judo performance? *International Journal of Sport Nutrition and Exercise Metabolism* 17:206–17.

Bahrke, M. S., et al. 1998. Anabolic-androgenic steroid abuse and performance-enhancing drugs among adolescents. *Child and Adolescent Psychiatric Clinics of North America* 7:821–38.

Ball, D., and Maughan, R. 1997. The effect of sodium citrate ingestion on the metabolic response to intense exercise following diet manipulation in man. *Experimental Physiology* 82:1041–56.

Baume, N., et al. 2006. Effect of multiple oral doses of androgenic anabolic steroids on endurance performance and serum indices of physical stress in healthy male subjects. *European Journal of Applied Physiology* 98:329–40.

Beedie, C., et al. 2006. Placebo effects of caffeine on cycling performance. *Medicine & Science in Sports & Exercise* 38:2159–64.

Bell, D., and Jacobs, I. 1999. Combined caffeine and ephedrine ingestion improves run times of Canadian Forces Warrior Test. *Aviation and Space Environmental Medicine* 70:325–29.

Bell, D., et al. 2002. Effect of ingesting caffeine and ephendrine on 10-km run performance. *Medicine & Science in Sports & Exercise* 34:344–49.

Bell, D., et al. 2001. Effect of caffeine and ephedrine ingestion on anaerobic exercise performance. *Medicine & Science in Sports & Exercise* 33:1399–1403.

Bents, R., and Marsh, E. 2006. Patterns of ephedra and other stimulant use in collegiate hockey athletes. *International Journal of Sport Nutrition and Exercise Metabolism* 16:636–43.

Beulens, J., et al. 2006. The effect of moderate alcohol consumption on fat distribution and adipocytokines. *Obesity* 14:60–66.

Bhasin, S., et al. 1996. The effects of supraphysiologic doses of testosterone on muscle size and strength in normal men. *New England Journal of Medicine* 335:1–7.

Bird, S., et al. 1995. The effect of sodium bicarbonate ingestion on 1500-m racing time. *Journal of Sports Sciences* 13:399–403.

Bishop, D., and Claudius, B. 2005. Effects of induced metabolic alkalosis on prolonged intermittent-sprint performance. *Medicine & Science in Sports & Exercise* 37:759–67.

Bouchard, N., et al. 2005. Ischemic stroke associated with use of an ephedra-free dietary supplement containing synephrine. *Mayo Clinic Proceedings* 80:541–45.

Brown, G., et al. 2004. Changes in serum testosterone and estradiol concentrations following acute androstenedione ingestion in young women. *Hormone and Metabolic Research* 36:62–66.

Brown, G., et al. 1999. Effect of oral DHEA on serum testosterone and adaptations to resistance training in young men. *Journal of Applied Physiology* 87:2274–83.

Bruce, C., et al. 2000. Enhancement of 2000-m rowing performance after caffeine ingestion. *Medicine & Science in Sports & Exercise* 32:1958–63.

Bui, L., et al. 2006. Blood pressure and heart rate effect following a single dose of bitter orange. *Annals of Pharmacotherapy* I40:53–57.

CARE Study Group. 2008. Maternal caffeine intake during pregnancy and risk of fetal growth restriction: A large prospective observational study. *BMJ* 337:a2332.

Cheuvront, S. et al. 1999. Effect of ENDUROX™ on metabolic responses to submaximal exercise. *International Journal of Sport Nutrition* 9:434–42.

Chopra, M., et al. 2000. Nonalcoholic red wine extract and quercetin inhibit LDL oxidation without affecting plasma antioxidant vitamin and carotenoid concentrations. *Clinical Chemistry* 46:1162–70.

Cohen, B., et al. 1996. Effects of caffeine ingestion on endurance racing in heat and humidity. *European Journal of Applied Physiology* 73:358–63.

Coiro, V., et al. 2007. Effects of moderate ethanol drinking on the GH and cortisol responses to physical exercise. *Neuro Endocrinology Letters* 28:145–8.

Colson, S., et al. 2005. Cordyceps sinensis- and Rhodiola rosea-based supplementation in male cyclists and its effect on muscle tissue saturation. *Journal of Strength and Conditioning Research* 19:358–63.

Costill, D., et al. 1978. Effects of caffeine ingestion on metabolism and exercise performance. *Medicine & Science in Sports* 10:155–58.

Dascombe, B., et al. 2010. Nutritional supplementation habits and perceptions of elite athletes within a state-based sporting institute. *Journal of Science and Medicine in Sport* 13:274–80.

Dean, S., et al. 2009. The effects of EGCG on fat oxidation and endurance performance in male cyclists. *International Journal of Sport Nutrition and Exercise Metabolism* 19:624–44.

De Bock, K., et al. 2004. Acute Rhodiola rosea intake can improve endurance exercise performance. *International Journal of Sport Nutrition and Exercise Metabolism* 14:298–307.

Del Coso, J., et al. 2009. Caffeine during exercise in the heat: Thermoregulation and fluid-electrolyte balance. *Medicine & Science in Sports & Exercise* 41:164–73.

Desbrow, B., and Leveritt, M. 2007. Well-trained endurance athletes' knowledge, insight, and experience of caffeine use. *International Journal of Sport Nutrition and Exercise Metabolism* 17:328–39.

Desbrow, B., and Leveritt, M. 2006. Awareness and use of caffeine by athletes competing at the 2005. Ironman Triathlon World Championships. *International Journal of Sport Nutrition and Exercise Metabolism* 16:545–58.

Dowling, E. et al. 1996. Effect of Eleutherococcus senticosus on submaximal and maximal exercise performance. *Medicine & Science in Sport & Exercise,* 28:482–89.

DuRant, R., et al. 1995. Anabolic-steroid use, strength training, and multiple drug use among adolescents in the United States. *Pediatrics* 96:23–28.

Earnest, C., et al. 2004. Effects of a commercial herbal-based formula on exercise performance in cyclists. *Medicine & Science in Sports & Exercise* 36:504–9.

Earnest, C. et al. 2000. In vivo 4-androstene-3, 17-dione and 4-androstene-3 beta, 17 beta-diol supplementation in young men. *European Journal of Applied Physiology* 81:229–32.

Eichenberger, P., et al. 2010. No effects of three-week consumption of a green tea extract on time trial performance in endurance-trained men. *International Journal for Vitamin and Nutrition Research* 80:54–64.

Engels, H., and Wirth, J. 1997. No ergogenic effect of ginseng (Panax ginseng C.A. Meyer) during graded maximal aerobic exercise. *Journal of the American Dietetic Association* 97:1110–15.

Engels, H., et al. 2003. Effects of ginseng on secretory IgA, performance, and recovery from interval exercise. *Medicine & Science in Sports & Exercise* 35:690–96.

Engels, H., et al. 2001. Effects of ginseng supplementation on supramaximal exercise performance and short-term recovery. *Journal of Strength and Conditioning Research* 15:290–95.

Essig, D., et al. 1980. Muscle glycogen and tri-glyceride use during leg cycling following caffeine ingestion. *Medicine & Science in Sports & Exercise* 12:109.

Faigenbaum, A. et al. 1998. Anabolic steroid use by male and female middle school students. *Pediatrics* 101:e6.

Foad, A., et al. 2008. Pharmacological and psychological effects of caffeine ingestion in 40-km cycling performance. *Medicine & Science in Sport & Exercise* 40:158–65.

Fraenkel-Conrat, H., and Singer, B. 1988. Nucleoside adducts are formed by cooperative reactions of acetaldehyde and alcohols: Possible mechanism for the role of alcohol in carcinogenesis. *Proceedings of the National Academy of Sciences* 85:3758–61.

French, C., et al. 1991. Caffeine ingestion during exercise to exhaustion in elite distance runners. *The Journal of Sports Medicine and Physical Fitness* 31:425–32.

Frost, L., and Vestergaard, P. 2005. Caffeine and risk of atrial fibrillation or flutter: The Danish Diet, Cancer, and Health Study. *American Journal of Clinical Nutrition* 81:578–82.

Ganmaa, D., et al. 2008. Coffee, tea, caffeine and risk of breast cancer: A 22-year follow-up. *International Journal of Cancer* 122:2071–78.

Gant, N., et al. 2010. The influence of caffeine and carbohydrate coingestion on simulated soccer performance. *International Journal of Sport Nutrition and Exercise Metabolism* 20:191–7.

Gaziano, J., et al. 1993. Moderate alcohol intake, increased levels of high-density lipoprotein and its subfractions, and decreased risk of myocardial infarction. *New England Journal of Medicine* 329:1829–34.

Graham, T. et al. 1998. Metabolic and exercise endurance effects of coffee and caffeine ingestion. *Journal of Applied Physiology* 85:883–89.

Green, G., et al. 2001. NCAA study of substance use and abuse habits of college student-athletes. *Clinical Journal of Sport Medicine* 11:51–56.

Greenway, F., et al. 2006. Dietary herbal supplements with phenylephrine for weight loss. *Journal of Medicinal Food* 9:572–78.

Gruenewald, P., et al. 2010. A dose-response perspective on college drinking and related problems. *Addiction* 105:257–69.

Haller, C., et al. 2004. Enhanced stimulant and metabolic effects of combined ephedrine and caffeine. *Clinical Pharmacology and Therapeutics* 75:259–73.

Hartgens, F., et al. 1996. Body composition, cardiovascular risk factors and liver function in long term androgenic-anabolic steroids-using bodybuilders three months after drug withdrawal. *International Journal of Sports Medicine* 17:429–33.

Hines, L., et al. 2001. Genetic variation in alcohol dehydrogenase and the beneficial effect of moderate alcohol consumption on myocardial infarction. *New England Journal of Medicine* 344:549–55.

Hodges, K., et al. 2006. Pseudoephedrine enhances performance in 1500-m runners. *Medicine & Science in Sports & Exercise* 38:329–33.

Hogervorst, E., et al. 2008. Caffeine improves physical and cognitive performance during exhaustive exercise. *Medicine & Science in Sports & Exercise* 40:1841–51.

Hogervorst, E., et al. 1999. Caffeine improves cognitive performance after strenuous physical exercise. *International Journal of Sports Medicine* 20:354–61.

Irwin, C., et al. 2011. Caffeine withdrawal and high-intensity endurance cycling performance. *Journal of Sports Sciences* 29:509–15.

Jacobs, L., et al. 2004. Effects of ephedrine, caffeine, and their combination on muscular endurance. *Medicine & Science in Sports & Exercise* 35:987–94.

Jenkins, N., et al. 2008. Ergogenic effects of low doses of caffeine on cycling performance. *International Journal of Sport Nutrition and Exercise Metabolism* 18:328–42.

Kelly, Y., et al. 2010. Light drinking during pregnancy: Still no increased risk for socio-emotional difficulties or cognitive deficits at 5 years of age? *Journal of Epidemiology and Community Health* Oct 5. [Epub ahead of print]

Kendrick, Z., et al. 1993. Effect of ethanol on metabolic responses to treadmill running in well-trained men. *Journal of Clinical Pharmacology* 33:136–39.

Kenny, A., et al. 2010. Dehydroepiandrosterone combined with exercise improves muscle strength and physical function in frail older women. *Journal of the American Geriatric Society* 58:1707–14.

King, D. et al. 1999. Effect of oral androstenedione on serum testosterone and adaptations to resistance training in young men. *JAMA* 281:2020–28.

Klatsky, A., et al. 2006. Coffee, cirrhosis, and transaminase enzymes. *Archives of Internal Medicine* 166:1190–95.

Kozak-Collins, K., et al. 1994. Sodium bicarbonate ingestion does not improve performance in women cyclists. *Medicine & Science in Sports & Exercise* 26:1510–15.

Leder, B. et al. 2000. Oral androstenedione administration and serum testosterone concentrations in young men. *JAMA* 283:779–82.

Linossier, M. et al. 1997. Effect of sodium citrate on performance and metabolism of human skeletal muscle during supramaximal cycling exercise. *European Journal of Applied Physiology* 76:48–54.

Lopez-Garcia, E., et al. 2008. The relationship of coffee consumption with mortality. *Annals of Internal Medicine* 148:904–14.

Lopez-Garcia, E., et al. 2006. Changes in caffeine intake and long-term weight change in men and women. *American Journal of Clinical Nutrition* 83:674–80.

Mann, K., et al. 2005. Neuroimaging of gender differences in alcohol dependence: Are women more vulnerable? *Alcoholism: Clinical & Experimental Research* 29:896–901.

McLellan, T., and Bell, D. 2004. The impact of prior coffee consumption on the subsequent ergogenic effect of anhydrous caffeine. *International Journal of Sport Nutrition and Exercise Metabolism* 14:698–708.

McNaughton, L., and Cedaro, R. 1992. Sodium citrate ingestion and its effects on maximal anaerobic exercise of different durations. *European Journal of Applied Physiology* 64:36–41.

McNaughton, L., and Thompson, D. 2001. Acute versus chronic sodium bicarbonate ingestion and anaerobic work and power output. *Journal of Sports Medicine and Physical Fitness* 41:456–62.

McNaughton, L., et al. 1999. Effects of chronic bicarbonate ingestion on the performance of high-intensity work. *European Journal of Applied Physiology* 80:333–36.

McNaughton, L., et al. 1999. Sodium bicarbonate can be used as an ergogenic aid in high-intensity, competitive cycle ergometry of 1 h duration. *European Journal of Applied Physiology* 80:64–69.

Meinhardt, U., et al. 2010. The effects of growth hormone on body composition and physical performance in recreational athletes: A randomized trial. *Annals of Internal Medicine* 152:568–77.

Michels, K., et al. 2005. Coffee, tea, and caffeine consumption and incident of colon and rectal cancer. *Journal of the National Cancer Institute* 97:282–92.

Mukamal, K., et al. 2006. Alcohol consumption and risk for coronary heart disease in men with healthy lifestyles. *Archives of Internal Medicine* 166:2145–50.

Mukamal, K., et al. 2003. Roles of drinking pattern and type of alcohol consumed in coronary heart disease in men. *New England Journal of Medicine* 348:109–18.

Naik, S., and Freudenberger, R. 2004. Ephedra-associated cardiomyopathy. *Annals of Pharmacotherapy* 38:400–03.

Naimi, T., et al. 2005. Cardiovascular risk factors and confounders among nondrinking and moderate-drinking U.S. adults. *American Journal of Preventive Medicine* 28:369–73.

Nair, K., et al. 2006. DHEA in elderly women and DHEA or testosterone in elderly men. *New England Journal of Medicine* 355:1647–59.

Namdar, M., et al. 2009. Caffeine impairs myocardial blood flow response to physical exercise in patients with coronary artery disease as well as in age-matched controls. *PLoS One* 4:e5665.

Neychev, V., and Mitev, V. 2005. The aphrodisiac herb Tribulus terrestris does not influence the androgen production in young men. *Journal of Ethnopharmacology* 101:319–23.

Norager, C., et al. 2005. Caffeine improves endurance in 75-yr-old citizens: A randomized, double-blind, placebo-controlled study. *Journal of Applied Physiology* 99:2302–06.

Oopik, V., et al. 2003. Effects of sodium citrate ingestion before exercise on endurance performance in well-trained college runners. *British Journal of Sports Medicine* 37:485–89.

Ostojic, S. 2006. Yohimbine: The effects on body composition and exercise performance in soccer players. *Research in Sports Medicine* 14:289–99.

Parcell, A., et al. 2004. Cordyceps Sinensis (CordyMax Cs-4) supplementation does not improve endurance exercise performance. *International Journal of Sport Nutrition and Exercise Metabolism* 14:236–42.

Paton, C., et al. 2001. Little effect of caffeine ingestion on repeated sprints in team-sport athletes. *Medicine & Science in Sports & Exercise* 33:822–25.

Pereira, M., et al. 2006. Coffee consumption and risk of type 2 diabetes mellitus: An 11-year prospective study of 28,812 postmenopausal women. *Archives of Internal Medicine* 166:1311–16.

Philip, P., et al. 2006. The effects of coffee and napping on nighttime highway driving: A randomized trial. *Annals of Internal Medicine* 144:785–91.

Plowman, S., et al. 1999. The effects of ENDUROX™ on the physiological responses to stair-stepping exercise. *Research Quarterly for Exercise and Sport* 70:385–88.

Potteiger, J., et al. 1996. The effects of buffer ingestion on metabolic factors related to distance running performance. *European Journal of Applied Physiology* 72:365–71.

Potteiger, J. et al. 1996. Sodium citrate ingestion enhances 30 km cycling performance. *International Journal of Sports Medicine* 17:7–11.

Price, M., et al. 2003. Effects of sodium bicarbonate ingestion on prolonged intermittent exercise. *Medicine & Science in Sports & Exercise* 35:1303–08.

Pritchard-Peschek, K., et al. 2010. Pseudoephedrine ingestion and cycling time-trial performance. *International Journal of Sport Nutrition and Exercise Metabolism* 20:132–8.

Rao, A., et al. 2005. The effects of combined caffeine and glucose drinks on attention in the human brain. *Nutritional Neuroscience* 8:141–53.

Rasmussen, B. et al. 2000. Androstenedione does not stimulate muscle protein anabolism in young healthy men. *Journal of Clinical Endocrinology and Metabolism* 85:55–59.

Raymer, G., et al. 2004. Metabolic effects of induced alkalosis during progressive forearm exercise to fatigue. *Journal of Applied Physiology* 96:2050–56.

Reis, J., et al. 2010. Coffee, decaffeinated coffee, caffeine, and tea consumption in young adulthood and atherosclerosis later in life: The CARDIA study. *Arteriosclerosis, Thrombosis, and Vascular Biology* 30:2059–66.

Richards, J., et al. 2010. Epigallocatechin-3-gallate increases maximal oxygen uptake in adult humans. *Medicine & Science in Sports & Exercise* 42:739–44.

Ritchie, K., et al. 2007. The neuroprotective effects of caffeine: A prospective population study (the Three City Study). *Neurology* 69:536–45.

Rogerson, S., et al. 2007. The effect of five weeks of Tribulus terrestris supplementation on muscle strength and body composition during preseason training in elite rugby league players. *Journal of Strength and Conditioning Research* 21:348–53.

Rogerson, S., et al. 2007. The effect of short-term use of testosterone enanthate on muscular strength and power in healthy young men. *Journal of Strength and Conditioning Research* 21:354–61.

Rudelle, S., et al. 2007. Effect of a thermogenic beverage on 24-hour energy metabolism in humans. *Obesity* 15:349–55.

Sattler, F., et al. 2009. Testosterone and growth hormone improve body composition and muscle performance in older men. *Journal of Clinical Endocrinology and Metabolism* 94:1991–2001.

Savitz, D., et al. 2008. Caffeine and miscarriage risk. *Epidemiology* 19:55–62.

Schabort, E., et al. 2000. Dose-related elevations in venous pH with citrate ingestion do not alter 40-km cycling time-trial performance. *European Journal of Applied Physiology* 83:320–27.

Schneiker, K., et al. 2006. Effects of caffeine on prolonged intermittent-sprint ability in team-sport athletes. *Medicine & Science in Sports & Exercise* 38:578–85.

Schroeder, E., et al. 2005. Six-week improvements in muscle mass and strength during androgen therapy in older men. *Journals of Gerontology. Series A, Biological Sciences and Medical Sciences* 60:1586–92.

Shave, R., et al. 2001. The effects of sodium citrate ingestion on 3,000-meter time-trial performance. *Journal of Strength and Conditioning Research* 15:230–34.

Siegler, J., and Hirscher, K. 2010. Sodium bicarbonate ingestion and boxing performance. *Journal of Strength and Conditioning Research* 24:103–8.

Skarpanska-Stejnborn, A., et al. 2009. The influence of supplementation with Rhodiola rosea L. extract on selected redox parameters in professional rowers. *International Journal of Sport Nutrition and Exercise Metabolism* 19:186–99.

Skinner, T., et al. 2010. Dose response of caffeine on 2000-m rowing performance. *Medicine & Science in Sports & Exercise* 42:571–6.

Smothers, B., and Bertolucci, D. 2001. Alcohol consumption and health-promoting behavior in a U.S. household sample: Leisure-time physical activity. *Journal of Studies on Alcohol* 62:467–76.

Spriet, D., et al. 1992. Caffeine ingestion and muscle metabolism during prolonged exercise in humans. *American Journal of Physiology* 262:E891–E898.

Stephens, T., et al. 2002. Effect of sodium bicarbonate on muscle metabolism during intense endurance cycling. *Medicine & Science in Sports & Exercise* 34:614–21.

Stevenson, E., et al. 2009. The effect of a carbohydrate-caffeine sports drink on simulated golf performance. *Applied Physiology, Nutrition, and Metabolism* 34:681–8.

Taaffe, D. et al. 1996. Lack of effect of recombinant human growth hormone (GH) on muscle morphology and GH-insulin-like growth factor expression in resistance-trained elderly men. *Journal of Clinical Endocrinology and Metabolism* 81:421–25.

Tarnopolsky, M., and Cupido, C. 2000. Caffeine potentiates low frequency skeletal muscle force in habitual and nonhabitual caffeine consumers. *Journal of Applied Physiology* 89:1719–24.

Todd, A., et al. 2007. Caffeine-induced changes in cardiovascular function during resistance training. *International Journal of Sport Nutrition and Exercise Metabolism* 17:466–77.

Tremblay, A., et al. 1995. Alcohol and a high-fat diet: A combination favoring overfeeding. *American Journal of Clinical Nutrition* 62:639–44.

Tunnicliffe, J., et al. 2008. Consumption of dietary caffeine and coffee in physically active populations: Physiological interactions. *Applied Physiology, Nutrition, and Metabolism* 33:1301–10.

Urhausen, A., et al. 2004. Are the cardiac effects of anabolic steroid abuse in strength athletes reversible? *Heart* 90:496–501.

van Gelder, B., et al. 2007. Coffee consumption is inversely associated with cognitive decline in elderly European men: The FINE Study. *European Journal of Clinical Nutrition* 61:226–32.

Van Montfoort, M., et al. 2004. Effects of ingestion of bicarbonate, citrate, lactate, and chloride on sprint running. *Medicine & Science in Sports & Exercise* 36:1239–43.

van Someren, K., et al. 1998. An investigation into the effects of sodium citrate ingestion on high-intensity exercise performance. *International Journal of Sport Nutrition* 8:356–63.

Verhoef, P., et al. 2002. Contribution of caffeine to the homocysteine-raising effect of coffee: A randomized controlled trial in humans. *American Journal of Clinical Nutrition* 76:1244–48.

Villareal, D., et al. 2000. Effects of DHEA replacement on bone mineral density and body composition in elderly women or men. *Clinical Endocrinology* 53:561–68.

Walker, T., et al. 2007. Failure of Rhodiola rosea to alter skeletal muscle phosphate kinetics in trained men. *Metabolism* 56:1111–17.

Wallace, M. et al. 1999. Effects of dehydroepi-androsterone vs androstenedione supplementation in men. *Medicine & Science in Sports & Exercise* 31:1788–92.

Wannamethee, S., et al. 2005. Alcohol and adioposity: Effects of quantity and type of drink and time relation with meals. *International Journal of Obesity* 29:1436–44.

Weng, X., et al. 2008. Maternal caffeine consumption during pregnancy and the risk of miscarriage: A prospective cohort study. *American Journal of Obstetrics and Gynecology.* January 28, epub ahead of print.

Whitehead, M., et al. 2007. The effect of 4 wk of oral Echinacea supplementation on serum erythropoietin and indices of erythropoietic status. *International Journal of Sport Nutrition and Exercise Metabolism* 17:378–90.

Wichstrøm, T., and Wichstrøm, L. 2009. Does sports participation during adolescence prevent later alcohol, tobacco and cannabis use? *Addiction* 104:138–49.

Wiles, J., et al. 1992. Effect of caffeinated coffee on running speed, respiratory factors, blood lactate and perceived exertion during 1,500-meter treadmill running. *British Journal of Sports Medicine* 26:116–20.

Williams, P. 1997. Interactive effects of exercise, alcohol, and vegetarian diet on coronary artery disease risk factors in 9242 runners: The National Runners' Health Study. *American Journal of Clinical Nutrition* 66:1197–206.

Willoughby, D. 2004. Effects of an alleged myostatin-binding supplement and heavy resistance training on serum myostatin, muscle strength and mass, and body composition. *International Journal of Sport Nutrition and Exercise Metabolism* 14:461–72.

Woolf, K., et al. 2008. The effect of caffeine as an ergogenic aid in anaerobic exercise. *International Journal of Sport Nutrition and Exercise Metabolism* 18:412–29.

Yarasheski, K., et al. 1993. Short-term growth hormone treatment does not increase muscle protein synthesis in experienced weight lifters. *Journal of Applied Physiology* 74:3073–76.

Yesalis, C., et al. 1997. Trends in anabolic-androgenic steroid use among adolescents. *Archives of Pediatric and Adolescent Medicine* 151:1197–1206.

Youngstedt, S. et al. 1998. Acute exercise reduces caffeine-induced anxiogenesis. *Medicine & Science in Sports & Exercise* 30:740–45.

Zhang, S., et al. 2007. Alcohol consumption and breast cancer risk in the Women's Health Study. *American Journal of Epidemiology* 165:667–76.

Ziemba, A. et al. 1999. Ginseng treatment improves psychomotor performance at rest and during graded exercise in young athletes. *International Journal of Sport Nutrition* 9:371–77.

Units of Measurement: English System— Metric System Equivalents

The Metric System and Equivalents

To measure ingredients, a standardized system known as the System Internationale (SI) has been established that is interpreted on an international basis. The SI is based on the metric system. However, in the United States we also employ another set of measure and weight, the English system. In the field of dietetics, both systems are employed. The following tables give the quantities of the measures besides stating equivalents. With this information it is possible to calculate in either system of measure and weight.

Household Measures (Approximations)

For easy computing purposes, the cubic centimeter (cc) is considered equivalent to 1 gram:

$$1 \text{ cc} = 1 \text{ gram} = 1 \text{ milliliter (ml)}$$

For easy computing purposes, 1 ounce equals 30 grams or 30 cubic centimeters.

1 quart	=	960 grams
1 pint	=	480 grams
1 cup	=	240 grams
1/2 cup	=	120 grams
1 glass (8 ounces)	=	240 grams
1/2 glass (4 ounces)	=	120 grams
1 orange juice glass	=	100–120 grams
1 tablespoon	=	15 grams
1 teaspoon	=	5 grams

Level Measures and Weights

1 teaspoon	=	5 cc or 5 ml
		5 grams
3 teaspoons	=	1 tablespoon
		15 cc
		15 grams
2 tablespoons	=	30 cc
		30 grams
		1 ounce (fluid)
4 tablespoons	=	1/4 cup
		60 cc
		60 grams
8 tablespoons	=	1/2 cup
		120 cc
		120 grams
16 tablespoons	=	1 cup
		240 grams
		240 ml (fluid)
		8 ounces (fluid)
		1/2 pound
2 cups	=	1 pint
		480 grams
		480 ml (fluid)
		16 ounces (fluid)
		1 pound
4 cups	=	2 pints
		1 quart
		960 cc
		960 ml (fluid)
		2 pounds
4 quarts	=	1 gallon

Units of Weight

		Ounce	Pound	Gram	Kilogram
1 ounce	=	1.0	0.06	28.4	0.028
1 pound	=	16.0	1.0	454	0.454
1 gram	=	0.035	.002	1.0	0.001
1 kilogram	=	35.3	2.2	1,000	1.0

Units of Volume

		Ounce	Pint	Quart	Milliliter	Liter
1 ounce	=	1.0	0.062	0.031	29.57	0.029
1 pint	=	16.0	1.0	0.5	473	0.473
1 quart	=	32.0	2.0	1.0	946	0.946
1 milliliter	=	0.034	0.002	0.001	1.0	0.001
1 liter	=	33.8	2.112	1.056	1,000	1.0

Units of Length

		Millimeter	Centimeter	Inch	Foot	Yard	Meter
1 millimeter	=	1.0	0.1	0.0394	0.0033	0.0011	0.001
1 centimeter	=	10.0	1.0	0.394	0.033	0.011	0.01
1 inch	=	25.4	2.54	1.0	0.083	0.028	0.025
1 foot	=	304.8	30.48	12.0	1.0	0.333	0.305
1 yard	=	914.4	91.44	36.0	3.0	1.0	0.914
1 meter	=	1,000	100	39.37	3.28	1.094	1.0

1 kilometer	=	1,000 meters	= 0.6216 mile
1 mile	=	1,760 yards	= 1.61 kilometers

Units of mechanical, thermal, and chemical energy (approximate equivalents)

	Foot-pounds	Kilogram-meters	Kilojoules	Watts*	Kilocalories	Oxygen**
1 foot-pound	1	0.138	0.00136	0.0226	0.00032	0.000064
1 kilogram-meter	7.23	1	0.0098	0.163	0.0023	0.00046
1 kilojoule	737	102	1	16.66	0.239	0.047
1 watt*	44.27	6.12	0.06	1	0.0143	0.0028
1 kilocalorie	3,088	427	4.18	0.00024	1	0.198
1 liter oxygen**	15,585	2,154	21.1	351.9	5.047	1

Note: Read all tables across, such as 1 watt equals 44.27 foot-pounds per minute; 1 foot-pound equals 0.0226 watt.

*Watts are units of power expressed per minute.

**Equivalents are based upon 1 liter of oxygen metabolizing carbohydrate. Energy equivalents would be slightly less on a mixed diet of carbohydrate, fat, and protein. For example, 1 liter of oxygen would equal only 4.82 kilocalories on such a mixed diet.

Approximate Caloric Expenditure per Minute for Various Physical Activities

When using this appendix, keep these points in mind.

A. The figures are approximate and include the resting energy expenditure (REE). Thus, the total cost of the exercise includes not only the energy expended by the exercise itself, but also the amount you would have used anyway during the same period. Suppose you ran for 1 hour and the calculated energy cost was 800 Calories. During that same time at rest, your REE may have been 75 Calories, so the net cost of the exercise is 725 Calories.

B. The figures in the table are only for the time you are performing the activity. For example, in an hour of basketball, you may exercise strenuously for only 35 to 40 minutes, as you may take time-outs and may rest during foul shots. In general, record only the amount of time that you are actually exercising during the activity.

C. The energy cost, expressed in Calories per minute, will vary for different physical activities in a given individual depending on several factors. For example, the caloric cost of bicycling will vary depending on the type of bicycle, going uphill and downhill, and wind resistance. Walking with hand weights or ankle weights will increase energy output. Energy cost for swimming at a certain pace will depend on swimming efficiency, so the less efficient swimmer will expend more Calories. Thus, the values expressed here are approximations and may be increased or decreased depending upon various factors that influence energy cost for a specific physical activity.

D. Not all body weights could be listed, but you may approximate by using the closest weight listed.

E. There may be small differences between males and females, but not enough to make a significant difference in the total caloric value for most exercises.

Body weight

Kilograms	45	48	50	52	55	57	59	61	64	66	68	70
Pounds	100	105	110	115	120	125	130	135	140	145	150	155

Sedentary activities

Lying quietly	1.0	1.0	1.1	1.1	1.2	1.3	1.3	1.4	1.4	1.5	1.5	1.5
Sitting and writing, card playing, etc.	1.2	1.3	1.4	1.5	1.5	1.6	1.7	1.7	1.8	1.8	1.9	2.0
Standing with light work, cleaning, etc.	2.7	2.9	3.0	3.1	3.3	3.4	3.5	3.7	3.8	3.9	4.1	4.2

Physical activities

Archery	3.1	3.3	3.5	3.6	3.8	4.0	4.1	4.3	4.5	4.6	4.8	4.9
Badminton												
Recreational singles	3.6	3.8	4.0	4.2	4.4	4.6	4.7	4.9	5.1	5.3	5.4	5.6
Social doubles	2.7	2.9	3.0	3.1	3.3	3.4	3.5	3.7	3.8	3.9	4.1	4.2
Competitive	5.9	6.1	6.4	6.7	7.0	7.3	7.6	7.9	8.2	8.5	8.8	9.1
Baseball												
Player	3.1	3.3	3.4	3.6	3.8	4.0	4.1	4.3	4.4	4.5	4.7	4.8
Pitcher	3.9	4.1	4.3	4.5	4.7	4.9	5.1	5.3	5.5	5.7	5.9	6.0
Basketball												
Half court	3.0	3.1	3.3	3.5	3.6	3.8	3.9	4.1	4.2	4.4	4.5	4.7
Recreational	4.9	5.2	5.5	5.7	6.0	6.2	6.5	6.7	7.0	7.2	7.5	7.7
Vigorous competition	6.5	6.8	7.2	7.5	7.8	8.2	8.5	8.8	9.2	9.5	9.9	10.2
Bicycling, level												
(mph) (min/mile)												
5 12:00	1.9	2.0	2.1	2.2	2.3	2.4	2.5	2.6	2.7	2.8	2.9	3.0
10 6:00	4.2	4.4	4.6	4.8	5.1	5.3	5.5	5.7	5.9	6.1	6.4	6.6
15 4:00	7.3	7.6	8.0	8.4	8.7	9.1	9.5	9.8	10.0	10.5	10.9	11.3
20 3:00	10.7	11.2	11.7	12.3	12.8	13.3	13.9	14.4	14.9	15.5	16.0	16.5
Bowling	2.7	2.8	3.0	3.1	3.3	3.4	3.5	3.7	3.8	3.9	4.1	4.2
Calisthenics												
Light type	3.4	3.6	3.8	4.0	4.1	4.3	4.5	4.7	4.8	5.0	5.2	5.4
Timed vigorous	9.7	10.1	10.6	11.1	11.6	12.1	12.6	13.1	13.6	14.1	14.6	15.1
Canoeing												
(mph) (min/mile)												
2.5 24	1.9	2.0	2.1	2.2	2.3	2.4	2.5	2.6	2.7	2.8	2.9	3.0
4.0 15	4.4	4.6	4.9	5.1	5.3	5.5	5.8	6.0	6.2	6.4	6.7	6.9
5.0 12	5.7	6.0	6.3	6.6	6.9	7.2	7.5	7.8	8.1	8.4	8.7	9.0
Dancing												
Moderately (waltz)	3.1	3.3	3.5	3.6	3.8	4.0	4.1	4.3	4.5	4.6	4.8	4.9
Active (square, disco)	4.5	4.7	5.0	5.2	5.4	5.6	5.9	6.1	6.3	6.6	6.8	7.0
Aerobic (vigorously)	6.0	6.3	6.7	7.0	7.3	7.6	7.9	8.2	8.5	8.8	9.1	9.4
Fencing												
Moderately	3.3	3.5	3.6	3.8	4.0	4.1	4.3	4.5	4.6	4.8	5.0	5.2
Vigorously	6.6	7.0	7.3	7.7	8.0	8.3	8.7	9.0	9.4	9.7	10.0	10.4
Football												
Moderate	3.3	3.5	3.6	3.8	4.0	4.1	4.3	4.5	4.6	4.8	5.0	5.2
Touch, vigorous	5.5	5.8	6.1	6.4	6.6	6.9	7.2	7.5	7.8	8.0	8.3	8.6
Golf												
Twosome (carry clubs)	3.6	3.8	4.0	4.2	4.4	4.6	4.7	4.9	5.1	5.3	5.4	5.6
Foursome (carry clubs)	2.7	2.9	3.0	3.1	3.3	3.4	3.5	3.7	3.8	3.9	4.1	4.2
Power-cart	1.9	2.0	2.1	2.2	2.3	2.4	2.5	2.6	2.7	2.8	2.9	3.0

APPENDIX B Approximate Caloric Expenditure per Minute for Various Physical Activities

Body weight

73	75	77	80	82	84	86	89	91	93	95	98	100
160	165	170	175	180	185	190	195	200	205	210	215	220
1.6	1.6	1.7	1.7	1.8	1.8	1.9	1.9	2.0	2.0	2.1	2.1	2.2
2.0	2.1	2.2	2.2	2.3	2.4	2.4	2.5	2.5	2.6	2.7	2.7	2.8
4.4	4.5	4.6	4.8	4.9	5.0	5.2	5.3	5.4	5.6	5.7	5.9	6.0
5.1	5.3	5.4	5.6	5.7	5.9	6.0	6.2	6.4	6.5	6.7	6.9	7.0
5.8	6.0	6.2	6.4	6.6	6.7	6.9	7.1	7.3	7.4	7.6	7.8	8.0
4.4	4.5	4.6	4.8	4.9	5.0	5.2	5.3	5.4	5.6	5.7	5.9	6.0
9.4	9.7	10.0	10.3	10.6	10.9	11.2	11.5	11.8	12.1	12.4	12.7	13.0
5.0	5.2	5.3	5.5	5.6	5.8	5.9	6.1	6.3	6.4	6.6	6.8	6.9
6.3	6.5	6.7	6.9	7.1	7.3	7.4	7.7	7.9	8.0	8.2	8.5	8.6
4.8	5.0	5.1	5.3	5.4	5.6	5.7	5.9	6.0	6.2	6.4	6.5	6.7
8.0	8.2	8.5	8.7	9.0	9.2	9.5	9.7	10.0	10.2	10.5	10.7	11.0
10.5	10.9	11.2	11.5	11.9	12.2	12.5	12.9	13.2	13.5	13.8	14.2	14.5
3.1	3.2	3.3	3.4	3.5	3.6	3.7	3.8	3.9	4.0	4.1	4.2	4.3
6.8	7.0	7.2	7.4	7.6	7.9	8.1	8.3	8.5	8.7	8.9	9.1	9.4
11.6	12.0	12.4	12.7	13.1	13.4	13.8	14.2	14.5	14.9	15.3	15.6	16.0
17.1	17.6	18.1	18.7	19.2	19.7	20.3	20.8	21.3	21.9	22.4	22.9	23.5
4.4	4.5	4.6	4.8	4.9	5.0	5.2	5.3	5.5	5.6	5.7	5.9	6.0
5.5	5.7	5.9	6.1	6.3	6.4	6.6	6.8	7.0	7.1	7.3	7.5	7.7
15.6	16.1	16.6	17.1	17.6	18.1	18.6	19.1	19.6	20.0	20.5	21.0	21.5
3.1	3.2	3.3	3.4	3.5	3.6	3.7	3.8	3.9	4.0	4.1	4.2	4.3
7.1	7.4	7.6	7.8	8.0	8.2	8.5	8.7	8.9	9.1	9.4	9.6	9.8
9.3	9.5	9.8	10.1	10.4	10.7	11.0	11.3	11.6	11.9	12.2	12.5	12.8
5.1	5.3	5.4	5.6	5.7	5.9	6.0	6.2	6.4	6.5	6.7	6.9	7.0
7.3	7.5	7.7	7.9	8.2	8.4	8.6	8.9	9.1	9.3	9.5	9.8	10.0
9.7	10.0	10.3	10.6	10.9	11.2	11.5	11.8	12.1	12.4	12.7	13.0	13.3
5.3	5.5	5.7	5.8	6.0	6.2	6.3	6.5	6.7	6.8	7.0	7.1	7.3
10.7	11.0	11.4	11.7	12.1	12.4	12.7	13.1	13.4	13.8	14.1	14.4	14.8
5.3	5.5	5.7	5.8	6.0	6.2	6.3	6.5	6.7	6.8	7.0	7.1	7.3
8.9	9.2	9.4	9.7	10.0	10.3	10.6	10.8	11.1	11.4	11.7	12.0	12.2
5.8	6.0	6.2	6.4	6.6	6.7	6.9	7.1	7.3	7.4	7.6	7.8	8.0
4.4	4.5	4.6	4.8	4.9	5.0	5.2	5.3	5.4	5.6	5.7	5.9	6.0
3.1	3.2	3.3	3.4	3.5	3.6	3.7	3.8	3.9	4.0	4.1	4.2	4.3

Body weight

	Kilograms	45	48	50	52	55	57	59	61	64	66	68	70
	Pounds	100	105	110	115	120	125	130	135	140	145	150	155
Handball													
Moderate		6.5	6.8	7.2	7.5	7.8	8.2	8.5	8.8	9.2	9.5	9.9	10.2
Competitive		7.7	8.0	8.4	8.8	9.2	9.6	10.0	10.4	10.8	11.1	11.5	11.9
Hiking, pack (3 mph)		4.5	4.7	5.0	5.2	5.4	5.6	5.9	6.1	6.3	6.6	6.8	7.0
Hockey, field		5.0	6.3	6.7	7.0	7.3	7.6	7.9	8.2	8.5	8.8	9.1	9.4
Hockey, ice		6.6	7.0	7.3	7.7	8.0	8.3	8.7	9.0	9.4	9.7	10.0	10.4
Horseback riding													
Walk		1.9	2.0	2.1	2.2	2.3	2.4	2.5	2.6	2.7	2.8	2.9	3.0
Sitting to trot		2.7	2.9	3.0	3.1	3.3	3.4	3.5	3.7	3.8	3.9	4.1	4.2
Posting to trot		4.2	4.4	4.6	4.8	5.1	5.3	5.5	5.7	5.9	6.1	6.4	6.6
Gallop		5.7	6.0	6.3	6.6	6.9	7.2	7.5	7.8	8.1	8.4	8.7	9.0
Horseshoes		2.5	2.6	2.8	2.9	3.0	3.1	3.3	3.4	3.5	3.7	3.8	3.9
Jogging (see Running)													
Judo		8.5	8.9	9.3	9.8	10.2	10.6	11.0	11.5	11.9	12.3	12.8	13.2
Karate		8.5	8.9	9.3	9.8	10.2	10.6	11.0	11.5	11.9	12.3	12.8	13.2
Mountain climbing		6.5	6.8	7.2	7.5	7.8	8.2	8.5	8.8	9.2	9.5	9.8	10.2
Paddle ball		5.7	6.0	6.3	6.6	6.9	7.2	7.5	7.8	8.1	8.4	8.7	9.0
Pool (billiards)		1.5	1.6	1.6	1.7	1.8	1.9	1.9	2.0	2.1	2.2	2.2	2.3
Racquetball		6.5	6.8	7.1	7.5	7.8	8.1	8.4	8.8	9.1	9.4	9.8	10.1
Roller skating (9 mph)		4.2	4.4	4.6	4.8	5.1	5.3	5.5	5.7	5.9	6.1	6.4	6.6
Running (steady state)													
(mph)	(min/mile)												
5.0	12:00	6.0	6.3	6.6	7.0	7.3	7.6	7.9	8.2	8.5	8.8	9.1	9.4
5.5	10:55	6.7	7.0	7.3	7.7	8.0	8.4	8.7	9.0	9.4	9.7	10.0	10.4
6.0	10:00	7.2	7.6	8.0	8.4	8.7	9.1	9.5	9.8	10.2	10.6	10.9	11.3
7.0	8:35	8.5	8.9	9.3	9.8	10.2	10.6	11.0	11.5	11.9	12.3	12.8	13.2
8.0	7:30	9.7	10.2	10.7	11.2	11.6	12.1	12.6	13.1	13.6	14.1	14.6	15.1
9.0	6:40	10.8	11.3	11.9	12.4	12.9	13.5	14.0	14.6	15.1	15.7	16.2	16.8
10.0	6:00	12.1	12.7	13.3	13.9	14.5	15.1	15.7	16.4	17.0	17.6	18.2	18.8
11.0	5:28	13.3	14.0	14.6	15.3	16.0	16.7	17.3	18.0	18.7	19.4	20.0	20.7
12.0	5:00	14.5	15.2	16.0	16.7	17.4	18.2	18.9	19.7	20.4	21.1	21.9	22.6
Sailing, small boat		2.7	2.9	3.0	3.1	3.3	3.4	3.5	3.7	3.8	3.9	4.1	4.2
Skating, ice (9 mph)		4.2	4.4	4.6	4.8	5.1	5.2	5.5	5.7	5.9	6.1	6.4	6.6
Skating, in-line (13 mph)		9.5	10.0	10.5	10.9	11.5	12.0	12.4	12.8	13.4	13.9	14.3	14.7
Skiing, cross-country													
(mph)	(min/mile)												
2.5	24:00	5.0	5.2	5.5	5.7	6.0	6.2	6.5	6.7	7.0	7.2	7.5	7.8
4.0	15:00	6.5	6.8	7.2	7.5	7.8	8.2	8.5	8.8	9.2	9.5	9.9	10.2
5.0	12:00	7.7	8.0	8.4	8.8	9.2	9.6	10.0	10.4	10.8	11.1	11.5	11.9
Skiing, downhill		6.5	6.8	7.2	7.5	7.8	8.2	8.5	8.8	9.2	9.5	9.9	10.2
Soccer		5.9	6.2	6.6	6.9	7.2	7.5	7.8	8.1	8.4	8.7	9.0	9.3
Squash													
Normal		6.7	7.0	7.3	7.7	8.0	8.4	8.7	9.1	9.5	9.8	10.1	10.5
Competition		7.7	8.0	8.4	8.8	9.2	9.6	10.0	10.4	10.8	11.1	11.5	11.9
Swimming (yards/min)													
Backstroke													
25		2.5	2.6	2.8	2.9	3.0	3.1	3.3	3.4	3.5	3.7	3.8	3.9
30		3.5	3.7	3.9	4.1	4.2	4.4	4.6	4.8	4.9	5.1	5.3	5.5
35		4.5	4.7	5.0	5.2	5.4	5.6	5.9	6.1	6.3	6.6	6.8	7.0
40		5.5	5.8	6.1	6.4	6.6	6.9	7.2	7.5	7.8	8.0	8.3	8.6

APPENDIX B Approximate Caloric Expenditure per Minute for Various Physical Activities

Body weight

| 73 | 75 | 77 | 80 | 82 | 84 | 86 | 89 | 91 | 93 | 95 | 98 | 100 |
160	165	170	175	180	185	190	195	200	205	210	215	220
10.5	10.9	11.2	11.5	11.9	12.2	12.5	12.9	13.2	13.5	13.8	14.2	14.5
12.3	12.7	13.1	13.5	13.9	14.3	14.7	15.0	15.4	15.8	16.2	16.6	17.0
7.3	7.5	7.7	7.9	8.2	8.4	8.6	8.9	9.1	9.3	9.5	9.8	10.0
9.7	10.0	10.3	10.6	10.9	11.2	11.5	11.8	12.1	12.4	12.7	13.0	13.3
10.7	11.0	11.4	11.7	12.1	12.4	12.7	13.1	13.4	13.8	14.1	14.4	14.8
3.1	3.2	3.3	3.4	3.5	3.6	3.7	3.8	3.9	4.0	4.1	4.2	4.3
4.4	4.5	4.6	4.8	4.9	5.0	5.2	5.3	5.4	5.6	5.7	5.9	6.0
6.8	7.0	7.2	7.4	7.6	7.9	8.1	8.3	8.5	8.7	8.9	9.1	9.4
9.3	9.5	9.8	10.1	10.4	10.7	11.0	11.3	11.6	11.9	12.2	12.5	12.8
4.0	4.2	4.3	4.4	4.5	4.7	4.8	4.9	5.2	5.2	5.3	5.4	5.6
13.6	14.1	14.5	14.9	15.4	15.8	16.2	16.6	17.1	17.5	17.9	18.4	18.8
13.6	14.1	14.5	14.9	15.4	15.8	16.2	16.6	17.1	17.5	17.9	18.4	18.8
10.5	10.8	11.2	11.5	11.8	12.1	12.5	12.8	13.1	13.5	13.8	14.1	14.5
9.3	9.5	9.8	10.1	10.4	10.7	11.0	11.2	11.6	11.9	12.2	12.5	12.8
2.4	2.5	2.6	2.6	2.7	2.8	2.9	2.9	3.0	3.1	3.2	3.2	3.3
10.4	10.7	11.1	11.4	11.7	12.0	12.4	12.7	13.0	13.4	13.7	14.0	14.4
6.8	7.0	7.2	7.4	7.6	7.9	8.1	8.3	8.5	8.7	8.9	9.1	9.4
9.7	10.0	10.3	10.6	10.9	11.2	11.6	11.9	12.2	12.5	12.8	13.1	13.4
10.7	11.1	11.4	11.7	12.1	12.4	12.8	13.1	13.4	13.8	14.1	14.5	14.8
11.7	12.0	12.4	12.8	13.1	13.5	13.8	14.3	14.6	15.0	15.4	15.7	16.1
13.6	14.1	14.5	14.9	15.4	15.8	16.2	16.6	17.1	17.5	17.9	18.4	18.8
15.6	16.1	16.6	17.1	17.6	18.1	18.5	19.0	19.5	20.0	20.5	21.0	21.5
17.3	17.9	18.4	19.0	19.5	20.1	20.6	21.2	21.7	22.2	22.8	23.3	23.9
19.4	20.0	20.7	21.3	21.9	22.5	23.1	23.7	24.2	24.8	25.4	26.0	26.7
21.4	22.1	22.7	23.4	24.1	24.8	25.4	26.1	26.8	27.5	28.1	28.8	29.5
23.3	24.1	24.8	25.6	26.3	27.0	27.8	28.5	29.2	30.0	30.7	31.5	32.2
4.4	4.5	4.6	4.8	4.9	5.0	5.2	5.3	5.4	5.6	5.7	5.9	6.0
6.8	7.0	7.2	7.4	7.6	7.9	8.1	8.3	8.5	8.7	8.9	9.1	9.4
15.3	15.7	16.2	16.8	17.2	17.6	18.1	18.7	19.1	19.5	20.0	20.6	21.0
8.0	8.3	8.5	8.8	9.0	9.3	9.5	9.8	10.0	10.3	10.6	10.8	11.1
10.5	10.9	11.2	11.5	11.9	12.2	12.5	12.9	13.2	13.5	13.8	14.2	14.5
12.3	12.7	13.1	13.5	13.9	14.3	14.7	15.0	15.4	15.8	16.2	16.6	17.0
10.5	10.9	11.2	11.5	11.9	12.2	12.5	12.9	13.2	13.5	13.8	14.2	14.5
9.6	9.9	10.2	10.5	10.8	11.1	11.4	11.7	12.0	12.3	12.6	12.9	13.2
10.8	11.2	11.5	11.8	12.2	12.5	12.9	13.2	13.5	13.9	14.2	14.6	14.9
12.3	12.7	13.1	13.5	13.9	14.3	14.7	15.0	15.4	15.8	16.2	16.6	17.0
4.0	4.2	4.3	4.4	4.5	4.7	4.8	4.9	5.1	5.2	5.3	5.4	5.6
5.6	5.8	6.0	6.2	6.4	6.5	6.7	6.9	7.1	7.2	7.4	7.6	7.8
7.3	7.5	7.7	7.9	8.2	8.4	8.6	8.9	9.1	9.3	9.5	9.8	10.0
8.9	9.2	9.4	9.7	10.0	10.3	10.6	10.8	11.1	11.4	11.7	12.0	12.2

Body weight

Kilograms		45	48	50	52	55	57	59	61	64	66	68	70
Pounds		100	105	110	115	120	125	130	135	140	145	150	155
Swimming (yards/min) (*continued*)													
Breaststroke													
20		3.1	3.3	3.5	3.6	3.8	4.0	4.1	4.3	4.5	4.6	4.8	4.9
30		4.7	5.0	5.2	5.4	5.7	5.9	6.2	6.4	6.7	6.9	7.1	7.4
40		6.3	6.7	7.0	7.3	7.6	8.0	8.3	8.6	8.9	9.3	9.6	9.9
Front crawl													
20		3.1	3.3	3.5	3.6	3.8	4.0	4.1	4.3	4.5	4.6	4.8	4.9
25		4.0	4.2	4.4	4.6	4.8	5.0	5.2	5.4	5.6	5.8	6.0	6.2
35		4.8	5.1	5.4	5.6	5.9	6.1	6.4	6.6	6.8	7.0	7.3	7.5
45		5.7	6.0	6.3	6.6	6.9	7.2	7.5	7.8	8.1	8.4	8.7	9.0
50		7.0	7.4	7.7	8.1	8.5	8.8	9.2	9.5	9.9	10.3	10.6	11.0
Table tennis		3.4	3.6	3.8	4.0	4.1	4.3	4.5	4.7	4.8	5.0	5.2	5.4
Tennis													
Singles, recreational		5.0	5.2	5.5	5.7	6.0	6.2	6.5	6.7	7.0	7.2	7.5	7.8
Doubles, recreational		3.4	3.6	3.8	4.0	4.1	4.3	4.5	4.7	4.8	5.0	5.2	5.4
Competition		6.4	6.7	7.1	7.4	7.7	8.1	8.4	8.7	9.1	9.4	9.8	10.1
Volleyball													
Moderate, recreational		2.9	3.0	3.2	3.3	3.5	3.6	3.8	3.9	4.1	4.2	4.4	4.5
Vigorous, competition		6.5	6.8	7.1	7.5	7.8	8.1	8.4	8.8	9.1	9.4	9.8	10.1
Walking													
(mph)	(min/mile)												
1.0	60:00	1.5	1.6	1.7	1.8	1.8	1.9	2.0	2.1	2.2	2.2	2.3	2.4
2.0	30:00	2.1	2.2	2.3	2.4	2.5	2.6	2.8	2.9	3.0	3.1	3.2	3.3
2.3	26:00	2.3	2.4	2.5	2.7	2.8	2.9	3.0	3.1	3.2	3.4	3.5	3.6
3.0	20:00	2.7	2.9	3.0	3.1	3.3	3.4	3.5	3.7	3.8	3.9	4.1	4.2
3.2	18:45	3.1	3.3	3.4	3.6	3.8	4.0	4.1	4.3	4.4	4.5	4.7	4.8
3.5	17:10	3.3	3.5	3.7	3.9	4.0	4.2	4.4	4.6	4.7	4.9	5.1	5.3
4.0	15:00	4.2	4.4	4.6	4.8	5.1	5.3	5.5	5.7	5.9	6.1	6.4	6.6
4.5	13:20	4.7	5.0	5.2	5.4	5.7	5.9	6.2	6.4	6.7	6.9	7.1	7.4
5.0	12:00	5.4	5.7	6.0	6.3	6.5	6.8	7.1	7.4	7.7	7.9	8.2	8.4
5.4	11:10	6.2	6.6	6.9	7.2	7.5	7.9	8.2	8.5	8.8	9.2	9.5	9.8
5.8	10:20	7.7	8.0	8.4	8.8	9.2	9.6	10.0	10.4	10.8	11.1	11.5	11.9
Water skiing		5.0	5.2	5.5	5.7	6.0	6.2	6.5	6.7	7.0	7.2	7.5	7.8
Weight training		5.2	5.4	5.7	6.0	6.2	6.5	6.8	7.0	7.3	7.6	7.8	8.1
Wrestling		8.5	8.9	9.3	9.8	10.2	10.6	11.0	11.5	11.9	12.3	12.8	13.2

Body weight

73	75	77	80	82	84	86	89	91	93	95	98	100
160	165	170	175	180	185	190	195	200	205	210	215	220
5.1	5.3	5.4	5.6	5.7	5.9	6.0	6.2	6.4	6.5	6.7	6.9	7.0
7.6	7.9	8.1	8.3	8.6	8.8	9.1	9.3	9.5	9.8	10.0	10.3	10.5
10.2	10.5	10.9	11.2	11.5	11.9	12.2	12.5	12.8	13.1	13.5	13.8	14.1
5.1	5.3	5.4	5.6	5.7	5.9	6.0	6.2	6.4	6.5	6.7	6.9	7.0
6.4	6.6	6.8	7.0	7.2	7.4	7.6	7.8	8.0	8.2	8.4	8.6	8.8
7.8	8.0	8.3	8.5	8.8	9.0	9.2	9.4	9.7	9.9	10.2	10.4	10.7
9.3	9.5	9.8	10.1	10.4	10.7	11.0	11.3	11.6	11.9	12.2	12.5	12.8
11.3	11.7	12.0	12.4	12.8	13.1	13.5	13.8	14.2	14.5	14.9	15.2	15.6
5.5	5.7	5.9	6.1	6.3	6.4	6.6	6.8	7.0	7.1	7.3	7.5	7.7
8.0	8.3	8.5	8.8	9.0	9.3	9.5	9.8	10.0	10.3	10.6	10.8	11.1
5.5	5.7	5.9	6.1	6.3	6.4	6.6	6.8	7.0	7.1	7.3	7.5	7.7
10.4	10.8	11.1	11.4	11.8	12.1	12.4	12.8	13.1	13.4	13.7	14.1	14.4
4.7	4.8	5.0	5.1	5.3	5.4	5.6	5.7	5.9	6.0	6.1	6.3	6.4
10.4	10.7	11.1	11.4	11.7	12.0	12.4	12.7	13.0	13.4	13.7	14.0	14.4
2.4	2.5	2.6	2.7	2.8	2.9	2.9	3.0	3.1	3.2	3.2	3.3	3.4
3.4	3.5	3.6	3.7	3.9	4.0	4.1	4.2	4.3	4.4	4.5	4.6	4.7
3.7	3.8	4.0	4.1	4.2	4.3	4.4	4.5	4.7	4.8	4.9	5.0	5.1
4.4	4.5	4.6	4.8	4.9	5.0	5.2	5.3	5.4	5.6	5.7	5.9	6.0
5.0	5.2	5.3	5.5	5.6	5.8	5.9	6.1	6.3	6.4	6.6	6.8	6.9
5.4	5.6	5.8	6.0	6.2	6.3	6.5	6.7	6.9	7.0	7.2	7.4	7.6
6.8	7.0	7.2	7.4	7.6	7.9	8.1	8.3	8.5	8.7	8.9	9.1	9.4
7.6	7.9	8.1	8.3	8.6	8.8	9.1	9.3	9.5	9.8	10.0	10.3	10.5
8.7	9.0	9.2	9.5	9.8	10.1	10.4	10.6	10.9	11.2	11.5	11.8	12.0
10.1	10.4	10.8	11.1	11.4	11.8	12.1	12.4	12.7	13.0	13.4	13.7	14.0
12.3	12.7	13.1	13.5	13.9	14.3	14.7	15.0	15.4	15.8	16.2	16.6	17.0
8.0	8.3	8.5	8.8	9.0	9.3	9.5	9.8	10.0	10.3	10.6	10.8	11.1
8.3	8.6	8.9	9.1	9.4	9.7	9.9	10.2	10.5	10.7	11.0	11.2	11.5
13.6	14.1	14.5	14.9	15.4	15.8	16.2	16.6	17.1	17.5	17.9	18.4	18.8

Self-Test on Drinking Habits and Alcoholism

Problem drinking often has its seeds in the teen years. Significant health consequences of this practice typically arise in adulthood. The following questionnaire was developed by the National Council on Alcoholism. With this assessment, you can determine whether you or someone you know might need help.

	Yes	No
1. Do you occasionally drink heavily after disappointment, after a quarrel, or when someone gives you a hard time?	____	____
2. When you have trouble or feel under pressure, do you drink more heavily than usual?	____	____
3. Have you ever noticed that you're able to handle liquor better than you did when you first started drinking?	____	____
4. Do you ever wake up the morning after you've been drinking and discover that you can't remember part of the evening before, even though your friends tell you that you didn't pass out?	____	____
5. When drinking with other people, do you try to have a few extra drinks when others won't know it?	____	____
6. Are there certain occasions when you feel uncomfortable if alcohol isn't available?	____	____
7. Have you recently noticed that when you begin drinking, you're in more of a hurry to get the first drink than you used to be?	____	____
8. Do you sometimes feel a little guilty about your drinking?	____	____
9. Are you secretly irritated when your family or friends discuss your drinking?	____	____
10. Have you recently noticed an increase in the frequency of memory blackout?	____	____
11. Do you often find that you wish to continue drinking after your friends say they've had enough?	____	____
12. Do you usually have a reason for the occasions when you drink heavily?	____	____
13. When you're sober, do you often regret things you have done or said while drinking?	____	____
14. Have you tried switching brands or following different plans to control your drinking?	____	____
15. Have you often failed to keep promises you've made to yourself about controlling or stopping your drinking?	____	____

	Yes	No
16. Have your ever tried to control your drinking by changing jobs or moving to a new location?	_____	_____
17. Do you try to avoid family or close friends while you're drinking?	_____	_____
18. Are you having an increasing number of financial and work problems?	_____	_____
19. Do more people seem to be treating you unfairly without good reason?	_____	_____
20. Do you eat very little or irregularly when you're drinking?	_____	_____
21. Do you sometimes have the shakes in the morning and find that it helps to have a little drink?	_____	_____
22. Have you recently noticed that you can drink more than you once did?	_____	_____
23. Do you sometimes stay drunk for several days at a time?	_____	_____
24. Do you sometimes feel very depressed and wonder whether life is worth living?	_____	_____
25. Sometimes after periods of drinking do you see or hear things that aren't there?	_____	_____
26. Do you get terribly frightened after you have been drinking heavily?	_____	_____

Interpretation

These are all symptoms that may indicate alcoholism. "Yes" answers to several of the questions indicate the following stages of alcoholism:

Questions 1–8:   Potential drinking problem

Questions 9–21:   Drinking problem likely

Questions 22–26:   Definite drinking problem

It is vital that people assess themselves honestly. If you or someone you know demonstrates some or a number of these symptoms, it is important to seek help. If there is even a question in your mind, go talk to a professional about it.

Reprinted courtesy of the National Council on Alcoholism and Drug Dependence.

Determination of Healthy Body Weight

A number of different techniques are utilized to determine a healthy body weight. The following three methods offer you an estimate of an appropriate body weight. Method A is based on the Body Mass Index (BMI). Method B is based on body-fat percentage. Method C, the waist circumference, does not determine a desirable body weight but provides an assessment of desirable body-fat distribution.

Method A

The BMI uses the metric system, so you need to determine your weight in kilograms and your height in meters. The formula is

$$\frac{\text{Body weight in kilograms}}{(\text{Height in meters})^2}$$

Dividing your body weight in pounds by 2.2 will give you your weight in kilograms. Multiplying your height in inches by 0.0254 will give you your height in meters.

$$\text{Your weight in kilograms} =$$

$$\frac{(\text{Your weight in pounds})}{2.2} = \underline{\hspace{1cm}}$$

$$\text{Your height in meters} =$$

$$(\text{Your height in inches}) \times 0.0254 = \underline{\hspace{1cm}}$$

$$\text{BMI} = \frac{\text{Body weight in kilograms}}{(\text{Height in meters})^2} = \underline{\hspace{1cm}}$$

Or you may use your weight in pounds and height in inches with the following formula:

$$\text{BMI} = \frac{\text{Body weight in pounds} \times 705}{(\text{Height in inches})^2}$$

A BMI range of 18.5 to 25 is considered to be normal, but a suggested desirable range for females is 21.3 to 22.1 and for males is 21.9 to 22.4. Individuals with BMI values between 25.0–29.9 are classified as overweight, those from 30.0–39.9 are classified as obese, and those 40 and above are classified as extremely obese. The higher the BMI, the greater the health risks faced by the individual, particularly diabetes, high blood pressure, and heart disease.

If you want to lower your body weight to a more desirable BMI, such as 22, use the following formula to determine what that weight should be; the weight is expressed in kilograms, so multiplying it by 2.2 will give you the desired weight in pounds.

$$\text{Kilograms body weight} =$$

$$\text{Desired BMI} \times (\text{Height in meters})^2$$

Here's a brief example for a woman who weighs 187 pounds and is 5'9" tall; her BMI calculates to be 27.7, so her weight poses a health risk. If she wants to achieve a BMI of 23, she will need to reduce her weight to 155 pounds.

$$\text{Kilograms body weight} = 23 \times (1.753)^2 = 70.6$$

$$70.6 \text{ kg} \times 2.2 = 155 \text{ pounds}$$

To calculate your desired body weight:

$$\text{Kilograms body weight} =$$

$$(\text{Your desired BMI}) \times (\text{Your height in meters})^2$$

$$\text{Kilograms body weight} = \underline{\hspace{1cm}} \times \underline{\hspace{1cm}}$$

$$\underline{\hspace{1cm}} \text{ kg} \times 2.2 = \underline{\hspace{1cm}} \text{ pounds}$$

Keep in mind that the BMI does not discriminate between muscle mass and body fat, so a high BMI may reflect an increased muscle mass and body fat may actually be relatively low. Conversely, an individual with a low BMI may

TABLE D.1 Generalized equations for predicting body fat

Measure the appropriate skinfolds for women (triceps, thigh, and suprailium sites) or men (chest, abdomen, and thigh sites) as illustrated in figures D.1–D.4. You may use either the appropriate formula or the appropriate table in appendix D to obtain the predicted body-fat percentage.

Women*	Men**
$BD = 1.0994921 - 0.0009929\,(X_1) + 0.0000023\,(X_1)^2 - 0.0001392\,(X_2)$	$BD = 1.10938 - 0.0008267\,(X_1) + 0.0000016\,(X_1)^2 - 0.0002574\,(X_2)$
BD = Body density	BD = Body density
X_1 = Sum of triceps, thigh, and suprailium skinfolds	X_1 = Sum of chest, abdomen, and thigh skinfolds
X_2 = Age	X_2 = Age
	To calculate percent body fat, plug into Siri's equation.

$$\left(\frac{4.95}{BD} - 4.5\right) \times 100$$

*From Jackson, A., Pollock, M., and Ward, A. 1980. Generalized equations for predicting body density of women. *Medicine & Science in Sports & Exercise* 12:175–182.
**Jackson, A., and Pollock, M. 1978. Generalized equations for predicting body density of men. *British Journal of Nutrition* 40:497–504.

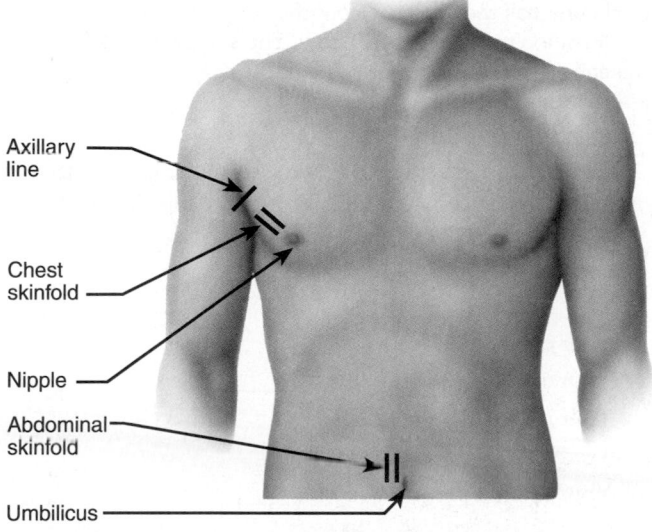

Axillary line
Chest skinfold
Nipple
Abdominal skinfold
Umbilicus

FIGURE D.1 The chest and abdomen skinfold. Chest—A diagonal fold is taken between the axilla and the nipple. Use a midway point. Abdomen—A vertical fold is taken about 2.5 centimeters (1 inch) to the side of the umbilicus.

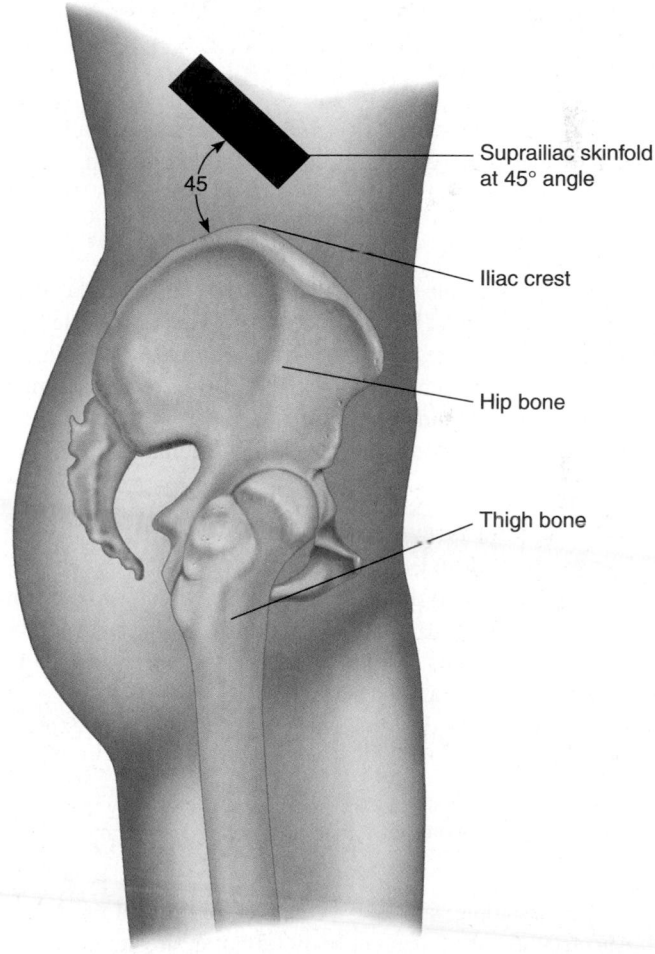

Suprailiac skinfold at 45° angle
Iliac crest
Hip bone
Thigh bone
45

FIGURE D.2 The suprailiac skinfold. A diagonal fold is taken at about a 45-degree angle just above the crest of the ilium.

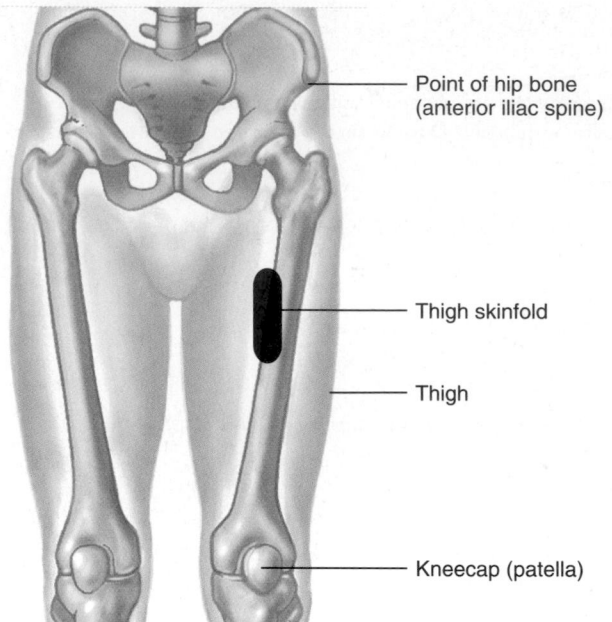

- Point of hip bone (anterior iliac spine)
- Thigh skinfold
- Thigh
- Kneecap (patella)

FIGURE D.3 The thigh skinfold. A vertical fold is taken on the front of the thigh midway between the anterior iliac spine and the patella.

have a higher level of body fat if muscle mass is small. The BMI also does not account for regional fat distribution.

Method B

For this method, you will need to know your body-fat percentage as determined by the procedure described in table D.1 or another appropriate technique. You will also need to determine the body-fat percentage you desire to have. You may use table 10.2 as a guideline.

You will need to do the following calculations for the formula:

1. Determine your current lean body weight (LBW). Multiply your current body weight in pounds by your current percent body fat expressed as a decimal (20 percent would be 0.20) to obtain your pounds of body fat. Subtract your pounds of body fat from your current weight to give you your lean body weight (LBW).
2. Determine your desired body-fat percentage and express it as a decimal.

$$\text{Desired body weight} = \frac{\text{LBW}}{1.00 - \text{Desired} \% \text{ body fat}}$$

As an example, suppose we have a 200-pound male who is currently at 25 percent body fat but desires to get down to 20 percent as his first goal. Multiplying his current weight by his current percent body fat yields 50 pounds of body fat ($200 \times 0.25 = 50$); subtracting this from his current weight yields a LBW of 150 ($200 - 50$). If we plug

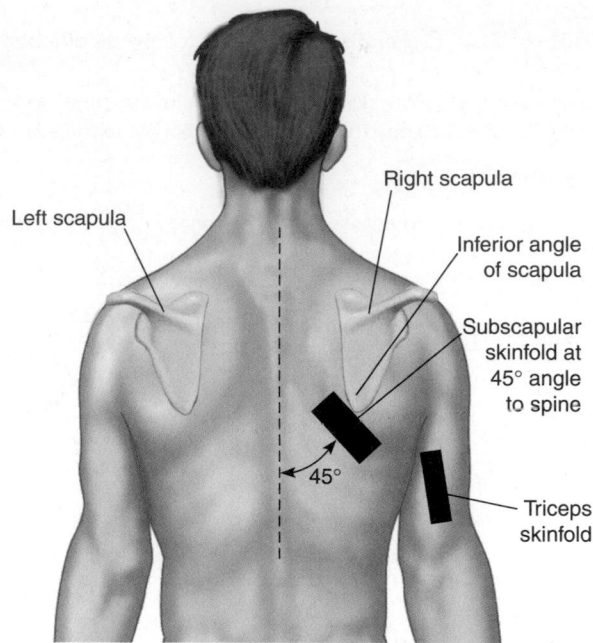

- Left scapula
- Right scapula
- Inferior angle of scapula
- Subscapular skinfold at 45° angle to spine
- 45°
- Triceps skinfold

FIGURE D.4 The triceps and subscapular skinfolds. In the triceps skinfold, a vertical fold is taken over the triceps muscle one-half the distance from the acromion process to the olecranon process at the elbow. The subscapular skinfold is taken just below the lower angle of the scapula, at about a 45-degree angle to the spinal column.

his desired percent of 20 into the formula, he will need to reach a body weight of 187.5 to achieve this first goal.

$$\text{Desired body weight} = \frac{150}{1.00 - 0.20} = \frac{150}{0.8} = 187.5$$

Your current body weight _____
Your current percent body fat _____
Your pounds of body fat _____
Your LBW _____
Your desired percent body fat _____

$$\text{Desired body weight} \frac{\text{LBW}}{1.00 - ?} = \underline{\hspace{1cm}} = \underline{\hspace{1cm}}$$

Method C

The waist circumference is a measure of regional fat distribution. Using a flexible (preferably metal) tape, measure the narrowest section of the bare waist as seen from the front while standing. Wear tight clothing. Do not compress skin and fat with pressure from the tape. The waist measurement may be used as a simple screening technique for abdominal obesity. Females with a waist of 35 inches or over, and men with a waist of 40 inches or over may be at increased risk.

Waist girth _____

In the following table, use both your BMI and waist measurement to evaluate your risk of associated disease.

Risk of associated disease according to BMI and waist size

BMI		Waist less than or equal to 40 in. (men) or 35 in. (women)	Waist greater than 40 in. (men) or 35 in. (women)
18.5 or less	Underweight	—	N/A
18.5 – 24.9	Normal	—	N/A
25.0 – 29.9	Overweight	Increased	High
30.0 – 34.9	Obese	High	Very high
35.0 – 39.9	Obese	Very high	Very high
40 or greater	Extremely obese	Extremely high	Extremely high

Note: Recent research suggests that waist sizes greater than 37 inches in men and 31.5 inches in women may increase health risks when accompanied by other conditions, such as high blood pressure.

Source: www.consumer.gov/weightloss.bmi.htm

Percent fat estimate for men: sum of chest, abdomen, and thigh skinfolds

Sum of skinfolds (mm)	Under 22	23–27	28–32	33–37	38–42	43–47	48–52	53–57	Over 57
				Age to last year					
8–10	1.3	1.8	2.3	2.9	3.4	3.9	4.5	5.0	5.5
11–13	2.2	2.8	3.3	3.9	4.4	4.9	5.5	6.0	6.5
14–16	3.2	3.8	4.3	4.8	5.4	5.9	6.4	7.0	7.5
17–19	4.2	4.7	5.3	5.8	6.3	6.9	7.4	8.0	8.5
20–22	5.1	5.7	6.2	6.8	7.3	7.9	8.4	8.9	9.5
23–25	6.1	6.6	7.2	7.7	8.3	8.8	9.4	9.9	10.5
26–28	7.0	7.6	8.1	8.7	9.2	9.8	10.3	10.9	11.4
29–31	8.0	8.5	9.1	9.6	10.2	10.7	11.3	11.8	12.4
32–34	8.9	9.4	10.0	10.5	11.1	11.6	12.2	12.8	13.3
35–37	9.8	10.4	10.9	11.5	12.0	12.6	13.1	13.7	14.3
38–40	10.7	11.3	11.8	12.4	12.9	13.5	14.1	14.6	15.2
41–43	11.6	12.2	12.7	13.3	13.8	14.4	15.0	15.5	16.1
44–46	12.5	13.1	13.6	14.2	14.7	15.3	15.9	16.4	17.0
47–49	13.4	13.9	14.5	15.1	15.6	16.2	16.8	17.3	17.9
50–52	14.3	14.8	15.4	15.9	16.5	17.1	17.6	18.2	18.8
53–55	15.1	15.7	16.2	16.8	17.4	17.9	18.5	19.1	19.7
56–58	16.0	16.5	17.1	17.7	18.2	18.8	19.4	20.0	20.5
59–61	16.9	17.4	17.9	18.5	19.1	19.7	20.2	20.8	21.4
62–64	17.6	18.2	18.8	19.4	19.9	20.5	21.1	21.7	22.2
65–67	18.5	19.0	19.6	20.2	20.8	21.3	21.9	22.5	23.1
68–70	19.3	19.9	20.4	21.0	21.6	22.2	22.7	23.3	23.9
71–73	20.1	20.7	21.2	21.8	22.4	23.0	23.6	24.1	24.7
74–76	20.9	21.5	22.0	22.6	23.2	23.8	24.4	25.0	25.5
77–79	21.7	22.2	22.8	23.4	24.0	24.6	25.2	25.8	26.3
80–82	22.4	23.0	23.6	24.2	24.8	25.4	25.9	26.5	27.1
83–85	23.2	23.8	24.4	25.0	25.5	26.1	26.7	27.3	27.9
86–88	24.0	24.5	25.1	25.7	26.3	26.9	27.5	28.1	28.7
89–91	24.7	25.3	25.9	26.5	27.1	27.6	28.2	28.8	29.4
92–94	25.4	26.0	26.6	27.2	27.8	28.4	29.0	29.6	30.2
95–97	26.1	26.7	27.3	27.9	28.5	29.1	29.7	30.3	30.9
98–100	26.9	27.4	28.0	28.6	29.2	29.8	30.4	31.0	31.6
101–103	27.5	28.1	28.7	29.3	29.9	30.5	31.1	31.7	32.3
104–106	28.2	28.8	29.4	30.0	30.6	31.2	31.8	32.4	33.0
107–109	28.9	29.5	30.1	30.7	31.3	31.9	32.5	33.1	33.7
110–112	29.6	30.2	30.8	31.4	32.0	32.6	33.2	33.8	34.4
113–115	30.2	30.8	31.4	32.0	32.6	33.2	33.8	34.5	35.1
116–118	30.9	31.5	32.1	32.7	33.3	33.9	34.5	35.1	35.7
119–121	31.5	32.1	32.7	33.3	33.9	34.5	35.1	35.7	36.4
122–124	32.1	32.7	33.3	33.9	34.5	35.1	35.8	36.4	37.0
125–127	32.7	33.3	33.9	34.5	35.1	35.8	36.4	37.0	37.6

From A. S. Jackson and M. L. Pollock, "Practical Assessment of Body Composition," May 1985, in *Physician and Sportsmedicine*. Reprinted with permission of McGraw-Hill, Inc.

Percent fat estimate for women: sum of triceps, suprailium, and thigh skinfolds

Sum of skinfolds (mm)	Age to last year								
	Under 22	23–27	28–32	33–37	38–42	43–47	48–52	53–57	Over 57
23–25	9.7	9.9	10.2	10.4	10.7	10.9	11.2	11.4	11.7
26–28	11.0	11.2	11.5	11.7	12.0	12.3	12.5	12.7	13.0
29–31	12.3	12.5	12.8	13.0	13.3	13.5	13.8	14.0	14.3
32–34	13.6	13.8	14.0	14.3	14.5	14.8	15.0	15.3	15.5
35–37	14.8	15.0	15.3	15.5	15.8	16.0	16.3	16.5	16.8
38–40	16.0	16.3	16.5	16.7	17.0	17.2	17.5	17.7	18.0
41–43	17.2	17.4	17.7	17.9	18.2	18.4	18.7	18.9	19.2
44–46	18.3	18.6	18.8	19.1	19.3	19.6	19.8	20.1	20.3
47–49	19.5	19.7	20.0	20.2	20.5	20.7	21.0	21.2	21.5
50–52	20.6	20.8	21.1	21.3	21.6	21.8	22.1	22.3	22.6
53–55	21.7	21.9	22.1	22.4	22.6	22.9	23.1	23.4	23.6
56–58	22.7	23.0	23.2	23.4	23.7	23.9	24.2	24.4	24.7
59–61	23.7	24.0	24.2	24.5	24.7	25.0	25.2	25.5	25.7
62–64	24.7	25.0	25.2	25.5	25.7	26.0	26.2	26.4	26.7
65–67	25.7	25.9	26.2	26.4	26.7	26.9	27.2	27.4	27.7
68–70	26.6	26.9	27.1	27.4	27.6	27.9	28.1	28.4	28.6
71–73	27.5	27.8	28.0	28.3	28.5	28.8	29.0	29.3	29.5
74–76	28.4	28.7	28.9	29.2	29.4	29.7	29.9	30.2	30.4
77–79	29.3	29.5	29.8	30.0	30.3	30.5	30.8	31.0	31.3
80–82	30.1	30.4	30.6	30.9	31.1	31.4	31.6	31.9	32.1
83–85	30.9	31.2	31.4	31.7	31.9	32.2	32.4	32.7	32.9
86–88	31.7	32.0	32.2	32.5	32.7	32.9	33.2	33.4	33.7
89–91	32.5	32.7	33.0	33.2	33.5	33.7	33.9	34.2	34.4
92–94	33.2	33.4	33.7	33.9	34.2	34.4	34.7	34.9	35.2
95–97	33.9	34.1	34.4	34.6	34.9	35.1	35.4	35.6	35.9
98–100	34.6	34.8	35.1	35.3	35.5	35.8	36.0	36.3	36.5
101–103	35.3	35.4	35.7	35.9	36.2	36.4	36.7	36.9	37.2
104–106	35.8	36.1	36.3	36.6	36.8	37.1	37.3	37.5	37.8
107–109	36.4	36.7	36.9	37.1	37.4	37.6	37.9	38.1	38.4
110–112	37.0	37.2	37.5	37.7	38.0	38.2	38.5	38.7	38.9
113–115	37.5	37.8	38.0	38.2	38.5	38.7	39.0	39.2	39.5
116–118	38.0	38.3	38.5	38.8	39.0	39.3	39.5	39.7	40.0
119–121	38.5	38.7	39.0	39.2	39.5	39.7	40.0	40.2	40.5
122–124	39.0	39.2	39.4	39.7	39.9	40.2	40.4	40.7	40.9
125–127	39.4	39.6	39.9	40.1	40.4	40.6	40.9	41.1	41.4
128–130	39.8	40.0	40.3	40.5	40.8	41.0	41.3	41.5	41.8

From A. S. Jackson and M. L. Pollock, "Practical Assessment of Body Composition," May 1985, in *Physician and Sportsmedicine.* Reprinted with permission of McGraw-Hill, Inc.

Exchange Lists for Meal Planning*

What Are Exchange Lists?

Exchange lists are foods listed together because they are alike. Each serving of a food has about the same amount of carbohydrate, protein, fat, and Calories as the other foods on that list. That is why any food on a list can be "exchanged" or traded for any other food on the same list. For example, you can trade the slice of bread you might eat for breakfast for one-half cup of cooked cereal. Each of these foods equals one starch choice.

Exchange Lists

Foods are listed with their serving sizes, which are usually measured after cooking. When you begin, you should measure the size of each serving. This may help you learn to "eyeball" correct serving sizes.

The following chart shows the amount of nutrients in one serving from each list.

The exchange lists provide you with a lot of food choices (foods from the basic food groups, foods with added sugars, free foods, combination foods, and fast foods). This gives you variety

Groups/Lists	Carbohydrate (grams)	Protein (grams)	Fat (grams)	Calories
Carbohydrate group				
Starch	15	3	1 or less	80
Fruit	15	—	—	60
Milk				
Skim	12	8	0–3	90
Low-fat	12	8	5	120
Whole	12	8	8	150
Other carbohydrates	15	varies	varies	varies
Vegetables	5	2	—	25
Meat and meat substitutes group				
Very lean	—	7	0–1	35
Lean	—	7	3	55
Medium-fat	—	7	5	75
High-fat	—	7	8	100
Fat group	—	—	5	45

*The Exchange Lists are the basis of a meal planning system designed by a committee of the American Diabetes Association and the American Dietetic Association. While designed primarily for people with diabetes and others who must follow special diets, the Exchange Lists are based on principles of good nutrition that apply to everyone.

© 1995 American Diabetes Association, Inc., American Dietetic Association.

in your meals. Several foods, such as dried beans and peas, bacon, and peanut butter, are on two lists. This gives you flexibility in putting your meals together. Whenever you choose new foods or vary your meal plan, monitor your blood glucose to see how these different foods affect your blood glucose level.

Most foods in the Carbohydrate group have about the same amount of carbohydrate per serving. You can exchange starch, fruit, or milk choices in your meal plan. Vegetables are in this group but contain only about 5 grams of carbohydrate.

A Word about Food Labels

Exchange information is based on foods found in grocery stores. However, food companies often change the ingredients in their products. That is why you need to check the Nutrition Facts panel of the food label.

The Nutrition Facts tell you the number of Calories and grams of carbohydrate, protein, and fat in one serving. Compare these numbers with the exchange information in this appendix to see how many exchanges you will be eating. In this way, food labels can help you add foods to your meal plans.

Ask your dietitian to help you use food label information to plan your meals, or read pages 61–66 for more tips on how to use food labels.

Getting Started!

See your dietitian regularly when you are first learning how to use your meal plan and the exchange lists. Your meal plan can be adjusted to fit changes in your lifestyle, such as work, school, vacation, or travel. Regular nutrition counseling can help you make positive changes in your eating habits.

Careful eating habits will help you feel better and be healthier, too. Best wishes and good eating with *Exchange Lists for Meal Planning.*

Starch List

Cereals, grains, pasta, breads, crackers, snacks, starchy vegetables, and cooked dried beans, peas, and lentils are starches. In general, one starch is:

- 1/2 cup of cereal, grain, pasta, or starchy vegetable
- 1 ounce of a bread product, such as 1 slice of bread
- 3/4 to 1 ounce of most snack foods. (Some snack foods may also have added fat.)

Nutrition tips

1. Most starch choices are good sources of B vitamins.
2. Foods made from whole grains are good sources of fiber.
3. Dried beans and peas are a good source of protein and fiber.

Selection tips

1. Choose starches made with little fat as often as you can.
2. Starchy vegetables prepared with fat count as one starch and one fat.
3. Bagels or muffins can be 2, 3, or 4 ounces in size, and can, therefore, count as 2, 3, or 4 starch choices. Check the size you eat.
4. Dried beans, peas, and lentils are also found on the Meat and Meat Substitutes list.
5. Regular potato chips and tortilla chips are found on the Other Carbohydrates list.
6. Most of the serving sizes are measured after cooking.
7. Always check Nutrition Facts on the food label.

One starch exchange equals
15 grams carbohydrate,
3 grams protein,
0–1 grams fat, and
80 Calories.

Bread

Bagel	1/2 (1 oz)
Bread, reduced-calorie	2 slices (1 1/2 oz)
Bread, white, whole wheat, pumpernickel, rye	1 slice (1 oz)
Bread sticks, crisp, 4 in. long × 1/2 in.	2 (2/3 oz)
English muffin	1/2
Hot dog or hamburger bun	1/2 (1 oz)
Pita, 6 in. across	1/2
Raisin bread, unfrosted	1 slice (1 oz)
Roll, plain, small	1 (1 oz)
Tortilla, corn, 6 in. across	1
Tortilla, flour, 7–8 in. across	1
Waffle, 4 1/2 in. square, reduced-fat	1

Cereals and grains

Bran cereals	1/2 cup
Bulgur	1/2 cup
Cereals	1/2 cup
Cereals, unsweetened, ready-to-eat	3/4 cup
Cornmeal (dry)	3 Tbsp
Couscous	1/3 cup
Flour (dry)	3 Tbsp
Granola, low-fat	1/4 cup
Grape-Nuts	1/4 cup
Grits	1/2 cup
Kasha	1/2 cup
Millet	1/4 cup
Muesli	1/4 cup
Oats	1/2 cup
Pasta	1/2 cup
Puffed cereal	1 1/2 cups
Rice milk	1/2 cup
Rice, white or brown	1/3 cup

Shredded Wheat .... 1/2 cup
Sugar-frosted cereal .... 1/2 cup
Wheat germ .... 3 Tbsp

Starchy vegetables

Baked beans .... 1/3 cup
Corn .... 1/2 cup
Corn on cob, medium ....1 (5 oz)
Mixed vegetables with corn, peas, or pasta .... 1 cup
Peas, green .... 1/2 cup
Plantain .... 1/2 cup
Potato, baked or boiled .... 1 small (3 oz)
Potato, mashed .... 1/2 cup
Squash, winter (acorn, butternut) .... 1 cup
Yam, sweet potato, plain .... 1/2 cup

Crackers and snacks

Animal crackers 8
Graham crackers, 2 1/2 in. square 3
Matzoh .... 3/4 oz
Melba toast .... 4 slices
Oyster crackers 24
Popcorn (popped, no fat added
    or low-fat microwave) .... 3 cups
Pretzels .... 3/4 oz
Rice cakes, 4 in. across 2
Saltine-type crackers 6
Snack chips, fat-free (tortilla, potato) .... 15–20 (3/4 oz)
Whole wheat crackers, no fat added .... 2–5 (3/4 oz)

Dried beans, peas, and lentils (Count as 1 starch exchange, plus 1 very lean meat exchange.)

Beans and peas (garbanzo, pinto,
    kidney, white, split, black-eyed) .... 1/2 cup
Lentils .... 1/2 cup
Lima beans .... 2/3 cup
Miso 🜂 .... 3 Tbsp
🜂 = 400 mg or more of sodium per serving.

Starchy foods prepared with fat (Count as 1 starch exchange, plus 1 fat exchange.)

Biscuit, 2 1/2 in. across 1
Chow mein noodles .... 1/2 cup
Corn bread, 2 in. cube ....1 (2 oz)
Crackers, round butter type 6
Croutons .... 1 cup
French-fried potatoes .... 16–25 (3 oz)
Granola .... 1/4 cup
Muffin, small ....1 (1 1/2 oz)
Pancake, 4 in. across 2
Popcorn, microwave .... 3 cups

Sandwich crackers, cheese or peanut butter filling 3
Stuffing, bread (prepared) .... 1/3 cup
Taco shell, 6 in. across 2
Waffle, 4 1/2 in. square 1
Whole wheat crackers, fat added .... 4–6 (1 oz)

Some food you buy uncooked will weigh less after you cook it. Starches often swell in cooking so a small amount of uncooked starch will become a much larger amount of cooked food. The following table shows some of the changes.

Food (starch group)	Uncooked	Cooked
Oatmeal	3 Tbsp	1/2 cup
Cream of Wheat	2 Tbsp	1/2 cup
Grits	3 Tbsp	1/2 cup
Rice	2 Tbsp	1/3 cup
Spaghetti	1/4 cup	1/2 cup
Noodles	1/3 cup	1/2 cup
Macaroni	1/4 cup	1/2 cup
Dried beans	1/4 cup	1/2 cup
Dried peas	1/4 cup	1/2 cup
Lentils	3 Tbsp	1/2 cup
Common measurements		
3 tsp = 1 Tbsp	4 ounces = 1/2 cup	
4 Tbsp = 1/4 cup	8 ounces = 1 cup	
5 1/3 Tbsp = 1/3 cup	1 cup = 1/2 pint	

Fruit List

Fresh, frozen, canned, and dried fruits and fruit juices are on this list. In general, one fruit exchange is:

- 1 small to medium fresh fruit
- 1/2 cup of canned or fresh fruit or fruit juice
- 1/4 cup of dried fruit

Nutrition tips

1. Fresh, frozen, and dried fruits have about 2 grams of fiber per choice. Fruit juices contain very little fiber.
2. Citrus fruits, berries, and melons are good sources of vitamin C.

Selection tips

1. Count 1/2 cup cranberries or rhubarb sweetened with sugar substitutes as free foods.
2. Read the Nutrition Facts on the food label. If one serving has more than 15 grams of carbohydrate, you will need to adjust the size of the serving you eat or drink.
3. Portion sizes for canned fruits are for the fruit and a small amount of juice.
4. Whole fruit is more filling than fruit juice and may be a better choice.

5. Food labels for fruits may contain the words "no sugar added" or "unsweetened." This means that no sucrose (table sugar) has been added.
6. Generally, fruit canned in extra light syrup has the same amount of carbohydrate per serving as the "no sugar added" or the juice pack. All canned fruits on the fruit list are based on one of these three types of pack.

One fruit exchange equals
15 grams carbohydrate and
60 Calories.

The weight includes skin, core, seeds, and rind.

Fruit

Apple, unpeeled, small	1 (4 oz)
Applesauce, unsweetened	1/2 cup
Apples, dried	4 rings
Apricots, canned	1/2 cup
Apricots, dried	8 halves
Apricots, fresh	4 whole (5 1/2 oz)
Banana, small	1 (4 oz)
Blackberries	3/4 cup
Blueberries	3/4 cup
Cantaloupe, small	1/3 melon (11 oz) or 1 cup cubes
Cherries, sweet, fresh	12 (3 oz)
Cherries, sweet, canned	1/2 cup
Dates	3
Figs, dried	1 1/2
Figs, fresh	1 1/2 large or 2 medium (3 1/2 oz)
Fruit cocktail	1/2 cup
Grapefruit, large	1/2 (11 oz)
Grapefruit sections, canned	3/4 cup
Grapes, small	17 (3 oz)
Honeydew melon	1 slice (10 oz) or 1 cup cubes
Kiwi	1 (3 1/2 oz)
Mandarin oranges, canned	3/4 cup
Mango, small	1/2 fruit (5 1/2 oz) or 1/2 cup
Nectarine, small	1 (5 oz)
Orange, small	1 (6 1/2 oz)
Papaya	1/2 fruit (8 oz) or 1 cup cubes
Peach, medium, fresh	1 (6 oz)
Peaches, canned	1/2 cup
Pear, large, fresh	1/2 (4 oz)
Pears, canned	1/2 cup
Pineapple, canned	1/2 cup
Pineapple, fresh	3/4 cup
Plums, canned	1/2 cup
Plums, small	2 (5 oz)
Prunes, dried	3
Raisins	2 Tbsp
Raspberries	1 cup
Strawberries	1 1/4 cup whole berries
Tangerines, small	2 (8 oz)
Watermelon	1 slice (13 1/2 oz) or 1 1/4 cup cubes

Fruit juice

Apple juice/cider	1/2 cup
Cranberry juice cocktail	1/3 cup
Cranberry juice cocktail, reduced-calorie	1 cup
Fruit juice blends, 100% juice	1/3 cup
Grape juice	1/3 cup
Grapefruit juice	1/2 cup
Orange juice	1/2 cup
Pineapple juice	1/2 cup
Prune juice	1/3 cup

Milk List

Different types of milk and milk products are on this list. Cheeses are on the Meat list and cream and other dairy fats are on the Fat list. Based on the amount of fat they contain, milks are divided into skim/very low-fat milk, low-fat milk, and whole milk. One choice of these includes:

	Carbohydrate (grams)	Protein (grams)	Fat (grams)	Calories
Skim/very low-fat	12	8	0–3	90
Low-fat	12	8	5	120
Whole	12	8	8	150

Nutrition tips

1. Milk and yogurt are good sources of calcium and protein. Check the food label.
2. The higher the fat content of milk and yogurt, the greater the amount of saturated fat and cholesterol. Choose lower-fat varieties.
3. For those who are lactose intolerant, look for lactose-reduced or lactose-free varieties of milk.

Selection tips

1. One cup equals 8 fluid ounces or 1/2 pint.
2. Look for chocolate milk, frozen yogurt, and ice cream on the Other Carbohydrates list.
3. Nondairy creamers are on the Free Foods list.
4. Look for rice milk on the Starch list.
5. Look for soy milk on the Medium-fat Meat list.

One milk exchange equals
12 grams carbohydrate and
8 grams protein.

Skim and very low-fat milk (0–3 grams fat per serving)

Skim milk	1 cup
1/2% milk	1 cup

1% milk .... 1 cup	Plain nonfat yogurt .... 3/4 cup
Nonfat or low-fat buttermilk .... 1 cup	Nonfat or low-fat fruit-flavored yogurt sweetened
Evaporated skim milk .... 1/2 cup	with aspartame or with a nonnutritive sweetener ..... 1 cup
Nonfat dry milk .... 1/3 cup dry	

Low-fat (5 grams fat per serving)

Whole milk (8 grams fat per serving)

2% milk .... 1 cup	Whole milk .... 1 cup
Plain low-fat yogurt .... 3/4 cup	Evaporated whole milk .... 1/2 cup
Sweet acidophilus milk .... 1 cup	Goat's milk .... 1 cup
	Kefir .... 1 cup

Other Carbohydrates List

You can substitute food choices from this list for a starch, fruit, or milk choice on your meal plan. Some choices will also count as one or more fat choices.

Food	Serving size	Exchanges per serving
Angel food cake, unfrosted	1/12th cake	2 carbohydrates
Brownie, small, unfrosted	2 in. square	1 carbohydrate, 1 fat
Cake, frosted	2 in. square	2 carbohydrates, 1 fat
Cake, unfrosted	2 in. square	1 carbohydrate, 1 fat
Cookie, fat-free	2 small	1 carbohydrate
Cookie or sandwich cookie with creme filling	2 small	1 carbohydrate, 1 fat
Cranberry sauce, jellied	1/4 cup	2 carbohydrates
Cupcake, frosted	1 small	2 carbohydrates, 1 fat
Doughnut, glazed	3 3/4 in. across (2 oz)	2 carbohydrates, 2 fats
Doughnut, plain cake	1 medium (1 1/2 oz)	1 1/2 carbohydrates, 2 fats
Fruit juice bars, frozen, 100% juice	1 bar (3 oz)	1 carbohydrate
Fruit snacks, chewy (pureed fruit concentrate)	1 roll (3/4 oz)	1 carbohydrate
Fruit spreads, 100% fruit	1 Tbsp	1 carbohydrate
Gelatin, regular	1/2 cup	1 carbohydrate
Gingersnaps	3	1 carbohydrate
Granola bar	1 bar	1 carbohydrate, 1 fat
Granola bar, fat-free	1 bar	2 carbohydrates
Hummus	1/3 cup	1 carbohydrate, 1 fat
Ice cream	1/2 cup	1 carbohydrate, 2 fats
Ice cream, light	1/2 cup	1 carbohydrate, 1 fat
Ice cream, fat-free, no sugar added	1/2 cup	1 carbohydrate
Jam or jelly, regular	1 Tbsp	1 carbohydrate
Milk, chocolate, whole	1 cup	2 carbohydrates, 1 fat
Pie, fruit, 2 crusts	1/6 pie	3 carbohydrates, 2 fats
Pie, pumpkin or custard	1/8 pie	1 carbohydrate, 2 fats
Potato chips	12–18 (1 oz)	1 carbohydrate, 2 fats
Pudding, regular (made with low-fat milk)	1/2 cup	2 carbohydrates
Pudding, sugar-free (made with low-fat milk)	1/2 cup	1 carbohydrate
Salad dressing, fat free ▮	1/4 cup	1 carbohydrate
Sherbet, sorbet	1/2 cup	2 carbohydrates
Spaghetti or pasta sauce, canned ▮	1/2 cup	1 carbohydrate, 1 fat
Sweet roll or Danish	1 (2 1/2 oz)	2 1/2 carbohydrates, 2 fats
Syrup, light	2 Tbsp	1 carbohydrate
Syrup, regular	1 Tbsp	1 carbohydrate
Syrup, regular	1/4 cup	4 carbohydrates
Tortilla chips	6–12 (1 oz)	1 carbohydrate, 2 fats
Vanilla wafers	5	1 carbohydrate, 1 fat
Yogurt, frozen, fat-free, no sugar added	1/2 cup	1 carbohydrate
Yogurt, frozen, low-fat, fat-free	1/3 cup	1 carbohydrate, 0–1 fat
Yogurt, low-fat with fruit	1 cup	3 carbohydrates, 0–1 fat

▮ = 400 mg or more sodium per exchange.

Nutrition tips

1. These foods can be substituted in your meal plan, even though they contain added sugars or fat. However, they do not contain as many important vitamins and minerals as the choices on the Starch, Fruit, or Milk list.
2. When planning to include these foods in your meal, be sure to include foods from all the lists to eat a balanced meal.

Selection tips

1. Because many of these foods are concentrated sources of carbohydrate and fat, the portion sizes are often very small.
2. Always check Nutrition Facts on the food label. It will be your most accurate source of information.
3. Many fat-free or reduced-fat products made with fat replacers contain carbohydrate. When eaten in large amounts, they may need to be counted. Talk with your dietitian to determine how to count these in your meal plan.
4. Look for fat-free salad dressings in smaller amounts on the Free Foods list.

One exchange equals
15 grams carbohydrate, or
1 starch, or 1 fruit, or 1 milk.

Vegetable List

Vegetables that contain small amounts of carbohydrates and Calories are on this list. Vegetables contain important nutrients. Try to eat at least 2 or 3 vegetable choices each day. In general, one vegetable exchange is:

- 1/2 cup of cooked vegetables or vegetable juice
- 1 cup of raw vegetables

If you eat 1 to 2 vegetable choices at a meal or snack, you do not have to count the Calories or carbohydrates because they contain small amounts of these nutrients.

Nutrition tips

1. Fresh and frozen vegetables have less added salt than canned vegetables. Drain and rinse canned vegetables if you want to remove some salt.
2. Choose more dark green and dark yellow vegetables, such as spinach, broccoli, romaine, carrots, chilies, and peppers.
3. Broccoli, brussels sprouts, cauliflower, greens, peppers, spinach, and tomatoes are good sources of vitamin C.
4. Vegetables contain 1 to 4 grams of fiber per serving.

Selection tips

1. A 1-cup portion of broccoli is a portion about the size of a light bulb.
2. Tomato sauce is different from spaghetti sauce, which is on the Other Carbohydrates list.
3. Canned vegetables and juices are available without added salt.
4. If you eat more than 4 cups of raw vegetables or 2 cups of cooked vegetables at one meal, count them as 1 carbohydrate choice.
5. Starchy vegetables such as corn, peas, winter squash, and potatoes that contain larger amounts of Calories and carbohydrates are on the Starch list.

One vegetable exchange equals
5 grams carbohydrate,
2 grams protein,
0 grams fat, and
25 Calories.

Artichoke
Artichoke hearts
Asparagus
Beans (green, wax, Italian)
Bean sprouts
Beets
Broccoli
Brussels sprouts
Cabbage
Carrots
Cauliflower
Celery
Cucumber
Eggplant
Green onions or scallions
Greens (collard, kale, mustard, turnip)
Kohlrabi
Leeks
Mixed vegetables (without corn, peas, or pasta)
Mushrooms
Okra
Onions
Pea pods
Peppers (all varieties)
Radishes
Salad greens (endive, escarole, lettuce, romaine, spinach)
Sauerkraut
Spinach
Summer squash
Tomato
Tomatoes, canned
Tomato sauce

Tomato/vegetable juice ▮
Turnips
Water chestnuts
Watercress
Zucchini

▮= 400 mg or more sodium per exchange.

Meat and Meat Substitutes List

Meat and meat substitutes that contain both protein and fat are on this list. In general, one meat exchange is:

- 1 oz meat, fish, poultry, or cheese
- 1/2 cup dried beans

Based on the amount of fat they contain, meats are divided into very lean, lean, medium-fat, and high-fat lists. This is done so you can see which ones contain the least amount of fat. One ounce (one exchange) of each of these includes:

	Carbohydrate (grams)	Protein (grams)	Fat (grams)	Calories
Very lean	0	7	0–1	35
Lean	0	7	3	55
Medium-fat	0	7	5	75
High-fat	0	7	8	100

Nutrition tips

1. Choose very lean and lean meat choices whenever possible. Items from the high-fat group are high in saturated fat, cholesterol, and Calories and can raise blood cholesterol levels.
2. Meats do not have any fiber.
3. Dried beans, peas, and lentils are good sources of fiber.
4. Some processed meats, seafood, and soy products may contain carbohydrate when consumed in large amounts. Check the Nutrition Facts on the label to see if the amount is close to 15 grams. If so, count it as a carbohydrate choice as well as a meat choice.

Selection tips

1. Weigh meat after cooking and removing bones and fat. Four ounces of raw meat is equal to 3 ounces of cooked meat. Some examples of meat portions are:
   - 1 ounce cheese = 1 meat choice and is about the size of a 1-inch cube
   - 2 ounces meat = 2 meat choices, such as
     1 small chicken leg or thigh
     1/2 cup cottage cheese or tuna
   - 3 ounces meat = 3 meat choices and is about the size of a deck of cards, such as
     1 medium pork chop
     1 small hamburger
     1/2 of a whole chicken breast
     1 unbreaded fish fillet
2. Limit your choices from the high-fat group to three times per week or less.
3. Most grocery stores stock Select and Choice grades of meat. Select grades of meat are the leanest meats.
4. Choice grades contain a moderate amount of fat, and Prime cuts of meat have the highest amount of fat. Restaurants usually serve Prime cuts of meat.
5. "Hamburger" may contain added seasoning and fat, but ground beef does not.
6. Read labels to find products that are low in fat and cholesterol (5 grams or less of fat per serving).
7. Dried beans, peas, and lentils are also found on the Starch list.
8. Peanut butter, in smaller amounts, is also found on the Fats list.
9. Bacon, in smaller amounts, is also found on the Fats list.

Meal planning tips

1. Bake, roast, broil, grill, poach, steam, or boil these foods rather than frying.
2. Place meat on a rack so the fat will drain off during cooking.
3. Use a nonstick spray and a nonstick pan to brown or fry foods.
4. Trim off visible fat before or after cooking.
5. If you add flour, bread crumbs, coating mixes, fat, or marinades when cooking, ask your dietitian how to count it in your meal plan.

Very lean meat and substitutes list (One exchange equals 0 grams carbohydrate, 7 grams protein, 0–1 grams fat, and 35 Calories.)

One very lean meat exchange is equal to any one of the following items.

Poultry: Chicken or turkey (white meat, no skin), Cornish hen (no skin) .... 1 oz
Fish: Fresh or frozen cod, flounder, haddock, halibut, trout; tuna fresh or canned in water .... 1 oz
Shellfish: Clams, crab, lobster, scallops, shrimp, imitation shellfish .... 1 oz
Game: Duck or pheasant (no skin), venison, buffalo, ostrich .... 1 oz

Cheese with 1 gram or less fat per ounce:

    Nonfat or low-fat cottage cheese .... 1/4 cup

    Fat-free cheese .... 1 oz

Other: Processed sandwich meat with 1 gram
or less fat per ounce, such as deli thin, shave meats,
chipped beef 🜹, turkey ham .... 1 oz

    Egg whites 2

    Egg substitutes, plain .... 1/4 cup

    Hot dogs with 1 gram or less fat per ounce 🜹 .... 1 oz

    Kidney (high in cholesterol) .... 1 oz

    Sausage with 1 gram or less fat per ounce .... 1 oz

Count as one very lean meat and one starch exchange.

    Dried beans, peas, lentils (cooked) .... 1/2 cup

🜹 = 400 mg or more sodium per exchange.

Lean meat and substitutes list (One exchange equals 0 grams carbohydrate, 7 grams protein, 3 grams fat, and 55 Calories.)

One lean meat exchange is equal to any one of the following items.

Beef: USDA Select or Choice grades of lean beef
    trimmed of fat, such as round, sirloin, and flank
    steak; tenderloin; roast (rib, chuck, rump);
    steak (T-bone, Porterhouse, cubed),
    ground round .... 1 oz

Pork: Lean pork, such as fresh ham; canned,
    cured, or boiled ham; Canadian bacon 🜹;
    tenderloin, center loin chop .... 1 oz

Lamb: Roast, chop, leg .... 1 oz

Veal: Lean chop, roast .... 1 oz

Poultry: Chicken, turkey (dark meat, no skin),
    chicken white meat (with skin), domestic
    duck or goose (well-drained of fat, no skin) .... 1 oz

Fish:

    Herring (uncreamed or smoked) .... 1 oz

    Oysters .... 6 medium

    Salmon (fresh or canned), catfish .... 1 oz

    Sardines (canned) .... 2 medium

    Tuna (canned in oil, drained) .... 1 oz

    Game: Goose (no skin), rabbit .... 1 oz

Cheese:

    4.5%-fat cottage cheese .... 1/4 cup

    Grated Parmesan .... 2 Tbsp

    Cheeses with 3 grams or less fat per ounce .... 1 oz

Other:

    Hot dogs with 3 grams or less fat per ounce ...... 1 1/2 oz

    Processed sandwich meat with 3 grams or
      less fat per ounce, such as turkey pastrami
      or kielbasa .... 1 oz

    Liver, heart (high in cholesterol) .... 1 oz

Medium-fat meat and substitutes list (One exchange equals 0 grams carbohydrate, 7 grams protein, 5 grams fat, and 75 Calories.)

One medium-fat meat exchange is equal to any one of the following items.

Beef: Most beef products fall into this category
    (ground beef, meatloaf, corned beef, short
    ribs, prime grades of meat trimmed of fat,
    such as prime rib) .... 1 oz

Pork: Top loin, chop, Boston butt, cutlet .... 1 oz

Lamb: Rib roast, ground .... 1 oz

Veal: Cutlet (ground or cubed, unbreaded) .... 1 oz

Poultry: Chicken dark meat (with skin), ground
    turkey or ground chicken, fried chicken
    (with skin) .... 1 oz

Fish: Any fried fish product .... 1 oz

Cheese: With 5 grams or less fat per ounce

    Feta .... 1 oz

    Mozzarella .... 1 oz

    Ricotta .... 1/4 cup (2 oz)

Other:

    Egg (high in cholesterol, limit to 3 per week) 1

    Sausage with 5 grams or less fat per ounce .... 1 oz

    Soy milk .... 1 cup

    Tempeh .... 1/4 cup

    Tofu .... 4 oz or 1/2 cup

High-fat meat and substitutes list (One exchange equals 0 grams carbohydrate, 7 grams protein, 8 grams fat, and 100 Calories.)

Remember these items are high in saturated fat, cholesterol, and Calories and may raise blood cholesterol levels if eaten on a regular basis. One high-fat meat exchange is equal to any one of the following items.

Pork: Spareribs, ground pork, pork sausage .... 1 oz

Cheese: All regular cheeses, such as American 🜹,
    cheddar, Monterey Jack, Swiss .... 1 oz

Other: Processed sandwich meats with 8 grams
    or less fat per ounce, such as bologna, pimento
    loaf, salami .... 1 oz

    Sausage, such as bratwurst, Italian, knockwurst,
    Polish, smoked .... 1 oz

    Hot dog (turkey or chicken) 🜹 1 (10/lb)

    Bacon .... 3 slices (20 slices/lb)

Count as one high-fat meat plus one fat exchange.

Hot dog (beef, pork, or combination) 🜹 1 (10/lb)

Peanut butter (contains unsaturated fat) .... 2 Tbsp

🜹 = 400 mg or more sodium per exchange.

Fat List

Fats are divided into three groups, based on the main type of fat they contain: monounsaturated, polyunsaturated, and saturated. Small amounts of monounsaturated and polyunsaturated fats in the foods we eat are linked with good health benefits. Saturated fats are linked with heart disease and cancer. In general, one fat exchange is:

- 1 teaspoon of regular margarine or vegetable oil
- 1 tablespoon of regular salad dressing

Nutrition tips

1. All fats are high in Calories. Limit serving sizes for good nutrition and health.
2. Nuts and seeds contain small amounts of fiber, protein, and magnesium.
3. If blood pressure is a concern, choose fats in the unsalted form to help lower sodium intake, such as unsalted peanuts.

Selection tips

1. Check the Nutrition Facts on food labels for serving sizes. One fat exchange is based on a serving size containing 5 grams of fat.
2. When selecting regular margarine, choose those with liquid vegetable oil as the first ingredient. Soft margarines are not as saturated as stick margarines. Soft margarines are healthier choices. Avoid those listing hydrogenated or partially hydrogenated fat as the first ingredient.
3. When selecting low-fat margarines, look for liquid vegetable oil as the second ingredient. Water is usually the first ingredient.
4. When used in smaller amounts, bacon and peanut butter are counted as fat choices. When used in larger amounts, they are counted as high-fat meat choices.
5. Fat-free salad dressings are on the Other Carbohydrates list and the Free Foods list.
6. See the Free Foods list for nondairy coffee creamers, whipped topping, and fat-free products, such as margarines, salad dressings, mayonnaise, sour cream, cream cheese, and nonstick cooking spray.

Monounsaturated fats list
(One fat exchange equals 5 grams fat and 45 Calories.)

Avocado, medium	1/8 (1 oz)
Nuts	
almonds, cashews	6 nuts
mixed (50% peanuts)	6 nuts
peanuts	10 nuts
pecans	4 halves
Oil (canola, olive, peanut)	1 tsp
Olives: ripe (black)	8 large
green, stuffed	10 large
Peanut butter, smooth or crunchy	2 tsp
Sesame seeds	1 Tbsp
Tahini paste	2 tsp

Polyunsaturated fats list
(One fat exchange equals 5 grams fat and 45 Calories.)

Margarine: stick, tub, or squeeze	1 tsp
lower-fat (30% to 50% vegetable oil)	1 Tbsp
Mayonnaise: regular	1 tsp
reduced-fat	1 Tbsp
Miracle Whip Salad Dressing®: regular	2 tsp
reduced-fat	1 Tbsp
Nuts, walnuts, English	4 halves
Oil (corn, safflower, soybean)	1 tsp
Salad dressing: regular	1 Tbsp
reduced-fat	2 Tbsp
Seeds: pumpkin, sunflower	1 Tbsp

= 400 mg or more sodium per exchange.

Saturated fats list* (One fat exchange equals 5 grams of fat and 45 Calories.)

Bacon, cooked	1 slice (20 slices/lb)
Bacon, grease	1 tsp
Butter: stick	1 tsp
reduced-fat	1 Tbsp
whipped	2 tsp
Chitterlings, boiled	2 Tbsp (1/2 oz)
Coconut, sweetened, shredded	2 Tbsp
Cream, half and half	2 Tbsp
Cream cheese: regular	1 Tbsp (1/2 oz)
reduced-fat	2 Tbsp (1 oz)
Fatback or salt pork, see below†	
Shortening or lard	1 tsp
Sour cream: regular	2 Tbsp
reduced-fat	3 Tbsp

*Saturated fats can raise blood cholesterol levels.

†Use a piece 1 in. × 1 in. × 1/4 in. if you plan to eat the fatback cooked with vegetables. Use a piece 2 in. × 1 in. × 1/2 in. when eating only the vegetables with the fatback removed.

Free Foods List

A *free food* is any food or drink that contains less than 20 Calories or less than 5 grams of carbohydrate per serving. Foods with a serving size listed should be limited to three servings per day. Be sure to spread them out throughout the day. If you eat all three servings at one time, it could affect your blood glucose level. Foods listed without a serving size can be eaten as often as you like.

Fat-free or reduced-fat foods

Cream cheese, fat-free .... 1 Tbsp
Creamers, nondairy, liquid.................................... 1 Tbsp
Creamers, nondairy, powdered .... 2 tsp
Margarine, fat-free .... 4 Tbsp
Margarine, reduced-fat... 1 tsp
Mayonnaise, fat-free .... 1 Tbsp
Mayonnaise, reduced-fat.. 1 tsp
Miracle Whip®, nonfat .... 1 Tbsp
Miracle Whip®, reduced-fat .... 1 tsp
Nonstick cooking spray
Salad dressing, fat-free.. 1 Tbsp
Salad dressing, fat-free, Italian .... 2 Tbsp
Salsa.. 1/4 cup
Sour cream, fat-free, reduced-fat .... 1 Tbsp
Whipped topping, regular or light.......................... 2 Tbsp

Sugar-free or low-sugar foods

Candy, hard, sugar-free.. 1 candy
Gelatin dessert, sugar-free
Gelatin, unflavored
Gum, sugar-free
Jam or jelly, low-sugar or light .... 2 tsp
Sugar substitutes†
Syrup, sugar-free... 2 Tbsp

†Sugar substitutes, alternatives, or replacements that are approved by the Food and Drug Administration (FDA) are safe to use. Common brand names include:

Equal® (aspartame)

Splenda® (sucralose)

Sprinkle Sweet® (saccharin)

Sugar Twin® (saccharin)

Sweet 'n Low® (saccharin)

Sweet One® (acesulfame K)

Sweet-10® (saccharin)

Drinks

Bouillon, broth, consommé ♦
Bouillon or broth, low-sodium
Carbonated or mineral water
Club soda
Cocoa powder, unsweetened................................... 1 Tbsp
Coffee
Diet soft drinks, sugar-free
Drink mixes, sugar-free
Tea
Tonic water, sugar-free

Condiments

Catsup .... 1 Tbsp
Horseradish
Lemon juice
Lime juice
Mustard
Pickles, dill ♦ .... 1 1/2 large
Soy sauce, regular or light ♦
Taco sauce... 1 Tbsp
Vinegar

Seasonings

Be careful with seasonings that contain sodium or are salts, such as garlic or celery salt, and lemon pepper.

Flavoring extracts
Garlic
Herbs, fresh or dried
Pimento
Spices
Tabasco® or hot pepper sauce
Wine, used in cooking
Worcestershire sauce

♦ = 400 mg or more of sodium per choice.

Combination Foods List

Many of the foods we eat are mixed together in various combinations. These combination foods do not fit into any one exchange list. Often it is hard to tell what is in a casserole dish or prepared food item. This is a list of exchanges for some typical combination foods. This list will help you fit these foods into your meal plan. Ask your dietitian for information about any other combination foods you would like to eat.

Food entrees	Serving size	Exchanges per serving
Chow mein (without noodles or rice)	2 cups (16 oz)	1 carbohydrate, 2 lean meats
Pizza, cheese, thin crust 🜚	1/4 of 10 in. (5 oz)	2 carbohydrates, 2 medium-fat meats, 1 fat
Pizza, meat topping, thin crust 🜚	1/4 of 10 in. (5 oz)	2 carbohydrates, 2 medium-fat meats, 2 fats
Pot pie 🜚	1 (7 oz)	2 carbohydrates, 1 medium-fat meat, 4 fats
Tuna noodle casserole, lasagna, spaghetti with meatballs, chili with beans, macaroni and cheese 🜚	1 cup (8 oz)	2 carbohydrates, 2 medium-fat meats

Frozen entrees	Serving size	Exchanges per serving
Entree with less than 300 calories 🜚	1 (8 oz)	2 carbohydrates, 3 lean meats
Salisbury steak with gravy, mashed potato 🜚	1 (11 oz)	2 carbohydrates, 3 medium-fat meats, 3–4 fats
Turkey with gravy, mashed potato, dressing 🜚	1 (11 oz)	2 carbohydrates, 2 medium-fat meats, 2 fats

Soups	Serving size	Exchanges per serving
Bean 🜚	1 cup	1 carbohydrate, 1 very lean meat
Cream (made with water) 🜚	1 cup (8 oz)	1 carbohydrate, 1 fat
Split pea (made with water) 🜚	1/2 cup (4 oz)	1 carbohydrate
Tomato (made with water) 🜚	1 cup (8 oz)	1 carbohydrate
Vegetable beef, chicken noodle, or other broth-type 🜚	1 cup (8 oz)	1 carbohydrate

🜚 = 400 mg or more sodium per exchange.

Fast Foods*

Food entrees	Serving size	Exchanges per serving
Burritos with beef 🜚	2	4 carbohydrates, 2 medium-fat meats, 2 fats
Chicken breast and wing, breaded and fried 🜚	1 each	1 carbohydrate, 4 medium-fat meats, 2 fats
Chicken nuggets 🜚	6	1 carbohydrate, 2 medium-fat meats, 1 fat
Fish sandwich/tartar sauce 🜚	1	3 carbohydrates, 1 medium-fat meat, 3 fats
French fries, thin	20–25	2 carbohydrates, 2 fats
Hamburger, large 🜚	1	2 carbohydrates, 3 medium-fat meats, 1 fat
Hamburger, regular	1	2 carbohydrates, 2 medium-fat meats
Hot dog with a bun 🜚	1	1 carbohydrate, 1 high-fat meat, 1 fat
Individual pan pizza 🜚	1	5 carbohydrates, 3 medium-fat meats, 3 fats
Soft-serve cone 🜚	1 medium	2 carbohydrates, 1 fat
Submarine sandwich 🜚	1 sub (6 in.)	3 carbohydrates, 1 vegetable, 2 medium-fat meats, 1 fat
Taco, hard shell 🜚	1 (6 oz)	2 carbohydrates, 2 medium-fat meats, 2 fats
Taco, soft shell	1 (3 oz)	1 carbohydrate, 1 medium-fat meat, 1 fat

🜚 = 400 mg or more of sodium per serving.

*Ask at your fast-food restaurant for nutrition information about your favorite fast foods. Also, see appendix F.

Calories, Percent Fat, Cholesterol, Sodium, and Dietary Fiber in Selected Fast-Food Restaurant Products*

Product	Calories	% Fat Calories	Cholesterol (mg)	Sodium (mg)	Dietary Fiber (g)
Arby's (www.arbys.com)					
Roast beef Classic	360	36	50	950	2
Beef'n Cheddar Classic	450	42	55	1,240	2
Chicken Cordon Bleu	490	39	85	1,600	2
Roast chicken club	460	35	65	1,440	2
Market Fresh roast turkey/swiss	500	44	75	1,510	8
Chopped side salad, Light Italian dressing	163	31	15	890	1
Burger King (www.burgerking.com)					
WHOPPER® Junior Sandwich	340	50	40	530	2
WHOPPER® Sandwich	670	54	75	980	4
WHOPPER Triple Sandwich	1,140	59	205	1,110	4
Onion rings (king size) with zesty dippy sauce	550	60	15	850	5
Vanilla milk shake, medium	520	28	55	420	0
BK veggie burger	410	35	5	1,030	7
Hardee's (www.hardees.com)					
Country Ham biscuit	440	53	35	1,710	0
French fries, large	470	40	5	1,640	5
Monster Thickburger	1,320	65	210	3,020	2
Cole slaw, small	170	53	10	140	2
Charbroiled chicken club sandwich	630	44	80	1,730	4
Apple turnover	270	44	5	260	1
KFC (www.KFC.com)					
Green beans	25	0	0	260	2
BBQ baked beans	210	7	0	780	8
Mashed potatoes with gravy	120	29	0	530	1
Breast (original recipe) without skin or dressing	160	22	85	580	0
Side breast (extra crispy)	420	52	110	1,250	0
Honey BBQ sandwich	320	11	70	770	3

*You may access the Website for any fast-food restaurant to obtain a detailed report on the nutrient content of all of their products.

Product	Calories	% Fat Calories	Cholesterol (mg)	Sodium (mg)	Dietary Fiber (g)
Long John Silver's (www.longjohnsilvers.com)					
Ultimate Alaskan pollock sandwich	530	45	55	1,500	3
Battered shrimp (3 pieces)	130	62	45	480	0
Grilled tilapia (1 piece)	110	18	55	250	0
Vegetable medley (4 ounces)	50	30	0	360	3
McDonald's (www.mcdonalds.com)					
Hamburger	250	32	25	520	2
Big Mac	540	48	75	1,040	3
Premium grilled chicken classic sandwich	350	23	65	820	3
Chicken McNuggets (6 pieces)	280	57	40	540	1
French fries (large)	500	44	0	350	6
Hotcakes with syrup	530	15	20	610	3
Egg McMuffin	300	37	260	820	2
Mango Pineapple Smoothie	350	4	5	65	3
Orange juice, large	280	0	0	5	0
Pizza Hut (www.pizzahut.com)					
Thin 'N Crispy cheese, 1 medium slice	190	37	25	550	1
Pan, cheese, Veggie Lover's medium slice	230	35	15	500	2
Fit N' Delicious diced chicken, red onion, green pepper	180	22	20	510	1
Personal pan pizza, pepperoni (whole pizza)	610	40	55	1,410	3
Cheese breadsticks (one)	170	35	15	390	1
Subway (www.subway.com)					
Subway Club (6 inches)	310	13	40	880	5
Turkey breast (6 inches)	280	11	20	810	5
Tuna deli (6 inches)	530	51	45	830	5
Veggie Delite (6 inches)	230	9	0	310	5
Sweet onion Chicken Teriyaki (6 inches)	380	11	50	900	5
Taco Bell (www.tacobell.com)					
Bean burrito, Fresco style	350	20	0	990	11
Soft taco, beef, regular	210	38	30	560	3
Soft taco, chicken, Fresco style	150	20	25	480	2
Fiesta taco salad	770	48	60	1,420	12
Chicken Quesadilla, regular	480	50	50	1,000	4
Wendy's (www.wendys.com)					
Junior hamburger	230	31	30	470	1
Ultimate Chicken grilled sandwich	360	17	80	1,110	2
Plain potato, baked	270	0	0	25	7
Potato with sour cream and chives	320	10	10	50	7
Caesar side salad	60	52	10	115	2
Caesar dressing	110	90	10	180	0
Chili (large)	310	26	60	1,330	10
Baja Fresh (www.bajafresh.com)					
Burrito Ultimo, steak	950	42	140	2,310	8
Burrito Mexicano, chicken	790	15	75	2,270	20
Grilled veggie burrito	800	38	65	1,880	16
Baja burrito, steak	850	49	125	2,260	7
Nacho burrito	1,250	30	145	3,200	23

Energy Pathways of Carbohydrate, Fat, and Protein

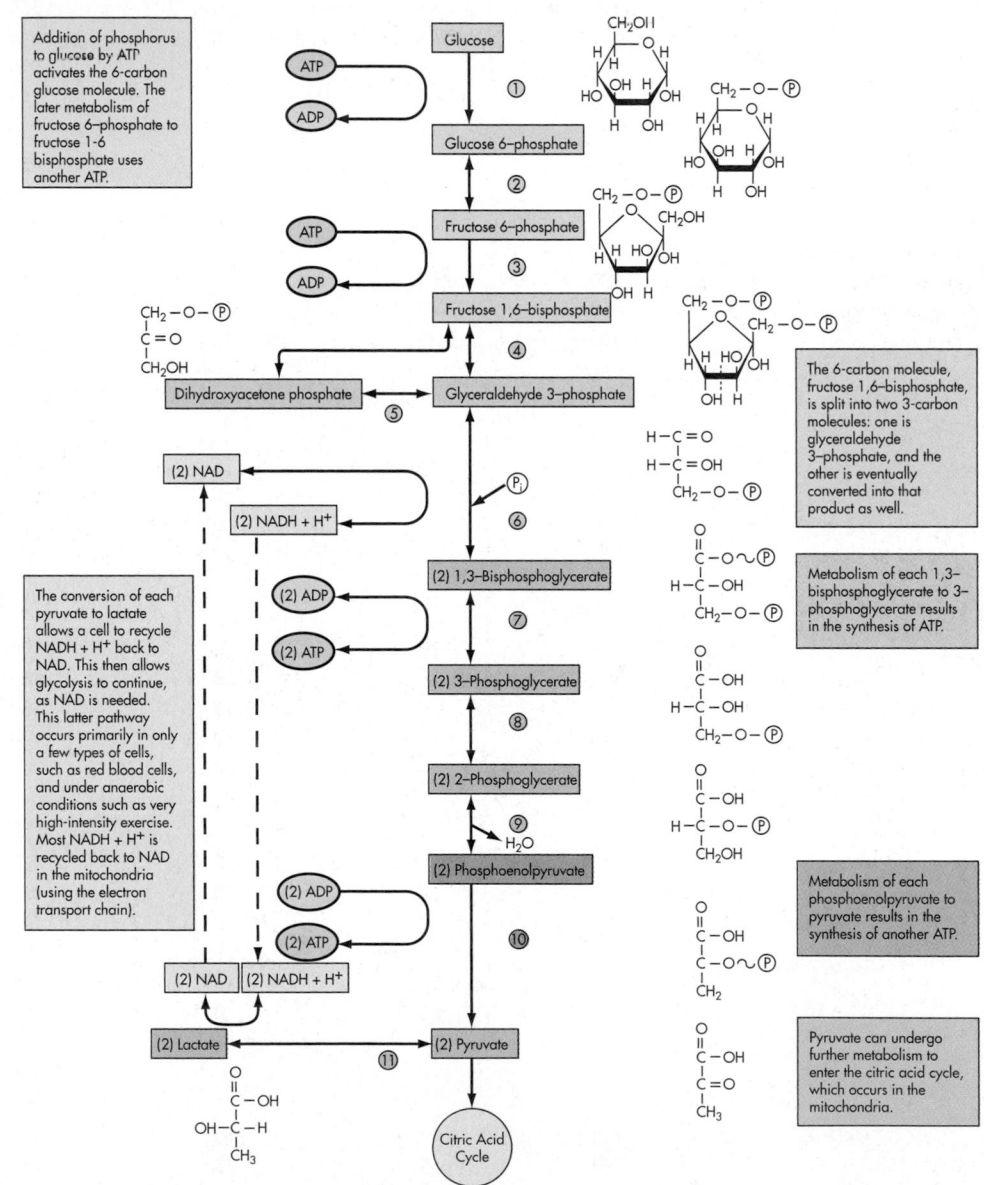

FIGURE G.1 Detailed depiction of the individual chemical reactions that comprise glycolysis—glucose to pyruvate. Glycolysis takes place in the cytosol of the cell. The enzymes in the cytosol that participate at the following steps are (1) hexokinase, (2) phosphohexose isomerase, (3) phosphofructokinase, (4) aldolase, (5) phosphotriose isomerase, (6) glyceraldehyde-3-phosphate dehydrogenase, (7) phosphoglycerate kinase, (8) phosphoglycerate mutase, (9) enolase, and (10) pyruvate kinase. Sometimes (11) lactate dehydrogenase is used to recycle NADH + H⁺ back to NAD (anaerobic glycolysis).℗ represents a phosphate group.

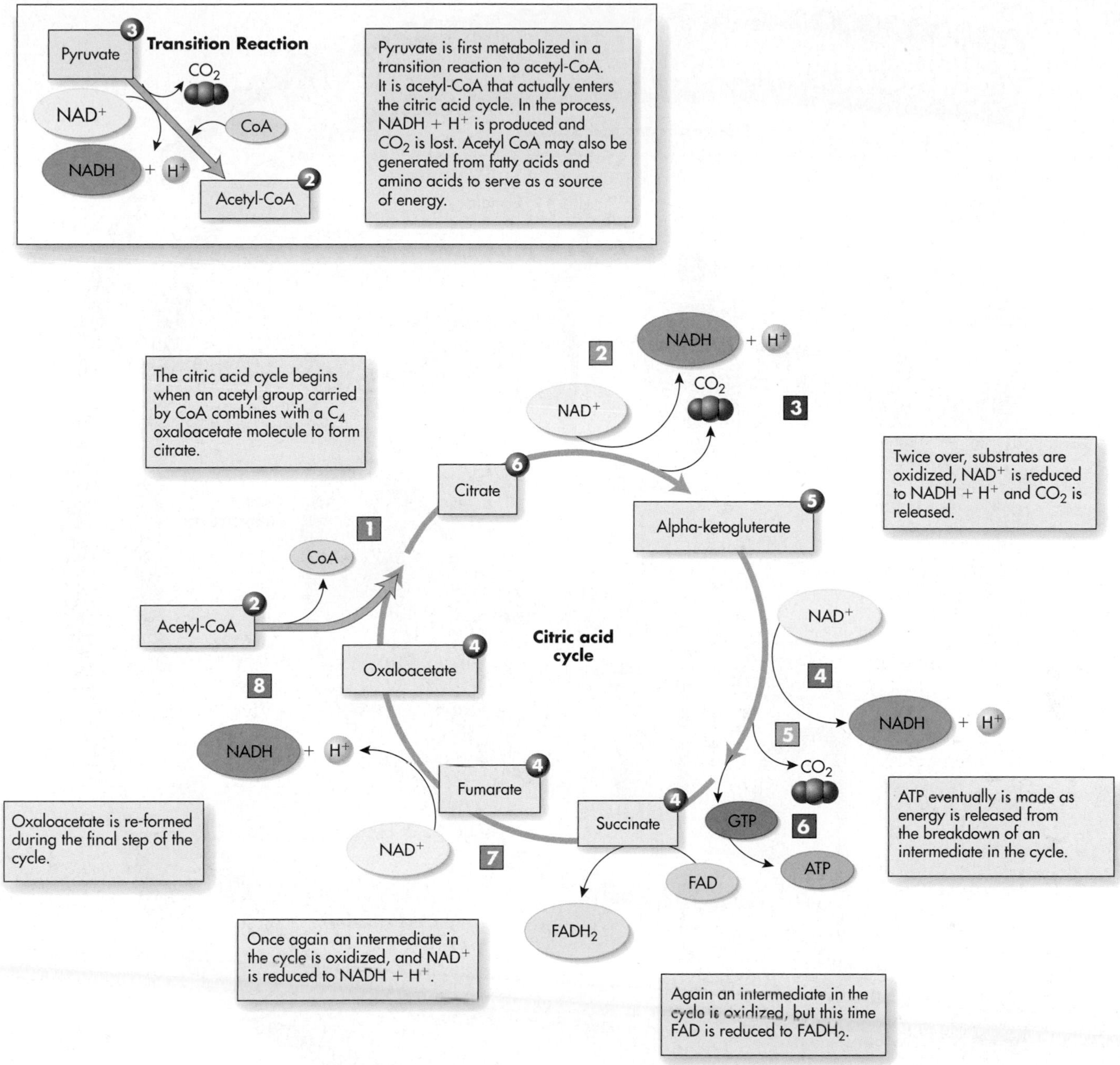

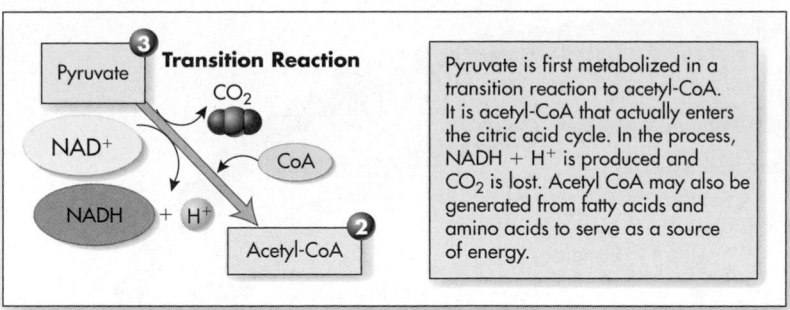

Transition Reaction

Pyruvate

CO_2

NAD^+

NADH + H^+

CoA

Acetyl-CoA

Pyruvate is first metabolized in a transition reaction to acetyl-CoA. It is acetyl-CoA that actually enters the citric acid cycle. In the process, NADH + H^+ is produced and CO_2 is lost. Acetyl CoA may also be generated from fatty acids and amino acids to serve as a source of energy.

The citric acid cycle begins when an acetyl group carried by CoA combines with a C_4 oxaloacetate molecule to form citrate.

NADH + H^+

CO_2

NAD^+

Citrate

CoA

Citric acid cycle

Acetyl-CoA

Oxaloacetate

Alpha-ketogluterate

Twice over, substrates are oxidized, NAD^+ is reduced to NADH + H^+ and CO_2 is released.

NAD^+

NADH + H^+

CO_2

GTP

ATP

ATP eventually is made as energy is released from the breakdown of an intermediate in the cycle.

Fumarate

Succinate

FAD

Oxaloacetate is re-formed during the final step of the cycle.

NADH + H^+

NAD^+

$FADH_2$

Once again an intermediate in the cycle is oxidized, and NAD^+ is reduced to NADH + H^+.

Again an intermediate in the cycle is oxidized, but this time FAD is reduced to $FADH_2$.

FIGURE G.2 The transition reaction and the citric acid cycle. The net result of one turn of this cycle of reactions (squares, steps 1–8) is the oxidation of an acetyl group to two molecules of CO_2 and the formation of three molecules of NADH + H^+ and one molecule of $FADH_2$. One GTP molecule also results, which eventually forms ATP. The citric acid cycle turns twice per glucose molecule. Note that oxygen does not participate in any of the steps in the citric acid cycle. It instead participates in the electron transport chain, where the vast majority of the ATP is formed (see figure G.3). The numbers in the circles represent the number of carbon atoms.

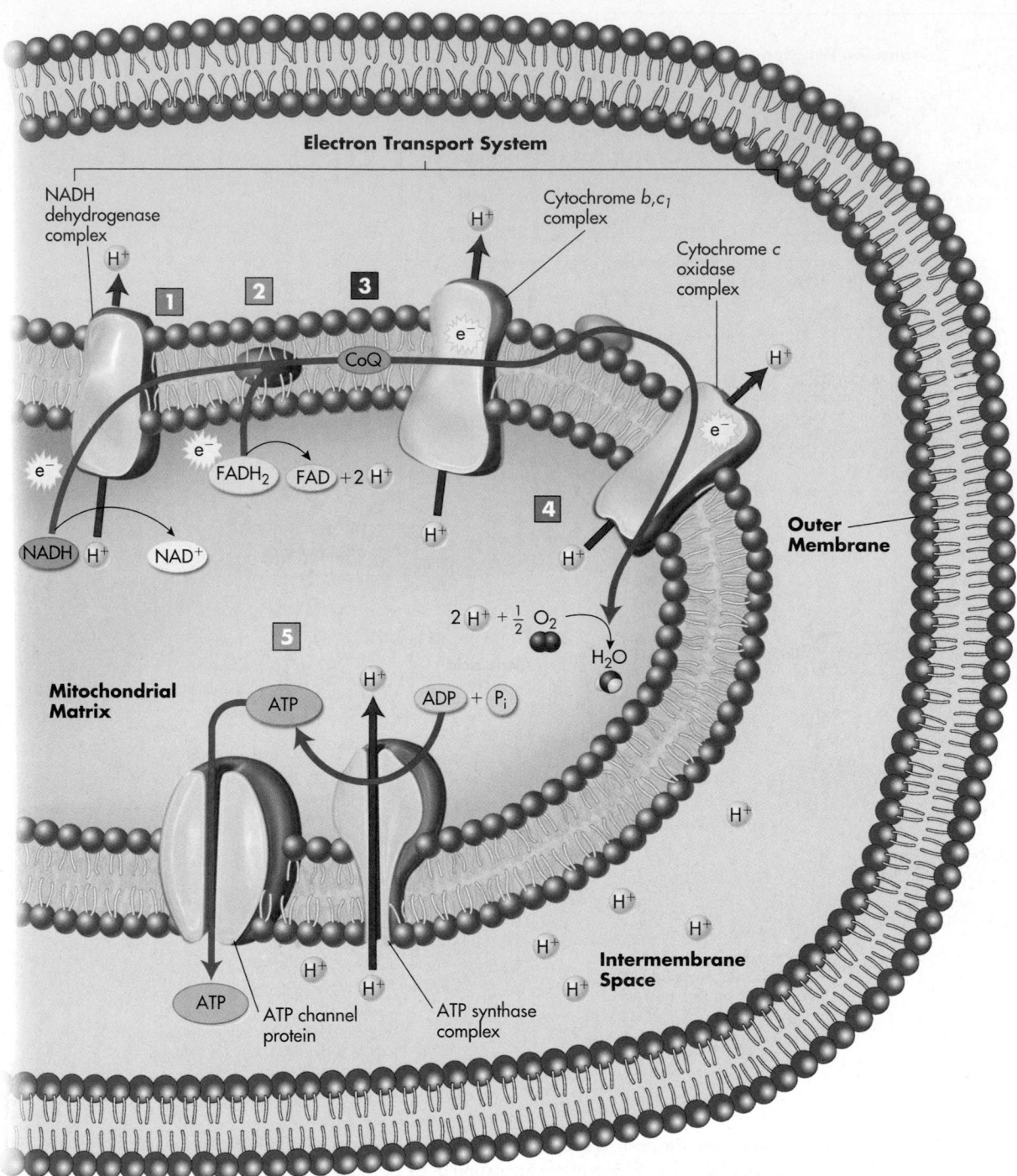

FIGURE G.3 Organization of the electron transport chain. As electrons move from one molecular complex to the other, hydrogen ions (H⁺) are pumped from the mitochondrial matrix into the intermembrane space (steps 1–4). (Note that each mitochondrion has an inner and outer membrane. Hydrogen ions flow down a concentration gradient from the intermembrane space into the mitochondrial matrix; ATP is then synthesized by the enzyme ATP synthase (step 5). ATP leaves the mitochondrial matrix by way of a channel protein.

Adipose Cells

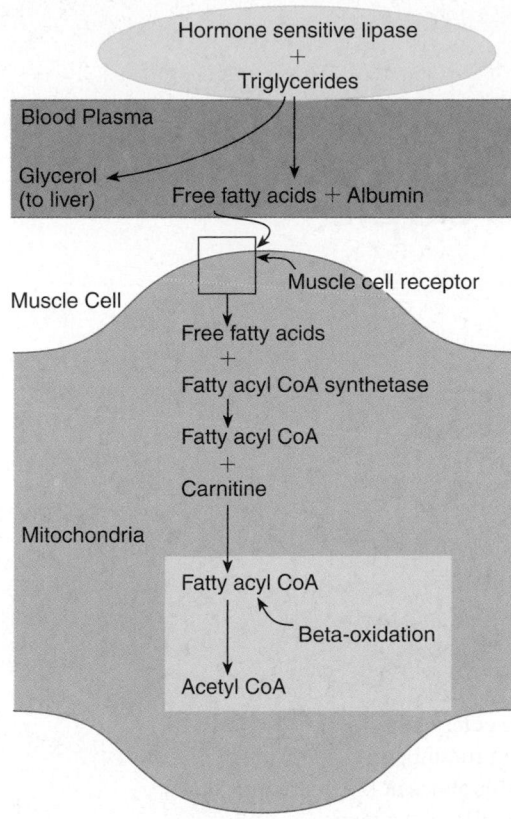

FIGURE G.4A Energy pathways for fatty acids. Triglycerides in the adipose tissue may be catabolized by hormone-sensitive lipase, with the fatty acids being released to the plasma and binding with albumin; the glycerol component is transported to the liver for metabolism. A receptor at the muscle cell transports the fatty acid into the muscle cell where it is converted into fatty acyl CoA by an enzyme (fatty acyl CoA synthetase). The fatty acyl CoA is then transported into the mitochondria with carnitine (in an enzyme complex) as a carrier. The fatty acyl CoA, which is a combination of acetyl CoA units, then undergoes beta-oxidation, a process that splits off the acetyl CoA units for entrance into the Krebs cycle.

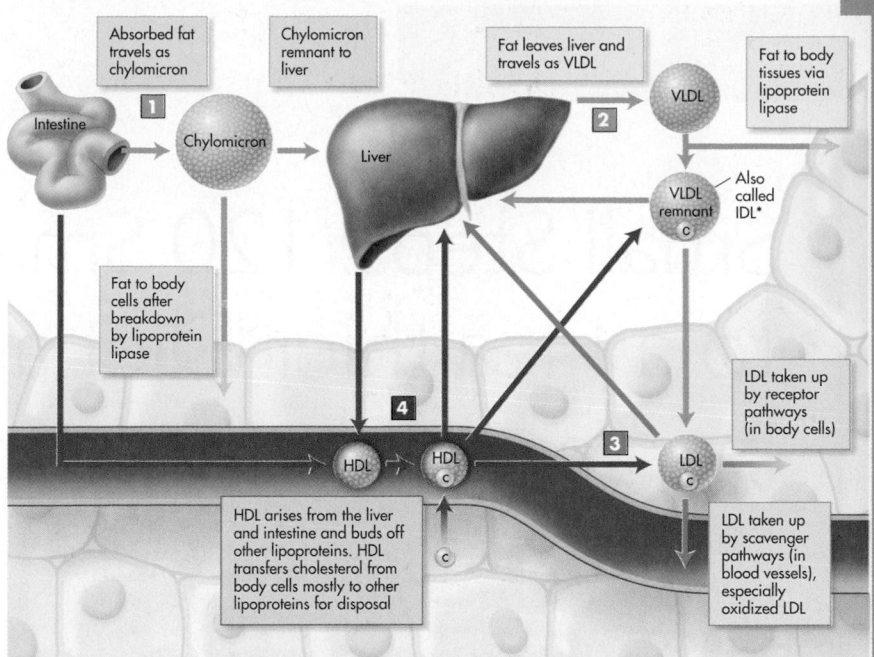

FIGURE G.4B Lipoprotein interactions. (1) Chylomicrons carry absorbed fat to body cells. (2) VLDL carries fat taken up from the bloodstream by the liver, as well as any fat made by the liver, to body cells. (3) LDL arises from VLDL and carries mostly cholesterol to cells. (4) HDL arises from body cells, mostly in the liver and intestine as well as from particles that bud off the other lipoproteins. HDL carries cholesterol from cells to other lipoproteins and to the liver for excretion.

*Intermediate Density Lipoprotein.

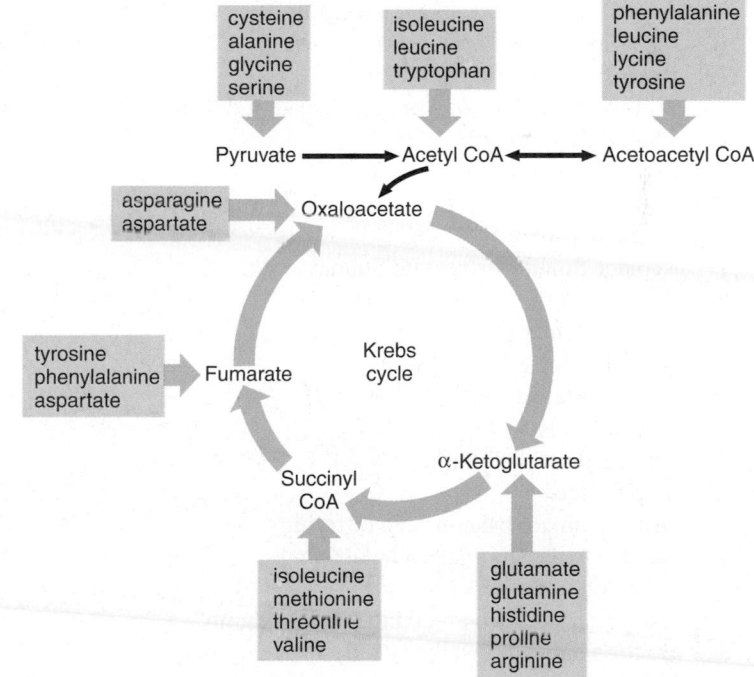

FIGURE G.5 Metabolic fates of various amino acids. Various amino acids, after deamination, may enter into energy pathways at different sites.

Small Steps: 120 Small Steps to a Healthier Diet and Increased Physical Activity

1. Walk to work.
2. Use fat-free milk over whole milk.
3. Do sit-ups in front of the TV.
4. Walk during lunch hour.
5. Drink water before a meal.
6. Eat leaner red meat & poultry.
7. Eat half your dessert.
8. Walk instead of driving whenever you can.
9. Take family walk after dinner.
10. Skate to work instead of driving.
11. Avoid food portions larger than your fist.
12. Mow lawn with push mower.
13. Increase the fiber in your diet.
14. Walk to your place of worship instead of driving.
15. Walk kids to school.
16. Get a dog and walk it.
17. Join an exercise group.
18. Drink diet soda.
19. Replace Sunday drive with Sunday walk.
20. Do yard work.
21. Eat off smaller plates.
22. Get off a stop early and walk.
23. Don't eat late at night.
24. Skip seconds.
25. Work around the house.
26. Skip buffets.
27. Grill, steam, or bake instead of frying.
28. Bicycle to the store instead of driving.
29. Take dog to the park.
30. Ask your doctor about taking a multivitamin.
31. Go for a half-hour walk instead of watching TV.
32. Use vegetable oils over solid fats.
33. More carrots, less cake.
34. Fetch the newspaper yourself.
35. Sit up straight at work.
36. Wash the car by hand.
37. Don't skip meals.
38. Eat more celery sticks.
39. Run when running errands.
40. Pace the sidelines at kids' athletic games.
41. Take wheels off luggage.
42. Choose an activity that fits into your daily life.
43. Try your burger with just lettuce, tomato, and onion.
44. Ask a friend to exercise with you.
45. Make time in your day for physical activity.
46. Exercise with a video if the weather is bad.
47. Bike to the barbershop or beauty salon instead of driving.
48. Keep to a regular eating schedule.
49. If you find it difficult to be active after work, try it before work.
50. Take a walk or do desk exercises instead of a cigarette or coffee break.
51. Perform gardening or home repair activities.
52. Avoid labor-saving devices.
53. Take small trips on foot to get your body moving.
54. Play with your kids 30 minutes a day.
55. Dance to music.
56. Keep a pair of comfortable walking or running shoes in your car and office.
57. Make a Saturday morning walk a group habit.
58. Walk briskly in the mall.
59. Choose activities you enjoy and you'll be more likely to stick with them.
60. Stretch before bed to give you more energy when you wake.
61. Take the long way to the water cooler.
62. Explore new physical activities.
63. Vary your activities, for interest and to broaden the range of benefits.

64. Reward and acknowledge your efforts.
65. Choose fruit for dessert.
66. Consume alcoholic beverages in moderation, if at all.
67. Take stairs instead of the escalator.
68. Conduct an inventory of your meal/snack and physical activity patterns.
69. Share an entrée with a friend.
70. Grill fruit or vegetables.
71. Eat before grocery shopping.
72. Choose a checkout line without a candy display.
73. Make a grocery list before you shop.
74. Buy 100% fruit juices over soda and sugary drinks.
75. Stay active in winter. Play with your kids.
76. Flavor foods with herbs, spices, and other low-fat seasonings.
77. Remove skin from poultry before cooking to lower fat content.
78. Eat before you get too hungry.
79. Don't skip breakfast.
80. Stop eating when you are full.
81. Snack on fruits and vegetables.
82. Top your favorite cereal with apples or bananas.
83. Try brown rice or whole wheat pasta.
84. Include several servings of whole-grain food daily.
85. When eating out, choose a small or medium portion.
86. If main dishes are too big, choose an appetizer or a side dish instead.
87. Ask for salad dressing "on the side."
88. Don't take seconds.
89. Park farther from destination and walk.
90. Try a green salad instead of fries.
91. Bake or broil fish.
92. Walk instead of sitting around.
93. Eat sweet foods in small amounts.
94. Take your dog on longer walks.
95. Drink lots of water.
96. Cut back on added fats or oils in cooking or spreads.
97. Walk the beach instead of sunbathing.
98. Walk to a co-worker's desk instead of e-mailing or calling them.
99. Carry your groceries instead of pushing a cart.
100. Use a snow shovel instead of a snow blower.
101. Cut high-Calorie foods like cheese and chocolate into smaller pieces and eat only a few pieces.
102. Use nonfat or low-fat sour cream, mayo, sauces, dressings, and other condiments.
103. Replace sugar-sweetened beverages with water and add a twist of lemon or lime.
104. Replace high-saturated fat/high Calorie seasonings with herbs grown in a small herb garden in your kitchen window.
105. Refrigerate prepared soups before you eat them. As the soup cools, the fat will rise to the top. Skim it off the surface for reduced-fat content.
106. When eating out, ask your server to put half your entrée in a to-go bag.
107. Substitute vegetables for other ingredients in your sandwich.
108. Every time you eat a meal, sit down, chew slowly, and pay attention to flavors and textures.
109. Try a new fruit or vegetable. (Ever had jicama, plantain, bok choy, starfruit, or papaya?)
110. Make up a batch of brownies with applesauce instead of oil or shortening.
111. Instead of eating out, bring a healthy, low-Calorie lunch to work.
112. Ask your sweetie to bring you fruit or flowers instead of chocolate.
113. Speak up for the salad bar when your co-workers are picking a restaurant for lunch, and remember Calories count, so pay attention to how much and what you eat.
114. When walking, go up the hills instead of around them.
115. Walk briskly through the mall and shop 'til you drop . . . pounds.
116. Clean your closet and donate clothes that are too big.
117. Take your body measurements to gauge progress.
118. Buy a set of hand weights and play a round of Simon Says with your kids. You do it with the weights; they do it without.
119. Swim with your kids.
120. Wear a SmallSteps bracelet to remind you to live a healthier lifestyle every day.

Source: www.SmallStep.Gov

Sample Menu for a 2,000-Calorie Food Pattern

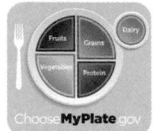

Sample menus for a 2,000 Calorie food pattern

Averaged over a week, this seven day menu provides all of the recommended amounts of nutrients and food from each food group.(Italicized foods are part of the dish or food that precedes it.)

Sample Menus for a 2000-Calorie Food Pattern

Use this 7-day menu as a motivational tool to help put a healthy eating pattern into practice, and to identify creative new ideas for healthy meals. Averaged over a week, this menu provides the recommended amounts of key nutrients and foods from each food group. The menus feature a large number of different foods to inspire ideas for adding variety to food choices. They are not intended to be followed day-by-day as a specific prescription for what to eat.

Spices and herbs can be used to taste. Try spices such as chili powder, cinnamon, cumin, curry powder, ginger, nutmeg, mustard, garlic powder, onion powder, or pepper. Try fresh or dried herbs such as basil, parsley, cilantro, chives, dill, mint, oregano, rosemary, thyme, or tarragon. Also try salt-free spice or herb blends.

While this 7-day menu provides the recommended amounts of foods and key nutrients, it does so at a moderate cost. Based on national average food costs, adjusted for inflation to March 2011 prices, the cost of this menu is less than the average amount spent for food, per person, in a four-person family.

DAY 1

BREAKFAST
Creamy oatmeal (cooked in milk):
- ½ cup uncooked oatmeal
- 1 cup fat-free milk
- 2 Tbsp raisins
- 2 tsp brown sugar

Beverage: 1 cup orange juice

LUNCH
Taco salad:
- 2 ounces tortilla chips
- 2 ounces cooked ground turkey
- 2 tsp corn/canola oil (to cook turkey)
- ¼ cup kidney beans*
- ½ ounce low-fat cheddar cheese
- ½ cup chopped lettuce
- ½ cup avocado
- 1 tsp lime juice (on avocado)
- 2 Tbsp salsa

Beverage:
1 cup water, coffee, or tea**

DINNER
Spinach lasagna roll-ups:
- 1 cup lasagna noodles(2 oz dry)
- ½ cup cooked spinach
- ½ cup ricotta cheese
- 1 ounce part-skim mozzarella cheese
- ½ cup tomato sauce*

1 ounce whole wheat roll
1 tsp tub margarine
Beverage: 1 cup fat-free milk

SNACKS
2 Tbsp raisins
1 ounce unsalted almonds

DAY 2

BREAKFAST
Breakfast burrito:
- 1 flour tortilla (8" diameter)
- 1 scrambled egg
- ⅓ cup black beans*
- 2 Tbsp salsa

½ large grapefruit
Beverage:
1 cup water, coffee, or tea**

LUNCH
Roast beef sandwich:
- 1 small whole grain hoagie bun
- 2 ounces lean roast beef
- 1 slice part-skim mozzarella cheese
- 2 slices tomato
- ¼ cup mushrooms
- 1 tsp corn/canola oil (to cook mushrooms)
- 1 tsp mustard

Baked potato wedges:
- 1 cup potato wedges
- 1 tsp corn/canola oil (to cook potato)
- 1 Tbsp ketchup

Beverage: 1 cup fat-free milk

DINNER
Baked salmon on beet greens:
- 4 ounce salmon filet
- 1 tsp olive oil
- 2 tsp lemon juice
- ⅓ cup cooked beet greens (sauteed in 2 tsp corn/canola oil)

Quinoa with almonds:
- ½ cup quinoa
- ½ ounce slivered almonds

Beverage: 1 cup fat-free milk

SNACKS
1 cup cantaloupe balls

DAY 3

BREAKFAST
Cold cereal:
- 1 cup ready-to-eat oat cereal
- 1 medium banana
- ½ cup fat-free milk

1 slice whole wheat toast
1 tsp tub margarine
Beverage: 1 cup prune juice

LUNCH
Tuna salad sandwich:
- 2 slices rye bread
- 2 ounces tuna
- 1 Tbsp mayonnaise
- 1 Tbsp chopped celery
- ½ cup shredded lettuce

1 medium peach
Beverage: 1 cup fat-free milk

DINNER
Roasted chicken:
- 3 ounces cooked chicken breast

1 large sweet potato, roasted
½ cup succotash (limas & corn)
1 tsp tub margarine
1 ounce whole wheat roll
1 tsp tub margarine
Beverage:
1 cup water, coffee, or tea**

SNACKS
¼ cup dried apricots
1 cup flavored yogurt (chocolate)

Sample Menus for a 2000-Calorie Food Pattern (cont'd)

DAY 4

BREAKFAST
1 whole wheat English muffin
1 Tbsp all-fruit preserves
1 hard-cooked egg
Beverage:
1 cup water, coffee, or tea**

LUNCH
White bean-vegetable soup:
1 ¼ cup chunky vegetable soup with pasta
*½ cup white beans**
6 saltine crackers*
½ cup celery sticks
Beverage: 1 cup fat-free milk

DINNER
Rigatoni with meat sauce:
1 cup rigatoni pasta (2 oz dry)
2 ounces cooked ground beef (95% lean)
2 tsp corn/canola oil (to cook beef)
*½ cup tomato sauce**
3 Tbsp grated parmesan cheese
Spinach salad:
1 cup raw spinach leaves
½ cup tangerine sections
½ ounce chopped walnuts
4 tsp oil and vinegar dressing
Beverage:
1 cup water, coffee, or tea**

SNACKS
1 cup nonfat fruit yogurt

DAY 5

BREAKFAST
Cold cereal:
1 cup shredded wheat
½ cup sliced banana
½ cup fat-free milk
1 slice whole wheat toast
2 tsp all-fruit preserves
Beverage:
1 cup fat-free chocolate milk

LUNCH
Turkey sandwich
1 whole wheat pita bread (2 oz)
3 ounces roasted turkey, sliced
2 slices tomato
¼ cup shredded lettuce
1 tsp mustard
1 Tbsp mayonnaise
½ cup grapes
Beverage: 1 cup tomato juice*

DINNER
Steak and potatoes:
4 ounces broiled beef steak
⅔ cup mashed potatoes made with milk and 2 tsp tub margarine
½ cup cooked green beans
1 tsp tub margarine
1 tsp honey
1 ounce whole wheat roll
1 tsp tub margarine
Frozen yogurt and berries:
½ cup frozen yogurt (chocolate)
¾ cup sliced strawberries
Beverage: 1 cup fat-free milk

SNACKS
1 cup frozen yogurt (chocolate)

DAY 6

BREAKFAST
French toast:
2 slices whole wheat bread
3 Tbsp fat-free milk and
⅔ egg (in French toast)
2 tsp tub margarine
1 Tbsp pancake syrup
½ large grapefruit
Beverage: 1 cup fat-free milk

LUNCH
3-bean vegetarian chili on baked potato:
¼ cup each cooked kidney beans, navy beans,* and black beans**
*½ cup tomato sauce**
¼ cup chopped onion
2 Tbsp chopped jalapeno peppers
1 tsp corn/canola oil (to cook onion and peppers)
¼ cup cheese sauce
1 large baked potato
½ cup cantaloupe
Beverage:
1 cup water, coffee, or tea**

DINNER
Hawaiian pizza
2 slices cheese pizza, thin crust
1 ounce lean ham
¼ cup pineapple
½ cup mushrooms
1 tsp safflower oil (to cook mushrooms)
Green salad:
1 cup mixed salad greens
4 tsp oil and vinegar dressing
Beverage: 1 cup fat-free milk

SNACKS
3 Tbsp hummus
5 whole wheat crackers*

DAY 7

BREAKFAST
Buckwheat pancakes with berries:
2 large (7") pancakes
1 Tbsp pancake syrup
¾ cup sliced strawberries
Beverage: 1 cup orange juice

LUNCH
New England clam chowder:
3 ounces canned clams
½ small potato
2 Tbsp chopped onion
2 Tbsp chopped celery
6 Tbsp evaporated milk
¼ cup fat-free milk
1 slice bacon
1 Tbsp white flour
10 whole wheat crackers*
1 medium orange
Beverage: 1 cup fat-free milk

DINNER
Tofu-vegetable stir-fry:
4 ounces firm tofu
¼ cup chopped Chinese cabbage
¼ cup sliced bamboo shoots
2 Tbsp chopped sweet red peppers
2 Tbsp chopped green peppers
1 Tbsp corn/canola oil (to cook stir-fry)
1 cup cooked brown rice (2 ounces raw)
Honeydew yogurt cup:
¾ cup honeydew melon
½ cup plain fat-free yogurt
Beverage:
1 cup water, coffee, or tea**

SNACKS
1 large banana spread with
*2 Tbsp peanut butter**
1 cup nonfat fruit yogurt

Notes:

*Foods that are reduced sodium, low sodium, or no-salt added products. These foods can also be prepared from scratch with no added salt. All other foods are regular commercial products, which contain variable levels of sodium. Average sodium level of the 7-day menu assumes that no salt is added in cooking or at the table.

**Unless indicated, all beverages are unsweetened and without added cream or whitener.

Italicized foods are part of the dish or food that precedes it.

Source: www.choosemyplate.com

624

Sample Menus for a 2000-Calorie Food Pattern (cont'd)

Average amounts for weekly menu:

Food group	Daily average over 1 week
GRAINS	6.2 oz eq
Whole grains	3.8
Refined grains	2.4
VEGETABLES	2.6 cups
Vegetable subgroups (amount per week)	
Dark green	1.6 cups per week
Red/Orange	5.6
Starchy	5.1
Beans and Peas	1.6
Other Vegetables	4.1
FRUITS	2.1 cups
DAIRY	3.1 cups
PROTEIN FOODS	5.7 oz eq
Seafood	8.8 oz per week
OILS	29 grams
CALORIES FROM ADDED FATS AND SUGARS	245 calories

Nutrient	Daily average over 1 week
Calories	1975
Protein	96 g
Protein	19% kcal
Carbohydrate	275 g
Carbohydrate	56% kcal
Total fat	59 g
Total fat	27% kcal
Saturated fat	13.2 g
Saturated fat	6.0% kcal
Monounsaturated fat	25 g
Polyunsaturated fat	16 g
Linoleic acid	13 g
Alpha-linolenic acid	1.8 g
Cholesterol	201 mg
Total dietary fiber	30 g
Potassium	4701 mg
Sodium	1810 mg
Calcium	1436 mg
Magnesium	468 mg
Copper	2.0 mg
Iron	18 mg
Phosphorus	1885 mg
Zinc	14 mg
Thiamin	1.6 mg
Riboflavin	2.5 mg
Niacin Equivalents	24 mg
Vitamin B6	2.4 mg
Vitamin B12	12.3 mcg
Vitamin C	146 mg
Vitamin E	11.8 mg (AT)
Vitamin D	9.1 mcg
Vitamin A	1090 mcg (RAE)
Dietary Folate Equivalents	530 mcg
Choline	386 mg

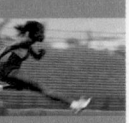

Glossary

A

Acceptable Daily Intake (ADI) The amount of a food additive an individual can consume without an adverse effect.

Acceptable Macronutrient Distribution Range (AMDR) A range of dietary intakes for carbohydrate, fat, and protein that is associated with reduced risk of chronic disease while providing adequate nutrients.

acclimatization The ability of the body to undergo physiological adaptations so that the stress of a given environment, such as high environmental temperature, is less severe.

acetaldehyde An intermediate breakdown product of alcohol.

acetic acid A naturally occurring saturated fatty acid; a precursor for the Krebs cycle when converted into acetyl CoA.

acetyl CoA The major fuel for the oxidative processes in the body, being derived from the breakdown of glucose and fatty acids.

acid-base balance A relative balance of acid and base products in the body so that an optimal pH is maintained in the tissues, particularly the blood.

acidosis A disturbance of the normal acid-base balance in which excess acids accumulate in the body. Lactic acid production during exercise may lead to acidosis.

acrylamide A cancer-causing agent that may be produced by prolonged, high-temperature cooking.

active transport A process requiring energy to transport substances across cell membranes.

activity-stat Center in the brain theorized to regulate daily physical activity.

acute exercise bout A single bout of exercise that will produce various physiological reactions dependent upon the nature of the exercise; a single workout.

added sugars Refined sugars added to foods during commercial food processing.

additives Substances added to food to improve flavor, color, texture, stability, or for similar purposes.

adenosine triphosphate *See* ATP.

Adequate Intake (AI) Recommended dietary intake comparable to the RDA, but based on less scientific evidence.

adipokines Substances released from adipose (fat) cells that function as hormones in other parts of the body.

Adonis complex A disturbed body image in which muscular individuals consider themselves too thin or not sufficiently muscular; also known as muscle dysmorphia.

adrenaline A hormone secreted by the adrenal medulla; it is a stimulant and prepares the body for "fight or flight."

aerobic Relating to energy processes that occur in the presence of oxygen.

aerobic glycolysis Oxidative processes in the cell that liberate energy in the metabolism of the carbohydrate glycogen.

aerobic lipolysis Oxidative processes in the cell that liberate energy in the metabolism of fats.

aerobic walking Rapid walking designed to elevate the heart rate so that a training effect will occur; more strenuous than ordinary leisure walking.

air displacement plethysmography (ADP) A procedure to measure body composition via displacement of air in a special chamber; comparable to water displacement in underwater weighing techniques to evaluate body composition.

alanine A nonessential amino acid.

alcohol A colorless liquid with depressant effects; ethyl alcohol or ethanol is the alcohol designed for human consumption.

alcohol dehydrogenase An enzyme in the liver that initiates the breakdown of alcohol to acetaldehyde.

alcoholism A rather undefined term used to describe individuals who abuse the effect of alcohol; an addiction or habituation that may result in physical and/or psychological withdrawal effects.

aldosterone The main electrolyte-regulating hormone secreted by the adrenal cortex; primarily controls sodium and potassium balance.

allithiamine A derivative of thiamine.

alpha-ketoacid Specific acids associated with different amino acids and released upon deamination or transamination; for example, the breakdown of glutamate yields alpha-ketoglutarate.

alpha-linolenic acid An omega-3 fatty acid considered to be an essential nutrient.

alpha-tocopherol The most biologically active alcohol in vitamin E.

alpha-tocopherol equivalent The amount of other forms of tocopherol to equal the vitamin E activity of one milligram of alpha-tocopherol.

AMDR *See* Acceptable Macronutrient Distribution Range.

amenorrhea Absence or cessation of menstruation.

amino acids The chief structural material of protein, consisting of an amino group (NH_2) and an acid group (COOH) plus other components.

amino group The nitrogen-containing component of amino acids (NH_2).

aminostatic theory A theory suggesting that hunger is controlled by the presence or absence of amino acids in the blood acting upon a receptor in the hypothalamus.

ammonia A metabolic by-product of the oxidation of glutamine; it may be transformed into urea for excretion from the body.

amylopectin A branched-chain starch.

amylose A straight-chain starch that is more resistant to digestion compared to amylopectin.

anabolic/androgenic steroids (AAS) Drugs designed to mimic the actions of testosterone to build muscle tissue (anabolism) while minimizing the androgenic effects (masculinization).

anabolism Constructive metabolism, the process whereby simple body compounds are formed into more complex ones.

anaerobic Relating to energy processes that occur in the absence of oxygen.

anaerobic glycolysis Metabolic processes in the cell that liberate energy in the metabolism of the carbohydrate glycogen without the involvement of oxidation.

anaerobic threshold The intensity of exercise at which the individual begins to increase the proportion of energy derived from anaerobic means, principally the lactic acid system. *Also see* steady-state threshold and onset of blood lactic acid (OBLA).

android-type obesity Male-type obesity in which the body fat accumulates in the abdominal area and is a more significant risk factor for chronic disease than is gynoid-type obesity.

androstenedione An androgen produced in the body that is converted to testosterone; marketed as a dietary supplement.

anemia In general, subnormal levels of circulating RBCs and hemoglobin; there are many different types of anemia.

angina The pain experienced under the breastbone or in other areas of the upper body when the heart is deprived of oxygen.

anion A negatively charged ion, or electrolyte.

anorexia athletica A form of anorexia nervosa observed in athletes involved in sports in which low percentages of body fat may enhance performance, such as gymnastics and ballet.

anorexia nervosa (AN) A serious nervous condition, particularly among teenage girls and young women, marked by a loss of appetite and leading to various degrees of emaciation.

anthropometry Use of body girths and diameters to evaluate body composition.

antibodies Protein substances developed in the body in reaction to the presence of a foreign substance, called an antigen; natural antibodies are also present in the blood. They are protective in nature.

antidiuretic hormone (ADH) Hormone secreted by the pituitary gland; its major action is to conserve body water by decreasing urine formation; also known as vasopressin.

antinutrients Substances in foods that can adversely affect nutrient status.

antioxidant A compound that may protect other compounds from the effects of oxygen. The antioxidant itself interferes with oxidative processes.

antipromoters Compounds that block the actions of *promoters,* agents associated with the development of certain diseases, such as cancer.

apolipoprotein A class of special proteins associated with the formation of lipoproteins. A variety of apolipoproteins have been identified and are involved in the specific functions of the different lipoproteins.

appestat Term used for the neural center in the hypothalamus that helps control appetite by stimulating either hunger or satiety.

appetite A pleasant desire for food for the purpose of enjoyment that is developed through previous experience; believed to be controlled in humans by an appetite center, or appestat, in the hypothalamus.

arginine An essential amino acid.

arteriosclerosis Hardening of the arteries; *also see* atherosclerosis.

ascorbic acid Vitamin C.

aspartame An artificial sweetener made from amino acids.

aspartates Salts of aspartic acid, an amino acid.

atherosclerosis A specific form of arteriosclerosis characterized by the formation of plaque on the inner layers of the arterial wall.

athletic amenorrhea The cessation of menstruation in athletes, believed to be caused by factors associated with participation in strenuous physical activity.

ATP Adenosine triphosphate, a high-energy phosphate compound found in the body; one of the major forms of energy available for immediate use in the body.

ATPase The enzyme involved in the splitting of ATP and the release of energy.

ATP-PCr system The energy system for fast, powerful muscle contractions; uses ATP as the immediate energy source, the spent ATP being quickly regenerated by breakdown of the PCr. ATP and PCr are high-energy phosphates in the muscle cell.

B

baking soda A commercial form of sodium bicarbonate.

basal energy expenditure (BEE) The basal metabolic rate (BMR) total energy expenditure over 24 hours.

basal metabolic rate (BMR) The measurement of energy expenditure in the body under resting, postabsorptive conditions, indicative of the energy needed to maintain life under these basal conditions.

Basic Four Food Groups Grouping of foods into four categories that can be used as a means to educate individuals on how to obtain essential nutrients. The four groups are meat, milk, bread-cereal, and fruit-vegetable.

bee pollen A nutritional product containing minute amounts of protein and some vitamins that has been advertised to be possibly ergogenic for some athletes.

behavior modification Relative to weight-control methods, behavioral patterns, or the way one acts, may be modified to help achieve weight loss.

beriberi A deficiency disease attributed to lack of thiamin (vitamin B$_1$) in the diet.

beta-alanine A nonessential amino acid, also labeled as β-alanine, that is a part of the peptides carnosine and anserine; beta-alanine is purported to have ergogenic potential.

beta-carotene A precursor for vitamin A found in plants.

beta glucan Gummy form of water-soluble fiber useful in reducing serum cholesterol; oats are a good source.

beta-oxidation Process in the cells whereby 2-carbon units of acetic acid are removed from long-chain fatty acids for conversion to acetyl CoA and oxidation via the Krebs cycle.

bile A fluid secreted by the liver into the intestine that aids in the breakdown process of fats.

bile salts Active salts found in bile; cholesterol is part of their structure.

binge eating disorder Condition in which individuals demonstrate some of the same behaviors as those with bulimia nervosa, such as eating more quickly and until uncomfortably full, but do not purge.

binge-purge syndrome An eating behavior characterized by excessive hunger leading to gorging, followed by guilt and purging by vomiting. *Also see* bulimia nervosa.

bioavailability In relation to nutrients in food, the amount that may be absorbed into the body.

bioelectrical impedance analysis (BIA) A method to calculate percentage of body fat by measuring electrical resistance due to the water content of the body.

bioengineered foods Foods modified by genetic engineering to produce desirable traits.

biotin A component of the B complex.

bisphosphonates Drugs used to inhibit bone resorption, but not mineralization, to help prevent bone loss and increase bone mineral density; Fosamax is one brand.

blood alcohol concentration (BAC) The concentration of alcohol in the blood, usually expressed as milligram percent.

blood alcohol level *See* blood alcohol concentration.

blood glucose Blood sugar; the means by which carbohydrate is carried in the blood; normal range is 70–120 mg/ml.

blood pressure The pressure of the blood in the blood vessels; usually used to refer to arterial blood pressure. *Also see* systolic blood pressure and diastolic blood pressure.

BMI *See* Body Mass Index.

BDNF *See* brain-derived neurotropic factor.

body image The image or impression the individual has of his or her body. A poor body image may lead to personality problems.

Body Mass Index (BMI) An index calculated by a ratio of height to weight, used as a measure of obesity.

body plethysmography A body composition technique using a special chamber to measure air displacement; similar to water displacement theory associated with underwater weighing.

brain-derived neurotropic factor (BDNF) Protein produced in the brain and other tissues that may promote growth and support of neurons.

branched-chain amino acids (BCAA) Three essential amino acids (leucine, isoleucine, and valine) that help form muscle tissue.

bread exchange One bread exchange in the Food Exchange System contains 15 grams of carbohydrate, 3 grams of protein, and 80 Calories.

brown fat A special form of adipose tissue that is designed to produce heat; small amounts are found in humans in the area of vital organs such as the heart and lungs.

buffer boosting Term associated with use of sodium bicarbonate as an ergogenic aid to increase the acid-buffering capacity of the blood.

bulimia nervosa An eating disorder involving a loss of control over the impulse to binge; the binge-purge syndrome.

bulk-up method A method of weight training designed to increase muscle mass; uses high resistance and moderate volume with many different muscle groups.

C

caffeine A stimulant drug found in many food products such as coffee, tea, and cola drinks; stimulates the central nervous system.

calciferol A synthetic vitamin D.

calcitriol The hormone form of vitamin D.

calcium A silver-white metallic element essential to human nutrition.

caloric concept of weight control The concept that Calories are the basis of weight control. Excess Calories will add body weight while caloric deficiencies will contribute to weight loss.

caloric deficit A negative caloric balance whereby more Calories are expended than consumed; a weight loss will occur.

Calorie A measure of heat energy. A small calorie represents the amount of heat needed to raise one gram of water one degree Celsius. A large Calorie (kilocalorie, KC, or C) is 1,000 small calories.

calorimeter A device used to measure the caloric value of a given food, or heat production of animals or humans.

calorimetry The science of measuring heat production.

carbohydrate-electrolyte solutions (CES) Fluids containing water, various forms of carbohydrate such as glucose and fructose, and various electrolytes such as sodium, chloride, and potassium, in a solution designed to maintain optimal hydration and energy during exercise. *See also* sports drinks.

carbohydrate loading A dietary method used by endurance-type athletes to help increase the carbohydrate (glycogen) levels in their muscles and liver.

carbohydrates A group of compounds containing carbon, hydrogen, and oxygen. Glucose, glycogen, sugar, starches, fiber, cellulose, and the various saccharides are all carbohydrates.

carcinogenicity The potential of a substance to cause cancer.

carnitine A chemical that facilitates the transfer of fatty acids into the mitochondria for subsequent oxidation.

carnosine A peptide found in muscle tissue theorized to possess ergogenic potential via its buffering effect on lactic acid during high intensity exercise; carnosine contains the nonessential amino acid beta-alanine.

catabolism Destructive metabolism whereby complex chemical compounds in the body are degraded to simpler ones.

catalase An enzyme that helps neutralize free radicals.

cation A positively charged ion or electrolyte.

cellulite A name given to the lumpy fat that often appears in the thigh and hip region of women. Cellulite is simply normal fat in small compartments formed by connective tissue, but may contain other compounds that bind water.

cellulose The fibrous carbohydrate that provides the structural backbone for plants; plant fiber.

Celsius A thermometer scale that has a freezing point of 0° and a boiling point of 100°; also known as the centigrade scale.

central fatigue Fatigue caused by suboptimal functioning of neurotransmitters, most likely in the brain.

cerebrospinal fluid (CSF) The fluid found in the brain and spinal cord.

chloride A compound of chlorine present in a salt form carrying a negative charge; Cl⁻, an anion.

cholecalciferol The product of irradiation of 7-dehydrocholesterol found in the skin. *Also see* vitamin D_3.

cholesterol A fat-like pearly substance, an alcohol, found in all animal fat and oils; a main constituent of some body tissues and body compounds.

choline A substance associated with the B complex that is widely distributed in both plant and animal tissues; involved in carbohydrate, fat, and protein metabolism.

chondroitin Formed in the body from amino acids and involved in cartilage formation; marked as a dietary supplement.

chromium A whitish metal essential to human nutrition; it is involved in carbohydrate metabolism via its role with insulin.

chronic fatigue syndrome Prolonged fatigue (over 6 months) of unknown cause characterized by mental depression and physical fatigue; may be observed in endurance athletes.

chronic training effect The structural and metabolic adaptations that occur in the body in response to exercise training over time; the adaptations are specific to the type of exercise, such as aerobic endurance training or resistance training.

chylomicron A particle of emulsified fat found in the blood following the digestion and assimilation of fat.

circuit aerobics A combination of aerobic and weight-training exercises designed to elicit the specific benefits of each type of exercise.

circuit weight training A method of training in which exercises are arranged in a circuit or sequence. May be designed with weight training to help convey an aerobic training effect.

cirrhosis A degenerative disease of the liver, one cause being excessive consumption of alcohol.

***cis* fatty acids** The chemical structure of unsaturated fatty acids in which the hydrogen ions are on the same side of the double bond.

citrulline An amino acid that may be converted in the body to arginine and hypothesized to possess ergogenic potential; citrulline is not needed to form any body tissues.

ciwujia A Chinese herb theorized to be ergogenic.

clinical obesity Obesity determined by a clinical procedure.

Clostridium A bacteria commonly involved in food poisoning.

cobalamin The cobalt-containing complex common to all members of the vitamin B_{12} group; often used to designate cyanocobalamin.

cobalt A gray, hard metal that is a component of vitamin B_{12}.

coenzyme An activator of an enzyme; many vitamins are coenzymes.

coenzyme Q10 *See* CoQ10.

colon The large intestine.

compensated heat stress A condition in which heat loss balances heat production, a set body temperature is maintained, and the individual can continue to exercise in warm environmental conditions.

complementary proteins Combining plant foods such as rice and beans so that essential amino acids deficient in one of the foods are provided by the other, in order to obtain a balanced intake of essential amino acids.

complete protein A protein that contains all nine essential amino acids in the proper proportions. Animal protein is complete protein.

complex carbohydrates A term used to describe foods high in starch, such as bread, cereals, fruits, and vegetables, as contrasted to simple carbohydrates such as table sugar.

concentric method A method of weight training in which the muscle shortens.

conduction In relation to body temperature, the transfer of heat from one substance to another by direct contact.

conjugated linoleic acid (CLA) Isomers of linoleic acid, an essential fatty acid. CLA is found in the meat and milk of ruminants, and is theorized to have health and exercise performance benefits, such as promotion of weight loss.

convection In relation to body temperature, the transfer of heat by way of currents in either air or water.

copper A reddish metallic element essential to human nutrition; it functions with iron in the formation of hemoglobin and the cytochromes.

CoQ10 A coenzyme involved in the electron transport system in the mitochondria.

core temperature The temperature of the deep tissues of the body, usually measured orally or rectally; *also see* shell temperature.

Cori cycle Cycle involving muscle breakdown of glucose to lactate, lactate transport via blood to the liver for reconversion to glucose, and glucose returning to the muscle.

coronary artery disease (CAD) Atherosclerosis in the coronary arteries.

coronary heart disease (CHD) A degenerative disease of the heart caused primarily by arteriosclerosis or atherosclerosis of the coronary vessels of the heart.

coronary occlusion Closure of coronary arteries that may precipitate a heart attack; occlusion may be partial or complete closure.

coronary risk factors Behaviors (smoking) or body properties (cholesterol levels) that may predispose an individual to coronary heart disease.

coronary thrombosis Occlusion (closure) of coronary arteries, usually by a blood clot.

cortisol A hormone secreted by the adrenal cortex with gluconeogenic potential, helping to convert amino acids to glucose.

creatine A nitrogen-containing compound found in the muscles, usually complexed with phosphate to form phosphocreatine.

crossover concept The concept that as exercise intensity increases, at some point carbohydrate rather than fat becomes the predominant fuel for muscle contraction.

cruciferous vegetables Vegetables in the cabbage family, such as broccoli, cauliflower, kale, and all cabbages.

CSSD Certification as a Specialist in Sports Dietetics; a certification program by the American Dietetic Association.

cyanocobalamin Vitamin B_{12}.

cysteine A breakdown product of cystine. It is also a sulfur-containing amino acid.

cystine A sulfur-containing amino acid.

cytochromes Any one of a class of pigment compounds that play an important role in cellular oxidative processes.

cytokine Small proteins or peptides produced in cells, such as adipokines by adipose tissue cells, that possess hormone-like functions on other cells in the body; the immune system secretes a number of different cytokines.

D

Daily Reference Values (DRVs) Recommended daily intakes for the macronutrients (carbohydrate, fat, and protein) as well as cholesterol, sodium, and potassium. On a food label, the DRV is based on a 2,000-Calorie diet.

Daily Value (DV) A term used in food labeling; the DV is based on a daily energy intake of 2,000 Calories, and for the food labeled presents the percentage of the RDI and the DRV recommended for healthy Americans. *See* RDI and DRV.

DASH diet The Dietary Approaches to Stop Hypertension diet plan that is designed to reduce or prevent an increase in blood pressure.

deamination Removal of an amine group, or nitrogen, from an amino acid.

dehydration A reduction of the body water to below the normal level of hydration; water output exceeds water intake.

dehydroepiandrosterone (DHEA) A natural steroid hormone produced endogenously by the adrenal gland. May be marketed as a nutritional sports ergogenic as derived from herbal precursors.

delayed onset of muscle soreness (DOMS) Term for the soreness in muscles experienced a day or two after strenuous eccentric exercise, such as running downhill. Prolonged, excessive eccentric exercise may lead to small muscle tears, and the pain is believed to occur during the repair process when swelling activates pain receptors.

depressant Drugs or agents that will depress or lower the level of bodily functions, particularly central nervous system functioning.

DHAP Dihydroxyacetone and pyruvate, the combination of two by-products of glycolysis.

DHEA *See* dehydroepiandrosterone.

Diabesity Term coined to highlight the relationship between the development of diabetes following the onset of obesity.

diabetes mellitus A disorder of carbohydrate metabolism due to disturbances in production or utilization of insulin; results in high blood glucose levels and loss of sugar in the urine.

diarrhea Frequent passage of a watery fecal discharge due to a gastrointestinal disturbance.

diastolic blood pressure The blood pressure in the arteries when the heart is at rest between beats.

dietary fiber Nondigestible carbohydrates and lignin that are intrinsic and intact in plants.

dietary folate equivalents (DFE) Used in estimating folate requirements, adjusting for the greater degree of absorption of folic acid (free form) compared with folate naturally found in foods. One microgram food folate equals 0.5 to 0.6 folic acid added to foods or as a supplement.

dietary-induced thermogenesis (DIT) The increase in the basal metabolic rate following ingestion of a meal. Heat production is increased.

Dietary Reference Intakes (DRI) Standards for recommended dietary intakes, consisting of various values. *See also* AI, EAR, RDA, AMDR, and UL.

dietary supplement A food product, added to the total diet, that contains either vitamins, minerals, herbs, botanicals, amino acids, metabolites, constituents, extracts, or combinations of these ingredients.

Dietary Supplement Health and Education Act (DSHEA) Act passed by the United States Congress defining a dietary supplement (*see* dietary supplement); legislation to control advertising and marketing.

2,3-diphosphoglyceride A by-product of carbohydrate metabolism in the red blood cell; helps the hemoglobin unload oxygen to the tissues.

disaccharide Any one of a class of sugars that yield two monosaccharides on hydrolysis; sucrose is the most common.

disordered eating Atypical eating behaviors such as restrictive dieting, using diet pills or laxatives, bingeing, and purging. In general, disordered eating behaviors occur less frequently or are less severe than those required to meet the full criteria for the diagnosis of an eating disorder.

dispensable amino acids *See* nonessential amino acids.

diuretics A class of agents that stimulate the formation of urine; used as a means to reduce body fluids.

diverticulosis Weak spots in the wall of the large intestine that may bulge out like a weak spot in a tire inner tube. May become infected, leading to diverticulitis.

DNA Deoxyribonucleic acid; a complex protein found in chromosomes that is the carrier of genetic information and the basis of heredity.

docasahexanoic acid (DHA) Docasahexanoic acid, an omega-3 fatty acid found in fatty fish.

dopamine A neurotransmitter secreted in the brain and involved in a number of functions, including sensations of pleasure. Decreased dopamine levels may be associated with Parkinson's disease.

doping Official term used by the WADA and the International Olympic Committee to depict the use of drugs in sports in attempts to enhance performance.

doubly labeled water technique A technique using labeled water to study energy metabolism.

dual energy X-ray absorptiometry (DEXA, DXA) A computerized X-ray technique at two energy levels to image body fat, lean tissues, and bone mineral content.

dumping syndrome Movement of fluid from the blood to the intestines by osmosis. May occur when a concentrated sugar solution is consumed in large quantities, causing symptoms such as weakness and gastrointestinal distress.

duration concept One of the major concepts of aerobic exercise; refers to the amount of time spent exercising during each session.

E

EAH *See* exercise-associated hyponatremia.

eating disorder A psychological disorder centering on the avoidance, excessive consumption, or purging of food, such as anorexia nervosa and bulimia nervosa.

eccentric method A weight-training method in which the muscle undergoes a lengthening contraction.

eicosanoids Derivatives of fatty acid oxidation in the body, including prostaglandins, thromboxanes, and leukotrienes.

eicosapentaenoic acid (EPA) An omega-3 fatty acid found in fatty fish.

electrolyte A substance that, when in a solution, conducts an electric current.

electrolyte solution A solution that contains ions and can conduct electricity; often the ions of salts such as sodium and chloride are called electrolytes; *also see* ions.

electron transfer system A highly structured array of chemical compounds in the cell that transport electrons and harness energy for later use.

element Relative to chemistry, a substance that cannot be subdivided into substances different from itself; many elements are essential to human life.

endocrine system The body system consisting of glands that secrete hormones, which have a wide variety of effects throughout the body.

energy The ability to do work; energy exists in various forms, notably mechanical, heat, and chemical in the human body.

English system A measurement system based upon the foot, pound, quart, and other nonmetric units; *also see* metric system.

enzyme A complex protein in the body that serves as a catalyst, facilitating reactions between various substances without being changed itself.

ephedra Term used for the plant *Ephedra sinica,* a source of ephedrine.

ephedrine A stimulant with somewhat weaker effects than amphetamine; found in some commercial dietary supplements; also known as ephedra.

epidemiological research A study of certain populations to determine the relationship of various risk factors to epidemic diseases or health problems.

epigenome A structure located just outside the genome that may be influenced by various factors, such as nutrients in the foods eaten; activates or deactivates DNA and subsequent genetic and cellular activity that may have either positive or negative health effects.

epinephrine A hormone secreted by the adrenal medulla that stimulates numerous body processes to enhance energy production, particularly during intense exercise.

epithelial cells The layer of cells that covers the outside and inside surfaces of the body, including the skin and the lining of the gastrointestinal system.

ergogenic aids Work-enhancing agents that are used in attempts to increase athletic or physical performance capacity.

ergogenic effect The physiological or psychological effect that an ergogenic substance is designed to produce.

ergolytic effect An agent or substance that may lead to decreases in work productivity or physical performance. *See also* ergogenic effect.

ergometer A device, such as a cycle ergometer, to measure work output in watts or other measures of work.

Escherichia A bacteria commonly involved in food poisoning.

essential amino acids Those amino acids that must be obtained in the diet and cannot be synthesized in the body. Also known as indispensable amino acids.

essential fat Fat in the body that is an essential part of the tissues, such as cell membrane structure, nerve coverings, and the brain; *also see* storage fat.

essential fatty acid Those unsaturated fatty acids that may not be synthesized in the body and must be obtained in the diet, e.g., linoleic fatty acid.

essential nutrients Those nutrients found to be essential to human life and optimal functioning.

ester Compound formed from the combination of an organic acid and an alcohol.

Estimated Average Requirement (EAR) Nutrient intake value estimated to meet the requirements of half the healthy individuals in a group.

Estimated Energy Requirement (EER) The daily dietary intake predicted to maintain energy balance for an individual of a defined age, gender, height, weight, and level of physical activity consistent with good health.

Estimated Minimal Requirement (EMR) Part of the RDA pertaining to the minimal daily requirement for sodium, chloride, and potassium.

Estimated Safe and Adequate Daily Dietary Intakes (ESADDI) Part of the previous RDA. Daily allowances for selected nutrients that are based upon available scientific evidence to be safe and adequate to meet human needs.

ethanol Alcohol; ethyl alcohol.

ethyl alcohol Alcohol; ethanol.

euhydration *See* normohydration.

evaporation The conversion of a liquid to a vapor, which consumes energy; evaporation of sweat cools the body by using body heat as the energy source.

exercise A form of structured physical activity generally designed to enhance physical fitness; usually refers to strenuous physical activity.

exercise-associated hyponatremia (EAH) Term associated with the decline in serum sodium levels during prolonged exercise with excessive fluid intake and/or sodium losses; *also see* water intoxication.

exercise frequency In an aerobic exercise program, the number of times per week that an individual exercises.

exercise intensity The tempo, speed, or resistance of an exercise. Intensity can be increased by working faster, doing more work in a given amount of time.

exercise metabolic rate (EMR) An increased metabolic rate due to the need for increased energy production; during exercise, the resting energy expenditure (REE) may be increased more than twenty-fold.

exercisenomics General term regarding the effects of exercise on genetic expression and resultant metabolic adaptations.

exercise sequence *See* principle of exercise sequence.

exercise stimulus The means whereby one elicits a physiological response; running, for example, can be the stimulus to increase the heart rate and other physiological functions.

exertional heat stroke Heat stroke that is precipitated by exercise in a warm or hot environment.

experimental research Study that manipulates an independent variable (cause) to observe the outcome on a dependent variable (effect).

extracellular water Body water that is located outside the cells; often subdivided into the intravascular water and the intercellular, or interstitial, water.

F

facilitated diffusion Process whereby glucose combines with a special protein carrier molecule at the membrane surface, facilitating glucose transport into the cell; insulin promotes facilitated diffusion in some cells.

faddism Relative to nutrition, the use of dietary fads based upon theoretical principles that may or may not be valid; usually used in a negative sense, as in quackery.

fasting Starvation; abstinence from eating that may be partial or complete.

fast-twitch fibers Muscle fibers characterized by high contractile speed.

fat exchange A fat exchange in the Food Exchange System contains 5 grams of fat and 45 Calories.

fat-free mass The remaining mass of the human body following the extraction of all fat.

fatigue A generalized or specific feeling of tiredness that may have a multitude of causes; may be mental or physical.

fat loading A term to describe practices used to maximize the use of fats as an energy source during exercise, particularly a low-carbohydrate, high-fat diet.

fat patterning The deposition of fat in specific areas of the human body, such as the stomach, thighs, or hips. Genetics plays an important role in fat patterning.

fats Triglycerides; a combination, or ester, of three fatty acids and glycerol.

fat substitutes Various substances used as substitutes for fats in food products; two popular brands are Simplesse and Olestra.

fatty acids Any one of a number of aliphatic acids containing only carbon, oxygen, and hydrogen; they may be saturated or unsaturated.

female athlete triad The triad of disordered eating, amenorrhea, and osteoporosis sometimes seen in female athletes involved in sports where excess body weight may be detrimental to performance.

female-type obesity *See* gynoid-type obesity.

ferritin The form in which iron is stored in the tissues.

fetal alcohol effects (FAE) Symptoms noted in children born to women who consumed alcohol during pregnancy; not as severe as fetal alcohol syndrome.

Fetal Alcohol Spectrum Disorders (FASD) The term used to describe birth anomalies associated with drinking alcohol while pregnant; refers to several conditions involving alcohol-related neurodevelopment disorders, birth defects, and other abnormalities in normal development. *See also* fetal alcohol syndrome and fetal alcohol effects.

fetal alcohol syndrome (FAS) The cluster of physical and mental symptoms seen in the child of a mother who consumes excessive alcohol during pregnancy.

fiber In general, the indigestible carbohydrate in plants that forms the structural network; *also see* cellulose.

First Law of Thermodynamics The law that energy cannot be created or destroyed; energy can be converted from one form to another.

flatulence Gas or air in the gastrointestinal tract, particularly the intestines.

fluoride A salt of hydrofluoric acid; a compound of fluorine that may be helpful in the prevention of tooth decay.

folacin Collective term for various forms of folic acid.

folate Salt of folic acid; form found in foods.

folic acid A water-soluble vitamin that appears to be essential in preventing certain types of anemia.

food additive *See* additives.

food allergy An adverse immune response to an otherwise harmless food. *Also see* food hypersensitivity.

food cultism Treating a particular food as if it possesses special properties, such as prevention or treatment of disease or improvement of athletic performance, usually without scientific justification.

Food and Drug Administration (FDA) Federal agency tasked with the responsibilities to monitor safety of foods and drugs sold in the United States.

Food Exchange System The system developed by the American Dietetic Association and other health groups that categorizes foods by content of carbohydrate, fat, protein, and Calories. Used as a basis for diet planning.

food hypersensitivity Term for some individuals who may develop clinical symptoms, such as migraine headaches, gastrointestinal distress, or hives and itching when certain foods are eaten.

food intolerance A general term for any adverse reaction to a food or food component not involving the immune system; an example is lactose intolerance.

food poisoning Foodborne illness caused by bacteria such as Salmonella, Escherichia, Staphylococcus, and Clostridium.

foot-pound A unit of work whereby the weight of 1 pound is moved through a distance of 1 foot.

Fosamax A commercial bisphosphonate product.

free fatty acids (FFA) Acids formed by the hydrolysis of triglycerides.

free radicals An atom or compound in which there is an unpaired electron; thought to cause cellular damage.

fructose A monosaccharide known as levulose or fruit sugar; found in all sweet fruits.

fruitarian A type of vegetarian who subsists solely on fruits, fruit products, and nuts.

fruit exchange One fruit exchange in the Food Exchange System contains 15 grams of carbohydrate and 60 Calories.

fTRP:BCAA ratio The ratio of free tryptophan to branched-chain amino acids; a high ratio is theorized to elicit fatigue in prolonged endurance events.

functional fiber Isolated, nondigestible carbohydrates that have beneficial effects in humans.

functional foods Food products containing nutrients designed to provide health benefits beyond basic nutrition.

G

galactose A monosaccharide formed when lactose is hydrolyzed into glucose and galactose.

gastric emptying The rate at which substances, particularly fluids, empty from the stomach; high gastric emptying rates are advisable for sports drinks.

generally recognized as safe (GRAS) A classification for food additives indicating that they most likely are not harmful for human consumption.

genomics The study of the entire genome of an individual or organism; human genomics attempts to determine DNA sequence and gene mapping. Human genomic research may lead to genetic modifications to enhance health of individuals; genomics may also be involved in gene doping, or sport performance enhancement with gene manipulation.

ghrelin Hormone released by an empty stomach to stimulate the appetite.

ginseng A general term for a variety of natural chemical plant extracts derived from the family Araliaceae; extract contains ginsenosides and other chemicals that may influence human physiology.

glucagon A hormone secreted by the pancreas; basically it exerts actions just the opposite of insulin, i.e., it responds to hypoglycemia and helps to increase blood sugar levels.

glucarate A compound found in cruciferous vegetables that is thought to block the actions of cancer causing agents.

glucogenic amino acids Amino acids that may undergo deamination and be converted into glucose through the process of gluconeogenesis.

gluconeogenesis The formation of carbohydrates from molecules that are not themselves carbohydrate, such as amino acids and the glycerol from fat.

glucosamine Formed in the body from amino acids and involved in cartilage formation; marketed as a dietary supplement.

glucose A monosaccharide; a thick, sweet, syrupy liquid.

glucose-alanine cycle The cycle in which alanine is released from the muscle and is converted to glucose in the liver.

glucose-electrolyte solutions Solutions designed to replace sweat losses; contain varying proportions of water, glucose, sodium, potassium, chloride, and other electrolytes.

glucose polymer A combination of several glucose molecules into a more complex carbohydrate.

glucostatic theory The theory that hunger and satiety are controlled by the glucose level in the blood; the receptors that respond to the blood glucose level are in the hypothalamus.

GLUT-4 Receptors in cell membranes that transport glucose from the blood to the cell interior.

glutathione peroxidase An enzyme that helps neutralize free radicals.

gluten intolerance A sensitivity to gluten; the immune system recognizes gluten as a foreign substance, but does not induce an allergic response.

glycemic index (GI) A ranking system relative to the effect that consumption of 50 grams of a particular carbohydrate food has upon the blood glucose response over the course of 2 hours. The normal baseline measure is 50 grams of glucose, and the resultant blood glucose response is scored as 100.

glycemic load (GL) A ranking system relative to the effect that eating a carbohydrate food has on the blood glucose level, but also includes the portion size. The formula is:

$$GL = \frac{(GI) \text{ (grams of non-fiber carbohydrate in one serving)}}{100}$$

Glycerate A commercial product containing glycerol; marketed to athletes.

glycerin *See* glycerol.

glycerol Glycerin, a clear syrupy liquid; an alcohol that combines with fatty acids to form triglycerides.

glycogen A polysaccharide that is the chief storage form of carbohydrate in animals; it is stored primarily in the liver and muscles.

glycogen-sparing effect The theory that certain dietary techniques, such as the use of caffeine, may facilitate the oxidation of fatty acids for energy and thus spare the utilization of glycogen.

glycolysis The degradation of sugars into smaller compounds; the main quantitative anaerobic energy process in the muscle tissue.

gout The deposit of uric acid by-products in and about the joints contributing to inflammation and pain; usually occurs in the knee or foot.

gram calorie A small calorie; *see* Calorie.

green tea A Chinese beverage that contains caffeine and other constituents, such as epigallocatechin gallate (EGCG), which are theorized to possess numerous health benefits.

gums A form of water-soluble dietary fiber found in plants.

gynoid-type obesity Female-type obesity; body fat is deposited primarily about the hips and thighs. *Also see* android-type obesity.

H

HDL High-density lipoprotein; a protein-lipid complex in the blood that facilitates the transport of triglycerides, cholesterol, and phospholipids. *Also see* HDL-cholesterol.

HDL-cholesterol High-density lipoprotein cholesterol; one mechanism whereby cholesterol is transported in the blood. High HDL levels are somewhat protective against CHD.

health-related fitness Those components of physical fitness whose improvement have health benefits, such as cardiovascular fitness, body composition, flexibility, and muscular strength and endurance.

Healthy Eating Index (HEI) USDA computerized dietary analysis to assess personal diets to provide an overall rating as related to health.

heat-balance equation Heat balance is dependent upon the interrelationships of metabolic heat production and loss or gain of heat by radiation, convection, conduction, and evaporation.

heat cramps Painful muscular cramps or tetany following prolonged exercise in the heat without water or salt replacement.

heat exhaustion Weakness or dizziness from overexertion in a hot environment.

heat index The apparent temperature determined by combining air temperature and relative humidity.

heat shock proteins Proteins released by the muscle, in response to increased temperature or exercise, that may (similar to the effect of cytokines) influence other body tissues and induce possible positive health effects.

heat stroke Elevated body temperature of 105.8°F or greater caused by exposure to excessive heat gains or production and diminished heat loss.

heat syncope Fainting caused by excessive heat exposure.

hematuria Blood or red blood cells in the urine.

heme iron The iron in the diet associated with hemoglobin in animal meats.

hemicellulose A form of dietary fiber found in plants. Differs from cellulose in that it may be hydrolyzed by dilute acids outside of the body. Not hydrolyzed in the body.

hemochromatosis Presence of excessive iron in the body resulting in an enlarged liver and bronze pigmentation of the skin.

hemoglobin The protein-iron pigment in the red blood cells that transports oxygen.

hemolysis A rupturing of red blood cells with a release of hemoglobin into the plasma.

hepatitis An inflammatory condition of the liver.

heterocyclic amines (HCA) Carcinogens formed in foods that have been charred by excess grilling or broiling.

hidden fat In foods, the fat that is not readily apparent, such as the high fat content of cheese.

high blood pressure *See* hypertension.

high-density lipoprotein *See* HDL.

high-fructose corn syrup A common high-Calorie sweetener used as a food additive; derived from the partial hydrolysis of corn starch.

histidine An essential amino acid.

HMB Beta-hydroxy-beta-methylbutyrate, a metabolic by-product of the amino acid leucine, alleged to retard the breakdown of muscle protein during strenuous exercise.

homeostasis A term used to describe a condition of normalcy in the internal body environment.

homocysteine A metabolic by-product of amino acid metabolism; elevated blood levels are associated with increased risk of vascular diseases.

hormone A chemical substance produced by specific body cells, secreted into the blood and then acting on specific target tissues.

hormone sensitive lipase (HSL) An enzyme that catalyzes triglycerides into free fatty acids and glycerol.

HR max The normal maximal heart rate of an individual during exercise.

HR reserve The mathematical difference, or reserve, between the resting HR and maximal HR. A percentage of this reserve may be added to the resting HR to determine exercise intensity.

human growth hormone (HGH) A hormone released by the pituitary gland that regulates growth; also involved in fatty acid metabolism; rHGH is a genetically engineered form.

hunger A basic physiological desire to eat that is normally caused by a lack of food; may be accompanied by stomach contractions.

hunger center A collection of nerve cells in the hypothalamus that is involved in the control of feeding reflexes.

hydrodensitometry Another term for the underwater weighing technique.

hydrogenated fats Fats to which hydrogen has been added, usually causing them to be saturated.

hydrolysis A mechanism for splitting substances into smaller compounds by the addition of water; enzyme action.

hypercholesteremia Elevated blood cholesterol levels.

hyperglycemia Elevated blood glucose levels.

hyperhydration The practice of increasing the body-water stores by fluid consumption prior to an athletic event; a state of increased water content in the body.

hyperkalemia An increased concentration of potassium in the blood.

hyperlipidemia Elevated blood lipid levels.

hyperplasia The formation of new body cells.

hypertension A condition with various causes whereby the blood pressure is higher than normal.

hyperthermia Unusually high body temperature; fever.

hypertonic Relative to osmotic pressure, a solution that has a greater concentration of solute or salts, hence higher osmotic pressure, in comparison to another solution.

hypertriglyceridemia Elevated blood levels of triglycerides.

hypertrophy Excessive growth of a cell or organ; in pathology, an abnormal growth.

hypervitaminosis A pathological condition due to an excessive vitamin intake, particularly the fat-soluble vitamins A and D.

hypoglycemia A low blood sugar level.

hypohydration A state of decreased water content in the body caused by dehydration.

hypokalemia A decreased concentration of potassium in the blood.

hyponatremia A decreased concentration of sodium in the blood.

hypothalamus A part of the brain involved in the control of involuntary activity in the body; contains many centers for neural control such as temperature, hunger, appetite, and thirst.

hypothermia Unusually low body temperature.

hypotonic Having an osmotic pressure lower than that of the solution to which it is compared.

I

IGF-1 *See* insulin-like growth factor.

incomplete protein Protein food that does not possess the proper amount of essential amino acids; characteristic of plant foods in general.

Index of Nutritional Quality (INQ) A mathematical means of determining the quality of any given food relative to its content of a specific nutrient.

indicator nutrients The eight nutrients which, if provided in adequate supply through a varied diet, should provide adequate amounts of the other essential nutrients: protein, vitamin A, thiamin, riboflavin, niacin, vitamin C, calcium, and iron.

indispensable amino acids *See* essential amino acids.

indoles Phytochemicals believed to help prevent various diseases.

infrared interactance Use of infrared technology to estimate body composition.

initial fitness level The physical fitness level of an individual prior to the onset of a physical conditioning program.

in-line skating An exercise-skating technique with specially designed shoes for use on sidewalks and similar surfaces.

inosine A nucleoside of the purine family that serves as a base for the formation of a variety of compounds in the body; theorized to be ergogenic.

inositol A member of the B complex, although its role in human nutrition has not been established; not classified as a vitamin.

INQ *See* Index of Nutritional Quality.

insensible perspiration Perspiration on the skin not detectable by ordinary senses.

insoluble dietary fiber Dietary fiber that is not soluble in water, such as cellulose. *Also see* soluble dietary fiber.

insulin A hormone secreted by the pancreas, involved in carbohydrate metabolism.

insulin-like growth factor (IGF-1) A growth factor found in the blood that resembles insulin; produced in response to growth hormone release.

insulin response Blood insulin levels rise following the ingestion of sugar and the resultant hyperglycemia; the insulin causes the sugar to be taken up by the muscles and fat cells, possibly creating a reactive hypoglycemia.

intercellular water Body water found between the cells; also known as interstitial water.

intermittent high-intensity exercise Short-term bouts of high-intensity exercise interspersed with short periods of recovery.

International Unit (IU) A method of expressing the quantity of some substance, such as vitamins, which is an internationally developed and accepted standard.

International Unit System (SI) *Le Systeme International d'Unite,* or the International System of Units; a system of measurement based upon the metric system.

interstitial water *See* intercellular water.

interval training A method of physical training in which periods of activity are interspersed with periods of rest.

intestinal absorption The rate at which substances, particularly fluids and nutrients, are absorbed into the body; a fast rate of intestinal absorption is a desirable characteristic of sports drinks.

intracellular water Body water that is found within the cells.

intravascular water Body water found in the vascular system, or blood vessels.

involuntary dehydration Unintentional loss of body fluids during exercise under warm or hot environmental conditions.

IOC International Olympic Committee.

iodine A nonmetallic element that is necessary for the proper development and functioning of the thyroid gland.

ions Particles with an electrical charge; anions are negative and cations are positive.

iron A metallic element essential for the development of several chemical compounds in the body, notably hemoglobin.

iron-deficiency anemia Anemia caused by an inadequate intake or absorption of iron, resulting in impaired hemoglobin formation.

iron deficiency without anemia A condition in which the hemoglobin levels are normal but several indices of iron status in the body are below normal levels.

irradiation Process whereby foods are subjected to ionizing radiation to kill bacteria.

ischemia Lack of blood supply.

isoflavones Phytochemicals believed to help prevent various diseases.

isokinetic Literally meaning "same speed"; in weight training an isokinetic machine is used to control the speed of muscle contraction.

isoleucine An essential amino acid.

isometric Literally meaning "same length"; in weight training the resistance is set so that the muscle will not shorten.

isotonic Literally meaning "equal tension or pressure"; in weight training the resistance is set so there is supposed to be equal tension in the muscle through a range of motion, but this is rarely achieved owing to movement of body parts. Isotonic also means equal osmotic pressures between two solutions.

J

jogging A term used to designate slow running; although the distinction between running and jogging is relative to the individual involved, a common value used for jogging is a 9-minute mile or slower.

joule A measure of work in the metric system; a newton of force applied through a distance of one meter.

K

ketogenesis The formation of ketones in the body from other substances, such as fats and proteins.

ketogenic amino acids Amino acids that may be deaminated, converted into ketones, and eventually into fat.

ketones Organic compounds containing a carbonyl group; ketone acids in the body, such as acetone, are the end products of fat metabolism.

ketosis The accumulation of excess ketones in the blood; because ketones are acids, acidosis occurs.

key-nutrient concept The concept that if certain key nutrients are adequately supplied by the diet, the other essential nutrients will also be present in adequate amounts. *Also see* indicator nutrients.

kidney stones Compounds in the pelvis of the kidney formed from various salts such as carbonates, oxalates, and phosphates.

kilocalorie (KC) A large Calorie; *see* Calorie.

kilogram A unit of mass in the metric system; 1 kilogram is the equivalent of 2.2 pounds.

kilogram-meter (KGM) A measure of work in the metric system whereby 1 kilogram of weight is moved through a distance of 1 meter; however, the joule is the recommended unit to express work.

kilojoule One thousand joules; one kilojoule (kJ) is approximately 0.25 kilocalorie.

Krebs cycle The main oxidative reaction sequence in the body that generates ATP; also known as the citric acid or tricarboxylic acid cycle.

L

lactic acid The anaerobic end product of glycolysis; it has been implicated as a causative factor in the etiology of fatigue.

lactic acid system The energy system that produces ATP anaerobically by the breakdown of glycogen to lactic acid; used primarily in events of maximal effort for one to two minutes.

lactose A white crystalline disaccharide that yields glucose and galactose upon hydrolysis; also known as milk sugar.

lactose intolerance Gastrointestinal disturbances due to an intolerance to lactose in milk; caused by deficiency of lactase, an enzyme that digests lactose.

lactovegetarian A vegetarian who includes milk products in the diet as a form of high-quality protein.

LDL Low-density lipoprotein; a protein-lipid complex in the blood that facilitates the transport of triglycerides, cholesterol, and phospholipids. *Also see* LDL-cholesterol.

LDL-cholesterol Low-density lipoprotein cholesterol; a mechanism whereby cholesterol is transported in the blood. High blood levels are associated with increased incidence of CHD.

lean body mass The body weight minus the body fat, composed primarily of muscle, bone, and other nonfat tissue.

lecithin A fatty substance of a class known as phospholipids; said to have the therapeutic properties of phosphorus.

legume The fruit or pod of vegetables including soybeans, kidney beans, lima beans, garden peas, black-eyed peas, and lentils; high in protein.

leptin Regulatory hormone produced by fat cells; when released into the circulation, it influences the hypothalamus to control appetite.

leucine An essential amino acid.

leukotrienes Eicosanoids that possess hormone-like activity in numerous cells in the body.

levulose Fructose.

lignin A noncarbohydrate form of dietary fiber.

limiting amino acid An amino acid deficient in a specific plant food, making it an incomplete protein; methionine is a limiting amino acid in legumes, whereas lysine is deficient in grain products.

linoleic acid An essential fatty acid.

lipase An enzyme that catabolizes fats into fatty acids and glycerol.

lipids A class of fats or fat-like substances characterized by their insolubility in water and solubility in fat solvents; triglycerides, fatty acids, phospholipids, and cholesterol are important lipids in the body.

lipoic acid A coenzyme that functions in oxidative decarboxylation, or removal of carbon dioxide from a compound.

lipoprotein A combination of lipid and protein possessing the general properties of proteins. Practically all the lipids of the plasma are present in this form.

lipoprotein (a) Serum lipid factor very similar to the LDL, being in the upper LDL density range and containing apolipoprotein (a); high levels are associated with increased risk for CHD.

lipoprotein lipase An enzyme involved in the metabolism of lipoproteins.

lipostatic theory The theory that hunger and satiety are controlled by the lipid level in the blood.

liquid meals Food in a liquid form designed to provide a balanced intake of essential nutrients.

liquid-protein diets Protein in a liquid form; a common form consists of protein predigested into simple amino acids.

liver glycogen The major storage form of carbohydrate in the liver.

long-chain fatty acids (LCFAs) Fatty acids containing chains with 12 or more carbons.

long-haul concept Relative to weight control, the idea that weight loss via exercise should be gradual, and one should not expect to lose large amounts of weight in a short time.

L-tryptophan One form of tryptophan. L is for levo (left), or the direction in which polarized light is rotated when various organic compounds are analyzed.

lycopene A carotenoid that serves as an antioxidant.

lysine An essential amino acid.

M

macrominerals Those minerals essential to human nutrition with an RDA in excess of 100 mg/day: calcium, magnesium, phosphorous, sodium, potassium, chloride.

macronutrient Dietary nutrient needed by the body in daily amounts greater than a few grams, such as carbohydrate, fat, protein, and water.

magnesium A white metallic mineral element essential in human nutrition.

magnetic resonance imaging (MRI) Magnetic-field and radio-frequency waves used to image body tissues; useful for imaging visceral fat.

ma huang A Chinese plant extract theorized to be ergogenic; contains ephedrine, a stimulant.

major minerals *See* macrominerals.

male-type obesity *See* android-type obesity.

malnutrition Poor nutrition that may be due to inadequate amounts of essential nutrients. Too many Calories leading to obesity is also a form of malnutrition. *Also see* subclinical malnutrition.

maltodextrin A glucose polymer that exerts lesser osmotic effects compared with glucose; used in a variety of sports drinks as the source of carbohydrate.

maltose A white crystalline disaccharide that yields two molecules of glucose upon hydrolysis.

manganese A metallic element essential in human nutrition.

maximal heart rate *See* HR max.

maximal heart rate reserve The difference between the maximal HR and resting HR. A percentage of this reserve, usually 60–90 percent, is added to the resting HR to get the target HR for aerobics training programs.

maximal oxygen uptake *See* VO_2 max.

meat exchange One very lean meat exchange in the Food Exchange System contains 0–1 gram of fat, 7 grams of protein, and 35 Calories; a lean meat exchange contains 3 grams of fat, 7 grams of protein, and 55 Calories; a medium-fat meat exchange has an additional 2 grams of fat and totals 75 Calories; a high-fat exchange has 5 additional grams of fat and totals 100 Calories.

Mediterranean diet A diet associated with reduced risk of cardiovascular disease attributed to olive oil, the primary source of dietary fat. However, other elements of the Mediterranean diet, such as seafood and vegetables, may also be associated with reduced CHD risk.

Mediterranean Food Guide Pyramid A food group approach to healthful nutrition that includes basic food groups, but also lists olive oil and wine as components of the diet.

medium-chain fatty acids (MCFAs) Fatty acids containing chains with 6–12 carbons.

medium-chain triglycerides (MCTs) Triglycerides containing fatty acids with carbon chain lengths of 6–12 carbons.

megadose An excessive amount of a substance in comparison to a normal dose of RDA; usually used to refer to vitamins.

menadione Vitamin K_3.

menoquinone The animal form of vitamin K.

MET A measurement unit of energy expenditure; one MET equals approximately 3.5 ml O_2/kg body weight/minute.

meta-analysis A statistical technique to summarize the findings of numerous studies in an attempt to provide a quantitatively based conclusion.

metabolic aftereffects of exercise The theory that the aftereffects of exercise will cause the metabolic rate to be elevated for a time, thus expending Calories and contributing to weight loss.

metabolic rate The energy expended to maintain all physical and chemical changes occurring in the body.

metabolic syndrome The syndrome of symptoms often seen with android-type obesity, particularly hyperinsulinemia, hypertriglyceridemia, and hypertension.

metabolic water The water that is a by-product of the oxidation of carbohydrate, fat, and protein in the body.

metabolism The sum total of all physical and chemical processes occurring in the body.

metalloenzyme An enzyme that must have a mineral component, such as zinc, to function effectively.

methionine An essential amino acid.

methylmercury An industrial waste product dumped in the seas that may accumulate in large fish; may lead to subsequent nerve damage in children or pregnant females who eat contaminated fish.

metric system A method of measurement based upon units of ten.

microgram One millionth of a gram (μg).

micronutrient Dietary nutrient needed by the body in daily amounts less than a few grams, such as vitamins and minerals.

milk exchange One skim milk exchange in the Food Exchange System contains 12 grams of carbohydrate, 8 grams of protein, a trace of fat, and 90 Calories. A low-fat exchange contains 120 Calories, whereas whole milk has 150 Calories.

milligram One thousandth of a gram.

millimole One thousandth of a mole.

mineral An inorganic element occurring in nature.

mitochondria Structures within the cells that serve as the location for the aerobic production of ATP.

mole One mole is the gram molecular weight of a compound, which is the quantity of a substance that equals its molecular weight.

molybdenum A hard, heavy, silvery-white metallic element.

monosaccharides Simple sugars (glucose, fructose, and galactose) that cannot be broken down by hydrolysis.

monounsaturated fatty acids (MUFAs) Fatty acids that have a single double bond.

morbid obesity Severe obesity in which the incidence of life-threatening diseases is increased significantly.

MPF factor Muscle protein factor; an unknown property of meat, fish, and poultry that facilitates the absorption of nonheme iron found in plant foods.

muscle dysmorphia *See* Adonis complex.

muscle glycogen The form in which carbohydrate is stored in the muscle.

muscle hypertrophy An increase in the size of the muscle.

myocardial infarction Death of heart tissue following cessation of blood flow; may be caused by coronary occlusion.

myoglobin An iron-containing compound, similar to hemoglobin, found in the muscle tissues; it binds oxygen in the muscle cells.

myokines Cytokines secreted by muscle tissue.

MyPlate The graphic and program, introduced in 2011, representing the healthful food guidelines presented by the United States Department of Agriculture.

MyPyramid The former graphic and program representing the healthful food guidelines presented by the United States Department of Agriculture. It was replaced by the new model, MyPlate, in 2011.

N

narcotic Any agent that produces insensibility to pain.

National Weight Control Registry A registry of individuals who have lost at least 30 pounds and have kept it off for a year.

Nautilus A brand of exercise equipment designed for strength-training programs; uses a principle to help provide optimal resistance throughout the full range of motion.

NCAA National Collegiate Athletic Association.

negative caloric balance A condition whereby the caloric output exceeds the caloric intake, thus contributing to weight loss.

negative nitrogen balance A condition in which dietary protein is insufficient to meet the nitrogen needs of the body. More nitrogen is excreted than is retained in the body.

net protein utilization (NPU) A technique used to assess protein quality.

neural tube defects (NTD) Birth defects involving incomplete formation of the neural tube in the spinal column of newborn children; may lead to paralysis; may be prevented by adequate folate intake.

neuropeptide Y (NPY) Neuropeptide produced in the hypothalamus; a potent appetite stimulant.

neutron activation analysis A sophisticated, noninvasive method of analyzing body structure and function.

newton A unit of force that will accelerate 1 kilogram of mass 1 meter per second.

NIAAA National Institute on Alcohol Abuse and Alcoholism.

niacin Nicotinamide; nicotinic acid; part of the B complex and an important part of several coenzymes involved in aerobic energy processes in the cells.

niacin equivalents (NE) A unit of measure of niacin activity in a food related to both the amount of niacin present and that obtainable from tryptophan; about 60 mg tryptophan can be converted to 1 mg niacin.

nickel A silvery-white metallic element.

nicotinamide An amide of nicotinic acid; niacin.

nicotinic acid Niacin.

nitrogen A colorless, tasteless, odorless gas comprising about 80 percent of the atmospheric gas; an essential component of protein that is formed in plants during their developmental process.

nitrogen balance A dietary state in which the input and output of nitrogen is balanced so that the body neither gains nor loses protein tissue.

nonessential amino acids Amino acids that may be formed in the body and thus need not be obtained in the diet; also known as dispensable amino acids. *See* essential amino acids.

nonessential nutrient A nutrient that may be formed in the body from excess amounts of other nutrients.

nonexercise activity thermogenesis (NEAT) Thermogenesis, or heat production by the body, that accompanies physical activity other than volitional exercise.

nonheme iron Iron that is found in plant foods; *see* heme iron.

nonprotein nitrogen Nitrogen in the body and foods that is associated with nonprotein compounds.

normohydration The state of normal hydration, or normal body-water levels, as compared with hypohydration and hyperhydration.

nutraceutical A nutrient that may function as a pharmaceutical when taken in certain quantities.

nutrient Substance found in food that provides energy, promotes growth and repair of tissues, and regulates metabolism.

nutrient density A concept related to the degree of concentration of nutrients in a given food; *also see* the related concept INQ.

nutrigenomics General term regarding the effects of nutrition on genetic expression and resultant metabolic adaptions.

nutrition The study of foods and nutrients and their effect on health, growth, and development of the individual.

nutritional labeling A listing of selected key nutrients and Calories on the label of commercially prepared food products.

O

obesity An excessive accumulation of body fat; usually reserved for those individuals who are 20–30 percent or more above the average weight for their size.

octacosanol A solid white alcohol found in wheat germ oil.

odds ratio (OR) A probability estimate; OR of 1.0 is normal.

Olestra A commercially produced substitute for dietary fat.

oligomenorrhea Intermittent periods of amenorrhea.

omega-3 fatty acids Polyunsaturated fatty acids that have a double bond between the third and fourth carbon from the terminal, or omega, carbon. EPA and DHA found in fish oils are theorized to prevent coronary heart disease.

omega-6 fatty acids Polyunsaturated fatty acids that have a double bond between the sixth and seventh carbon from the terminal, or omega, carbon. Linoleic acid is an essential omega-6 fatty acid.

OmniHeart diet The Optimal MacroNutrient Intake diet, consisting of *healthy* carbohydrates, *healthy* fats, and *healthy* proteins designed to reduce risks of cardiovascular disease, particularly high blood pressure.

onset of blood lactic acid (OBLA) The intensity level of exercise at which the blood lactate begins to accumulate rapidly.

oral contraceptives Birth control pills used to prevent conception.

oral rehydration therapy (ORT) Fluids balanced in nutrients that help restore normal hydration levels in the body and prevent excessive dehydration.

organic foods Foods that are stated to be grown without the use of man-made chemicals such as pesticides and artificial fertilizers.

orlistat A prescription drug for weight loss that blocks the digestion of dietary fat.

osmolality Osmotic concentration determined by the ionic concentration of the dissolved substance per unit of solvent.

osmoreceptors Receptors in the body that react to changes in the osmotic pressure of the blood.

osmotic pressure A pressure that produces a diffusion between solutions that have different concentrations.

osteomalacia A disease characterized by softening of the bones, leading to brittleness and increased deformity; caused by a deficiency of vitamin D.

osteoporosis Increased porosity or softening of the bone.

overload principle *See* principle of overload.

overtraining syndrome Symptoms associated with excessive training, such as tiredness, sleeplessness, and elevated heart rate.

overweight Body weight greater than that which is considered normal; *also see* obesity.

ovolactovegetarian A vegetarian who also consumes eggs and milk products as a source of high-quality animal protein.

ovovegetarian A vegetarian who includes eggs in the diet to help obtain adequate amounts of protein.

oxalates Salts of oxalic acid, which are found in green leafy vegetables such as spinach and beet greens.

oxidized LDL An oxidized form of low-density lipoprotein that has increased atherogenic potential.

oxygen consumption The total amount of oxygen utilized in the body for the production of energy; it is directly related to the metabolic rate.

oxygen system The energy system that produces ATP via the oxidation of various foodstuffs, primarily fats and carbohydrates.

P

paidotribe Individual who served as a personal trainer in ancient Greece to advise athletes on proper diet and exercise training programs.

pangamic acid A term often associated with "vitamin B_{15}," the essentiality of which has not been established; often contains calcium gluconate and dimethylglycine.

pantothenic acid A vitamin of the B complex.

para-aminobenzoic acid (PABA) Although not a vitamin, often grouped with the B complex.

partially hydrogenated fats Polyunsaturated fats that are not fully saturated with hydrogen through a hydrogenation process; *also see trans* fatty acids.

peak bone mass The concept of maximizing the amount of bone mineral content during the formative years of childhood and young adulthood.

pectin A form of soluble dietary fiber found in some fruits.

pellagra A deficiency disease caused by inadequate amounts of niacin in the diet.

pentose A simple sugar containing five carbons instead of six as in glucose.

peptides Small compounds formed by the union of two or more amino acids; known also as dipeptides, tripeptides, and so on, depending on the number of amino acids combined.

perceptual-motor activities Physical activities characterized by the perception of a given stimulus and culminating in an appropriate motor, or movement, response.

periodization A technique applied to resistance training, as well as other forms of exercise training, that modifies the amount of exercise stress placed on the individual over the course of time. Various cycles, such as the microcycle, mesocycle, and macrocycle, are designed to allow the body to adapt to exercise stress in ways beneficial to performance enhancement.

peripheral vascular disease Atherosclerosis or blockage of the peripheral arteries.

pernicious anemia A severe progressive form of anemia that may be fatal if not treated with vitamin B_{12}. Usually caused by inability to absorb B_{12}, not a dietary deficiency of B_{12}.

pescovegetarian A vegetarian who eats fish, but not poultry, or other animal meats.

pesticides Poisons used to destroy pests of various types, including plants and animals.

pH The abbreviation used to express the level of acidity of a solution; a low pH represents high acidity.

phenylalanine An essential amino acid.

phenylketonuria (PKU) Congenital lack of an enzyme to metabolize phenylalanine, an essential amino acid. May lead to mental retardation if not detected early in life.

phosphagens Compounds such as ATP and phosphocreatine that serve as a source of high energy in the body cells.

phosphates Salts of phosphoric acid, purported to possess ergogenic qualities.

phosphatidylserine Like phosphatidylcholine, a naturally occurring phospholipid found in cell membranes; as a dietary supplement, it is theorized to possess ergogenic potential.

phosphocreatine (PCr) A high-energy phosphate compound found in the body cells; part of the ATP-PCr energy system.

phospholipids Lipids containing phosphorus that in hydrolysis yield fatty acids, glycerol, and a nitrogenous compound. Lecithin is an example.

phosphorus A nonmetallic element essential to human nutrition.

phosphorus:calcium ratio The ratio of calcium to phosphorus intake in the diet; the normal ratio is 1:1.

photon absorptiometry An analytical, noninvasive technique designed to assess bone density.

phylloquinone Vitamin K; essential in the blood clotting process.

physical activity Any activity that involves human movement; in relation to health and physical fitness, physical activity is often classified as structured and unstructured.

Physical Activity Level (PAL) Increase in energy expenditure through physical activity based on energy expended through daily walking mileage or equivalent activities; National Academy of Sciences lists four PAL categories: sedentary, low active, active, and very active.

Physical Activity Pyramid A guide to weekly physical activity, including aerobic endurance, muscular strength and endurance, and flexibility.

Physical Activity Quotient (PA) Coefficient used to calculate estimated energy requirement (EER) based on categories of physical activity level (PAL).

physical conditioning Methods used to increase the efficiency or capacity of a given body system so as to improve physical or athletic performance.

physical fitness A set of abilities individuals possess to perform specific types of physical activity. *Also see* health-related fitness and sports-related fitness.

phytates Salts of phytic acids; produced in the body during the digestion of certain grain products; can combine with some minerals such as iron and possibly decrease their absorption.

phytochemicals Chemical substances, other than nutrients, found in plants that are theorized to possess medicinal properties to help prevent various diseases.

phytoestrogens Phytochemicals that may compete with natural endogenous estrogens; believed to help prevent certain forms of cancer associated with excess estrogen activity in the body.

picolinate A natural derivative of tryptophan; commercially it is bound to chromium as a means of enhancing chromium absorption.

plaque The material that forms in the inner layer of the artery and contributes to atherosclerosis. It contains cholesterol, lipids, and other debris.

platelet aggregability Function of platelets to promote clumping together of red blood cells.

polypeptides A combination of a number of simple amino acids; *also see* peptides.

polysaccharide A carbohydrate that upon hydrolysis will yield more than ten monosaccharides.

polyunsaturated fatty acid Fat that contains two or more double bonds and thus is open to hydrogenation.

positive caloric balance A condition whereby caloric intake exceeds caloric output; the resultant effect is a weight gain.

Positive Health Lifestyle A lifestyle characterized by health behaviors designed to promote health and longevity by helping to prevent many of the chronic diseases afflicting modern society.

postabsorptive state The period after a meal has been absorbed from the gastrointestinal tract; in BMR tests it is usually a period of approximately 12 hours.

potassium A metallic element essential in human nutrition; it is the principal cation present in the intracellular fluids.

power Work divided by time; the ability to produce work in a given period of time.

power-endurance continuum In relation to strength training, the concept that power or strength is developed by high resistance and few repetitions, whereas endurance is developed by low resistance and many repetitions.

PRE Progressive resistive exercise.

pre-event nutrition Dietary intake prior to athletic competition; may refer to a 2- to 3-day period prior to an event or the immediate pre-event meal.

premenstrual syndrome (PMS) A condition associated with a wide variety of symptoms during the time prior to menses.

principle of exercise sequence Relative to a weight-training workout, the lifting sequence is designed so that different muscle groups are utilized sequentially so as to be fresh for each exercise.

principle of overload The major concept of physical training whereby one imposes a stress greater than that normally imposed upon a particular body system.

principle of progressive resistance exercise (PRE) A training technique, primarily with weights, whereby resistance is increased as the individual develops increased strength levels.

principle of recuperation A principle of physical conditioning whereby adequate rest periods are taken for recuperation to occur so that exercise may be continued.

principle of specificity of training The principle that physical training should be designed to mimic the specific athletic event in which one competes. Specific human energy systems and neuromuscular skills should be stressed.

Pritikin program A dietary program developed by Nathan Pritikin, which severely restricts the intake of certain foods like fats and cholesterol and greatly increases the consumption of complex carbohydrates.

profile of mood states (POMS) An inventory to evaluate mood states such as anger, vigor, etc.

proline A nonessential amino acid.

promoters Substances or agents necessary to support or promote the development of a disease once it is initiated.

proof Relative to alcohol content, proof is twice the percentage of alcohol in a solution; 80-proof whiskey is 40 percent alcohol.

prostaglandins Eicosanoids that possess hormone-like activity in numerous cells in the body.

proteases Enzymes that catalyze proteins.

protein Any one of a group of complex organic compounds containing nitrogen; formed from various combinations of amino acids.

protein-Calorie insufficiency A major health problem in certain parts of the world where the population suffers from inadequate intake of protein and total Calories.

protein complementarity The practice among vegetarians of eating foods together from two or more different food groups, usually legumes, nuts, or beans with grain products, in order to ensure a balanced intake of essential amino acids.

Protein Digestibility Corrected Amino Acid Score (PDCAAS) A scientific measure used to assess the quality of protein in foods with values from 1.0 to 0.0, with 1.0 being the highest quality.

protein hydrolysate A high-protein dietary supplement containing a solution of amino acids and peptides prepared from protein by hydrolysis.

protein-sparing effect An adequate intake of energy Calories, as from carbohydrate, will decrease somewhat the rate of protein catabolism in the body and hence spare protein. This is the basis of the protein-sparing modified fast, or diet.

proteinuria The presence of proteins in the urine.

provitamin A Carotene, a substance in the diet from which the body may form vitamin A.

Prudent Healthy Diet A diet plan based upon healthful eating principles that is designed to help prevent or treat common chronic diseases in the United States, Canada, and Mexico, particularly cardiovascular disease and cancer.

psyllium A plant product that contains both water-soluble and insoluble dietary fiber.

purines The end products of nucleoprotein metabolism, which may be formed in the body; they are nonprotein nitrogen compounds that are eventually degraded to uric acid.

pyridoxal A component of the vitamin B group.

pyridoxamine A part of the vitamin B group; an analog of pyridoxine.

pyridoxine A component of the vitamin B complex, vitamin B_6.

pyruvate The end product of glycolysis. Under aerobic conditions it may be converted into acetyl CoA, whereas under anaerobic conditions it is converted into lactic acid.

PYY Peptide YY (PYY), a gut hormone fragment produced by the intestines; affects neurons in the hypothalamus to reduce appetite and food intake.

Q

quackery Misrepresentation of the facts to deceive the consumer.

quality Calories Calories in foods that are accompanied by substantial amounts of nutrients. Skim milk contains quality Calories, as it provides considerable amounts of protein, calcium, and other nutrients, whereas cola drinks provide similar Calories but no nutrients.

quercetin A dietary flavonol, part of polyphenolic compounds that functions as an antioxidant and may also be an anti-inflammatory agent.

R

radiation Electromagnetic waves given off by an object; the body radiates heat to a cool environment.

radura International symbol of radiation; used on labels for irradiated foods.

rating of perceived exertion (RPE) A subjective rating, on a numerical scale, used to express the perceived difficulty of a given work task.

reactive hypoglycemia A decrease in blood glucose caused by an excessive insulin response to hyperglycemia associated with a substantial intake of high-glycemic-index foods.

Recommended Dietary Allowances (RDA) The levels of intake of essential nutrients considered to be adequate to meet the known nutritional needs of practically all healthy persons.

recommended dietary goals Dietary goals for U.S. citizens that have been established by a U.S. Senate subcommittee on nutrition; goals stress dietary reduction of fat, cholesterol, salt, and sugar, and increase of complex carbohydrates.

recuperation principle *See* principle of recuperation.

Reference Daily Intakes (RDIs) Used in food labeling as the recommended daily intake for protein and selected vitamins and minerals. It replaces the old U.S. RDA (United States Recommended Daily Allowance).

regional fat distribution Deposition of fat in different regions of the body. *See also* android- and gynoid-type obesity.

relative humidity The percentage of moisture in the air compared to the amount of moisture needed to cause saturation, which is taken as 100.

relative risk (RR) A probability estimate; RR of 1.0 is normal.

relative-weight method A method of determining obesity by comparing the weight of an individual to standardized height and weight tables.

repetition maximum (RM) In weight training, the amount of weight that can be lifted for a specific number of repetitions.

repetitions In relation to weight training or interval training, the number of times that an exercise is done.

resistin An adipokine secreted by adipose tissue that is thought to increase insulin resistance and may be the link between obesity and development of type 2 diabetes.

resting energy expenditure (REE) The energy required to drive all physiological processes while in a state of rest.

resting metabolic rate (RMR) *Also see* BMR and REE.

retinol Vitamin A.

retinol equivalent (RE) and retinol activity equivalent (RAE) Measures of vitamin A activity in food as measured by performed vitamin A (retinol) or carotene (provitamin A). 1 RE or RAE equals 1 microgram of retinol or 3.3 IU.

rHGH *See* human growth hormone.

riboflavin Vitamin B_2, a member of the B complex.

ribose A five-carbon sugar found in several body compounds, such as riboflavin.

risk factor Associated factor that increases the risk for a given disease; for example, cigarette smoking and lung cancer.

RNA Ribonucleic acid; nuclear material involved in the formation of proteins in cells.

RRR-alpha-tocopherol One of the two major forms of vitamin E; serves as the basis for the RDA.

RRR-gamma-tocopherol One of the two major forms of vitamin E.

running Although the distinction between running and jogging is relative to the individual involved, a common value used for running is 7 mph or faster.

S

saccharide A series of carbohydrates ranging from simple sugars (monosaccharides) to complex carbohydrates (polysaccharides).

saccharine An artificial sweetener made from coal tar.

Salmonella A bacteria commonly involved in food poisoning.

sarcopenia Loss of muscle mass associated with the aging process.

satiety center A group of nerve cells in the hypothalamus that responds to certain stimuli in the blood and provides a sensation of satiety.

saturated fatty acid Fat that has all chemical bonds filled.

SCAN Sports and Cardiovascular Nutritionists, a practice group of the American Dietetic Association focusing on applications of nutrition to sport and wellness.

scurvy A deficiency caused by a lack of vitamin C in the diet; symptoms include weakness, bleeding gums, and anemia.

SDA Specific dynamic action; often used to represent the increased energy cost observed during the metabolism of protein in the body. *Also see* dietary-induced thermogenesis and TEF.

Seasonal affective disorder (SAD) Symptoms associated with various seasons of the year, e.g., depression in winter months.

secondary amenorrhea Cessation of menstruation after the onset of puberty; primary amenorrhea is the lack of menstruation prior to menarche.

Sedentary Death Syndrome (SeDS) Term associated with a sedentary lifestyle and related health problems that predispose to premature death.

selenium A nonmetallic element resembling sulfur; an essential nutrient.

semivegetarian An individual who refrains from eating red meat but includes white meat such as fish and chicken in a diet stressing vegetarian concepts.

serotonin A neurotransmitter in the brain; may induce a sense of relaxation and drowsiness, possibly associated with fatigue; may also depress the appetite.

serum lipid level The concentration of lipids in the blood serum.

set-point theory The weight-control theory that postulates that each individual has an established normal body weight. Any deviation from this set point will lead to changes in body metabolism to return the individual to the normal weight.

sets In weight training, a certain number of repetitions constitutes a set; for example, a lifter may do three sets of six repetitions per set.

settling-point theory Theory that the body weight set point may be increased or decreased through interactions of genetics and the environment; an environment rich in high-fat foods may lead to a higher set point so that the body settles in at a higher weight and fat content.

shell temperature The temperature of the skin; *also see* core temperature.

short-chain fatty acids (SCFAs) Fatty acids with chains containing fewer than six carbons.

sibutramine A prescription drug for weight loss that suppresses the appetite by affecting brain neurotransmitters.

silicon A nonmetallic element.

simple carbohydrates Usually used to refer to table sugar, or sucrose, a disaccharide; may refer also to other disaccharides and the monosaccharides.

Simplesse A commercially produced fat substitute derived from protein.

skinfold technique A technique used to compute an individual's percentage of body fat; various skinfolds are measured and a regression formula is used to compute the body fat.

sling psychrometer A device that incorporates both a dry-bulb and wet-bulb thermometer, thus providing a heat-stress index incorporating both temperature and relative humidity.

slow-twitch fibers Red muscle fibers that have a slow contraction speed; designed for aerobic-type activity.

Smilax A commercial plant extract theorized to produce anabolic effects.

soda loading Term associated with use of baking soda (sodium bicarbonate) as an ergogenic aid.

sodium A soft metallic element; combines with chloride to form salt; the major extracellular cation in the human body.

sodium bicarbonate $NaHCO_3$; a sodium salt of carbonic acid that serves as a buffer of acids in the blood, often referred to as the alkaline reserve.

sodium citrate A white powder used as a blood buffer; *see also* sodium bicarbonate.

sodium loading Consumption of excess amounts of sodium; endurance athletes may use sodium loading in attempts to increase plasma volume, improve blood flow, and enhance aerobic endurance.

soluble dietary fiber Dietary fibers in plants such as gums and pectins that are soluble in water.

specific dynamic action *See* SDA.

specific heat The amount of energy or heat needed to raise the temperature of a unit of mass, such as 1 kilogram of body tissue, 1 degree Celsius.

specificity of training *See* principle of specificity of training.

sports anemia A temporary condition of low hemoglobin levels often observed in athletes during the early stages of training.

sports bars Commercial food products targeted to athletes and physically active individuals containing various concentrations of carbohydrate, fat, and protein; some products contain other nutrients, such as antioxidants.

sports drinks Popular term for various glucose-electrolyte fluid replacement drinks.

sports gels Commercial food products targeted to athletes; consist primarily of carbohydrate in a gel form.

sports nutrition The application of nutritional principles to sport with the intent of maximizing performance.

sports-related fitness Components of physical fitness that, when improved, have implications for enhanced sport performance, such as agility and power.

sports supplements Dietary supplements marketed to athletes and physically active individuals.

spot reducing The theory that exercising a specific body part, such as the thighs, will facilitate the loss of body fat from that spot.

standard error of measurement or estimate A measure of variability about the mean. Sixty-eight percent of the population is within one standard error above and below the mean, while about 95 percent is within two standard errors.

standardized exercise An exercise task that conforms to a specific standardized protocol.

Staphylococcus A bacteria commonly involved in food poisoning.

steady state A level of metabolism, usually during exercise, when the oxygen consumption satisfies the energy expenditure and the individual is performing in an aerobic state.

steady-state threshold The intensity level of exercise above which the production of energy appears to shift rapidly to anaerobic mechanisms, such as when a rapid rise in blood lactic acid exists. The oxygen system will still supply a major portion of the energy, but the lactic acid system begins to contribute an increasing share.

sterols Substances similar to fats because of their solubility characteristics; the most commonly known sterol is cholesterol.

stimulus period In exercise programs, the time period over which the stimulus is applied, such as a HR of 150 for 15 minutes.

storage fat Fat that accumulates and is stored in the adipose tissue; *also see* essential fat.

strength-endurance continuum In relation to strength training, the concept that power or strength is developed by high resistance and few repetitions and that endurance is developed by low resistance and many repetitions.

structured physical activity A planned program of physical activities usually designed to enhance physical fitness; often referred to as exercise.

subclinical malnutrition A nutrient-deficiency state in which no clinical signs of the nutrient deficiency are observable, but other nonspecific symptoms such as fatigue may be present.

subcutaneous fat The body fat found immediately under the skin; evaluated by skinfold calipers.

sucrose Table sugar, a disaccharide; yields glucose and fructose upon hydrolysis.

sulfur A pale yellow nonmetallic element essential in human nutrition; component of the sulfur-containing amino acids.

sumo wrestling A form of wrestling in Japan.

superoxide dismutase An enzyme in body cells that helps neutralize free radicals.

Syndrome X *See* metabolic syndrome.

synephrine A dietary supplement marketed for fat loss; synephrine is derived from a fruit plant known as bitter orange. Used as an alterative to ephedra, or ephedrine.

systolic blood pressure The blood pressure in the arteries when the heart is contracting and pumping blood.

T

target heart rate range In an aerobic exercise program, the heart-rate level that will provide the stimulus for a beneficial training effect.

taurine A vitamin-like compound synthesized from amino acids, mainly methionine and cysteine.

teratogen Any substance that can interfere with the normal development of the embryo or fetus; may lead to various birth defects.

testosterone The male sex hormone responsible for male secondary sex characteristics at puberty; it has anabolic and androgenic effects.

thermic effect of exercise (TEE) Increased muscular contraction produces additional heat.

thermic effect of food (TEF) The increased body heat production associated with the digestion, assimilation, and metabolism of energy nutrients in a meal just consumed.

thermogenesis The production of heat; metabolic processes in the body generate heat constantly.

thiamin Vitamin B$_1$.

threonine An essential amino acid.

threshold stimulus The minimal level of exercise intensity needed to stimulate gains in physical fitness.

thromboxanes Eicosanoids that possess hormone-like activity in numerous cells in the body.

thyroxine A hormone secreted by the thyroid gland that is involved in control of the metabolic rate.

tin A white metallic element.

tocopherol Generic name for an alcohol that has the activity of vitamin E.

Tolerable Upper Intake Level (UL) The highest level of daily nutrient intake likely to pose no adverse health risks.

tonicity Tension or pressure as related to fluids; fluids with high osmolality exhibit hypertonicity, whereas fluids with low osmolality exhibit hypotonicity.

total body electrical impedance A sophisticated method of measuring the resistance provided by water in the body as a means to predict body composition.

total body fat The sum total of the body's storage fat and essential fat stores.

total daily energy expenditure (TDEE) The total amount of energy expended during the day, including REE, TEF, and TEE.

total fiber Sum of dietary fiber and functional fiber.

trabecular bone The spongy bone structure found inside the bone, as contrasted with the more compact bone on the outside.

trace minerals Those minerals essential to human nutrition that have an RDA less than 100 mg.

trans **fatty acids** Unsaturated fatty acids in which the hydrogen ions are on opposite sides of the double bond.

triglycerides One of the many fats formed by the union of glycerol and fatty acids.

triose A simple sugar having three carbon atoms.

tryptophan An essential amino acid.

Type I muscle fiber The slow-twitch red fiber that provides energy primarily by the oxygen system.

Type IIa muscle fiber The fast-twitch red fiber that provides energy by both the oxygen system and the lactic acid system.

Type IIb muscle fiber The fast-twitch white fiber that provides energy primarily by the lactic acid system.

tyrosine A nonessential amino acid.

U

ubiquinone *See* CoQ10.

uncompensated heat stress A condition in which heat loss is insufficient to offset heat production during exercise in the heat, the body temperature continues to rise, and exhaustion eventually occurs.

uncoupling protein (UPC) A protein believed to stimulate thermogenesis in fat tissues; uncouples thermogenesis with the production of ATP, so no ATP is generated in this process.

underwater weighing A technique for measuring the percentage of body fat in humans.

United States Recommended Daily Allowances *See* U.S. RDA.

Universal Gym A brand name for exercise equipment, particularly weights for strength development.

unsaturated fatty acids Fatty acids that contain double or triple bonds and hence can add hydrogen atoms.

unstructured physical activity Many of the normal, daily physical activities that are generally not planned as exercise, such as walking to work, climbing stairs, gardening, domestic activities, and games and other childhood pursuits.

urea The chief nitrogenous constituent of urine and the final product of the decomposition of proteins in the body.

uric acid A crystalline end product of purine metabolism; commonly involved in gout and the formation of kidney stones.

USDA United States Department of Agriculture.

USOC United States Olympic Committee.

U.S. RDA The United States Recommended Daily Allowances; the RDA figures used on labels, representing the percentage of the RDA for a given nutrient contained in a serving of the food. The U.S. RDA are now known as the Reference Daily Intake (RDI).

V

valine An essential amino acid.

Valsalva phenomenon A condition in which a forceful exhalation is attempted against a closed epiglottis and no air escapes; such a straining may cause the person to faint.

vanadium A light gray metallic element.

vanadyl sulfate A salt form of vanadium; marketed for its anabolic potential.

vascular water The body water contained in the blood vessels; a part of the extracellular water.

vasodilation An increase in the size of the blood vessels, usually referring to the arterial system.

vasopressin *See* antidiuretic hormone (ADH).

vegan Vegetarian who eats no animal products.

vegetable exchange One vegetable exchange in the Food Exchange System contains 5 grams of carbohydrate, 2 grams of protein, and 25 Calories.

vegetarian One whose food is of vegetable or plant origin; *also see* lactovegetarian, ovovegetarian, ovolactovegetarian, pescovegetarian, semivegetarian, and vegan.

ventral tegmental area (VTA) One of the oldest parts of the brain; a group of neurons that integrates input from various neural centers and helps to control basic human needs by secreting neurotransmitters, such as dopamine, to other parts of the brain.

very-low-Calorie diet (VLCD) A diet containing less than 800 Calories per day.

very low-density lipoprotein *See* VLDL.

visceral fat The deep fat found in the abdominal area; measurement of this fat requires special techniques, such as MRI.

vitamin, natural Often referred to as a vitamin derived from natural sources; i.e., food in nature; contrast with vitamin, synthetic.

vitamin, synthetic An artificial vitamin commercially produced from the separate components of the vitamin.

vitamin A Retinol, an unsaturated aliphatic alcohol; fat soluble.

vitamin B_1 Thiamin; the antineuritic vitamin.

vitamin B_2 Riboflavin.

vitamin B_6 Pyridoxine and related compounds.

vitamin B_{12} Cyanocobalamin.

vitamin B_{15} Not a vitamin but marketed as one; usual composition is calcium gluconate and dimethylglycine (DMG).

vitamin C Ascorbic acid; the antiscorbutic vitamin.

vitamin D Any one of related sterols that have antirachitic properties; fat soluble.

vitamin D_3 The prohormone form of vitamin D, also known as cholecalciferol, formed in the skin by irradiation from the sun. Released into the blood and eventually converted by the kidney to the hormone form of vitamin D.

vitamin deficiency Subnormal body-vitamin levels due to inadequate intake or absorption; specific disorders are linked with deficiencies of specific vitamins.

vitamin E Various forms of tocotrienols and tocopherols; fat soluble.

vitamin K The antihemorrhagic, or clotting vitamin; fat soluble.

vitamins A general term for a number of substances deemed essential for the normal metabolic functioning of the body.

VLDL Very low-density lipoproteins; a protein-lipid complex in the blood that transports triglycerides, cholesterol, and phospholipids; has a very low density. *Also see* HDL-cholesterol and LDL-cholesterol.

voluntary dehydration Intentional loss of body fluids in attempts to reduce body mass for sports competition; techniques include exercise, sauna, and diuretics.

VO_2 max Maximal oxygen uptake; measured during exercise, the maximal amount of oxygen consumed reflects the body's ability to utilize oxygen as an energy source; equals the cardiac output times the arteriovenous oxygen difference.

W

WADA The World Antidoping Agency, which develops and enforces regulations against the use of prohibited performance-enhancing substances by athletes in international sport competition.

waist circumference The circumference of the waist at its most narrow point as seen from the front; used as a measure of regional adeposity.

warm-down A phase after an exercise session during which the individual gradually tapers the level of activity—for example, by jogging slowly after a fast run.

warm-up Low-level exercises used to increase the muscle temperature and/or stretch the muscles prior to a strenuous exercise bout.

water A tasteless, colorless, odorless fluid essential to life; composed of two parts hydrogen and one part oxygen (H_2O).

water intoxication Consumption of excessive amounts of water leading to dilution of body electrolytes. *See also* hyponatremia.

watt A unit of power in the SI; one watt equals about 6 kilogram-meters per minute.

WBGT Index Wet-bulb globe thermometer index; a heat-stress index based upon four factors measured by the wet-bulb globe thermometer.

weight cycling Repetitive loss and regain of body weight; often called yo-yo dieting.

wet-bulb globe thermometer A device that takes into account the various factors determining heat stress: air temperature, air movement, radiation heat, and humidity.

wheat germ oil Oil extracted from the embryo of wheat, high in linoleic fatty acid, vitamin E, and octacosanol.

work Effort expended to accomplish something; in terms of physics, force times distance.

X

xerophthalmia Dryness of the conjunctiva and cornea of the eye, which may lead to blindness if untreated; caused by a deficiency of vitamin A.

xylitol A sugar alcohol that may be obtained from fruits.

Y

yohimbine A plant extract theorized to stimulate testosterone production and elicit anabolic effects.

Z

zinc A blue-white crystalline metallic element essential to human nutrition.

zone diet A high-protein diet plan; the 40-30-30 plan consisting of 40 percent Calories from carbohydrate, and 30 percent each from protein and fat.

Photo Credits

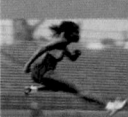

Chapter 1

Page 2 & 3: © Fruits & Vegetables, OS1/PhotoDisc/Getty RF; 1.4: © R-F Website/Getty RF; Table 1.1: © Supporting Cast: Teens, OS39/PhotoDisc/Getty RF; 1.8: © Corbis RF; p. 18 (left): © Fruits & Vegetables, OS1/PhotoDisc/Getty RF; p. 18 (right): © Sporting Goods, OS25/PhotoDisc/Getty RF; p. 19: © Fruits & Vegetables, OS1/PhotoDisc/Getty RF; 1.11: © Mauro Femariello/Photo Researchers

Chapter 2

Page 39: © Fruits & Vegetables, OS1/PhotoDisc/Getty RF; Fig 2.2 (All): © Greg Kidd and Joanne Scott; p. 42: © Supporting Cast: Teens, OS39/PhotoDisc/Getty RF; 2.3: Courtesy U.S. Department of Agriculture, U.S. Department of Health and Human Services; Table 2.4 (all): © Fruits & Vegetables, OS1/PhotoDisc/Getty RF; 2.5: © DV023/Digital Vision/Getty RF; p. 48 (left): © Supporting Cast: Teens, OS39/PhotoDisc/Getty RF; p. 48 (right): © Fruits & Vegetables, OS1/PhotoDisc/Getty RF; 2.7 (left): © The McGraw-Hill Companies, Inc. Sabina Dowell, photographer; 2.7 (right): © Greg Kidd and Joanne Scott; 2.8: © Brian Leatart /FoodPix/Getty; 2.9: © The McGraw-Hill Companies, Inc. Sabina Dowell, photographer; p. 60 & 61: © Supporting Cast: Teens, OS39/PhotoDisc/Getty RF; 2.11: © The McGraw-Hill Companies, Inc. Sabina Dowell, photographer; 2.12: © Vol. 67 PhotoDisc/Getty RF; p. 77 (left): © Supporting Cast: Teens, OS39/PhotoDisc/Getty RF; p. 77 (right): © Market Fresh, OS49/PhotoDisc/Getty RF; Table 2.19 (all): © Fruits & Vegetables, OS1/PhotoDisc/Getty RF

Chapter 3

Fig 3.3: © Samual Ashfield/SPL/Photo Researchers; 3.4: © Delicious Delights/Corbis RF; 3.6: © People in Sports/Corbis RF; p. 99: © Supporting Cast: Teens, OS39/PhotoDisc/Getty RF; Table 3.4 (all): © Supporting Cast: Teens, OS39/PhotoDisc/Getty RF; 3.14: © Yoav Levy/Phototake; p. 105: © Supporting Cast: Teens, OS39/PhotoDisc/Getty RF; 3.16: © Vol. 10 PhotoDisc/Getty RF; p. 106 (right): © Sporting Goods, OS25/PhotoDisc/Getty RF; p. 108: © Supporting Cast: Teens, OS39/PhotoDisc/Getty RF

Chapter 4

Page 134: © Market Fresh, OS49/PhotoDisc/Getty RF; p. 138: © Rubberball/Getty RF; p. 148: © Jupiterimages RF; p. 151: © Market Fresh, OS49/PhotoDisc/Getty RF; p. 154: © Familiar Objects, OS57/PhotoDisc/Getty RF; p. 158: © The McGraw-Hill Companies, Inc. Jill Braaten, photographer; p. 161: © Food and Dining, Vol. 12/PhotoDisc/Getty RF

Chapter 5

Page 185: © Rubberball/Getty RF; p. 191: © Corbis RF; p. 194 (left): © Corbis RF; p. 194 (right): © Supporting Cast: Teens, OS39/PhotoDisc/Getty RF; 5.17: © Vol. 12 PhotoDisc/Getty RF

Chapter 6

Fig 6.3: © The McGraw-Hill Companies, Inc. John Thoeming, photographer; p. 231: © Rubberball/Getty RF

Chapter 7

Page 277: © Health and Well Being, Vol. 67/PhotoDisc/Getty RF; p. 286 & 289: © Fruits & Vegetables, OS1/PhotoDisc/Getty RF; p. 292: © Market Fresh, OS49/PhotoDisc/Getty RF; p. 294: © Child's Play, OS47/PhotoDisc/Getty RF; p. 298 & 308: © Sporting Goods, OS25/PhotoDisc/Getty RF

Chapter 8

Page 321: © Vol. 111 PhotoDisc/Getty RF; p. 329: © Sports & Fitness, Vol. 103/Corbis RF; p. 335: © American Food Basics, Vol. 4/Corbis RF; p. 346: © Sports & Fitness, Vol. 103/Corbis RF

Chapter 9

Page 365: © John Lund/Drew Kelly/Blend Images RF; p. 367: © People in Sports/Corbis RF; p. 371: © The McGraw-Hill Companies, Inc.; p. 382: © Fruits & Vegetables, OS1/PhotoDisc/Getty RF; p. 396: © BrandXPictures/PunchStock RF; 9.12: © Tony Duffy/Getty

Chapter 10

Fig 10.2: Rick O'Quinn/University of Georgia; 10.3: Photo courtesy of Life Measurement Instruments; p. 423: © Mediscan/Corbis; p. 424: © Sports & Fitness, Vol. 103/Corbis RF; p. 439: © Sporting Goods, OS25/PhotoDisc/Getty RF; p. 440 & 443: © Sports & Fitness, Vol. 103/Corbis RF

Chapter 11

Page 471: © Sports & Fitness, Vol. 103/Corbis RF; 11.4 (golf ball): © Vol. 127/Corbis RF; 11.4 (tennis ball): © Sporting Goods, OS25/PhotoDisc/Getty RF; 11.4 (yo-yo): © Corbis RF; 11.4 (mouse): © Vol. 127/Corbis RF; 11.4 (baseball): © Sporting Goods, OS25/PhotoDisc/Getty RF; 11.4 (fist): © OS02/PhotoDisc/Getty RF; 11.6: © Digital Vision/Getty RF; p. 490: © Sports & Fitness, Vol. 103/Corbis RF; 11.11: © Stockbyte/PunchStock RF; p. 500: © Sports & Fitness, Vol. 103/Corbis RF

Chapter 12

Page 522: © Food Collections/Getty RF; p. 525: © Sports & Fitness, Vol. 103/Corbis RF; 12.4: © Vol. 51/PhotoDisc/Getty RF

Chapter 13

Page 550: © Contemporary Cuisine, Vol. 30/PhotoDisc/Getty RF; 13.4: © Vol. 66/PhotoDisc/Getty RF; 13.5: © The McGraw-Hill Companies, Inc. Lars A. Niki, photographer; p. 560: © Contemporary Cuisine, Vol. 30/PhotoDisc/Getty RF; 13.6: © Vol. 59/PhotoDisc/Getty RF; 13.7 & 13.8: © The McGraw-Hill Companies, Inc. Jill Braaten, photographer; 13.10: © Sports & Fitness CD/Corbis RF; 13.12: © The McGraw-Hill Companies, Inc. Jill Braaten, photographer

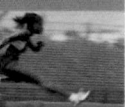

Index

A

AAHPERD (American Alliance for Health, Physical Education, Recreation, and Dance), 4
AAS. *See* Anabolic/androgenic steroids
Absorption of nutrients, 93, 126
  carbohydrates, 126–127
  of dietary fat, 179–181
  of proteins, 223–224
Accelerometer, 90–91
Acceptable Macronutrient Distribution Range (AMDR), 40, 221, 472
  macronutrient percentages, 42
Acclimatization, 401, 402
Acesulfame-K, 158
ACSM. *See* American College of Sports Medicine
Active category, 110, 463
Active transport, 126
Activity-stat, 429
Adaptations, 101
  loss of, 5
Adaptive thermogenesis, 428
Added sugar, 124–125, 158, 481
  healthful dietary guidelines for, 52
Additives. *See* Food additives
Adenosine triphosphate (ATP)
  ATP-PCr system, 95–96
  defined, 94
  electron transport chain and, 618
  lactic acid system, 96
  oxygen system, 96–97
  stored in body, 94, 95
  supplements, 334
Adequate Intake (AI), 40
ADH (antidiuretic hormone), 368
Adipokines, 7, 435, 436, 437–438
  defined, 182
Adiponectin, 7
Adolescents, 9. *See also* Children
Adonis Complex, 518
Advertising, nutritional quackery and, 22–24
Aerobic capacity, 97, 98
Aerobic endurance exercise
  caffeine and, 557
    high-protein diets and improved performance, 237–238
    protein metabolism and training, 228–229

Aerobic exercise, 9
  amount needed for health benefits, 8
  benefits of, other than weight loss, 490
  caffeine and, 557
  circuit aerobics, 539
  equipment for, 107
  low muscle glycogen, 137–138
  mode of, 491
  protein as energy source during, 226
  recommendation guidelines, 9
  resting energy expenditure (REE) and, 489–490
  warm-down, 496
  warm-up, 495–496
  for weight loss, 488–490, 507
Aerobic glycolysis, 96, 97, 98
Aerobic lipolysis, 97, 98
Aerobic power, 97, 98
Aerobic system, 96
Aerobic walking, 501
Age
  exercise benefits and, 6
  exercise recommendation guidelines and, 9–10
  fat as energy source during exercise and, 186
  physical performance and nutritional recommendations, 82
  resting energy expenditure and, 101
  tolerating exercise in heat, 400–401
Aggression, 551
AHA. *See* American Heart Association
AI (Adequate Intake), 40
Air displacement plethysmography (ADP), 422
Alanine, 219
Alcohol, 472, 547–555
  blood alcohol concentration, 548
  Calories per gram, 92–93
  cholesterol-lowering recommendations, 206, 209
  dehydration and, 402
  in energy drinks, 551, 560
  ergogenic effects
    energy source, 549
    exercise metabolism, 549
    psychological processes, 549–550

    ergolytic effects, 549
  health effects, 406, 550–555
    alcohol dependence, 553
    Alzheimer's disease, 554
    binge drinking, 550, 551, 552
    cancer, 552
    cardiovascular disease, 552, 554
    coronary heart disease, 552, 554
    dementia, 554
    fetal alcohol spectrum disorders, 552–553
    liver disease, 550–551
    obesity, 432, 553
    positive effects, 553–555
    psychological problems, 551–552
    sick quitters, 554
    stroke, 554
  healthful dietary guidelines for, 14, 52
  historical perspective on, 547
  limiting, for weight loss, 472
  metabolism of, 547–548
  nutrient content of typical alcoholic beverage, 547
  obesity and, 553
  permissibility of in competition, 550
  proof, 547
  social drinking effects, 550
  in weight-gain diets, 523
  in weight-loss diets, 482
Alcohol consumption, 2
Alcohol Use Disorders Identification Test (AUDIT), 553
Alcoholism, 553
  self-test on, 596–597
Aldosterone, 371
Alimentary canal, 126–127
Allium sulfides, 59
Alpha-ketoacid, 224
Alpha-linoleic acid, 178
Alpha-linolenic acid, 203–206
Alpha-tocopherol, 281–283
Alzheimer's disease, 2
  alcohol and, 554
  antioxidant supplements to prevent, 307
  caffeine and, 562
AMA. *See* American Medical Association
AMDR (Acceptable Macronutrient Distribution Range), 39, 221, 472

Amenorrhea, 232
  athletic, 331
  exercise-induced, 209
  female athlete triad, 331, 446–447
  secondary, 331
American Alliance for Health, Physical Education, Recreation, and Dance (AAHPERD), 4
American College of Sports Medicine (ACSM), 4
American Diabetes Association, 6
American Heart Association (AHA), 4
American Medical Association (AMA), 6
Amines, 246
Amino acids. *See also specific amino acids*
  consumption of individual, 259–260
  defined, 218
  dietary, 219
  ergogenic aspects of, 238–256
  essential, 219, 222
  functions and effects, 226
  glucogenic, 224
  ketogenic, 224
  metabolism of, 619
  nonessential, 219
  supplementation, 226
Aminostatic theory, 427
Ammonia, 224, 227
Amylase, 126
Anabolic/androgenic steroids (AAS), 21, 570–572
  defined, 570
  health risks of, 571
  legality of, 569, 572
Anabolic hormones, 569–573
Anabolism, 99
Anaerobic capacity, 96, 98
Anaerobic exercise
  caffeine and, 557–558
  low muscle glycogen, 138
  sodium bicarbonate and, 566
Anaerobic glycolysis, 96, 137
Anaerobic power, 96, 98, 247
Anderson, Richard, 346
Android-type obesity, 437–439
Androstenedione, 572
  defined, 573
  as ergogenic aid, 21, 572, 573
  permissibility of, 573
Anemia
  iron-deficiency, 339, 341
  pernicious, 289, 290
  sports, 230–231, 340–341

Median Heights and Weights and Recommended Energy Intake

Category	Age (years) or condition	Weight (kg)	Weight (lb)	Height (cm)	Height (in)	REE[a] (kcal/day)	Average energy allowance (kcal)[b] Multiples of REE	Per kg	Per day[c]
Infants	0.0–0.5	6	13	60	24	320		108	650
	0.5–1.0	9	20	71	28	500		98	850
Children	1–3	13	29	90	35	740		102	1,300
	4–6	20	44	112	44	950		90	1,800
	7–10	28	62	132	52	1,130		70	2,000
Males	11–14	45	99	157	62	1,440	1.70	55	2,500
	15–18	66	145	176	69	1,760	1.67	45	3,000
	19–24	72	160	177	70	1,780	1.67	40	2,900
	25–50	79	174	176	70	1,800	1.60	37	2,900
	51+	77	170	173	68	1,530	1.50	30	2,300
Females	11–14	46	101	157	62	1,310	1.67	47	2,200
	15–18	55	120	163	64	1,370	1.60	40	2,200
	19–24	58	128	164	65	1,350	1.60	38	2,200
	25–50	63	138	163	64	1,380	1.55	36	2,200
	51+	65	143	160	63	1,280	1.50	30	1,900
Pregnant	1st trimester								+0
	2nd trimester								+300
	3rd trimester								+300
Lactating	1st 6 months								+500
	2nd 6 months								+500

[a]REE is resting energy expenditure; see chapter 3 for explanation. Calculation is based on food and Agriculture Organization equations, then rounded.
[b]In the range of light to moderate activity, the coefficient of variation is ± 20 percent. Thus, for an individual with an average energy allowance of 2,500 Calories per day, the typical range might be 2,000–3,000, which is plus or minus 500 Calories (0.20 × 2,500). See chapter 3 for an expanded discussion of energy requirement based upon physical activity levels.
[c]Figure is rounded.

Dietary Reference Intakes (DRIs): Tolerable Upper Intake Levels (UL[a]), Vitamins

Food and Nutrition Board, Institute of Medicine, National Academies

Life stage group	Vitamin A (μg/d)[b]	Vitamin C (mg/d)	Vitamin D (IU/d)	Vitamin E (mg/d)[c,d]	Vitamin K	Thiamin	Riboflavin	Niacin (mg/d)[d]	Vitamin B$_6$ (mg/d)	Folate (μg/d)[d]	Vitamin B$_{12}$	Pantothenic Acid	Biotin	Choline (g/d)	Carotenoids[e]
Infants															
0–6 mo	600	ND[f]	1,000	ND	ND	ND	ND	ND	ND	ND	ND	ND	ND	ND	ND
7–12 mo	600	ND	1,500	ND	ND	ND	ND	ND	ND	ND	ND	ND	ND	ND	ND
Children															
1–3 y	600	400	2,500	200	ND	ND	ND	10	30	300	ND	ND	ND	1.0	ND
4–8 y	900	650	3,000	300	ND	ND	ND	15	40	400	ND	ND	ND	1.0	ND
Males, Females															
9–13 y	1,700	1,200	4,000	600	ND	ND	ND	20	60	600	ND	ND	ND	2.0	ND
14–18 y	2,800	1,800	4,000	800	ND	ND	ND	30	80	800	ND	ND	ND	3.0	ND
19–70 y	3,000	2,000	4,000	1,000	ND	ND	ND	35	100	1,000	ND	ND	ND	3.5	ND
>70 y	3,000	2,000	4,000	1,000	ND	ND	ND	35	100	1,000	ND	ND	ND	3.5	ND
Pregnancy															
≤18 y	2,800	1,800	4,000	800	ND	ND	ND	30	80	800	ND	ND	ND	3.0	ND
19–50 y	3,000	2,000	4,000	1,000	ND	ND	ND	35	100	1,000	ND	ND	ND	3.5	ND
Lactation															
≤18 y	2,800	1,800	4,000	800	ND	ND	ND	30	80	800	ND	ND	ND	3.0	ND
19–50 y	3,000	2,000	4,000	1,000	ND	ND	ND	35	100	1,000	ND	ND	ND	3.5	ND

[a]UL = The maximum level of daily nutrient intake that is likely to pose no risk of adverse effects. Unless otherwise specified, the UL represents total intake from food, water, and supplements. Due to lack of suitable data, ULs could not be established for vitamin K, thiamin, riboflavin, vitamin B$_{12}$, pantothenic acid, biotin, or carotenoids. In the absence of ULs, extra caution may be warranted in consuming levels above recommended intakes.

[b]As preformed vitamin A only.

[c]As α-tocopherol; applies to any form of supplemental α-tocopherol.

[d]The ULs for vitamin E, niacin, and folate apply to synthetic forms obtained from supplements, fortified foods, or a combination of the two.

[e]β-Carotene supplements are advised only to serve as a provitamin A source for individuals at risk of vitamin A deficiency.

[f]ND = Not determinable due to lack of data of adverse effects in this age group and concern with regard to lack of ability to handle excess amounts. Source of intake should be from food only to prevent high levels of intake.

SOURCES: Dietary Reference Intakes for Calcium, Phosphorus, Magnesium, Vitamin D, and Fluoride (1997); Dietary Reference Intakes for Thiamin, Riboflavin, Niacin, Vitamin B$_6$, Folate, Vitamin B$_{12}$, Pantothenic Acid, Biotin, and Choline (1998); Dietary Reference Intakes for Vitamin C, Vitamin E, Selenium, and Carotenoids (2000); and Dietary Reference Intakes for Vitamin A, Vitamin K, Arsenic, Boron, Chromium, Copper, Iodine, Iron, Manganese, Molybdenum, Nickel, Silicon, Vanadium, and Zinc (2001). These reports may be accessed via www.nap.edu.